W9-CER-851

FUNDAMENTALS OF NURSING

Sixth Edition

FUNDAMENTALS OF NURSING

The Humanities and the Sciences in Nursing

LuVerne Wolff, R.N., M.A.

Formerly Consultant, College of
Nursing, Arizona State University, Tempe, Arizona;
Research Associate, Institute of Research
and Service in Nursing Education, Teachers
College, Columbia University, New York.

Marlene H. Weitzel, R.N., Ph.D.

Associate Professor
College of Nursing
The University of Texas at El Paso
El Paso, Texas

Elinor V. Fuerst, R.N., M.A.

Formerly Educational Consultant,
Muhlenberg Hospital School of
Nursing, Plainfield, N. J.; Assistant
Professor of Nursing, Cornell
University—New York Hospital School
of Nursing, New York.

J. B. LIPPINCOTT COMPANY

PHILADELPHIA   NEW YORK   TORONTO

To our parents

ISBN: 0-397-54234-8

Library of Congress Catalog Card Number 78-31576

Printed in the United States of America

2 4 6 8 9 7 5 3

Library of Congress Cataloging in Publication Data

Lewis, LuVerne Wolff.
  Fundamentals of nursing.

  Fifth ed. by E. V. Fuerst, L. Wolff, and M. H. Weitzel.
  Includes bibliographies.
  1. Nursing. I. Weitzel, Marlene H., joint author. II. Fuerst, Elinor V., joint author.
III. Title
RT41.F85 1979   610.73   78-31576
ISBN 0-397-54234-8

Contents

Preface

This book was prepared primarily for students in basic programs of education for nursing. However, it can serve well as a reference for students in other types of educational programs for nursing as well as for the practicing nurse.

The purpose of the book is to present content which is fundamental to the practice of nursing. The content is designed to be applicable to persons of various ages who have nursing needs which are met in different settings. It is intended to be useful when caring for persons who have a wide variety of pathological conditions. It is also designed to be appropriate when caring for persons with no known illness for whom the goal of nursing care is to maintain wellness and prevent illness. While no particular age, setting, or health state is the focus of this book, examples citing these specifics are often used to illustrate application of content.

The sixth edition of this text represents a major revision. The authors have incorporated considerable new material and have updated previous content. These revisions are intended to reflect changes in contemporary society and nursing practice. Some examples of revised and new content will be cited.

- As with previous editions, this text continues to place emphasis on the use of principles, rather than empirical knowledge, when planning and giving nursing care. Considerable new information is presented that offers sound rationales for nursing practice.

- This text continues to stress the holistic approach when offering the patient nursing care. Man cannot be separated into psychosocial and physiological entities. Similarly, man is constantly subjected to environmental influences, and hence, a patient is best considered in the context of the environment whence he came.

- The nursing process, based on general systems theory, is again presented in this edition. However, the content has been revised and simplified with the intent that it will be more helpful to the reader. *The application of the nursing process is illustrated in most chapters of the text.*

- The emphasis on the nurse being accountable for her practice continues. The nurse is expected to provide care which is based on objective information and sound reasoning and which produces observable results. Accountability for each part of the nursing process and of total nursing care is presented as an integral part of nursing.

- Health maintenance and disease prevention are stressed throughout the book. In the past, health professionals were largely concerned with the treatment of disease and the care of the sick. Without ignoring these important aspects of comprehensive health care, nursing is assuming a leadership role in promoting health and preventing disease, which is reflected in this text. The content is intended to help the learner develop a commitment to the importance of health maintenance and disease prevention as well as an understanding of the basic techniques used to accomplish them.

• Participation of the consumer in his health care has become prominent in recent years. The nursing process, as presented in this text, stresses the active role of the consumer in planning his nursing care. In addition, patient teaching by the nurse is emphasized throughout. Including family members in teaching programs is also stressed. The purpose of teaching is to help the consumer participate in his care and to be able to act independently whenever possible. Health teaching also illustrates respect for the patient's right to know about the care he receives.

• The increased knowledge of developmental characteristics throughout life provides health practitioners with a basis for identifying and meeting health care needs for persons of all ages. The nurse uses this information to determine problem areas and to provide nursing care which is consistent with the patient's developmental characteristics. A new chapter is included in this edition which summarizes physiological and psychosocial characteristics over the life span. Common health problems associated with each age period are included.

• The concepts of homeostasis and adaptation are not new. However, increased applications of the concepts are being made in the health professions. Nursing care is intended to provide and support adaptive mechanisms which contribute to homeostasis of the patient. A new chapter discussing the concepts is included in this edition.

• This nation is demonstrating evidence of moving from a position of promoting a common culture to one of encouraging citizens to retain their distinctive cultural beliefs and practices. Cultural influences have been shown to influence health significantly. Nursing has been actively involved in identifying important cultural influences and in planning for ways of incorporating them in professional health care. In this edition, information regarding the major culture and subcultures of this country has been included. The nurse can use this information to provide effective care for persons with different cultural backgrounds.

• The physical examination and physical assessment are becoming recognized as essential when offering consumers comprehensive health care. Extensive knowledge and skills acquired through study and experience are necessary to be proficient in these areas. However, the basis for such proficiency is an understanding of the appropriate techniques to assess physical health and of the specific characteristics for which one is observing. Introductory and basic information which is believed to be appropriate for beginning students in nursing is included in this text.

• Behavioral objectives are a new addition to this edition. They are included at the beginning of each chapter. The objectives are intended to help the reader determine mastery of content in each chapter.

• Much of the illustrative material in this edition is new. Many photographs have been replaced and new ones have been added. Some new tables and diagrams have also been included.

• The references and situations for supplemental library study have been updated. The majority have not appeared previously. An effort was made to use a variety of sources, but those which are believed to be readily accessible to most students. The references and supplementary library study sections in each chapter can serve a variety of purposes. Some present material in greater depth than was possible to incorporate in the text. Others present material that may be under debate today. Occasionally, a study situation presents material that may be considered tangential to content in the book but which may be of particular interest to at least some readers. They will also help the student expand her knowledge. Sources used for the sections describing supplemental library study are not repeated in the references at the end of the chapter.

• Here are some additional examples of new and revised content included in this edition. The discussion of emergency resuscitation has been expanded and included in a separate chapter. Behavior modification as a teaching technique has been introduced. Techniques, such as those used when caring for patients with a fracture, a tracheotomy, and an ileal conduit, have been added. The hospice movement and living wills are discussed. Content describing commonly used over-the-counter drugs has been added to many chapters. The chapters in Unit I have been revised to reflect the new roles and responsibilities being assumed by nurses, changing ethical and legal implications, and the rights and viewpoints of health care consumers. The most recent recommendations from the Center for Disease Control are included in discussions dealing with infection control. The section on problem-oriented recording has been updated and expanded. Material on blood transfusions and blood extracts has been enlarged and updated. The number of terms in the glossaries has been increased. Information concerning common diagnostic tests and the nurse's role in preparing the patient has also been updated and enlarged.

There are numerous ways in which content can be arranged. A final decision often must be made arbitrarily, with the realization that every arrangement presents advantages and disadvantages. The final arrangement of chapters arrived at does not imply a suggested course outline. Rather, it is hoped that the arrangement lends itself to easy adaptation to meet the reader's needs. A particular unit may be considered as a whole, using the several chapters in the sequence offered. The advantage of this approach is that new words are defined in the chapter the first time they are used. Chapters may also be considered without regard to the particular unit or sequence in which they are placed. When the chapters are dealt with in a different sequence from that presented and terms which have been defined earlier are encountered, the reader merely has to check the index to find where the definition is located.

Decisions had to be made also concerning in which chapter certain content should be placed. One example concerns the care of a patient having gastric or duodenal suction. Since helping to meet nutritional and fluid needs of such a patient is an important objective of care, the content was placed in Chapter 19.

Some literature and certain health agencies differentiate between the words client and patient. Both terms are described in Chapter 1. The term "patient," rather than "client," continues to be used in this text when speaking of individuals or groups receiving health care. While recognizing that either term could be used, patient was selected since most health personnel continue to use it. Also, consistent use of one term appeared to add to the ease of reading.

We recognize that there are an increasing number of men in nursing and we encourage and welcome their entering the field. However, for the sake of clarity and convenience, we have continued to use the feminine pronoun, except in a few instances, when referring to the nurse and the masculine pronoun, in most instances, when referring to the patient. They have no other significance.

It is our sincere hope that this text will make positive contributions to educational programs in nursing and will serve the nurse in her practice in society today. The ultimate goal of the book will have been achieved when high-quality nursing care is provided.

Acknowledgments

The authors wish to express gratitude to these persons who made important contributions during the preparation of this edition. Grace Stoebner Labaj, R.N., M.S.N., Associate Professor of Nursing, Mary Hardin-Baylor College, Belton, Texas, who helped with Chapter 22; Shannon Perry, R.N., M.S., Mesa, Arizona; who helped with Chapters 9 and 23; Barbara M. Petrosino, R.N., M.S.N., Assistant Professor of Nursing, The University of Texas at Austin, Austin, Texas, who helped with several chapters; Marjorie S. VanderLinden, R.N., M.S.N., Assistant Professor of Nursing, Arizona State University, Tempe, Arizona, who helped with Chapter 26; Margaret Wallace, R.N., Ph.D., Assistant Professor of Nursing, Incarnate Word College, San Antonio, Texas, who helped with Chapter 6; Grace Whitis, R.N., M.S.N., Associate Professor of Nursing, Mary Hardin-Baylor College, Belton, Texas, who helped with Chapter 21.

These three clergymen reviewed the sections on religion in Chapter 7. The Reverend William C. Brooks, Associate Pastor, Saint Louis Catholic Church, Austin, Texas; The Reverend Philip A. Gangsei, Prince of Peace Lutheran Church, Phoenix, Arizona; and Rabbi Zalman Levertov, Executive Director, Chabad-Lubavitch, Tempe, Arizona.

We wish to thank the members of the undergraduate faculty of the College of Nursing, Arizona State University, Tempe, Arizona, who did much of the basic work on the nursing process from which Chapter 4 was developed.

The following book was used extensively for the preparation of Chapter 9: Doris Cook Sutterley and Gloria Ferraro Donnelly, *Perspectives in Human Development: Nursing Throughout the Life Cycle,* J. B. Lippincott Company, Philadelphia, 1973.

Our photographers were Ted Hill, Scottsdale, Arizona; Donald Lawson, Austin Texas, who also prepared several sketches; and Michael Patrick, Austin, Texas.

We wish to thank those who served as models in photographs and assisted in arranging for photography, especially Frances M. Brummeler, Instructor for Unit Support, Good Samaritan Hospital, Phoenix, Arizona; Emily Cornett, R.N., Ph.D., Associate Professor of Nursing, The University of Texas at Austin, Austin, Texas; Rozanne Thatcher, R.N., M.S.N., Assistant Professor of Nursing, The University of Texas at Austin, Austin, Texas; and the staff of the Learning Center, The University of Texas at Austin, Austin, Texas.

We wish to thank these facilities where some of the photographs were taken: Good Samaritan Hospital, Phoenix, Arizona; Kivel Nursing Home, Phoenix, Arizona; Salina Activity Center, Austin Texas; Scottsdale Christian Home, Scottsdale, Arizona; and Seton Medical Center, Austin, Texas.

Barbara Poley, R.N., Ph.D., provided typing assistance and helped with the preparation of references.

David T. Miller, Managing Editor, Nursing Department, J. B. Lippincott Company, Philadelphia, offered valuable editorial assistance and guidance.

We extend a special thank you to our family members and friends who displayed patience and understanding and offered support during the preparation of this edition.

unit I
Nursing and the Consumer of Health Services

1. The Role of the Nurse
2. Ethical and Legal Considerations in Nursing
3. The Consumer of Health Care Services

1

BEHAVIORAL OBJECTIVES

When content in this chapter has been mastered, the student will be able to

Define the terms appearing in the glossary.

Describe nursing, using at least six aspects that typify nursing practice today.

Discuss briefly a nurse's professional rights, including her right to withdraw from the care of a patient.

Describe the health care team and briefly discuss how it functions.

Explain the four common services ordinarily included when describing comprehensive health care and give at least one example of each.

Describe the underlying philosophy of the concept of continuity of care.

List at least ten trends which are currently influencing nursing practice and explain how each one is affecting nursing practice.

Describe several ways in which nursing services are administered. Indicate the method of organization that is currently having strong influence on nursing practice.

The Role of the Nurse

GLOSSARY

Accountability: Answerable and responsible for one's conduct.

Biomedical Engineering: Engineering concerned with the use of technology in the delivery of health care.

Biopsychosocial: A term used to describe the wholeness of man; it connotes the interwoveness of the biological, psychological, and social aspects of the human organism.

Certified Registered Nurse: A registered nurse who has met certain criteria as determined by a professional national organization which qualifies her for advanced and specialized practice.

Client: Any person receiving services from a health practitioner. The term is most commonly used when describing care in an ambulatory setting, especially when health maintenance rather than illness care is the primary service being offered.

Clinical Nurse Specialist: A nurse who, by reason of expertise in a clinical speciality, assumes primary responsibility for nursing practice and its effects on health care. Synonym for nurse clinician.

Consumer: One who uses a service or commodity. A health care consumer is one who uses health care services.

Continuing Education: Formal or informal education offered to nurses who have completed basic educational programs in nursing.

Continuity of Care: A continuum of health care, whether the person receiving it is in a state of wellness or illness.

Demography: The science of population statistics.

Dependent Function: An action of the nurse which cannot be executed without a physician's order.

Empirical Knowledge: Knowledge gained primarily from experience or observation.

Expanded Role: A role which has enlarged or increased in size.

Health Care: The total of all services offered by the various health disciplines.

Health Care Team: An organization of health practitioners representing various professions who work collaboratively in planning and administering health care services.

Health Practitioner: One engaged in the practice of dispensing health care services.

Holism: The tendency in nature to produce an organism from units or systems but which functions as a whole.

Independent Function: An action of the nurse which can be executed without a physician's order.

Nurse Clinician: A nurse who, by reason of expertise in a clinical speciality, assumes primary responsibility for nursing practice and its effects on health care. Synonym for clinical nurse specialist.

Nursing Team: A group of technical and professional nursing personnel under the leadership of a qualified nurse, having the goal of providing comprehensive nursing care.

Patient: Any person, well or ill, receiving services from a health practitioner.

Patient Advocate: One who intercedes for or works on behalf of the patient.

Peer Review: The study of one's conduct by another person of the same profession, ability, and rank.

Physician Assistant: One who works as a physician extender. Abbreviated PA.

Physician Extender: One who assumes certain medical care responsibilities delegated by a physician.

Primary Care Nursing: Nursing practice that offers a person his first contact with health care services and assumes responsibility for continuing care by the nurse in cooperation with other health personnel whose services the person requires.

Third Party Payment: Expenditures for health care not paid by the consumer but by a third party, such as an insurance company or a governmental agency.

INTRODUCTION

Nursing today is far removed from nursing of the past which was concerned primarily with the physical care of the sick and disabled. Nursing was task- and illness-oriented. Its chief concern was doing something *to* and *for* the patient but rarely with the patient.

Nursing has changed and continues to do so at an extraordinarily rapid rate. This chapter looks at some of the changes in nursing practice and the role of the nurse in the health care system.

Concepts related to health and illness are described in Chapter 10. In this chapter, they are used in their popular context.

NURSING DESCRIBED

Nursing is concerned with the care of people. Generally, the recipient of nursing care is called a *patient,* that is, any person, well or ill, who is receiving nursing care. Recently the term *client* has often been used to describe the recipient of nursing care. The differentiation between client and patient is not clear-cut. The word patient usually conjures up the image of a sick person who accepts a dependent role as he seeks help from health professionals. Hospitals refer to their populations as patients as do physicians and their employees who see persons in private offices. The word client tends to imply that the person seeking health care services plays an active role and works with health professionals from whom he seeks an assist as he strives to maintain or regain health. At present the term is most often used by nurses when speaking of persons receiving care in an ambulatory setting, ~~walking~~ especially when health maintenance rather than illness care is the primary service being offered. Since most health personnel continue to use the word patient and for ease of reading, this text will use the word patient although it is recognized that either patient or client could be used.

A *consumer* is a person who uses a service. A health care consumer is one who uses health care services.

The person giving nursing care is most often called the nurse. There are some who would prefer that the professional nurse be called a nurse practitioner. Their primary premise is that the term would help destroy the old image of the nurse as a task- and illness-oriented person subservient to medical and institutional bureaucracy. Those opposed to the use of the term point out that it may lead to confusion and that, although the role of the nurse has changed over the years, her title need not. This text will continue to use the word nurse when speaking of the person giving nursing care.

Nursing offers health care services that are directed toward maintaining and promoting health and helping persons cope in the best way possible with the problems of daily living, illness and injury, disability, and death. Nursing is becoming increasingly health-oriented although the care of the sick is still one of its important functions. The nursing role that once included a minimum of health teaching and counseling of patients and their families with regard to health maintenance is now gaining increased attention. The nurse's role that once took limited responsibility in the rehabilitation of the ill and handicapped now implements restorative regimens extensively.

Generally, nursing involves close, personal contact with the recipients of care. It is usually offered on a one-to-one basis. However, many nurses offer services to groups of people, such as families, or neighborhoods.

Nursing is offered on a continuing basis. Care does not begin and end in any one setting, such as the hospital. Rather, through all of life, during health and sickness, nursing services are offered to help consumers maintain healthful behavior, avoid and minimize disease and disability, and restore persons to their best health potential. Continuity of care is defined and discussed later in this chapter.

Nursing is committed to personalized services for all persons without regard to color, creed, or social or economic status. It includes caring for the young and the old, the rich and the poor, the dirty and the clean. A basis for nursing is a belief in the value of every person. Competent nursing practice demonstrates this belief by seeing that a person's health needs are met in a manner that shows concern for him as a unique individual.

Nursing is concerned with services that take into account the wholeness of man. The human being is a physiological as well as a psychological and sociological organism and the three are inextricably interwoven to function as one whole. The term *holism,* which means that nature tends to produce an organism from units or systems but which functions as a whole, is often used to describe the concept of wholeness. A term frequently used in nursing literature to describe the wholeness of man is *biopsychosocial.*

Promoting health by teaching and counseling the patient and his family is assuming an increasing significance in nursing. This changing emphasis from care of the sick only to care aimed at maintaining and promoting health also has resulted in nurses working in a wide variety of settings. Although hospitals are the largest single employer of nurses, they also work in schools, industries, private homes, community health agencies, clinics, physicians' offices, convalescent and nursing homes, day care centers, residential treatment centers, health maintenance organizations, private and group practices, the armed forces, and so on.

In some instances, the nurse functions as a *patient advocate;* that is, she either works indirectly on behalf of a person or intercedes for him. For example, the nurse who lobbies in the legislature in support of programs which benefit the consumer of health care functions as a patient advocate, as does the nurse who seeks a specific service of other health practitioners on behalf of the patient, the nurse who intercedes for the patient by helping him obtain services from various community health agencies, and the nurse who interprets the patient's needs to his family. A nurse becomes an advocate also as she plans the patient's total health care while she articulates the services of all disciplines represented in a health care team.

Nursing recognizes that individuals are members of families. It is of little value to help someone when he must return to a family environment that is nonsupportive of health. Families exist in neighborhoods, communities, and the nation as a whole and nursing has committed itself to service these environments as well. Nursing cannot be everything to everyone, nor can it expect to cure all ills that jeopardize health. However, nursing is committed to promoting individual, family, neighborhood, city, and national health goals in the best manner possible.

Nursing is caring. It is wanting to help somebody who is considered important and to be there when needed. Benjamin Franklin once said that want of care does us more damage than want of knowledge and many nurses would wish to endorse his statement. Many articles in nursing periodicals have described the difference caring made in a person's response when he entered the health care system. One of them appears in the Supplemental Library Study near the end of this chapter. Caring has been a characteristic of nursing since its inception and continues to be fervently guarded.

THE NURSE'S RIGHTS

Nurses enjoy the same rights that society in general accords to all humans, and statements and explorations concerning these rights are appearing more often in nursing literature. But in addition, it is generally agreed that nurses have professional rights too. A nurse who has done considerable research in this area summarized nurses' professional rights as follows:

1. The right to find dignity in self-expression and self-enhancement through the use of our special abilities and educational background.
2. The right to recognition for our contribution through the provision of an environment for its practice, and proper, professional economic rewards.
3. The right to a work environment which will minimize physical and emotional stress and health risks.
4. The right to control what is professional practice within the limits of the law.
5. The right to set standards for excellence in nursing.
6. The right to participate in policy making affecting nursing.
7. The right to social and political action in behalf of nursing and health care.*

Does a nurse have a professional right *not* to do something when she holds her own beliefs or when she feels incompetent to handle a particular health care problem? According to most authorities, nurses do have the right to withdraw in such situations, but only under certain conditions. The Michigan State Nurses' Association prepared a resolution on this issue which has become a guide for other states:

RESOLVED, That the nurse practitioner has the responsibility to inform employers, present and prospective, of her educational preparation, experience, clinical competencies and those ethical beliefs which would affect her practice, and be it,

RESOLVED, That the nurse practitioner has the responsibility to alter, adjust to or withdraw from situations which are in conflict with her preparation, competencies and beliefs, and be it,

RESOLVED, That the employer shall provide the resources through which health services are made available to the recipient, and be it.

RESOLVED, That the nurse practitioner has the right and responsibility to collaborate with her/his employer to create an environment which promotes and assures the delivery of optimal health services, and be it further,

RESOLVED, That the nurse has the right to expect that her/his employer will respect her/his competencies values and individual differences as they relate to her/his practice.†

Note that in this resolution the recipient of care is not neglected when a nurse withdraws. To omit care when a nurse feels incapable of providing it for whatever reason would be a grave injustice to the patient.

---

*Fagin, Claire M. "Nurses' Rights." *American Journal of Nursing,* 75:84, January 1975.
†Fagin, Claire M. "Nurses' Rights." *American Journal of Nursing,* 75:82, January 1975.

COMPREHENSIVE HEALTH CARE

Health care is the total of all services offered by the various health disciplines. It is comprehensive and continuing in nature. Figure 1–1 illustrates the *health care team*. Note that the consumer of health care is the center of focus. A variety of health personnel work interdependently and collaboratively to help meet the needs of persons who enter the health care system. Each group of professionals has specific skills and knowledge to offer the consumer of health care: the nurse offers care that helps an individual achieve and maintain health; the physician focuses on diagnosing pathological conditions and prescribes appropriate medical treatment; the nutritionist plans appropriate care in relation to dietary needs; the physical therapist offers rehabilitation services; and so on. The general term *health practitioner* is often used to describe anyone engaged in the practice of dispensing health care services.

The question is often asked, who is the captain of a team offering total health care? Any health practitioner may assume leadership, depending on the needs of the consumer. For example, when meeting nutritional needs is of prime concern, a nutritionist may take a leadership role. When a patient is acutely ill and needs medical care, the physician may guide the team. Nurses assume leadership when a person is being helped to maintain or regain his state of health with various nursing intervention measures, such as health teaching, comfort measures, and restorative support. The emphasis of the health team is on health. True, caring for the ill remains an important part of total health care but it is no longer considered the only concern of

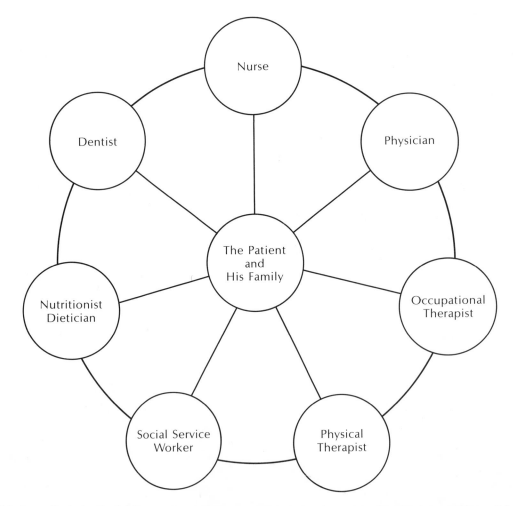

Figure 1–1   This figure illustrates the health care team whose members represent a variety of professions working collaboratively and interdependently to help meet the needs of the patient.

persons working in today's health care system. This change in emphasis from only illness care to health care has had a marked influence on the practice of nursing and will be described more fully later in this chapter.

Comprehensive health care is generally considered to consist of four services: the promotion of health, the prevention of disease, the detection and treatment of disease, and rehabilitation. To list and describe these services does not imply that any one of them is an entity unto itself; in fact, it is difficult to determine exactly where one service ends and another begins since all are related in many ways. In certain instances good rehabilitation practices promote health and thereby prevent disease and disability. Practices that promote health often prevent disease. Techniques that promote health and prevent disease have often improved as a result of improved methods of diagnosing and treating disease.

Nor should it be assumed that health personnel usually are concerned only with a part of these services. Many practitioners contribute to all areas of health care services. For example, each service is of major concern to nurses, and the various ways in which nurses contribute to them are discussed throughout this text.

Sometimes comprehensive health care is further described as being primarily personal or environmental in nature. For instance, a neighborhood can be thought of as a health care consumer. The well-being of the neighborhood can be assessed and it can be offered comprehensive health care containing the same four services listed above. While personal and environmental health services cannot be separated in practice, some distinction can be made in describing them, as the following discussion illustrates.

The Promotion of Health

Health promotion includes the support and development of mental as well as physical health programs. Psychologists and psychiatrists have studied individual responses to stress and strain in considerable detail. From such studies, programs that help to cope with the demands of everyday living are enabling more persons to enjoy better mental and social well-being. The numerous counseling programs are also services that promote good mental health.

The promotion of physical health may be seen in the field of nutrition. Basic food requirements of the body have been well-established. Animal experimentation as well as scientific observation of the dietary customs of humans have shown the effects of both poor and good

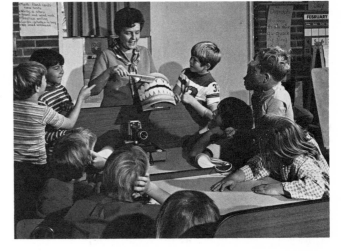

Figure 1–2 Nursing is concerned with promoting health. This school nurse has captured the attention of the children as she demonstrates the proper method of brushing teeth.

eating habits. Through intensive educational programs, nutritionists and their allied co-workers have contributed immeasurably to health promotion by helping people learn how to select proper foods.

The development of park systems throughout our country is one type of environmental program that promotes the health of our citizens. Recreation and activity are recognized as important health factors. The regulations concerning the use of parks are designed to keep them "healthy" for persons wishing to use them.

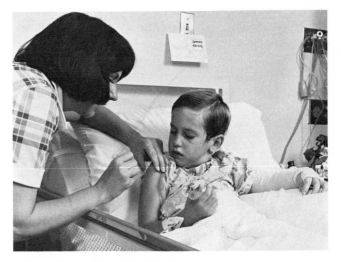

Figure 1–3 The nurse plays an important role in disease prevention. This child was hospitalized with an arm injury. The nurse noted that he had not received a booster DTP (Diphtheria, Tetanus, Pertussis) injection recently and advised that he receive it.

Prevention of Disease

Despite health promotion efforts, disease still attacks man, and science is constantly at work to discover and utilize measures that will aid illness prevention. Fortunately, in many instances, the challenges of disease prevention have been well met. Certain communicable diseases that were prevalent in this country as recently as a few decades ago are now almost nonexistent, due primarily to a nationwide development of immunization programs. Examples are smallpox, diphtheria, and poliomyelitis. Other diseases, such as typhoid fever, have been reduced to a minimum by means of sanitation measures.

Several trends are apparent in preventive health care. One is an attempt to identify early signs of chronic diseases. Preventive measures can then help to decrease the ravages of disability and physical deterioration long before they occur. For example, many of the deteriorating effects of asthma and emphysema can be decreased by early detection and health care regimens, including health education, that diminish progression of these illnesses.

A second trend is increased interest in health problems of the elderly in our population. A great deal of research has been done on the aging process. Some of the common occurrences in the elderly, such as dimming vision and hearing, are now being considered as normal results of aging, rather than as abnormalities or illnesses per se. Also, health practitioners have become increasingly interested in preparing people for those years when it may be necessary to adapt to a new way of life with different but still challenging interests.

A third trend is a marked increase in concern for environmental factors that may cause illness. For example, the interest in air, water, and noise pollution, and their effects on health are front-page news almost daily. Legislating and lobbying to enact measures to promote healthful environments are increasing throughout the country. The promotion of safe working conditions is another example of concern for environmental factors affecting the health of employees. Vacations and rest periods are recognized as important factors in industrial programs to help prevent bodily insult from unrelieved stress and strain.

Still another trend is an effort to locate persons whose health is at risk. Measures usually include screening techniques accompanied by educational programs. These measures have proven effective in disease prevention as well as early disease detection.

Detection and Treatment of Disease

The detection and treatment of disease remain essential responsibilities of health practitioners. In nursing, traditionally, the nurse's role has been one of caring for the ill, and that responsibility remains today. Through her observations and skills in carrying out and supervising nursing care, much of which is very complicated in nature, the nurse plays a critical role in the detection and treatment of disease. Also, the nurse often assists in research programs, and in many instances her contributions have made it possible to move forward more rapidly in disease detection and treatment.

Disease detection and treatment are also noted by persons who have studied the environment of our society. For instance, a neighborhood, like an individual, may be considered to be sick. Poor housing may be one factor contributing to the illness of a neighborhood. Housing facilities that provide for privacy as well as for family sociability and that are hygienic can lead to a cure for conditions that could otherwise take their toll in personal illness.

Rehabilitation

Although rehabilitation has been concerned primarily with restoring a disabled person to his best possible health, a much broader concept is accepted today: rehabilitation is an important aspect of all health care. It is concerned with both emotional and physical disa-

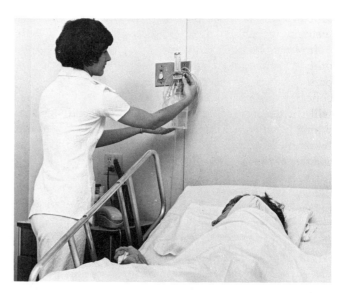

Figure 1-4 Nursing includes caring for the ill. This nurse is monitoring oxygen therapy required by this acutely ill patient.

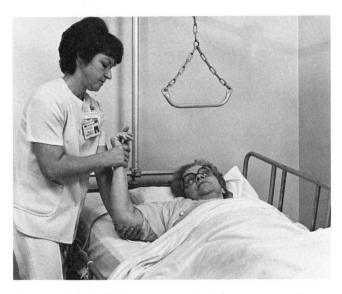

Figure 1–5   Rehabilitation is an important part of nursing. The nurse is performing range of motion exercises so that the patient can use the trapeze to help herself move about in bed and be better prepared for eventual self-care.

bility, and encompasses all ages and occupational groups. For example, it is not limited to that time when a patient may be helped with muscle reeducation in order that he may learn new skills that enable him to regain economic and social usefulness.

Rehabilitation begins with the earliest contact with any person receiving health care. It includes all elements of care and continues throughout the period of illness and thereafter until the person is restored to wellness.

In previous times it was believed that nurses and other health practitioners should provide complete personal care for the patient, even though his physical condition did not necessarily warrant such care. Caring will always be important, but the best care is that which guides the patient toward independence. Rehabilitation is in progress when the patient is taught or assisted to help himself so that he loses neither the desire for self-sufficiency nor the abilities required for day-to-day living. Participation in a program of self-help provides the physical and mental stimulation that contributes to wellness. Self-care also improves patient morale and dignity. Most patients experience great satisfaction and a sense of personal worth as they gradually regain their ability to care for themselves and to make whatever adjustments in living that illnesses or disabilities necessitate.

An environment can also be rehabilitated and many examples could be cited. The present efforts to clean up dirty water in "dead" lakes and streams and then to restock them with plant and animal life characteristic of the natural environment are measures to rehabilitate those lakes and streams for the general good of society.

CONTINUITY OF CARE

Continuity of care is a continuum of care, whether the person is in a state of health or illness. It is implemented by the smooth transfer and follow-up among the comprehensive health care services and among health practitioners and health facilities. It means that any type of care—maintenance, preventive, curative, or rehabilitative—will be available to everyone as required. In far too many instances, persons may be dropped from the rosters of health practitioners or health facilities when an immediate problem has been solved. There has been a decided lack of follow-up to observe results of care given and to offer other types of needed care, either related or unrelated to the problem that initially brought the person to a health practitioner. Implicit in a philosophy of comprehensive health care is the concept of continuity in those services.

The following example will illustrate. A teacher referred a child to the school nurse because the child was having a reading problem. The school nurse examined the child and noted poor focusing of eyes with strabismus (cross-eyes). She referred the child to an eye clinic for evaluation. Surgery was recommended and the child was hospitalized for the surgical procedure. The hospital referred the child to a community health agency. A community health nurse visited the child at home, supervised his home care, and recommended his return to school at the appropriate time. Upon return to school, the nurse followed the child's progress to determine whether the surgical procedure had helped solve the reading problem. Many more people may be involved in any one situation, but this example shows the continuity of the child's care.

The example also shows the importance of health care team personnel working together. A health care team may consist of any number of people with varying skills and educational preparation, but it needs coordination to achieve high-quality care with communications carefully planned among team members. Community health facilities also need to plan together so that unnecessary duplication and gaps in services can be minimized. Methods of communicating among health practitioners that help assure continuity of care are discussed in Chapter 5.

TRENDS INFLUENCING NURSING PRACTICE

There are strong currents in nursing and in society that are influencing nursing practice. Nursing cannot remain static and continue practice that is based solely on tradition without threatening its very existence and relevance. Some trends and the manner in which they are affecting nursing are briefly discussed here.

The Emphasis on Health Promotion

Many factors have no doubt influenced the present concern with health promotion. Possibly one of the greatest influences has been the skyrocketing costs of illness care. It has been estimated that the cost of caring for persons with heart diseases is approximately $3 billion annually. The incidence of heart diseases could be cut in half, it is believed, with proper health promotion and early disease detection. The cost of hospital and medical care has far exceeded the rate of inflation in this country in the last few decades with the result that illness care is economically intolerable for many people. Research has clearly shown that such high costs could be pared if people were helped to maintain their health and prevent illness and disability. Nursing has taken a leadership role in this area and now emphasizes health promotion. Even during periods of illness when nurses work to help patients regain health, the emphasis and concern with care that will eventually support health is maintained.

The general public, as well as health practitioners, now accepts the philosophy that health is a fundamental right of everyone. This philosophy has been best demonstrated in practice as health maintenance has become the core of health care. It is also demonstrated in thinking of wellness as being a great deal more than just not being ill. This concept will be discussed in Chapter 10.

Autonomy of Nursing

Nursing has traditionally labored under hospital and medical bureaucracy. As recently as this midcentury, much education for nursing was given by physicians in hospital settings and nurses had little voice in their practice. A marked change is evident as nurses are removing the yokes of the past and demanding their independence with the right to govern their own practice. And nursing is beginning to receive recognition from other health practitioners and the public for planning and executing nursing services.

Many responsibilities accompany autonomy. If nurses want self-government, they must assume *accountability* for their practice; that is, they must be ready to answer for their conduct in nursing practice. Nurses recognize that they are certainly accountable to the persons for whom they are caring. In addition, they are accountable to themselves and their peers and to professional standards of nursing care as determined by nurses.

Nurses have defined standards of care for some time. However, the public seemed skeptical of health care services and demanded to have quality and cost controls. The United States Congress passed legislation in the mid 1970s calling for some Professional Service Review Organizations (PSRO) to help safeguard the quality of health care while still holding down health care costs. With their belief in autonomy, nurses hold that only they can describe standards of nursing care, and peer review of practice has become increasingly common. *Peer review* is the study of one's practice by another person of the same profession, ability, and rank. Peer review is also seen as a way to implement the standards for nursing practice developed under the aegis of the American Nurses' Association Congress for Nursing Practice and its Divisions on Practice.

The striving for autonomy requires that nurses function on a sound knowledge base. Through research, nursing is actively working to establish its own body of scientific knowledge. Much of the research is being put to use more quickly than in the past as studies attain a higher level of competency and as nursing literature helps to disseminate research findings. A noted trend in research is cooperative study when several institutions, cities, and even states work together. Research in nursing is on the increase and it is being supported by both governmental and private funds.

Nurses are striving for more autonomy through legislative action. This will be discussed more fully later in this chapter and also in Chapter 2.

As autonomy grows, nurses are increasingly working as agents of change in the health care system rather than as the handmaidens of others and they are assuming full responsibility for the care they plan and give.

The Power of Nursing

There are approximately $1\frac{1}{4}$ million nurses in the United States. Roughly 700,000 to 800,000 are gainfully employed in the profession. Nurses are increasingly aware of the strength they have in numbers and are using it effectively to influence health care. As one nursing educator stated, this number of nurses has the power to get us from where we now are in the health care system to where we wish to be in order to offer consumers quality health care. Leadership lies primarily in the American Nurses' Association and its state associations although only about one-fifth of the nurses in this country are members.

The Nurses Coalition for Action in Politics, commonly called N-CAP, is the political arm of the American Nurses' Association. The director of N-CAP described its function thus: "Political action is a program to elect to public office people who share our views on public policy, a program to seek out good candidates, to endorse them, to give them campaign money and volunteers, and to do everything we possibly can do to help them win elective office."* In 1976, for the first time, nurses endorsed and worked for the election of candidates for the Congress of the United States. Approximately 90 percent of the candidates supported by N-CAP won election. State nurses' associations are also developing political action committees to work at state levels.

The power of nursing has become evident also in matters of federal legislation on health care. For example, nurses are being asked to serve on committees dealing with topics related to health care and they are being called upon for testimony in Congress when bills affecting health are being considered. As another example, in the mid-1970s, the then President Ford vetoed a bill that would have denied nursing millions of dollars in support of educational programs for nursing. Legislative committees of the American Nurses' Association joined forces to convince representatives in Congress for the need to override the President's veto. Nurses believed that health care in this nation would suffer by the loss of money to support education for nursing. Congress defeated the veto mainly because of the lobbying efforts of countless numbers of nurses. At state and local levels too, the power of nursing is being used more and more with the result that nurses are gaining their place as an autonomous and equal profession in the health care system.

The Knowledge Explosion

Scientific research has uncovered new knowledge at a tremendously rapid pace. Consider for a moment a few relatively recent applications of new knowledge that have changed our way of living dramatically: space

exploration, the computer, and communication via satellites. Or consider these scientific advances more closely associated with health: organ transplants, the "pill" and other new drugs, the laser beam, and the sophisticated hardware used in electronic monitoring systems.

In the social sciences, great strides have been made in attempting to understand and predict human behavior, an important area of knowledge for health practitioners. Thus, knowledge related to values, attitudes and prejudices, social mobility, and ethnic, social, and cultural backgrounds is utilized by health practitioners in designing care that is appropriate and acceptable to each individual and more in accordance with his own life-style.

Nurses must know more in order to function effectively, efficiently, and safely in today's world, and in more settings than previously. However, as in other areas of study, it is impossible to acquire all of the knowledge available and appropriate to nursing. Educational programs in nursing are responding to the knowledge explosion in several ways.

Educators and practitioners know that *empirical knowledge,* which is gathered primarily from experience and observation only, and the memorization of procedures and routines are no longer adequate. The result has been that educational programs are increasingly teaching scientific principles that will guide practice for all possible circumstances. For example, the nurse who has learned what equipment she will use and what steps she will take in the procedure of administering a cleansing enema to an adult patient in a particular hospital is helpless in any other setting or with other types of patients. However, the nurse who understands the scientific principles involved (introduction of a solution into the colon to stimulate peristalsis) can function anywhere, using appropriate equipment on hand.

Education for nursing places more emphasis than previously on applying knowledge from the behavioral sciences. Concern for a person who is a unique human being, demands a knowledge of human behavior. This approach emphasizes the person being served and is being applied increasingly when there is concern for a biopsychosocial being.

There appears to be no evidence that the knowledge explosion is about to diminish. This requires that *continuing education,* education offered to nurses who have completed basic education programs in nursing, be a part of every practitioner's life in order that she be up-to-date and competent. Continuing education includes workshops, conferences, and agency inservice

*"N-CAP Slates ERA Program During ANA Convention." *American Journal of Nursing,* 76:712, May 1936.

education programs. Chapter 2 contains additional discussion of the trend to make continuing education mandatory.

The knowledge explosion has made it increasingly necessary for specialization in nursing. Educational programs have responded accordingly. Those offered in institutions of higher learning grant degrees upon successful completion of master's and doctoral requirements. In addition, there are many formal and informal nondegree educational offerings which further the preparation of specialized practitioners in nursing. This trend toward specialization has been accomplished with greater emphasis on clinical nursing. It is different from the specialization that once was almost entirely limited to administration or teaching in nursing. For example, there are nurses who prepare to work in cardiac and coronary units, respiratory units, hemodialysis units, community mental health centers, adult ambulatory clinics, and well-baby and well-child clinics. Clinical practitioners are being prepared in increasing numbers in various specialties, such as gerontology which deals with aging, oncology which focuses on cancer, neonatology which concentrates on the newborn, family practice, and midwifery. These nurses are often called *clinical nurse specialists* or *nurse clinicians*.

Another way in which nursing is moving to qualify experienced registered nurses for advanced and specialized nursing care is to provide for certification. In 1977, the definition of certification adopted by the Interdivisional Council on Certification of the American Nurses' Association was as follows: "Certification is the documented validation of specific qualifications demonstrated by the individual registered nurse in the provision of professional nursing care in a defined area of practice."*

Qualifications for certification vary somewhat but generally include having had a license to practice nursing for two years, practicing in an area in which certification is sought, passing an examination, having evidence of continuing education and satisfactory work experience, references, and presenting evidence of case studies or of innovative projects. Certification is valid for five years.

Nurses who meet certification requirements are usually called *certified registered nurses*. Well over a thousand nurses had been certified by the American Nurses' Association in 1976. Various other organizations also certify registered nurses.

---

* "ANA Certification Council Approves New Definition to Reflect Current Goals." (News) *American Journal of Nursing,* 77:1390, September 1977.

Demographic Changes

Demography is the science of population statistics. Population statistics include life expectancy rates, mortality rates, population shifts, marriage and divorce rates, and birth rates.

The population is increasing in the United States which means more people are in need of health care services. Life expectancy has increased, resulting in more older people in our population. Older persons and youngsters create increased demands on health practitioners since it has been observed that both these groups tend to require more health services than other age groups.

There has been a change in population patterns with more people moving to urban and suburban areas, although some reports indicate that in selected areas this trend may be reversing somewhat. Many persons, especially the elderly, are electing to live in regions with favorable weather. The rural areas, especially those that are sparsely populated, are often isolated from adequate health care facilities or practitioners.

Family and community structures are also changing. Today's population is more mobile than in the past, resulting in weakening neighborhood and community support to family life. Divorce rates have increased, resulting in more single-parent homes. More people live alone than was true in the past. And so on.

Nursing is responding to demographic changes in various ways. More educational offerings and programs of many varieties are evident. Recruitment is helping to attract more persons to a career in nursing. Nursing, once almost entirely limited to Caucasian women, now welcomes men and non-Caucasians to its ranks. Recruitment of inactive nurses has been on the increase. Health services, often with governmental support, are being extended to remote areas of this country, and nurses are increasingly attracted to positions in these areas. In order to utilize nurses more efficiently, careful scrutiny has resulted in delegating non-nursing tasks that once occupied much of the nurse's time to nonnursing personnel.

The Increasingly Knowledgeable Consumer

A better educated population, with more knowledge of health and with easy access to numerous communications media dispensing increasing amounts of health information, has resulted in a more knowledgeable consumer. At least two results are evident: the consumer is demanding more health care and he is demanding high-quality health care. This means that nurses, just like other health practitioners, must be better educated and prepared if consumer demands are to be satisfied. This, nursing is attempted to do. Chapter 3 will further discuss the health demands of the consumer and the implications these have for health practitioners.

The Women's Liberation Movement

Nursing traces its origins to orders, often religious in nature, that expected unending service and unquestioned obedience to superiors. Nursing was a woman's occupation, and the nurse's role was that of a mother surrogate who nurtured those who were ill and helpless. A nurse would have been considered unworthy if she asked for something for herself or if she questioned authority. Men are increasingly choosing nursing as a career, but most nurses are still women. However, men are joining women to change the traditional image of the nurse and of women in general.

Today's woman is taking steps to free herself for independent action and thought. She seeks social, economic, political, and educational equality with men. Through legislative channels she is demanding equality as a legal right, not as a privilege granted only by those who voluntarily choose to recognize her as an individual and equal. Some contemporary commentators have said that women are in the midst of a social revolution. Through the women's liberation movement and with considerable determination, women are fighting prejudice and oppression and progressing toward liberation.

The goals of the women's liberation movement are legitimate goals for women in nursing too. These goals include such rights as equality and dignity, pursuit of life goals, access to leadership positions, economic rewards commensurate with their contributions to society, and self-determination. Attaining these goals requires cohesiveness and a unified spirit which nursing is learning to attain and use. Nurses are willing to assume responsibility for their conduct and are beginning to assume a new self-identity. They are in the process of consciousness-raising, of publicizing their cause, of becoming more assertive, and of demanding recognition for the worth of their unique contributions to the nation's health care.

Economic and General Welfare Programs in Nursing

Many authorities believe that nursing's failure from its inception to take aggressive steps to assure economic and general welfare benefits has proven to be a stum-

bling block to progress toward full autonomy and social recognition. The costs of nursing services are rarely calculated in relation to nursing's contribution to the health care system. Except for private duty nurses and nurses in private practice, patients and insurance carriers have not reimbursed nurses for services rendered. Rather, institutions, and often physicians, have made decisions concerning economic benefits without regard to input from nurses. There is evidence that this situation is changing.

The American Nurses' Association has worked to improve economic and general welfare programs for decades and has been able to make considerable progress. The ANA welcomed amendments to the Taft-Hartley Act to ensure protective collective bargaining activities for employees (except management personnel) in nonprofit health care agencies. The Act states that employees have the right to bargain collectively through representatives of their own selection. While there have been differences of opinion concerning details in the intent of the law, most nurses accept collective bargaining as a way not only to improve their own economic security and general welfare, but also to effectively upgrade health care.

Nurses are also actively seeking to change present policies concerning payment for nursing services. *Third party payment* is presently the most common way for providing reimbursement for health care. The consumer does not pay directly for most of his care; insurance carriers, including governmental reimbursement programs, pay for the consumer's care. Nursing services are not reimbursed as a separate part in these third party payments. Rather, the employers of nurses (health institutions, physicians, and others) are paid and they in turn reimburse nurses for services rendered. Generally this has meant that nurses have little or no control over their economic and general welfare programs. It is hoped that within the not too distant future, direct reimbursement will replace present payment policies.

In addition, nurses are continuing to work to change laws presently affecting their education and licensure. This type of legislation, indirectly at least, influences economic and general welfare programs also. Legislation in nursing will be discussed more fully in Chapter 2.

Technological Advances in Health Care

Nursing is becoming enmeshed with *biomedical engineering,* a relatively new field that is concerned with the increasing use of technology in the delivery of health care. More sophisticated equipment is being developed to assist the health care team. Monitoring equipment and kidney dialysis machines are two examples. Another is the computer which can be used to assist with such nursing responsibilities as recording, developing care plans, and staff scheduling. Inevitably, biomedical engineering will expand and broaden and the nurse who fails to keep in step with the trend will soon fall short of competent practice. However, all machines have limitations and cannot replace the personal and continued contact that nurses have with consumers of health care services.

The Human Rights Movement

The tendency for each person to be concerned primarily with only his own welfare is rapidly disappearing. Society today is looking closely at the moral and ethical quality of its actions and motives. This trend has resulted in a closer scrutiny of what may be considered as morally right or wrong in our relations with others. Concern for the poor, the lonely, the criminal, the alcoholic, the drug addict, the unemployed and unemployable, the neglected, and the underdog in society is evident throughout the country. Isolating and forgetting the down-and-outer, the wrongdoer, or the misfit to a hopeless life of despair and frustration irritate a responsible social conscience.

A national concern for human rights, born of discrimination, has become a reality within the last few decades. The human rights movement has improved the lot of many people, including women, children, homosexuals, racial minorities, the handicapped, prisoners, the poor, and other groups as well.

Many nurses have joined various human rights movements. Their efforts often improved their own lot, but also that of the consumers of health care. Further discussion of the rights of the patient will be included in Chapter 3.

Since its beginning, nursing has demonstrated interest in caring for all persons needing care, regardless of the circumstances of the individual. The human rights movement has helped strengthen nursing's long-standing commitment to care that demonstrates compassion and understanding and accepting the consumer as the person he is.

The Expanding Role of the Nurse

The trends just discussed have had a marked influence on the role of the nurse. It is often described as an *expanded role,* that is, one which has enlarged or increased in size. The nurse no longer serves only other health practitioners. Nor do her services consist of little more than technical skills. Rather, as described earlier, she has enlarged her role to give care that will help meet the total needs of consumers of health services.

This expanded role of the nurse has developed largely as a result of consumer demands. Everyone tends to insist on more and better care. To fill gaps, nurses have stepped in to take the responsibility for total health care with a resulting expanded role.

The expanded role of the nurse should not be confused with that of the *physician extender*. Such a person, also called a *physician assistant,* or PA, takes over certain medical care responsibilities delegated by the physician. It could be said that the PA works to "extend the physician's arm." The expanded role of the nurse focuses on the provision of *nursing* care that is unique and different from medical care.

ADMINISTERING NURSING SERVICES

As stated earlier in this chapter, the health care team was developed as a means to organize, coordinate, and dispense health care services. Nursing too often organizes a team of personnel to help carry out nursing care. The team leader plans, supervises, and evaluates the total team effort. Characteristically, a *nursing team* is headed by a qualified nurse who has as her assistants other nurses as well as practical nurses, nursing assistants, nursing aides, home health aides, nursing volunteers, clerical assistants, and the like.

There are some persons who refer to dependent and independent functions of the nurse and have described the administration of nursing services with these functions in mind. *Dependent functions* of the nurse are those which are not executed without a physician's order. For example, a nurse does not prescribe and administer drugs without a physician's order. *Independent functions* are those which can be carried out by a nurse without a physician's order. Tending to the hygienic needs of a patient is a responsibility of the nurse that does not require a physician's order.

Many nurses are objecting to a description of independent and dependent functions in the manner just described. These nurses say nursing is its own profession, self-regulating, self-determining, and separate from other health disciplines. Hence, nursing's functions are independent of other health professionals.

While dependent and independent functions are still described in some literature, the terms appear to be losing popularity.

A more recent term that is having an impact on the nurse's role in the administration of health care services is primary care. The nurse offering primary care is often called a primary care nurse or primary nurse. *Primary care nursing* is described as continuing nursing responsibility for a person during all stages of illness and wellness. A primary nurse begins contact with the person at his point of entry into the health care system. She continues to assume responsibility for his total care, using other health disciplines and social and health agencies as required by the patient.

When a person requires hospitalization, a primary nurse becomes responsible for his care. The hospital primary nurse admits the patient, plans his 24-hour care, sees to it that the patient's plan of care is executed, does health teaching, and plans for discharge and continuing care after hospitalization.

Primary care nurses are professional practitioners who are accountable for their practice, demonstrate leadership and ability to work interdependently with other health professionals, assess and diagnose a patient's nursing needs, and manage, develop, implement, and evaluate nursing care. Primary care nursing usually results in the nurse speaking of those to whom she gives care as "my patients" and her patients speak of the primary nurse as "my nurse." According to primary care nurses, the result has been an interpersonal relationship that fosters a high quality of nursing care.

CONCLUSION

Nurses constitute the largest single group of health personnel in the United States. Still, with ever-increasing demands for their services, more nurses are needed. In addition, the scope and range of nursing's responsibilities in meeting the health care needs of society mean assuming increased responsibility, developing effective collaboration with other health practitioners, and supporting new and promising methods for delivering health care services more effectively.

SUPPLEMENTAL LIBRARY STUDY

1. This chapter pointed out the importance of caring. The following article describes its importance in nursing care:

    Domstead, D. J. "With Mr. J—We Didn't Know Where to Begin." *Nursing 77,* 7:28–29, August 1977.

    How did the nurses demonstrate caring for Mr. J.? To what does the author give credit when Mr. J. began showing signs of caring about himself? Describe at least three types of physical care included in the patient's plan of care. Describe several ways in which the students and their instructor communicated with Mr. J. before he started speaking.

2. The following article describes collaboration between a nurse and a physician who were co-directors of a comprehensive child care center:

    Thomstad, Beatrice, et al. "Changing the Rules of the Doctor-Nurse Game." *Nursing Outlook,* 23:422–427, July 1975.

    What backgrounds did the nurse and physician bring to their working relationship which made it difficult for both of them to work in an interdependent and collaborative manner? What "rules" did the nurse follow in order to gain the support of parents so that treatment and follow-up care of children being seen in the clinic were observed? After following new "rules" in the nurse-physician-parent relationship, what did the authors list and describe as improvements in the health care services they offered?

3. The following article describes a form of independent nursing practice:

    Whitson, Betty Jo, et al. "Complemental Nursing." *American Journal of Nursing,* 77:984–988, June 1977.

    On what premise was the type of nursing care described in this article based? What effect did it make on the patient when she could say that Ms. Hartley was "my nurse"? What did the nurse consider to be the rewarding aspects of complemental nursing? How does the type of nursing described here compare with primary care nursing as described in this chapter?

4. The editor of the *American Journal of Nursing* describes the danger of using poor semantics with regard to medical and nursing practice in the following editorial:

    Schorr, Thelma M. "Watch Those Words!" (Editorial) *American Journal of Nursing,* 77:805, May 1977.

    Ms. Schorr stated that the term physician extender has no meaning in relation to the nurse practitioner. Describe how you would support this statement. Summarize the testimony given by an American Nurses' Association official to the Senate Committee on Agriculture and Forestry. According to the editorial, what stands in the way of needed health care services for many people who live in rural areas?

2

BEHAVIORAL OBJECTIVES

When content in this chapter has been mastered, the student will be able to

Define the terms appearing in the glossary.

State the essence of the American Nurses' Association and the International Code for Nurses.

Explain why ethical issues in health care services are more complex today than was true in the past.

List four sources of laws and give an example of one law derived from each source.

Indicate the primary purpose of nurse practice acts.

Describe briefly the four types of programs that presently prepare nursing personnel for licensure and the New York State Nurses' Association proposed legislation for 1985. Include how the proposal will influence the state's educational programs and licensure procedures.

Summarize the National League for Nursing's position on collegiate programs that have no major in nursing but are being offered to enrolled nursing students and registered nurses.

Describe one current legislative trend related to each of the following: continuing education, certification, and institutional licensure.

Give an example of each of the following wrongs: tort, crime, malpractice, slander, libel, false imprisonment, invasion of privacy, assault, battery, fraud.

Explain why students in nursing have been held legally responsible for their nursing practice.

Briefly discuss how each of the following laws influences nurses: good samaritan laws; drug abuse laws; the Food, Drug, and Cosmetic Act; and the Occupational Safety and Health Act.

Describe the basic legal requirements of a will.

State the principle upon which the defense of the accused is based in this country.

Ethical and Legal Considerations in Nursing

GLOSSARY

Administrative Law: A law made by administrative or executive agencies of the government.

Assault: A threat, or an attempt, to make bodily contact with another person without that person's consent.

Battery: An assault that is carried out.

Civil Law: A rule that regulates relationships among people. Synonym for private law.

Common Law: A law resulting from court decisions that is then followed when other cases involving similar circumstances and facts arise. Common law is as binding as civil law.

Constitutional Law: A law stated in the federal and state constitutions.

Continuing Education: Planned educational experiences offered nurses who have completed basic educational programs in nursing.

Crime: An offense against persons or property. The act is considered to be against the government, referred to in a lawsuit as "The People" and the accused is prosecuted by the state.

Defamation: Wrongs of slander and libel.

Defendant: A person accused of a tort or crime.

Ethics: Judgments concerning right and wrong conduct.

Expert Witness: A person having special training or experience who assists a judge and jury in their decision-making process.

False Imprisonment: Unjustifiable retention or prevention of the movement of another person without proper consent.

Felony: A crime punishable by imprisonment in a state or federal penitentiary for more than one year. Felony is also described as a crime of deeper offense than a misdemeanor.

Fraud: Willful and purposeful misrepresentation that could cause, or has caused, loss or harm to persons or property.

Good Samaritan Law: A law that holds physicians and nurses harmless when undertaking to aid a person in emergency situations.

Invasion of Privacy: A wrong that invades the right of a person to be let alone.

Jurisprudence: The philosophy or science of law.

Law: A rule of conduct established and enforced by the government of a society.

Lawsuit: A legal action in a court of law.

Libel: An untruthful written statement about a person that subjects him to ridicule or contempt.

Litigation: The process of a lawsuit.

Malpractice: An act of negligence as applied to a professional person, such as a physician, nurse, or dentist.

Mandatory Nurse Practice Act: A law that requires a nurse to be licensed in order to practice nursing.

Manslaughter: Second-degree murder.

Misdemeanor: A crime, of lesser offense than a felony, punishable by fines or imprisonment, usually for less than one year, or both.

Murder: The illegal killing of another person.

(First-degree murder: Murder with malice aforethought.)

(Second-degree murder: Murder without previous deliberation, sometimes called manslaughter.)

Negligence: Performing an act that a reasonably prudent person under similar circumstances would not do, or failing to perform an act that a reasonably prudent person under similar circumstances would do.

Permissive Nurse Practice Act: A law that allows the licensed nurse to call herself a registered nurse but does not require that the nurse be licensed to practice.

Plaintiff: A person or government bringing a lawsuit against another.

Precedent: The first case that sets down a common law.

Private Law: A rule that regulates relationships among people. Synonym for civil law.

Privileged Communication: Information that need not be revealed in court by the person receiving it.

Public Law: A rule that regulates relationships between individuals and their government.

Respondeat Superior: The master-servant rule that states that an employer is legally liable for his employee's acts.

Responsibility: An obligation to perform some act for which one can be held accountable.

Right: A claim to a particular privilege.

Slander: An untruthful oral statement about a person that subjects him to ridicule or contempt.

Standard of Care: A description of conduct that illustrates what a reasonably prudent person would have done, or would not have done, under similar circumstances.

Stare Decisis: A Latin phrase meaning "Let the decision stand." **Stare decisis** is the basis for common law.

Statutory Law: A law enacted by a legislative body.

Testator: One who makes a will.

Tort: A wrong committed by a person against another person or his property.

Waiver: A legal provision that gives up a right or claim.

INTRODUCTION

As indicated in Chapter 1, accountability for practice has become a generally accepted principle in nursing. In the past, physicians and hospitals assumed much more responsibility for a nurse's action than is true today. However, as the nurse's role expanded, and as it continues to do so, the responsibility of being accountable for her action increased for the nurse and assumed increased ethical and legal implications.

There is a public trust involved when health practitioners administer health care services. Society rightfully expects practitioners to assume responsibility for giving services that are skillfully done and executed with sound judgment. To offer less violates that public trust.

A detailed discussion of ethical and legal aspects of nursing generally is included in curricula of schools of nursing at the time students are nearing graduation. Hence, the discussion here will be brief. However, because certain ethical and legal considerations involve nurses from the time they begin their education in nursing, it seems appropriate to include an early overview.

ETHICS, RIGHTS, AND RESPONSIBILITIES: CODES OF ETHICS FOR NURSES

The word *ethics* originates from the Greek word *ethos.* It is concerned with judgments on what is right or wrong conduct. An important word in this definition is judgment. For example, an ethical issue is involved concerning when to stop life-saving measures if a patient is dying since no habitual code of conduct has been defined in this matter in our culture. Some say ethics is what we *ought* to do when society does not have a law or a rule to describe what we should do.

The ethics of various professions are described in codes. Through its code, each professional group sets standards of practice for its members. An ethical code derives from the dignity and rights of the patient as a person and indicates acceptance of the trust and of the responsibility the patient places in the profession. It is based on respecting the values and circumstances of those nursing serves.

The code of ethics for nurses adopted by the American Nurses' Association in 1950 and revised periodically since then consists of 11 statements.

A copy of the code and an interpretation of each of the 11 statements can be obtained from the American Nurses' Association or from state nurses' associations.

Code for nurses

1 The nurse provides services with respect for human dignity and the uniqueness of the client unrestricted by considerations of social or economic status, personal attributes, or the nature of health problems.
2 The nurse safeguards the client's right to privacy by judiciously protecting information of a confidential nature.
3 The nurse acts to safeguard the client and the public when health care and safety are affected by the incompetent, unethical, or illegal practice of any person.
4 The nurse assumes responsibility and accountability for individual nursing judgments and actions.
5 The nurse maintains competence in nursing.
6 The nurse exercises informed judgment and uses individual competence and qualifications as criteria in seeking consultation, accepting responsibilities, and delegating nursing activities to others.
7 The nurse participates in activities that contribute to the ongoing development of the profession's body of knowledge.
8 The nurse participates in the profession's efforts to implement and improve standards of nursing.
9 The nurse participates in the profession's efforts to establish and maintain conditions of employment conductive to high quality nursing care.
10 The nurse participates in the profession's effort to protect the public from misinformation and misrepresentation and to maintain the integrity of nursing.
11 The nurse collaborates with members of the health professions and other citizens in promoting community and national efforts to meet the health needs of the public.

Code for Nurses with Interpretive Statements. American Nurses' Association, Kansas City, Missouri, 1976, p. 3.

The code of ethics for nurses adopted in 1973 by the International Council of Nurses is shown on page 19.

While these codes have served well, shortcomings have been described. One nursing author has suggested that nurses might do well to develop a personal code of ethics to use in addition to the two described here. Her criticisms of the present codes and suggestions for a personal code are included in the Supplemental Library Study at the end of this chapter.

A *right* is a claim to a particular privilege. For example, adults in the United States who have met certain legal requirements have a right to vote. A *responsibility* is an obligation on the part of a person to perform some act for which he becomes accountable. Tending to the hygienic needs of a helpless patient is a responsibility in nursing.

Nurses are becoming increasingly concerned with the rights of the individual and nurses' responsibilities when research using humans as subjects is conducted. The American Nurses' Association Commission on

---

1973 Code for nurses
ETHICAL CONCEPTS APPLIED TO NURSING

The fundamental responsibility of the nurse is fourfold: to promote health, to prevent illness, to restore health and to alleviate suffering.

The need for nursing is universal. Inherent in nursing is respect for life, dignity and rights of man. It is unrestricted by considerations of nationality, race, creed, colour, age, sex, politics or social status.

Nurses render health services to the individual, the family and the community and coordinate their services with those of related groups.

Nurses and People
The nurse's primary responsibility is to those people who require nursing care.

The nurse, in providing care, respects the beliefs, values and customs of the individual.

The nurse holds in confidence personal information and uses judgment in sharing this information.

Nurses and Practice
The nurse carries personal responsibility for nursing practice and for maintaining competence by continual learning.

The nurse maintains the highest standards of nursing care possible within the reality of a specific situation.

The nurse uses judgment in relation to individual competence when accepting and delegating responsibilities.

The nurse when acting in a professional capacity should at all times maintain standards of personal conduct that would reflect credit upon the profession.

Nurses and Society
The nurse shares with other citizens the responsibility for initiating and supporting action to meet the health and social needs of the public.

Nurses and Co-Workers
The nurse sustains a cooperative relationship with co-workers in nursing and other fields.

The nurse takes appropriate action to safeguard the individual when his care is endangered by a co-worker or any other person.

Nurses and the Profession
The nurse plays the major role in determining and implementing desirable standards of nursing practice and nursing education.

The nurse is active in developing a core of professional knowledge.

The nurse, acting through the professional organization, participates in establishing and maintaining equitable social and economic working conditions in nursing.

"The ICN Meets in Mexico City." *American Journal of Nursing*, 73:1351, August 1973.

Nursing Research points out that the relationship between patient and nurse as described in codes for nurses applies also in situations involving research. There are elements of trust and respect for the individual that must remain inviolate. The Commission has prepared position statements for two sets of rights. The first set concerns the rights of qualified nurses to conduct research and to have access to information in their investigations. The other set deals with the rights of persons who participate in the research and is described thus:

> The relationship of trust between patient and nurse has always been an essential element of the professional code of ethics. In research, the relationship of trust between subject and investigator requires that the investigator assume special obligations to safeguard the subject in several ways. The subject needs to be assured that his rights will not be violated without his voluntary and informed consent. Secondly, the investigator guarantees that no risk, discomfort, invasion of privacy, or threat to personal dignity beyond that initially stated in describing the subject's role in the study will be imposed without further permission being obtained. Finally, the subject is assured that if he does not wish to participate in the study, he will neither be subjected to harassment nor will the quality of his care be influenced by this decision.*

---

* *Human Rights Guidelines For Nurses in Clinical and Other Research.* American Nurses' Association, Kansas City, Missouri, 1975, pp. 1–2.

Words such as ethics, rights, and responsibilities are relatively easy to define. However, issues often fall into grey areas when, in practice, all terms become involved. For example, when a patient is judged terminally ill, is it ethically correct to halt life-saving procedures? Does the patient in this type of situation have a right to assist with decision-making about his care? What responsibilities do health care professionals have in the matter?

Time was when decisions involving ethical issues were fairly easy to make. But they are becoming more complex because of such factors as the increased use of machines and techniques to prolong life, the legalization of abortions, the increased knowledge related to genetic and molecular biology, in vitro transplants, and research using humans as subjects. Science has reached the point of no longer being free of value judgments. Ethical issues ultimately raise questions of values and cannot be based solely on logic or "common sense."

Without ethical guidelines, health care becomes dehumanized and loses sight of the uniqueness of each individual and his rights as a human being. There is no easy answer for what to do in every situation in which an ethical issue is at stake. While ethical codes offer help, each situation usually must be judged on its own merits. However, a commitment to ethical standards of practice is an essential part of nursing as is the commitment to respecting the rights and dignity of the person receiving health care.

DEFINITION OF LAW

A *law* is a rule of conduct established and enforced by the government of a society. Laws are applicable to the people living in a governmental jurisdiction, such as the city, county, state, and country, over which authority is exercised by that government. Laws are intended chiefly to protect the rights of the public. For example, nurse practice acts are intended primarily to protect the public and secondarily, to protect the nurse. Of particular importance is the fact that laws are not only promulgated by governmental processes, but are also enforceable by authority of that government.

Laws may be regarded as standards of conduct. They make it possible for people to live together peacefully. The philosophy or science of law is called *jurisprudence*.

Public law is a law in which the government is directly involved. It regulates the relationships between individuals and the government. Also, an important body of public law describes the powers of the government in authority. (*Private law,* also called *civil law,* regulates the relationships among people. Civil law includes laws relating to contracts, ownership of property, the practice of nursing, medicine, pharmacy, dentistry, and so on.)

SOURCES OF LAWS

There are four main sources of laws or rules of conduct in our country: constitutions, legislatures, the judiciary system, and administrative regulations.

Constitutions

In any society there must be an authoritative body if chaos is to be prevented. Although authority comes from the people, each individual relinquishes certain rights in order that a form of government can be established and given the authority to govern. The government is charged with the responsibility of maintaining order and protecting the general welfare of its people.

Federal and state constitutions indicate how their governments are created and given authority. These constitutions state the principles and provisions for establishing specific laws. Although they contain relatively few laws (called *constitutional laws*), they are constant guides to legislative bodies. In our country each state constitution directs the governing of a specific geographic area, but it can in no way violate principles set down in the federal constitution.

Although individuals relinquish certain rights in order that a government can be created, constitutions are not without their limits. For example, the first ten amendments of the federal constitution are called the Bill of Rights. These amendments restrict the passage of laws that infringe on certain basic liberties, such as freedom of worship, freedom of speech, freedom from unwarranted search and seizure of our homes and persons, and so on. Each state constitution sets similar limitations.

The Legislatures

Under the federal constitution our government has created legislative bodies that are responsible for enacting laws. These bodies are called the Congress at the federal level and legislatures at the state level. Certain legislative bodies at the local level, such as county and municipalities, may be established also. A *statutory law* is a law enacted by a legislative body. Statutory laws must be in keeping with the federal constitution and, within each state, with that state's constitution as well. Nurse practice acts are statutory laws.

The Judiciary System

Our government provides for a judiciary system which is responsible for reconciling controversies and conflicts. It interprets legislation as it has been applied in specific instances and makes decisions concerning law enforcement. Over the years, a body of law known as *common law* has grown out of these accumulated judiciary decisions.

Common law is based on the principle of *stare decisis,* or "Let the decision stand." In other words, once a decision has been made in a court of law, that decision becomes the rule to follow when other cases involving similar circumstances and facts arise. The case that first sets down the rule by decision is called a *precedent*. Court decisions can be changed, but only when strong justification exists. Common law helps prevent one set of rules from being used to judge one person and another set to judge another person in similar circumstances.

Common law directly related to nursing exists.

Under common law, students in hospital-controlled schools of nursing have been considered employees of the hospital.

Administrative Regulations

One responsibility of the executive branch of our government is to execute the law of the land. Executive power resides in the president of the United States, the governors of the states, and the mayors, or their equivalents, at the municipal level. These chief executive officers administer various agencies that, among other things, are responsible for law enforcement. These agencies have power to make administrative rules and regulations in conformity with enacted law. The rules and regulations act as laws and are enforceable, just as any law in the country. They are called *administrative laws.*

Federal administrative agencies include the Federal Trade Commission, the Federal Communications Commission, and the Interstate Commerce Commission. Boards of nursing are administrative agencies at the state level, and a municipal administrative agency is a city's board of health.

NURSE PRACTICE ACTS

It has been pointed out that federal and state constitutions provide governments that we as individuals charge with the responsibility of securing the public welfare. Legislative bodies have used this principle to enact laws that control certain occupational and professional groups. In other words, to secure public welfare, laws governing these groups are designed to prevent incompetent persons from practicing by establishing minimum standards which qualified practitioners must meet. In general, the goal of these laws is accomplished through two channels: schools preparing practitioners must maintain certain minimum standards of education, and graduates of the educational programs may be licensed only after satisfactory completion of an examination. In addition, these laws include certain other requirements, such as citizenship.

Nursing is one group operating under state statutory laws that were designed in keeping with federal and state constitutional principles to promote the general welfare. The first law in the United States dealing with the practice of nursing was enacted in 1903 in North Carolina. At present there are nurse practice acts in the 50 states, the District of Columbia, Puerto Rico, Guam, Samoa, and the Virgin Islands.

Laws vary considerably from state to state. Some laws define nursing, while others describe what a nurse may or may not do in the practice of nursing. In some states the law requires that a nurse be licensed to practice; such a law usually is referred to as a *mandatory nurse practice act.* In other states, the law allows the licensed nurse to call herself a registered nurse or an RN but does not require that the nurse be licensed to practice. Such a law is called a *permissive nurse practice act.* In states having permissive nurse practice acts, many health agencies have a policy of not employing unlicensed nurses. While these agencies are entitled to have such a policy, this policy does not change the fact that the laws in those states do not require licensure to practice nursing.

In most states, the administrative agency that has power to make regulations regarding nurse practice acts is the state board of nursing. In a few states, the board of nursing acts in an advisory capacity to an agency that is ultimately responsible for the enforcement of the nurse practice act. The regulations made by these boards or their equivalent become laws in themselves, as previously described. Some typical responsibilities include determining minimum standards for education of nurses, setting requirements for licensure, and deciding when a nurse's license may be suspended or revoked.

Nurses who actively supported and worked hard for enactment of nurse practice acts deserve much credit. But modifications in earlier laws continue. For example, a change, actively being sought in many states, would broaden the legal definition of nursing in order that nurses may assume greater responsibilities legally as their roles expand. In some states, this has already been accomplished. In others, legislation is still pending.

EDUCATION FOR NURSING AND PROPOSED LEGISLATION

At present, several kinds of state-approved educational programs for preparing nurses for licensure exist in this country.

Practical/Vocational Programs

One type of state-approved program prepares practical/vocational nurse personnel. Upon completing a course of study, usually one to one and a half years, the graduate is eligible to write the practical or vocational nurse licensing examination. These programs are administered in different kinds of settings—hospitals, high schools, vocational schools, and others.

Associate Degree Programs

Seven associate degree programs in nursing were started in this country in the early 1950s. By 1979, there were well over 600 associate degree programs. Most are located in community colleges, and courses of study can be completed within two years. The primary purpose of these programs has been to prepare nurses capable of practicing at a technical level under the supervision of a professional registered nurse. Graduates of these programs are awarded an associate degree in nursing and are eligible to write the registered nurse licensure examination.

Diploma Programs

The total number of diploma schools of nursing in the United States has been dropping in recent years although these schools continue to prepare a large number of students for registered nurse licensure. Diploma programs are usually offered by hospitals and ordinarily can be completed within a three-year period. A diploma is earned upon completing the course of study and the graduate of a diploma program is eligible to write the registered nurse licensure examination.

Baccalaureate Programs

Baccalaureate programs in nursing are graduating approximately 25,000 nurses each year. The programs are offered by both senior colleges and universities and can be completed in about four years. A baccalaureate degree in nursing is earned upon completion of the course, and graduates are eligible to write the registered nurse licensure examination. In addition to programs leading to baccalaureate degrees in nursing, many institutions of higher education also offer master's and doctoral programs.

Graduates of associate degree, diploma, and baccalaureate degree programs in nursing write identical examinations for registered nurse licensure although the goals of these three types of programs vary considerably. Often, employers of nurses, the general public, and nurses themselves have been confused concerning appropriate roles in nursing for persons graduated from very different types of programs. The confusion has often influenced the role of the practical/vocational nurse as well. As a result, nurses are now exploring ways in which all nursing personnel can be prepared and licensed in a manner that will more accurately describe their appropriate roles, improve the quality of education for nursing, end much present confusion, and ultimately improve the quality of health care in this country.

In 1965, the American Nurses' Association supported the position of many nurse educators when it proposed that basic education for nursing be placed in educational institutions. Since then, many hospital-controlled schools gf nursing have ceased functioning and many more programs for nursing have been opened in college and university settings.

The New York State Nurses' Association has now proposed to carry this trend of placing programs for nursing in educational institutions one step further. In a striking move, it proposed legislation that would make a baccalaureate degree in nursing the minimum requirement for professional nursing licensure by 1985. It also proposed that there be a second level of nursing and that programs to prepare these persons should lead to an associate degree in nursing. Graduates of these programs would be eligible to write a licensure examination but one which would be different in intent from the examination for persons qualified to become registered nurses. New York State's licensed practical nurse organization has endorsed this proposed legislation.

Titles for nursing personnel to be graduated from these two New York State Nurses' Association proposed programs are still unclear, according to nursing leaders presently discussing the proposal. Graduates of associate degree programs might be called practical nurses, technical nurses, or registered associate nurses. Graduates of baccalaureate programs would be called registered nurses, professional nurses, or registered professional nurses. The proposed legislation has separate definitions for the two types of nurses.

A *waiver* is a legal provision that gives up a right or claim. For example, when a new licensure bill becomes law, in order to avoid prejudice against persons licensed under a previous law, a waiver exempts these persons from having to comply. This type of waiver is often called a "grandfather clause." According to the New York State Nurses' Association proposal, anyone licensed before January 1, 1984 would not need to meet the degree requirements and would be waivered in for one of the two licenses.

There are obstacles to the passage of the proposed

bill, but the New York State Nurses' Association is optimistic that it will become law by 1985. Other states are following this proposed legislation carefully and some are presenting conferences at local levels to discuss the pros and cons of the bill. Many nurses believe that when legislation of this nature becomes a law in New York, other states will rapidly follow with similar legislation.

The New York State Nurses' Association has shown leadership and considerable courage in making a new path for education for nursing and for nursing as a whole. Chapter 1 described nursing's drive for autonomy and the political power nurses have. Nurses in New York are illustrating both in their actions.

Another issue related to education for nursing deserves mention, although legislation is not being proposed at the present time. There has been concern about degree programs for nurses that do not have a major in nursing. The National League for Nursing, which is the professional accrediting body for various educational programs in nursing, has taken a stand against these programs, as the following statement indicates:

> The National League for Nursing notes with concern the growth in the number of collegiate programs that have no major in nursing but are designed to appeal specifically to potential and enrolled nursing students and registered nurses. Unfortunately, the publicity about these programs leads students to believe that degree programs with no major in nursing offer preparation for advanced positions in nursing and/or provide the base needed for further education in nursing when this is *not* the case.
>
> The programs in question lead to associate or baccalaureate degrees in such fields as applied science, biology, education, health science, occupational therapy, psychology, sociology, and community or health arts. The collegiate programs may provide the student with increased knowledge in the specified area of the major, but they do not offer additional preparation in nursing. Therefore, the nurse may encounter difficulty in pursuing graduate study in nursing.
>
> The National League for Nursing believes the misguidance of the students occurs when publicity about these programs:
>
> 1. Implies that a major in another field is equivalent to a major in nursing as preparation for nursing practice—*when it is not.*
> 2. Implies that they are acceptable as a base for further education in nursing—*when they are not.*
> 3. Implies that they lead to advancement in employment—*which in many instances they do not.*
> 4. Implies that because only graduates of NLN-accredited nursing programs are awarded credit, the degree programs are therefore approved by NLN—*which they are not.**

Not all nurses support the National League for Nursing stand on this issue. However, prospective students are well-advised to consider promotional literature carefully before making a decision on career goals, according to the League.

LEGISLATION ON CONTINUING EDUCATION, CERTIFICATION, AND INSTITUTIONAL LICENSURE

Many health disciplines have been criticized because licensure laws have not made provisions to assure continued competency after a license to practice has been granted. Because of the knowledge explosion, changing roles in many health professions, and the public's general disillusionment with health care, some type of action seemed necessary. *Continuing education,* that is, planned educational experience offered to nurses who have completed basic education programs in nursing, has been offered as a solution.

Nursing has supported continuing education programs for many years. However, these offerings were usually attended on a voluntary basis. When attendance was made mandatory by employees, nurses often complained that the programs were inadequate and useless. Others said there were insufficient qualified nurses to teach. Nursing has begun to take steps to help assure continued competency and to assist in the development of better continuing educational experiences. In addition, many states are taking legislative action to make continuing education mandatory for the renewal of licenses.

The American Nurses' Association Commission on Nursing Education, through its Council on Continuing Education, developed a national program to assist states with their continuing education programs. There is also a national accrediting board that evaluates the programs. These efforts, it is hoped, will eventually help assure nurses that they are attending worthwhile programs.

In 1977, the *American Journal of Nursing* began featuring a self-study program for continuing education. A test is taken during or after study, the results of which can be sent to the agency or person of the nurse's choice, for continuing education credit. This innovative program should be of particular help to

---

*"A Statement of Concern About Associate and Baccalaureate Degree Programs for Nurses That Have No Major in Nursing." *Nursing Outlook,* 25:484, August 1977.

those nurses who, for whatever reason, find it impossible to attend continuing education programs.

Each year, more states are requiring continuing education for licensure renewal. State boards of nursing or their equivalent are usually charged with such responsibilities as approving programs, specifying credit or unit values, approving licensure renewal when nurses have met the requirements, and so on. The boards often seek advice from state nurses' associations concerning the quality of continuing educational offerings. It is predicted that the trend to legislate mandatory continuing education for licensure renewal will continue despite sufficient initial opposition in some states to kill bills in legislative committees.

Certification of registered nurses was discussed in Chapter 1. Washington became the first state to pass a law allowing nurses authorized by its Board of Nursing to prescribe legend (prescription) drugs. The Board's plan was to approve nurses for this expanded role who were certified registered nurses and, hence, qualified for specialization and advanced practice. Many believe that this type of legislation is likely to spread to other parts of the country.

Several years ago, proposals were made to replace state licensure for nurses with institutional licensure. Proponents of the plan believed that institutions, such as hospitals, should license nurses since they would be better able to determine continued competency in nursing than state boards of nursing. Nursing in general deplored these proposals and worked hard to prevent their becoming a legal reality. At present, there appears to be a dwindling interest in institutional licensure. However, the experience has illustrated how nursing remains constantly alert to efforts which, opinion holds, will decrease nursing autonomy and which in the long run would be detrimental to providing consumers with competent health care services.

TORTS AND CRIMES

A *tort* is a wrong committed by a person against another person or his property. In most instances, the court in a civil case, that is, a case involving a tort, will settle damages with money but rarely by imprisonment. Torts may be intentional or unintentional acts of wrongdoing. A person committing an intentional tort is considered to have knowledge of the permitted legal limits of his words or acts. Violating these limits is grounds for prosecution.

A *crime* is also a wrong against a person or his prop-

erty, but the act is considered to be against the public as well. In a criminal case, the government, called "The People", prosecutes the offender. When a crime is committed, the factor of intent to commit wrong is present. A crime is punished either by fines or imprisonment or both.

An act generally considered a tort may, because of its severity, be classed as a crime. For example, gross negligence that demonstrates the offender guilty of complete disregard for another's life may be tried as both civil and criminal action. It is then prosecuted under criminal as well as civil law. By its very nature, a wrong tried as a crime implies a more serious offense with more legal implications than a tort.

There are specific laws that define action of violators of such laws as crimes. For example, failure to observe the Federal Food, Drug and Cosmetic Act may constitute a crime, whether there was intent or not.

Negligence and Malpractice

Negligence is defined as performing an act that a reasonably prudent person under similar circumstances would not do, or conversely, failing to perform an act that a reasonably prudent person under similar circumstances would do. As the definition implies, an act of negligence may be an act of omission or commission.

In order to determine negligence, a *standard of care* is devised by deciding what a reasonably prudent person would or would not have done, under similar circumstances. To assist juries and judges, standards of care are given in testimony by an *expert witness*. An expert witness is a person having special training or experience that assists a judge and jury in their decision-making process. In instances involving nursing practice, a nurse may be requested to act as an expert to describe what standards of care could be expected under similar circumstances. The expert witness is not called upon to testify either for or against the person charged with negligence. He merely describes standards of care to assist the court in arriving at its decision.

Two important additional items are involved in determining negligence: knowing that failure to observe the standard of care could cause harm and demonstrating that harm resulted because of improper care.

Table 2–1 offers guidelines for understanding negligence. Giving medications is used as an example in the table. The following are other negligent acts often committed by nurses:

• Being careless with a patient's personal belongings, such

TABLE 2-1   Guidelines on negligence*

ELEMENTS OF LIABILITY	EXPLANATION	EXAMPLE—GIVING MEDICATIONS
Duty to use due care (defined by the standard of care)	The care which should be given under the circumstances (what the reasonably prudent nurse would have done)	A nurse should give medications: accurately and completely and on time
Failure to meet standard of care (breach of duty)	Not giving the care which should be given under the circumstances	A nurse fails to give medications: accurately or completely or on time
Foreseeability of harm	Knowledge that not meeting the standard of care will cause harm to the patient	Giving the wrong medication or the wrong dosage or not on schedule will probably cause harm to the patient
Failure to meet standard of care (breach) *causes* injury	Patient is harmed because proper care is not given	Wrong medication causes patient to have a convulsion
Injury	Actual harm results to patient	Convulsion or other serious complication

Adapted from Springer, Eric W., editor. *Nursing and the Law.* Aspen Systems Corporation, Pittsburgh, 1970, p. 4.
* Professional negligence is malpractice.

as clothing, jewelry, dentures, and eyeglasses, which results in damage or loss of the articles.

- Failing to see that a hospitalized patient's call signal is answered. The patient may then try to take care of his own need and injure himself in the attempt.

- Failing to use proper protective measures with resulting injury to the patient, such as neglecting to take proper steps to avoid an accident with fire in the presence of oxygen therapy and failing to remove faulty equipment from use.

- Failing to carry out orders for treatments and medications correctly, to report untoward signs and symptoms, and to investigate a questionable order before carrying it out when its execution results in harm to the patient.

Malpractice is the term generally used to describe negligence of professional personnel. One authority stated that malpractice is a limited term. Negligence is all-inclusive. In other words, malpractice and negligence are not two separate torts, but one and the same. What is necessary to constitute an act of negligence is essential to constitute an act of malpractice.

Slander and Libel

Slander and libel are sometimes called the wrongs of *defamation*. Slander is an untruthful oral statement about a person that subjects him to ridicule or contempt. Libel is the same, except that the statement is in writing, signs, pictures, or the like. Thus false statements that indicate someone is unfit for the practice of his profession can be either slander or libel. Falsely accusing someone of committing a crime constitutes slander or libel. Nurses who make false statements about their patient or their co-workers run the risk of being sued for slander or libel.

A person charged with slander or libel is not liable if he can prove that his oral or written statement is true. Also, *privileged communication* is legally acceptable defense for defamation. Privileged communication protects information exchanged between certain people, and the information need not be disclosed in a court of law. Communication between an attorney and his client has long been recognized as privileged. Many states have statutes that recognize privilege in a physician–patient or a priest–communicant communication. A few specifically mention nurses in their laws. Privilege is based on the supposition that professional persons cannot give adequate care without the person's complete disclosure of facts related to his problems. Privileged communication is a complex subject, but the nurse should at least be aware of the existence of laws on confidential information coming to her knowledge when attending patients.

False Imprisonment

Unjustifiable retention or preventing the movement of another person without proper consent can constitute *false imprisonment*. The indiscriminate and thoughtless use of restraints is an act that can constitute false imprisonment. Only a reasonable amount of restraint should be used in circumstances that warrant restraint. Occasionally a delicate balance of judgment is required in the use of restraints.

A person cannot be held legally against his will for his failure to pay for services rendered. Nor can he be legally forced to remain in a health agency, such as a hospital, if he is sound of mind, even when health practitioners believe the person should remain for additional care. Health agencies have special forms to use in such cases which the person signs indicating he will not hold the agency responsible for any harm that may result from his leaving. A mentally ill patient or a person with certain communicable diseases can legally be kept in an agency if he presents a danger to society.

Invasion of Privacy

The U.S. Supreme Court has interpreted the right against invasion of privacy as inherent in the federal constitution. The Fourth Amendment, it held, was an effort to protect citizens by giving them the right of privacy and the right to be let alone.

Necessary exposure of a patient by procedures essential to his care is not grounds for invasion of privacy. However, if a patient is exposed to the public, either personally or through pictures or recordings, the person responsible for the exposure can be held liable. This does not hold if the patient has given consent for the exposure. Unauthorized exposure even after death may constitute invasion of privacy.

Health practitioners should recognize that unnecessary exposure of patients, while moving them through health agency corridors or while caring for them in shared rooms, can constitute invasion of privacy. Talking with patients in areas that are not soundproof can constitute unnecessary exposure. Personnel who gossip or discuss information concerning patients with persons not entitled to the information may be charged with invasion of privacy. Information on patients' records is considered confidential and should not be discussed with unauthorized persons. Special care to protect a patient's privacy is recommended in the use of tape recorders, Dictaphones, computer banks, and so on. Nurses who prepare written or oral class assignments are advised to conceal the identity of patients in order to prevent invasion of privacy. Nurses carrying out research are also encouraged to take precautions to protect the anonymity of patients.

Assault and Battery

Assault is a threat, or an attempt, to make bodily contact with another person without that person's consent. *Battery* is an assault that is carried out. Every person is granted freedom from bodily contact by another unless consent has been granted. In the field of health, a person operated on without his consent can sue the surgeon, or the health agency involved, or both. Health personnel cannot force persons to do things or submit to care against their will, unless consent has been granted, without fear of legal suit.

Every individual has the right to be free from inva-

sion of his person. For health practitioners, an awareness of this principle and of requirements for consent is extremely important. Table 2–2 offers guidelines on consent.

TABLE 2–2 Guidelines on consent

WHAT IS IT	PERMISSION TO TOUCH	
When it is needed or not needed	Needed: Routine hospital services, diagnostic procedures and medical treatment Any nonroutine medical or surgical treatment	Not needed: Emergency *if:* immediate threat to life or health experts agree that it's an emergency patient unable to consent and legally authorized person can't be reached Action in response to a complication during an operation if legally authorized person can't be reached When patient voluntarily submits
Consequences of not having consent	Nurse and doctor may be liable for battery Hospital is liable for battery because it has a duty to protect patients or it's responsible for its employees' actions	
Criteria for valid consent	Written (oral, if can be proved in court) Signed by patient or person legally responsible for him Patient (or signer) understands the nature of the procedure, the risks involved and probable consequences Procedure performed was one consented to	
Who signs	Patient signs when able Others sign When patient is physically unable, legally incompetent, a minor, unless married or self-supporting When patient's reproductive capability will be ended, spouse should sign	
Failure to sign	A patient has the right to refuse, but should sign a release form as proof of his refusal A hospital may request a court order to act when a patient's refusal endangers his life	

Adapted from Springer, Eric W., editor. *Nursing and the Law.* Aspen Systems Corporation, Pittsburgh, 1970, p. 29.

Fraud

Fraud is willful and purposeful misrepresentation that could cause, or has caused, loss or harm to persons or property. Misrepresentation of a product is a common fraudulent act. In nursing, persons fraudulently misrepresenting themselves in order to obtain a license to practice may be prosecuted under nurse practice acts. Also, misrepresenting the outcome of a procedure or treatment may constitute fraud.

Table 2–3 aids in understanding intentional torts.

CRIMINAL ACTS

A *crime* is an offense against persons or property. It is a more serious offense than a tort and is considered to be against the government representing the people. Hence, in a lawsuit, the plaintiff, that is, the one bringing suit, is called "The People" and the accused is prosecuted by the state.

In most states, criminal law is statutory law and only infrequently, common law. Crimes are classified as *felonies* or *misdemeanors.* Misdemeanors are less serious crimes than felonies. Felonies are punishable by imprisonment in a state or federal penitentiary for more than one year. Misdemeanors are commonly punishable with fines or imprisonment for less than one year, or both.

First-degree murder is illegally killing another person with malice aforethought. *Second-degree murder* is killing another person without previous deliberation. In some states, second-degree murder is called *manslaughter.* First- and second-degree murders are felonies.

A person practicing nursing or medicine unlawfully and whose patient dies as a result can be tried for the felony of manslaughter. Additional crimes include rape, mayhem, robbery, accessories to crime, extortion, and blackmail.

ADDITIONAL LAWS OF INTEREST TO NURSES

The Nursing Student's Legal Status

In hospital-controlled programs, the nursing student has been considered an employee of the agency. The student is responsible for her own act of negligence if injury to a patient results. The hospital can also be held

TABLE 2–3 Intentional torts important to the nurse

LEGAL TERM	DEFINITION	EXAMPLE
Assault*	Placing a person in fear of being touched without his consent	Threatening to hit someone
Battery*	Actually touching someone without his consent	Hitting someone
False imprisonment	The unlawful detention of a person against his wishes	Keeping a patient hospitalized until he has paid his bill
Invasion of privacy	Violation of a person's right to be left alone and to have certain personal matters kept out of the public view	Taking pictures of a malformed child without parental permission
Defamation	Injuring the good name of another person by telling falsehoods about him to a third person	
Libel	Written defamation	Writing that someone is a thief
Slander	Oral defamation	Saying someone is a thief

Adapted from Springer, Eric W., editor. *Nursing and the Law.* Aspen Systems Corporation, Pittsburgh, 1970, p. 52.
* They usually occur together so the popular term for such a wrong is "Assault and Battery." But either act may occur separately: threatening to strike somebody, an assault; touching someone without consent or warning, a battery without assault.

liable under the principle of *respondeat superior,* which states that an employer is responsible for his employee's acts. The status of students enrolled in college and university programs is not clear since there appears to be no evidence of the status having been defined in a court of law.

Patients harmed by student acts may also bring suit for damages against an instructor-supervisor. An instructor-supervisor can be held responsible for reasonable and prudent supervision of students. Through student assignments, she is vouching for fitness and competency. If standards of supervision are violated, negligence may be charged. If students feel their assignments are beyond their competency, it is recommended that they call attention to this to the instructor-supervisor responsible for the assignment.

This is the way one author discussed student negligence:

"Although it may seem a harsh rule at first, a student nurse is held to the standard of a competent professional nurse in the performance of nursing duties. In several judicial decisions, the courts have indicated that anyone who acts as a nurse by performing duties customarily performed by professional nurses is held to the standards of a professional nurse . . . From the patient's point of view, it would be unfair to deprive him of the opportunity to recover from the injury because the hospital uses students to provide nursing care to him.*

It is strongly recommended that nursing students carry professional liability insurance which is often called malpractice insurance. Schools generally do not have such insurance coverage for students. A health agency in which the student gives care *may* have insurance, but the student may find the coverage unsatisfactory to her. Investigation of the policy is urged. After studying the policy, the student may feel more secure if she has her own insurance also. Insurance is available from commercial insurance companies. It is also available through the National Student Nurses' Association. For graduate nurses, insurance is available through the American Nurses' Association. The company with whom the nurse insures provides legal defense when a suit is brought and also pays the defendant's claim if the insured is found guilty. Personal professional liability insurance also protects the insured when the person is away from his place of work. An employer's policy will not. For example, if a nursing student assisted in an emergency in a neighbor's home, an agency's policy would not offer her liability protection. Nor would an agency's policy protect a nurse who is "moonlighting" as a private duty nurse.

Good Samaritan Laws

Good samaritan laws are designed to hold physicians and nurses, and others in some states, unaccountable when they undertake to give aid to persons in emergency situations. For example, if a nurse or physician happens onto the scene of an auto accident, either may give emergency care as it appears necessary without fear of legal suit, unless care is given in a grossly negligent manner.

Forty-eight states, Kentucky and Missouri excepting, and Washington D.C. have good samaritan laws although the laws vary considerably. Nurses are covered in some states, while in others, they are not. So far, there appears to be no common law resulting from

decisions based on these statutes. As a result, the manner in which these laws would be interpreted in a court case remains speculative. Many laws give certain persons immunity, and some provide standards of care in emergency situations with phrases such as actions in "good faith" or actions "without gross negligence." These descriptions of standards and the immunities would appear to decrease likelihood of liability and, hence, tend to encourage health practitioners to render assistance at the scene of an emergency.

No person has a legal obligation to help another and a health practitioner, as any other person, may choose to help or to leave the scene of an emergency. However, in many situations, there would appear to be an ethical responsibility to assist. When health practitioners do assist and consent is not possible prior to giving care, they are expected to use good judgment in determining whether an emergency exists and to give care that a reasonably prudent person with a similar background and in a similar circumstance would give.

Drug Abuse Laws

The Harrison Narcotic Act of 1914 was the first federal law which attempted to prevent drug abuse. Several amendments were added. The Comprehensive Drug Abuse Prevention and Control Act of 1970 replaced the previous act and its amendments. The Federal Bureau of Narcotics and Dangerous Drugs (BNDD) of the U.S. Department of Justice enforces this 1970 Act. States also have laws to further regulate drug abuse. Violators of federal and state laws are prosecuted either under federal or state law as indicated. Wrong acts are considered as acts of crime.

Drug abuse laws provide for the registration of those who may prescribe drugs, such as physicians, dentists, and veterinarians. Nurses ordinarily act under the supervision of a registered person in the eyes of the laws and, hence, are not required to be registered to administer prescribed drugs. Drug abuse laws are specific and violations are serious offenses.

Federal Food, Drug, and Cosmetic Act

Among other things, this act is concerned with non-narcotics, such as hypnotic and barbiturate drugs, and with certain other "dangerous" drugs. Only qualified persons, such as physicians and dentists, may prescribe drugs described in this law. The nurse's role relates to the administration of these drugs.

---

*Springer, Eric W., editor. *Nursing and the Law*. Aspen Systems Corporation, Health Law Center, Pittsburgh, 1970, p. 8.

Occupational Safety and Health Act

The Occupational Safety and Health Act of 1970, popularly known as OSHA, set legal standards in an effort to "assure safe and healthful working conditions for men and women." The Act is intended to reduce work-related injuries and illnesses. It has had an impact on health agencies and has increased the responsibilities of many nurses. The following situations require careful consideration because of threats to worker safety: the use of isolation techniques for patients with infectious diseases and the management of contaminated equipment and supplies; the use of radiation, sound or radio waves, infrared, ultraviolet, and laser beams; the use of electrical equipment; and the use of chemicals, such as those that are toxic or flammable. The law is specific concerning its application and fines can be severe when infractions are noted. Nurses can assist in implementing this law by promoting health and safety precautions wherever they work. Nurses employed in industrial settings have a particularly important role in conforming to the law's requirements. Later in this text, there will be descriptions of recommended safety measures when, for example, nurses are working with patients who are isolated because of infectious diseases or are receiving oxygen therapy.

Laws Related to Wills

State laws regulate requirements for a will. Nurses sometimes are asked to witness a will. By so doing, the nurse, indicates that the will was signed by the *testator,* the person who made the will in which he describes intentions he wishes to be carried out upon his death. Also, the witness indicates that to the best of his knowledge, the testator was of sound mind and acted voluntarily.

Wills occasionally specify intention concerning autopsies and organ donations. Consent necessary when wills do not specify wishes will be discussed in Chapter 26. So also will the "living will."

DEFENSE OF THE ACCUSED

A *lawsuit* is a legal action in a court. *Litigation* is the process of a lawsuit. The person or government bringing suit against another is called the *plaintiff.* The one being accused of a tort or crime is called the *defendant.* The defendant has every opportunity in our courts of law to defend himself and certain specific defenses for torts and crimes have already been mentioned. Philosophically, a defendant is presumed innocent unless proven guilty. Recent U.S. Supreme Court decisions, some of which gained considerable publicity, were predicated on the tenet that in our country every effort shall be directed toward justice for the accused. Hence, being accused of a tort or a crime does not necessarily imply guilt.

CONCLUSION

Graduate and student nurses, as individuals and as members of their profession, are legally and ethically responsible for their acts and are committed to the promotion of the public welfare. While discussion on the legal and ethical aspects of nursing is necessarily brief in this text, the reader is urged to study references and news media reports, especially reports appearing in nursing periodicals, to keep informed and up-to-date on the legal and ethical components of nursing.

SUPPLEMENTAL LIBRARY STUDY

1. The following article describes several legal responsibilities of the nurse:

    Creighton, Helen. "Your Legal Risks in Nursing Coronary Patients: How You Can (And Should) Minimize Them." (Career Guide) *Nursing 77,* 7:65–68, 70–71, January 1977.

    List the legal responsibilities of nurses as stated in this article and briefly describe how you can safeguard yourself with regard to each of the responsibilities. Describe what the author meant when she said that there are risks as well as rewards when a nurse specializes in some area of nursing care.

2. Scientific advances often present ethical problems, according to the following article:

    Silva, Mary Cipriano. "Science, Ethics, and Nursing." *American Journal of Nursing,* 74:2004–2007, November 1974.

    List three or four nursing situations in which an ethical issue may be involved other than those noted by the author. According to Ms. Silva, what limitations do most professional codes have? Describe the nature of a personal code of ethics suggested by this author.

3. The following author describes the legislative process on pages 109 and 110 in this publication:

    Anderson, Edith H. "The Political Context and Process of Health Legislation." In Madeleine Leininger and Gary Buck, editors. *Health Care Dimensions: Fall 1974 Health Care Issues.* F. A. Davis Company, Philadelphia, 1974, pp. 107–116.

    Describe how an idea becomes a bill and finally a law. List

two or three national health issues described by the author. What strategies for change does she recommend?

4. The following editorial focuses on a problem that can arise when two members of a health care team hold different views concerning the scope of their respective practices:

Lewis, Edith P. "The Right to Inform." (Editorial) *Nursing Outlook*, 25:561, September 1977.

In this instance, on what aspect of the nurse's practice was she found guilty in a court of law? What implication does this court decision have on the scope and limits of nursing practice and how is this implication at variance with present views on professional nursing practice?

5. It is common for nurses to act as witnesses when patients sign consent forms before surgery and certain other medical procedures. A nurse writes that a signed consent form in certain cases can be without legal substance.

"Profile: Avice Kerr, RN" *Nursing 75*, 5:15, July 1975.

In order to be of legal value, what essential ingredient must be present when a patient signs a consent form? What right does a patient have before signing such a form? Describe how Miss Kerr has acted in the role of an advocate in her work.

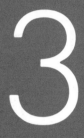

3

BEHAVIORAL OBJECTIVES

When content in this chapter has been mastered, the student will be able to

Define the terms appearing in the glossary.

List at least eight objections that consumers are voicing in relation to health care services.

Describe briefly the content of the American Hospital Association's bill of rights for patients.

Summarize at least six expectations most consumers hold regarding nursing care.

Describe how most health care services are financed in this country.

State at least two pros and two cons related to proposed national health insurance plans.

Summarize briefly the main points made by the American Nurses' Association in its resolution on national health insurance.

List at least ten problems of health-illness that have been largely solved in this country since the turn of the century.

List at least ten problems of health-illness that have largely evaded solution to date in this country.

Discuss briefly the implications an aging population in this country has in terms of health-illness care.

Describe how the American life-style stands in the way of increased longevity and health.

Identify at least ten current trends which demonstrate efforts that are being taken to meet common demands of consumers of health care.

The Consumer of Health Care Services

GLOSSARY

Life Expectancy: The average number of years a person at a given age can be expected to live.

Life Span: The length of time that it is possible for a member of a species to live.

Longevity: The length or duration of life.

Morbidity: The incidence of disease or pathological condition in a poulation.

Mortality: The ratio of deaths to a population.

Paraprofessional: A health worker who is prepared to assist professional health personnel.

INTRODUCTION

Until recently, the consumer of health care services has been largely ignored, although he was known to have dissatisfactions and unmet needs. He was excluded from research and planning for health care services and was offered primarily what health personnel thought he needed and wanted. But now his voice is being heard throughout the country. This chapter describes some of the consumer's complaints and problems related to health care and efforts that are being taken to meet the consumer's needs.

THE CONSUMER SPEAKS

The United States enjoys the largest number of health care workers in proportion to the total population in the world. About 44 million people are employed in health-related work. Approximately 8 percent of our gross national product, or over $600 for every American, is spent each year for health care services, and the total expenditures continue to rise. It is estimated that, by the early 1980s, the total amount of money spent each year on health care will exceed $200 billion. This country has advanced technologically at a fantastic rate. Yet, ironically, it is suffering from what many consider to be a health care crisis.

It is possible that the consumer has started a new social movement with regard to health care. He is beginning to exert what he considers to be his right to high-quality health care and is demanding that he receive it at a price he can afford. He does not see himself as helpless. He is no longer satisfied to be told what he needs and wants. He does not want to be stripped of his dignity and identity, and he resents invasions of his privacy. He asks for courtesy and information concerning his care. Health care still remains largely disaster- and illness-oriented and too concerned with treating parts rather than the whole person. The consumer resents this sort of care. To summarize, the consumer is concerned about the high cost of health care, the inability to get services in some areas of the country, the lack of respect for his rights, and neglect by health personnel in helping him stay well. He wants more knowledge about his care, insists that he too should help make decisions concerning the care he receives, and shows interest in helping himself to stay well.

The Citizen's Board of Inquiry into Health Services for Americans had as its purpose the study of America's health services from the viewpoint of the consumer.

The Board found the consumer to be vocal and frank. Although its report was published early in the 1970s, a review of current literature reveals that the situation apparently has not changed appreciably for the consumer of health care services in this country. The report summarized the voice of the consumer as follows:

- Most Americans do not have adequate health care; they have crisis care. They obtain health services only when sickness or injury forces them to muster the money and risk the obstacles and humiliations.
- Once a decision is made to seek care, many Americans have no choice of where or from whom to seek it, and those with a choice usually have available no reasonable basis for decision.
- Having decided where to go for care, the patient must still overcome a variety of obstacles before he receives services.
- On arriving at a hospital or other health care facility, the patient may discover that he must "buy a ticket" (receipt for payment) before receiving any services.
- The persistent patient who overcomes the barriers to care may find himself treated with indignity and insensitivity.
- Sometimes the line between insensitivity and poor quality care is blurred. A patient's persistent attempts to get more careful attention may have negligible or negative results.
- The patient often discovers that the medical services he has received are more expensive than he had expected, and that the insurance for which he has paid so dearly affords him only minimal coverage.
- Many of the same barriers that deterred the patient from seeking care in the first place interfere with his following through on the medical advice and recommendations he receives.
- With all the anger and the difficulties, people will still do what they feel they must to get needed health care. While there is great frustration, sometimes even desperation, there is little apathy.*

The consumer has learned what constitutes quality care from many sources—education, the news media, travel, and so on. He has gained confidence to ask questions concerning the services he is receiving. He is aware of his power at the polls and his right to quality care at a price he can afford. He may well be the greatest spur to better health care that this country has ever experienced.

THE CONSUMER'S BILL OF RIGHTS

The consumer's demand for what he believes he is due when he enters the health care system has resulted in

---

* *Heal Yourself.* Report of the Citizens Board of Inquiry Into Health Services for Americans, pp. 1–13.

statements frequently referred to as the patient's bill of rights. As early as 1959, the National League for Nursing drafted a patient's bill of rights which, according to reports, is being updated and revised. The 1959 version includes such rights as the patient's right to receive quality and continuing nursing care to regain or maintain health and his right to have care that is sensitive to his needs and feelings, instructions on how he can help himself to stay well, and personal matters related to his care kept confidential.

Another notable effort occurred when the American Hospital Association described a patient's bill of rights as follows:

The American Hospital Association presents a Patient's Bill of Rights with the expectation that observance of these rights will contribute to more effective patient care and greater satisfaction for the patient, his physician, and the hospital organization. Further, the Association presents these rights in the expectation that they will be supported by the hospital on behalf of its patients, as an integral part of the healing process. It is recognized that a personal relationship between the physician and the patient is essential for the provision of proper medical care. The traditional physician–patient relationship takes on a new dimension when care is rendered within an organizational structure. Legal precedent has established that the institution itself also has a responsibility to the patient. It is in recognition of these factors that these rights are affirmed.

1. The patient has the right to considerate and respectful care.

2. The patient has the right to obtain from his physician complete current information concerning his diagnosis, treatment, and prognosis in terms the patient can be reasonably expected to understand. When it is not medically advisable to give such information to the patient, the information should be made available to an appropriate person in his behalf. He has the right to know by name the physician responsible for coordinating his care.

3. The patient has the right to receive from his physician information necessary to give informed consent prior to the start of any procedure and/or treatment. Except in emergencies, such information for informed consent should include but not necessarily be limited to the specific procedure and/or treatment, the medically significant risks involved, and the probable duration of incapacitation. Where medically significant alternatives for care or treatment exist, or when the patient requests information concerning medical alternatives, the patient has the right to such information. The patient also has the right to know the name of the person responsible for the procedures and/or treatment.

4. The patient has the right to refuse treatment to the extent permitted by law, and to be informed of the medical consequences of his action.

5. The patient has the right to every consideration of his privacy concerning his own medical care program. Case discussion, consultation, examination, and treatment are confidential and should be conducted discreetly. Those not directly involved in his care must have the permission of the patient to be present.

6. The patient has the right to expect that all communications and records pertaining to his care should be treated as confidential.

7. The patient has the right to expect that within its capacity a hospital must make reasonable response to the request of a patient for services. The hospital must provide evaluation, service, and/or referral as indicated by the urgency of the case. When medically permissible, a patient may be transferred to another facility only after he has received complete information and explanation concerning the needs for and alternatives to such a transfer. The institution to which the patient is to be transferred must first have accepted the patient for transfer.

8. The patient has the right to obtain information as to any relationship of his hospital to other health care and educational institutions insofar as his care is concerned. The patient has the right to obtain information as to the existence of any professional relationships among individuals, by name, who are treating him.

9. The patient has the right to be advised if the hospital proposes to engage in or perform human experimentation affecting his care or treatment. The patient has the right to refuse to participate in such research projects.

10. The patient has the right to expect reasonable continuity of care. He has the right to know in advance what appointment times and physicians are available and where. The patient has the right to expect that the hospital will provide a mechanism whereby he is informed by his physician or a delegate of the physician of the patient's continuing health care requirements following discharge.

11. The patient has the right to examine and receive an explanation of his bill regardless of source of payment.

12. The patient has the right to know what hospital rules and regulations apply to his conduct as a patient.

No catalogue of rights can guarantee for the patient the kind of treatment he has a right to expect. A hospital has many functions to perform, including the prevention and treatment of disease, the education of both health professionals and patients, and the conduct of clinical research. All these activities must be conducted with an overriding concern for the patient and, above all, the recognition of his dignity as a human being. Success in achieving this recognition assures success in the defense of the rights of the patient.

The American Hospital Association bill of rights has been widely disseminated and the consumer is beginning to assert his right to know what is happening to him when he enters the health care system.

Two federal acts have also had repercussions in the health care system: the 1967 Freedom of Information Act and the 1974 Privacy Act. These laws were en-

*Source: A Patient's Bill of Rights, American Hospital Association, Chicago; 1973. Reprinted with the permission of the American Hospital Association.

acted primarily to open general government records to individuals described in them, but medical records were cited also. Patients in health agencies operated by the federal government, the Veteran's Administration, for example, and patients receiving Medicare are now entitled to see their records. The specifics of the laws are unclear and there is no concise opinion as yet on the interpretation of parts of these two acts. Nevertheless, the trend is apparent—consumers are demanding their right to know about their health care and are seeking legislation to support this right.

Physicians traditionally have been held responsible for informing patients about their health care. However, nurses are involved in this matter also and most believe they too have a responsibility to inform consumers about their care. In some situations, physicians have refused to give certain information to patients which nurses felt the patients had a right to know. In such instances, the problem may be ethical as well as legal. Nurses have reported that withholding information often leads to anxiety and worry which, they believe, can frequently be more detrimental to health than appropriate disclosure of information.

WHAT THE CONSUMER EXPECTS OF THE NURSE

When a consumer submits to the care of members of the health professions, he has expectations about the behavior and abilities of those caring for him. This has been demonstrated by investigation and from what patients have written in articles and books, letters to editors of newspapers and periodicals, and so on.

Health care consumers expect the nurse to be professionally competent. This has been found to be especially true of technical skills. Consumers are apt to doubt the competence of a nurse who seems unsure of equipment she is using. A casually spoken thought, like "I can't seem to get this to work," does little for a person's confidence in the nurse. It is not surprising that a patient questioned his physician about his pulse rate after the nurse who came to take it kept shaking her watch and said she wondered if it was working correctly. But people are quick to compliment the nurse who carries out a procedure with deftness and self-assurance. One frequently hears patients speak of the nurse who gives "good shots."

Consumers expect nurses to be serious about their work. Human emotions can be contagious; hence, patients tend to enjoy having persons who are cheerful, but still obviously sincere, care for them. Patients often

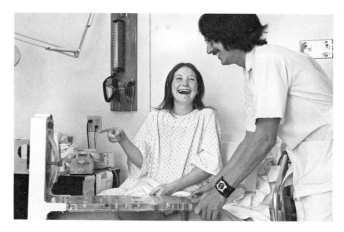

Figure 3–1   This patient enjoys a few moments of fun playing with a miniature pinball machine. The nurse, who took time to share the game with the patient, can help to relieve anxiety through such incidents, but he is still serious about his work.

enjoy sharing a humorous experience with the nurse, as illustrated in Figure 3–1. Humor can often relieve anxiety, stress, and anger and help to develop warm relationships when used appropriately. The give-and-take of humorous incidents can often serve therapeutic ends. However, when any individual overuses humor, he may be using it as a cover-up for distress too great to accept. The alert nurse will wish to learn to recognize humor that is used as an escape from reality.

While humor is appreciated, it is the rare person who accepts frivolity or casualness. Some patients may find it disturbing to see nurses in groups chatting and laughing. Families also find it disconcerting when nursing personnel laugh and talk outside a room in which someone is ill or deeply concerned with his health problem. In such situations, the nurse might well be serious-minded about her work but her behavior may cause the patient and his family to be critical.

Consumers expect nurses to be thoughtful, understanding, and accepting of them. They are critical of behavior that is punitive or judgmental. Calling a person by his name is a thoughtful and, often, a long-remembered act. It is not that nurses are always expected to *do* or *say* something. Just remaining with a person for a few minutes to listen to what he has to say, or holding his hand for a few seconds, is a great contribution to his comfort and well-being.

When patients are unable to care for themselves, they expect the nurse to assist them in meeting their hygienic needs. Although the nurse may assign other nursing personnel to assist with these responsibilities, the patient still expects the nurse to know about them.

For example, they expect to be bathed when they feel unable to do so for themselves. Placing a basin of water in front of a one-day postoperative patient who has had major surgery and telling him that it is good to be active would be regarded as gross insensitivity.

Patients can be made unhappy by having their hair left uncared for when they cannot care for it themselves. Grooming is important to the male patient also, and many express discomfort when not shaven. They do not like visitors to see them in a state that is embarrassing to them. Helping a patient to maintain normal bladder and bowel functioning is appreciated because neglect in these matters usually brings with it many disturbing physiological, as well as possible psychological, problems.

There may be times when the patient wishes to be too dependent on the nurse, and as a result, restorative care may suffer. This must be guarded against, but when a patient needs assistance, he expects the nurse to anticipate and to meet his needs.

Health care consumers expect nurses to orient them to the health care facility. Nearly everyone is afraid of the unknown, and to be left alone without orientation can be a frightening experience. Courtesies that help persons feel that they are respected help in developing a desirable therapeutic climate in which to care for them.

Consumers expect to receive an explanation of their care and they wish to have their questions answered. Not knowing and understanding what is being done is a vexing and frightening experience. Apprehension is increased by unfamiliar sounds, nursing jargon, and an array of strange equipment. Health practitioners who ignore this aspect of care are often referred to as cruel, unkind, and thoughtless.

Consumers wish to be a partner with health practitioners in planning their care. This facet of care has been described earlier but its importance cannot be overstressed. One goal of health care is to help persons attain maximum functioning with the best possible use of capabilities. It can well become an elusive goal if consumers are excluded when health care is planned.

Consumers expect nurses to ensure their privacy to the greatest extent possible. While asking personal questions, conducting physical examinations, and carrying out treatments, privacy can still be provided. For example, the nurse who walked into a four-bed hospital unit and loudly asked, "How many of you have had bowel movements today?" demonstrated little respect for the patients' privacy. Families have complained when community health nurses have visited their homes without an appointment. Some persons consider it an invasion of privacy to be called by their first names. People resent an invasion of privacy when, during examintions and treatments, nursing personnel have been careless about unnecessary exposure. Patients have also been critical of personnel who invade privacy when they enter a hospital room without first knocking.

Legal implications when invasion of privacy occurs were discussed in Chapter 2. In the eyes of the law, invasion of privacy may constitute a tort.

Privacy means different things to different people. The person's age, sex, the influence of his childhood rearing, the cultural and socioeconomic class of which he is a member, all play a role in the concept of privacy held by the consumer of health care. Nursing care can be enhanced when various concepts of privacy are respected and when purposeful efforts are made to protect consumers from unnecessary invasion of privacy.

THE FINANCING AND DELIVERY OF HEALTH CARE SERVICES

Two closely related problems of great concern to most consumers of health care are the high cost of care and the poor delivery of health services. The impoverished cannot afford the care they need. Even with increased affluence, persons not considered at poverty levels are finding that health care is rapidly becoming more elusive, more expensive, and out of their financial reach. Many people may feel they could afford at least maintenance care, but paying for crisis care is another matter. Also, health needs will continue to be poorly met if services are not available or accessible to the consumer, cost notwithstanding.

The Financing of Health Care Services

Time was when health care services were paid for by the individual. This method is still used for the payment of much ambulatory medical and dental care, for many medications, and for the use of health facilities, such as hospitals, to the extent that insurance or government revenues do not cover expenses. Usually, services are rendered by solo health practitioners—physicians, nurses, dentists, osteopaths, and others—although services may be offered through a group of practitioners working together but on the same fee-for-service basis.

Voluntary health insurance plans, or indemnity insurance, constitute a sizeable source of health care financing in the United States. About 90 percent of the population under 65 years of age has insurance for hospital and surgical care and approximately half are covered for some physican service. Preventive services, such as routine eye and dental care, are not covered by most insurance plans, although some now are beginning to offer such care.

Blue Cross and Blue Shield plans were among the first programs to offer prepaid health plan insurance. For a specific cost, or premium, that is paid regularly, these plans agree with subscribers to furnish certain services when they are needed. Blue Cross contracts with its member hospitals to pay for services at an agreed upon rate. Blue Shield functions similarly except the subscriber prepays for physician services. Blue Cross and Blue Shield are nonprofit corporations; they pay for specific hospital and physician services in accordance with the subscriber's contract.

Commercial insurance companies were quick to follow Blue Cross and Blue Shield with prepaid hospital and medical insurance. However, they pay in dollars rather than in services contracted with hospitals and physicians. The amount depends on the insured's contract. There are other differences between Blue Cross and Blue Shield and commercial insurance health policies but the major one is that the former pay for contracted services while the latter pay in dollars.

Another type of prepaid health plan, somewhat different from traditional health insurance, provides health services by a group of health practitioners who are employed by the plan and who use health facilities contracted by the plan. These plans originated in this country at the turn of the century in the mining and railroad industries and were known as contract practice. Two common plans that often serve as models for others today are the Kaiser-Permanente Medical Care Program in California and the Greater New York Plan in the east, often called HIP, for Health Insurance Plan.

Another prepaid group plan that offers personnel and facilities to its members is the health care corporation, or health maintenance organization—HMO. As the name suggests, the stated purpose is to furnish health promotion services that are paid for in advance on an insurancelike basis by either the member or his employee or both. The emphasis of HMOs has been on health promotion and maintenance although they offer illness care also. Those that have been in existence long enough to accumulate statistics have demonstrated fewer hospital admissions for illness care and less recourse to the use of expensive facilities than, for example, persons with indemnity insurance in which admission to a hospital may be the only way to receive benefits.

The two groups with the most health problems and with the least resources for paying for care are ordinarily not covered, at least to any great extent, by private health insurance or plans such as the HMOs—the poor and the elderly. Medicare and Medicaid were introduced to help serve these people. Medicare is a nationwide health insurance program for people of 65 and over, although it also covers some individuals under 65. For example, certain people who need kidney transplants qualify for Medicare regardless of age. Medicare is available to persons who pay for this insurance but it can be purchased without regard for income. Medicaid is a federally aided, state-operated and administered program which provides benefits for low-income persons in need of health care. It does not cover all poor but only persons who qualify in one of various categories, such as a person covered under welfare payment programs. Most states have adopted Medicaid, and it is estimated that approximately 25 million people used Medicaid monies in 1975. The amount has no doubt increased since then. Medicare and Medicaid are authorized by titles of the Social Security Act. Both contain various provisions or restrictions, but in general, the purposes are similar: to help the elderly and poor obtain health care at a reduced cost or, in the case of Medicaid, without cost. Although these programs have had problems and have not always met their original goals, they have increased the amount of health care available for a large sector of our population.

Health care costs continue to rise and on the average of as much as one and one-half times the rise in the annual cost of living in this country. It has been estimated that the average American works one month each year to pay for his health care needs. Many factors contribute to the high cost of care: poor health maintenance with a resulting need for expensive illness- and crisis-oriented care; increased use of highly sophisticated technology and expensive equipment; the increasing number of elderly in our population who, according to studies, require about two and one-half times more health care than younger persons; the preparation of many professional specialists whose skills often are being used by consumers when needs could be met just as adequately and more economically by general practitioners and *paraprofessionals,* that is, those prepared to assist professional health personnel; the duplication of health care facilities, especially hospitals, in areas where one facility could more economically furnish specialized services; the use of hospitals when ambulatory or home settings could be used satisfactorily from a health standpoint; the use of medical and surgical procedures that, according to investigations, are often unnecessary; and care of a quality that sometimes compounds a health problem. Still other factors could be mentioned but these are among those most frequently cited.

Attempts have been made to tackle these cost-increasing practices, sometimes by voluntary efforts and sometimes by government intervention. For example, nursing is certainly one profession that is making concerted efforts to prepare personnel better equipped to promote and maintain the consumer's health in order to help decrease needs for expensive curative care. There is evidence that other health disciplines are also taking steps to increase teaching related to health promotion in their educational programs. More students in all of the health disciplines are encouraged to prepare for practice as generalists rather than as specialists. Much more home care of the ill and many more ambulatory settings for minor health problems are becoming available to the consumer. Hospitals are being used less for diagnostic purposes and simple medical and surgical procedures that can be more economically carried out in offices and clinics. Hospital patients are discharged more quickly and better prepared through teaching to care for themselves while convalescing at home. There has been more emphasis on using paraprofessionals to better advantage. The National Health Planning and Resources Development Act created a network of Health System Agencies (HSAs) with authority to review and approve or disapprove of health agencies' plans for additions and expansions to avoid duplication of services. The PSROs, discussed in Chapter 1, and Utilization Review (UR) Committees are attempting to identify unnecessary and poor quality practices which increase the cost of health care as well as jeopardize the consumer.

Despite various insurance and aid programs and efforts to cut costs of health care, some persons are still without adequate care in this country for financial reasons. Either they are not eligible for any existing program or they cannot afford to pay what is necessary for proper health care. As a result, the momentum for a national health insurance program appears to be gaining. The federal government is being looked to for help so that everyone can obtain health care by using a financing system resembling the one used by Medicare and Medicaid.

Those opposed to national health insurance believe that the costs would not be adequately controlled, and hence, would be prohibitively expensive. They also argue that experience with Medicare and Medicaid has shown that quality of care would also likely suffer or at least fail to improve health maintenance care.

Those supporting national health insurance argue that present methods of financing health care are inadequate and that in a democratic society everyone has the right to have whatever health care services he needs regardless of his economic status.

The American Nurses' Association has supported national health insurance. Here is a description of its position and resolution:

For many years the American Nurses' Association has recognized health care as a basic human right. The Association has looked upon prepayment insurance systems as an effective way to guarantee that people will seek and receive care. Further, the Association has recognized the impact of health insurance plans on the systems for delivery of health care. What health insurance pays for determines to an increasingly great extent what people receive in terms of quantity and quality of care.

National health insurance is on the horizon. When it comes, the demand for services will grow to the extent the program provides payment for services. The character of the insurance benefits and the payment systems will determine to a great extent what services health care systems provide, to whom they provide services, the quality of these services, and how and where services are delivered.

Preparation for the advent of national health insurance, and the concerns of the nursing profession in this regard have pervaded Association priorities and programs in recent years.

ANA demands that there be a national system of health insurance benefits that would guarantee comprehensive health services to all people. Comprehensive services in this context mean the total range of health care services: preventive, health maintenance, diagnostic services, treatment, and protective services. If health care as a right is to be realized in this country, government must insure that health care is universal, covering every person, and that coverage is compulsory for every person so that all share in the costs according to their circumstances.

The American Nurses' Association needs to be clear as to its beliefs about the issues in a national health insurance plan so that legislative proposals can be evaluated in detail; and the profession left free to deal with these issues rather than with any current bill in its entirety.

Therefore, the following resolution is being presented to clarify positions on the issues in what has long been supported by ANA, a national health insurance program.

Resolution on National Health Insurance

WHEREAS, health, a state of physical, social and mental well-being is a basic human right, and

WHEREAS, government at all levels must act to insure that health care services are provided for all citizens, and

WHEREAS, there is a need for integrated systems to deliver comprehensive health care services that are accessible and acceptable to all people without regard to age, sex, race, social or economic condition, and

WHEREAS, there is need for a national program designed to correct serious inadequacies in present health care delivery systems, and

WHEREAS, nursing care is an essential component of health care; therefore, be it

RESOLVED, that the American Nurses' Association aggressively work for the enactment of legislation to establish a program of national health insurance benefits, and be it further

RESOLVED, that the national health program guarantee coverage of all people for the full range of comprehensive health services, and be it further

RESOLVED, that the national health program clearly recognize the distinctions between health care and medical care; and that the plan provide options in utilization of health care services that are not necessarily dependent on the physician, and be it further

RESOLVED, that nursing care be a benefit of the national health program, and be it further

RESOLVED, that the data systems necessary for effective management of the national insurance program protect the rights and privacy of individuals, and be it further

RESOLVED, that the plan include provisions for peer review of services that will protect the right and the responsibility of each health care discipline to monitor the practice of its own practitioners, and be it further

RESOLVED, that there continue to be a system of individual licensure for the practice of nursing, and be it further

RESOLVED, that provision be made for consumer participation in periodic evaluation of the national health insurance program, and be it further

RESOLVED, that the national health program be financed through payroll taxes, payment of premiums by the self-employed, and purchase of health insurance coverage for the poor and unemployed from general tax revenues, and be it further

RESOLVED, that ANA strongly urge the designation of nurses as health providers in all pending or proposed legislation on national health insurance.*

Many authorities are stating that spending still more money on health care costs will only compound present problems. They suggest that while present efforts to cut costs and provide better insurance coverage may be necessary, the best hope for the future lies in promoting health, preventing illness, teaching people to take more responsibility for maintaining their own health, and minimizing occupational and environmental hazards to health. Nurses, along with other health professionals,

---

* "ANA Convention '74." *American Journal of Nursing,* 74:1262–1263, July 1974.

will always need to care for the sick and injured, but the role of the future must certainly include much more active concern for helping to keep people well.

The Delivery of Health Care Services

This country enjoys high-quality science and technology in relation to health care and more health practitioners and facilities in proportion to population than any other place in the world. However, there is a marked maldistribution of both health facilities and personnel. This means that certain people, whether they can afford it or not, cannot obtain health care. Health practitioners tend to congregate in affluent metropolitan areas for a variety of reasons. Persons living in rural areas and inner cities where needs tend to be the greatest are generally without adequate care. Incentives of various types have been offered to health practitioners so that they would serve the rural and inner city areas but success has not been notable.

Poor distribution of health facilities and personnel is closely related to the cost of care. Can paraprofessionals be prepared at less cost than professionals and adequately meet certain health maintenance services that are now sparingly offered in far too many areas of the United States? Can the consumer be taught health maintenance so that demands for illness care can be reduced? Many requests for professional health care involve problems that do not require specialized and sophisticated care and treatment, uncomplicated upper respiratory infections, for example. Can consumers be taught to meet their own needs in these instances and learn to recognize when they do indeed need the care of a professional? Are there incentives that remain untried to attract more health professionals as well as paraprofessionals to offer care in underserviced areas?

Various approaches are presently being used to try to help improve delivery of health services. The hospital, once the center of the health care system, is being used less while newer types of health facilities have increased in number. A few nurses, individually or in groups, are offering health care through independent practice and sometimes in less well-served areas. Ambulatory care centers are handling many of the simpler health problems, such as the need for minor surgical procedures and care for simple injuries. The Health Insurance Association of America recently recommended that ambulatory care centers should be available in every community since those in existence have met many health needs well and economically, and often in areas removed from hospital health centers.

Neighborhood health centers are springing up in many deprived areas and ordinarily have a wider array of services than ambulatory care centers. Personnel often include social workers and community health practitioners. Various types of clinics and day care centers are helping to dispense health services to underserviced areas. The growing number of nursing homes are helping to meet needs of the elderly and are often located in areas that are quite accessible to the consumer.

Unfortunately, some insurance plans do not include care obtained in some of the facilities just described, but coverage is tending to increase. However, it is believed that these types of facilities can eventually offer continuous and comprehensive health care to many people now geographically removed from the metropolitan hospitals.

The final answers on how to deliver and finance quality health care to everyone are still largely illusive. But the interest and strong demands for change are apparent everywhere. Consensus is that some form of national health insurance and better delivery of services are forthcoming. Nurses will wish to keep abreast of the news on these issues since the impact on nursing will certainly be substantial.

THE CONSUMER'S HEALTH-ILLNESS PROBLEMS: SOLVED AND UNSOLVED

Available statistics reflect, at least in an indirect manner, the status of health-illness in the nation and offer guidance in health program planning. Several familiar terms are used to describe these statistics. A *morality rate* describes the ratio of deaths to a population. A *morbidity rate* describes the incidence of disease or pathological conditions in a population. *Longevity* is the length or duration of life. *Life span* is the length of time that is possible for a member of a species to live. In humans, this is presently about 100 years. *Life expectancy* is the average number of years a person at a given age can expect to live; it is based on mortality statistics.

The infant mortality rates reflect improvements in the United States, as Figure 3-2 illustrates. Yet, 14 countries report even lower infant mortality rates than does the United States. These statistics pose interesting questions to health practitioners seeking solutions to infant mortality. Also, note that nonwhite infants died at a rate not far from double that for white infants in America as late as 1974 when the last comparable figures were available.

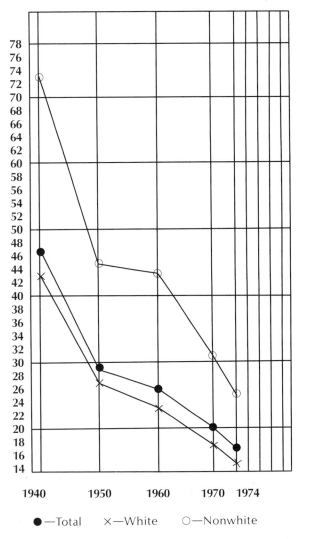

Figure 3-2 Infant mortality rates for white, nonwhite, and total deaths per 1,000 live births in the United States. (Statistical Abstract of the U.S., 1976. U.S. Department of Commerce, Bureau of the Census.)

Respiratory illnesses account for 54 percent of morbidity due to acute causes in this country. Between 40 and 60 percent of our population suffers at least one chronic health problem and about 14 percent of the total population has limited activity as a result of a chronic health problem. There are marked differences in limitations among various age groups. For example, about 4 percent of the population under 17 years of age is limited but in the over-65 age group, nearly 50 percent has limitations.

Figure 3-3 illustrates life expectancy in the United States. Most gains in life expectancy were made in the first half of this century when cures or methods of

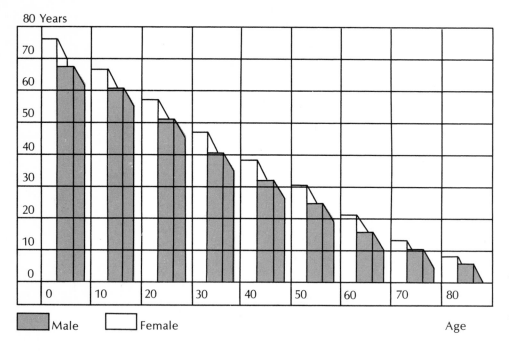

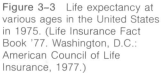

Figure 3–3 Life expectancy at various ages in the United States in 1975. (Life Insurance Fact Book '77. Washington, D.C.: American Council of Life Insurance, 1977.)

control for many of the greatest killers of youth and middle age were found. Safe water and food supplies have practically eliminated in some areas, and greatly reduced in others, such diseases as typhoid fever, vitamin deficiencies, and certain infant diarrheas. Vaccinations and immunizations and the use of antibiotics have served to control most infectious diseases. Early detection programs have been important in the control of such diseases as tuberculosis and some cancers. Modern drug and surgical procedures have added to life expectancy in many instances. Still, despite successful U.S. world leadership in many areas, certain other countries, Sweden, Bulgaria, and Ireland being examples, have longer life expectancy rates. Another revealing statistic is that nonwhite Americans have a life expectancy five to six years shorter than that of white Americans.

Scientists are unsure why the gap between male and female life expectancy exists although many believe it is due to genetic differences. The gap causes social and health problems because of the large number of women who are widowed and living alone and often in poverty. Some research has shown that the lonely person is more likely prey to illness since divorced as well as widowed persons experience more illness than the married. This finding supports psychological theory that human relationships are basic to good health.

Authorities state that a primary cause for the low rank of the United States in life expectancy, as compared with other countries, is failure to deliver health services adequately. Also, many segments of society, particularly the poor, have not had adequate nutrition. Other experts point out that violent deaths in the United States, such as suicides and homicides, are another reason. Motor vehicle accidents also play an important role in decreasing life expectancy. However, it is believed that these accident rates have fallen recently due primarily to the national 55–mile-an-hour speed limit.

Despite greater life expectancy, efforts to increase the life span have been largely ineffectual. After reaching a certain age, the individual's ability to fight illness and injury diminishes. There is considerable research underway on the process of aging. When methods can be found to slow the aging process, the human life span may increase.

The decrease in untimely deaths and the increase in life expectancy have resulted in more elders in the U.S. population. Figure 3–4 illustrates the population in various age groups in 1972 and as predicted for 1990. Note the increase in the percentage of people in the 65-years-and-over category. The number of people 65 years and older is expected to reach about 26.8 million by 1985, 29 million by 1990, and 30.6 million by the turn of the century. Although chronic diseases affect all age groups, invalidism and dependency due to chronic illness are particularly prevalent in the older age groups, and the public is becoming increasingly active in supporting programs leading to their solution.

The population shift from rural to urban areas continues today, although the most marked shift occurred shortly after World War II. The social importance of this shift has sparked much interest and underlies the health needs of large sectors of people. Overcrowding, poor housing, and often inability to find work are a few conditions that exist in crowded urban areas and that result in poor health. Ironically, many of the poor, urban dwellers live almost next door to fine medical centers in large cities and yet do not receive even minimum health care because of inability to pay for it.

The number of poor persons in our population remains distressingly high despite a continued rise in family income and government aid. As can be expected, these persons characteristically have higher morbidity and mortality rates than the more affluent.

While many diseases have been checked, many still remain unconquered. Figure 3–5 illustrates the ten leading causes of death in the United States. Since 1968, all causes of death were down except malignant diseases and cirrhosis of the liver. In all age groups except for ages 34 to 44, deaths due to heart disease were down. The greatest increases in deaths due to malignancies were for lung and other respiratory cancers. The upsurge is most often linked to the continued use of cigarettes by Americans and their use is increasing, especially among teenagers and women. Of all malignancies classified according to where they occur, only cancers of the genital organs decreased. Credit for this drop is usually given to early detection screening of women with the Papanicolaou (Pap) test. The increase in deaths from cirrhosis of the liver is believed due to the excess use and abuse of alcohol. The United States has the highest rate of alcoholism in the world.

Figure 3–6 illustrates the death rate in the United States in 1975. The overall drop in the death rate in

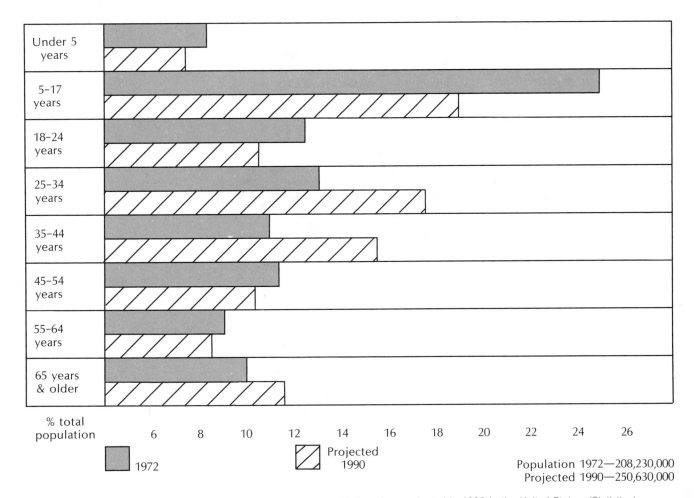

Figure 3–4 Percentage of the total population in age groups in 1972 and as projected in 1990 in the United States. (Statistical Abstract of the U.S., 1976. U.S. Department of Commerce, Bureau of the Census.)

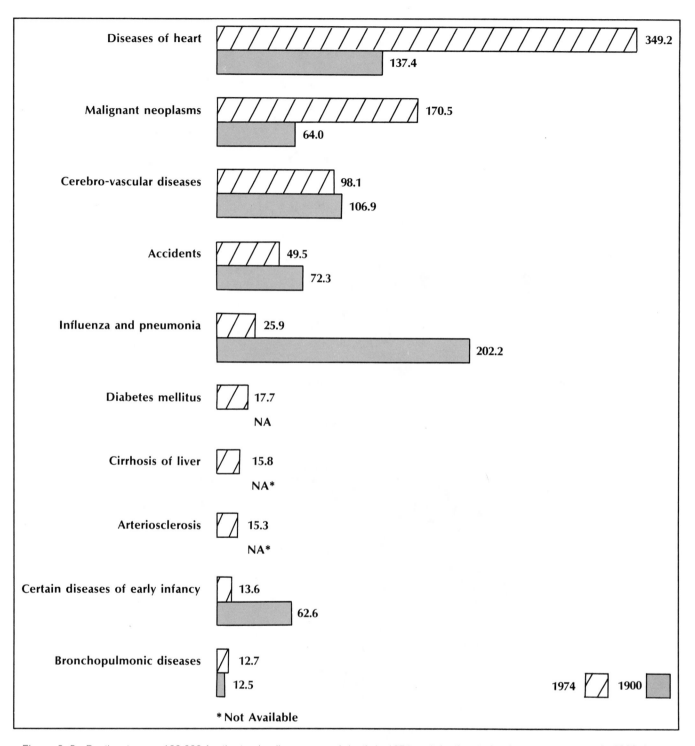

Figure 3–5 Death rates per 100,000 for the ten leading causes of death in 1974 and death rate for these same causes in 1900, in the United States. (Statistical Abstract of the U.S., 1976. U.S. Department of Commerce, Bureau of the Census.)

an effort to serve more people more effectively. Research continues to study causes of premature death, aging, and unconquered illness.

The goal of high-quality care for everyone may still be a dream, but efforts to reach it are numerous and commendable. Still, much has to be done, and this remains one of the biggest challenges facing health practitioners today.

CONCLUSION

Comprehensive health care services with facilities and personnel to provide them for everyone is of national concern. The need for them has often been described as having reached crisis proportions. Statistics indicate that while scientific knowledge continues to grow, its incorporation into health care practices still leaves much to be desired. This is particularly true of health maintenance, of the promotion of wellness, of making sophisticated modern care techniques available to more people, and of reaching all persons in our population.

The consumer who now knows his rights and is making his demands known can no longer be ignored. Health practitioners who fail to listen are not meeting their obligation of providing services for all. Mankind appears to have a need for societal control and is intolerant of impediments that stand in his way. Consumers may be frustrated, but they are no longer apathetic.

SUPPLEMENTAL LIBRARY STUDY

1. The following article presents a philosophical viewpoint on the ethical and technical issues involved when the right to health care for everyone becomes a goal:

    Page, Benjamin B. "The Right to Health Care." *Current History,* 73:5–8, 34, July–August 1977.

    What does the author describe as a violation of the health provider's rights if the right to health care for everyone becomes an actuality? What alternatives to scientific medicine does this author present as needing further investigation to help solve present-day problems related to health care?

2. As this chapter pointed out, the consumer of health care is concerned about services he receives. The following article describes some consumer concerns:

    Hoover, Eleanor Links. "Far Out: Treating the Whole Body Instead of the Diseased Part," *Human Behavior,* 6:14–15, July 1977.

    What struck the author as the primary conclusion most persons attending holistic medical conferences in California reached in relation to health care? What did these conferences pinpoint as the two leading causes of poor health? What primary dietary changes have occurred in the United States in the last century, according to this article?

3. The following article presents some of the issues related to national health insurance:

    Bowman, Rosemary Amason and Culpepper, Rebecca Clark.

    "National Health Insurance: Some of the Issues." *American Journal of Nursing,* 75:2017–2021, November 1975.

    What type of national health insurance program do the authors believe will eventually be put into action? Discuss briefly several contradictions in opinion concerning national health insurance held by health professionals and by consumers which these authors believe must be resolved. What proposals do they offer to resolve differences in opinion?

4. There are people who believe we are facing a crisis in health care in this country today. The following article explains further:

    Ramey, Irene G. "The Crisis in Health Care: Fact or Fiction." In Leininger, Madeleine and Buck, Gary, editors. *Health Care Dimensions: Fall 1974 Health Care Issues.* F. A. Davis Company, Philadelphia, 1974, pp. 17–27.

    What differentiation does the author make between health care and medical care? What does she consider to be the three major health care problems contributing to the health care crisis? After studying this chapter, what additional problems would you add to those given by Dr. Ramey? Describe at least three recommendations the author makes to help solve problems currently contributing to a crisis in health care in this country today?

References For Unit I

CHAPTER 1

Aiken, Linda H. "Primary Care: The Challenge for Nursing." *American Journal of Nursing,* 77:1828–1832, November 1977.

Bakke, Kathy. "Primary Nursing: Perceptions of a Staff Nurse." *American Journal of Nursing,* 74:1432–1434, August 1974.

Billings, Gloria. "ANA in the Nation's Capital." *American Journal of Nursing,* 75:1182–1183, July 1975.

Bowar-Ferres, Susan. "Loeb Center and Its Philosophy of Nursing." *American Journal of Nursing,* 75:810–815, May 1975.

Bowman, Rosemary Amason and Culpepper, Rebecca Clark. "Power: R$_x$ for Change." *American Journal of Nursing,* 74:1053–1056, June 1974.

"Caring Makes the Difference." *Nursing 75,* 5:34–39, November 1975.

Ciske, Karen L. "Primary Nursing: Evaluation." *American Journal of Nursing,* 74:1436–1438, August 1974.

Despres, Leon M. "A Lawyer Explains What The National Labor Relations Act Really Says." *American Journal of Nursing,* 76:790–794, May 1976.

Fagin, Claire M. "Nurses' Rights." *American Journal of Nursing,* 75:82–85, January 1975.

Haase, Patricia T. "Pathways to Practice—Part I." *American Journal of Nursing,* 76:806–809, May 1976.

Haase, Patricia T. "Pathways to Practice—Part II." *American Journal of Nursing,* 76:950–954, June 1976.

Hannah, Kathryn J. "The Computer and Nursing Practice." *Nursing Outlook,* 24:555–558, September 1976.

Hauser, Mary Alice. "Initiation Into Peer Review." *American Journal of Nursing,* 75:2204–2207, December 1975.

Kelly, Lucie Young. "Credentialing of Health Care Personnel." *Nursing Outlook,* 25:562–569, September 1977.

Kelly, Lucie Young. *Dimensions of Professional Nursing.* Edition 3. Macmillan Publishing Co., Inc., New York, 1975, 573 p.

Kinlein, M. Lucille. "The Self-Care Concept." *American Journal of Nursing,* 77:598–601, April 1977.

Kitzman, Harriet, "The Nature of Well Child Care." *American Journal of Nursing,* 75:1705–1708, October 1975.

Levine, Eugene. "What Do We Know About Nurse Practitioners?" *American Journal of Nursing,* 77:1799–1803, November 1977.

Maas, Meridean, et al, "Nurse Autonomy: Reality Not Rhetoric." *American Journal of Nursing,* 75:2201–2208, December 1975.

Mauksch, Ingeborg G. and Rogers, Martha E. "Nursing Is Coming of Age . . . Through the Practitioner Movement: Pro: Con." *American Journal of Nursing,* 75:1834–1843, October 1975.

"N-CAP Slates ERA Program During ANA Convention." *American Journal of Nursing,* 76:712, May 1976.

"Nurses and Nursing's Issues." *American Journal of Nursing,* 75:1848–1859, October 1975.

Page, Marjorie. "Primary Nursing: Perceptions of a Head Nurse." *American Journal of Nursing,* 74:1435–1436, August 1974.

Partridge, Kay B. "Nursing Values in a Changing Society." *Nursing Outlook,* 26:356–360, June 1978.

Pollok, Clementine S., et al. "Students' Rights." *American Journal of Nursing,* 76:600–603, April 1976.

Raheja, Krishna K. "Nursing in Transition." *Nursing Forum,* 15:413–417, Number 4, 1976.

Ramphal, Marjorie. "Peer Review." *American Journal of Nursing,* 74:63–67, January 1974.

Schorr, Thelma M. "Encounter." (Editorial) *American Journal of Nursing,* 75:1979, November 1975.

Schorr, Thelma M. "Qualified to Care." (Editorial) *American Journal of Nursing,* 77:1287, August 1977.

Smoyak, Shirley A. "Is Practice Responding to Research?" *American Journal of Nursing,* 76:1146–1150, July 1976.

"The "Rights" Explosion Splintering America?" (Special Report) *U. S. News & World Report,* 83:29–32, October 31, 1977.

Thomstad, Beatrice, et al. "Changing the Rules of the Doctor-Nurse Game." *Nursing Outlook,* 23:422–427, July 1975.

White, Susan. "The Expanded Role for Nurses." *Nursing 77,* 7:90–93, October 1977.

CHAPTER 2

Althouse, Harold L. "How OSHA Affects Hospitals and Nursing Homes." *American Journal of Nursing,* 75:450–453, March 1975.

"ANA Certification Council Approves New Definition to Reflect Current Goals." (News) *American Journal of Nursing,* 77:1390, 1393, September 1977.

"A Statement of Concern About Associate and Baccalaureate Degree Programs for Nurses That Have No Major in Nursing." *Nursing Outlook,* 25:484, August 1977.

Bullough, Bonnie. "Influences on Role Expansion." *American Journal of Nursing,* 76:1476–1481, September 1976.

Bullough, Bonnie, Editor. *The Law and the Expanding Nursing Role.* Appleton-Century-Crofts, New York, 1975, 211 p.

Code for Nurses With Interpretive Statements. American Nurses' Association, Kansas City, Missouri, 1976, 20 p.

"Ethics." (A Special AJN Feature) *American Journal of Nursing,* 77:845–876, May 1977.

Human Rights Guidelines for Nurses in Clinical and Other Research. American Nurses' Association, Kansas City, Missouri, 1975, 11 p.

Kelly, Lucie Young, *Dimensions of Professional Nursing,* Edition 3. Macmillan Publishng Co., Inc., New York, 1975, 573 p.

Kelly, Lucie Young. "Keeping Up With Your Legal Responsibilities." *Nursing 76,* 6:81–93, March 1976.

Kelly, Lucie Young. "Nursing Practice Acts." *American Journal of Nursing,* 74:1310–1319, July 1974.

Larocco, Susan Arendt. "The Time for Mandatory Continuing

Education is Now." (Speaking Out) *Nursing 77,* 7:16, 19, October 1977.

McGriff, Erline P. and Simms, Laura L. "Two New York Nurses Debate the NYSNA 1985 Proposal," *American Journal of Nursing,* 76:930–935, June 1976.

"Mandatory CE Signed Into Law in New Mexico; Close to Law in Some States, Killed in Others." (News) *American Journal of Nursing,* 77:1100, 1119, July 1977.

Nathanson, Iric. "Getting a Bill Through Congress." *American Journal of Nursing,* 75:1179–1181, July 1975.

"N.Y. Nurses Mobilize to Push "1985 Proposal" After State Legislator Threatens to Delay Action." (News) *American Journal of Nursing,* 77:1093, 1117, 1119, July 1977.

Perry, Shannon E. "If You're Called as an Expert Witness." *American Journal of Nursing,* 77:458–460, March 1977.

Peterson, Paul and Guy, Joan S. "Should Institutional Licensure Replace Individual Licensure?" *American Journal of Nursing,* 74:444–447, March 1974.

Rabb, J. Douglas. "Implications of Moral and Ethical Issues for Nurses." *Nursing Forum,* 15:168–179, Number 2, 1976.

Schorr, Thelma M. "Securing Licensure." (Editorial) *American Journal of Nursing,* 75:1131, July 1975.

Schorr, Thelma M. "The New York Plan." (Editorial) *American Journal of Nursing,* 75:2141, December 1975.

"Some Washington RN's May Prescribe Drugs." (News) *American Journal of Nursing,* 77:1383, 1393, September 1977.

Springer, Eric W., Editor. *Nursing and the Law.* Aspen Systems Corporation, Health Law Center, Pittsburgh, 1970, 188 p.

"Survey Shows Slow But Strong Movement in States Toward Mandatory Continuing Education." (News) *American Journal of Nursing,* 78:766, 802, 804, 808, 810, May 1978.

"The ICN Meets in Mexico City." *American Journal of Nursing,* 73:1344–1359, August 1973.

CHAPTER 3

"A Consumer Speaks Out About Hospital Care." (Anonymous) *American Journal of Nursing,* 76:1443–1444, September 1976.

Alfano, Genrose J. "There Are No Routine Patients." *American Journal of Nursing,* 75:1804–1807, October 1975.

Chopoorian, Teresa and Craig, Margaret Mabrey. "PL93–641: Nursing and Health Care Delivery." *American Journal of Nursing,* 76:1988–1991, December 1976.

Davis, Elizabeth. "Funding Rural Nurse Practitioner Care." *Nursing Outlook,* 25:628–631, October 1977.

Etzioni, Amitai. "National Health Insurance: Can We Afford It?" (Public Affairs) *Human Behavior,* 6:9–10, May 1977.

Greeley, John T. *National Health Care: Yes & No.* Pamphlet Publication, Cincinnati, Ohio, 1977, 39 p.

Heal Yourself. Report of the Citizens Board of Inquiry Into Health Services For Americans, 92 p.

Jennings, Carole P. and Jennings, Thomas F. "Containing Costs Through Prospective Reimbursement." *American Journal of Nursing,* 77:1155–1159, July 1977.

Judd, Leda R. "Federal Involvement in Health Care After 1956." *Current History,* 72:201–206, 227, May/June 1977.

Kelly, Lucie Young. "The Patient's Right to Know." *Nursing Outlook,* 24:26–32, January 1976.

"Loneliness Can Kill You: Companionship as Preventive Medicine." (Behavior) *Time,* 110:45, September 5, 1977.

Long, Edna S. "How To Survive Hospitalization." *American Journal of Nursing,* 74:486–488, March 1974.

Mauksch, Ingeborg G. "On National Health Insurance." *American Journal of Nursing,* 78:1322–1327, August 1978.

Novello, Dorothy Jean. "The National Health Planning and Resources Development Act." *Nursing Outlook,* 24:354–358, June 1976.

Rice, Dorothy P. "Health Facilities in the United States." *Current History,* 72:211–214, 230, May/June 1977.

Scheffler, Richard M. and Paringer, Lynn. "The Nation's Health Today." *Current History,* 72:193–195, 229, May/June 1977.

Schorr, Thelma M. "It's Vent-My-Spleen Time." (Editorial) *American Journal of Nursing,* 75:1287, August 1975.

Sobel, Lester A., Editor. *Health Care: An American Crisis.* Facts On File, Inc., New York, 1976, 189 p.

Welch, Cathryne A. "Health Care Distribution and Third-Party Payment for Nurses' Services." *American Journal of Nursing,* 75:1844–1847, October 1975.

unit II
The Methodology of Nursing

4

BEHAVIORAL OBJECTIVES

When content in this chapter has been mastered, the student will be able to

Define terms appearing in the glossary.

Explain the primary differences between the nursing process based on the problem-solving technique and the nursing process based on general systems theory.

Describe briefly general systems theory.

Indicate why it is appropriate to describe the nursing process as an open system.

Describe the various steps that are necessary in order to carry out the four parts of the nursing process: data collection, assessment, planning nursing care, and nursing intervention. Give an example of each of these steps.

Identify several commonly noted problems, possible causes of these problems, and suggested remedies related to carrying out data collection, assessment, planning nursing care, and nursing intervention.

The Nursing Process

GLOSSARY

At risk: An individual or situation exposed to sufficient risk factors that the likelihood of a health problem is great.

Behavioral objective: A statement describing desired behavior and conditions under which behavior is to occur.

Closed system: A system which does not interact with its environment.

Evaluation: The measurement of success or failure.

Feedback: The procedure of placing certain information back into a system.

Goal: An aim or end. Synonym for objective.

Health state profile: An organized record of the initial information collected about the individual's health.

Input: The material or information which enters a system.

Interview: A purposeful conversation, generally in a face-to-face meeting.

Interviewee: The person from whom information is sought.

Interviewer: The person seeking information in an interview.

Medical diagnosis: A physician's statement describing a patient's pathological condition.

Negative assessment: A judgment that the patient is having a health-threatening problem with which he is unable to deal independently.

Norm: An accepted measure, model, or pattern which can be used for comparison. Synonym for standard.

Nursing assessment: The nurse's judgment about the patient's health state.

Nursing care plan: A guide for the provision of nursing care.

Nursing diagnosis: A statement, based on a negative nursing assessment, describing a specific problem related to a person's state of health. The problem is potentially responsive to nursing intervention.

Nursing intervention: The actions performed by the nurse intended to assist a patient with his particular health-related problem.

Nursing order: A written statement of nursing action which is to be performed.

Nursing process: A set of acts that are directed toward the goal of helping a patient achieve or maintain well-being; its parts (data collection, assessment, planning nursing care, and nursing intervention) occur in sequence, are interrelated, and are dynamic.

Objective: An aim or end. Synonym for goal.

Observation: The taking in of information through the senses.

Open system: A system which interacts with its environment.

Output: The end product of a system.

Positive assessment: A judgment that describes the patient's strengths which allow him to make independent adjustments to achieve or maintain his desired state of health.

Response: A reaction to a stimulus.

Risk factor: A hazard that has a high potential for resulting in a problem.

Standard: An accepted measure, model, or pattern which can be used as a basis for comparison. Synonym for norm.

System: A set of interrelated or interacting things or parts forming a unified whole.

Validation: The act of confirming or certifying.

INTRODUCTION

Traditionally, nursing practice focused on the actions of nurses. These actions were based mostly on custom and common sense. While nurses were sincere, their actions were not always necessarily structured, deliberate, based on scientific evidence, and individualized to the needs of the consumer of health care.

In recent years, as nursing has struggled to assume its place as an independent profession that is accountable to the consumer, there has been a concerted effort to develop a more systematic and rational pattern for the practice of nursing. The nursing process has evolved as the frame of reference for nursing practice. The American Nurses' Association Congress for Nursing Practice developed the following Standards of Practice to guide the performance of nursing, and these standards have been integrated into the nursing process:

  I. The collection of data about the health status of the client/patient is systematic and continuous. The data are accessible, communicated, and recorded.

  II. Nursing diagnoses are derived from health status data.

  III. The plan of nursing care includes goals derived from the nursing diagnoses.

  IV. The plan of nursing care includes priorities and the prescribed nursing approaches or measures to achieve the goals derived from the nursing diagnoses.

  V. Nursing actions provide for client/patient participation in health promotion, maintenance, and restoration.

  VI. Nursing actions assist the client/patient to maximize his health capabilities.

  VII. The client's/patient's progress or lack of progress toward goal achievement is determined by the client/patient and the nurse.

  VIII. The client's/patient's progress or lack of progress toward total achievement directs reassessment, reordering of priorities, new goal setting, and revision of the plan of nursing care.*

These general standards have been made more specific for particular types of nursing practice by the various Divisions on Practice of the American Nurses' Association.

DEFINITION OF THE NURSING PROCESS

A *process* is defined as a set of actions leading to a particular goal. The actions in a process occur in sequence, are interrelated, and are dynamic.

*American Nurses' Association, *Standards of Nursing Practice*. Kansas City, Missouri, 1973. Reprinted with permission.

The *nursing process* is a set of actions used to determine, plan, and implement nursing care. The purpose of the nursing process is to provide care that will help the consumer attain and maintain his best possible state of health. The parts of the nursing process are carried out in sequence, are interrelated, and are dynamic.

While some nursing literature describes the nursing process as having five or six parts, most authors list four basic components: assessment, planning, implementation, and evaluation.

Assessment includes such nursing activities as collecting data about the person who is to receive care, identifying health problems of the person by analyzing data that were collected, and ranking the person's health problems so that those requiring immediate action are met before those that may not be as urgent.

Planning involves the development of a guide that is frequently called a nursing care plan. This plan ordinarily includes goals of nursing care and nursing intervention measures that will be used to meet these goals.

Implementation is the carrying out of nursing measures described in the nursing care plan.

The final step ordinarily is called evaluation. In this part, the effectiveness of care the person receives is judged. Evaluation tells the nurse whether her care has been effective, in which case the goals of nursing care have been met. If evaluation indicates that goals are not being met, adjustments in care are made. Possibly, more information about the patient is necessary, or perhaps the nursing care plan was inappropriate for the particular patient. Another possibility is that implementation of nursing care may have been poorly executed.

This has been a brief summary of the nursing process as some persons describe it. It is based primarily on the techniques of problem-solving.

In this text, general systems theory is used as the basis upon which to develop the nursing process. Using this approach, the nurse's activities are continually being evaluated from the moment data collection starts until nursing intervention is no longer deemed necessary. This continuing evaluation provides the nurse with information so that she can adjust her efforts as she proceeds to better meet the unique needs of each patient. In addition, the purpose of the nursing process is evaluated after all the parts have been examined.

The nursing process described in this chapter has four parts: data collection, assessment, planning of nursing care, and nursing intervention. A characteristic of a process is that all its parts are interrelated and influence the whole. Because of this interrelatedness, it is difficult to break a process into parts for examination.

A process is somewhat like a movie. To stop the projector gives a still picture which can be viewed more closely. However, each picture tells only one portion of the story and it loses meaning when isolated from the whole. For discussion purposes, each part of the nursing process will be described later in this chapter. But always remember that while studying the parts is useful for learning, the process must be put together in order to understand the whole process "story."

GENERAL SYSTEMS THEORY

Since the nursing process described later is based on general systems theory, a brief description of this theory will be helpful to an understanding of the nursing process.

A *system* is a set of interrelated or interacting parts which form a unified whole. For example, a railroad system has parts such as trains, tracks, stations, and signals. Each part has its own purpose, each is related to all other parts, and all, functioning together, form the unified whole, the railroad system. Most systems are composed of lesser systems commonly called subsystems, or simply, parts. In the railroad system, the train may be thought of as one part. It too has parts: the engine, caboose, freight cars, passenger cars, and so on. Each part of the train is related to all other parts of the train, and the sum of these parts is equal to the whole, the train. Each part has its purpose: the train carries freight and passengers; the tracks carry the train, and so on. The purpose of the railroad system, transportation of passengers and freight, is achieved when the purpose of each part has been met.

Input is the material or information which enters a system. It is used in whatever manner is appropriate to achieve the purpose of the system. Assume you wish to select a dessert for a dinner party you are giving. You would need certain information, such as the number of people attending your party, the amount of time you have to prepare a dessert, the amount of money you can afford to spend, and preferences of your guests. That information is the input for your system.

Output is the end product of a system. In the above example, the output of the system is the selection of dessert that you will prepare and serve to your guests.

Evaluation is the measurement of success or failure. General systems theory uses continuous evaluation; that is, there is not a separate part devoted to evaluation. The nursing process in this text also does not consider evaluation separately since it is constantly functioning in the entire system.

How does one evaluate in order to determine success or failure? Standards of measurement are specific descriptions of the expectations of the system's output. Remember the county fairs when favorite baked goods were entered and prizes were awarded for the best goods? The judges of the pies, for example, decided that pies should be judged on the basis of appearance, texture of the crust and the filling, and taste. These standards served as standards of measurement. They are often called criteria in general systems theory.

In systems theory, how does one use the information one obtains after comparing the output of a system or one of its parts with standards? In other words, how does one use the results of evaluation in systems theory? It is used in the procedure called *feedback*. If the output of the system does not meet standards, that information is fed back into the system and appropriate modifications are made. If evaluation demonstrates that the purpose of the system is being achieved, this information is fed back into the system to tell the operator to continue with the action until the purpose of the system is met. The latter feedback tells the operator that he is on the right track. If evaluation demonstrates that the purpose of the system has been achieved, the system can be terminated.

Recall the example in which systems theory was used to select a dessert. After comparing your selection with standards, assume you became aware that the dessert selected was inappropriate since you did not have time to prepare it. That information—lack of sufficient time to prepare dessert—is fed back into your system. The selection process and feedback will continue until you find a dessert that meets all of the criteria you have set. If feedback tells you that you are on the right track, you continue your search in the manner you have been using. When the dessert that meets your standards is selected, the systems process is discontinued since you have then achieved your purpose.

Systems are of two types. A *closed system* does not interact with its environment. A chemical reaction occurring under controlled conditions is a system in which there is no interaction with the environment. An *open system* is one that interacts with its environment. There is an exchange of information, matter, or energy between the system and its environment.

The nursing process is an open system. Human beings are constantly being influenced by their environment; therefore, environmental influences may affect the nursing process at any point and necessitate changes since it is an open system. For example, a nurse who has been supervising a woman's prenatal care will need

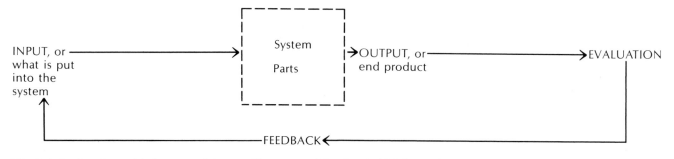

Figure 4-1   A system exists to accomplish a specific purpose. It has input which is acted upon within the system to produce output. The output is evaluated and the conclusion is returned to the system in the form of feedback. The broken lines indicate that the system is open and constantly interacts with the environment.

to make adjustments when the woman reports that her husband has just learned he has pulmonary tuberculosis. A nurse may need to make certain modifications in her care of a family when she learns that one of its teenaged members is using illegal drugs. A community health program will be influenced by the effects of a flood in the community. A hospitalized patient learns that his father is seriously ill and his nursing care requirements change when the patient demonstrates anxiety and concern. A spell of dry, windy weather may influence the care of a patient who has hay fever.

Figure 4-1 illustrates an open general system and Figure 4-2 illustrates the nursing process. A comparison of these figures shows that the nursing process is based on general systems theory and that both interact with the surrounding environment. The nursing process diagram also indicates that input for the nursing process is the state of the person's health as it currently exists. Output of the nursing process is the resulting state of the person's health.

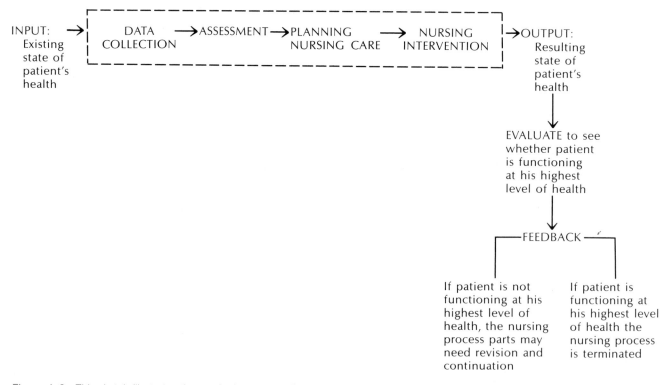

Figure 4-2   This sketch illustrates the nursing process and its parts. The broken lines indicate that the system is open and constantly interacting with the environment. It is not possible for a diagram to convey the dynamic nature of a process. However, the nursing process, like all processes, is active and ongoing.

DATA COLLECTION

Data collection consists of gathering information about the person who is seeking care. The purpose of gathering data is to assemble information about a person's state of health which can be used for providing necessary nursing care. Information about the person serves as input for the data collection part of the nursing process.

Selecting Appropriate Data

Analyzing a situation that involves humans can be a complicated and difficult procedure because of man's complex nature. Data gathering concerning a person would be endless if one wished to amass every piece of information that could be found. Before starting, the nurse needs to ask, what data are appropriate in *this* person's situation?

Appropriate data are relevant data; that is, they have a bearing upon, an influence on, or some connection with the situation under consideration. There is no hard and fast rule for deciding which information is relevant. Here are some questions, the answers to which will help in the selection of relevant data.

Who is the person? What is his name, age, sex, marital status, occupation, education, economic status, and the like?

Why is the person being considered for nursing care? Is he ill? Does he know he has a health problem? Is he presumably well? Data which would be relevant for a woman in labor would differ from information about an adolescent who is being prepared for an appendectomy. Relevant data for a middle-aged man found to be overweight during an annual physical examination will be different from data the nurse needs when caring for an elderly woman who has just lost her spouse.

What factors in this person's life are influencing his present health status? For example, if a person's occupation involves strenuous lifting, it would be relevant to learn how well-acquainted the person is with the principles of body mechanics. If a mother is concerned about her child's weight, it would be appropriate for the nurse to learn what knowledge the mother has of normal weight and growth patterns for children of her youngster's age.

The patient may be an individual, a family, a neighborhood, a community, or others. A person may be encountered in a variety of settings, such as in a hospital, a community health center, a clinic, a physician's office, or at home. When a community is the nurse's responsibility, she might be concerned with all persons living in a housing development, a neighborhood, or a governmental area such as a county, city, or state.

The nurse's general knowledge helps her to select appropriate data. For example, she learns that cow's milk contains no iron and that babies who do not have iron-containing food added to their diets before their maternal supply is depleted will generally develop anemia. This knowledge helps the nurse to determine what information is pertinent for a one-year-old child's diet.

Because people interpret new situations by drawing upon past experiences, the nurse will attempt to gather data from the patient's past experiences that may influence his present situation. Thus, the manner in which a person coped with an emergency appendectomy three years ago may influence his response to surgery today. The manner in which a community organized itself to promote polio immunizations would undoubtedly be significant when plans are being made to implement a veneral disease education program for the same community.

The nurse's own past experiences also influence her observations, and she should be careful not to jump to conclusions. For example, a nurse had an experience with an elderly lady, with disheveled hair, who said she had no interest in her personal appearance. When the nurse next cared for an elderly patient with uncombed hair, she concluded that the patient was uninterested in her personal appearance. Had she investigated further, she would have learned that the second patient could not comb her hair because of arthritis in her shoulders.

Sources of Data

Two factors should guide the nurse when she considers sources of data: accuracy and economy. Data can be collected from a variety of sources, but using those from which the most accurate information can be acquired in the least amount of time and with the least effort is most economical.

Generally, the person is an accurate and economical source of information and most people are eager and willing to provide information that they believe will be useful in their health care. There are instances when the patient is unable or unwilling to participate in data collection because of age, illness, or state of mind. If so, alternative sources must be used. There are also situations in which the patient may unintentionally or deliberately give inaccurate information. Even though data are incorrect, it may be important for the nurse to obtain this information from the patient as a means to better understand him (Fig. 4–3).

Current records prepared by health practitioners and those kept by health agencies the person has visited in the past are additional important sources of data. It is suggested that the nurse review available information early when gathering data—in some instances before her first contact with the patient. Then, she will wish to confirm and amplify data obtained from other sources and return to the patient as necessary. Using available data helps to prevent the gathering of duplicate information. People who are asked the same questions again and again become understandably annoyed and fatigued. It is a waste of everyone's time, and the patient may begin to distrust the health practitioner's interest in and ability to care for him.

Other persons who know the patient often are helpful. Family members and close friends often can make meaningful and useful contributions. Care must be taken, however, to determine that the patient does not object to information being gathered from these sources and that these other persons wish to participate. A clear understanding by the patient, his family, and friends of the confidential nature of the data is also important.

Other health practitioners frequently secure data that are useful to the nurse's purpose. Physicians, social workers, physical therapists, nursing personnel, and others often have information which is mutually helpful when shared. Conferences are important in the process of sharing and exchanging these data.

Methods of Collecting Data

The methods used for collecting information should also be governed by accuracy and economy. The most common methods for gathering data used in nursing are interviewing and observation.

An *interview* is a purposeful conversation, generally in a face-to-face meeting. At least two persons engage in conversation. The *interviewer* seeks information and the *interviewee* is the person from whom information is sought. Interviewees include the patient, another health practitioner, and people of personal significance to the patient. When gathering data about a neighborhood or family, the interview is ordinarily conducted with representatives of the neighborhood or family. There will be further discussion of interviewing in Chapter 6.

Observation is the taking in of information through the senses of vision, hearing, smell, touch, and taste.

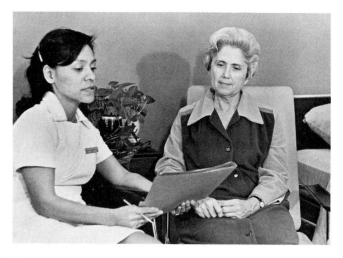

Figure 4–3 The nurse is reviewing the data-collection form with the patient before she starts to record information. Showing the patient the form and explaining that the information will be used for assessing and planning nursing care generally helps the patient to understand the purpose of data collection and to participate more readily.

Data gathered by this method should be objective so that they can be confirmed by others.

Visual observation includes physical characteristics, facial expressions, behavioral responses to interactions with others, and so on. Observations made through hearing include coughing, breathing, and noise in a particular neighborhood. Smell or olfactory observations include odors from wound drainage, garbage, foods, auto emission fumes, and so on. Touch or tactile observations include comparative skin temperatures and the shape, texture, and size of body organs. Taste is the least commonly used sense for data collection. However, there have been instances when babies have been diagnosed as having cystic fibrosis by the salty taste of perspiration when they were kissed.

Instruments are often employed in the collection of data. The stethoscope, ophthalmoscope, electrocardiograph, thermometer, and scales are commonly used as observational tools. Laboratory analyses of body tissues, fluids, and environmental elements are also useful aids. Chapter 15 will include a discussion of instruments commonly used during the physical examination.

A variety of forms for the collection of data has been developed that offer the nurse guidelines on information to collect and schemes for organizing data. Some of them are intended for use with hospitalized patients while others are better suited for well individuals. There are those designed for persons with particular types of pathology. Still others are intended for specific age groups or for use with families.

These forms are developed for typical or average persons. Since each person is unique, forms must be adapted to fit the particular situation. They serve only as guides for the nurse. As the nurse becomes more skillful, she may wish to develop her own form. This is acceptable and often encouraged since it helps the nurse incorporate her personality and manner of thinking into her professional practice.

Samples of forms for collecting data are illustrated in Figures 4–4, 4–5, and 4–6. Others are included in some of the references at the end of this chapter. Still others will be found in health agencies.

Collecting and Recording Data

Collecting data is a deliberate and conscious act and the nurse needs to set aside a specific time and place for the procedure. The time should be when persons involved are sufficiently free from other concerns and distrac-

tions to concentrate on the task. The actual amount of time will vary. Ten to 15 minutes may be all that is necessary in some circumstances while an hour or more may be necessary in others. Information may be gathered in several meetings. Generally, the initial interview will take more time than subsequent meetings when the collection of only supplemental information is necessary.

Sometimes a patient may wish to discuss his greatest concern first, and if the nurse does not allow him to do so, he may be reluctant to talk about other topics. At other times the nurse may find the patient so threatened by a particular problem that he is unable to discuss it until after he has tested the nurse with less threatening subjects.

The primary purpose for recording information about the patient is to prevent loss and distortion of information and to have it available so that it can be examined and studied later. Some nurses do their recording during the interview or while observing and others take notes which they later use to write a report.

Areas	Subjective/Objective Data
Client perceptions of: Current health status Goals Needed/usable services **Functional Abilities:** Breathing/circulation Elimination Emotional/cognitive Mobility/safety Nutrition Hygiene/grooming Sensory input Sexuality Sleep/rest **Resources and Support Systems:** Environmental Personal/social Other	

Figure 4–4 This guide for collecting data illustrates categories which the nurse uses as reminders to prevent omitting any area of information. She formulates her own questions in any order she wishes from the listing on the left and records the data she collects on the right. This form could be used for persons of varying ages, states of health, and in different settings.

A. *Patient's understanding of illness and for hospitalization:*
   1. Why did it become necessary for you to come to the hospital or go to the doctor?_____
   2. What do you think caused you to get sick?_____
   3. What does your doctor say caused you to get sick?_____
   4. What have you been told about what to expect here?_____
   5. How do you feel about it?_____
   6. Have you been told how long you are likely to be here? How long?_____
   7. With whom do you live?_____
   8. Who is the most important person(s) to you?_____
   9. What effect has your coming here had on your family (or closest person)?_____
   10. Will they be able to visit?_____
   11. How do you expect to get along after you leave the hospital?_____
B. *Comfort and Maintenance:*
   1. Comfort
      a. Pain/Discomfort
         1) Have you had any pain or discomfort recently? Yes_____ No_____
            If yes, explain:_____
         2) What did you do to relieve the pain/discomfort?_____
         3) Did it help? How much?_____
         4) If you have pain/discomfort while here what would you like the nurse to do to relieve it?
            _____

      b. Rest/Sleep
         1) Do you usually have trouble getting to sleep or staying asleep?
            Yes_____ No_____
         2) What would you like us to do to help you get the rest and sleep you need while in the
            hospital?_____
      c. Hygiene
         1) Do you need help with your bath while here? Yes_____ No_____
            Hair?_____
            Tub or shower?_____
            How often do you usually like to bathe?_____
            What time of day?_____
         2) Do you need help with your teeth? Yes_____ No_____
            How?_____
         3) Do you use anything on your face or skin (lotions, astringents)?_____
   2. Safety and Ambulation
      a. Ambulation
         1) Do you have any problems walking or moving about?
            Yes_____ No_____
            If yes, explain:_____
         2) How do you feel about staying in bed while here?_____
         3) Do you know how much the doctor wants you in or out of bed while you are here?___
            _____

      b. Eyesight
         1) Do you have any difficulty with your eyesight? Yes_____ No_____
            If yes, explain:_____
      c. Hearing
         1) Do you have any trouble with your hearing? Yes_____ No_____
            If yes, explain:_____
   3. Fluids
      1) How much liquid do you drink each day when you are well?_____
      2) What liquids do you like to drink?
         Water:_____ Coffee:_____
         Milk:_____ Tea:_____
         Fruit Juice:_____ Soft Drinks:_____
      3) What fluids do you dislike?_____
      4) Do you drink alcoholic beverages? Yes_____ No_____
         If yes, explain:_____
   4. Oral Hygiene
      a. Teeth/Mouth
         1) What is condition of your teeth and gums?_____
         2) Do you wear dentures or partial plates?_____
         3) Do you have any trouble eating because of your teeth? Yes_____ No_____
            If yes, explain:_____
         4) Do you have any soreness or swelling in your mouth? Yes_____ No_____
            If yes, explain:_____

b. Diet
   1) Has your illness made any difference in your eating? Yes_____ No_____
      If yes, explain:_____
   2) What foods do you usually eat?_____
   3) Are there any foods you do not eat? Yes_____ No_____
      If yes, explain:_____
   4) Are you on a special diet? Yes_____ No_____
      If yes, what kind?_____
      Did you have any problems with your diet? Yes_____ No_____
      If yes, explain:_____
   5) Do you believe yourself to be overweight or underweight? Yes_____ No_____
      If yes, explain (how much and why):_____

5. Elimination
  a. Bowels
    1) How often do your bowels usually move?_____
    2) What time of day?_____
    3) Do you take a laxative? _____ or an enema?_____
                  Regularly_____ Regularly_____
                  Frequently_____ Frequently_____
                  Occasionally_____ Occasionally_____
                  Never_____ Never_____
      What kind?_____
    4) Do you do anything else to help you have a bowel movement?
                                         Yes _____
                                         No _____
      If yes, explain:_____
    5) Has being sick changed your bowel functions? Yes_____ No_____
      If yes, explain:_____
    6) Do you ever have any difficulty with your urine or passing your urine?
      Yes_____ No_____ If yes, explain:_____
      What do you do about it?_____

6. Aeration
   1) Have you ever had any difficulty with your breathing? Yes_____ No_____
      If yes, explain:_____
   2) Has being sick caused any changes in your breathing? Yes_____ No_____
      If yes, explain:_____

7. Sex and close relationships (Ask according to marital status and appropriateness to the patient)
   1) (If married) Has being sick caused you any problems with your being a
      husband_____ wife _____ Yes_____ No_____
      father_____ mother_____ Yes_____ No_____
      If yes, explain:_____
      (If single and appropriate) Has being sick made any difference in your relationships with other
      people, including close relationships with the opposite sex. Yes_____ No_____
      If yes, explain:_____
   2) (If appropriate) Has being sick caused any change in your sexual functioning (sex life?)
      Yes_____ No_____ If yes, explain:_____
   3) Do you expect your sex life to be changed in any way after you leave the hospital?
      Yes_____ No_____ Don't know_____ If yes, explain:_____
   4) Do you expect your ability to function as a husband, wife, father, mother, or in a social
      relationship to be changed in any way after you leave the hospital? Yes_____ No_____
      Don't know_____ If yes, describe:_____

C. *Other*
  1. Do you have any allergies? Yes_____ No_____
    If yes, what kind?_____
    How have you managed?_____
    To what extent does the allergy handicap you?_____
  2. How far did you go in school?_____
    Can you read and write? (Ask only if indicated) Yes_____ No_____
  3. Is there anything else you wish to tell me that would help with your nursing care?_____

Figure 4–5 This guide for collecting data is quite specific and contains preformulated questions. It is intended for use with hospitalized adult patients. The nurse may rephrase the questions or omit those that are inappropriate or have been answered by a response to a previous question. (Mayers, Marlene Glover: *A Systematic Approach to the Nursing Plan*. Appleton-Century-Crofts, 1972, pp. 240–243.)

1. PRODUCTIVITY, RELAXATION, SLEEP

00☐ I usually enjoy my work.
01☐ I seldom feel tired and rundown (except after strenuous work).
02☐ I fall asleep easily at bedtime.
03☐ I usually get a full night's sleep.
04☐ If awakened, it is usually easy for me to go to sleep again.
05☐ I rarely bite or pick at my nails.
06☐ Rather than worrying, I can temporarily shelve my problems and enjoy myself at times when I can do nothing about solving them immediately.
07☐ I feel financially secure.
08☐ I am content with my sexual life.
09☐ I meditate or center myself for 15 to 20 minutes at least once a day.

2. PERSONAL CARE AND HOME SAFETY

10☐ I take measures to protect my living space from fire and safety hazards (such as improper sized fuses and storage of volatile chemicals).
11☐ I have a dry chemical fire extinguisher in my kitchen and at least one other extinguisher elsewhere in my living quarters. (If very small apartment, kitchen extinguisher alone is adequate).
12☐ I regularly use dental floss and a soft toothbrush.
13☐ I smoke less than one pack of cigarettes or equivalent cigars or pipes *per week.*
14☐ I don't smoke at all (if this statement is true, mark item above true as well).
15☐ I keep an up-to-date record of my immunizations.
16☐ I have fewer than three colds per year.
17☐ I minimize my exposure to sprays, chemical fumes, or exhaust gases.
18☐ I avoid extremely noisy areas (or wear protective ear plugs).
19☐ I am aware of changes in my physical or mental state and seek professional advice about any which seem unusual.

WOMEN

100☐ I check my breasts for unusual lumps once a month.
101☐ I have a Pap test annually.

MEN

102☐ If uncircumcised, I am aware of the special need for regular cleansing under my foreskin.
103☐ If over 45, I have my prostate checked annually.

3. NUTRITIONAL AWARENESS

20☐ I eat at least one uncooked fruit or vegetable each day.
21☐ I have fewer than three alcoholic drinks (including beer) per week.
22☐ I rarely take medications, including prescription drugs.
23☐ I drink fewer than five soft drinks per week.
24☐ I avoid eating refined foods or foods with sugar added.
25☐ I add little salt to my food.
26☐ I read the labels for the ingredients of the foods I buy.
27☐ I add unprocessed bran to my diet to provide roughage.
28☐ I drink fewer than three cups of coffee or tea (with the exception of herbal teas) a day.
29☐ I have a good appetite and maintain a weight within 15% of my ideal weight.

4. ENVIRONMENTAL AWARENESS

30☐ I use public transportation or car pools when possible.
31☐ I turn off unneeded lights or appliances.
32☐ I recycle papers, cans, glass, clothing, books, and organic waste (mark true if you do at least three of these).
33☐ I set my thermostat at 68° or lower in winter.

34□ I use air conditioning only when necessary and keep the thermostat at 76° or higher.
35□ I am conscientious about wasted energy and materials both at home and at work.
36□ I use nonpolluting cleaning agents.
37□ My car gets at least 18 miles per gallon. (If you don't own a car, check this statement as true).
38□ I have storm windows and adequate insulation in attic and walls. (If you don't own your home or live in a mild climate, check this statement as true).
39□ I have a humidifier for use in winter. (If you don't have central heating check this statement as true).

5. PHYSICAL ACTIVITY

40□ I climb stairs rather than ride elevators.
41□ My daily activities include moderate physical effort (such as rearing young children, gardening, scrubbing floors, or work which involves being on my feet, etc.).
42□ My daily activities include vigorous physical effort (such as heavy construction work, farming, moving heavy objects by hand, etc.).
43□ I run at least one mile twice a week (or equivalent aerobic exercise).
44□ I run at least one mile four times a week or equivalent (if this statement is true, mark the item above true as well).
45□ I regularly walk or ride a bike for exercise.
46□ I participate in a strenuous sport at least once a week.
47□ I participate in a strenuous sport more than once a week (if this statement is true, mark the item above true as well).
48□ I do yoga or some form of stretching-limbering exercise for 15 to 20 minutes at least twice per week.
49□ I do yoga or some form of stretching exercise for 15 to 20 minutes at least four times per week (if this statement is true, mark the item above true as well).

6. EXPRESSION OF EMOTIONS AND FEELINGS

50□ I am frequently happy.
51□ I think it is OK to feel angry, afraid, joyful, or sad.
52□ I do not deny my anger, fear, joy, or sadness, but instead find constructive ways to express these feelings most of the time.
53□ I am able to say "no" to people without feeling guilty.
54□ It is easy for me to laugh.
55□ I like getting compliments and recognition from other people.
56□ I feel OK about crying, and allow myself to do so.
57□ I listen to and think about constructive criticism rather than react defensively.
58□ I would seek help from friends or professional counselors if needed.
59□ It is easy for me to give other people sincere compliments and recognition.

7. COMMUNITY INVOLVEMENT

60□ I keep informed of local, national and world events.
61□ I vote regularly.
62□ I take interest in community, national, and world events and work to support issues and people of my choice. (If this statement is true, mark both items above true as well.)
63□ When I am able, I contribute time or money to worthy causes.
64□ I make an attempt to know my neighbors and be on good terms with them.
65□ If I saw a crime being committed, I would call the police.
66□ If I saw a broken bottle lying in the road or on the sidewalk, I would remove it.
67□ When driving, I am considerate of pedestrians and other drivers.
68□ If I saw a car with faulty lights, leaking gasoline, or another dangerous condition, I would attempt to inform the driver.
69□ I am a member of one or more community organizations (social change group, singing group, club, church, or political group).

8. CREATIVITY, SELF-EXPRESSION

70☐ I enjoy expressing myself through art, dance, music, drama, sports, etc.
71☐ I enjoy spending some time without planned or structured activities.
72☐ I usually meet several people a month who I would like to get to know better.
73☐ I enjoy touching other people.
74☐ I enjoy being touched by other people.
75☐ I have at least five close friends.
76☐ At times I like to be alone.
77☐ I like myself and look forward to the future.
78☐ I look forward to living to be at least 75.
79☐ I find it easy to express concern, love, and warmth to those I care about.

9. AUTOMOBILE SAFETY

☐ If you don't own an automobile and ride less than 1,000 miles per year in one, enter 7 in the box at left and skip the next 11 questions. (If you ride more than 1,000 miles per year but don't own a car, answer as many statements as you can and show this copy to the car's owner.)
80☐ I never drink when driving.
81☐ I wear a lap safety belt at least 90% of the time that I ride in a car.
81a☐ I wear a shoulder-lap belt at least 90% of the time that I ride in a car. (If this statement is true, mark the item above true as well.)
82☐ I stay within 5 mph of the speed limit.
83☐ My car has head restraints on the front seats and I keep them adjusted high enough to protect myself and passengers from whiplash injuries.
84☐ I frequently inspect my automobile tires, lights, etc. and have my car serviced regularly.
85☐ I have disc brakes on my car.
86☐ I drive on belted radial tires.
87☐ I carry emergency flares or reflectors and a fire extinguisher in my car.
88☐ I stop on yellow when a traffic light is changing.
89☐ For every 10 mph of speed, I maintain a car length's distance from the car ahead of me.

10. PARENTING

☐ If you don't have any responsibility for young children, enter 7 in the box at left and skip the next 10 questions. (If some of the questions are not applicable because your children are no longer young, answer them as you would if they were youngsters again.)
90☐ When riding in a car, I make certain that any child weighing under 50 pounds is secured in an approved child's safety seat or safety harness similar to those sold by the major auto manufacturers.
91☐ When riding in a car, I make certain that any child weighing over 50 pounds is wearing an adult seat belt/shoulder harness.
92☐ When leaving my child(ren), I make certain that the person in charge has the telephone numbers of my pediatrician or a hospital for emergency use.
93☐ I don't let my children ride escalators in bare feet or tennis shoes.
94☐ I do not store cleaning products under the sink or in unlocked cabinets where a child could reach them.
95☐ I have a lock on the medicine cabinet or other places where medicines are stored.
96☐ I prepare my own baby food with a baby food grinder—thus avoiding commercial foods.
97☐ I have sought information on parenting and raising children.
98☐ I frequently touch or hold my children.
99☐ I respect my child as an evolving, growing being.

Figure 4–6 This guide for the collection of data contains checklists, and is intended to be completed by the well adult. The nurse can then amplify or clarify information as needed in an interview. (Adapted from *Wellness Inventory* with permission, © 1977 John W. Travis, M.D., 42 Miller Avenue, Mill Valley, CA 94941. The entire *Wellness Inventory* is available for purchase from the above address.)

TABLE 4–1   Common problems of data collection, possible causes of problems, and suggested remedies

PROBLEM	POSSIBLE CAUSES	SUGGESTED REMEDIES
Irrelevant or duplicate data collected.	Failure to identify specific purpose of data collection. Failure to review available patient records. Using inappropriate tools for data collection.	Determine specific purpose of data collection for each patient. Consider existing data before initiating collection. Consider modifying data collection tool or selecting alternative.
Pertinent data omitted.	Not following up on clues during data collection.	Identify potentially relevant factors in advance of collection.
Erroneous or misinterpreted data collected.	Failure to observe carefully and/or validate during data collection.	Sharpen observation skills by independently observing the same situation with a peer and compare notes afterward. Role play several validation techniques.
Too little data acquired from patient.	Failure to establish sufficient rapport or use appropriate communication techniques with client. Failure to know what information is wanted.	Review and practice communication techniques discussed in Chapter 5. Role play several explanations of purpose of data collection. Identify general data desired before collection.
Health state profile inappropriately organized.	Use of inappropriate tools for data collection.	Consider modifying tool for data collection or select an alternative tool.

respiratory diseases established for urban areas. Comparing a child's daily dietary intake with a dietary norm established for adults is also an irrelevant norm. A relevant norm in this instance would be one established for healthy children.

When the health state profile describes a general or broad item, a relevant norm is one that is also general or broad in nature. For example, the health state profile indicates that the patient is completely immobile in bed. A relevant standard would be the fact that immobility has been observed to contribute to cardiovascular, respiratory, gastrointestinal, motor, urinary, metabolic, and psychosocial dysfunctioning.

A more specific item requires a more specific standard for comparison. For example, a diagnostic test indicates that a six-year-old child's white blood cell count is 22,000 per cu. mm. of blood. An appropriate standard for comparison would be a norm that describes the average number of white blood cells per cu. mm. of blood normally found in healthy children of that age.

Standards also must be reliable. Standards accepted by health professionals when making assessments are usually based on data collected from large numbers of persons. Normal ranges of physiological functioning and developmental characteristics for various age groups have been identified in this way. Typical reactions to trauma and therapy have been formulated after studying large numbers of people. Generally, the more data, the more reliable a standard is believed to be. However, standards are subject to change as more information and knowledge become available.

There are numerous sources of standards. Many standards can be found in the literature. Many practicing nurses have developed practical and helpful standards that focus on particular types of patients with whom they have had extensive contact. The patient himself may be a source of standards. For example, the manner in which a person faces a stressful situation becomes a standard when assessing his present behavior. However, such a standard applies only to the one individual. Theories sometimes serve as standards. Erik Erikson's theory of the psychosocial developmental tasks of man through the life span is one example. This theory will be discussed more fully in Chapter 9. Theories which have been developed concerning the stages of dying and grieving also can be used as standards. They will be discussed in Chapter 26.

There is another source of standards which health professionals have been using more extensively in recent years. Through research, predictions can be made about hazards with which a person lives. Hazards that have a high potential for resulting in health problems are called *risk factors*. When an individual is exposed to sufficient risk and the likelihood of health problems seems good, the person is said to be *at risk*. Risk factors are used to identify potential problems so that close observations can be maintained and preventive or early treatment can be initiated. In relation to the probability of developing breast cancer, being Caucasian and over 40 years of age, having a mother or sister with breast cancer, never having borne children, and experiencing an early onset of menopause are risk factors.

The Social Readjustment Rating Scale is a tool that helps identify persons at risk in relation to adjusting to changes in their lives. It is illustrated and explained in

RANK	LIFE EVENT	LCU VALUE
1	Death of spouse	100
2	Divorce	73
3	Marital separation	65
4	Jail term	63
5	Death of close family member	63
6	Personal injury or illness	53
7	Marriage	50
8	Fired at work	47
9	Marital reconciliation	45
10	Retirement	45
11	Change in health of family member	44
12	Pregnancy	40
13	Sex difficulties	39
14	Gain of new family member	39
15	Business readjustment	39
16	Change in financial state	38
17	Death of close friend	37
18	Change to different line of work	36
19	Change in number of arguments with spouse	35
20	Mortgage over $10,000	31
21	Foreclosure of mortgage or loan	30
22	Change in responsibilities at work	29
23	Son or daughter leaving home	29
24	Trouble with in-laws	29
25	Outstanding personal achievement	28
26	Wife begin or stop work	26
27	Begin or end school	26
28	Change in living conditions	25
29	Revision of personal habits	24
30	Trouble with boss	23
31	Change in work hours or conditions	20
32	Change in residence	20
33	Change in schools	20
34	Change in recreation	19
35	Change in church activities	19
36	Change in social activities	18
37	Mortgage or loan less than $10,000	17
38	Change in sleeping habits	16
39	Change in number of family get-togethers	15
40	Change in eating habits	15
41	Vacation	13
42	Christmas	12
43	Minor violations of the law	11

Figure 4-8 The Social Readjustment Rating Scale is an example of a tool used by health practitioners for identifying persons at risk for developing health problems. The scale is based on the premise that change requires adjustment, and excessive adjusting is a causative factor in illness. A value has been assigned to common changes in one's life called life change units or LCUs. The LCU values are an indication of the amount of adjusting required by each change. The sum of the LCUs is an indication of the total amount of adjusting required of an individual at a particular time. The higher the cumulative score, the greater the amount of adjustment required, and the greater the likelihood of life crisis within one to two years, including health problems. An LCU score of 150 to 199 is felt to be an indicator of probable mild life crisis. A score of 200 to 299 is predictive of moderate life crisis, and a score of 300 or more is a predictor of major life crisis. (Holmes, Thomas H. and Rahe, Richard H.: "The Social Adjustment Rating Scale." *Journal of Psychosomatic Research* 11:216, August 1967, Copyright © 1967, Pergamon Press, Ltd.)

Figure 4-8. The Apgar Scoring Chart, illustrated in Figure 4-9, is another tool containing standards that are useful for assessing the newborn and identifying infants who are at risk.

Making an Assessment

After a standard is selected, the nurse is ready to compare the health state profile with that standard. The process of comparing involves bringing items together so they can be examined. The purpose is to draw conclusions about the items being compared with the norm.

During assessment, if a person appears to meet a standard, the nurse concludes that the person has a strength in that particular area and this strength contributes to his level of wellness. An assessment that describes a person's strengths, that is, his ability to make satisfactory independent adjustments to achieve or maintain his desired state of health, is often called a *positive assessment.* When it appears that a person does not meet certain standards, the nurse concludes that the person most probably has a limitation in this aspect of his level of wellness and needs professional services. This type of conclusion is often called a *negative assessment* and indicates that the person is having a health-threatening problem which he is unable to handle independently. Unfortunately, in too many instances, nurses tend only to look at negative assessments without considering positive assessments. A far better practice is to use the person's strengths in assisting him to meet needs which may exist. Also, identifying strengths tends to promote a less biased picture of the person than does identification of health problems only. For example, assume that a person is hard of hearing. This information will be important to consider in planning his nursing care. Assume that the same person's profile indicates that his eyesight is excellent. The nurse can then consider this as a strength and build upon it when helping the person to solve at least some problems he may have because of his hearing limitation.

Another type of assessment may have predictive value; that is, the nurse anticipates that something may occur. For example, a patient displays signs of a wound infection, but laboratory results show that his white blood cell count has not increased as is usual when an infection of this nature is present. The nurse concludes that the body is apparently not building up normal defenses to combat the infection. She then predicts certain problems, such as a longer wound-healing pe-

SIGN	0	1	2
Heart rate	Absent	Slow (Less than 100)	Over 100
Respiratory effort	Absent	Slow irregular	Good, crying
Muscle tone	Flaccid	Some flexion of extremities	Active motion
Reflex irritability	No response	Cry	Vigorous cry
Color	Blue, pale	Body pink Extremities blue	Completely pink

Figure 4–9 The Apgar Scoring Chart is an example of a tool used for identifying newborns who are at risk. The nurse observes each of the five signs one minute after delivery and again at five minutes. The infant is scored on each sign following each observation. After each observation, the scores are totaled and then assessed by comparing them with a scale that accompanies the chart. The maximum score is 10. A score of 7 to 10 indicates the infant's condition is good and no special action needs to be taken. A score of 4 to 6 means the baby is in fair condition and certain recommended procedures should be followed. A score of 3 or less means the baby is in serious condition and emergency measures are needed. It should be noted that the Apgar tool was developed for use with Caucasian babies. A change in skin color is difficult to observe in black and other dark-skinned infants. In these babies changes in the color of the mucous membrane is generally easier to detect than the skin.

riod than would normally be expected. This has many implications for nursing care, such as those related to the patient's diet, fluid intake, urinary output, mobility, and so on.

Assume that a well child's health state profile is compared with certain developmental norms. The nurse concludes that the child is developing normally. She can then predict that barring unusual illness or injury, this child will most likely continue to develop normally.

The following are some assessments a nurse might make:

The patient *is* or *is not* independently capable of

- adapting his fluid intake appropriately to meet increased demands resulting from his infection and an elevated temperature.
- controlling his anxiety to make it possible to learn how to care for himself.
- modifying his sleep requirements sufficiently to cope with his postoperative discomfort.
- altering his life-style to include necessary dietary changes.

Validating the Nursing Assessment

The purpose of validation is to minimize the occurrence of errors, biases, and misinterpretations. The nurse seeks confirmation of the person's strengths and problem areas. Usually it is not practical or possible to validate all nursing assessments. However, the more that are validated, the more effective nursing care planning is likely to be. Because of the potential for human error in each step of the assessment process, a high percentage of validations is recommended, especially for beginners. With more experience, the nurse may become more selective when she validates.

The patient is a good source for validating some of the nursing assessment statements. If a patient is unable to confirm the statements because of age or degree of illness, family members can sometimes do so. Some statements cannot be validated by the patient or family because of lack of knowledge. Patient's records can sometimes also be used for validation. Some statements can be validated by other nurses or by the physician, dietitian, and others. Views of authorities on a particular subject may be useful validators. If the nurse takes care to be objective, her own past experiences can sometimes be used for validation.

While the primary purpose of validation is to ensure the accuracy of judgments upon which nursing care will be planned and provided, it has an additional benefit for the nurse. Validation can provide immediate positive or negative evidence of her judgment skills. Either result can be helpful in her continued efforts to perfect her nursing skills.

Stating Nursing Diagnoses and Establishing Their Priorities

A nursing diagnosis is the end product of the assessment part of the nursing process. A *nursing diagnosis* is a statement that describes a specific problem related to a person's state of health and is based on a negative nursing assessment. A nursing diagnosis implies that the problem is potentially responsive to nursing intervention measures. Some authors define the nursing diagnosis as the nursing problem, nursing need, or nursing difficulty.

Nursing diagnoses are of various types. One type describes an individual's lack of ability to meet his own health needs. For example, a patient may be too ill to feed himself. Another type of diagnosis describes a situation in which an individual is unaware of an actual or potential health problem. For instance, a mother may not know that a child's sore throat caused by streptococci can predispose the youngster to rheumatic fever and possible heart damage. A third type describes activities that are detrimental to an individual's well-being. A person who habitually takes laxatives may depress his own intestinal activity to a serious degree.

The purpose of the nursing diagnosis is to pinpoint a health problem so that specific planning and intervention measures may be used to alleviate the problem. Hence, including the specific cause of the problem in the nursing diagnosis is helpful whenever possible. Here are some nursing diagnoses based on the examples of nursing assessments given on page 69:

- The patient has an inadequate fluid intake to meet increased demands because of arthritic disability in her hands.

- The patient is experiencing anxiety associated with misunderstandings about his medical treatment which is impeding his learning of self-care skills.

- The patient is sleepless due to discomfort associated with recent surgery.

- The patient is failing to incorporate required dietary changes into his life-style because of the threat to his self-concept.

The term diagnosis is most commonly associated with physicians. A *medical diagnosis* refers to a patient's pathological condition. Other health practitioners also may diagnose. Physical therapists identify skeletal and motor malfunctioning; social workers point out social and psychological problems; nutritionists uncover dietary deficiencies. A patient may have several different and valid health-related diagnoses at the same time from various health practitioners.

If a person has more than one nursing diagnosis, which is frequently the case, it is recommended that these diagnoses be ranked in order of priority. This procedure offers guidance when planning nursing care. Health problems which endanger the person's life, such as acute respiratory or circulatory failure, receive highest priority. Problems of lesser urgency are ranked lower. The ranking depends on the significance of the problem in relation to well-being and life itself.

If the patient is able to participate, his consideration for ranking priorities should be taken into account. Often the effectiveness of the entire nursing process is jeopardized when the nurse ignores what the patient feels is important.

Unless the nursing diagnosis deals with a problem that can be remedied immediately, the diagnosis is usually recorded. This practice makes it available for later reference by the diagnosing nurse and other nurses and health personnel.

HEALTH STATE PROFILE EXCERPT–

Pale, 30-pound, 11-month-old baby. Birth weight of 7 pounds. Mother reports worry, frustration, and embarrassment because baby continually fussy and irritable. Usually takes 6 to 8 8 oz. bottles of cow's milk with added Karo syrup/day. Mother interpreted baby as not liking solid foods because child spit them out at only feeding at which they were offered. First child for mother who has had no contact with other babies before. Mother has sixth-grade education and no extended family members immediately available.

STANDARDS–

Cow's milk contains little or no iron. Stored fetal iron supply is normally depleted in four to six months. Birth weight should approximately triple by one year of age. Tongue manipulation for swallowing solid foods and adjustment to different food textures and tastes are learned behaviors for which neuromuscular development exists by approximately four months of age. Maternal behaviors are also learned.

NEGATIVE ASSESSMENTS–

Child's diet not adequate for developmental needs. Mother lacks knowledge and skills of child care.

POSITIVE ASSESSMENT–

Mother concerned about child.

NURSING DIAGNOSIS–

Nutritional deficiency in child because diet limited to cow's milk due to mother's insufficient knowledge and skills.

Figure 4–10 This example of assessment shows the health state profile and standards which are compared to determine the positive and negative nursing assessments. The statement of the nursing diagnosis is the end product of assessment.

Figure 4–10 shows the development of nursing diagnoses. This example is intended to be illustrative and is not necessarily all-inclusive of a particular person's situation.

Evaluation and Feedback

The end product of assessment is the nursing diagnosis. The nurse should judge the diagnosis for appropriateness and objectivity.

Answers to the following questions will help test objectivity. Does the diagnosis reflect the person's present health status? Are all relevant factors in the person's situation considered? Is each diagnosis logical and valid? Is the diagnosis based on existing evidence?

Appropriate nursing diagnoses should reflect the sum of the person's health problems and should be potentially useful to the nurse for planning nursing care. Appropriateness means that an effort has been made to identify all of the person's problems that are amenable to nursing measures and that priorities have been established with regard to the urgency of the problems.

If the nursing diagnoses are objective and appropriate, the nurse proceeds to plan nursing care. If the nursing diagnoses do not satisfy objectivity and appropriateness, the nurse has two options. She either repeats the assessment or gathers supplemental data. For example, if her evaluation tells her she has used an inappropriate standard when she studied the person's health state profile, she returns to the process of selecting an appropriate standard. If, on the other hand, evaluation illustrates that her data appear inaccurate or incomplete, she returns to gather more data.

Figure 4–11 on page 72 summarizes the assessment part of the nursing process.

Common Problems of Assessment

Problems have been identified in relation to assessment from experiences of students in nursing. Some of the more common ones, their possible causes, and suggested remedies are given in Table 4–2.

PLANNING NURSING CARE

A plan is a scheme or guide for action. A *nursing care plan* is a guide for action used when giving someone nursing care. The purpose of planning nursing care is to develop a guide for helping the person attain and maintain wellness. The plan is based on nursing diagnoses which were the end products of assessment and is designed to build on the person's strengths as they were determined during assessment.

Determining and Writing Objectives of Nursing Care

An *objective* is an aim or an end. Effort is exerted to attain the aim so as to help the person regain or maintain health. For example, a person feels hungry; his problem is securing something to eat. Therefore, he directs his efforts toward the objective of obtaining food in the kitchen or at the hamburger stand. The word *goal* is often used as a synonym for the word objective.

After determining problems that require nursing services and establishing priorities, the nurse next states objectives of nursing care. The objective describes the behavior one wishes to occur and the conditions under

TABLE 4–2 Common problems of nursing assessment, possible causes of problems, and suggested remedies

PROBLEM	POSSIBLE CAUSES	SUGGESTED REMEDIES
Difficulty locating appropriate standards.	Standards used by the nurse and those found in the literature are frequently not clearly identified as appropriate standards.	Develop a technique for collecting standards that will be useful, i.e., underline them in textbooks, record them on indexed file cards, and the like.
Assessments made without adequate support.	Failure to go through the logical process of making a comparison of data and standard before drawing a conclusion.	Practice writing out the steps in making assessments a few times, until it is an habitual way of thinking.
Strengths of the patient omitted.	Oversight and negligence due to emphasis on the patient's health problems	Consciously practice identifying strengths of the patient until it is a habit.
Nursing diagnoses stated in inappropriate manner for planning effective nursing care.	Failure to differentiate nursing and medical diagnoses, and identify patient difficulties which are within the realm of nursing.	Identify the difficulty or problem specified in some acceptable examples of medical and nursing diagnoses. Compare the identified problems until their distinctiveness is clear.

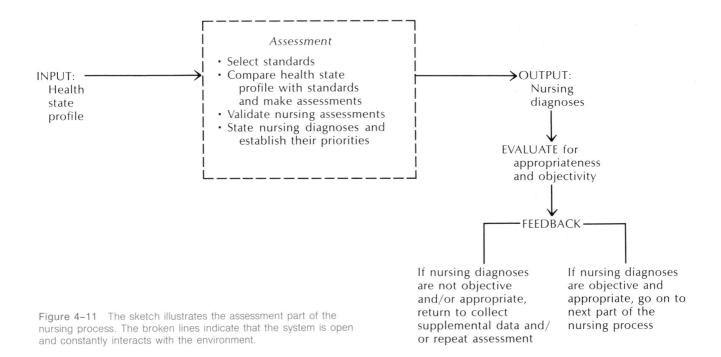

Figure 4-11   The sketch illustrates the assessment part of the nursing process. The broken lines indicate that the system is open and constantly interacts with the environment.

which one wishes the behavior to occur. This type of objective is often called a *behavioral objective*. For example, consider the patient who is hospitalized and has just had a leg amputation. The major objective of nursing care states that the patient will be employable and that employment will be satisfactory to both the employer and employee. When the objective is attained, the patient's behavior will demonstrate that he is fully employable; this is the behavior one wishes to occur. The person will be not only employable, but also employed; this is the condition under which one wishes the behavior to occur. The person's behavior on the job will be satisfactory to the person and to the employer; this states further conditions of the behavior.

Objectives may be short-term or long-term. Usually long-term objectives tend to cover a larger area than short-term objectives. The objective of care stated above for the patient with the leg amputation is a long-term objective.

While long-term objectives are necessary and useful when planning patient care, the more precise short-term objectives which lead the way to the long-term objectives are especially important. Short-term objectives illustrate exactly what should be accomplished along the way and show even small increments of progress. Since short-term objectives are usually quicker to attain, the patient as well as the nurse can enjoy the satisfactions of observing progress enroute. In

addition, there is less likelihood of the patient being off track and reinforcing poor habits on the way to the long-term goal. An additional advantage of stating short-term goals is that they are much easier to adjust in order to plan care that will meet an individual's needs as they change from day to day or week to week.

For the patient with an amputation cited above, short-term goals will aid in directing the course toward the desired end more accurately and precisely.

- To move from sitting to standing position with assistance of nurse.
- To move from sitting to standing position without assistance.
- To stand for five minutes at side of bed with support of nurse.
- To stand for five minutes at side of bed with support of chair or table.
- To stand for ten minutes with the aid of crutches.
- To walk ten steps with crutches with nurse's assistance.
- To walk ten steps with crutches without assistance.
- To apply artificial leg correctly with nurse's assistance.
- To apply artificial leg correctly within ten minutes without assistance.
- To stand unassisted on artificial leg for five minutes.
- To walk ten steps unassisted with artificial leg. And so on.

The above objectives are expressed as activities the patient will be able to do in a relatively short time, unless complications occur. It will be relatively simple to evaluate the progress the patient makes at each step and to recognize when additional time is necessary before the patient can proceed to the next. The advantage of short-term objectives is that one is able to identify problems at their onset so that the patient does not reinforce poor learning or become frustrated while exerting efforts to reach his long-term goals.

Objectives which are stated clearly and concisely and which are realistic in terms of specific, expected behavior are important for communicating a plan of action to other members of the health care team. Reconsider the patient with the leg amputation. Think about this objective: the patient will be able to stand. Stand where and how? Stand with or without assistance? For how long? It can be seen that the objective just stated hampers communication among health practitioners concerning the patient's progress. Without clear communication, health team members cannot reinforce each other's efforts.

Identifying Alternatives of Nursing Care and Selecting the Type of Care Which Will Best Meet Objectives

An alternative offers a choice of things. The nurse will identify various kinds of nursing measures that could be used to meet the objectives and then will select from those alternatives the care which she believes will best meet the objectives. Some alternatives may be unrealistic, and therefore, will not be considered. A person has many options; for example, when traveling from New York to San Francisco, he may travel by bus, plane, bicycle, on foot, automobile, and so on. However, if he wishes to make the trip when he has business one day in New York and business in San Francisco two days later, any choice other than using a plane is unrealistic.

Options may be unrealistic because of such limitations as lack of available time, skilled personnel, or financial resources. In some instances, an agency's policies may act as a restraint. Thus, a nurse may think that a relative might be of great assistance if allowed to stay overnight with a hospitalized patient. When the agency's policies forbid the practice, the nurse will seek an alternative method to accomplish the goal. A patient unable to get in and out of a tub may use a shower bath as a substitute. When a patient is on a low cholesterol diet and does not care for fish, one alternative is to use chicken as a substitute.

In considering the various nursing care alternatives to accomplish an objective, the nursing assessment with

its conclusions describing the patient's strengths is often very helpful in making a final choice. A patient who is demonstrating difficulty in adjusting to blindness may have family members who are willing to assist him to gain as much independence as possible. The nurse will wish to use this information in assisting the patient. A nurse can build on a patient's manual dexterity when he is now required to administer his own injections. Or, the nurse can make the most of a patient's good respiratory functioning after a laryngectomy (removal of the voice box) in assisting the patient in learning to speak again.

Involving the patient when choices are made is essential when selecting appropriate care for achieving a particular objective. Many times a patient will have his own ideas on how best to achieve an objective. For example, an arthritic patient may tell the nurse that he can feed himself and carry out his prescribed exercises more effectively if he can soak in a tub of warm water first. Community leaders in a neighborhood may have had a previous, successful experience with publicizing a visit of a mobile chest x-ray unit to the area by distributing information through school children and through signs in the grocery stores. The nurse who fails to consider this experience may find her alternative of using other publicity media unsuccessful in achieving the goal.

Involving other nursing and health team members is also recommended when selecting care for a particular person. This practice often serves to reinforce each other's efforts. Also, an alternative one person may propose may generate still more ideas from others. A proposal for care that has not been successful when used by one nurse may enable another to make a choice.

Knowledge of the person's cultural and religious backgrounds is useful in selecting care, such as dietary customs observed by practicing Orthodox Jews. Certain cultures stress close physical contact between mother and child in their child-rearing customs; others practice a good deal of physical restraint. These examples may remind the nurse that her own cultural and religious customs may be inappropriate as norms when selecting care for patients holding different beliefs from her own. Chapter 7 will discuss cultural and religious considerations when planning nursing care.

Unfortunately, there is no absolute certainty that a particular action will result in successfully achieving nursing care objectives in the best manner possible. What may be successful for one person may not be for another. Efforts are being made to establish a statistical basis for predicting the probability of success. As this work continues, the appropriate selection of nursing measures will become increasingly more accurate and will also no doubt lead to the increased use of computers in planning nursing care. Figure 4–12 shows one method that can be used to assist the nurse when selecting measures that are likely to succeed in meeting a nursing care objective.

The nurse, together with the patient, makes a final decision on the best way to meet an objective by selecting the care that has the greatest probability of resulting in desirable effects. Identifying alternatives and selecting best ways to meet an objective are stimulating and challenging experiences. Sometimes, the most effective way to give care is not the most obvious.

NURSING DIAGNOSIS–

Nutritional deficiency in child because diet limited to cow's milk due to mother's insufficient knowledge and skills.

NURSING CARE OBJECTIVE–

Child will eat minimum of 8 oz. solid food per day from mother within one week.

ALTERNATIVE NURSING MEASURES–

1– Demonstrate technique for holding and feeding child.
2– Describe neuromuscular development of tongue.
3– Have mother observe other babies being fed.
4– Provide printed material about feeding children solid food.
5– Describe different techniques for feeding children.
6– Provide correction and reinforcement while observing mother feeding child.

Nursing Measures	Probability of Success	Acceptability to Patient
1*	Moderate	High
2	Low	Moderate
3	Low	High
4	Low	Moderate
5	Low	High
6*	High	High

* Nursing measures decided upon for implementation.

Figure 4–12   A method for selecting nursing measures is demonstrated using the nursing diagnosis example from Figure 4–10. The nurse rates the alternative nursing measures according to their probability of success for the particular patient and for their acceptability to the patient. The measure(s) with the greatest combined success probability and acceptability are then selected for implementation. Ideally both the success and acceptability ratings for the alternatives selected would be high. In practice, this ideal often does not exist. A measure with a high probability of success and a low acceptability to the patient is generally not likely to be effective, nor is the reverse situation. For these reasons probability of success and acceptability to the patient are both considered when selecting nursing measures.

It requires creativity and ingenuity to look for alternative methods of care and avoid giving stereotyped care to everyone. However, the rewards of individualized service are well worth the efforts.

Writing Nursing Orders

Nursing orders are written on the basis of the nursing care selected for a particular person. A *nursing order* tells what nursing care is to be done. It is particularly important that these orders be spelled out clearly and concisely. Carefully written nursing orders are essential to promote communications among team members in order that patient needs will be met as planned. A few examples will illustrate.

A hospitalized patient with an elevated body temperature needs a larger than usual fluid intake to prevent dehydration, a condition of a deficiency in body water. One nursing order states, "Force fluids." A better and much more precise order would read, "Offer 200 ml. of fluid every two hours while patient is awake to a total of 3,000 ml. intake in each 24-hour period." Another patient had a nursing order that read, "Increase activity." A preferable way to state the order is, "Have patient walk length of hall three times a day."

A community health nurse wrote this nursing order for the children in a family, "Have children immunized." A better order would have stated the names of each child needing immunization, the exact type of immunization needed for each, and when the immunization was to be done.

A good nursing order is a written order. Depending on memory and on verbal communication of nursing orders is not safe. Oral orders may be forgotten, misunderstood, or incorrectly interpreted.

Developing a Nursing Care Plan

A *nursing care plan* is a written guide or scheme for giving nursing care. Usually, health agencies have their own nursing care plan forms, which are helpful and the use of which is encouraged. Many suggestions for forms appear in the nursing literature and descriptions of various kinds of forms can be found in the references at the end of this chapter.

Figures 4–13 and 4–14 illustrate two nursing care plans. It must be remembered that the information called for on any agency form may not be appropriate or complete for every patient. Therefore, the nurse will use the form but will make whatever adjustments are indicated for each patient.

NAME: *Mrs. Mary Cawkins*

DATE ADMITTED: *7/8*   ADMISSION WEIGHT: *122 lbs.*

DATE OF BIRTH: *4/13/11* AGE: *68* SEX: *F* NATL'.: *Am.*

REMARKS: *Lives alone; Been generally well and active; Poor appetite; Mentally alert and responsive*

DIAGNOSIS: *Cerebrovascular accident, right-sided paralysis, left-sided weakness*

NEXT OF KIN: *Joan Lawson, Daughter*

ADDRESS: *1383 Elm Dr., City*   PHONE: *481-0836*

LOCAL ADDRESS: *Same*   LOCAL PHONE: *Same*

RELIGION: *Protestant*   LAST RITES ___   CRITICAL LIST ___

ALLERGIES: *None known*

NURSING CARE PLAN

INDIVIDUAL NEEDS	POSSIBLE SOLUTIONS
<u>Nursing Diagnosis</u> — *Probable circulatory impairment resulting in decubitus ulcers (bedsore) unless immobility and bladder control improved.*	*Nursing Prescription*
OBJ. #1 — *Adequate circulation while paralyzed to maintain intact skin.*	1. *Reposition at least every 2 waking and 4 sleeping hrs. Alternate between rt. and lt. lateral and face-lying positions. Permit pt. to select positions so long as each is assumed a minimum of twice during each 24 hr. period.*
	2. *Massage back and bony prominence areas at time of each position change.*
	3. *Reinforce explanation of purpose and plan at each repositioning.*
OBJ. #2 — *Regain urinary control within one week (7/15) demonstrated by use of bedpan at regular intervals and no evidence of urinary incontinence.*	1. *Position pt. on bedpan at her request and/or immediately after awakening and meals, before retiring, and at least every 2 waking and every 4 sleeping hrs.*
	2. *Assist pt. to drink minimum of 3-4 ozs. fluid 20-30 mins. before each planned daytime bedpan use.*
	3. *Provide privacy and remind pt. to concentrate on urination while on the bedpan. Run water faucet within hearing range while on bedpan. Remove bedpan promptly after use or within 10 mins.*

Figure 4–13   This example of a nursing care plan is intended for a patient who has experienced a cerebrovascular accident (stroke) and is at risk for developing decubitus ulcers (bedsores).

Evaluation and Feedback

The final phase in the process of planning nursing care is to evaluate the plan by judging how well it relates to the nursing diagnoses and whether it is acceptable to the patient.

Assume that when the nurse gathers data, she learns that a patient has certain sensitivities (allergies). The nursing diagnosis states that the patient has a high degree of sensitivity to varied determined and undetermined substances. One objective of care is that the patient avoid sensitivity reactions during hospitalization. Then, nursing care would include actions to avoid common substances to which the patient may be sensitive. The nursing care plan includes one nursing order stating that a nondetergent soap be used when bathing the patient. A relationship can readily be seen between the nursing diagnosis and the nursing care plan.

During evaluation, the nurse will also wish to answer the question: Do the nursing orders utilize the strengths of this patient as these strengths are stated in the nursing assessment? If they do not, an appropriate relationship between assessment and planning may be questionable.

Evaluation to determine whether the plan is acceptable to the patient is usually a relatively easy step. The nurse will wish to consult with the patient initially. There will be times when the patient believes a plan is satisfactory but decides later that it is unacceptable. In such instances, a modification in the plan is made. If the patient is unable to help evaluate the plan, a member of the family may be consulted (See Figure 4–15 on page 77.)

DATE	PROB #	PROBLEMS	RES.	EXPECTED OUTCOME	DEADLINES	PLAN OF ACTION	SIG.
7/23	1	Overweight		Lose 30# by adhering to Wt. Watcher's Diet	5 mos.	Refer to convenient Wt. Watcher's Center. Check on wt. reduction progress monthly.	
7/23	2	Lack of regular exercise		Walk 1/2 mile daily.	2 wks.	Check on progress of incorporating walking plans into daily activities. Check effect of increased exercise on blood pressure and pulse.	
7/23	3	Lack of planning for changes in life style which will result from retirement in 9 mos.		Initiate discussion of plans for use of time, maintenance of social relationships, health care, and living arrangements after retirement.	1 mo.	Provide pamphlet and recommend book on retirement preparation. Promote discussion of his plans regarding changes in life style./K.Lee, RN	

NAME Robert H. Johnson   SEX M   BIRTH DATE 1/16/15
ADDRESS 814 Main Ave., City   PHONE 462-1103   INITIAL VISIT 7/23

Figure 4-14 This example of a nursing care plan has been designed for a well person who needs some assistance in areas which contribute to the maintenance of his state of health. Note tht this form differs from Figure 4-13.

A community health nurse developed a nursing care plan with a family. The man and his wife stated that the plan they and the nurse had devised was acceptable: one of the children was to be evaluated by a private psychiatrist. However, before the youngster saw the psychiatrist, the parents changed their minds and told the nurse that the plan was unacceptable. The alternative in this case was to use a mental health clinic instead, a plan with which the parents concurred.

When evaluation of the nursing care plan indicates it is unsatisfactory, the nurse retraces her steps. She decides to redo her plan or go back to previous parts of the nursing process. In the latter case, she may gather more data or may use different standards for assessing. If evaluation of the nursing care plan indicates that it is satisfactory, the nurse goes on to the next part of the nursing process which is nursing intervention.

Figure 4-16 summarizes the part of planning nursing care in the nursing process.

Common Problems of Planning Nursing Care

Problems have been identified in relation to the planning of nursing care from experiences of students in nursing. Some of the more common ones, their possible causes, and suggested remedies are given in Table 4-3 on page 78.

NURSING INTERVENTION ✓

To intervene means to come between. For example, a labor arbitrator intervenes to help settle a strike. He comes between an employer and an employee. *Nursing intervention,* sometimes called nursing care, consists of actions taken by the nurse to assist a patient. She comes between a problem and its resolution by carrying out actions to solve the problem. The purpose of intervention is to render care that helps solve the patient's health problem.

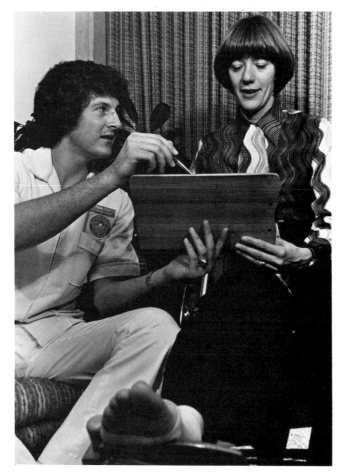

Involvement of the patient to the greatest extent possible is important when giving nursing care. It often has been demonstrated and described in nursing literature that expressions of patient satisfaction are directly proportional to the patient's involvement in his care. Whether the nurse is caring for an individual, a family, or a community, there is a sense of accomplishment when the patient participates. Patient involvement takes more time, but in the long run, the expenditure of time is worthwhile and generally helps the patient to become more independent to meet his own needs.

Putting the Nursing Care Plan into Action

The information contained in the nursing care plan becomes the basis for action. The nature of the action varies but each nursing measure should be performed with the intent of achieving the objectives of nursing care.

The principle of maintaining the patient's individuality is considered during nursing intervention. There

Figure 4–15 The nurse is reviewing the proposed nursing care plan with the patient to determine if it is acceptable.

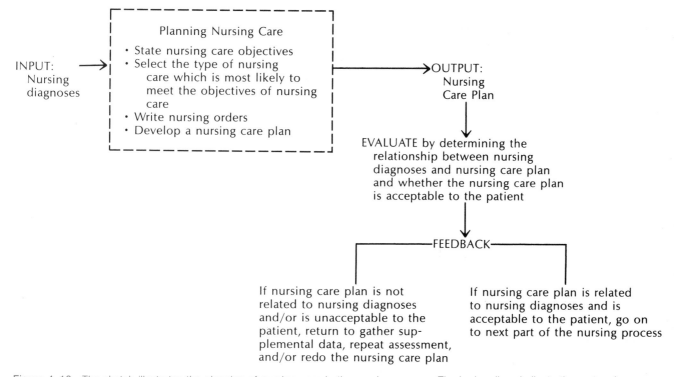

Figure 4–16 The sketch illustrates the planning of nursing care in the nursing process. The broken lines indicate the system is open and constantly interacting with the environment.

TABLE 4–3 Common problems in the planning of nursing care, possible causes of problems, and suggested remedies

PROBLEM	POSSIBLE CAUSES	SUGGESTED REMEDIES
Nursing care objective stated too generally to be useful for directing or evaluating nursing care.	Objective fails to include specific description of desired patient behavior.	Review each nursing care objective formulated with the following questions: What behavior should the patient exhibit when the goal is achieved? How and under what circumstances should this behavior occur?
Failure to develop nursing care objectives from specified nursing diagnoses.	Does not relate nursing assessment process to planning process.	Check each nursing care objective for a related nursing diagnosis, and each nursing diagnosis for related nursing objective(s).
Failure to write nursing orders clearly.	Uses ambigious and nonspecific words and phrases.	Ask a peer or other appropriate person to review a nursing care plan you've prepared and to interpret the nursing orders. If not interpreted as intended, request corrective suggestions.
Patient not appropriately involved in planning.	Uncomfortable with notion of acting *with* patients, instead of acting *on* or *for* them. Unskilled in techniques of involving others, while remaining in control of planning.	Reconsider definition of the purpose of a helping relationship and of nursing. Role play several techniques for involving patients in nursing care planning.

may be times when the nurse will make on-the-spot decisions in order to keep care individualized. For example, a nurse may be teaching a mother the essentials of a balanced diet for her family. She may find that it seems better to use a chart picturing the essentials of a balanced diet for this patient before presenting information in printed form. In another instance, a patient may appear to prefer reading something first before studying about it from a chart or discussing it during an interview. Or, a patient needs to exercise her arm following a mastectomy (removal of a breast). She may prefer doing the exercise after lunch rather than before, and she is allowed to do so.

While patient involvement is important, care must be exercised to avoid inappropriate demands on the patient. Some patients may be frightened or fearful of involvement. Others may accept involvement only out of fear of being labeled "uncooperative." Refusal may cause the patient to fear that the nurse may retaliate. Sensitivity to the patient's feelings, with encouragement and support, are important as the nurse promotes patient involvement with his care.

Another precaution when involving patients with their care is to be sure that adjustments in care suggested by the patient will not interfere with objectives. A patient may wish to postpone learning how to administer his own insulin until after he has returned from a vacation. This arrangement may be unwise if postponement represents a threat to the control of his disease.

Still one more precaution should be observed. While modifying nursing care measures, it is important that the scientific basis for care has not been violated. For example, the nurse may alter the placement of the adhesive securing a dressing to accommodate the patient. However, her action is not justified if the technique then causes contamination of the dressing and wound. In such instances, it is important for the nurse to explain to the patient why she cannot accommodate the patient's wishes.

Identifying Responses of the Patient to Nursing Care

A *response* is a reaction to a stimulus. A person's reactions of joy could be his response to the stimulus of seeing a long-time friend unexpectedly.

Identifying responses to nursing care requires deliberate efforts to detect reactions of the patient to the care he received. Reviewing the objectives of care will aid the nurse to identify responses that indicate change has occurred. For example, an objective of care stated that the patient's intestinal elimination will occur on a daily basis within two weeks of beginning a bowel-training program. The patient's responses to the training program are relatively easy to see: bowel elimination occurs or it does not in the manner stated in the objective. Other responses or changes in the patient may be more subtle and difficult to note. How a patient feels about adjustments he may need to make in his activities of daily living following a heart attack is difficult to gauge. The nurse will have to form her impressions from a number of clues.

The methods used to identify patient responses to

nursing care are those used when gathering data. The nurse needs to know what she is looking for with regard to patient responses; she must be alert to any clues, the subtle as well as the obvious; and she must be objective in her appraisal of patient responses to care. The following examples show how nurses identified patient responses to care.

A nurse is caring for a patient who is nauseated and vomiting. He is unable to retain fluids or food. The objective of care is that there will be less nausea and vomiting and an increase in fluid intake to 2,000 ml. within 24 hours. Once appropriate care has been given, the nurse will identify the responses of this patient to it in several ways. She may ask the patient to compare his current feelings about nausea with previous ones. If he states he feels no nausea and if there has been no vomiting, his responses to care have been demonstrated. The nurse will also observe the patient's appearance to detect changes in his skin coloring, his facial expressions, his mannerisms, and so on. The pale appearance of his skin has disappeared; his facial muscles appear relaxed; he no longer wants an emesis basin at his side. In addition, the nurse notes that the patient's oral intake has reached 2,000 ml. during the last 24 hours; his urinary output has increased; his body temperature and his pulse and respiratory rates are within normal ranges; and laboratory reports indicate that his blood chemistry findings are within normal ranges.

Assume now that instead of the responses just described, the patient demonstrates the following signs: he states he still feels nauseated and he continues to vomit; he insists he needs an emesis basin at his side at all times; he appears pale and his facial muscles are tense. Also, the patient states he feels "bloated" and the nurse observes that his abdomen is distended (swollen); he is urinating much less than would be expected of an adult, and he is refusing fluids and food; his body temperature is elevated and his respiratory and pulse rates do not fall within normal ranges; laboratory reports indicate that his blood chemistry findings do not fall within normal ranges. These responses obviously indicate that care measures were unsuccessful.

Evaluation and Feedback

To evaluate care, the nurse should look for evidence to indicate that nursing care objectives have been or are being met. Reconsider for a moment the patient who was nauseated and vomiting. The objectives of nursing care for this patient were met in the first instance. When in the second instance, the patient's nausea and vomiting continued, his fluid intake failed to meet the objective, and he displayed additional signs that served as clues that his condition was becoming worse. The objective of care was not being met. This example shows the importance of stating objectives of nursing care in precise and specific terms so that the nurse can clearly determine whether or not objectives were reached and the extent to which they have been reached.

The nurse should also determine whether care has been acceptable to the patient. This can be discussed with him, or if he is unable to participate, the nurse may observe his reaction or involve his family in a discussion of his care.

When evaluation of the patient's responses indicates objectives of care are being met and care has been acceptable, the nurse continues with the care. When objectives have been met, the measures are terminated. If objectives have not been met, the nurse collects supplemental data, takes steps to reassess the patient's condition, modifies the nursing care plan, and/or adapts nursing care measures so that they will meet the objectives.

Figure 4–17 on page 80 summarizes nursing intervention in the nursing process.

Since nursing intervention is the final part of the nursing process, when it is terminated, the nursing process purpose is evaluated. The following questions can be considered: Is the person functioning at his highest level of wellness? If so, the entire nursing process is concluded. If not, is the problem one that is potentially responsive to nursing care? If so, process parts may need to be revised and continued.

Common Problems of Nursing Intervention

Problems have been identified in relation to nursing intervention from experiences of students in nursing. Some of the more common ones, their possible causes, and suggested remedies are given in Table 4–4 on page 81.

SUMMARY OF THE NURSING PROCESS

While carrying out the collection of data, the nurse

- identifies data that she believes is appropriate about the person who is to receive care.

- determines sources of data and selects an appropriate guide for assisting with the collection of data.

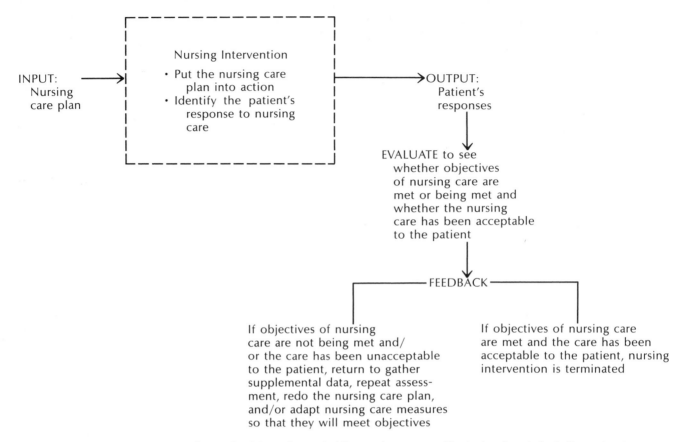

Figure 4–17 This sketch illustrates the nursing intervention part of the nursing process. The broken lines indicate the system is open and constantly interacts with the environment.

- uses various methods to collect and record data for the person's health state profile.
- validates data in order that they will be free of error, bias, and misinterpretation.
- determines that data are appropriate and accurate and proceeds to assess. Or, if data prove to be inaccurate or inappropriate, continues to collect supplemental data so that the person's health state profile is appropriate and accurate before assessing.

While assessing, the nurse

- selects relevant and reliable standards and draws conclusions by comparing the person's health state profile with the standards.
- validates the nursing assessments in order to minimize error, bias, and misinterpretation.
- states the patient's nursing diagnoses and lists them in order of their priority.

- determines that the nursing diagnoses are appropriate and accurate and proceeds to planning nursing care. Or, if nursing diagnoses prove to be inappropriate or inaccurate, collects supplemental data and/or repeats the assessment process.

While planning nursing care, the nurse

- determines areas where the patient requires nursing care and estabishes their priorities.
- states objectives of nursing care.
- identifies alternatives of nursing care and selects the type of care which is most likely to meet the objectives of nursing care.
- writes nursing orders on the basis of the nursing care that was selected.
- develops a nursing care plan.
- evaluates the nursing care plan by judging whether it relates to the nursing diagnoses and whether it is accept-

TABLE 4–4   Common problems related of intervention, possible causes of problems, and suggested remedies

PROBLEM	POSSIBLE CAUSES	SUGGESTED REMEDIES
Appropriate intervention which does not result in meeting nursing care objectives provided.	Supportive climate not adequate, and-/or nursing actions not sufficiently adapted to individual patient because the primary focus is on the learner rather than on the patient.	Review and practice techniques of anticipated nursing actions in advance so primary attention can be focused on the patient rather than on performance of the nursing actions.
Nursing actions inappropriately performed.	Nursing orders or nursing care objective(s) not clear or specific enough. Unfamiliar with scientific basis of technique or necessary skills for its performance.	Review nursing care plan following intervention for need for revisions. Critique performance of nursing actions. Review and practice as needed.
Inappropriate conclusions about the effectiveness of nursing actions drawn.	Failure to observe and use patient responses to nursing actions as a basis for determining effectiveness. Often conclusions are erroneously based on the nurse's intentions.	Before performing nursing actions, review specific patient responses to be observed.

able to the patient. Or, if the plan is not related to nursing diagnoses or is not acceptable to the patient, collects supplemental data, reassesses, and/or repeats planning of nursing care.

During nursing intervention, the nurse

- puts the nursing care plan into action while involving the patient as much as possible.
- identifies the patient's responses to the care given.
- evaluates nursing care by judging whether it has met objectives of nursing care and whether it is acceptable to the patient.
- terminates measures if objectives of nursing care have been met.
- if objectives of nursing care are not being met or if care is unacceptable to the patient, collects supplemental data, reassesses, modifies the nursing care plan, and/or adjusts nursing intervention measures.

CONCLUSION

The nursing process may seem complicated and in some ways, possibly it is since the human being is complex. On the other hand, following the nursing process is less laborious than describing it. Think about the baby's first struggle to learn to walk or the school child's efforts to learn how to do long division when studying arithmetic. Once the skills are learned, they can be carried out easily and without painful awareness of each step in the process. Proficiency in the use of the nursing process will develop with practice and with increased clinical knowledge so that the end result will be individualized, high-quality nursing care.

SUPPLEMENTAL LIBRARY STUDY

1. The author of the following article expresses concern about nurses losing sight of the purpose and interaction of the nursing process parts:

   Monken, Sally Speth. "After Assessment—What Then?" *The Nursing Clinics of North America,* 10:107–120, March 1975.

   Read the author's brief description of the parts of the nursing process and study the case study example when she applies them for Mrs. Boland. While the approach varies from the one presented in this chapter and you may not be familiar with all of the clinical information, try to identify examples of how the diagnoses are related to the assessments and goals. Are the orders stated clearly enough so you could carry them out?

2. The amount of published literature has expanded dramatically in every field. Hence, the professional health practitioner must develop techniques for rapidly finding the information needed. The author of the following article makes some suggestions which should be helpful to the learner in locating information necessary to apply the nursing process:

   Taylor, Susan D. "How To Search the Literature." *American Journal of Nursing,* 74:1457–1459, August 1974.

   What sources does the author suggest for identifying journal literature on a particular topic? What computerized retrieval system is recommended? What three basic guidelines for conducting a literature search does the author suggest?

3. Locating standards for the assessment part of the nursing process is often a difficult task for the beginning student. The following book is one resource containing general standards appropriate for many types of situations:

   Nordmark, Madelyn T. and Rohweder, Anne W. *Scientific Foundations of Nursing.* Edition 3. J. B. Lippincott Company, Philadelphia, 1975, 426 p.

   Practice identifying standards by selecting those which are pertinent to a patient for whom you have recently cared.

   Sources with more specific standards are found in the following references which deal with adult development:

Diekelmann, Nancy. *Primary Health Care of the Well Adult.* McGraw-Hill Book Company, New York, 1977, 243 p.

Hayter, Jean. "Biologic Changes of Aging." *Nursing Forum,* 13:289–308, Number 3, 1974.

Review them for useful standards for the next adult for whom you provide care. You may also wish to consider the data collection tools in Chapter 16 of the book authored by Diekelmann for your use.

4. This chapter indicated that there are varied types of data-collection tools available. The following authors provide examples of useful guides for specific circumstances:

Aspinall, Mary Jo. "Development of a Patient-Completed Admission Questionnaire and Its Comparison with the Nursing Interview." *Nursing Research,* 24:377–381, September–October 1975.

MacVicar, Mary G. and Archbold, Pat. "A Framework for Family Assessment in Chronic Illness." *Nursing Forum,* 15:180–194, Number 2, 1976.

Tinkham, Catherine W. "The Plant as the Patient of the Occupational Health Nurse." *The Nursing Clinics of North America,* 7:99–107, March 1972.

Is each guide helpful in collecting information about the characteristics of a patient, the reason for which he is being considered for nursing care, and the factors influencing his health situation?

5. The following reference is concerned with the stating of objectives:

Smith, Dorothy M. "Writing Objectives as a Nursing Practice Skill." *American Journal of Nursing,* 71:319–320, February 1971.

What does the author identify as the two purposes of nursing care objectives? What three difficulties are described as being common in the writing of behavioral objectives? Do the objectives you write avoid these pitfalls?

5

BEHAVIORAL OBJECTIVES

*When content in this chapter has been mastered, the
student will be able to*

Define terms appearing in the glossary.

Describe the major purpose of communications
among health practitioners.

Explain at least three characteristics of effective
communications. Give two examples of information
to be exchanged that illustrate each characteristic.

List eight guides which assist in preparing patient
records that meet legal standards.

Identify at least three forms which are included in the
nurses' section, physicians' section, and special
department section of the traditional patient record.
Give an example of information found on each form.

Explain the primary difference between traditional
patient records and problem-oriented records.

Discuss the four major parts of the problem-oriented
record.

Explain the meaning of the acronym SOAP and
provide an example of each part.

Define the purpose of quality assurance programs.

Describe the purpose of and method for conducting
a nursing audit.

Identify three purposes of classifying nursing
diagnoses.

Communications Among Health Practitioners

GLOSSARY

Audit: The systematic review of patient records for the purpose of objectively evaluating the care that has been received.

Communication: The exchange of information.

Concurrent Audit: The review and evaluation of patient records while the patients are receiving care.

Confer: To consult with someone in order to exchange ideas or to seek information, advice, or instructions from another.

Direct: To guide or order.

Nomenclature: A system of names used in a branch of learning or activity.

Patient Record: A health care agency's compilation of a person's health care information. Synonyms are patient chart, health record, health care record, and client record.

Problem-Oriented Record: A patient record which is organized according to the person's specific health problems. Abbreviated POR.

Refer: To send or direct someone for action or help.

Report: To give an account of something that has been seen, heard, done, or considered.

Retrospective Audit: The review and evaluation of patient records after the patients are no longer receiving care.

INTRODUCTION

The importance of effective communications among health practitioners is a basic assumption underlying the contents of this book. As discussed in the previous chapter, communications are essential to the functioning of the nursing process.

The reader will note that Chapter 6 is also concerned with communications, but it focuses on communications between the nurse and the person to whom she is giving care. This chapter will center on communications among health practitioners.

THE PURPOSE OF COMMUNICATIONS AND METHODS COMMONLY USED FOR COMMUNICATING AMONG HEALTH PRACTITIONERS

The primary purpose of *communications* among health practitioners is to improve the care of the person by exchanging information that will promote coordination and continuity of care and result in a harmonious blending of whatever services the person requires. Effective communications will enable personnel to supplement and complement each other's services and to avoid duplication, omissions, and unnecessary overlaps in care.

Consider the person being cared for by a variety of health practitioners, as illustrated in Figure 5–1. A smooth transfer of responsibility and coordination of care is important. For the hospitalized and acutely ill patient, communications may be necessary at frequent intervals, including change-of-shift time. When the patient receives services from various departments in the hospital, such as the x-ray, operating room, laboratory, and physical therapy departments, good communications will coordinate the services of personnel. Communications among health practitioners when the patient is discharged from a hospital remain important as the individual turns to community agencies offering health services, such as a visiting nurse service, the health office at work or school, or an extended care facility. This same person, at home or while hospitalized, may require services of a social worker; a physical, recreational, speech or an occupational therapist; a clergyman; a person from a homemaker service, and others.

Communications occur in face-to-face meetings and through such indirect means as tape recordings and the telephone.

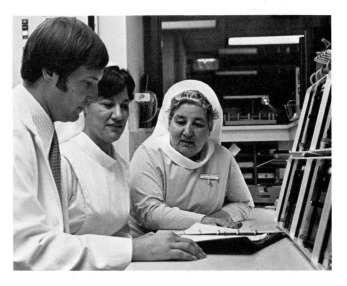

Figure 5–1 The importance of health team colleagues exchanging information in relation to a patient has been discussed often in this text. Here, a social worker, a nurse, and a physician discuss the best way to coordinate their plans for a patient being cared for in the coronary care unit who will face problems when he is ready to return to his home and family. Even during the acute phase of the patient's illness, groundwork is being laid to provide for continuity of care.

Speaking directly to someone has several advantages. One can transmit an immediate message, as well as its interpretation when indicated. Also, there is the added advantage of exchanging nonverbal messages that are often conveyed by tone, facial expressions, gestures, and so on. Nonverbal communications and their important role in information exchange are discussed in Chapter 6.

A face-to-face meeting for the purpose of exchanging information has disadvantages too. The people communicating must be in the same place at the same time and have the time available for communicating then and there. Also, there generally is no permanent record of the information exchanged for use at a later date.

Telephone communications and messenger-relayed information, while direct, have limitations. Telephone communications cannot convey most forms of nonverbal communications; only tone of voice, voice inflections, and the like, can be noted. A messenger also does not necessarily carry the original sender's nonverbal messages, and the information may become garbled in delivery. While messenger and telephone communications have some of the advantages of face-to-face meetings, they also have the disadvantages described in the preceding paragraph.

A common type of face-to-face communication occurs in groups, as for example, when team members confer, when health practitioners visit patients during rounds, or when a formal case presentation is made. Informal face-to-face meetings concerning patient care sometimes take place over a cup of coffee or during a meal.

Indirect communications, such as using the written word or a tape recorder, have several advantages over face-to-face communication. The information can be exchanged at times convenient for the people involved and a record is available for later use. However, a disadvantage is that the sender of the message is not in a position to judge whether his message was interpreted as he intended it to be.

In general, communications among health personnel fall into four categories: reporting, directing, conferring, and referring.

To *report* is to give an account of something that has been seen, heard, done, or considered. For instance, hospital nurses report a summary of patients' care and conditions at the change-of-shift time or when they have completed their care, as seen in Figure 5–2. The report may be tape recorded or given in a face-to-face meeting. It is provided for the nurse who assumes responsibility for continuing care of the patient. Several references for this chapter provide suggestions for appropriate information to include in these reports.

Nurses also report to physicians. A nurse might report when a signifiant change occurs in a patient's condition. Perhaps his level of consciousness or the location or intensity of pain has changed. Or, a nurse may report when an anticipated response to a therapeutic measure has or has not occurred.

To *direct* is to guide or order. A nurse uses nursing orders to guide nursing care activities. The physician's order directs personnel concerning the care he wishes his patient to receive. An assignment sheet directs personnel to those activities for which they are responsible. When communication involves a directive, it is important to tell who does what and when. Often, directives are given verbally. However, written directives are much safer because they lessen the likelihood of errors and misunderstandings.

To *confer* is to consult with someone to exchange ideas or to seek information, advice, or instructions from another. A nurse may consult with another nurse, as when a team leader consults with a clinical specialist about a particular patient's care. A school nurse may consult with a child's teacher or a psychologist about a behavior problem. A community health nurse and

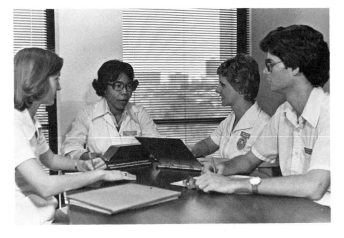

Figure 5–2 Members of the nursing staff often communicate in conferences as illustrated here. These nurses are discussing the nursing care of patients in order to help assure coordination and continuity of their efforts.

physician may confer about a patient's activity regimen. Health practitioners also confer in order to validate information. Both nursing and health team members confer in groups to plan and coordinate patient care. Often such conferences are also used for instructing students and practitioners.

To *refer* is to send or direct someone for action or help. The process of sending or guiding someone to another source for assistance is called a *referral*. A referral may be used among health agencies. A patient may be referred by a hospital to a community health nursing service for assistance with home care. A school nurse may refer a student to a hospital emergency room. A community health nurse may refer a problem she encounters in a neighborhood to the department of health for action. A referral may be used within a particular agency also; for example, a hospital outpatient clinic may refer a patient to the hospital's inservice facilities. A woman may be referred by a prenatal clinic to the agency's postpartum clinic after delivery.

The nurse's role as the patient's advocate was discussed in Chapter 1. Nurses often function in this capacity when they use referrals to seek assistance in meeting the patient's various needs. Thus the nurse may obtain services for a patient through a referral to an agency's dietary department or to a community social service agency or a home health care service. In such instances, the nurse will wish to discuss the referral with the patient so that he knows of the plan and gives his permission for the nurse to initiate action on his behalf.

Most health agencies have policies related to referrals. An agency may have a special form that personnel are to use when making referrals. The policies usually indicate who may initiate a referral, how it is to be done, and so on.

It can be seen that referrals are especially important in providing continuity of care for persons needing a variety of services. It is essential, then, that health practitioners to whom a person is referred be given information that is most useful to other practitioners and to do so with a minimum of break in its continuity. The key question is: What would I want to know about this patient if I were the person who had to continue his care at this point? The patient must of course know and approve of a referral to another agency or other health personnel for care.

Both direct and indirect communications may be used in any one or all of the four categories described above. Also, one communication experience may have parts that fall into each of these four categories. A nurse and a physician may report, direct, confer, and/or refer in a face-to-face meeting or through a patient's record.

Communications designed to inform and challenge health practitioners also improve the care of the consumer. Such communications are generally transmitted verbally and through publications, although audio and video tape recordings, television, and satellite transmissions are also being used. The exchange of information may be confined to persons within a particular agency or expanded to include individuals on local, state, national, and international levels.

Communications can convey as well as generate new ideas and they can also invite constructive criticism. Ideas are exposed for critical analysis, further testing, and additional refining.

Communications dealing with the improvement of health care may occur among individuals who share common interests. For example, two nurses who are concerned with the care of persons with similar health problems, such as adjustment to chronic diseases, may discuss observations, theoretical explanations, proposals for improving care, and ways of testing their ideas.

The presentation of new ideas concerning nursing care and the results of research are discussed at various meetings and conferences. Such organizations as the American Nurses' Association, the National League for Nursing, the Association of Operating Room Nurses, the American Association of Critical Care Nurses, and many others promote the communication of various ways to improve nursing care. Multidisciplinary orga-

nizations, such as the American Public Health Association and the Joint Practice Commission, encourage efforts to communicate ideas among various health disciplines.

Publications sponsored by various organizations and by commercial publishers communicate ideas for the consideration of health practitioners. Research and experiences are reported, problems and questions are posed, and ideas are challenged as well as supported. Large numbers of practitioners are kept informed through publications. For this reason, literature is one of the most productive means of communication for the improvement of health care.

CHARACTERISTICS OF EFFECTIVE COMMUNICATIONS

Volumes have been written about effective communications. A brief summary of essential characteristics of effective communications will be presented here.

To be effective, the information to be exchanged should be presented so that it is easily understood and free from doubt and confusion. The meaning of the information should be obvious.

Using terms that are understood in the same way by the sender and receiver is a basic rule. Words that are ambiguous or have more than one meaning can cause confusion and misunderstanding. If there is no commonly understood word or phrase available, a description and definition need to be provided by the sender. For instance, words indicating amount or quality may have different interpretations. "Slowly," "rapidly," "large," and "moderate" have many meanings. An indication of precise rate or amount is preferable.

The information to be exchanged should be specific. For example, if a patient requires assistance, the communication should indicate the type of assistance needed, as well as the activities in which he needs the assistance. Or, if a new technique is being communicated, it must be described well enough so that the receiver can duplicate it exactly if he so chooses.

Information presented to others should be well-organized. It should proceed logically and should not be composed of disconnected pieces of information that are the receiver's job to organize. Planning is ordinarily required in order to organize information to be presented to others. The sender needs to ask himself, what is the message I intend to convey? What is the most logical way to convey it?

Effective communications require that the information be objective, accurate, and factual. The sender should attempt to convey what actually exists. When it is necessary to communicate an interpretation, this should be made obvious and the basis on which the interpretation was made should be available also. If information that will substantiate an interpretation is present, the receiver can come to his own conclusion and compare it with the sender's message for verification.

To achieve efficiency, it is best to keep information to be exchanged as brief and concise as possible. This means that effort should be taken to eliminate irrelevant words that will result in the receiver having to hunt for meanings. Communications may never occur if a sender clutters information with irrelevancies.

One means for increasing brevity and clarity of communications among health practitioners has been the use of abbreviations and symbols. Some of the more common ones are listed in Table 5–1. Others will be included in Chapters 15 and 24. Symbols and abbreviations are acceptable in some agencies. However, the nurse is cautioned to use only those approved by the agency in which she cares for patients. The use of unfamiliar abbreviations and symbols can create confusion, misunderstandings, and serious errors.

PATIENT RECORDS

A *patient record* is an agency's compilation of a person's health care information. A patient record is often called a patient chart. In ambulatory settings, it is sometimes called a health record, health care record, or a client record.

An accurate record serves as a valuable means of communication among health practitioners. It is also a permanent accounting of an individual's health state and care. Since the dates of entries are specified, it has value as an historical record even years later when information becomes pertinent to an individual's current health and care. Patients' records are also used to help improve health care. Quality assurance programs which are discussed later in this chapter use records for this purpose.

Traditionally, records have not been available to consumers of health care. Several factors are responsible for a present trend that allows consumers access to their records: greater understanding of health needs and problems by the consumer, increased interest by consumers to participate in their health care, and growing respect for the rights of the consumer. It is expected that this trend will continue.

TABLE 5–1 Abbreviations and symbols commonly used by health practitioners

ā	before
abd	abdomen
ad lib	as desired
ASHD	arteriosclerotic heart disease
AMA	against medical advice
BM	bowel movement
BPH	benign prostatic hypertrophy
BRP	bathroom privileges
C	Celsius (centigrade)
c̄	with
CA	cancer
CBC	complete blood count
CO_2	carbon dioxide
c/o	complains of
COPD	chronic obstructive pulmonary disease
CPR	cardiopulmonary resuscitation
CVA	cerebrovascular accident
dc	discontinue
Dx	diagnosis
EKG (ECG)	electrocardiogram
F	Fahrenheit
GI	gastrointestinal
GU	genitourinary
h/o	history of
hs	hour of sleep
I & O	intake and output
lt	left
neg	negative
noc	night
NPO	nothing per os (nothing by mouth)
O_2	oxygen
OOB	out of bed
p̄	post (after)
P	pulse
PE	physical examination
post op	postoperative
pre op	preoperative
prep	preparation
PT	physical therapy
pt	patient
rt	right
R	respirations
Rx	treatment
s̄	without
stat	at once
SOB	short of breath
Sx	symptoms
TPR	temperature, pulse, and respirations
T	temperature
UA	urinalysis
WNL	within normal limits
x	times
>	greater than
<	less than
↑	increase
↗	increasing
↓	decrease
↙	decreasing
2°	secondary to
=	equal
≠	unequal

Patient records are generally composed of various agency forms on which information pertaining to the individual has been recorded. The forms are usually placed in a binder or folder where health practitioners have easy access to them.

Most agencies have specific policies about patient records. For example, because the record contains personal information, agencies have policies about maintaining the confidentiality of the record. They also have policies that indicate which personnel are responsible for the recording on each form and may describe the order in which forms are to appear in the record. Additional policies concern the frequency with which entries are to be made; whether routine care is to be recorded; the manner in which health personnel identify themselves after making an entry; which types of abbreviations are acceptable; and the manner in which an error in recording is handled. The nurse should familiarize herself with the policies and observe them as described by the agency in which she is giving care.

In the past, records have generally been written but there has been a trend in recent years to use mechanical devices for preparing and storing records. The dictaphone is used in some agencies for dictating material which is later transcribed and entered into the permanent record. Computer print-outs produced from information entered into a computer become part of the patient's record in some agencies. Computers are also used for the storage and easy retrieval of patient records. Audio and video tape recordings occasionally become part of the patient's record.

While there are differences among records, all contain identifying information. A form called a face sheet or admission sheet is ordinarily used. The form is generally prepared by clerical personnel but in some agencies health care personnel may be expected to prepare it. The identifying information generally includes the following items: the patient's legal name, current address, identification number, age, birthdate, sex, marital status, religious preference, occupation and employer, person to notify in an emergency, and the next of kin. Often, the following information is entered on this form also: date and time of admission or of the first contact with the patient; name of health practitioner, the service or the clinic responsible for care; reason for admission; dates of previous admissions; information concerning how financial responsibility is to be handled; and discharge information. The identifying information is available to all health practitioners as a preliminary means of acquainting them with the patient.

Patient Records as Legal Documents

Patient records can be used as legal documents and entered into courts for evidence. The patient's record can play an important role in implicating or absolving health practitioners charged with improper care. The record can also be used in accident or injury claims by the patient.

The nurse should record her observations and actions carefully to provide an accurate record because it may be used in litigations. Care must be taken to record only relevant information in order to protect the patient's privacy. Properly acquired written consents for therapies are another important part of the record. Improper consents can result in assault and battery charges. The use of verbal, rather than written, orders also has legal implications. Local policy and law will guide the nurse in executing verbal orders. In the past, problems have arisen primarily from verbal orders given to nurses by physicians.

The following guidelines will help the nurse to prepare records that are acceptable legal documents:

- Entries should be factual and accurate.
- Entries should be legible.
- Entries should include the date and time.
- Entries should be signed. Generally, the first initial, the last name, and the person's title are required, such as M. Jones, RN.
- Dittos or erasures are not permitted. A single line should be drawn through an incorrect entry; the word, error, should be written beside an incorrect entry; the entry should be rewritten correctly; and the person making and correcting the error should identify herself.
- Blank or partially blank lines are not permitted. A single line is drawn through unused space. Blank spaces can raise doubt about the addition of entries made later.
- Only approved abbreviations and symbols should be used.
- Each page of the record should be identified with the patient's name.
- Entries should clearly and specifically show how a health practitioner fulfilled responsibility to the patient.

Traditional Patient Records

While the specifics vary among agencies, the general characteristics of the traditional patient record have remained the same for many years. Entries in the traditional patient record are organized according to the source of information. Sections of the record are designated for nurses and physicians and for laboratory, x-ray, and other special services. Entries are entered chronologically with the most recent being nearest the front of each section.

Nurses' Section.   In the nurses' section of the traditional record, one commonly finds nurses' notes, graphic sheets, medication forms, and checklists. In addition, the nursing history and nursing care plan may be part of the record. Or, they both may be kept separately from the record. There may also be additional nursing forms to accommodate the needs of particular patients in some health agencies.

Nurses' notes contain narrative statements specifying the nursing care received by the patient and descriptions of his responses to care. These statements should focus on the nursing diagnoses. In addition, nurses' notes include a constant updating of pertinent observations of the patient. Figure 5–3 shows one type of nurses' notes.

Graphic sheets, medication forms, and checklists are designed for ease and rapidity of recording nursing observations or actions which are of a recurring nature. For instance, graphic sheets commonly provide a place to record blood pressure, temperature, respiratory and pulse rates, weight, and other measurements so that they can be compared over a period of time. Figure 5–4 on page 92 shows a sample of a graphic sheet.

Checklists are forms for recording nursing activities that are performed on a routine basis. Space for recording nursing actions related to personal hygiene, elimination, activity, fluid and food intake are commonly provided. Such checklists are concise and convenient but they may need to be supplemented with entries in the nurses' notes when the patient's condition warrants. Figure 5–5 on page 93 illustrates a checklist.

Medication forms are also provided for rapid recording. Generally, the name and dosage of regularly administered medications are recorded initially. Thereafter, only the time and identification of the person administering the drugs is recorded. The patient's response to the medication or any other pertinent information is recorded in the nurses' notes. In

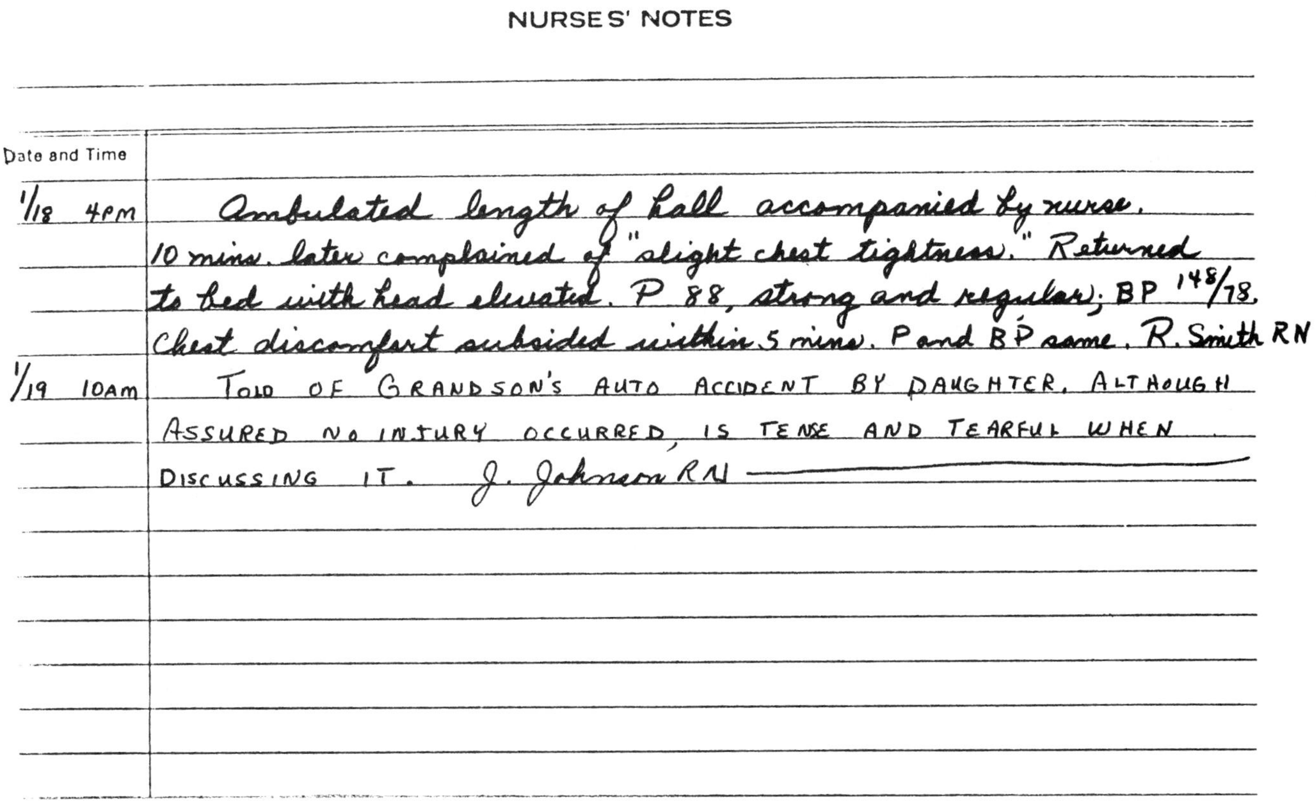

NURSES' NOTES

Date and Time	
1/18 4PM	Ambulated length of hall accompanied by nurse. 10 mins. later complained of "slight chest tightness." Returned to bed with head elevated. P 88, strong and regular; BP 148/78. Chest discomfort subsided within 5 mins. P and BP same. R. Smith RN
1/19 10AM	TOLD OF GRANDSON'S AUTO ACCIDENT BY DAUGHTER. ALTHOUGH ASSURED NO INJURY OCCURRED, IS TENSE AND TEARFUL WHEN DISCUSSING IT. J. Johnson RN

Figure 5–3   This is a sample of nurses' notes as they would appear in a traditional patient record.

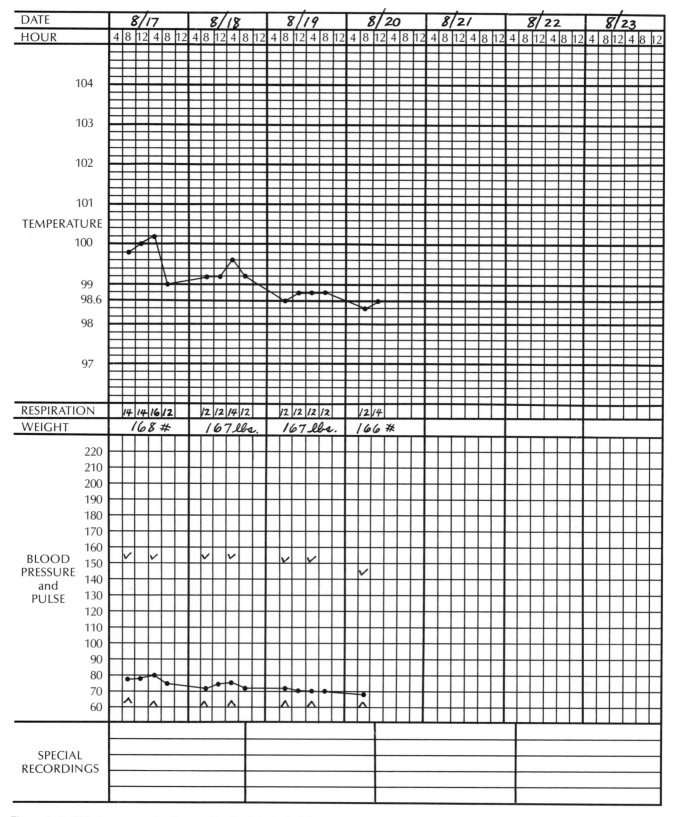

Figure 5–4   This is an example of a graphic sheet, typical of the type used in traditional patient records.

Date 9/15	7-3	3-11	11-7	Remarks	Remarks
Diet Type					
SOFT	✓	✓			
How Taken	FAIR	WELL		DOESN'T NORMALLY EAT BREAKFAST.	
Activity	OOB	OOB	SLEPT	AMBULATED IN HALLWAY X3 / SHIFT	
Urine	✓	✓	✓	TO BR q̄ 2 - 3 HRS.	
Stool	✓	0	0	SOFT FORMED, TO BR.	
Side Rails	0	0	✓		
Dr. Visited	✓			DR. M. JENSEN IN 10 A.M.	
Intake — Oral	640cc	520	200		
Intake — I.V.	—	—	—		
Intake —					
Intake —					
Intake — Total	640	520	200		
Output — Urine	—	—	—	NOT MEASURED.	
Output — Drainage	—	—	—		
Output —					
Output —					
Output — Total					
24 Hr. Intake	1360 CC.				
24 Hr. Output	—				

Date	7-3	3-11	11-7	Remarks	Remarks
Diet Type					
How Taken					
Activity					
Urine					
Stool					
Side Rails					
Dr. Visited					
Intake — Oral					
Intake — I.V.					
Intake —					
Intake —					
Intake — Total					
Output — Urine					
Output — Drainage					
Output —					
Output —					
Output — Total					
24 Hr. Intake					
24 Hr. Output					

Figure 5-5 This is an example of a checklist, typical of the type used in traditional patient records.

MEDICATIONS↓ DATES	5/20	5/21	5/22	5/23	5/24
Digoxin 0.25mg. daily→	RJ 8 AM	RJ 8 am	8 AM CR		
Aldomet 250mg. tid	RJ 8 RJ 8 8 LT	RJ 8 RJ 8 8 MK	8 CR 8 CR 8 GO		
Unicap ī cap Daily	RJ 8 AM	RJ 8 AM	8 AM CR		
Colace 100mg. cap. HS	HS LT	HS MK	HS GO		

Figure 5-6 This is an example of a form often used for recording medications a patient has received.

some agencies, only medications taken orally or non-narcotic drugs are recorded on medication forms. Other medications are entered in the nurses' notes. Figure 5-6 illustrates a medication form.

Physicians' Section. Several parts of the physicians' section of the record, are of particular interest to the nurse. The medical history and physical examination, the physician's progress notes, and the physician's order sheet contain information which is useful in planning and providing nursing care.

The medical history and physical examination contain information about the patient's present medical condition, previous illnesses, and the family medical history. In addition, the physician's confirmed or tentative diagnosis and often his therapeutic plans are included. The physician's progress notes contain a chronological commentary of the physician's interpretation of the patient's pathology and his response to medical therapy.

The order sheet contains the directives specified by the patient's physician that are to be carried out by others. For example, orders for medications and treatments to be administered by the nurse are recorded here, as well as directives for diagnostic x-ray and laboratory examinations, physical therapy treatments, and so on.

Special Department Sections. Hospital departments other than nursing and medical have sections in the patient's record for recording information. This information is also of interest to the nurse as a source of data that can be used for planning nursing care. For example, patient records have a section where laboratory test results can be found and these results are often important to the nurse. Other departments include the dietary, physical therapy, inhalation therapy, and social service departments. Often the recording indicates the care provided and the practitioner's interpretation of the patient's responses to the care.

Problem-Oriented Records

Another type of record used in many health agencies is the *problem-oriented record* which is a patient record that is organized according to the person's specific health problems. The record, abbreviated POR, was originated by Dr. Lawrence Weed in the 1960s. Extensive literature describing the POR is available. Several references at the end of this chapter describe it in detail. Only a brief summary will be presented here.

The POR is organized around the patient's problems rather than around sources of information as is the case with traditional records. All health practitioners record on the same form. Supporters of the POR believe this practice focuses the attention of health care personnel on solving the patient's problems cooperatively, and therefore, it has the potential of improving the quality of care.

There are four major parts in the problem-oriented record: the data base, the problem list, the initial plans, and the progress notes.

Data Base. The data base is the compilation of all initial patient information that is collected. It includes the nurse's health state profile, the physician's medical history and physical examination, the social history, and initial diagnostic test results. Data that are collected through interview and observation by various health practitioners are brought together in one place.

Problem List. The problem list itemizes major aspects of the patient's life which require health care attention. The list results from an analysis of data collected by health practitioners caring for the patient. The single listing is filed at the beginning of the record and serves as the organizer for the remainder of the record.

Ideally, the problem list is planned to be a permanent organizing scheme for the patient's health care for the remainder of his life. Solved problems are not removed from the list but the date of their resolution is noted. New problems are listed as they become apparent. Figure 5–7 illustrates a problem list.

Initial Plan. The initial plan outlines the beginning steps to be taken for each problem. The initial plan may include specific therapy, diagnostic tests, patient education programs, and so on. Modifications of the initial plan are incorporated in the progress notes. All health practitioners may contribute to the initial plan depending on the patient's particular problems.

Number	Patient Problem	Date Identified	Date Resolved
1	GI hemorrhage	8/13	8/16
2	Anemia 2° hemorrhage	8/15	
3	Dehydration 2° to hemorrhage	8/16	
4	Worry about hospitalization expenses	8/16	
5	Duodenal ulcer	8/16	

Figure 5–7 This example of a problem list in a problem-oriented record illustrates the recording of a patient's health problems and the dates they were identified. The date is also noted when a problem has been resolved. In some agencies, the problems are numbered as they are in this example.

Progress Notes. The POR progress notes are of three types: narrative, flowsheets, and discharge. Entries on each refer to the problems specified in the problem list and can be made by any of the health practitioners.

The narrative progress notes follow what is known as the SOAP format. SOAP is an acronym. S refers to subjective information reported by the patient; O to objective observations by health practitioners; A to assessments drawn from new subjective and objective information; and P to further plans for action related to the patient's problems. Figure 5–8 gives a sample of narrative progress notes.

Flowsheets are used for recording information that is monitored over a time—hours, weeks, months, and years. The flowsheet provides data for comparing a

#2, ANEMIA
S– Pt states she feels "so weak and tired."
O– Pale skin and oral mucous membrane.
 BP 94/48; P 92, irregular.
 Hemoglobin 9.8 Gms./100 ml.
A– Anemia 2° to blood loss continues.
P– Whole blood transfusion.
 Will recheck hemoglobin after transfusion.

#3, DEHYDRATION
S– Pt states she doesn't "want to drink too much because I don't want to be a bother for the nurses. You know I need help to go to the BR."
O– Lips cracked, oral mucous membrane dry, skin turgor poor. Eyes sunken; Urine concentrated.
A– Not comfortable with dependence.
P– Put commode at bedside. Empty regularly. Offer assistance.

#4, WORRY
S– Pt states she's concerned about the hospital expenses.
O– Tense facial expression. Speaks in short sentences.
A– Financial concerns causing increased stress.
P– Request Social Service consultation.

Figure 5–8 This example contains excerpts from narrative progress notes of a problem-oriented record. It illustrates how the acronym SOAP is used as a guide. These notes were developed from Figure 5–7 which listed the patient's health problems.

person's status at one point in time with his status later. Biopsychosocial behavior, developmental changes, responses to treatment, and evidence of learning are types of information recorded on flowsheets. Periodic conclusions or summaries of the flowsheet information may be entered in the narrative notes. Figure 5–9 illustrates a flowsheet.

Discharge notes are the entries made in the record at the time an episode of the patient's care is terminated. The SOAP format is used to address each problem and state its level of resolution. Referrals and other discharge recommendations are included in the plan for unresolved or partially solved problems.

The nursing process as described in Chapter 4 and problem-oriented records supplement each other. The part of the nursing process dealing with the collection of data contributes to the POR data base. Assessment can be used in developing the POR problem list. Planning care is necessary for the segment on planning for problem resolution. Intervention is essential for acquiring information recorded in the POR progress notes.

QUALITY ASSURANCE PROGRAMS

In recent years, there has been concerted effort to improve the quality of health care by systematically and objectively evaluating care that has been given by various health practitioners. Professional Standards and Review Organizations, as described in Chapter 1, have been developed as one means to help improve health care. The work of these organizations has the assurance of high-quality care as its primary objective.

Audit and observation are the two most commonly used techniques for implementing quality assurance programs in nursing. An *audit* is a systematic review of patient records for the purpose of evaluating the care that has been received. Standards that describe quality care are used to evaluate care that was actually given. In a nursing audit, the nursing history, the nursing care plan, the nursing intervention measures that were used, and the patient's responses to nursing care are ordinarily reviewed and evaluated.

An audit can be retrospective or concurrent. A *retrospective audit* reviews and evaluates records after individuals are no longer receiving care. A *concurrent audit* reviews and evaluates records while persons are receiving care. At this point in the development of quality assurance programs, retrospective audits are more prevalent than concurrent audits.

Most nursing audits sample data from records after they have been placed in categories. Such categories include records of persons with diabetes mellitus, persons with colostomies or ileostomies, and persons within a certain age range. Nursing audits are generally conducted at regular intervals, usually monthly. In some agencies, computer data retrieval systems are used to assist with the procedure of auditing.

Observation has not been generally used to the same extent as the nursing audit in quality assurance programs. However, tools are being developed for observing the nurse as she provides care over a period of time. The observations can be carried out continually over several hours or for specified intervals over a period of weeks or months. The quality of the nurse's performance is then rated according to standards that describe quality care.

	10:00 A.M.	10:30 A.M.	11:00 A.M.	11:30 A.M.	12:00 P.M.	12:30 P.M.
Transfusion Flow Rate						
TPR						
BP						
Restlessness						
Back Pain						
Site Inflammation						
Other Untoward Signs						

Figure 5–9   This is an example of a flowsheet used in problem-oriented records. It is used for recording observations made during the time a patient is receiving a blood transfusion. The patient is monitored every 30 minutes and the observations are recorded so that they can be compared with each other.

Tools have also been developed for observing a patients' responses to nursing care. In some situations, patients' opinions solicited verbally and through questionnaires are also included as a part of quality assurance programs.

Effective communication, between health practitioners are a basic requisite for the success of quality assurance programs. Communications between nurses are essential for developing and refining professional standards and measurement tools, documenting patient information, coordinating nursing care efforts, evaluating nursing performance, transmitting evaluation results, and initiating improvement programs. For communications to be supportive of quality assurance programs, they must be objective and accurate and arise from a commitment to the patient's welfare.

CLASSIFYING NURSING DIAGNOSES

In an attempt to increase consistency in terminology and thereby improve communications, efforts are being made to standardize and classify nursing diagnoses. The National Group for Classification of Nursing Diagnoses has coordinated the work. The goal of the group is to develop a *nomenclature* which is a system of names used in a branch of learning or activity. In nursing, nomenclature is being developed that will describe patient problems most frequently identified by nurses. This task includes specifying diagnoses commonly made by nurses, determining consistent descriptive terminology for each diagnosis, classifying the diagnoses, and developing an abbreviation or numbering system for computerization of the information.

Classifying diagnoses would provide consistency of meaning and simplify communications among nurses and other health practitioners. A nursing diagnosis nomenclature is also expected to provide a logical foundation for relating research results to each other and strengthening the scientific basis of nursing. It is also anticipated that standardization of terminology will enhance the collecting of statistics which demonstrates the contributions of nursing to total health care.

Efforts to classify nursing diagnoses are described in reports of the Nursing Diagnosis Conferences which are listed in the references at the end of this unit. Completion of the project will require many years, but with these efforts, nursing is making another step in helping to improve this nation's health care and in contributing to its own professional growth.

CONCLUSION

Effective communications are essential for the use of the nursing process and for the efficient functioning of the health and nursing teams. Communications alone cannot produce well-coordinated, high-quality, and continuous care, but lack of good communications can very often result in inferior health care.

SUPPLEMENTAL LIBRARY STUDY

1. Using commonly understood terms is one of the recommended ways for promoting effective communications. The following author presents some varied definitions of terms used in the nursing process:

    Bloch, Doris. "Some Crucial Terms in Nursing: What Do They Really Mean?" *Nursing Outlook,* 22:689–694, November 1974.

    Review the author's definitions and compare them with the ones presented in this text. How are they alike and how are they different?

    The following article describes some reactions to the Bloch article:

    Vincent, Pauline. "Some Crucial Terms in Nursing—A Second Opinion." *Nursing Outlook,* 23:46–48, January 1975.

    Do you agree with this author's suggestion about the need for defining nursing and health? How do you define these terms?

2. Computers are affecting the daily lives of everyone. The following author suggests ways in which the computer is affecting nursing practice:

    Hannah, Kathryn J. "The Computer and Nursing Practice." *Nursing Outlook,* 24:555–558, September 1976.

    Identify the five ways the author believes computers can improve the quality of patient care.

3. In the article listed below, the author suggests that the problem-oriented record replace the typical nursing care plan:

    McCloskey, Joanne Comi. "The Problem-Oriented Record vs the Nursing Care Plan: A Proposal." *Nursing Outlook,* 23:492–495, August 1975.

    Identify the pros and cons of implementing her suggestions in a setting where you have clinical practice.

4. There are dangers involved in almost every endeavor. The following authors discuss the pitfalls of peer review and the classification of nursing diagnoses:

    Bircher, Andrea U. "On the Development and Classification of Diagnoses." *Nursing Forum,* 14:10–29, Number 1, 1975.

    Ramphal, Marjorie. "Peer Review." *American Journal of Nursing,* 74:63–67, January 1974.

    Identify dangers these authors describe and indicate the remedies they offer for avoiding them.

References For Unit II

CHAPTER 4

Aspinall, Mary Jo. "Nursing Diagnosis—The Weak Link." *Nursing Outlook,* 24:433–437, July 1976.

Baer, Ellen D., et al. "How to Take a Health History." *American Journal of Nursing,* 77:1190–1193, July 1977.

Bower, Fay Louise. *The Process of Planning Nursing Care: A Model for Practice.* Edition 2. The C. V. Mosby Company, Saint Louis, 1977, 153 p.

Byers, Virginia B. *Nursing Observation.* Edition 2. Wm. C. Brown Company Publishers, Dubuque, Iowa, 1973, 106 p.

Carrieri, Virginia Kohlman and Sitzman, Judith. "Components of the Nursing Process." *The Nursing Clinics of North America,* 6:115–124, March 1971.

Eggland, Ellen Thomas. "How to Take a Meaningful History." *Nursing 77,* 7:22–30, July 1977.

Fuller, Dorothy and Rosenaur, Janet Allan. "A Patient Assessment Guide." *Nursing Outlook,* 22:460–462, July 1974.

Glatt, Carol R. "How Your Hospital Library Can Help You Keep Up In Nursing." *American Journal of Nursing,* 78:642–644, April 1978.

Goodwin, Judy Ozbolt and Edwards, Bernadine Symons. "Developing a Computer Program to Assist the Nursing Process: Phase 1—From Systems Analysis to an Expandable Program." *Nursing Research,* 24:299–305, July/August 1975.

Gordon, Marjory. "Nursing Diagnoses and the Diagnostic Process." *American Journal of Nursing,* 76:1298–1300, August 1976.

Grier, Margaret R. "Decision Making about Patient Care." *Nursing Research,* 25:105–110, March/April 1976.

Gulbrandsen, Mary Wachter. "Guide to Health Assessment." *American Journal of Nursing,* 76:1276–1277, August 1976.

Hazzard, Mary Elizabeth. "An Overview of Systems Theory." *The Nursing Clinics of North America,* 6:385–393, September 1971.

House, Mary J. "Devising a Care Plan You Can Really Use." *Nursing 75,* 5:12–14, July 1975.

Krall, Mary Louise. "Guidelines for Writing Mental Health Treatment Plans." *American Journal of Nursing,* 76:236–237, February 1976.

Lewis, Lucile. *Planning Patient Care.* Edition 2. Wm. C. Brown Company Publishers, Dubuque, Iowa, 1976, 209 p.

Little, Dolores E. and Carnevali, Doris L. *Nursing Care Planning.* Edition 2. J. B. Lippincott Company, Philadelphia, 1976, 325 p.

McCloskey, Joanne Comi. "The Nursing Care Plan: Past, Present, and Uncertain Future—A Review of the Literature." *Nursing Forum,* 14:364–482, Number 4, 1975.

Mayers, Marlene Glover. *A Systematic Approach to the Nursing Care Plan.* Appleton-Century-Crofts, New York, 1972, 304 p.

Mundinger, Mary O'Neil and Jauron, Grace Dotterer. "Developing a Nursing Diagnosis." *Nursing Outlook,* 23:94–98, February 1975.

Nicholls, Marion E. "Quality Control in Patient Care." *American Journal of Nursing,* 74:456–459, March 1974.

"Patient Assessment: Taking a Patient's History." (Programmed Instruction) *American Journal of Nursing,* 74:293–324, February 1974.

Sparks, Susan M. "Letting the Computer Do the Work." *American Journal of Nursing,* 78:645–647, April 1978.

Turnbull, Sister Joyce. "Shifting the Focus to Health." *American Journal of Nursing,* 76:1985–1987, December 1976.

Yura, Helen and Walsh, Mary B. *The Nursing Process: Assessing, Planning, Implementing, Evaluating.* Edition 3. Appleton-Century-Crofts, New York, 1978, 288 p.

CHAPTER 5

Bloch, Doris. "Evaluation of Nursing Care in Terms of Process and Outcome: Issues in Research and Quality Assurance." *Nursing Research,* 24:256–263, July/August 1975.

Cook, Margo and McDowell, Wanda. "Changing to an Automated Information System." *American Journal of Nursing,* 75:46–51, January 1975.

Gebbie, Kristine M., Editor. *Summary of the Second National Conference: Classification of Nursing Diagnoses.* Clearinghouse—National Group for Classification of Nursing Diagnoses, Saint Louis, 1976, 180 p.

Gebbie, Kristine M. and Lavin, Mary Ann, Editors. *Classification of Nursing Diagnoses: Proceedings of the First National Conference.* The C. V. Mosby Company, Saint Louis, 1975, 171 p.

Gebbie, Kristine M. and Lavin, Mary Ann. "Classifying Nursing Diagnoses." *American Journal of Nursing,* 74:250–253, February 1974.

Hanna, Karolyn Klammer. "Nursing Audit at a Community Hospital." *Nursing Outlook,* 24:33–37, January 1976.

Hirsch, Irma Lou. "Evolution of the Audit." *American Journal of Nursing,* 75:961, June 1975.

Jacobson, Sylvia R. "A Study of Interprofessional Collaboration." *Nursing Outlook,* 22:751–755, December 1974.

Kerr, Avice H. "Nurses' Notes: 'That's Where the Goodies Are'." *Nursing 75,* 5:34–41, February 1975.

Lynaugh, Joan E. and Bates, Barbara. "The Two Languages of Nursing and Medicine." *American Journal of Nursing,* 73:66–69, January 1973.

Mezzanotte, E. Jane. "Getting It Together for End-of-Shift Reports." *Nursing 76,* 6:21–22, April 1976.

Nelson, Marilyn. "Suggestions on Taping Records." *American Journal of Nursing,* 74:899, May 1974.

Pepper, Ginette A. "Bedside Report: Would It Work For You?" *Nursing 78,* 8:73–74, June 1978.

Phaneuf, Maria C. *The Nursing Audit: Self-regulation in Nursing Practice.* Edition 2. Appleton-Century-Crofts, New York, 1976, 204 p.

Phaneuf, Maria C. and Wandelt, Mabel A. "Quality Assurance in Nursing." *Nursing Forum,* 13:328–345, Number 4, 1974.

Rinaldi, Leena Aalto and Kelly, Barbara. "What to Do After the Audit Is Done." *American Journal of Nursing,* 77:268–269, February 1977.

Roy, Sister Callista. A Diagnostic Classification System for Nursing." *Nursing Outlook,* 23:90–94, February 1975.

Wandelt, Mabel A. and Ager, Joel W. *Quality Patient Care Scale.* Appleton-Century-Crofts, New York, 1974, 82 p.

Wandelt, Mabel A. and Stewart, Doris Slater. *Slater Nursing Competencies Rating Scale.* Appleton-Century-Crofts, New York, 1975, 101 p.

Weed, Lawrence L. *Medical Records, Medical Education, and Patient Care: The Problem-Oriented Record as a Basic Tool.* Year Book Medical Publishers Inc., Chicago, 1971, 297 p.

Wiggins, Addie and Carter, Joan H. "Evaluation of Nursing Assessment and Intervention in the Surgical ICU." *The Nursing Clinics of North America,* 10:121–144, March 1975.

Wiley, Loy. "Whadda Ya Say at Report?" *Nursing 75,* 5:73, 75–76, 78, October 1975.

Will, Marilyn B. "Referral: A Process, Not a Form." *Nursing 77,* 7:44–45, December 1977.

Zimmer, Marie J., Guest Editor. "Symposium on Quality Assurance." *The Nursing Clinics of North America,* 9:303–379, June 1974.

unit III
Basic Concepts in the Practice of Nursing

BEHAVIORAL OBJECTIVES

When content in this chapter has been mastered, the student will be able to

Define terms appearing in the glossary.

Explain how the gratification of human needs relates to the helping relationship.

Describe at least four characteristics of the helping relationship.

Identify three phases of the helping relationship. Provide an example of appropriate patient behaviors for each phase.

Describe how the expressive and functional factors contribute to an effective helping relationship.

Identify four essential requirements for communication to occur.

Explain at least five principles of communication which are used in the helping relationship.

Illustrate at least four techniques which tend to promote effective communication and four techniques which tend to inhibit effective communication.

The Helping Relationship and Communication Skills

GLOSSARY

Cliche: A trite, stereotyped phrase.

Expressive Factor: The behaviors in a social interaction that influence the person's emotional tone and indirectly move him toward his goal.

Functional Factor: The behaviors in a social interaction that directly move a person toward his goal. Synonyms include utilitarian factor and instrumental factor.

Helping Relationship: An interaction of individuals which sets the climate for movement of the participants toward common goals.

Hierarchy of Needs: A process or system that places requirements or necessities in an order or rank.

Hierarchy: A process or system that places things or persons in graded order or rank.

Language: A prescribed way of using words; a means of expressing throughts or feelings.

Nonverbal Communication: An exchange of information without the utilization of words.

Open-ended Comment: A verbal response that gives a general lead or broad opening to communication.

Rapport: A feeling of mutual trust experienced by persons in a satisfactory relationship.

Reflective Comment: A verbal response that repeats what a person has said or describes what he appears to be feeling.

Relationship: An interaction of individuals over a period of time.

Semantics: The study of the meaning of words.

Social Interaction: The reciprocal action or behavior of persons which results from their influence on each other.

Symbol: A sign that represents an idea or concept.

Touch: The tactile sense.

Verbal Communication: An exchange of information using words.

INTRODUCTION

Nursing is concerned with assisting or facilitating another person to function at his highest potential. The nurse provides assistance to another individual within the helping relationship. Communication skills are the vehicle the nurse uses to provide the assistance. This chapter will discuss the helping relationship and the nurse's use of communication skills within this context.

NEED GRATIFICATION OF THE HUMAN ORGANISM

Maslow's theory of the human organism's hierarchy of needs is important for an understanding of the helping relationship because the gratification of certain needs has been observed when effective relationships exist. The word *hierarchy* is defined as a process or system that places things or persons in a graded order or rank. A *hierarchy of needs* is the placement of requirements or necessities for human functioning in order of importance. The following discussion will illustrate.

When a particular physiological need in the hierarchy of human needs is being met with a relative degree of satisfaction, other less important needs take precedence. Thus, when an individual is extremely thirsty, he makes every effort possible to satisfy the need for fluid which is high in the hierarchy of physiological needs. Once his thirst has been satisfied, he becomes occupied with some other need. The need may be physiological, as for food, or, if this has been satisfied, a psychosocial need, as for love and affection, may emerge.

Psychosocial needs may also wholly dominate behavior as an individual seeks to meet them. The person whose life is in danger will use every ounce of ingenuity and strength to satisfy the need for survival, for example, when confronted by a person wielding a gun, by a blazing fire, or by a raging body of water. Until the immediate need for survival and safety has been met, physiological needs or lesser ranking psychosocial needs will play little part in what he does.

Psychologists and sociologists have described the psychosocial needs of the human organism in much of their literature. While there are some differences of opinion among them, these are some common phrases which Maslow uses to describe basic psychosocial needs: the need for security and survival; the need for belongingness, love, and affection; the need for self-respect and self-esteem; the need for self-fulfillment and self-actualization; the need to know and understand; and the need for aesthetics. When these needs are thwarted, humans tend to feel lonely, friendless, and rejected. They experience feelings of fear, weakness, and inferiority; they often feel dejected, anxious, and depressed. The gratification of these and other human needs often involves assistance provided by another person.

THE HELPING RELATIONSHIP

A *relationship* may be defined as an interaction of individuals over a period of time. A *helping relationship* is an interaction which sets the climate for movement of the participants toward common goals. The goals have arisen out of human needs. Therefore, need gratification occurs as the result of a successful helping relationship. A helping relationship exists among many persons who provide and receive assistance in meeting human needs.

When a nurse and patient are involved in a helping relationship, the nurse assists the patient to achieve goals that allow his human needs to be satisfied. In other words, the nurse is the helper, and the patient is the person being helped. The helping relationship between the nurse and patient is sometimes called the nurse-patient or the nurse-client relationship.

The goals of a helping relationship between a nurse and a patient are determined cooperatively and defined in terms of the patient's needs. Broadly speaking, common goals might include increased independence for the person, greater feelings of worth, and improved physical well-being. Depending on the goal, the nurse selects nursing care activities that will move the person toward the goal. As the patient's needs and goals change, so do the nursing care activities.

It is acknowledged that the nurse also has human needs which must be met. However, the helping relationship between the nurse and the patient is focused on the patient's needs.

The helping relationship is intangible, and therefore, difficult to describe, but most authorities agree that it has the following characteristics. It is dynamic. Both the person providing the assistance and the person being helped are active participants, to the extent that each is able. It is purposeful and time-limited. This means that there are specific goals which are intended to be accomplished within a certain amount of time.

Within the helping relationship, the person providing the assistance assumes the dominant role. The helping person must also assume responsibility for presenting himself and his helping abilities as honestly as possible. He should not convey the idea that he can provide more assistance than he is capable of offering.

The difference between a helping relationship and a friendship must be emphasized. Needs of both participants are generally considered in a friendship. In the helping relationship, only the needs of the person receiving the help are of concern. A friendship may grow out of a helping relationship, but this is separate from the purposeful, time-limited interaction described as a helping relationship.

Carl R. Rogers, an eminent psychotherapist, has described the helping relationship. Rogers has pointed out several factors he has found important after years of service to people who have come to him for help.

First, the person offering the help must be knowledgeable about himself. The practitioner must be aware of his own needs, feelings, and sentiments. An understanding of self, Rogers believes, makes one a genuine person, and the patient perceives such a person as dependable and real, characteristics necessary in establishing a helping relationship.

Second, the relationship between practitioner and patient is characterized by feelings of acceptance and a warm attitude. The patient and practitioner must feel a mutual respect and trust.

Third, it is important that the patient be allowed to be free to explore himself without fear of being judged. The relationship will usually deteriorate when the practitioner sits in judgment or places himself as the authority with all of the right answers.

Fourth, Rogers believes that a good helping relationship provides a climate in which the patient can develop motivation to change, to grow, to mature, and to cope with his problems in a more satisfactory manner. It is a climate in which the patient's strengths are used to capitalize on his inner resources.

The reader is referred to the book in the references at the end of this unit in which Rogers discusses the helping relationship.

The helping relationship is ordinarily described as having three phases: the orientation phase, the working phase, and the termination phase. A discussion of each follows. Ideally, the helping relationship between the patient and the nurse is initiated when the nurse starts the data-gathering part of the nursing process. However, it can also be initiated at other times.

ORIENTATION PHASE OF THE HELPING RELATIONSHIP

In the orientation phase, the tone and guidelines for the relationship are established. The nurse and patient meet and learn to identify each other by name. It is especially important that the nurse introduce herself to the patient. It may even be helpful for her to write her name for him. Failure to do so may result in the patient becoming confused and mistrustful because of the number of health agency personnel with whom most patients come in contact.

Following the introductions, the roles of both persons in the relationship are clarified. It has been observed that a successful relationship is more likely to occur when there is a known and accepted division of labor among participants and when there is leadership present. In the nurse-patient relationship, the roles of the nurse and the patient constitute a division of labor, and the nurse, by virtue of her role, generally assumes leadership. Consider the situation in which a misunderstanding concerning roles occurred due to poor cooperative planning between a hospitalized patient and nurse. A nurse who was otherwise competent failed to convey to the patient the importance of initiating self-care. As a result, the patient felt that the nurse was refusing to assume her proper role of leadership and administer his personal care without his assistance. He appeared dejected and commented: "The nurse doesn't like me and won't give me the care I need."

Leadership does not mean control in the restrictive or manipulative sense. The importance of including the patient in planning his care has been discussed several times in this text. When cooperative planning occurs with consideration of patient needs, a labor division between nurse and patient is more likely to be mutually satisfactory. Leadership here implies taking the initiative in enlisting the patient's point of view.

After the roles of the nurse and patient are clarified, an agreement or contract about the relationship is established. The agreement is usually a simple verbal exchange. Or, occasionally it may be a written document, especially if the relationship extends over a long period. Elements in the agreement include the goals of the relationship, location, frequency, and length of the contacts, and the duration of the relationship. Depending on the purpose of the relationship, the agreement may also include the way in which personal information which the patient may divulge will be handled.

During the orientation phase, it may also be part of

the nurse's responsibility to orient the patient to the health agency, its facilities, admission routines, and the like. If so, she identifies this as one of the goals of the particular contact.

Specific routines and policies vary among agencies. The nurse needs to familiarize herself with those of the agency in which she gives care. Regardless of the particular details which may be included in the health agency orientation, the nurse's concern for the psychological and physiological comfort of the patient should be paramount. Seeking care from a health agency is a frightening experience for many persons. Assisting the patient to feel familiar and at ease in the setting can be an important prelude to assisting him to function at his highest potential.

WORKING PHASE OF THE HELPING RELATIONSHIP

The working phase occurs when concerted effort is exerted by both participants to achieve their common goal. Interaction is the essence of this phase.

Social interaction is a reciprocal form of behavior. It is action by one person that produces action in another, and so on. In other words, behavioral activity of one person stimulates behavioral activity in another.

Why should we be interested in the psychosocial aspects of the nurse–patient relationship? One social scientist stated it well: "The nurse's traditional patient care role includes motivating the patient to care for himself, and cooperating with those aiding him toward a cure. Motivation is psychological, and it is through social interaction with the patient that the nurse can affect the patient's motivation."*

Study of social interaction is concerned with a variety of factors, two of which are of special concern to this discussion of the working phase of the helping relationship: the functional factor, sometimes called the utilitarian or instrumental factor, and the expressive factor.

The *functional factor* refers to direct action that is taken to move people toward a goal. Two examples will illustrate. An elderly patient has a poor appetite and the goal is for him to increase his food intake. The nurse discusses the idea of small, more frequent meals with the patient. With the patient's approval, the nurse

makes the necessary arrangements. A mother explains to a school nurse that she cannot afford dental care recommended for her child although she would like to have the work done. The nurse asks if a referral to a social agency for financial assistance would be acceptable. With the mother's permission, the nurse contacts the agency. Arranging for the patient's meals and contacting the social agency are direct actions or functional factors.

The *expressive factor* refers to an emotional state. An emotional state may be described by many words—feelings, drives, attitudes, sentiments, and so on. The words sentiments and feelings will be used here. When sentiments and feelings between persons are unsatisfactory, they often cannot work cooperatively toward achieving a common goal. When sentiments and feelings are satisfactory, the persons can usually work together. In the examples in the preceding paragraph, satisfactory sentiments and feelings between the nurse and patients might have been the key aspects. The person's relationship with the nurse may have allowed the elderly individual to respond positively to the small, more frequent meals without feeling as though he was being treated as a child. The mother's feelings about the nurse may have allowed her to accept financial assistance for the dental care without feeling degraded. Satisfactory interaction preserves the integrity of individuals while promoting an atmosphere characterized by minimum fear, anxiety, distrust, and tension. Persons feel harmonious and contented with each other as they work cooperatively to reach common goals.

The functional and expressive aspects of social interaction must both be present. In a successful helping relationship, they function harmoniously and interdependently as the nurse and patient work toward their common goals. For example, the teaching program the nurse designs may have flawless organization, content, and teaching methods and it may be acceptable to the patient; that is, the functional element is satisfactory. However, unless the relationship is one in which the participants feel good and which is characterized by warmth, understanding, and acceptance of each other, teaching may fail because of lack of concern for the expressive factor in the interaction.

Behavioral scientists have observed that when a relationship is satisfactory, social interactions of a similar nature tend to be repeated and continued. When a helping relationship is unsatisfactory, further social interactions tend to be avoided. For instance, a patient

---

* "Social and Psychological Aspects of the Nurse's Role—Introduction." In Skipper, James K. Jr. and Leonard, Robert C., editors. *Social Interaction and Patient Care.* J. B. Lippincott Company, Philadelphia, 1965, p. 3.

began to break clinic appointments. He had not appeared to lack interest in his health when he began visiting the clinic. When a community health nurse called on the patient at home, he said, "The nurse at the clinic seems too busy; she just doesn't seem to care if I come or go. I don't like to go to that clinic." The lack of satisfactory interaction between the nurse and the patient discouraged him from continuing the relationship, even at the expense of his health. Had the interaction been satisfactory, breaking appointments probably would not have been a problem.

The emotional tone in interaction usually is heightened when a crisis occurs. Sentiments often become very intense between health practitioners and patients when patients are faced with urgent situations. When the interaction is positive during crises, the resultant feelings can serve as great assists in the helping relationship after a crisis subsides. It is easy to forget the importance of the expressive factor in social interaction in a crisis when the functional factor may necessarily take precedence. But even in a crisis, the expressive factor in interaction remains important. Consider a surgical patient.

Most patients view surgery as a crisis. There are many technical tasks involved in preparing a patient for surgery, and it is important that they be done correctly; for example, forgetting to remove a patient's dentures could result in serious respiratory complications. However, if during preparation for surgery the nurse neglects the expressive factor in her relationship with the patient, she may allow the patient's fears and anxieties to become intensified and diminishes the chances for cooperative postoperative relationships.

People are not void of sentiments as they enter social interactions. In the helping relationship, both the nurse and the patient bring their sentiments from past experiences to the new relationship. They will be reflected in the new relationship and play a role in the behavior of the participants also.

In summary, the successful working phase of the helping relationship results in gratification of some of the patient's human needs. The nurse and patient work cooperatively toward common goals and the sentiments of both are positive. The patient *feels* better as a result of interactions with the nurse and his improved feelings can often be discerned by observing his behavior. Inflections in the tone of voice, the manner in which he holds his head, the stride of his walk, the movements of his hands, the glimmerings of hope in his eyes, or a smile are examples.

TERMINATION PHASE OF THE HELPING RELATIONSHIP

The termination phase occurs when the conclusion of the initial agreement is acknowledged. This may happen at change-of-shift time, when the patient is discharged, when a nurse leaves on vacation, or when she departs an agency for employment elsewhere. The patient and nurse examine the goals of the helping relationship for indications of their attainment or for evidence of progress toward the goals. If the goals have been reached, this fact should be acknowledged. Such acknowledgment generally results in a feeling of satisfaction for both the patient and nurse. If the goals have not been reached, the progress can be acknowledged and either the patient or the nurse may make suggestions for future efforts.

There ordinarily are feelings associated with the termination of a helping relationship. If the goals have been met, there is often regret about the ending of a satisfying relationship, even though a sense of accomplishment persists. If the goals have not been completely achieved, the patient may experience anxiety and fear about the future. Whatever his feelings, the patient should be encouraged to express his emotions about the termination.

There are various ways of preparing for the termination of the helping relationship. The thoughtful nurse can set the stage for the patient to establish a helping relationship with another nurse, if this is appropriate. The nurse can assist the patient transferring from one agency to another or from one unit in an agency to another by offering explanations concerning the transfer. In some instances, the nurse may introduce the patient to personnel about to care for him. Termination has been planned for when a teaching program has been used effectively. For instance, the new mother will be less fearful of going home when nursing personnel have taught her how to care for herself and for her newborn baby. The patient will usually feel a sense of effectiveness and competency when he has been included in planning a program of rehabilitation that readies him for adjustments required in his activities of daily living. This is especially true of patients with chronic diseases and permanent physical handicaps.

Occasionally, termination of the helping relationship for some persons produces emotional reactions. The person may feel angry; he may feel rejected by the nurse; he may deny that a relationship ever really existed; he may feel depressed and helpless. Should such reactions occur, the nurse should help and support the person rather than make him feel guilty or wrong for having these views. However, emotional reactions of this sort are less likely to occur if the person has been involved with establishing goals and has been helped to anticipate termination of the helping relationship.

Table 6–1 summarizes the behaviors of patients during the three phases of an effective helping relationship. The relationship sets the climate for more effective functioning of the patient. Communication skills are the tools the nurse uses within the helping relationship. The remainder of this chapter will discuss communication skills.

COMMUNICATION AS A VEHICLE FOR THE HELPING RELATIONSHIP

The exchange of information in communication occurs through hearing, seeing, tasting, smelling, and touching. Everything one does or uses has communicative value—one's work, the house one lives in, the food one eats, the clothes one wears. All that impinges on our senses—a glance, a wink of the eye, a touch, the spoken word, a gesture, the fragrance of one's cologne—communicates something. In other words, we communicate in a variety of ways through talking, signaling, writing, gesturing, drawing, singing, and dancing.

The process of communication begins when one person begins a relationship with another. Unless people communicate, no sort of relationship develops between them. Communication is the means for a relationship between persons. The example of two strangers sitting next to each other in a theater demonstrates physical closeness without any type of relationship necessarily developing between them. However, if during the movie these two people exchange words or glances, that is, communicate, a relationship comes into existence. Whether the communication is verbal (one makes a comment to the other) or nonverbal (one frowns at the other for eating popcorn loudly), hostile or friendly does not matter, a human relationship is there. Hence, communication is behavior. It involves both physical and mental activity and provides for an exchange of ideas, attitudes, thoughts, and feelings.

Communication is the vehicle by which a nurse learns to know a patient as a person, to determine his needs, and to work with him in meeting those needs. It can be seen that communication is not an end in itself. Rather, it is the means to attain the goals of the helping relationship. The requirement for communication is continuous since patient needs change as one need is met and other needs emerge. Consider the nursing care designed for a pregnant woman. Her care while she is in the prenatal period is quite different from that during labor and delivery. Her needs, and hence, her nursing care, change again during the postpartum period. Continuous communication is the means to attain the constant goal of assisting a woman to attain and maintain optimum physical and psychological functioning during three very distinct and different periods in her life. Without adequate communication, her health care may be ineffective.

TABLE 6–1 Summary of typical patient behaviors during the three phases of an effective helping relationship

ORIENTATION PHASE	WORKING PHASE	TERMINATING PHASE

1. The patient will call the nurse by name.
2. The patient will accurately describe the roles of the participants in the relationship.
3. The patient and nurse will establish an agreement about:
  a) Goals of the relationship.
  b) Location, frequency, and length of the contacts.
  c) The duration of the relationship.
	1. The patient will actively participate in the relationship.
	2. The patient will respond positively to both functional and expressive factors of the nurse's behavior.
		1. The patient will participate in identifying the goals accomplished, or the progress made toward goals.
		2. The patient will verbalize his feelings about the termination of the relationship.

ESSENTIAL REQUIREMENTS FOR COMMUNICATION TO OCCUR

If communication is to occur, there must be a message delivered from one person to another. A gesture indicating where a visitor to a hospital may find a particular patient may not be seen. A letter may be lost in the mail. A child playing too far from home may not hear his mother's call. These illustrations demonstrate a breakdown in communication: a message was sent but not delivered to the intended receiver.

If one mumbles while talking, speaks too softly or too rapidly, if there are noises in the room, if the intended receiver is not listening, and so on, what has been said may not be heard. Sometimes, patients have been reprimanded because they failed to follow instructions for taking medications at home when they probably did not clearly hear the instructions. For many people, especially the very ill or the elderly, it may be necessary to ask, "Did you hear me?" or "Was that clear?"

If communication is to occur, when a message is sent, it must get the attention of the receiver. A letter that has arrived at its destination must be read. Commercials on television and radio often are sent at a higher decibel level than the programs they interrupt. This technique is intended to catch the attention of the audience. The patient's call light is a signal for a nurse, but the communication fails if the light does not catch the nurse's attention. Preoccupation with other thoughts may divert attention. Thus, a patient may be so afraid of giving himself injections that his attention is diverted when the nurse attempts to teach him the procedure. Without an attentive receiver, effective communication is not possible.

The sending and receiving of messages usually cannot be separated distinctly, since both often go on simultaneously. For example, assume that a nurse is talking with an individual who is describing his headache. While the person talks, the nurse listens and receives the message. But at the same time, she may be sending messages to the person by the expression on her face and her actions as he speaks, such as drumming her fingers impatiently. The patient and the nurse both receive messages while transmitting them. Stop for a moment and consider any conversation with another person. One soon realizes that the exchange of messages is constant and simultaneous. Hence, communication is a reciprocal process, and an experience in which both the sender and the receiver of messages participate simultaneously.

If communication is to occur, once a message has been sent and received, it must be interpreted. Interpretation by the receiver is based on his past experience. If the sender and receiver have had different experiences in terms of the message being sent, a breakdown in communication can result. The sign language of the deaf cannot be interpreted by one inexperienced in this form of communication. A person listening to a message spoken in a language unfamiliar to him cannot interpret the sender's message. Pain means one thing to a person who has suffered a great deal, but it may mean something quite different to one who has experienced little. The grief of death may have relatively little meaning to a person who has not experienced the loss of a loved one.

Consider many of the adjectives used commonly in everyday conversations. What is a *big* car? A *small* child? A *good* meal? A *poor* movie? An *expensive* garment? A *high* temperature? A *rapid* pulse rate? Unless the sender's and receiver's past experiences are similar in relation to the manner in which these adjectives are used, effective communication is impossible.

It is of utmost importance for the nurse to use words that the patient can understand. A nurse speaking to a patient who is to have a blood test would not be of much help if she said, "You are fasting this A.M., since you'll have a VP for a BUN." She is more likely to convey a clearer message to the patient if she tells him that his breakfast will be delayed until after a blood sample has been taken, that the doctor wishes a study of his blood and that taking food may alter the blood findings. Often nurses tend to forget that most patients are not familiar with medical and nursing jargon.

If communication is to occur, the message must be stated in words having a common meaning to the sender and the receiver. The study of the meaning of words is called *semantics.* To persons speaking the same language, identical words may have entirely different meanings. For example, the word "democracy" means one thing to most people in the Western world but something quite different in the Eastern world, even when a common language is being used. Communication using such words as liberty, freedom, fraternity, love, and hate will fail unless the sender and receiver attach common meanings to these words. A 45-year-old will be lost in a conversation with a teenager unless he knows current teenage jargon.

VERBAL AND NONVERBAL COMMUNICATIONS

Communications can be either verbal or nonverbal. *Verbal communication* uses the spoken word. Technically, reading and writing may be considered forms of verbal communication but this chapter will consider the spoken word.

Verbal communication depends upon language. *Language* is a prescribed way of using words so that people can share information effectively. Language includes a common definition of words being used, as well as a method of arranging words in a certain order to convey the message. The development of language represented a great step forward in the history of communication, for it enabled everyone using the same language to share information more readily.

Nonverbal communication is the exchange of messages without the use of words. It is what is *not* said. Individuals communicate through the use of facial expressions, as illustrated in Figure 6–1, body movements, tone of voice, gait, and so on. Crying and moaning are oral, but not verbal, communications.

Nonverbal communication is more likely to be in-

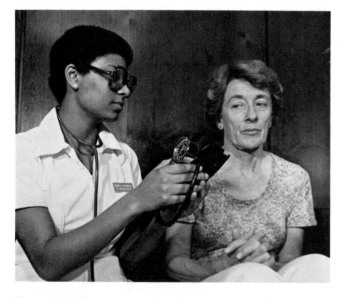

Figure 6–1   The nurse must be alert to the nonverbal, as well as the verbal, communication of the patient. This patient's facial expression and posture seem to be sending a message that she is anxious. Is she unfamiliar with the equipment and technique for determining blood pressure? Is she worried about the level of her blood pressure? Or, is she fearful for some other reason? The nurse needs to receive the message, interpret it, and validate her interpretation before she can determine what action may alleviate the patient's anxiety.

voluntary, and therefore, less under the control of the person conveying the message than is verbal communication. Hence, nonverbal communication is generally considered as being a more nearly accurate expression of true feelings. How many times have we asked or been asked, "What's wrong?", when obvious appearance and behavior showed that all was not well. The great pantomimist Marcel Marceau and many of the stars of silent motion pictures illustrate in their performances that the power of the body in action and facial expressions can carry innumerable messages in very dramatic ways.

Nonverbal communication occurs concurrently with verbal communication. There is a proverb that goes: "What you do speaks so loud I cannot hear what you say." For instance, the words "hello" and "good-bye" can be said in ways that imply another's presence in either the best or the worst thing that could have happened.

As another example, a patient may joke about his preoperative tests and be casual about his impending surgery, but his expressions do not fool the observant nurse who notes that he is in and out of bed, is unable to sit and read, makes frequent trips to the telephone booth, and gets out of the corridor whenever he sees a stretcher coming along.

There are several forms of nonverbal communication that are sometimes used in nursing. A *symbol* is a sign that represents an idea or concept. The national flag of a country is a well-known symbol. The symbol ♀ means female while the symbol ♂ means male. Doodlings have been demonstrated to have communicative value with some patients.

Signals can carry information. Most hospitals use a light as a signal when the patient wishes a nurse. Most health agencies have a fire alarm system, such as a siren or bell, to alert everyone to the danger of fire.

The messages of communication cannot always be assumed to mean what the receiver, upon first glance, believes them to mean. True meanings may be camouflaged. A person may say he is ill and wishes to leave a meeting; he may simply be bored but uses illness as an excuse to leave. A child may say he does not wish to eat because he has no appetite; the real meaning of his behavior may be that he is seeking attention. In other words, things may not always be what they appear to be.

Validation is important in order that true feelings and meanings can be discerned. Validation is a two-way street. The nurse will wish to validate what she believes the patient is communicating to her as well as validate that the patient is receiving accurate messages from her.

TOUCH AS A MEANS OF COMMUNICATION

Touch, the tactile sense, has been studied seriously as a form of nonverbal communication only within the last three decades or so. Anthropologists have been largely responsible for sparking interest in the sense of touch after learning that it has played and continues to play an important role in various cultures. Their investigations have further shown that tactile experiences are largely shaped by familial, regional, class, and cultural influences. Such factors as age and sex also play a role in developing meanings that are associated with touch. These influences individualize the meaning of touch. In other words, touch expresses very personal behavior and it means different things to different people. Two men embracing upon meeting is usual behavior in some cultures; in others, shaking hands is more common. Tactile experiences between people of different sexes can have different meanings from tactile experiences between people of the same sex.

Touch can be used to carry a variety of messages: comfort, love, affection, security, anger, frustration, aggression, excitement, any number of emotional reactions. Figure 6–2 illustrates touch in a nursing situation.

As stated earlier, authorities agree that nonverbal communication is more expressive in conveying the quality and intent of attitudes and feelings than is verbal communication, and touch is one of the most effective nonverbal ways of expressing them. Consider the youngster who defies his parent's verbal admonition and facial expressions to prepare for bed. The message may not be completely grasped until the parent's hand firmly touches his shoulder and steers the youngster to the stairway.

Because of its personal nature, assigning meanings to touch can be complicated and should be done with caution. According to investigations, there can well be differences in interpreting the meaning of touch as much as 50 percent of the time. A patient gloomily told a nurse that his children no longer cared for him because they had not visited him for several weeks. The nurse wished to express comfort and understanding when she patted the patient softly on his shoulder. The patient may have assumed the nurse's gesture meant that she did not consider his complaint to be significant. Anxiety may result when a patient does not

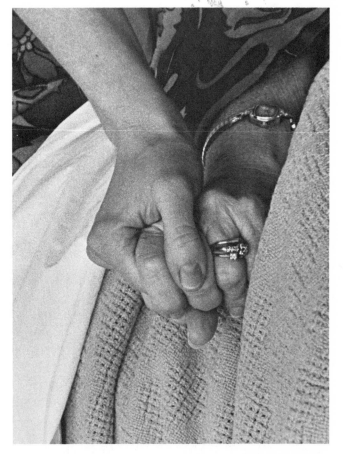

Figure 6–2 A reassuring hand clasp uses touch to convey a message. Sometimes touch can be a more effective way of expressing concern and interest than verbal communication.

know or understand the meaning of a tactile gesture or when he simply dislikes being touched. It must be remembered that specific tactile gestures do not have universal meanings, and hence, the use of touch requires care and forethought.

Touch is more highly developed at birth than any of the other sense organs. According to research, tactile experiences of infants and young children appear essential for the normal development of the self and awareness of others. Many nurses and mothers have been reconsidering and changing child care that minimized body contact and touch. Note the emergence in the popularity of the rocking chair in hospital pediatric units and in many homes.

Physical closeness between patient and nurse is an essential of nursing. There is much use of hands and touching patients when nursing care is given. For example, the nurse who firmly holds the hand of a patient who is anxious and fearful may help to convey understanding and willingness to help. She has transmitted feelings of interest and concern. Dexterity and sureness in the use of her hands may help the nurse to assure a patient of the nurse's expertise, as when administering an injection, palpating the abdomen, assisting a patient to walk, or giving the patient a bath. One patient remarked that a nurse's hands gave love when the nurse rubbed her back. By holding a crying child securely in her arms, the nurse offers the child security and affection. Numerous other illustrations might be given. However, these few help to show that when nursing intervention includes the judicious use of touch, it can be an important means of communicating in the helping relationship.

PRINCIPLES OF COMMUNICATION

Psychological well-being requires that individuals have an adequate means for communicating with others. Human beings are social creatures as well as biological organisms. Psychologists and sociologists have demonstrated that social interactions among people are required to fulfill some of their most elemental psychosocial needs, such as love, affection, recognition, and desirability. Communication is basic to human relationships and nursing care is dependent on helping relationships. Without communication, an individual is in isolation. Without it, nursing intervention to meet patients' needs is generally less effective.

Communication is influenced by the patient's age, mental and physical capabilities, socioeconomic class, culture, interests, and other variables. No one approach will fit all patients. Communicating with a hospitalized patient about the importance of nourishment is quite different from communicating with a well person in her home concerning a nourishing diet for her family. The use of certain slang expressions may be acceptable when communicating with an adolescent but quite unacceptable when communicating with a middle-aged executive.

The following description illustrates certain mannerisms having a cultural basis. A communication problem resulted when the nurse failed to understand these mannerisms.

A community health nurse visited a mother and her newborn in the hogan of a Navajo Indian family. The purpose of the nurse's visit was to check on the baby's progress and to make plans for treatment of a minor birth defect. The baby appeared well cared for and the mother indicated concern about his welfare. However, the nurse noted that as she described the preparation for the baby's surgery, the mother continually looked down or away from the nurse. At the conclusion of the discussion, the mother thanked the nurse for the visit but still never looked directly at the nurse.

When the nurse returned to her office, she discussed the visit with her supervisor. She told the supervisor that the mother was polite and considerate but she ". . . never once looked me in the eye and acted as though she didn't hear a word I said." The supervisor, familiar with the Navajo culture, explained that looking another person in the eye is considered rude and disrespectful by many American Indians. They believe that to gaze into another person's eyes is to see into his soul, and this act is a significant invasion of privacy. With this additional understanding of the mother's culture and mannerisms, the nurse returned to the home a week later. The mother had followed the instructions for preparation of the baby. She had indeed heard and understood all the nurse had said.

Silences are a meaningful part of communication. Silence has many meanings. The patient may be rejecting the nurse and refusal to speak may be defiant and mean, "I have nothing to say to you!" It may be that the patient is exploring his feelings, and speaking at that time may disrupt his thoughts. Silence can be used as a retreat, and hence, as an escape from a threat. The person who refuses to discuss a fear may be using silence to avoid an unpleasant emotion. Silence may be a sign of comfort to close friends, or a husband and wife may observe silence and yet be communicating many things. Silence may be discussed in due time with the individual, especially if the nurse wishes to validate her speculation on its meaning.

Fear of silence sometimes leads to too much talking by the nurse. Whatever the cause of silence, too much talking may mean that the person's problems cannot be identified and explored. Also, excessive talking usually places the focus on the nurse, rather than on the patient where it should be. A verse in the third chapter of the Book of Ecclesiastes in the Bible states this idea well: There ". . . is a time for every matter under heaven: . . . a time to keep silence, and a time to speak; . . ."

Listening is an essential part of communication. Listening is an active process involving hearing and interpretation of what is being said. It requires attention and concentration in order to sort out, evaluate, and validate clues that are the aids to understanding real meanings in what the person is saying. It requires forgetting about oneself and thinking of the speaker.

Listening selectively, or hearing only what one wants to hear, limits communication. All of us, including patients and nurses, are guilty at times of hearing only what each wants to hear. No one likes to hear bad news; no one wants to hear that he must give up some of the pleasures of life; nor do we want to hear that there are difficult times ahead.

Pretending to listen and responding impulsively when someone is speaking are barriers to communication. It is a rare speaker who is insensitive to an attitude of apathy, boredom, lack of interest, or feigned attention on the part of a listener.

Observation is an essential part of communication. Observation is an active process involving seeing and interpreting. It is an especially useful validating tool. For example, a nurse suspected that a patient was afraid to hear the results of certain blood tests he had had, but the patient kept saying that the tests were not important. However, the nurse observed the patient pacing back and forth in the corridor while appearing to be in deep thought. Observing the patient's behavior helped validate the nurse's clue that the patient was possibly fearful and his asserting that he was not appeared to be a cover-up for his true feelings.

Information essential to understanding a person and his problems can best be obtained when communication has a purpose and when it focuses on the individual. To illustrate, if a nurse realizes that knowing something about a patient's usual daily activities will aid her in planning his care, she plans her communications with the patient accordingly.

Social conversations are useful as a display of friendliness and politeness, but generally of limited value in understanding the patient.

A common pitfall is to focus communication on an activity of the nurse rather than on the patient. A nurse missed an important clue concerning the patient's feelings in this conversation:

PATIENT: I don't know why these injections scare me but they do.

NURSE: Let's hurry and get this shot done. Then you won't have time to worry.

Had the nurse posed this question, "You are afraid of these injections?", after the patient made the remark, she would have been focusing on the patient rather than on the procedure.

While being attentive to the patient, the nurse will wish to keep her own feelings to herself. Also, questions that tend to make the patient feel his answers must fit the nurse's expectations are of little value in attempting to understand the patient.

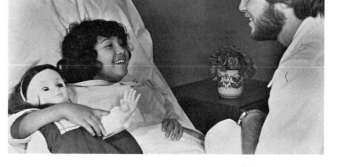

Figure 6–3 This nurse and young patient seem to be sharing an enjoyable moment. The nurse has apparently established rapport with the child and they share a mutual trust.

The above principle can be further elaborated by adding that effective nurse-patient communications depend on attitudes of sincere interest in and concern for the patient. Patients are quick to ascertain when personnel are going through the motions of appearing to care. Failure to listen is failure to be concerned. The attribute of *caring* in nursing has been discussed earlier in this text. This feeling of caring and concern arises out of a mutual trust and is sometimes called *rapport*. Note the rapport that appears to be present in Figure 6–3. It is an essential in promoting effective nurse-patient communications.

Still another elaboration of the above principle is that effective communication is promoted when the nurse remains nonjudgmental. Patients tend to feel safe when they are allowed to express their feelings without being judged and condemned. A patient was heard to say, "I think I have a right to be afraid of this operation." The nurse would be nonjudgmental and respect that right by responding to the comment by saying, "Tell me what you think has made you afraid."

Consider the nurse who noted that a young woman was crying. The nurse's comment was, "You aren't acting very grown-up. How do you think your husband would feel if he saw you crying like that?" The nurse judged the patient as being immature, and the hostility she seemed to be displaying could end effective communication.

A variety of techniques have been observed to promote effective communication. The following discussion will describe some of these techniques.

A comfortable environment promotes effective

communication. This is one in which both the patient and the nurse are at ease. Such items as suitable furniture, proper lighting, and moderate temperature are important. Also, effective relationships are enhanced when the atmosphere is relaxed and unhurried. If the nurse seems preoccupied and "on the run," or if the patient is ill at ease for fear of missing visitors or because he has another commitment, communications are impaired. When possible the nurse will wish to sit down while speaking with the patient and in a place so that she and the patient can see and hear each other without strain.

Providing for privacy is important. It may not always be possible to carry on conversations with just the patient and the nurse in a room. However, every effort should be made to provide sufficient privacy so that conversations cannot be overheard by others.

Any distracting influence is likely to interfere, such as preoccupation with personal matters, extremes of emotions, intrusions, and so on. Also, as stated earlier in this chapter, communication depends on a common understanding of the words and symbols that are being used in the communication process.

Cliché-type statements generally are to be avoided. A *cliché* is a stereotyped, trite, or pat answer. Most of them tend to indicate no cause for anxiety or concern or lack of interest in what has been said. Typical clichés are "Everything will be all right"; "Don't worry, you will be all right"; or "Your doctor knows best." Cliché-type statements fail to respond to what the patient is trying to say and, hence, tend to block communication. While often they are used to reassure a patient, they have little or no effect on doing so.

In certain instances, clichés can serve a purpose. Occasionally they may be used to break the ice when conversation begins. However, even then they lose their effectiveness unless the patient feels the nurse is really interested. For example, one of the most common clichés is "How do you feel?" If the person has any reason to suspect that the nurse is not sincerely interested in how he feels, effective communication is difficult.

Questions that can be answered by simply saying "yes" or "no" and questions containing the words, "why" and "how" generally elicit little information. Questions that can be answered by "yes" or "no" tend to cut off further information, even when the individual might well wish to go on. The question, "Did you have a good day?", almost begs for a noncommital sort of answer which tells the listener very little.

Questions using "why" and "how" tend to intimi-

date the patient. The question, "Why were you not tired enough to sleep?", might better be stated by asking, "What were you doing while you were unable to sleep?"

A comment that repeats what a person has said or describes what he appears to be feeling tends to encourage him to talk and describe more. A comment of this nature is called a *reflective comment*. It is one of the most common communication tools. The following are reflective comments:

PATIENT: I surely wish I knew why I feel so blue today.
NURSE: You are saying that you feel blue . . .

or

PATIENT: My children certainly have been pests lately.
NURSE: Your children are annoying you?

Obviously the use of the reflective comment can be overdone. If the patient concludes that the nurse is employing a technique mechanistically, communication will end.

Broad openings or general leads often help to encourage persons to go on. Comments of this nature are called *open-ended comments*. They often serve as the bridge to continued conversations. Such comments as "And after that . . ."; "And then?"; "You were saying . . ."; or sometimes a nod of the head while saying "Yes . . ."; "Uh-huh"; or "Oh . . ." effectively encourages further conversation.

Comments that help to place events into meaningful sequences or to demonstrate cause-and-effect relationships aid in promoting helpful communications. The question, "When did you start feeling bad?" helps to put events into chronological order. The question, "You started feeling bad yesterday after you forgot to take your medicine?" may determine a possible cause-and-effect relationship.

Questions that appear to probe for information tend to cut off communication. Patients who are made to feel as though they are receiving the "third degree" become resentful and will usually clam up and try to avoid further communication. Although the nurse may feel she needs more information, it is better to follow the patient's lead. Letting him take the initiative allows him to delve more deeply at a time when he is ready. The person who says, "Let's get to the bottom of this," is likely to destroy conversation unless the patient feels like facing the real cause of a problem.

Comments that indicate that the nurse might not have understood tend to encourage clarification for both the nurse and the patient. Interrupting the patient may be necessary but should be done with care in order to avoid breaking a train of thought. Also, interrupting should be done politely in order not to offend the speaker. However when opportune moments arrive in the conversation, interrupting for clarification is important, for failure to explore may result in failure to understand. Comments asking for clarification include "I don't follow you"; "About whom are you speaking?"; and "Are you saying that listening to music takes your mind off things?"

Listening and observing for themes in nonverbal and verbal communications aid in understanding the speaker. Following are suggested questions the nurse will wish to keep in mind when communicating with patients. What are the repeated themes in the person's speech and behavior? What topics does the individual tend to avoid? What subjects tend to make the individual shift the conversation to other topics? What inconsistencies and gaps appear in the person's conversation? Answers to these questions are useful tools in understanding the patient and in determining his problems.

THE INTERVIEW

An interview was defined in Chapter 4 as a purposeful conversation. It is generally conducted for the purpose of collecting information and can be either formal or relatively informal. An interview may be considered as a special type of communication.

When the nurse is interviewing a person, it is especially important that she identify herself and indicate the purpose of the interview. Many persons have never been interviewed by a nurse and tend to become both confused and reluctant when they do not know the intent of the interview. If the nurse takes the time to explain how the information collected will be used to identify and to meet the individual's nursing needs, most persons will participate readily.

The confidentiality with which the information will be treated should be established. The nurse indicates to whom the information collected in the interview will be available. The person should know he has the right to specify the individuals who have access to the information. Failure to take this factor into account can be considered a breech of the person's right to privacy.

Conducting an effective interview incorporates principles of communication and techniques described earlier in this chapter. The nurse who is interviewing a person should take care to select an appropriate setting for the interview, establish rapport with the individual, use words that have a common meaning to the interviewer and interviewee, listen and observe for clues to further significant information, and validate information as necessary. In terms of the social interaction, the functional factor of a successful interview often results in gathering information essential for high-quality nursing care. The expressive factor of an effective interview strengthens the helping relationship. Figure 6–4 illustrates several principles for successful interviewing.

SPECIAL PROBLEMS OF COMMUNICATION

Nurses can expect to encounter certain communication problems during the course of their practice that will require special attention. Whatever the situation, however, the same principles of communication discussed above will apply.

Communicating with the deaf, the blind, and the mute person are examples. Writing may be used with the deaf person when gestures are insufficient, unless someone is available to interpret if the person uses sign language. The blind person requires adaptations in care when sight ordinarily is used during the communication process. It is often helpful to ask the patient or members of his family what means of communication have been found to be most effective. Nursing care for the deaf, the blind, or the mute patient will also include consideration and respect for how the patient feels about his physical limitation.

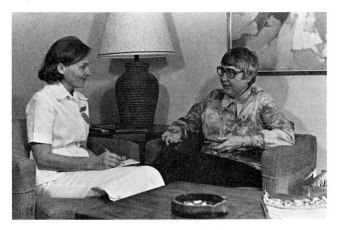

Figure 6–4 This patient's living room is apparently a comfortable environment for the nurse to conduct an interview. The patient seems to feel relaxed and at ease communicating with the nurse.

Another special problem is communicating with a person who speaks a language which is not understood by the nurse. Using an interpreter is a great assist, but, with effort, a great deal can be accomplished by using various forms of nonverbal communication. Publications with translation of common health-related terms also are available.

An interesting and helpful learning situation is to practice communicating with an associate who role-plays the patient with special communication problems. Some of the references for this chapter will offer suggestions also.

The nurse caring for a patient who is unconscious will want to remember that the patient sometimes still is able to hear and to feel touch. Communicating with the seriously ill patient will be discussed further in Chapter 26.

COMMUNICATING WITH GROUPS

Nurses communicate with groups when teaching patients with common interests or needs, such as teaching diabetics, pregnant women, school children, tuberculous patients, patients with colostomies, and so on.

Communicating with groups of people is somewhat different from communicating with just one other person. The same principles discussed earlier in this chapter apply except that instead of thinking in terms of one person, one considers a cluster of individuals having certain commonalities, such as a topic of common interest.

Individual differences among group members are to be considered, but these usually can best be handled in a one-to-one relationship after a group presentation when a particular problem arises. Using question periods after a general presentation of whatever material is set forth can help also to meet individual differences.

CONCLUSION

The helping relationship provides the climate for the nurse to assist the patient to grow to his fullest capacity. Paramount to the success of the helping relationship is the effective use of communication skills by the nurse. Effective communication assists one to learn to know another person for what he is. Communication consists of hearing as well as speaking, and especially of hearing what others want to say. There are many who feel that the true essence of nursing, and possibly its most important element, lies in the nurse's use of communication skills in the expressive role of the helping relationship.

SUPPLEMENTAL LIBRARY STUDY

1. The following article elaborates the gratification of human needs through the helping relationship by describing a patient situation:

    Walke, Mary Anne Kelly. "When a Patient Needs to Unburden His Feelings." *American Journal of Nursing,* 77:1164–1166, July 1977.

    What were the clues the nurse identified as indicating that the patient's safety needs were threatened? How did the patient demonstrate his movement to independence and self-esteem needs, after his safety needs were met? Can you identify some of the communication techniques the nurse used?

2. In Chapter 4 of the following book, the helping process is described in eight stages:

    Brammer, Lawrence M. *The Helping Relationship: Process and Skills.* Prentice-Hall, Inc., Englewood Cliffs, New Jersey, 1973, pp. 47–68.

    How do the author's eight stages relate to the three phases of the helping relationship discussed in this chapter? Can you identify overlaps? Can you identify additional ideas presented in the book?

3. The author of the following article recommends that the nurse listen for themes in her communications with patients:

    Hein, Eleanor C. "Listening." *Nursing 75,* 5:93–96, 98–102, March 1975.

    What does the author suggest as the meaning of the theme of self-effacement? of poverty? of "me"? of wellness? of loneliness? of loss? and of humor? Have you identified any of these themes in your communications with patients?

4. The following article examines the concept of touch as it relates to nonverbal communication:

    Barnett, Kathryn. "A Theoretical Construct of the Concepts of Touch As They Relate to Nursing." *Nursing Research,* 21: 102–110, March–April 1972.

    Note the proposals for future research on page 109. Recall nursing care you have given recently. Were any of these propositions supported or rejected by your observations in relation to touch?

7

BEHAVIORAL OBJECTIVES

When content in this chapter has been mastered, the student will be able to

Define terms appearing in the glossary.

Describe general religious practices of Judaism.

Describe general religious practices of Christianity.

Describe at least five practices of religious denominations which are often related to health care.

Compare and contrast typical cultural practices in the white middle-class, black, Spanish-speaking, American Indian, and Oriental cultures.

Compare and contrast the cause of illness as typically assigned by the white middle-class, black, Spanish-speaking, American Indian, and Oriental cultures.

Identify at least five examples of folk medicine practices of various cultures described in this chapter.

Describe at least ten examples of how nurses and other health practitioners can provide care which incorporates the patient's religious and cultural beliefs and practices.

Religious and Cultural Considerations in Nursing Practice

GLOSSARY

Caring Practices: The protecting and assisting activities which are related to health and performed as a part of a culture.

Culture: The beliefs, values, and behavior patterns which are common to a group and transmitted to succeeding generations.

Ethnocentrism: The preoccupation with one's own culture that leads one to judge other cultures as inferior.

Folk medicine practices: The methods and techniques of health care which are a traditional part of a culture.

Professional medicine: The methods and techniques of health care which are based on formal study and scientific research and are provided by various health disciplines.

Subculture: A group within a culture that does not hold all beliefs of the larger culture or gives them different significance.

Transcultural nursing: The comparative study of cultural beliefs and practices regarding health and their relationship to nursing.

INTRODUCTION

Religious and cultural beliefs and practices influence the lives of most persons. Often the way an individual thinks, his values, and his behavior are partially determined by his religious and cultural influences. Because of this, it is important that the nurse have an understanding of differing beliefs and practices if she is to offer consumers individualized health care.

The variations of religious and cultural beliefs and practices are numerous, and no one can possibly understand them all. However, the nurse is encouraged to become familiar with the major characteristics of at least the most common religions and cultures with which she comes in contact in her practice.

The reader is cautioned to be aware that persons with whom she comes in contact may not possess any or all of the characteristics of a particular religious faith or cultural group, even when they are members of that faith or group. Both religion and culture are subject to wide personal interpretation and practice. Stereotyping individuals according to their religious or cultural background is frequently both inaccurate and unjust. Each person is unique and must be considered separately by the nurse.

The discussion of religions and cultures in this text gives a general overview which is intended to provide a framework for understanding. The reader is encouraged to seek additional information from the extensive literature on religions and cultures which is available in most libraries. Some references which are believed to be helpful are included at the conclusion of this unit. The reader is also cautioned that even authorities in the fields of religion and culture have differing interpretations about some aspects of these subjects.

RELIGION, HEALTH, AND ILLNESS

The word *religion* has been defined in many different ways. Some scholars define it as a belief in a God or gods, others as a way of living rather than a way of believing. In a general sense, religion is perhaps best defined as man's attempt to understand his relationship with the universe about him. It provides an orderly relation between man and his surroundings. This chapter will focus on Judaism and Christianity, the most commonly practiced religions in the United States.

Religious beliefs and practices are associated with all aspects of man's life, including health and illness. Relationships with others, daily living habits, required and prohibited behaviors, and the general frame of reference for thinking about oneself and the world are some of the aspects of a person's life commonly influenced by religion.

The nurse must be aware that certain practices generally associated with health care may have religious significance for an individual. For example, many religions prescribe dietary requirements and restrictions. Acceptable birth control practices are determined by some religious faiths, as are some types of medical treatments.

It is also common for many persons to seek support from their religious faith during times of stress. This support is often vital to the acceptance of an illness, especially if the illness brings with it a prolonged period of convalescence or indicates a questionable outcome. Prayer, devotional reading, and other religious practices often do for the person spiritually what protective exercises do for the body physically.

The values derived from religious faith cannot be enumerated or evaluated easily. However, the effects attributable to faith are constantly in evidence to health workers. Persons have been known to endure extreme physical distress because of strong faith. Patients' families have taken on almost unbelievable rehabilitative tasks because they had faith in the eventual positive results of their effort. Some of the greatest personal triumphs over disease and injury are recorded not in medical or nursing texts but in biographical literature. A health team composed of every type of expert in medicine can bring an ill person only to a certain phase of recovery. The effort to take that which has been "repaired" and to develop it to its fullest must come from the individual. Even though not all patients are faced with major problems because of illness, all are in need of maintaining a constructive and hopeful attitude. Spiritual support is often the key to the hope and determination that helps them, and it is a real comfort to many persons to be able to adhere closely to their religious practices during illness.

The presence of a Bible, a prayer book, rosary beads, or other religious objects among the patient's personal items is significant. It may well be that he spends a portion of each day in devotional reading, meditation, or prayer. Although some persons may have no objection to praying or meditating in the presence of others, other individuals may prefer privacy. Inasmuch as hospitalized patients may feel that a request for privacy may not be understood, it is a thoughtful gesture if the suggestion is initiated by the nurse.

Many hospitals have chapels in which patients may worship, and in some instances regular services are held for various denominations. When regular services are not held, patients are permitted to worship in the chapel at their convenience. Frequently, it is through the consideration of members of the nursing staff that patients are made aware of such facilities.

There are times when religious beliefs conflict with prevalent health care practices. For example, the doctrine of the Jehovah's Witnesses prohibits blood transfusions. In the Islamic religion, man is regarded as largely helpless in controlling his environment and illness is accepted as his fate rather than something against which action might be taken. Some Navajo Indians use a lengthy religious ceremony to "cure" certain diseases, such as tuberculosis. For some people, illness is viewed as punishment for sin, and, therefore, inevitable.

Such beliefs may require the health worker to modify a treatment plan to accommodate the person's religion. In some instances, acknowledgment of the individual's religious convictions and efforts by health practitioners to accommodate his beliefs can result in quality health care without violating the person's religious practices. In other situations, an objective explanation of alternative treatments and the predicted consequences of each may help the individual to determine the therapy he wishes to accept. This type of decision may require the assistance of the person's religious advisor. Whatever the person's decision about his health care, the nurse should remember that each individual is unique and that he has a right to pursue his own convictions, even though they may differ from those of the health care provider. Every mentally competent person has the right to accept or refuse therapy as he chooses.

THE CLERGYMAN'S ROLE ON THE HEALTH TEAM

Because physical recovery is closely related to mental attitude and emotional stability, the patient's religious counselor plays a key role on the health team. He may provide comfort, support, and guidance for the patient and his family. There are instances when he serves as an associate to the physician and the nurse by interpreting

therapy and its value to the patient and his family. He may very well be the person who helps the patient to accept various phases of care. The clergyman may also clarify the person's beliefs to the health team members.

In many large hospitals, clergymen of various faiths are available at any time of the day or night. When the patient is in a hospital near his own community, the clergyman from his own church or synagogue may also visit, and generally this is a satisfying experience for the patient.

The hospital nurse can be helpful to a clergyman by greeting him and helping him to locate his parishioner or congregant when he comes to visit. She may assist by determining whether the patient is able to receive a call from the clergyman. Having him enter the room at an inopportune moment can be embarrassing to both clergyman and patient.

Preparations of the patient's room for the clergyman's call may vary. The room should be orderly and free from unnecessary equipment and items. There should be a seat for the clergyman at the bedside or near the patient so that both can be comfortable during the visit. If a sacrament is to be administered, the top of the bedside table should be free of items and covered with a clean white cover. If the patient is in a unit having several patients, he may appreciate having the bed curtains drawn to provide some degree of privacy. In addition, the nurse may ask the clergyman if there is any further way in which she can be of assistance.

JUDAISM

Judaism teaches the unity of God, and that God is the creator and source of all life. Each person is free to choose between good and evil. Man is considered a child of God. Unlike Christianity and some religions of the Near East, Judaism does not hold resurrection and immortality as a central concept. Nor does it accept the divinity of Christ. One rabbi states that the aim of Judaism is salvation of humanity in history rather than salvation of the soul in the hereafter. Salvation is found by fulfilling social responsibilities. Death is considered part of the continuance of birth, growth, and decay.

The spiritual adviser of the Jewish faith is the rabbi. There are three forms of Judaism: Reform, Conservative, and Orthodox. Reform Judaism is more liberal than the other two in its thinking, whereas Orthodox Judaism is the most traditional of the three. Conservative Judaism finds its place more or less between Reform and Orthodox Judaism.

The Jewish Sabbath and Holy Days

The Sabbath begins on Friday at sundown and ends on Saturday at sundown. It is a day for rest and worship. For the patient who observes the Sabbath, treatments and procedures should be postponed if postponement will not harm the patient.

In Judaism, New Year's Day is called Rosh Hashanah and usually occurs in September. Rosh Hashanah is the beginning of a ten-day period for reflections and consideration of life and its problems. The period ends with the Day of Atonement or Yom Kippur.

Hanukkah usually occurs in December. It is a festival recalling ancient resistance to tyranny and is a time of rejoicing and giving of gifts.

Passover occurs in the spring and is observed for seven days. It is a festival of redemption that recalls the departure of the Jews from Egypt.

There are additional Jewish holy days but the ones just mentioned are observed most commonly.

Dietary Practices

Dietary practices are important for the nurse to understand, especially when she is caring for patients who observe Conservative or Orthodox Judaism. Reform Judaism does not hold these practices as relevant. Because dietary practices vary in Judaism, and also occasionally among Jews practicing the same form of Judaism, the nurse should consult with the patient, a family member, or a rabbi, if questions arise.

Dietary regulations permit the eating of meat of kosher animals and fowl. Animals are considered kosher if they are ruminants and have divided hooves, such as cows, goats, and sheep. Kosher fowl are primarily those that are not birds of prey, such as chickens, ducks, and geese. Fowl and animals are slaughtered, dressed, and prepared in a prescribed manner in order to be considered kosher. Fish are considered kosher if they have both scales and fins, such as salmon, tuna, sardines, carp. Shellfish, such as shrimp and lobster, are not acceptable. Fish do not have to be slaughtered and dressed in a prescribed manner.

Fish and meat products, such as oils and fats, milk and milk products, and eggs are considered kosher if they are from the above-mentioned animals. Plant or vegetable oils are acceptable.

Milk products may not be eaten with or immediately following meat products. An interval of six hours must elapse between eating meat and milk products. Meat products, on the other hand, may be eaten after milk products after an interval of only a few minutes. If a patient is having both meat and milk products during the same meal, serve the products separately, first the milk products and then the meat.

Fish may be eaten with dairy products if prepared with a nonmeat shortening or if broiled.

Kosher foods may not be prepared in utensils used for the preparation of nonkosher foods unless they have been cleansed in a prescribed manner. Fruits and vegetables that have been steamed or cooked in nonkosher utensils are permissible if nonkosher sauce, gravy, or shortening are omitted.

For the patient who is in the hospital and observing dietary practices, the following suggestions are helpful. Use paper dishes for serving food; substitute fresh vegetables and fruits for leavened products; if kosher meat or fish is unavailable, use an acceptable protein substitute, such as milk products or eggs.

During Passover, leavened products, such as bread, cake, cookies, noodles, or beverages containing grain alcohol, are not used. The nurse may suggest that the family bring matzos (unleavened bread product) for the patient.

If a Jewish patient's observance of dietary practices interferes with his medical regimen, Jewish law permits modifications. Before proceeding with modifications, the nurse should consult with the patient, a member of his family, or a rabbi.

Circumcision

Male Jewish infants are required to be circumcised on the eighth day after birth. However, the rite may be postponed for as long as necessary if the infant's health does not permit it at that time. The mohel, that is, a professional circumciser, may perform it or, in some instances, it may be done by a Jewish surgeon while a rabbi attends. A quorum of ten men attends the ceremony, if available. However, a quorum is not necessary for religious circumcision.

Death and Preparation for Burial

There are appropriate prayers for the dying patient. Also, if the patient and family so desire, a service of confession and prayer may be observed as death approaches. Preferably the rabbi is present for this—if not the patient's own rabbi, then one associated with the health agency.

A patient who has died may be washed and covered

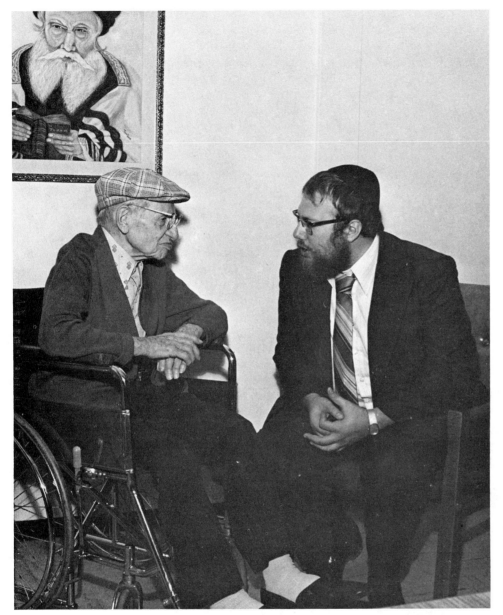

Figure 7–1 The rabbi's visit is important for this gentleman who is a resident in a geriatric center. The man explained that he wears his cap at all times because it was a custom in his culture.

with a clean cloth. Should a Jewish patient who has no kin to claim the body die, a rabbi should be contacted immediately.

Reform and Conservative Jews do not object to post-mortem examination. They consider an autopsy to be a means by which medical knowledge learned from the dead can be helpful to the living. Either the patient gives consent for autopsy before death or the family grants such permission after the patient has died.

CHRISTIANITY: ROMAN CATHOLICISM AND PROTESTANTISM

Christianity teaches the trinity of God; that is, there are three persons in one God: God the Father, God the Son, and God the Holy Spirit. God the Father is considered the creator and the source of life. The Son of God is Jesus Christ, who came into the world in human form, suffered, and died for the salvation of all men.

Christianity holds resurrection and immortality as a central concept. Although social responsibility is important in Christianity, salvation is found through faith in the triune God. However, the two go together—faith and good works.

In the United States, most Christians are Roman Catholics or Protestants. The spiritual adviser in the Roman Catholic faith is the priest. For Protestants the spiritual adviser is called a minister, pastor, or preacher.

Sundays and Holy Days

Most Christians observe Sunday as a day for worship. An exception is the Seventh Day Adventist, who sets aside Saturday for worship.

Although many holy days are observed in the various faiths in Christianity, two are held in common and are familiar to almost everyone.

Christmas is observed in most places in the world on December 25. It is celebrated as the day on which Christ was born. The day is a joyous one and a time for giving gifts in memory of Christ's birth.

In the spring, Christians observe Lent and the Easter season. Easter occurs in March or April. The six-week period prior to Easter is called Lent and the Friday before Easter is Good Friday.

Lent is a time for contemplation on the sufferings and death of Christ. Many Christians make personal sacrifices during Lent as a symbol of humility and in memory of Christ's suffering. These sacrifices may involve some type of fasting, which may need to be taken into account during periods of illness, especially if it interferes with the medical regimen. Good Friday is a day of sorrow when the Christian recalls the agonizing death of Christ on the cross.

Easter marks the end of the Lenten period and is a day of great rejoicing. It commemorates the day when Christ arose from the dead. Belief in His resurrection confirms the Christian tenet that Christ is the Son of God.

Roman Catholicism

In the care of Roman Catholic patients, the nurse will find it necessary to be acquainted with the following sacraments: baptism, reconciliation, holy communion, and the anointing of the sick. Sacraments in the Catholic faith, by virtue of the fact that they are accepted as having been instituted by Christ, are believed to have the power to produce the effect that each signifies.

The Sacrament of Baptism. Since a nurse may be present during the delivery of a child or the miscarriage of a living fetus, it is imperative that she understand that, for a Catholic family, any child in danger of death must be baptized. At the time of death most Catholics desire to be in the state of grace, free from serious sin. It is mainly by means of the sacraments that sin is absolved and grace given. Baptism is the first sacrament and removes the first, or original, sin deriving from Adam and Eve. To the Catholic, this is essential for salvation.

If a priest is not available, the nurse or the doctor should administer the sacrament of baptism. It is preferred that a Catholic nurse or doctor administer the sacrament, but if a Catholic is not available, anyone having the use of reason may do so. It is necessary that the person conferring the sacrament have the intention of doing what the Catholic Church desires and use the proper form. The procedure is as follows: while pouring plain water over the forehead so that it flows upon the skin, say, "I baptize you in the name of the Father, and of the Son, and of the Holy Spirit."

Since baptism may be conferred when there is possible danger to the child's life, and since the family may not be aware of it, the fact that the sacrament of baptism was conferred should be recorded on the infant's chart and in the chaplain's baptismal roster if there is one in the health agency. If a priest confers the baptism, he will notify the family that it has been done. If the child is baptized by someone other than a priest, the priest should be informed; then he can discuss it with the parents.

The Sacrament of Reconciliation. The sacrament of reconciliation involves the confessing of one's sins against God and fellow man and asking for His forgiveness. It is often called *penance* or *confession*. The priest hears the person's confession and offers assistance and counseling to help the penitent avoid future sins. God absolves the sorrowful penitent of his sins through the priest. Since a person wishes to be free of sin before receiving other sacraments, reconciliation is often sought before such sacraments are administered, although it may be desired at other times also.

The Sacrament of Holy Eucharist or Holy Communion. Holy Communion is the most revered of all sacraments of the Catholic faith. According to Catholic belief, the eucharist is the Body and Blood of Jesus Christ, under the appearance of bread and wine. Most Catholics in danger of death desire to receive communion if possible. As necessary, confession precedes communion. To prepare to receive communion, Catholics, except those

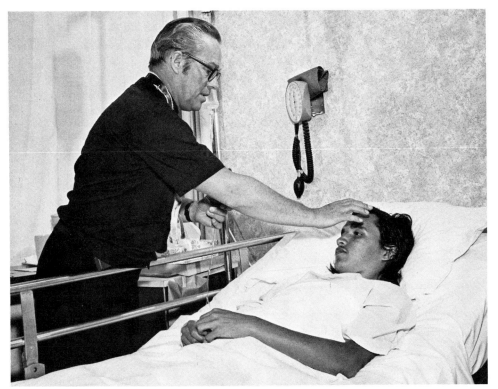

Figure 7-2   The priest administers the sacrament of the anointing of the sick to this young Mexican-American patient who is being prepared for surgery.

in danger of death, may wish to fast from solid food. The fast is of one hour's duration. A person is not required to fast from water or medications.

If communion is to be administered in the patient's room, the patient should be made comfortable and the room prepared as described earlier. The patient should be provided with privacy so that he may pray and prepare himself for the sacrament.

The Sacrament of the Anointing of the Sick.   The sacrament of the anointing of the sick has been changed somewhat since the 1962–1965 Second Vatican Council. The rite now encourages that the sacrament be administered to ill persons who are not in immediate danger of death. Also, the rite emphasizes that any person who must undergo surgery for a reason that has caused the person to be seriously or critically ill may be given the benefit of the sacrament of the sick. In addition, this sacrament may now be offered to those whose life forces are growing weaker simply because of age, even though death *may* be remote. The sacrament can be administered to groups of persons as well, such as, a group of residents living in a nursing home.

When administering the sacrament, the priest anoints the person's forehead and the palms of the hands with holy oil. The prayers used are designed to help the sick endure their suffering, recover their health, and, in case of death, attain salvation.

When the patient appears to be dying, he may wish to receive communion if he is conscious and capable of swallowing. If time appears short, communion is given first and then, if still possible, the patient receives the sacrament of the anointing of the sick. Confession before communion is said, if desired.

The changed rite for anointing of the sick eliminates the previous practice of anointing the dead. Instead the priest offers a prayer of forgiveness for sins and commends the person to the mercy of God. If there is any doubt that the person is dead, the priest, using his discretion, may anoint the person conditionally. In the case of an unconscious person, it is encouraged that a priest administer the anointing of the sick when he has reasonable assurance that the person would desire the benefits of this sacrament, if he were capable of requesting it.

Protestantism

The Protestant faith embraces a large number of denominations. Some of the religious groups that are active today originated before the Reformation, and others have developed since then apart from the Reformation influence. While certain doctrines are common to most of these denominations, there are individual practices and interpretations which give each a distinct pattern of its own.

While some denominations employ certain sacraments that are similar to those in the Catholic faith, others reject the concept of sacraments and observe baptism and communion as ordinances that are means of grace but not of salvation. Others, such as the Friends (Quakers), reject both ordinances and sacraments.

The Sacrament or Ordinance of Baptism. Some Protestant faiths hold that baptism should be performed in infancy. The Baptists, the Disciples of Christ, and some others believe that the ordinance of baptism should not be administered before the person reaches the age of accountability. If a child of Protestant parents is in danger of dying, the nurse should ask whether the parents wish to have the child baptized. If the parents wish it and a Protestant minister is not available, the child may be baptized as follows: a baptized nurse who has understanding of and belief in the act that she is about to perform may baptize the baby by pouring water continously over the baby's forehead and saying the following words, "I baptize thee in the name of the Father, and of the Son, and of the Holy Spirit. Amen." The baptism is recorded on the child's chart by the person performing it and the parents are informed as soon as convenient.

The Sacrament or Ordinance of Communion. In most Protestant faiths, communion is administered less frequently than in the Catholic faith. However, many Protestant patients request it prior to surgery or during a period of illness. It represents the body and the blood of Christ which were sacrificed for the remission of sin. Before the arrival of the minister, the room should be properly prepared and the patient given privacy so that he has an opportunity for prayer and self-examination.

OTHER RELIGIOUS BELIEFS

While it is impractical to discuss all faiths in this text, the nurse should be aware that other religious beliefs also have a direct influence on health care. For example, Seventh Day Adventists are generally vegetarians. Members of the Church of Jesus Christ of Latter-Day Saints, or Mormons as they are commonly called, do not use tobacco, alcohol, or caffeinated drinks.

Christian Scientists believe healing is a religious function and have their own healers and sanitariums. However, they may seek medical attention for childbirth and fractures, although they do not use medications. Vaccinations and inoculations are also generally not acceptable to Christian Scientists.

Pentecostalism is often interdenominational and may include various Christian denominations as well as persons of the Jewish faith. Pentecostalism frequently

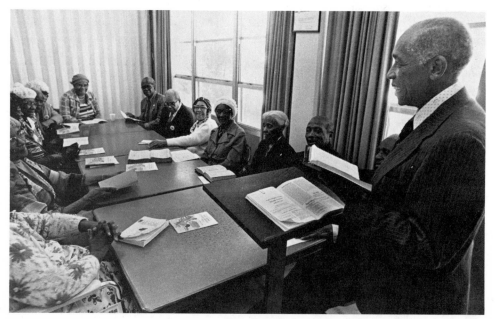

Figure 7–3 A group of retired persons gather for their weekly Bible study. (Photographer, Michael Patrick, Austin, Texas.)

includes spiritual healing or the "laying on of hands" and "speaking in tongues."

Some churches leave decisions about birth control and abortion up to the individual. Other denominations, such as the Greek Orthodox, Roman Catholic, and the Church of Jesus Christ of Latter-Day Saints, have specific teachings on birth control and abortion.

In her education and working career, the nurse may also have contact with still other religious beliefs. Hinduism, Buddhism, Shintoism, Confucianism, and Islam are other major world religions. If the nurse has contact with a person of a faith with which she is unfamiliar, she should acknowledge this fact. Through reading, discussion with the person, his family, and clergymen, she can learn about the basic tenets of the faith and how they may affect health care.

Persons who do not choose to be affiliated with any particular religious faith are referred to as *unchurched.* Many unchurched persons believe religion is a personal and nonsectarian matter and practice their beliefs privately.

An *atheist* is a person who denies the existence of a God while an *agnostic* is one who holds that nothing is known about the existence of a God. The agnostic and the atheist are guided by philosophies of living that do not include a religious faith. Nevertheless, they too deserve respect for what they choose to believe just as do those who accept a particular religious creed.

CULTURES AND SUBCULTURES

Culture is defined as the beliefs, values, and behavior patterns which are common to a group and transmitted to succeeding generations. The scientific study of the origin of cultural characteristics of population groups is carried out by the cultural anthropologist. Cultural characteristics have a wide-ranging influence on individual lives. Therefore, it is important for the nurse to be familiar with the cultural backgrounds of the persons with whom she has frequent contact. For example, habits of daily living, such as those involving sleeping, eating, personal hygiene, work, social interactions, health practices, child-rearing, expressions of feelings, kinship relations, and roles of persons of various ages, are almost always influenced by the culture in which an individual lives.

Cultures are frequently composed of subcultures. A *subculture* is a group within a culture that does not hold all beliefs of the larger culture or gives them different significance. American subcultures, for example, are almost infinitely diversified according to such factors as region, education, occupation, income, social class, and so on. Moreover, each individual is the product of a number of subcultures, every one of which will affect his behavior to some degree.

The following are examples of what some authorities consider to be subcultures in America. There are those who describe a subculture of poverty in the United States. Persons living in poverty have often been observed to hold certain common attitudes, such as lack of trust and understanding of individuals from other subcultures, because they have often been treated in a dehumanizing way. They often share a feeling of powerlessness and resignation about their lives. Also the communes which sprang up across the country during the 1960s are often thought of as a subculture. Life in a commune is usually very dependent on nature for livelihood and the attitudes its members hold regarding such things as family life, rearing of children, education, and the like, are very different from other subcultures. There have been descriptions of rural and urban subcultures, the subculture of the industrial worker, the subcultures of different age groups, and even the subcultures of various types of institutions, such as hospitals.

Biological traits of population groups are generally studied separately from cultural traits. Physical anthropologists conduct research into man's biological origins and characteristics. There is general agreement that biological traits of a group are the result of genetic responses to environmental influences and living habits over generations. Living habits are intertwined with cultural traits and, in that sense, culture exerts some influence on biological traits.

The majority of citizens in the United States, including the majority of health care providers, are white and members of the middle socioeconomic class. Hence, health care standards and practices have generally been oriented toward the white middle-class culture.

In recent years more health care practitioners are being recruited from minority cultures. In addition, effort is being made by members of the health care disciplines to become more aware of cultural variations and to incorporate them in their health care practices. For instance, studies have been done which show racial differences in characteristics of growth and development of children. Black infants and young children typically develop motor coordination earlier than do white children. This fact is being incorporated in assessment standards. Typical values of the Oriental culture make it difficult for the Chinese woman who is pregnant to accept care from a male physician. Female physicians and midwives are providing more acceptable prenatal care in some settings. Continued efforts and increasing numbers of health care workers from minority cultures will undoubtedly bring about more modifications in health care in response to cultural differences.

TRANSCULTURAL NURSING

In recent years an increased emphasis has been placed on the influence of culture on nursing care. *Transcultural nursing* is a relatively new field which focuses on the comparative study of cultural beliefs and practices regarding health and their relationship to nursing.

Dr. Madeleine Leininger, a nurse anthropologist, has been especially instrumental in promoting research in transcultural nursing and in stimulating related programs of study. According to Leininger, the purpose of studying transcultural health practices is to develop a greater understanding of man's behavior with regard to his health. By identifying traditional and contemporary health practices of varying cultures, commonalities may emerge. Leininger believes that combining the knowledge of patterns of transcultural practices with technological advances can result in improved health and nursing care for persons of many cultures.

Providing health care that takes cultural factors into consideration is a complex and difficult task. Leininger identifies several problems which often present obstacles. Typically, health care workers lack sufficient knowledge about cultural differences to understand how their professional practice needs to be altered to be acceptable to persons of another culture. Extensive time and effort are necessary to acquire an understanding of the whole social structure of a culture and the place of health care in the structure. Individuals, including health care workers, who enter a new culture generally experience feelings of discomfort and uncertainty which is called culture shock. Consciously or unconsciously, health care workers have frequently forced their own cultural views about health on persons with differing beliefs and values. Some suggestions for dealing with these problems are made later in this chapter. For further assistance, the reader is also encouraged to pursue the writings of Leininger and others who are active in this field. Some of their writings are included in the references at the end of this unit.

Transcultural nursing is concerned with the caring and folk medicine practices of cultures. *Caring practices* are the protecting and assisting activities which are related to health and performed as a part of a culture. *Folk medicine practices* are the methods and techniques of health care which are a traditional part of a culture. Almost all cultures have been found to have some type of caring and folk medicine practices. Some are highly organized and others are very informal. Caring practices are considered to be the responsibility of certain family members in some cultures. In other cultures, specific persons who are not necessarily family members are prepared and designated to carry out the caring tasks.

Some folk medicine practices have been found to have a scientifically supported basis. Others have no known scientific basis, but for people who practice them, their value to health is significant. Caring and folk medicine practices are an important part of the total culture and are intertwined with other cultural values, beliefs, and practices. They also frequently overlap with religious practices.

Folk medicine practices are utilized by many persons. They are most often found where large numbers of persons from a particular culture live, such as in inner cities and rural areas. In these settings, other cultural practices which support folk medicine are usually prevalent also. It should be remembered that cultural traditions, including folk medicine practices, can be found in the homes of persons who do not live in inner cities or rural areas. Understanding these influences helps in understanding individuals and their behavior.

Many persons of various cultures use both professional medicine and folk medicine. *Professional medicine* refers to the methods and techniques of health care which are based on formal study and scientific research and are provided by the various health disciplines. Many individuals believe folk medicine is specific for some types of health problems while professional medicine deals with others.

The United States has more varied cultures and subcultures than any other country in the world. The sheer numbers and variations are staggering. Further complexity is added by the blending and combining that occurs because of cross-cultural influences. In order to familiarize nursing students with the most prevalent cultures in the United States, brief discussions of some outstanding characteristics of the majority and four minority cultures follow. The four minority cultures which will be discussed have been defined by the federal government. They are the black, Spanish-speaking, American Indian, and Oriental cultures. There are also subcultures within each of these minority cultures.

The majority culture in this country is the middle socioeconomic class. Originally, this class consisted of Caucasians and was called the Anglo-Saxon middle class. The term referred to the geographical and hereditary origin as well as the socioeconomic status of its members. Within recent years, some persons of other than Anglo-Saxon origin have become a part of the large middle class in the United States. However, as a group, it is still primarily composed of Caucasians. This chapter uses the term white middle class to mean the majority culture in the United States while cautioning the reader that some nonwhites do exist within this group. It is also readily acknowledged that many subcultures exist within the predominantly white middle class.

Not all persons who are members of a particular cultural group necessarily believe or practice all aspects of the culture. Also because of the overlaps among cultures within this country, probably few individuals can be considered culturally pure. Therefore the nurse must guard against stereotyping individuals according to their cultural backgrounds.

WHITE MIDDLE-CLASS CULTURE

A belief in individualism is usually prevalent throughout the white middle class. The characteristics of this belief are interpreted differently. However, they generally include the ideas that adults are expected to be responsible in activities related to society's welfare and the individual has rights which deserve protection. Individuals are expected to take initiative and to function relatively independently. A person's right to privacy is considered important.

Achievement is generally prized in the white middle-class culture. The value placed on achieving promotes high standards of performance, competition, efficiency, productivity, and progress. It results in an emphasis on time, mechanization, newness, scientific thinking, formal education, and the future. Scientific causes are usually assigned to health problems and detailed, technical explanations are expected from health practitioners. The value placed on achievement and its correlates is thought by some authorities to be at least partially responsible for some health problems of middle-class persons, such as some cardiovascular and

gastrointestinal diseases, some forms of cancer, auto accidents, suicides, mental illness, and alcoholism.

Vigorousness or ideal health is assigned high value by most white middle-class persons. Youth is generally valued over old age. Body defects and handicaps are carefully avoided or repaired whenever possible. Health care is most frequently sought from professional practitioners and generally includes extensive preventive measures. Some authorities describe persons of the white middle-class culture as excessively dependent on professional medicine. Folk medicine practices of the middle class have not generally been described. However, in one sense, prevalent self-diagnosis and the generous use of over-the-counter drugs might be considered common folk medicine practices in this culture. In addition, fad diets and the extensive use of health clubs and exercise facilities might also be called white middle-class folk medicine practices.

Cleanliness, orderliness, and attractiveness are common values of the white middle class. A great deal of time, energy, and money are spent on perfecting external appearances. It has been said that middle-class Americans have almost made a fetish of soap and water rituals. Fashionable wearing apparel, homes, and automobiles are among prized possessions. Neatness and organization are also considered important characteristics.

Generally, the nuclear family is most valued by the white middle class. Grandparents and other extended family members are not necessarily abandoned, but the home life, activities, plans, and concerns most often focus on the nuclear family. Prevalent family mobility also results in geographical separation of the extended family. The emphasis on the nuclear family and the division of the extended family result in extensive middle-class purchasing of personal services, such as child care, care of the elderly and ill, and household assistance. In some cultures, these tasks are usually performed by extended family members.

Most members of the white middle class have a Protestant background. Whether they actually accept this religious orientation or not, the associated Puritan ethic is generally prevalent. The cultural characteristics of individualism, achievement, and cleanliness and orderliness are thought to be rooted in this Puritan heritage.

These are a few characteristics of the white middle-class culture which influence the behavior of the majority of persons in this country. It has been estimated that approximately 40 percent of the population in the United States belongs to this group.

BLACK CULTURE

The black culture typically retains some characteristics of its African origins, although the American heritage of nearly all blacks in the United States goes back more than 300 years. The black culture is significantly influenced by poverty. As a result of the effects of slavery and discrimination, a large percentage of blacks have lived in the lowest socioeconomic class for generations.

Persons from the black culture are generally present-oriented. Their concerns and efforts are focused on day-to-day happenings rather than on the past or the future. It is hypothesized that long endurance of the conditions of poverty and repression have had this effect.

Personal appearance is of particular importance to most blacks. Grooming, especially hair care and wearing apparel, reflects the fact that self-worth in the black culture is often related to appearance.

Close family relationships usually exist between several generations and extended family members of blacks. Families ordinarily maintain close and supportive relations even after children are grown. Members of black communities also often have kinshiplike ties with individuals who are not blood relatives but who are associated through church and organizational or social groups. Both family and community relationships are supportive and usually very important to the black person at times of crisis and joy in his life. Daily living activities often revolve around family and community relationships.

Religion generally plays an important role in the black culture. It usually is a blend of traditional and Christian influences. Expressions of religious beliefs are frequently emotional and permit obvious manifestations of happiness, sadness, or anxiety. Especially at times of stress, black persons are frequently comforted by praying, singing, or chanting together. Members of the black clergy are generally highly respected members of the black community and play an important role in both community and family activities and problems. Churches often provide emotional support and tangible assistance, especially for elderly and ill members of the community.

Folk Medicine Beliefs and Practices

Traditional folk medicine practices vary extensively in the black culture and generally are combined with religious beliefs. They are probably carried out more frequently in inner city and rural areas but can be found throughout the black culture. Folk medicine practices are typically based on a general belief that events are classified into natural and unnatural categories. Natural events are predictable and are in harmony with God. Unnatural events are unpredictable, in disharmony with God, and often the work of the devil.

Natural illnesses are frequently thought to result from God's punishments for sin or a lack of faith. They can be cured by repentance, faith healers, the use of home remedies, and professional medicine. Unnatural events are particularly frightening because of their unpredictability. When an illness is classified as unnatural, it is generally felt to be the result of a supernatural power possessed by a witch or a spirit. Such illnesses are believed to be cured only by appropriate supernatural means.

Unnatural powers which result in harm are variously called rootwork, voodoo, hoodoo, or hexes. The harmful effects are removed by the use of various ceremonies and rituals, frequently involving mixtures of particular herbs or roots believed to have supernatural powers. Spiritualists, herb doctors, root doctors, conjurers, and skilled elder family members may be called upon to cure unnatural illnesses. At times, both unnatural and natural illnesses may exist simultaneously and, therefore, folk and professional medicine practices are used at the same time.

Common Health Problems

Because of the prevalence of poverty in the black culture, health problems resulting from inadequate sanitation, nutrition, and housing are frequent. Lead poisoning, respiratory infections, tuberculosis, and infant and maternal death rates are greater than in the majority population. The frequent inaccessibility of adequate health care has also resulted in the failure to seek anything but acute illness care. Therefore, the incidence of some disabling and chronic conditions is high.

Genetic characteristics are also thought to be responsible for certain health problems in blacks. Hypertension is seen more frequently in blacks than nonblacks and probably is the greatest single health problem. The precise biological cause of hypertension is unknown. Sickle cell anemia is a hereditary blood disease which is prevalent among blacks, although it is also found among some other cultural groups. It is thought to result from an environmental resistance to malaria acquired in Africa many generations ago.

In recent years an enzyme deficiency among blacks and some other cultural groups has been discovered. The enzyme is essential for the digestion of lactose, a major constituent of milk, and makes black persons tolerate milk poorly.

Skin disorders of some types are more common among blacks. Inflammation of hair follicles, various types of dermatitis, and excessive growths of scar tissue (keloids) are also frequent problems.

SPANISH-SPEAKING CULTURE

The Spanish-speaking culture in the United States is primarily composed of three subcultures—Mexican-American, Hispanic, and Puerto Rican. Mexican-Americans are the largest Spanish-speaking subculture and are called Chicanos in some parts of the country. They have a Mexican and Indian heritage and the majority of them reside in the Southwest. The Hispanics or Spanish-Americans are descendents of the early Spanish settlers and American Indians. The largest number live in New Mexico and Colorado. Puerto Ricans have a Spanish and black heritage and live primarily on the east coast.

The Mexican-American, Hispanic, and Puerto Rican subcultures are distinctive in origin and characteristics, but they share some common elements which will be the focus of the discussion here. When having contact with persons from these subcultures, it is important for the nurse to realize that they consider themselves separate and distinct groups.

In the Spanish-speaking culture, the family is generally the primary unit of society and is extremely important. The welfare of the family is more highly valued than that of the individual and often takes precedence if a choice must be made. The husband traditionally is the primary decision-maker for the family. The family unit includes the extended family as well as the godparents or co-parents (*compadres*). All family members are expected to show concern and respect for each other and especially for the elders of the family.

Because English may not be spoken or is a second language for the Spanish-speaking, many of these persons tend to isolate themselves in their own communities. Poverty is generally prevalent. Because younger members often involve themselves with the majority culture, their strong commitment to the family and their cultural background frequently causes a value conflict for them.

Religion is generally a fundamental part of the culture of Spanish-speaking persons. Roman Catholicism is the predominant faith and religious practices play a significant part in their lives. Persons of the traditional Spanish-speaking culture generally believe God gives health and allows illness for a reason. Illness may be viewed as a punishment or as a cross to bear. They further believe that an unbending faith in God is essential for recovery from illness. Praying for health and the endurance to tolerate illness, and for special blessings of patron saints are often part of daily religious practices. Formal religious teachings and practices are also influenced by mystical beliefs.

Persons from the Spanish-speaking culture generally believe in the necessity of a balance between man and nature for health to exist. Natural illnesses result from an imbalance in God's natural world. Supernatural illness is the result of Satan and his followers.

Folk Medicine Beliefs and Practices

Besides natural illness, there are several specific types of supernatural illnesses. *Mal ojo,* or evil eye sickness, is believed to be the result of a spell cast by someone who excessively admires a person or desires something of the individual. It most often occurs in children and is characterized by vomiting, diarrhea, fever, and restlessness. It is believed to be preventable when the admiring person touches the child while admiring him. It is treated by prayers and specific rituals.

Caida de la mollera, or *mollera caida,* is a common illness of babies and results in sunken eyes and fontanels, diarrhea, vomiting, and irritability. It is believed to be caused by dropping the child or by suddenly withdrawing the nipple from his mouth. Treatment includes applications of various substances to the skin.

Susto is an illness induced by fright or an emotional trauma. It is thought to be caused by fear and frequently follows the loss of a loved one. Typically the person has difficulty sleeping and eating and is anxious and tense. Treatment may include prayer and the use of certain herbs and rituals.

Empacho is a childhood digestive illness and is thought to be caused by eating bad food. A ball of food is believed to be caught in the stomach. Massage and a special diet may be used as treatment.

Mal puesta is an illness induced by a hex. It can be caused by a *brujo,* or male witch, or other malicious persons. A *bruja* is a female witch.

There is generally an older family member who

initially treats mild illnesses within the home. Various herbs and home remedies are often used effectively.

A *curandero* (male) and a *curandera* (female) are healers by virtue of divine blessing. They use prayer, rituals, herbs, and massages to treat illnesses but do not use countermagic against witches. The *curandero* generally treats *susto* and *mal ojo* as well as other illnesses, but usually will not treat someone who is critically ill. He often refers seriously ill persons for professional medical care. The *curandero* generally includes the family in his treatment. He works closely with the individual and helps the patient use his own energies and resources to recover. His individualized treatment and the ability to communicate in Spanish, both of which are frequently unavailable in professional health care, make him highly regarded in this culture.

The *espiritualisto* is a male spiritualist healer who has the ability to predict the future, communicate with spirits, and remove hexes. The *espiritualisto* counters the influence of the *brujo*. An *espiritualista* is a female spiritualist healer.

Folk healers are generally highly respected in Spanish-speaking communities. Their assistance is often sought first or simultaneously with practitioners of professional medicine.

Common Health Problems

Like other minority groups, Spanish-speaking persons have a high incidence of health problems associated with poverty. Inadequate medical care is thought to be responsible for a higher incidence of death from rheumatic fever, pneumonia, and influenza than in the majority population. Poor nutrition and the lack of prenatal care also result in a higher mortality rate for infants and new mothers than is seen in the white middle-class culture.

The incidence of diabetes mellitus and its complications among Mexican-Americans is prevalent. At present, it is unclear whether the cause is genetic or nutritionally induced. Interestingly, Mexican-American mortality rates resulting from cancer and cardiovascular diseases are lower than those for the majority population.

Parasitic diseases, such as dysentery, malaria, filariasis, and hookworm, are particularly common among Puerto Ricans, and generally result from inadequate sanitary conditions and general poor health. The incidence of tuberculosis is also higher among Puerto Ricans than among the majority population.

The lactose enzyme deficiency resulting in poor digestion of milk is less common than in blacks, but it is also found among Spanish-speaking people.

AMERICAN INDIAN CULTURE

The American Indian culture is composed of several hundred different subcultures called tribes. Each tribe has its own language, traditions, beliefs, and practices. While each tribe is distinctive, there are commonalities which will be discussed here.

American Indians are found throughout the United States although the majority live in the West. About half of the million Indians in the United States live on the more than 200 reservations. Most of the others live in urban and suburban areas. The majority of those on reservations live in isolated areas and exist in poverty.

Most American Indian tribes share a belief in the importance of the natural balance or harmony which exists in man and between man and his environment. Imbalance often results in illness. Health care practices are frequently closely associated with religious and supernatural beliefs. God is the giver and cause of life, and therefore, illness is related to Him. Microorganisms are not generally acknowledged as a cause of disease.

The belief system of American Indians generally includes a cyclic notion of birth, living, and death. Man experiences the natural cycles himself and is a part of the same cycle which involves the world in which he lives. In this perspective, time is also cyclical and tends to have more of a natural basis, rather than clock subdivisions of hours and minutes.

Sharing is an extremely important value in the American Indian culture. Little importance is attached to material possessions except as they can be shared with others.

Extended family and tribal kinship relations are important to most American Indians. Several generations, as well as great aunts and uncles, cousins, and tribally related individuals, are often involved in making decisions, rearing children, providing support and assistance, and in sharing good fortunes and problems.

Folk Medicine Beliefs and Practices

Most American Indian tribes have folk medicine beliefs and practices which incorporate the supernatural and natural. There is generally a health practitioner in the extended family who is consulted initially about illness. There may also be someone in the community who has had experience in caring for the sick and whose assist-

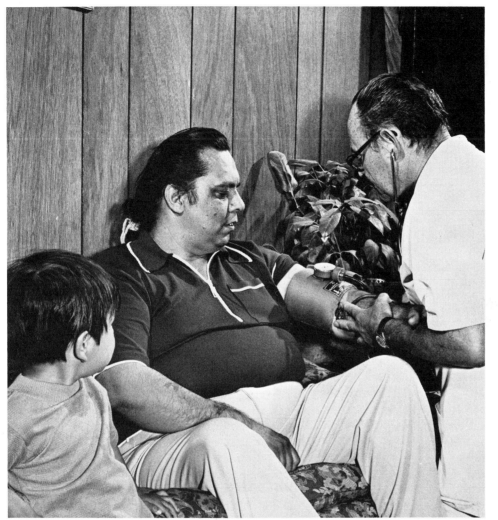

Figure 7-4 This American Indian exemplifies cross-cultural influences. He lives in an urban area and dresses in a middle-class manner, but he continues to wear his hair in the traditional Indian style.

ance is sought. Both of these individuals commonly use various home remedies, herbs, and plants in their treatment.

The tribal medicine man is a person who has had special preparation in the use of natural herbal and medicinal curing as well as supernatural cures which incorporate religious beliefs. His services are an important part of Indian health care. Herbs, plants, heat, massage, and other techniques are all used effectively by the medicine man. Interestingly, hundreds of the plants and herbs originally discovered by the American Indians are now scientifically accepted and used in various forms by practitioners of professional medicine.

Additional substances believed to have supernatural powers, such as cornmeal, pollens, and evergreens, are used in healing ceremonies. Depending on the tribe,

the ceremonies may include chants, sings, fasting, meditation, masks, dances, and sandpaintings. Professional medicine is also frequently used simultaneously with the medicine man's cures. In fact, in recent years efforts have been made to incorporate traditional Indian folk medicine and professional medicine in such a way as to complement each other in the care of American Indian patients in the Southwest.

Common Health Problems

A number of health problems consistent with living in poverty are prevalent among American Indians. The incidence of tuberculosis, malnutrition, and communicable diseases, and maternal and infant mortality rates are higher than in the majority population.

High rates of suicide in young persons and alcoholism are two major health problems. They are thought to result partially from living in poverty and the conflict which exists between the values of the American Indian and the majority culture. The cause of a high incidence of diabetes mellitus, hypertension, and gallbladder disease among the American Indian is uncertain. Both genetic and environmental factors are being considered.

ORIENTAL CULTURE

The beliefs and practices of the Oriental culture originated in the countries of eastern Asia. The countries include China, Japan, Korea, Vietnam, and the Philippine Islands. The subcultures of each of these countries are distinctive. However, there are some shared characteristics which will be discussed here.

For various historical reasons, the Chinese subculture has had a greater influence than any other single country on the Oriental culture. Most Orientals in this country live in urban areas on either coast although some can be found in other parts of the nation.

The Oriental culture is generally influenced by an Eastern philosophy which is somewhat similar to the American Indian beliefs. The universe is believed to be composed of interacting entities. Energy for regulating the universe comes from the opposing forces of Yin and Yang. For harmony to exist, Yin and Yang must be in balance. Yin is the negative, dark, cold, and empty force. Yang is the positive, light, warm, and full force. When an imbalance exists, an increase in the opposite force is needed to counterbalance it and restore equilibrium.

The extended family and the individual's lineage or ancestry are generally important in the Oriental culture. Persons from several generations often live together, or at least in close proximity, and the family is revered as an institution. The father is usually the major figure in the family. The welfare of the family is generally valued above the individual and children are reared according to their sex and place of birth in the family line. This pattern results in each person having a feeling of commitment and belonging to the family. However, the relationships are not primarily emotional as is characteristic of some other cultures. A strong sense of self-respect and the importance of self-control to avoid personal and family disgrace are considered to be important values. Sharing among family members and respect for age are also characteristic of the Oriental culture.

Folk Medicine Beliefs and Practices

Consistent with the Eastern philosophy of balance, health is believed to result from equilibrium between the opposing forces of Yin and Yang. Illness occurs when the balance is not present. Health care is oriented toward maintaining or reestablishing the necessary balance. Meditation, diet, herbalism, acumassage, acupressure, acupuncture, and spiritual healing are important in Oriental folk medicine.

Meditation is used to prevent or control strong emotional feelings. It is believed that it retains or restores emotional balance between Yin and Yang.

Dietary practices are based on the classification of foods as Yin (cold) and Yang (hot) but the cold and hot designations do not necessarily relate to the temperature of the food. A healthy diet consists of a mixture of Yin and Yang foods, such as meat and vegetables. Excesses of any type of food are discouraged. A Yin illness is treated with Yang foods and a Yang illness is treated with Yin foods. For instance, an infection, a Yang illness, is treated with a Yin food, such as melon. A Yin disease, such as cancer, is treated with Yang foods, such as meat or chicken. The classification of Yin and Yang foods is traditional and passed down through the culture. As far as is known, there is no complete listing recorded in writing.

Herbs are used extensively for their various medicinal qualities. Many of them have been demonstrated to have a scientifically supported basis. An herbalist is an Oriental folk medicine practitioner who prescribes various combinations of herbs on the basis of his diagnosis. He uses the patient's symptoms and his observations of the person's physiological functioning as the basis for his diagnosis.

Acumassage, acupressure, and acupuncture are therapeutic techniques based on the premise of energy balance. Certain points on the body are located on the meridians or energy pathways. If the energy flow is out of balance, treatment of the pathway may be necessary to restore the energy equilibrium. Acumassage is a technique of manipulating points along the energy pathways. Acupressure is a technique for compressing the energy pathway points. Acupuncture is a technique in which fine needles are inserted into the body at energy pathway points. The purpose of acumassage, acupressure, and acupuncture is to restore the disturbed

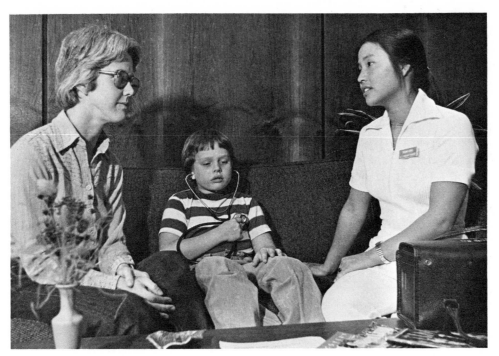

Figure 7-5 This Oriental nurse and her patients demonstrate that persons of differing cultures can learn to respect and appreciate each other's beliefs and values.

energy balance. The various Oriental subcultures have different names and techniques for these healing practices, but their purpose and general approaches are similar. In recent years these practices have been investigated and used more extensively in professional medicine in this country.

Spiritual healing is the use of psychic energies and auras to heal another person; and is generally associated with religious practices. Spiritual healing often has different names and techniques in the varying subcultures but all involve the transferring of healing energies from one person to another. The use of psychic energies in healing, usually without religious associations, is also being investigated in professional medicine in the United States.

Common Health Problems

The incidence of health problems associated with poverty are greater among Oriental persons than among the majority population. Tuberculosis, other communicable diseases, and malnutrition are prevalent. A lactose enzyme deficiency resulting in poor tolerance for milk and milk products is common among Orientals.

Suicide, especially among females, and various forms of mental illness occur more frequently among Orientals than among the majority population. It is felt that the conflict associated with the contrast between the traditional Oriental culture and the majority culture in this country is an important factor in emotional and mental illnesses among Orientals.

IMPLICATIONS FOR NURSING

Religious and cultural differences have implications for nursing since the patient and his behavior are affected by his religious and cultural background. The nurse needs to take the patient's background into account when collecting data, identifying nursing care needs, and planning for meeting them, if her care is to have maximum effectiveness. Care that is in conflict with the patient's values and practices will often be unacceptable to him. If he does accept it, the care may even be harmful since resulting feelings of guilt and of alienation from his religious and cultural group are likely to threaten his well-being.

At one time, religious and cultural beliefs and practices, especially of minority persons, were generally ignored or openly contradicted by health care practitioners. Such approaches often resulted in the person's refusal of care or only temporary adherence to the prescribed treatment. Also, ignoring or contradicting a person's religion or culture often had the effect of discouraging his return for follow-up or future professional health care. It is now believed preferable to incorporate factors from the patient's religious and cultural practices in health care whenever possible and when the practices are not considered harmful to his health.

For the nurse to provide nursing care that is consistent with the patient's religious and cultural background, she needs to be aware of the significance these influences have on people's lives. A good way for the nurse to become sensitive to the influence of religion and culture on the lives of others is to become conscious of their role in her own life. The nurse is encouraged to objectively examine her own beliefs, values, practices, and family experiences to become aware of religious and cultural influences in her personal life. As the nurse becomes more sensitive to the importance of these factors in her own life, an increasing awareness of her right to adhere to the beliefs and practices she wishes often occurs. Simultaneously, it usually becomes easier to acknowledge other people's rights to hold and practice their particular beliefs even when they are different from one's own.

A careful analysis of one's personal life can also help to identify one's biases. It is sometimes difficult to be aware of negative feelings about persons who have different beliefs. Or, if one is aware of negative feelings, the basis for the feelings may be unclear without careful self-examination.

After the nurse is aware of the significance of religious and cultural influences on people's lives, she needs to appreciate the differences in religions and cultures. Learning to appreciate these differences requires that the nurse make concerted and conscientious effort to study different religions and cultures. Studying factual information included in the literature that describes various religions and cultures is a good place to start.

The nurse should make an effort to learn as much as possible about the whole belief system of the religion or culture being studied. When isolated beliefs or practices are examined out of context, their significance is frequently difficult to understand. Prejudice, bias, fear, and discomfort can develop easily when misunderstanding exists. This may be a prime example of the old adage that a little bit of knowledge can be a dangerous thing.

A study of religion and culture requires an accepting nonjudgmental, and objective attitude. An approach that presumes one's own religion or culture as the best defeats appreciation of others. In every society, people learn, as part of their religion and culture, what is important and what is not, what is moral and what is wrong, and what behaviors are expected. While these concepts are important to all persons, judging people of other religions and cultures by one's own standards leads to failure and inappropriate conclusions in attempting to understand others.

A preoccupation with one's own culture that leads one to judge all but one's own as inferior is called *ethnocentrism*. A certain amount of ethnocentrism is necessary to the survival of a society. Without it, increasing personal conflicts and alienation could result. However, if one is studying other cultures, ethnocentrism defeats the purpose of investigation. The same can be said of religion.

To acquire an appreciation of religious and cultural differences requires that the nurse sincerely desire to understand how religions and cultures are distinctive. She then conscientiously observes and listens. Techniques that help in observing and listening have been discussed earlier in this text. They are important tools for studying different religions and cultures.

Many nurses serve a family, a neighborhood, or a community. They can acquire knowledge of religion and cultural differences as they develop skills in observing and listening during their visits. Nurses employed in schools, clinics, physicians' offices, hospitals, industries, and so on, are well-advised to visit the patient's homes whenever possible, and the neighborhoods whence their patients come.

As the nurse learns about different religions and cultures, discussion with patients, family members, clergymen, and others in the community can be helpful. Since some persons, especially those of minority religions and cultures, have often been belittled and subjected to ridicule and insults, they may be hesitant to discuss their beliefs and practices. The topic must be approached carefully. If the nurse is motivated by sincerity, respect, and concern for the individual, her attitude will generally convey this and the person will usually respond. On the other hand, if her motivation is mere curiosity and her attitude is one of condescension, she will likely receive little or no response.

Providing nursing care which is compatible with the patient's religious and cultural background requires further sensitivity on the part of the nurse. She has to be sensitive to the patient's individuality and demonstrate respect for him as a person. She can convey these attitudes unconsciously through her tone of voice, facial expression, the way she touches the patient, and her general approach.

The manner in which the nurse handles a patient's

personal belongings conveys her unspoken feelings. For example, the nurse who belittles or insists on removing an herb bag which is fastened to the patient's clothing or a religious medal worn around his neck is inconsiderate. Or, the nurse who places the patient's prayer book where he cannot reach it and who acts in a patronizing manner toward his prayer shawl tells the patient a great deal.

Incorporating the person's religious and cultural beliefs and practices in his health care requires effort. The following paragraphs describe some specific ways in which nurses and other health workers can accommodate the religious and cultural preferences of persons in their care.

The nurse should make it as easy as possible for the hospitalized patient to carry out his religious practices as long as they do not significantly disturb other patients. The nurse can adjust some routines to accommodate the patient's religious practices. Often she can delay the patient's meal easily if the patient wishes to fast before receiving communion. She can adjust the timing of personal hygiene measures to accommodate the visit of a clergyman. She may be able to offer a private area for the patient's use for religious rituals. This may be especially important when several persons are praying aloud or when singing is involved.

While the ill person who is confined at home generally has family members or friends who can assist with arranging for the clergyman's visits, this is not always the case. The community health nurse may initiate a discussion with the person about whether he would like a visit from his clergyman. If so, the nurse may contact the clergyman or ask someone else to do so.

In some instances, the patient may need the assistance of a respected family member, clergyman, or folk medicine practitioner to accept health care services with which he is unfamiliar. Acknowledging the role of the person's religious leader or folk medicine practitioner in his life can be an important way of building trust. If invited, clergymen or folk practitioners can work closely with professional health practitioners in the interest of the patient and his family. Such efforts can promote mutual understanding, respect, and cooperation.

Religious and cultural dietary practices of patients can often be accommodated by health practitioners. Dietary departments in many hospitals supply patients with meals consistent with special diet practices. Families may be encouraged to bring food from home for patients with particular preferences when this practice does not violate hospital policy. Teaching patients and families about therapeutic diets can also be done within the framework of particular religious and cultural practices.

While the nurse is encouraged to provide an explanation of her care for all individuals, she may find that persons of some cultural backgrounds will tend to need more detailed explanations than others. She may also find persons from some cultures initially tend to be more eager to participate in nursing care planning than others. It should be remembered that explanations and participation are perceived differently in varying cultures. The nurse needs to adjust her approaches to the individual patient.

The nurse often must take into consideration the cultural role of the person in the family who makes most of the important decisions. In some cultures, it is the husband or father while in others, it is the grandmother or other respected elder. To ignore this fact or to proceed with nursing care which is not approved by this person can result in conflict or ignoring what has been taught. The nurse should be certain this person is involved in the nursing care planning.

In cultures where the family is of greater significance than the individual, the nurse must be aware that expensive and lengthy health care measures may not be implemented if they are interpreted to be inconsistent with the good of the family. She may need to make certain that the well-being of the entire family is considered in these situations.

For persons whose cultural backgrounds place little importance on the future, health care which focuses on prevention and early detection of illness may require special emphasis. For example, it may be more important for the nurse to stress the short-range effects of the treatment of asymptomatic hypertension for some patients than to focus on the long-range care.

The combination of folk medicine and professional medicine is considered beneficial for some persons. Some health care practitioners who deal with persons who use folk medicine extensively are adapting health care measures so that they are not in conflict with the individual's beliefs and are still scientifically sound. For instance, there are numerous folk remedies containing herbs and plants which are therapeutic. Many commercial medications include the same basic ingredients. The person may prefer to use the folk remedies and he may do so. However, it is important for the professional practitioner to know what substances the person is taking to avoid overdoses or incompatibility when both traditional remedies and prescribed drugs are being used simultaneously. Only when the person feels he will not be ridiculed is he likely to indicate that he is receiving both types of health care at once.

Accommodations for other cultural practices are being made in some health care facilities. For instance, adjustments are made in some hospitals to accommodate visits from extended family members. The family members can often be involved in the patient's care in ways that are significant to them and to the patient, such as bathing or feeding the patient.

Some persons of Oriental and Spanish-speaking cultures believe that the pores of a mother remain open after delivery for a period of time, usually 30 days. During this time it is believed harmful for the mother to take a tub bath or shower. Accommodations for sponge bathing are not difficult to provide for these individuals.

Those persons who believe that magic, hexes, and spells cause illness are frequently hesitant to reveal their beliefs for fear of being humiliated. However, they will often respond if they are asked if they know what made them sick or how they became sick, as long as the nurse is sincere and respectful and does not belittle their beliefs. This information is helpful in understanding the patient and in planning care that takes these beliefs into consideration. Such patients can often accept professional medical care along with folk medicine care. For example, persons who believe in imitative magic find a knife under the bed "to cut the pain" to be reassuring. The practice does not conflict with simultaneous use of professional pain relief measures. Such professional and folk medicine can often have a complementary effect.

When there is no known scientific basis for a folk remedy, the professional practitioner may consider it to have no therapeutic value, but it may be culturally important for the person to continue with the remedy. Experience has shown that when the nurse and other professional practitioners express their disapproval of folk practices, it generally does not cause the individual to stop believing in or using folk medicine. Rather, it merely causes him to become more secretive about his folk practices and alienates him further from the professional health care system. When a disparity between folk and professional medicine becomes obvious, it is usually preferable for the nurse to explain that professional medicine has a different basis and is practiced differently from folk medicine.

When an occasional folk remedy is felt to be harmful to the health of the individual, the professional practitioner may face a difficult situation. The question arises—To what extent has any person the right to change another's cultural practice? The question has produced much debate. Some scholars will say that just as we accept the right of man to his own religious beliefs, we must also accept the right of a man to other aspects of his culture. They would add that no one has a right to deliberately change the cultures of others.

Those who feel there is sometimes good reason for attempting to produce cultural change hold that it is justified *under certain circumstances*. They feel that individual rights are not violated when people are given accurate and sufficient knowledge concerning alternative behavior so that they can make an intelligent choice without coercion. This principle seems to be especially applicable in the field of health.

The nurse must keep in mind that health practices are a part of the overall culture and that changing them may have widespread implications for the individual. An accurate understanding of these implications is essential before such a change is encouraged. The nurse also needs to be prepared to put forth sufficient time and effort to provide the necessary support and reinforcement for the patient if a change in a health practice with a cultural basis is considered necessary.

There are times when some recommended health care measures may simply not be acceptable to the individual for religious or cultural reasons. Every effort should be made to be certain that the patient has a clear understanding of the factors involved and that the professional practitioner accurately perceives the specific objection. In some instances, satisfactory modifications or alternative measures can be developed. If not, the individual's right to refuse care should be respected.

CONCLUSION

This chapter has emphasized that religious and cultural practices and beliefs affect everyone's behavior. An understanding of an individual's religious and cultural background will assist the nurse to develop more acceptable and effective nursing care. It often requires extra time and ingenuity to integrate certain religious and cultural beliefs with professional medicine. Efforts to do so are consistent with nursing's commitment to respect the beliefs and practices of others while promoting their welfare and well-being.

SUPPLEMENTAL LIBRARY STUDY

1. The following articles are a series describing major religious practices adhered to by persons of various faiths:

Richards, Flora. "What They Believe and Why: Part 1. Roman Catholics, Jehovah Witnesses, and Christian Scientists."

Nursing Mirror and Midwives Journal, 144:65–66, April 14, 1977.

Richards, Flora. "What They Believe and Why: Part 2. The Jewish Faith." *Nursing Mirror and Midwives Journal,* 144:64, April 21, 1977.

Richards, Flora. "What They Believe and Why: Part 3. Muslims, Hindus, and Buddhists." *Nursing Mirror and Midwives Journal,* 144:67, April 28, 1977.

Can you discuss in your own words the basis for each of the practices described?

2. The following authors describe a chaplaincy program in a hospital:

Morris, Karen L. and Foerster, John D. "Team Work: Nurse and Chaplain." *American Journal of Nursing,* 72:2197–2199, December 1972.

In what specific ways do the authors indicate the nurse can assist the chaplain? How do they say the chaplain can assist the nurse? How can they both assist the patient with his spiritual needs in the hospital described?

3. The following article describes some of the folk beliefs and practices of Filipino-Americans which pertain to health:

McKenzie, Joan L. and Chrisman, Noel J. "Healing Herbs, Gods, and Magic: "Folk Health Beliefs Among Filipino-Americans." *Nursing Outlook,* 25:326–329, May 1977.

What is the meaning of the three folk medicine practices of flushing, heating, and protecting? What is the significance of eye contact to the Filipino person, as described by the authors?

4. This chapter has focused primarily on the differences in beliefs and practices as they pertain to patients. Nurses are also influenced by their religious and cultural backgrounds. The following articles describe two studies conducted on nurses from different cultures:

Bhanumathi, Patinhara Pokkiarath. "Nurses' Conceptions of 'Sick Role' and 'Good Patient' Behaviour: A Cross-Cultural Comparison." *International Nursing Review,* 24:20–24, January/February 1977.

Davitz, Lois J., et al. "Suffering As Viewed In Six Different Cultures." *American Journal of Nursing,* 76:1296–1297, August 1976.

How did the nurses from various cultures differ in their perceptions of pain? How did the nurses' expectations of patients differ? What are some of the ways the authors indicate these differences influence nursing care? Have you considered how your perception of pain and expectations of patients influence your nursing care?

5. It will be noted that terms which refer to a specific religion or culture were not defined in the glossary of this chapter.

Instead, as part of your study, define this sampling of religious and cultural terms:

Religion	*Curandero*
Rosh Hashanah	Medicine man
Judaism	Yin
Christianity	Yang
Kosher	Supernatural
Atheist	Spiritualist
Minister	Rootwork
Priest	Hex
Rabbi	Herbs
Mal ojo	Herbalist
Caida de la mollera	Spiritual healing

8

BEHAVIORAL OBJECTIVES

When content in this chapter has been mastered, the student will be able to

Define the terms appearing in the glossary.

List five principles of learning and give an example that illustrates the use of each.

Describe the general objective of health teaching.

Describe five conditions which promote learning.

State two assumptions upon which behavior modification is based.

Describe several intervention measures that promote behavior modification.

Discuss at least three objections that some people express concerning the use of behavior modification and describe how its advocates answer these objections.

The Nurse's Role in Teaching and Behavior Modification

GLOSSARY

Affective Learning: The acquiring of new attitudes, values, and appreciations.

Aversive Stimulation: The use of a painful or unpleasant event to modify behavior.

Behavior Modification: A teaching technique which is based on operant conditioning and used to change behavior.

Cognitive Learning: The acquiring of new understandings.

Learn: To add to one's store of knowledge; to have one's behavior change as the result of an experience.

Motivation: The desire to act.

Motor Learning: The acquiring of new physical skills.

Operant Theory of Learning: A theory that holds that certain behavior tends to reinforce learning. Synonym for reinforcement theory.

Readiness: Being able or being in due condition to respond only in certain ways.

Reinforcement Theory: A theory that holds that certain behavior tends to reinforce learning. Synonym for operant theory of learning.

Teach: To assist another to learn; to impart knowledge.

INTRODUCTION

From the beginning, nurses recognized the importance of health teaching. Through the years, promoting health through teaching and helping persons develop healthful habits of daily living have grown in significance so that today they are preeminent parts of nursing.

Various influences have increased the nurse's concern with helping people to follow healthful life-styles. For example, the consumer of health services has become more knowledgeable about his health. With this awareness, he has come to demand more information about attaining and maintaining well-being. Also, with the increase in longevity and in the incidence of chronic diseases, teaching has become especially important in promoting maximum well-being for the chronically ill and aged. Research, too, has promoted the position of teaching in nursing. Studies have shown that preoperative teaching and encouragement have resulted in fewer complications, less need for pain relievers, and less anxiety during the postoperative period.

When greater emphasis was placed on patients assuming self-care activities, the nurse's role as a promoter of health increased steadily. At one time, patients had almost everything done for them by the nurse. Now nurses are helping patients to learn to do as much as possible for themselves. As the values of increased activity and decreased bed rest have been noted, authorities in physical medicine and rehabilitation have concluded that too much tender loving care is harmful.

This text has emphasized the importance of including the patient in planning his health care and respecting his right to make decisions concerning his life. When the patient is taught and learns alternative behaviors and their consequences, he can then make more intelligent decisions. There is no place in nursing for coercing persons or demanding that they do as they are told. Teaching depends on patient participation as well as imparting knowledge to help him understand the options available to him and to help him overcome attitudes that may stand in the way of changing behavior, if change is his desire.

As with other types of nursing care, the nursing process is used to determine, plan, and implement teaching. By gathering and assessing data on the person to be taught, the nurse determines areas in which teaching is indicated. Next, she prepares a teaching plan with the patient. The teaching plan is then put into action.

PRINCIPLES OF LEARNING AND IMPLICATIONS FOR TEACHING

To *learn* is to add to one's knowledge, the word knowledge being used here in its broadest sense. To *teach* is to help someone to learn. Learning is said to have occurred when an experience changes the learner's behavior. This change may be in certain understandings the learner has gained, which is called *cognitive learning*. Or it may occur in physical skills he has acquired, which is called *motor learning;* or in attitudes, values, and appreciations, which is called *affective learning*. When a person provides an experience that results in a change in the learner's behavior, that person has taught and may be called the teacher.

Innumerable opportunities exist for teaching in the practice of nursing. There are times when the nurse plans and participates in formal teaching of an individual or a group of persons. But most often, teaching in nursing occurs spontaneously and informally, such as when the nurse teaches oral hygiene or care of the skin during the bathing procedure.

While teaching may often occur on the spur of the moment, it is still recommended that teaching follow a definite plan. If one teaches haphazardly and without organization or planning, one cannot attain success except by sheer accident.

The nurse cannot afford to overlook the fact that many patients learn from observing the examples she sets. Thus, the nurse visiting in a home is often teaching when the family observes her covering her mouth and nose, should she sneeze or cough, and washing her hands before beginning her work. On the other hand, the nurse in the clinic is teaching negatively if she displays obvious symptoms of an upper respiratory infection while advising a mother to keep her children at home when they have colds. In teaching, actions and words must be consistent.

How do we learn? Educational psychologists have explored this question for years, and while differences of opinions on certain aspects exist, there is general agreement on some principles that guide the learning process. Teaching depends on or is guided by principles of learning.

The goal of the learner directs his learning efforts as he strives for a consequence he wishes to attain. When learning is in progress, the learner is attempting to satisfy what he sees as his need. For example, a child may desire a cookie that is in a jar outside of his reach; to satisfy this desire, he must learn how to reach the jar. A college football star can remain on the team if his scholastic average is above a certain rating; to attain his goal, he must do well in classes. A bride wishes to please her husband by serving delicious meals; to achieve her wish, she learns to cook.

Assume that a nurse wishes to teach a mother the care of her newborn infant. Most new mothers are excited about caring for their babies, and, although they may be somewhat apprehensive, they recognize the need and have the desire to learn. However, often an individual's goals cannot be defined clearly, and in some cases the person may even attempt to conceal them. Consider a patient who may not seem to be interested in doing certain things for himself or in learning self-care activities. Although he may never admit it, his real goal could be to remain dependent if he has learned to find satisfaction in having things done for him, or continuing in a state of "ill health" helps him remain away from an unsatisfactory work situation.

This concept concerning the goal or need in learning has implications for the teacher. The focus is on the learner's goals, not the teacher's. The goal of the learner may not always be easy to discern, but it is important for the teacher to attempt to identify it. For instance, if the nurse wishes to teach a patient measures that will promote normal elimination so that his daily use of laxatives will not be necessary, her efforts will be in vain unless the patient feels he has a need for the teaching. Therefore, it is important for the nurse to discern the patient's goal or help him to develop learning goals that have personal meaning when she begins her teaching program.

Every person has certain capabilities and limitations that determine or set boundaries for what he can do. One aspect of this is what psychologists refer to as *readiness*. Readiness is influenced by many factors, some of the more common ones of which are discussed here.

The stage of illness the patient is experiencing will influence his readiness to learn. A patient who has just learned that he has diabetes is not ready to be taught how to administer his insulin until he has accepted his diagnosis and recognizes the importance of taking insulin (Fig. 8–1). Also, the acutely ill patient is rarely ready for participation in a teaching program.

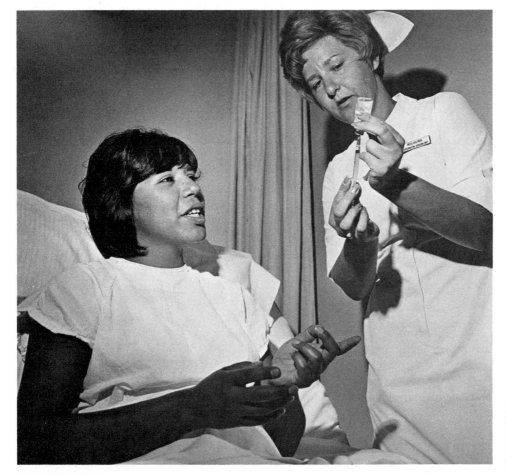

Figure 8–1 Instruction is given to the patient who will be managing at home. This patient is learning how to prepare and give herself an injection.

An individual's intellectual capacity will affect his ability to learn. If he is well-endowed and if he puts his inheritance to good use, the learner can assimilate much in little time. The person who is limited may never learn as much and often needs to spend considerable time in achieving what he does learn.

The degree to which an individual has matured physically and emotionally will influence his readiness for learning. For example, most children learn to walk between the ages of 12 to 16 months; prior to this period, their musculoneurological maturity is insufficient to permit them to learn to walk, and attempts to teach them to do so result in failure.

Physical maturity is easier to determine than emotional maturity, since the former can be judged, to a large extent, in relation to the individual's chronological age. Estimating emotional maturity is a different matter, and simply judging it on the basis of chronological age sometimes leads to false conclusions. The young adult presently dependent on a wheelchair may have sufficient physical maturity to have learned the skills of a mechanic, but he may not demonstrate sufficient emotional maturity to see why he should bother with the rehabilitation that eventually will give him the ability to earn his own living.

An individual's previous experiences will affect the learning process. Certain cultures believe that a person is not ill unless he feels and looks ill. Assume that it has been found on a routine examination that a person reared in such a culture has pulmonary tuberculosis and positive sputum but that the disease has not progressed to the point that the patient feels and looks sick. Unless a nurse knows and understands what this patient has learned from his culture, it may be difficult or even impossible to teach him to care for himself in order that he may regain health and refrain from exposing his family and friends to the disease.

Consider the person who practices poor oral hygiene because he has learned an attitude of indifference. As he stated it, "My father never went to a dentist in his life. Anyway, I've never heard of anyone who died because he lost his teeth." This attitude can be expected to block learning of oral hygiene.

Chapter 7 discussed cultural change and pointed out suggestions to promote attitudinal change, when in the eyes of health practitioners, change seems desirable. But, as indicated, care must be exercised. How much *right* do we have to change a person's choice in the way he wishes to live or die? When a patient's health becomes a menace to others, certain legal implications exist that may involve forcing a patient to do something. States have laws requiring the treatment of persons with active pulmonary tuberculosis who have contact with others because of the communicable implications of disease. But this force is different from teaching that offers persons alternatives to present behavior.

A person's previous educational experiences play a vital role in his learning. A patient who is a college graduate with a major in human physiology may be ready for information that a patient who is also a college graduate but has a major in English literature may be in no position to understand. Or, consider teaching two patients how to irrigate their wounds, one is a college graduate, the other has reached only the tenth grade. Despite the difference in their educational experiences, and other things being equal, the nurse may teach both in a very similar manner. The amount of formal education that an individual has does not necessarily indicate his ability to learn; some very intelligent people have not had educational opportunities. But the nature of either a formal education or self-teaching to which an individual has been exposed can influence his readiness for learning.

Some people may find security in having the goal of *not* knowing something. Thus, a patient's apparent lack of interest in learning about his illness may be the result of the patient's experiencing a sense of security in not knowing. He may be refusing or may not be able to recognize a reality that is stressful to him.

Learning in one situation can prepare a learner for a new situation when he recognizes similarities between the two. Psychologists have debated transfer of learning for many years. Research has proven that at least some long-held theories were incorrect. For example, investigation showed that although concentration is important in the study of Greek, one's power of concentration is not necessarily improved by studying Greek. However, there are situations that are considered favorable for learning transfer. Assume that a nurse is caring for a patient with an amputation who has not lived with or known anyone who has had an amputation. The teaching program for this patient might be quite different from one used for a patient whose father also had an amputation. In the latter instance, much learning could be transferred.

Consider an example of learning through error. A child began vomiting, had a low-grade fever, and complained of generalized abdominal discomfort. The mother sought medical attention. It so happened that she had had similar symptoms when she was a college student and cared for herself, thinking she had the flu.

When she eventually saw a physician, she learned she had appendicitis and emergency surgery was necessary. The mother learned from her illness how *not* to respond to symptoms she now observed in her child. Inappropriate behavior in one situation led to appropriate behavior in another similar situation.

Learning from previous experiences that is transferred to new situations requires recognizing relationships between the old and the new situations. A student is about to learn how to do a venipuncture (entering a vein with a needle). In previous classes, she has learned how to administer a medication intramuscularly. By being aware of a relationship between intramuscular injections and venipunctures, she can transfer learning. The process begins by directing attention to the past experience of administering an intramuscular injection. Then, relating the past situation to the present one, she notes that there are similarities between the two techniques. Then the *differences* are taught. Thus, the known services as the springboard for entry into the unknown.

When behavior changes during learning, the learner evaluates the consequences of his behavior by deciding that the new behavior satisfies or thwarts attainment of his goals. If it is satisfying, he will be motivated to learn more. Evaluation of the response usually is an unconscious experience; that is, the learner rarely expresses this response nor is he consciously aware of it. The student in nursing usually feels satisfaction and pleasure after learning how to give an injection. However, she may be quite unaware of having evaluated her response.

If the learner decides that his new response is unsatisfactory, one of two things is likely to occur. The learner either will try again and modify his response until he experiences satisfaction, or he may feel thwarted by the unsatisfactory results and become frustrated and discouraged. He may give up further trying, at least temporarily if not permanently.

Assume that a nurse is teaching a patient to use crutches. On his first try he may use the crutches sufficiently well to find satisfaction, even though his skill is far from perfect. He is encouraged to use the crutches again at the earliest opportunity. A second person learning crutch-walking may find little to be happy about in his early trials and become frustrated, but he eagerly attempts it again, until he does learn to use them with satisfaction. But a third patient, unable to use crutches with any success on his first try, becomes frustrated, stating that he is perfectly happy using a wheelchair and refuses further practice. The first patient experienced sufficient satisfaction to be

stimulated to further learning; the second was dissatisfied but the dissatisfaction became a challenge to try again; and the third was dissatisfied, frustrated, and willing to give up.

Motivation promotes learning. *Motivation* is the desire to act. Motivation comes from within the individual and is essential for learning to occur. External incentives can stimulate motivation. Some persons have sufficient motivation for learning. Others may need incentives provided by the nurse to stimulate their motivation to learn.

Readiness for learning is a prime factor in the motivating process. Learning is generally stimulated when the educational offering is challenging but not beyond the learner's ability to comprehend. Respect for the learner's previous experiences and building on them tend to stimulate interest and promote learning.

The experience of satisfaction when learning occurs promotes additional learning. Most people enjoy success, and one success encourages another. When the teacher recognizes achievement with a smile and a word of praise, the learner generally responds favorably and continues to learn more. Psychologists call this encouragement process the *reinforcement* or *operant theory of learning*. It is used in behavior modification which will be discussed later in this chapter.

When learning has not been accomplished and the learner's goal is thwarted, the teacher will wish to take another look at the person and at the teaching plan. The setting of goals and the readiness of the learner may require further study, and possible adaptation in the teaching program can be made. Repeated attempts to teach a particular thing may prove motivating provided learning can be expected to succeed on subsequent tries. Possibly failure can be turned to success by improving the conditions for learning. The patient's failure to inject himself successfully may be turned to success when the nurse suggests that the patient try it while sitting on a firm chair rather than on the edge of a bed. Perhaps too much is being taught too fast, and the learner is not experiencing satisfaction by having mastered one thing at a time. Perhaps the goals were unrealistic.

Sometimes, pointing out small degrees of success and giving the learner praise and encouragement help to stimulate him to further learning. It is safer to begin with small segments of relatively easy teaching so that the learner may enjoy satisfaction. Then, the amount and the speed can be geared to the learner's ability and interest.

Additional factors that tend to motivate the learner

will be discussed in the section entitled, "Conditions That Promote Learning."

TEACHING OBJECTIVES, CONTENT, AND EVALUATION

The objective of health teaching is to help a person to attain and maintain well-being. While this broad objective remains, a narrower objective is more useful for specific teaching situations.

Learning has occurred when behavior changes. Therefore, it is best to state an objective of teaching in behavioral terms so that the nurse and the patient can determine learning progress more accurately. Behaviorally stated objectives were discussed in more detail in Chapter 4.

Assume that a nurse wishes to assist a patient who has had a heart attack to achieve maximum functioning. As a first step, the nurse will probably discuss the patient with his physician. She will wish to become acquainted with the physician's philosophy of care for the patient, as well as with the specific medical regimen. She learns that a low-cholesterol diet has been prescribed. Now she can state an objective of teaching more specifically and in behavioral terms. The objective is for the patient to select and adhere to a diet low in cholesterol.

Once an objective has been defined, the nurse will determine content; that is, she will acquire information necessary for the patient to know in order to select and eat the prescribed diet. Answers to the following questions will help the nurse to know what content to include in her teaching program. Why is the diet advised? What do words used in a description of the diet mean, such as cholesterol and specifically *low* cholesterol? What is the relationship between the patient's illness and the diet being recommended? Which kinds of food are advised and which are not? What low cholesterol menus are appetizing to the patient and still nutritious? How should the foods be prepared? How can the patient adapt his eating habits and still eat away from home with comfort and ease?

While the nurse establishes objectives of the teaching program and selects content, she will wish to keep the principles described in the learning process in mind. As she does, answers to additional questions will become pertinent content as she individualizes her teaching for each patient or each group of patients. Consider the patient in the previous example. What attitudes does he have about eating and diet restrictions? Do cultural factors in his background have influence on content? If he is a married man, should his wife be included in his teaching program? If so, what adaptations in the content and objectives may be necessary when she also becomes a learner in the situation?

The teaching program can be evaluated when the nurse observes the extent to which the patient follows his diet. If he follows it, the learning goals have been achieved. If he does not, the nurse will then attempt to identify areas where he is unsuccessful and take another look at her teaching program. Thus, if the patient follows his diet except when eating out, there are several possibilities the nurse should investigate. Possibly the patient did not understand (learn) how to adapt his diet when eating away from home. Perhaps, he did not learn that "at all times" meant at those times when he ate away from home also. Or his attitude may be one of 'living it up" while socializing. In the latter instance, the patient may not be sufficiently impressed with the possible consequences of deviating from the diet. Or, he may be denying them.

To attempt to teach without objectives is like buying an airline ticket without a destination. Even in informal teaching, an objective is important in order to plan and execute a successful teaching program. Once objectives are stated, the content and an evaluation plan can be developed.

It is important to record the progress the patient makes during the teaching program, just as it is necessary to record other nursing care activities that have been carried out. If this is not done, there is the possibility that the teaching started by one nurse may never be completed, or that the patient may be taught the same thing by a succession of different personnel—both possibilities irritating to the patient.

CONDITIONS THAT PROMOTE LEARNING

Learning can occur under adverse conditions, but ideally the environment should help stimulate interest in learning. The following environmental factors should be considered.

Establishing Satisfactory Helping Relationships

Teaching can be enhanced when the nurse and the learner have a warm and accepting relationship. The feeling, tone, and attitude of the person teaching are often more important than many other environmental considerations. If the learner senses that the teacher is interested in him and trying to help him, he will be more receptive and stimulated. However, if he senses urgency or a superior or condescending attitude, the nurse's teaching will have little or no effect.

Providing a Comfortable Environment

The learner as well as the nurse should be comfortable. Suitable chairs, adequate lighting, and good venilation add to the comfort. Privacy is desirable.

Using Teaching Aids

Many health agencies have audiovisual aids available for teaching. In some instances, the agency allows the use of their equipment outside of the agency, for example, when the nurse is teaching a neighborhood or community group. These aids include filmstrips and slides. Television and radio often offer good teaching programs to assist nurses in their teaching programs.

Many agencies have a variety of teaching aids. One type is illustrated in Figure 8–2. Typical voluntary agencies that offer literature the nurse will often find helpful are American Cancer Society, American Heart Association, Kenny Rehabilitation Institute, and the American Foundation for the Blind.

The U.S. Government Printing Office is the source of a large variety of teaching material. State and local governmental agencies also have material available for teaching purposes.

Libraries are another good source of teaching aids. They often have not only books, pamphlets, and periodicals, but also films, slides, and posters for borrowing.

Many companies with health-related products have charts, booklets, and similar material that can be used in teaching programs. Although such material is sometimes prepared primarily to aid in promoting the company's product, most of it is helpful when used judiciously.

Equipment for demonstrations is a helpful teaching aid. For example, if the nurse wishes to teach a mother how to bathe her newborn baby, she should have equipment similar to that which the mother may use at home to demonstrate the procedure.

Programmed instruction has become popular as an aid to teaching. The program offers information and periodically quizzes the learner. If the learner answers questions correctly, he goes on with the program. If he answers incorrectly, he is given additional information

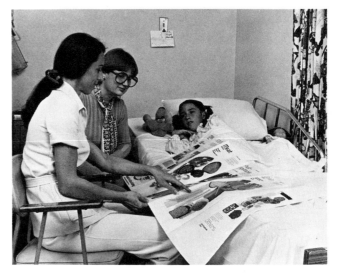

Figure 8–2 The nurse is teaching the essentials of a well-balanced diet with the mother of a child convalescing from a respiratory tract infection. Note the illustrative material the nurse is using with apparent effectiveness in this situation.

before he proceeds. Some of the programmed instruction available on the market can be appropriately used for patient teaching.

Being Free from Distractions

A distracted person rarely is able to utilize learning opportunities to a maximum. Teaching a hospitalized patient during visiting hours can hardly be expected to be beneficial when the patient may have visitors waiting for him. The same is true if he knows that he is to be called to the x-ray department at any moment.

Outside the hospital setting, this principle also holds true. For instance, the housewife who is coping with immediate domestic problems is not able to concentrate on learning.

Using Various Teaching Methods

The stimulating teacher arouses the person's desire to learn when she uses a variety of appropriate methods in an interesting and skillful way. Some settings may limit variety of methods, but almost always, the imaginative nurse can find ways to supplement the spoken word. Methods include the use of audiovisual aids, printed materials, charts, graphs, demonstrations, and so on. Even using the nurse's freehand sketches can make the material come alive. Teaching groups rather than only individuals adds variety. Including a patient with a particular experience as a teacher is often interesting to a group. Using resource people is another method. The nutritionist, for instance, can be included in certain parts of a program designed to teach patients who require special diets. Puppets have been used effectively with children. Using a variety of methods tends to stimulate interest and relieve the monotony of using only "teaching by telling," an approach that sometimes tends to focus more on the nurse than on the patient.

Most persons will agree readily that whatever teaching method is used, the teacher should have her instruction organized. It has been said that learning and bewilderment may differ only in terms of organization. However, organization does not mean rigidity. Flexibility in teaching methods to capture the enthusiasm of the learner is as essential as organization.

DESCRIPTION OF BEHAVIOR MODIFICATION

Behavioral modification is a teaching technique for dealing with behavioral problems of humans. It helps persons modify behavior that stands in the way of well-being to behavior that promotes health.

Teaching and behavior modification are not in conflict. Rather, principles of teaching and learning remain relevant when one uses the technique of behavior modification. Thus, in order to be successful, the person who wishes to change his behavior should have honest, complete, and accurate information about techniques to be used and why behavior modification may be a useful technique. This information can be shared while using the principles and techniques of teaching described earlier in this chapter.

The work of B. F. Skinner, a psychologist who developed the theory of operant conditioning, is the basis for behavior modification. It was first used in this country in hospitals for the mentally ill to help patients change socially undesirable behavior. However, it is now used in many settings, including industry, schools, clinics, home teaching programs, and hospitals, where acutely ill patients receive care.

Behavior modification is based on two assumptions. One is that human behavior is learned, the good as well as the bad. One learns to talk, walk, read, enjoy, socialize, smoke, overeat, and abuse drugs. Habits one uses in the course of living are learned forms of behavior.

A second assumption is that human behavior can be modified. If one learns a particular way of behaving,

one can also learn to change or modify that behavior.

One way to modify behavior is to eliminate the behavior that stands in the way of well-being. Smoking cigarettes has been linked with various types of lung pathology. Assume that a cigarette smoker has developed early signs of emphysema, a respiratory condition that interferes with the proper exchange of oxygen and carbon dioxide in the alveoli of the lungs and which is aggravated by smoking. The person's behavior, smoking, can often be eliminated by using techniques of behavior modification.

Human behavior can be modified also by strengthening behavior that is conducive to well-being. Assume that the cigarette smoker has stopped smoking recently after many years of heavy cigarette use. Behavior modification techniques can be used to strengthen his new habit of *not* smoking so that he will be less tempted to slip back to his old ways of behaving. This will be discussed in more detail later in this chapter.

As with other types of nursing care, the nursing process is observed when behavior modification techniques are used. Data gathering is used to learn to know the person. What is his way of behaving in everyday life? Which of his behaviors are related to his present or to potential health problems? What is his age, educational and occupational background?

It is best when behaviors are described as specifically as possible rather than in global terms. Assume that a nurse is caring for a person who is overweight. Here are some data about specific behaviors which she will wish to gather: the person consumes about 3,000 calories daily; his diet is proportionately high in carbohydrate content; he eats three meals a day and snacks most afternoons and every evening; his usual snacks are peanuts, pretzels, and candy; he does no daily exercising; he weighs 73.85 kg. or 198 pounds; and he wishes to lose weight.

The nurse then assesses by selecting standards to identify the person's strengths and problem areas. The standards are determined from a knowledge of what behaviors are conducive to well-being and what behaviors stand in the way of well-being.

The overweight person described above has a heart disease, and from her knowledge, the nurse knows that excess weight is aggravating the heart's ability to function at its best potential. The nurse determined that the person was 10.2 kg. or 30 pounds overweight when she compared his present weight with that which is recommended for persons of his physical stature and age. She also assesses that the person is concerned about being overweight and is motivated to do something about it. In this case, his attitude is identified as a strength when the nurse plans his care.

A plan for behavior modification is then developed with the cooperation of the person who wishes to change his behavior, and specific objectives of the program are defined. The plan will describe intervention measures that are intended to help the person modify his behavior.

For the overweight person, the objective will be to lose .373 kg. or 1 pound of weight each week for about 30 weeks. From her knowledge of nutrition, the nurse recognizes that for this person, a well-balanced diet of 2,000 calories daily will maintain his weight. In order to lose weight, he must consume fewer than 2,000 calories. She realizes that too rapid weight loss using crash and fad diets will not promote health. A well-balanced diet containing 1,500 calories each day will be used. This means that in a week's time, this person's caloric intake will be 3,500 calories less than he requires to maintain his weight and this number of calories is equivalent to approximately .373 kg. or 1 pound of weight. The plan also includes changing other behavior, such as eliminating snacking with high-caloric foods, eating a diet with proportionately fewer carbohydrates, including some exercise in his daily living, and so on. The final step is to put the plan into action.

INTERVENTION MEASURES THAT PROMOTE BEHAVIOR MODIFICATION

A primary requisite for promoting behavior modification is that the person be involved, just as is true of all types of nursing care. When he is not aware of behavior that interferes with well-being and has not helped develop the plan and objectives for behavior modification, the plan has little chance of succeeding. Involving the person in such a program has important ethical implications also, as will be discussed later in this chapter.

Behavior modification requires that desirable behavior be reinforced and undesirable behavior be ignored. A common tendency is to call attention to undesirable behaviors. Reprimanding is often used. For example, the person who stopped smoking had been harassed by friends and family each time he lit a cigarette. Ironically, people rarely comment about change in behavior when a person cuts down and finally stops smoking. The same observation has been reported by persons who were overeating, failing to follow thera-

peutic regimens, neglecting good habits of personal hygiene, and so on. In behavior modification programs, those behaviors which the nurse and her patient are attempting to increase are reinforced by rewards. The theory is that behavior which is rewarded will be repeated and strengthened while behavior which is ignored will decrease in frequency and will finally be eliminated.

Authorities state that any reinforcement for desirable behavior is best when it is administered consistently, immediately after the desired behavior has occurred, and with honesty and sincerity. The person who is attempting to lose weight is praised immediately and sincerely each time the scale indicates a weight loss. Reinforcement is not postponed until the final objective is reached; nor is attention called to backsliding with undesirable behavior when it occurs.

Reinforcements by using rewards for desirable behavior are varied. In hospitals for the mentally ill, reinforcements often include tokens for desired behavior that can be "spent" for extra privileges, such as additional time for watching television, listening to the radio, and visiting with friends and family members. Rewards of extra privileges have also been found effective in helping mentally retarded children work at academic tasks. Placing gold stars on a chart has been used to reinforce desired behavior in the classroom when the student has completed homework, done well in an examination, been prompt for classes, and so on. Being able to watch a graph that shows progress, such as when a person is working to lose weight, has been an effective reward for many persons. A person who seeks others with whom to socialize will respond to extra time a nurse spends chatting with him as a reward for desirable behavior. Verbal praise given in sincerity and honesty is an effective reward for many persons.

Self-reward has been used in certain instances. The person who stopped smoking reinforces his behavior by using money he is not spending on cigarettes to buy something that he would enjoy. Figure 8–3 illustrates a group identifying other ways to reward themselves for stopping smoking. A person who has lost weight rewards himself by purchasing a new wardrobe.

Some authorities describe the use of what some call punishment as an intervention measure in behavior modification. A painful or unpleasant event used to modify behavior is usually called *aversive stimulation*. For example, the mother uses aversive stimulation when she spanks her youngster who is hitting and biting another child.

It has been observed by some that the use of aversive

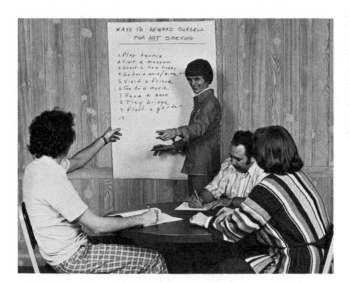

Figure 8-3 This group has been using behavior modification techniques to stop smoking. They are listing various ways in which they can reward themselves to reinforce their new habit of not smoking.

stimulation tends to interfere with the helping relationship, and this may suppress rather than modify behavior. Also, most persons find aversive stimulation, such as spanking, distasteful to use. However, those who describe its use recommend that it be combined with positive reinforcements, such as rewards or tokens for desired behavior.

When a youngster is observed to be hurting another with hitting and biting as described above, another approach is to hold the child so that he cannot touch the one he is attacking. This is followed by involving the child in activity he enjoys, such as playing with a ball, and he is praised for play that does not hurt others. Restraining the child is a type of aversive stimulation. But the intervention measure of restraint is accompanied by praise when the child is rewarded for desired behavior. Aversive stimulation used in this manner becomes more acceptable intervention for most persons. Some smoke cessation programs use aversive stimulation, such as the application of a small electrical shock each time the person lights a cigarette. Good results have been reported by some people. However, the shock is accompanied by praise when smoking is stopped and the person also has agreed to the use of shock as a means of reaching his goal.

The following example describes how behavior modification was used in a nursing situation. The patient wished to eat without assistance so that he could become independent but frustration thwarted his efforts. Note that the first few sentences imply data gathering and assessment although the words are not used. A plan with the objective of increasing self-feeding was devised with the patient to modify behavior and intervention measures that included selective reinforcements were used. The patient was involved during the process.

Mr. Y was an elderly stroke patient who experienced difficulty feeding himself. After many difficulties and failures, he gave up trying. His nurse sat down with him and worked out a treatment plan to increase self-feeding behavior. She needed a unit of eating behavior that was much more precise than the general statement, "he does not feed himself." She chose as the movement cycle the mouthful, defined as loading a fork or spoon, moving it to the mouth, unloading it, and returning it to the food or the table. It was now possible to specify how much or little self-feeding Mr. Y accomplished. For two meals the nurse counted the number of movement cycles carried out by the patient. That gave the baseline, or starting point, for the efforts at changing his self-feeding behavior, which in this case was zero. The nurse also determined that Mr. Y was capable of feeding himself, even though it was a bit arduous for him. She then worked out a treatment plan with him involving the use of reinforcers made contingent upon the target behavior, self-feeding. She chose perhaps the most natural and available of reinforcers in that situation, the mouthful. Each time he took a mouthful, she would help him with a mouthful. In subsequent meals, she reduced the reinforcement schedule. She expected him to take an increasing number of mouthfuls for each mouthful she delivered. Figure 8-4 shows what happened.*

ETHICAL CONSIDERATIONS AND BEHAVIOR MODIFICATION

There are those who believe that behavior modification coerces persons to do what they do not wish to do. An ethical issue is involved, they contend, because behavior modification manipulates people. As was pointed out earlier, the person should be involved and agree with the plan and objectives of care before proceeding with behavior modification. He should not become someone to manipulate but one working cooperatively for goals he wishes to reach. This basic approach of involving the person limits threats to personal freedom and infringement on human rights.

---

*Berni, Rosemarian and Fordyce, Wilbert E. *Behavior Modification and the Nursing Process.* Edition 2. The C. V. Mosby Company, St. Louis, 1977, pp. 27-28.

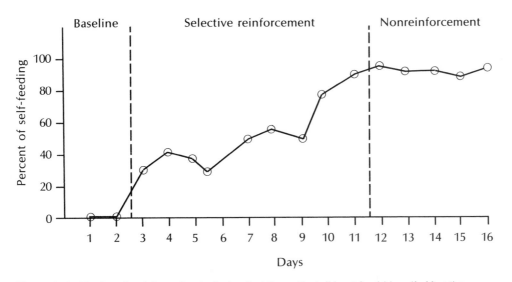

Figure 8–4 The baseline information indicates that the patient did not feed himself. After the nurse reinforced the patient's self-feeding by offering help with a mouthful of food after he took a mouthful, she gradually reduced reinforcement. During this reduced or selective reinforcement as it is described in the graph, note how the patient gradually increased self-feeding. When the reinforcement was stopped, the patient was approaching the goal of eating for himself. (Berni, Rosemarian and Fordyce, Wilbert E.: *Behavior Modification and the Nursing Process*, edition 2. St. Louis, The C. V. Mosby Company, 1977, p. 28.)

Another issue that has often been presented is that incentives which reinforce desired behavior amount to bribery, which for most persons, is a repugnant way to change behavior. Yet, in everyday living, incentives that act to reinforce desired behavior are numerous. Compliments on grooming encourage one to tend to one's appearance. We usually respond positively when our salary is increased and favorable comments are made about the quality of our work. Most would agree that these rewards reinforce desirable behavior. Bribing someone is more aptly used when speaking of asking someone to perform a behavior that is illegal or unethical. When the person is involved in a program of behavior modification and indicates and agrees that he wishes to reach a particular goal for his own well-being, the ethical issues of bribery and behavior manipulation generally cease to be troublesome.

The use of punishment as aversive stimulation has been raised as an ethical issue by some people. The word punishment has many interpretations. It may mean the technique of restraining a person likely to harm another, but it is also used in reference to the incarceration of the law breaker and such techniques of punishment as solitary confinement. Those who describe aversive stimulation in behavior modification recommend its use in selected instances. They hold that

it is a satisfactory technique when the person willingly subscribes to its proper use, is aware of its purpose, and understands how it functions to help him reach his desired goal. It must be made clear that no one advocates any type of aversive stimulation that may possibly be harmful to the person for whom it will be used.

There are several references for this chapter which describe behavior modification in more detail for those interested in further reading on the subject. Also, a situation in which behavior modification was used by nurses caring for a terminally ill patient is given in the Supplemental Library Study.

CONCLUSION

Teaching and helping persons modify behavior are highly individualistic and creative matters. When we recall persons who have most influenced our lives, we see that they were often very different from one another. But most often, they were people who held that the important person in the teaching-learning situation was the learner. The nurse who is enthusiastic in her efforts to help those she serves, keeps the learner's needs foremost, and uses sound principles to guide her action generally is most successful.

SUPPLEMENTAL LIBRARY STUDY

1. The following articles describe two very different teaching methods:

    Hester, Judy. "Food for Thought." (Tips & Timesavers) *Nursing 77,* 7:88, October 1977.

    "Turning on Jan in the Middle of the Night." (Creative Care Unit) *American Journal of Nursing,* 76:1951, December 1976.

    Indicate how Ms. Hester's and Ms. Horsman's ideas could be modified and used in other health-teaching situations.

2. Some people find it difficult to promote discussion during health teaching. The following article discusses possible causes when learner participation is lacking:

    Eaton, Sharon, et al. "Discussion Stoppers in Teaching." *Nursing Outlook,* 25:578–583, September 1977.

    What 11 discussion stoppers do the authors describe? In each case, indicate how these discussion stoppers can be corrected or avoided.

3. The following article offers a wide variety of methods and techniques to improve health teaching:

    Murray, Ruth and Zentner, Judith. "Guidelines for More

Effective Health Teaching." *Nursing 76,* 6:44–53, February 1976.

How is significant learning defined and what conditions foster it, according to these authors? Briefly discuss what the authors refer to as prohibitors in health teaching. The authors believe that a wellness orientation rather than a pathological orientation is important when nurses teach. Why?

4. The following article describes how behavior modification was used to alter undesirable behavior:

Whitman, Helen H. and Lukes, Shelby J. "Behavior Modification for Terminally Ill Patients." *American Journal of Nursing,* 75:98–101, January 1975.

Describe how the nurses involved the patients in their plans of care. Review the seven guidelines the authors offer when working out a plan of intervention to modify behavior. Are these guidelines compatible with the discussion in this chapter? Where do they differ?

Margaret L. Fong and Joyce Dingeldein wrote letters critical of the above article. Their letters appear in the *American Journal of Nursing,* 75:948, June 1975. Do you agree or disagree with the criticisms offered by these two persons? In which way do you agree or disagree?

9

BEHAVIORAL OBJECTIVES

When content in this chapter has been mastered, the student will be able to

Define terms appearing in the glossary.

Describe Erikson's theory of developmental tasks that are characteristic of each age group throughout the life span.

Summarize ten generalizations that are related to human growth and development.

Discuss major physiological and psychosocial growth and developmental tasks for each of the age periods. Give one or two examples that illustrate typical changes which occur during the various periods of life.

List at least twelve common sexual myths and describe briefly the facts that refute them.

Identify at least eight current trends which are influencing the traditional family structure and organization.

List at least three reasons why the family's survival is believed to be secure.

Discuss how knowledge of changes in the individual that occur during the life span have implications for nursing, using the nursing process as a guide.

List three examples of how knowledge of changes in an individual during the various periods of life can be used by the nurse in a health promotion program.

Identify a reaction to illness and several common illnesses that the nurse can expect to occur most often in persons in each of the age groups.

Nursing Through the Life Span

GLOSSARY

Asexuality: Exhibiting no apparent interest in sex.

Autosexuality: Sexual behavior that focuses on the self.

Bisexuality: Having sexual feelings for persons of both sexes.

Body Image: The way one perceives his physical attributes.

Climacteric: The age of menopause; decline and cessation of reproductive capacities in women. The term is sometimes used also when speaking of physiological and psychosocial changes occurring in men during middle adulthood.

Cognition: Perceiving and responding by an individual to the world about him.

Developmental Task: An accomplishment that an individual normally seeks to complete during each of the various age periods of man.

Ego: The conscious self; consciousness of the self.

Extended Family: The nuclear family and grandparents, aunts, uncles, and cousins.

Family: A small group of people which is bound by ties and which accepts responsibility for child-rearing.

Gay: A homosexual.

Heterosexuality: Having sexual feelings for a person of the opposite sex.

Homosexuality: Having sexual feelings for a person of the same sex.

Lesbian: A female homosexual.

Masturbation: Playing with and handling the genitals, as applied to children. Erotic stimulation of the genitals, as applied to adults.

Nuclear Family: The immediate family unit consisting of mother, father, and children.

Perception: Taking in with the mind; the act of knowing that involves reception, sensation, and interpretation of an environmental stimulus.

Physiological Development: The growth and functioning of the various body systems and organs.

Psychology: The study of human behavior in relation to needs, motives, thought processes, and emotions.

Psychosocial: A consideration of the interrelatedness of psychological and sociological concepts or variables in human behavior.

Self-Image: The way one perceives himself to be. Body image is sometimes used as a synonym although body image more correctly refers to a person's physical attributes.

Sociology: The study of human relations in terms of how individuals associate with one another in various groups.

Superego: The conscience; that part of the self concerned with ethical and moral standards.

INTRODUCTION

Nursing offers services to persons of all ages. This chapter will summarize some of the major changes that occur during the life cycle in order to provide the nurse with basic knowledge concerning human growth and development.

There was a time when it was believed that fetal development meant only physiological maturation. However, doubts have arisen because research now suggests that much more than physiological growth occurs in utero. This chapter will not explore growth and development prior to birth. Speciality texts are recommended for readers interested in findings concerning intrauterine life.

Ideally, the individual should be viewed in a holistic manner. The parts that make up the whole are inextricably related and behavior cannot be predicted on the basis of any particular part. Also, no part of the life span makes much sense without looking at the full life cycle. However, for the sake of discussion, seven periods in the life span are presented here. The normal physiological and psychosocial growth and development of each period will be discussed. Communication, the self-image, and human sexuality are discussed in sections dealing with psychosocial development. Some readers may have preferred that some of these topics be considered as physiological developmental tasks. This difference in preference illustrates how interrelated physiological and psychosocial development can be.

This chapter's material applies to normal, healthy individuals. There are factors which may influence normal growth and development but they will not be discussed here. Such factors include illness, physical and mental handicaps, birth defects, and environmental hazards.

It will be noted that age ranges are given for each of the periods through which one passes from birth to death. These ages are approximations only. Some persons may experience growth and development more or less rapidly than others and still be considered normal in terms of the total life cycle.

While physical development does not vary widely among various cultures, psychosocial development may. The material in this chapter focuses on the American middle-class culture since this group represents the largest number of people in the United States. The reader is cautioned that psychosocial development may be quite different in other cultural groups both within the United States and outside of this country. For example, Mead found that psychosocial develop-ment of teenagers was very different in the foreign cultures she studied from teenage development observed in the United States. Chapter 7 discussed culture and implications for nursing, and hence, further discussion will not be included here.

THE NATURE OF HUMAN GROWTH AND DEVELOPMENT

The process of aging begins with conception when the sperm fertilizes the ovum and ends with the death of the individual. Growing older, a life experience common to all living beings, is not an uphill movement with growing up until adulthood, a plateau during adulthood, and a decline during the later years of life. Rather, every age period of man has ascents, plateaus, and declines. Growth is a continuous evolution through life. When the strengths, potentials, needs, and developmental tasks of individuals of all ages are recognized, a firm base upon which to plan measures to help promote health and overcome health problems has been laid.

Study of the physiology and anatomy of man probably began with the earliest medicine man when he became interested in how the body works. Study of the psychological and sociological aspects of man began primarily within the last century or so. Possibly Sigmund Freud could be considered the founder when, during the late nineteenth and early twentieth century, he studied man through psychoanalysis. Charlotte Bühler in the second and third decade of this century was the first to conduct extensive research in psychosocial development. A great advance was made in the 1950s when Erik Erikson presented his theory of the eight stages in the psychosocial development of man. Many behavioral scientists followed whose research added to our general understanding of the human being. Jean Piaget developed theories of cognition. Alfred Adler and Rudolph Dreihers stressed the influence of social groups, especially during the years of childhood. Robert J. Havighurst studied human behavior in terms of developmental tasks and its implications for education. Harry S. Sullivan studied interpersonal relationships and Lawrence Holberg's interest lay in moral development. Alfred Kinsey, William Masters, and Virginia Johnson concentrated on adult sexuality. Margaret Mead explored cultural influences on human growth and development. Bernice Neugarten and James Birren studied the aging process. There are still others who have made important contributions.

Many of the concepts developed by the persons just mentioned are integrated in the material presented here.

The following are definitions of terms that will be used in the remainder of this chapter.

Physiological development is the growth and functioning of the various body systems and organs.

Psychology is concerned with understanding a wide range of human experiences, including needs and motives of humans, their thought processes, their feelings, and their emotions. Psychologists study how our senses work, the learning process, and why and how people become happy and unhappy.

Sociology is the study of human relations, that is, how humans associate with one another in groups of various kinds. The groups include the family, school, church, work, neighborhood, community, and so on. Sociologists study the causes of both individual and group behavior that arise when there is human social contact.

Psychology and sociology are often classed as behavioral sciences. The term *psychosocial* is often used when speaking of concepts from both psychology and sociology and denotes their interrelatedness.

Perception is a taking in with the mind; it is the act of knowing and involves reception, sensation, and interpretation of an environmental stimulus. Some psychologists, notably Piaget, used the term *cognition* to mean an individual's perceiving and responding to the world about him.

Self-image is the way an individual perceives himself to be. It includes the physical as well as psychosocial aspects of the personality, such as emotions, moods, status, perceptions of how others as well as the self views the total person, and feelings of worth or inadequacy and of acceptance or rejection. Such expressions as "I-ness," "wholeness feelings," "the mirrored self," "photographic self," and "this is the *real* me," are often used to further describe self-image.

Some persons use the term *body-image* as a synonym for self-image. The literature is beginning to differentiate between the two terms and uses body-image to mean the person's physical attributes.

Erikson used the term *developmental tasks* extensively in his theory of human development. He defined it as an individual's attempt to accomplish balance between two opposites. He also used the word "versus" (vs) between the two opposites when he described developmental tasks. He did not imply that one of the two opposites had to be present. Rather, Erikson explained that it is necessary to experience some of both of the opposites in life, but, during each state of development, the individual strives for a balance that allows for eventual growth for positive achievment. Erikson explained that when the developmental task typical of a particular period in life was not accomplished, the person could not proceed to subsequent tasks without first reaching positive achievement of an earlier developmental task. He described psychosocial development in terms of these tasks. Many persons have used developmental tasks in a broader sense than did Erikson and have described physiological as well as psychosocial tasks in life. Erikson's theory of developmental tasks is integrated into the section on psychosocial growth and development for each period in the life span. It is illustrated in Figure 9–1 on page 158.

Certain generalizations about the nature of human growth and development can be made.

Growth and development are complex. There are many processes that comprise human growth and development, all interrelated with each other. This generalization supports the concept that man strives for wholeness throughout the life span.

Growth and development are both quantitative and qualitative. Continuously adding to quantity would result in grossness and chaos. But the body constantly differentiates and becomes selective in what it will support and maintain, both in a physical and a psychosocial sense, as it strives for constancy and stability. The body differentiates and alters in a complex yet organized and qualitative manner.

Growth and development are continuous and orderly. Growth and development begin at conception and end with death. There is no time during life when growth and development are static and they are orderly and organized even during periods of decline. Because of this, is it possible to describe characteristic patterns for the different stages in life through which man passes.

There are regular trends in the direction of growth and development. There are three trends in the direction of physical growth that can be observed. Growth begins in the upper part of the body and proceeds downward and from the middle of the body outward. Examples will be given later in this chapter. Growth also is symmetrical, with the right side of the body growing simultaneously with the left side. Erikson's theory, as illustrated in Figure 9–1, points out trends in psychosocial development.

The tempo of growth and development is uneven. Although orderly and organized, growth and development proceed unevenly. Physical growth is very rapid during the age of infancy, slower during childhood,

TRUST vs. MISTRUST Birth to approximately 18 months	This stage forms the base of subsequent personality. The quality of the relationship between infant and primary caretaker is important.
AUTONOMY vs. SHAME/DOUBT Approximately 18 months to 4 years	With trust, the infant can now discover his own behavior. The toddler becomes assertive and wants to explore himself and his environment.
INITIATIVE vs. GUILT Approximately 4 to 6 years	Language and good locomotion gives the youngster ability to expand imagination. The development of conscience begins.
INDUSTRY vs. INFERIORITY Approximately 6 to 12 years	The school child begins to differentiate between work and play. He learns to enjoy his work for the pleasures he gains from it.
IDENTITY vs. DIFFUSION Approximately 12 to 18 years	The adolescent is learning about who he is, where he wants to go, and what he wishes to do with his life. He is putting it all together for adulthood.
INTIMACY vs. ISOLATION Approximately 18 to 40 years	The young adult is concerned with establishing sexual intimacy which is usually centered around marriage. Final career choices become important.
GENERATIVITY vs. STAGNATION Approximately 40 to 65 years	The concern in middle adulthood is to contribute something of lasting value to youth and society. Adjusting to a change in sexual activity becomes important.
INTEGRITY vs. DESPAIR Approximately 65 years and older	Accepting one's life for what it was and enjoying what has been promotes integrity. Feeling useful and enjoying respect are important.

Figure 9–1   This is a summary of Erik Erikson's theory of psychosocial development. When the critical issues at each stage of life are resolved, the individual goes on to the next stage, although some back sliding may occur at times. When a critical issue remains unresolved, the individual ordinarily has difficulties in adjusting to the next stage in life.

and again rapid during adolescence. Also, it varies among individuals. Maturation does not occur at the same time for every person. This is true of both physical and psychosocial development.

Different aspects of growth and development occur at different rates. For example, muscular development varies with age, as does sexual maturity.

The rate and pattern of growth and development can be modified. Nutrition is one factor that can very definitely affect patterns of growth. Another factor that appears to influence growth is the quality and quantity of loving care an infant receives. Experiences early in life are known to have far-reaching effects on an individual's later development.

There are critical periods in growth and development. To illustrate this generalization, it has been noted that certain diseases, rubella being one, can have a profound effect on the development of the fetus. The same disease does not have a marked effect later in life, unless complications occur. If psychosocial developmental tasks are not accomplished at certain times in life, a later age period may be complicated by psychological problems.

There is a tendency for an organism to seek its maximum potential for development. Maximum potential is difficult to determine for each individual. There is a genetic quality which cannot be surpassed. But the environment of the individual plays a crucial role in maximizing the individual's hereditary potential. When factors that are completely unrelated to genetics are overwhelming, genetic potential cannot be attained.

Each individual grows and develops in his own unique way. No two persons are exactly alike, not even identical twins. The individual's uniqueness results from an interplay between hereditary and environmental influences and individuality can be observed throughout the life span.

THE NEWBORN AND THE INFANT: BIRTH TO APPROXIMATELY 18 MONTHS

Physiological Growth and Development

The human being begins with the union of a sperm and an ovum and progresses to become organically independent and remarkably competent in a relatively

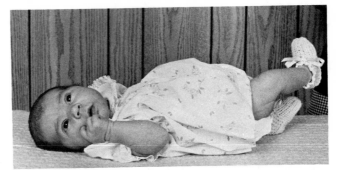

Figure 9–2 This healthy, full-term newborn is six days old. The sudden flash of light startled her. Note the Moro or startle reflex: she draws up her legs and brings her arms forward. She is alert and is making visual contact with the light near the camera. Even at this early age, her parents have dressed her in feminine-appearing clothes.

brief time. The most profound physical change at birth occurs when the newborn's independent respiratory process begins. The circulatory, hepatic, and renal functions also are initiated in a manner that promotes physiological life although they have been functioning in utero.

The period when organic independence is reached is followed by the stage of infancy when much stabilization of physiological processes occurs. The maturation of the central nervous system is especially important for an increased stabilization of the body systems. Infancy is a period when survival is still at stake, but gradually, the baby achieves considerable physiological stabilization.

The average newborn weighs approximately 3.2 to 3.7 kg. (7 to 8 pounds) and is ordinarily 47.5 to 52.5 cm. (19 to 21 inches) in length. The newborn's head is large in relation to the rest of its body. Figure 9–2 illustrates a normal full-term newborn.

A young infant will gain as much as an ounce a day but this rate and caloric needs decline beginning at approximately six to eight months of age. The average infant trebles his birth rate by the age of one year while his length increases by about 50 percent. The head grows only slightly in comparison with the rest of the body. This results in a relative change in head and trunk proportions. It can be noted when comparing Figure 9–2 with Figures 9–4 and 9–5 on pages 162 and 163.

The newborn's proportion of body fluids when compared with body weight is as much as 77 percent, the highest it will be during life. As a result, water and caloric requirements are relatively high and the new-born will suffer quickly when intake is inadequate or improper since physiological stability, though competent, is fragile.

The amount of body fluids gradually declines. By approximately one year of age, the proportion approaches that of an adult. There is a greater water turnover in an infant and the proportion of body surface is large in relation to body size when compared with that of older children and adults. Hence, fluid intake remains critical during this period. By the end of infancy, the basal metabolism rate is still high—about twice that of an average healthy adult.

Blood values change between birth and the end of infancy. Red and white cells and hemoglobin values are high in the newborn. They drop during the first four to six months of life. The red cells and hemoglobin then gradually increase to approximate adult levels by late childhood. White cells reach adult levels by as early as late infancy.

The body temperature of the newborn and infant is labile and responds quickly to environmental conditions. This is due to the proportionately large body surface and unstable temperature control. Temperature stability develops by late infancy. Normal body temperature is considered to be approximately 37°C. (98.6°F.) throughout life.

The pulse rate of the newborn is rapid; that is, it is as high as 110 to 160 beats per minute. It gradually decreases but remains relatively high during infancy. The respiratory rate of a newborn can normally vary between 35 and 60 per minute but drops to approximately 30 during infancy. Blood pressure is low, approximately 85/60 mm. Hg at birth, and remains relatively low during infancy. It increases gradually and reaches adult levels at about the beginning of adolescence.

Although all of the body's neurons are present at birth, the central nervous system is not fully developed, and hence, coordination and neurological integration are immature. This immaturity results in uncoordinated, purposeless movements, tremors, and an easily aroused startling response. As high cerebral centers begin to mature, more meaningful behavior develops during infancy. The newborn's eyes cannot accommodate at birth, but the baby can see. He can hear soon after birth when the eustachian tubes open and are free of fluid. Tactile senses are present. There are strong startle or Moro, rooting (turning the mouth to the nipple), swallowing, sucking, grasping, blinking,

coughing, sneezing, and yawning reflexes present at birth. Figure 9–3 illustrates the rooting and grasping reflexes in the newborn. The newborn sleeps most of the time and tends to lie in the fetal position.

The infant gradually decreases his sleeping time so that by the end of this period, he will sleep about 12 hours in each 24-hour period. Napping is necessary to prevent undue fatigue.

Central nervous system maturation during infancy includes a marked increase in interneural connections and in the complexity of axon and dendrite structure. Conductive time becomes more rapid also as nerve fibers and cellular membranes mature. There is increased sensitivity to stimuli from an ever-enlarging environment which now also begins to take on meaning. The infant can use his hands by the end of this period in a manipulative manner, as can be seen when he plays with building blocks, scribbles with crayons, and tries to feed himself. Figure 9–4 on page 162 illustrates the infant's ability to feed himself.

During the age of infancy, teeth erupt and a change in eating habits occurs. The infant begins to take soft foods and eventually lumpy to solid foods which he can chew before swallowing.

The gastrointestinal tract is not fully developed at birth. There is poor cardiac sphincter control in the stomach which results in the ease of regurgitating feedings. Processes of elimination are present but involuntary.

Sphincter control soon develops and the muscular system matures sufficiently so that control of urinary and intestinal elimination can be expected to be developing by the time infancy ends. The development of the musculoskeletal system progresses from the head downward and from the central part of the body outward to the periphery. To illustrate, control of head movements occurs before control in the use of arms and finally the legs. General arm and leg movements occur first; then there is gradual control of the hands and feet and eventually the fingers and toes. Growth is symmetrical, that is, the right and the left sides of the body grow simultaneously and at the same rate.

The newborn's muscle tone is good but motion in response to stimuli is limited, random, purposeless, and global. The newborn is incapable of moving himself and cannot change his position on his own although he can move if his feet are placed against a solid surface.

It is during infancy that the human begins his exploration of the world about him. Rapid maturation of the neuromuscular system leads to progress in controlling and handling the body. The infant learns to crawl,

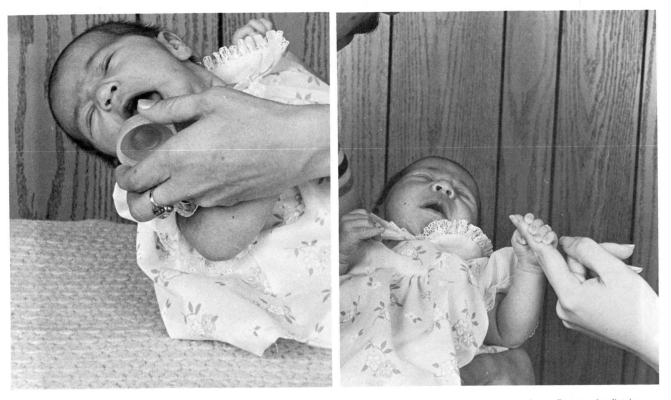

Figure 9–3   The newborn in the photo on the left demonstrates the rooting reflex as she opens her mouth and turns her head toward the nipple that had touched her cheek. In the photo on the right, the newborn shows the grasping reflex as she firmly circles her fingers around her mother's forefinger.

then walk, and eventually run. As a result, the baby begins to experiment in reaching goals beyond self. He is still clumsy but he becomes very active.

Psychosocial Growth and Development

There is evidence that the newborn who is indifferent to such individual characteristics as age, appearance, and gender, is very sensitive and responsive to an emotional environment. He has need for love and feelings of belongingness and reciprocal relationships. The newborn responds positively to gentle care by parents and other significant persons in his environment who are relaxed and comfortable in their roles. He responds to touch, cuddling, and warmth. He relaxes with rhythmic motions, such as occurs when rocking him. He appears to have need for security and physical closeness and dislikes openness, bright lights, and loud noises.

The ability to develop psychosocial skills is present at birth and develops rapidly during infancy. At birth, we see a competent but dependent human who is busy establishing organic independence and ready to begin the process of becoming a psychosocial being.

During infancy, the central psychosocial developmental task is to develop basic trust as opposed to mistrust. For this to occur, the infant's world needs to be dependable, consistent, and have much sameness of experiences. From trust of others grows a sense of trust in the self. The mother, who is usually the primary caretaker, and infant relationship is important at this time as the infant tends to reject others for her. When the mother or other primary caretakers demonstrate a sensitivity to the baby's needs, show genuine affection, and provide gentle care, trust grows. When this quality of care is absent or in short supply, mistrust with fear and suspicion flourish. As trust in others and the self develops, the infant can learn to be away from the familiar for short periods without feelings of panic.

The infant begins to perceive differences in various sensations. For example, he will know food satisfies hunger and water quenches thirst. He experiences pleasure with accomplishment when he reaches a goal, such as the joy when he takes his first steps alone.

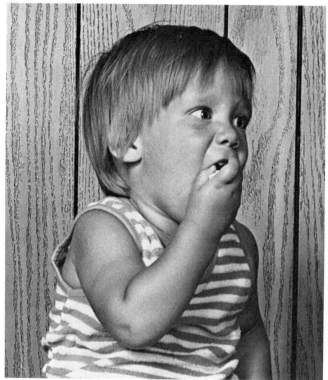
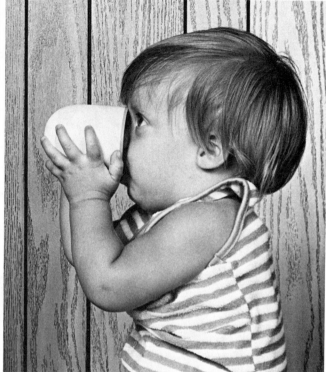

Figure 9–4   This infant is about one year old. He is eager to get the food into his mouth and does so with his fingers and hand. He is able to hold his cup for himself for drinking. Compare this figure with Figure 9–2 on page 159. Note that the infant's head is smaller than the head of a newborn when compared with total body size. The infant has hair that replaced the fine dark hair typically noted in the newborn.

Communication. Physiological development along with locomotion and the development of rudimentary communication skills are inextricably associated with psychosocial development. Locomotion leads to a gradual weaning from mother and other caretakers. Verbal and nonverbal communications propel the infant into a social world. The maturing process of the central nervous system ushers the beginning of meaningfulness to stimuli received from the environment and increased perceptive development.

The baby's attention span is short. However, some discipline can be accepted during the latter part of infancy, especially when balanced with an environment that provides safe and appropriate opportunities to explore, find, examine, and know.

During infancy, the baby can receive as well as express emotional feelings. For example, the infant responds to affection, tension, anger, and fear and can also demonstrate these emotional feelings.

The language of the newborn is crying which he will use when discomforts are present, such as fatigue, hunger, and temperature variations. When physical needs are being met and when the infant receives affectionate parenting, crying has been observed to be minimum.

Early in infancy, the baby uses and responds to sounds by smiling, cooing, and eventually laughing. The infant's social world expands rapidly when he begins to say words at approximately six to eight months of age. By the end of infancy, two or three words may be joined so that the beginning of sentence structure is apparent. The infant also learns the meaning of simple gestures and facial expressions. Thus, both verbal and nonverbal communications continue to develop during this period and many new windows to the world have been opened. By one year, the infant makes expressive sounds that become more distinct and begins to respond to his own name, knows familiar people, and expresses shyness in the presence of the unfamiliar. The words of the infant are mostly nouns. One exception to this statement is the word "no" which most infants late in this period use with ease, frequency, and vehemence as they begin their drive for independence.

Self-Image. The newborn is apparently without body-image and self-image. There is no evidence that he has emotional feelings about his physical and psychosocial being. A differentiation between self and nonself begins during infancy. By the end of this period, the blur between the self and others clears and a rapid development of self-image has been initiated.

During infancy, concepts of an intact body are not believed to be present. The infant's anxieties and crying associated with a nursing procedure, such as an injection, are probably due to fear of an unfamiliar setting and the possibility of separation from the mother rather than fear of mutilation or pain.

The infant is still essentially mother bound. However, the father becomes an important figure during this period and studies have shown that he can be just as caring and loving of infants and sensitive to their needs as the mother. The infant is most content in a familiar home environment, although he may begin to take small steps away from persons in his usual world.

The infant responds to the spoken word, smiles, and enjoys being held and cuddled. A healthy self-image can best be developed at this age by consistent, caring, and affectionate parenting.

Sexuality. Environmental influences on sexuality begin at birth. An appropriate male or female name is chosen and clothes differentials are generally made. The color of choice is pink for girls and clothing is selected that reflects femininity. Note the clothing of the newborn girl in Figure 9–2. The color for boys is blue and clothing is more tailored and masculine in appearance. Soon, hair styles are different. Even play activity is planned differently. Very early in life, girls are given dolls and boys receive trucks and balls. Figure 9–5 illustrates typical play for boy infants. Parents begin to praise behavior that is considered to be consistent with femininity or masculinity.

Even during infancy, sexual differences can be noted in terms of behavior. Girl babies tend to cry more than boy babies. Girls tend to jabber more and earlier than boys, and girls appear to have better use of small muscles than boys. Reasons for these observed differences are still not clear and conclusive. Does the infant re-

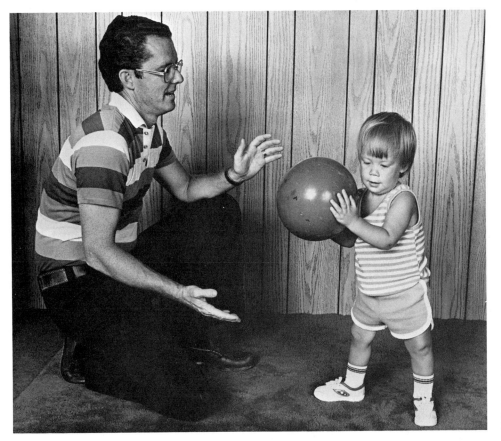

Figure 9–5 Father begins play typical for boys with his son. This infant is beginning to stand and take steps. Note his stance with his feet well separated. The position gives the infant a wide base of support for standing.

spond to its gender because of environmental or genetic influences or both?

During infancy, the sex organs are normally dormant although an erect penis or clitoris may be observed. However, these erections probably are without sexual significance. Actions of affection, such as cuddling, touching, and talking to the baby by caring, meaningful persons are believed to promote healthful sexual development.

Infancy is a period of phenomenal growth and development. From the relatively helpless newborn emerges a dynamic, active individual who is taking steps into an ever-enlarging world.

Common Health Problems of the Newborn and Infant

There are several problems of gestation which ordinarily require the help of health practitioners at the time of birth. Some of the more common ones are incompatability between the blood group of the mother and her infant; congenital malformations, such as cleft palate and cleft lip, spina bifida acculta, Down's syndrome, congenital syphilis, and congenital drug addiction. During infancy, typical health problems brought to the attention of health practitioners include the following: feeding problems, including malnutrition; respiratory infections; gastroenteritis; skin disorders, such as diaper rash, contact dermatitis, prickly heat, and candida albicans (monilia); and child abuse.

THE TODDLER AND THE PRESCHOOLER: APPROXIMATELY 18 MONTHS TO 6 YEARS

Physiological Growth and Development

There is a slowing of the physical growth processes during the toddler and preschool years. As described earlier, an infant trebles his birth weight by approximately one year of age. Between then and age six, he will approximately double his one-year weight. The chubby toddler grows slowly but steadily to a lean body build with muscle tissue development and loss of fat tissue by school age. His height at six years will be about 100 to 120 cm. (40 to 45 inches).

The child's appetite may taper, but because these are years of great physical activity, caloric needs remain relatively high. All of the temporary teeth will have appeared although some may be lost by age six. The

consistency of the child's diet resembles that of an adult by the latter part of this period.

The neuromuscular system continues to mature. The head approaches its adult size. Toilet-training can be completed. Manual dexterity and eye and hand coordination become good. Excellent locomotion results in this age of high activity levels.

The central nervous, cardiovascular, and respiratory systems mature as do the blood and lymph systems. They will not have reached the full stability of adulthood but will have made great and steady strides in that direction.

Many mothers call the toddler years the terrible two's and the expression seems warranted in terms of locomotion. The age is characterized by almost continuous motion, activity, walking, running, climbing, and jumping as the youngster seeks to explore his environment. Energy seems endless. The sense of danger is slower to develop, and hence, the toddler is normally a dynamo without fears of peril, as Figure 9–6 illustrates. A frequent "No!" demonstrates eagerness to find independence. The great zest for living of both the toddler and the preschooler accompanies an ever-expanding need to reach new goals. Hence, these children need a stimulating but safe environment.

Psychosocial Growth and Development

The period between infancy and school age is characterized by a tremendous growth in the development of the self and independence. The growth, while steady, requires many experiences and experiments and backsliding may occur at times. Such words as capricious, unpredictable, and stubborn, may be used to describe the youngster while he strives for personal and social maturity. The development of language and cognitive skills during this period is crucial. It is through the use and understanding of words that the child eventually finds peace with himself and in the world. Reality, memory, a sense of time and space, and an understanding of causality begin development during this period.

During toddlerhood until approximately four years of age, the child works to establish autonomy. The trust of infancy propels the child to stand alone although there is confusion as autonomy develops. He is still dependent on his primary caretakers and is mostly pleasure bound, but he wants his independence, too. Note the pleasure and independence the toddler shows in Figure 9–7. As many parents say, it is "I this," and "I that," constantly. The conflict between dependence tonomy. Cognitive skills are present that help the child make discriminations which allow him to know his body, its ability, his impulses, and his autonomous self.

After toddlerhood, between approximately three or four and six years of age, there is marked intellectual and emotional growth when initiative builds on autonomy. Now there is reality with planning and attacking a particular task for the sake of a goal. Play becomes something with meaning and occurs cooperatively with others. Prior to this time, play is often described as parallel or solitary; that is, youngsters play next to each other but not with each other. The term intrusive has been used to describe the preschool child's activities since he tends to thrust himself at other people, into his physical environment, and into the unknown with fantasy and dreams. Initiative will be replaced by guilt when he is made to feel that his behavior is silly, unnecessary, a nuisance, or without reason or logic. The child then fears contemplated behavior and psychosocial growth becomes stunted.

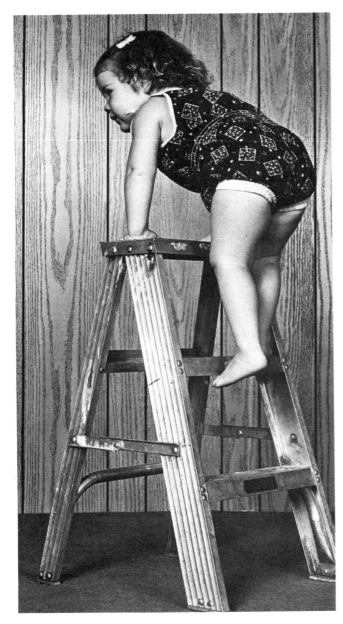

Figure 9–6 The toddler has much energy, is constantly on the go, and has little fear of danger. It is especially important to provide a safe yet stimulating environment for the toddler.

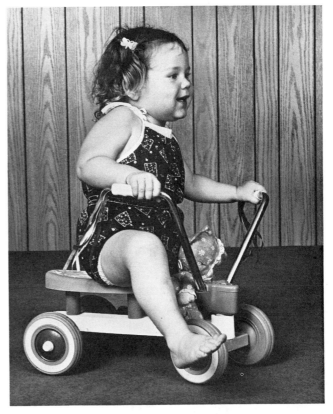

Figure 9–7 This toddler is happy with her ability to move around easily and quickly and to maneuver her toy. Note the chubbiness which is characteristic of the age.

and independence is often described as an inability to decide when to hold onto something and when to let go. These conflicting feelings, if not resolved, are likely to result in feelings of shame and doubt. The youngster then tends to turn against himself. An environment with parents who recognize the toddler's feelings and which offers firm reassurances is important to help the toddler struggling with the developmental task of au-

During the preschool years, the *ego,* or consciousness of the self, is strengthened and the superego develops. The *superego* is the conscience and is concerned with ethical and moral thought. The child begins to internalize moral and ethical standards by beginning to perceive right and wrong. A toddler has little concern for the feelings of others; the preschool child begins to have feelings for those about him.

Communication. Speech readiness appears late in infancy. The development of language progresses from having a vocabulary of a few words to using a thousand words or more by the age of six. There is an almost insatiable curiosity with frequent use of the word why. A recognition of time relationships with knowledge of the past, present, and future is reflected in the selection of words. Interest span, which is very short early in this period, lengthens and the ability to postpone gratification grows to a considerable extent.

Self-Image. During toddlerhood and the preschool years, importance is given to the body and its various parts. However, the child is unable to comprehend how the parts of the body function to make up the whole. As a result, during these years, an intact body becomes especially important. The preschooler may think, for example, that a needle introduced into a vein means that he will have a permanent opening from which he will lose his blood. He may have difficulty during toddlerhood "giving up" excreta which he feels is part of his body. A broken bone may signify the loss of an arm or leg in the mind of a preschooler. An adult may think of a tonsillectomy as a simple procedure, but the preschooler may associate it with a threat of permanent mutilation. The fear of health care measures during this age is very frequently believed to be related to the child's struggle to maintain an intact body and preserve his self-image.

Sexuality. Most authorities believe that the years between approximately two and five or six are critical in terms of sexual identity. In most cultures, the mother is the all important figure during infancy, but during this period, the significance of the father increases and his presence is important for proper sexual growth. Behavior that demonstrates a boy is acting like a boy and a girl like a girl is usually reinforced and praised as the child takes on the appearance and emotions of the parent of the same sex. Figure 9–8 illustrates. Traditionally, dependency in girls has been reinforced while aggression in boys has been supported and encouraged.

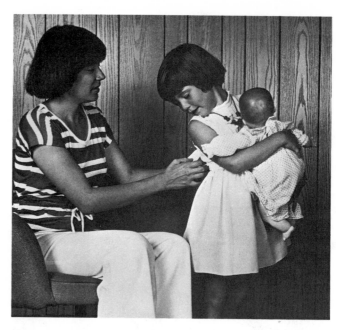

Figure 9–8   The preschooler learns femininity and masculinity from parents. Here, mother dresses her five year old daughter to reflect femininity. A piece of jewelry is worn and the child carries her doll which has been important to her since toddlerhood. Note that this youngster has a lean appearance. She has lost the chubbiness typically seen in toddlers.

The curiosity of this age includes an interest in the body, including the genitals. There is often play involving make-believe doctor when the body is examined. Another common type of play is imitating the family: the boy is the father, the girl is the mother, and a doll that is cuddled, rocked, and wheeled about, is the baby.

By the time a child reaches school age, it is generally agreed that sexuality has been internalized and preferences for sexual partners that will be part of adulthood have been established. Playing with and handling the genitals is considered to be a normal, not an injurious act. The term *masturbation* is often used for this type of playing. However, it should be noted that for adults, the term is used somewhat differently and is then usually defined as erotic stimulation of the genitals. When parents view childhood masturbation as normal activity in which pleasure is derived from stimulation of the skin, and when they handle the situation accordingly, the child is not likely to feel guilt and shame about it.

From the egocentric, active, jabbering, forever-on-the-go age of the toddler follows the preschooler who leaves this period as a fairly well-socialized youngster with strengthened autonomy and physical and psychosocial skills necessary to begin school.

Common Health Problems of the Toddler and Preschooler

Accidents are the leading cause of death in children from approximately one to 14 years of age. About one-third of all deaths during the toddler and preschool years are due to automobile accidents, and about one-fifth to fires and burns. Poisonings due to a variety of agents are another important accidental cause of death in this age group.

Infections of many sorts are common during the toddler and preschool years. Upper respiratory infections and associated complications, such as otitis media, account for about half of the acute illnesses between about two and six years of age. Other types of infections that are common during this period include communicable diseases, such as chicken pox, measles, and mumps; skin infections, such as impetigo; and central nervous system infections (the meningitides). Allergic diseases of various sorts, such as asthma, are commonly seen during these years. Surgical treatment of certain congenital anomalies often is carried out in preschool years, two examples being repairs of cleft palates and heart anomalies.

MIDDLE CHILDHOOD: APPROXIMATELY 6 TO 12 YEARS

Physiological Growth and Development

By the time a child reaches school age, he is sturdy, strong, and lean. He will be tall, average or short for his age since height now is influenced primarily by hereditary factors. His physical growth during middle childhood is relatively slow but steady. The appetite and caloric needs have decreased due to a drop in activity and growth rate. Eating which was previously used simply to satisfy hunger now becomes more of a social event, and having meals with peers takes on significance. By the end of this period, the body will be approaching adult levels of basal metabolism rate, vital signs, most blood values, proportion of body fluids, and so on. Physiological stability is well-developed.

During school years, the temporary teeth are lost and replaced by permanent teeth. The child normally sleeps well, eats somewhat sparingly, and has less activity when compared with the toddler and preschooler.

The typical physical characteristics of the school-age child are his good to excellent locomotion and manipulative power. These are years when neuromuscular skills are coordinated and perfected. He has overcome clumsiness and reaches agility. Purposeless activity decreases and feats of doing become important. Note the enthusiasm of using neuromuscular skills shown in Figure 9–9.

Psychosocial Growth and Development

Primary tasks of development during the school years include increasing independence from home and parents, socialization with peers, and a move from egocentricity to outer-world interest. There is emphasis on doing, succeeding, and accomplishing. Learning now becomes important for its own sake and for increasing autonomy.

As the school-age youngster's ego strengthens, his sense of conscience grows simultaneously, giving him better control of the world and himself. The child can accept reality when he sees he now has some control of his environment. A scale of values also develops. Although striving for independence, he also likes to know what is, and what is fair or unfair. These are years of rituals and games with an endless number of rules by which to guide behavior. Figure 9–10 illustrates.

The school-age child is industrious, as is shown in

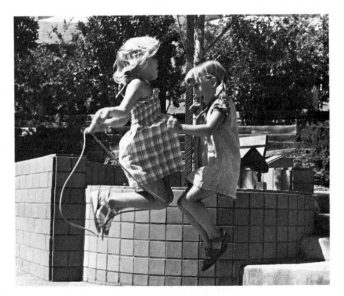

Figure 9–9 These two school-age children are obviously enjoying the fun of rope-skipping. School-age children are typically agile and like participating in physical activity that tests their neuromuscular and skeletal development.

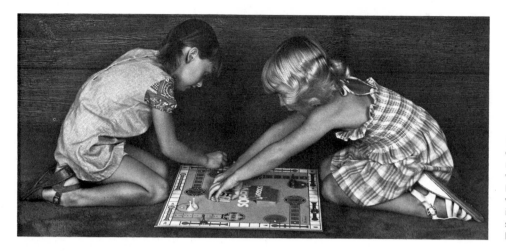

Figure 9–10 Much time was devoted to describing various rules of this game before play was underway. This is typical behavior of children of this age who are striving for independence but who still want safe limits to help guide their behavior.

Figure 9–11. He wishes to do, succeed, and feel a sense of accomplishment and competency. The exuberance and randomness of earlier years become channeled and he now can separate work from play. When industry cannot thrive, the child develops a sense of inferiority and inadequacy, and if he gives up, he may experience feelings of mediocrity and despair.

While the home environment continues to be important, agencies in the community, such as the school and the church, begin to have significant influence during this period of development. It is now that the child becomes aware of his origins, including such factors as race, religion, ethnic background, and economic status. These understandings along with emotional overtones that usually accompany them are likely to follow the youngster throughout his life. The child begins to feel inferior when his origins appear to be more important than his accomplishments and industriousness in the judgment of others.

Communication. When the youngster reaches school age, he has a good foundation for the use of verbal communication and the use of nonverbal communication is present and developing rapidly. The vocabulary expands and there is a growing interest in the meaning of word forms, symbolism, logic, verbal expression, and grammar. Reading now becomes a tool and most school-age children enjoy reading as a hobby and diversion, as well as a skill needed for learning.

Self-Image. During middle childhood, youngsters internalize a sense of being trusted and loved, and hence, tend to look upon themselves as being competent and trustworthy. In other words, they learn to have faith in themselves and their bodies. Dependency on parents

lessens as they gain control of their environment. During these years, a concept of the self and the differences between the self and others become strong. School-age children still have a blurred understanding of how the body functions but their self-image and interest in body intactness are well-developed. They begin to make comparisons of themselves with others and often

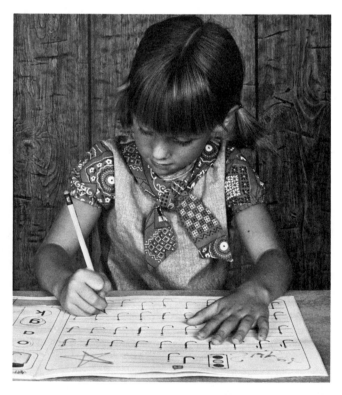

Figure 9–11 This school-age child is industrious and completely engrossed in her school work. She likes her work and enjoys a sense of having done well.

find differences that most adults may not even see. The interest in what may seem unimportant minutiae appears to strengthen the self-image.

Sexuality. Earlier in life, the child may have experienced conflicting feelings about his interest in one or the other parent. During middle childhood, the conflict resolves and a period of calmness develops with regard to sexuality. There tends to be an attachment to the parent of the opposite sex.

Peer relationships become important as the youngster pushes for autonomy and independence from parents and other adults. Boys and girls tend to separate and socialize with members of their own sex. This behavior helps differentiation of gender and shores up male and female identity and self-image that began in earlier years. Also, it has been observed that this repetition of behaving, of wanting to be only with members of the same sex produces mastery, in this case, mastery of the self-image. Nevertheless, there is an awareness of members of the opposite sex and interest in sexual matters. Boys say they hate girls and vice versa, when actually they are interested in each other but in a self-conscious way. Interest in how life is created is strong.

While school years were once characterized as a period of sexual latency, it is now believed that almost the opposite is true. Interest in sex diversifies and generalizes and new thoughts and feelings about sexual matters become internalized. It is a time when authorities believe the child's natural curiosity should be satisfied by answering questions honestly and to the extent the child wishes and can understand. As one psychologist said, during middle childhood, education concerning sexuality is important and when the youngster is not receiving instructions to satisfy his curiosity in the home or school, he will find answers elsewhere.

The physical and psychosocial developmental accomplishments of middle childhood may seem less dramatic than development during the ages immediately prior to and following these years. Nevertheless, the child has accomplished a great deal, and well, when he has a firm ego identity, a secure self-image, a feeling of independence, and physical integrity. He is ready to move on to the more tumultuous years of adolescence.

Common Health Problems During Middle Childhood

Accidents are the chief cause of death during middle childhood and most involve automobiles, bicycles, and water. Rheumatic fever is the most common cause of death from a heart disease between ages five and 24.

As in earlier years, various types of infection are common, examples being the communicable diseases, upper respiratory infections, urinary tract infections, and appendicitis. Lice infestation which spreads rapidly in the school environment is frequently noted and often difficult to contain.

Other health problems encountered during these years include renal diseases, such as nephrotic syndrome; juvenile diabetes mellitus; cystic fibrosis; and muscular dystrophy. Dental caries and irregularities in the spacing of teeth are significant health problems of this age.

ADOLESCENCE: APPROXIMATELY 12 TO 18 YEARS

Physiological Growth and Development

Adolescence is a period of marked growth which will end abruptly by age 18 or 19. As one person stated, growth is rushing to a halt. The body reaches almost full stature and the various body organs and systems attain maturity.

It is during adolescence that the secondary sex characteristics appear and reproductive maturity arrives. Endocrine changes during adolescence are primarily responsible for the growth spurt and adult sexuality. Girls tend to experience sexual maturity a year or two earlier than boys. Puberty begins at about age 10 or 11 for girls and age 12 or 13 for boys. Most girls start menstruating between 13 and 15 years of age.

Crash diets, especially among teenage girls, and food fads are common among adolescents so that proper nutrition is a matter of concern. Many parents claim their teenagers who are not dieting eat constantly, everything, and anytime, practices which help provide sufficient calories to support the teenager's growth spurt. This is common following middle childhood when growth is slower and appetites seem jaded. The adolescent sleeps like an adult.

Most persons think of the adolescent as being clumsy which would appear to be a decline in locomotive abilities. It is generally believed that since there is a sudden and rapid growth spurt during these years, the adolescent needs time to learn how to handle his body again. Until he does, he is likely to stumble, drop articles and run into things. When he becomes accustomed to his larger body frame, agility returns.

By late in this period, the adolescent has developed full muscular control and coordination. He moves about with grace and litheness. Witness the ease with which most mature adolescents are able to participate in various sports.

Psychosocial Growth and Development

Adolescents are concerned with sexuality, independence, and self-identity and are beginning to think about a career choice. The six years or so prior to adulthood are characterized by turmoil, for the teenager as well as for his family. Previous generations of adolescents were concerned primarily with *doing,* such as contributing to the economy and working for a secure future. Today's young people are more occupied with expressing themselves by "doing one's thing", as Figure 9-12 illustrates, and living for now with less concern for the future. Parents and other adults who are willing to give the adolescent room to grow as an individual are usually more successful than those who wish the youngster to be a miniature of themselves. Inquisitions and asking for submission will take away from the teenager's creativity and the emotional stability he needs to tackle the adult world. Although the young person still wants limits set, self-discipline replaces the discipline of others and he wants to make his own mistakes from which he can grow. He wants affection but independence from parents. Probably most of all, the adolescent needs empathetic listening with expressions of understanding to help overcome his anxieties as he struggles to resolve the developmental tasks characteristic of his age. He finds adult efforts unacceptable when the adult minimizes his problem, offers cliché solutions to his questions, gives self as an example, expresses pity, and puts him down.

The primary psychosocial task during adolescence is the drive for self-identity. Before settling on a career, adolescents must resolve who they are in the eyes of themselves and the world. The teenager seems dissatisfied with his home life, is often moody, daydreams, wants the things he fears, considers advice as bossing and offers of help as interference, and feels unique as the only person with troubles. Add to this the strong and clannish peer relationships, the striving to be midstream in whatever is the "in" thing to do—all of which are believed to be parts of the process for developing a secure self-identity. It may seem paradoxical that while the youngster seeks independence and individuality, he still wants to be exactly like his peers. But his behavior is easier to understand when one realizes

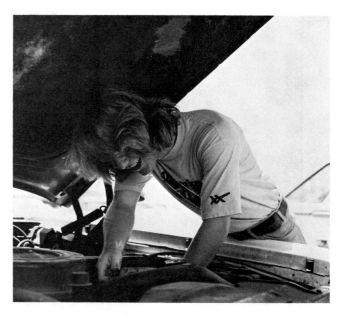

Figure 9-12   Many adolescent boys enjoy tinkering with cars and strive for independence and the power they feel when owning and driving their own car.

that his peers offer him support and the opportunity to try out behavior on them which helps promote independence from adults. The behaviors just described do not seem bizarre when they are interpreted as the youngster's great endeavor to be himself and yet different from his elders. When youth fails to resolve the task of establishing self-identity, the teenager falls into the trap of role diffusion which is frequently associated with delinquency and lawlessness.

In terms of cognitive skills, the adolescent approaches an adult level of intellectual functioning, and he has the intellectual capacities with which he will proceed during life. He is capable of inductive and deductive reasoning, causality, logic, abstract thinking, reflective thought, and empathy. He relates well to both the past and the future. He is developing an ethical system and an ideology. The superego grows and functions to guide his future.

Communication.   Communication skills are well-developed during this period and there is a good understanding of semantics. The teenager often seems unwilling to talk with parents and is secretive about his activities. This is related more to the young person's psychosocial development than to communication skills, although many adults might have doubts.

The teenager is especially communicative with peers. This may well be more talk than communication. It is

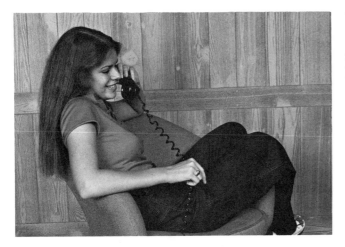

Figure 9-13 The telephone gives the teenager many opportunities for long talk sessions with peers. Ideas can be exchanged without fear of criticism while self-identity develops.

very probable that the seemingly endless telephoning, as illustrated in Figure 9-13, and talk sessions are of special importance in helping the adolescent learn self-identity. The talking serves as a mirror as the young person tries to find answers to questions concerning who he is and where he fits into the world. He is bouncing off ideas on peers since he feels comfortable with them and can expect their acceptance of his behavior.

Self-Image. Adolescence begins with seemingly little interest in the body. It is difficult to get the young man to bathe and comb his hair. Both girls and boys tend to be somewhat sloppy and uninterested in general appearance, although this is more prominent in the male. But this soon changes as both boys and girls become very interested and concerned about their body-image and become proud of their bodies. Now, getting them away from their bathroom mirrors becomes difficult and a hair brush sometimes seems to be an anatomical extension of the hand.

There are noticeable difficulties as the adolescent struggles to cope with rapid growth, sexual maturity, and the development of a self-image, but they are gradually integrated and an improved and intact self-image eventually appears. The adolescent is neither a child nor an adult and he seems to be trying desperately to put himself together. As though to add to the problem, the body reaches physiological maturity before psychological maturity. This is a period of negativism and a time when youth loves what adults hate. These characteristics help the adolescent to find his own identity as he strives to avoid being like his elders.

Sexuality. An important developmental task during adolescence occurs in relation to sexuality. As described earlier, preferences for a sexual partner are believed to develop during the preschool years. Adolescence is a period of great sexual awareness and there is progression to a consolidation and strengthening in preferred relationships. Figure 9-14 illustrates a typical teenage relationship.

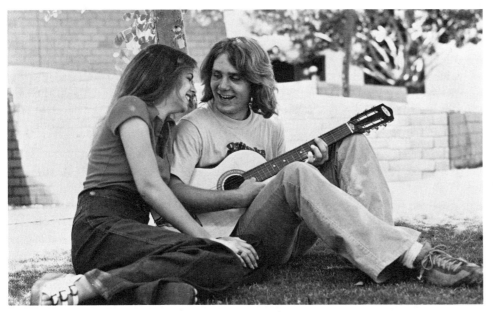

Figure 9-14 Relating with members of the opposite sex takes on meanings that add to self-identity during adolescence. These two young people appear to be enjoying each other's company and the fun of music during relaxing moments together.

The adolescent is very sensitive to his body and the new feelings of sexuality which often involve guilt and fear. For the boy especially, sexuality becomes very demanding and urgent. Masturbation is relatively common and conversation is laced with talk of sexual conquests.

With descriptions of explicit sex being readily available in the various media and better dissemination of knowledge of contraceptive devices, including the "pill," sexual activity appears to be more common among teenagers than once was the case. One study conducted in the early 1970s found that nearly half of the single girls queried were sexually active before the age of 20 and four-fifth of adult married women interviewed had premarital sexual experiences during adolescence and immediately following that period. Interestingly enough and despite popular opinion, research has indicated that promiscuity is not generally condoned among adolescents. It has also been observed that the father of a baby born to an unmarried adolescent most often is a person with whom the mother has had a relatively long-standing and exclusive relationship.

Many persons say that the cure for adolescence is five years. The rebellious and anxious adolescent progresses to the disciplined person with a good self-identity, relative independence from his family, and ideas on a career choice. He has achieved a developmental stage so that he is ready to accept the responsibilities and appreciate the joys of adulthood.

Common Health Problems During Adolescence

From a statistical point of view, the stage of adolescence is the healthiest and the death rate is low. The most frequent causes of death are vehicular accidents, suicide, and homicide.

Psychosomatic disorders, that is, conditions involving an interrelationship between psychological and physiological processes, are relatively common during adolescence. Sometimes, a pathological condition, such as gastric and duodenal ulcers, can be found and treated. But the psychological turmoil of the teenager that accompanies the condition is another matter. Headaches, abdominal pain, and various symptoms of a nonspecific nature are not uncommon.

Skin problems, especially acne, plague most adolescents. Typical infectious diseases of the age include infectious mononucleosis; hepatitis, especially among persons abusing injectable drugs; and venereal diseases.

Malnutrition due to fad diets is frequently seen. Young girls often seek help because of menstrual difficulties and pregnancy. There is an increasing problem of alcoholism among teenagers, and it is during these years that the illicit use of drugs often begins.

EARLY ADULTHOOD APPROXIMATELY 18 TO 40 YEARS

Physiological Growth and Development

Adulthood has often been thought of as years of plateauing, a time for living and functioning but not necessarily a time for growing and changing. However, this is a false assumption since physiologically and psychosocially, the years between about 20 and 65 are filled with many tasks and changes in living. There are developmental years also as some aspects of life begin to decline and appropriate adjustments must be made while other aspects of life move to greater heights.

Maximum physiological and intellectual maturity is attained between approximately 20 and 30 years of age. Physiological regression begins shortly after that. It has been estimated that the body's organs and systems lose approximately 1 percent of their efficiency each year beginning between 30 and 35 years of age.

Early adulthood is characterized by maximum neuromuscular development and coordination and greatest efficiency in the use of the body. Note the professional athletes who ordinarily come into their best years during the time of early adulthood. As with the other systems of the body, the musculoskeletal and nervous systems begin a slow decline in the 30s and tapering continues more or less steadily through late adulthood and into the age of the elderly. Cognitive skills are well-honed but are more likely to reach their peak during later adulthood.

Psychosocial Growth and Development

During early adulthood, the individual is eager to experience intimacy which is reflected in his selection of a mate. During adolescence, sexual activity was usually practiced for the sake of identifying the self. Now, sexual relationships are established for building a loving and lasting intimacy. Ethical and moral standards and ideologies become solidified as the adult makes various selections—mate, having children, career—and learns to accept the good along with the bad. When these needs for intimacy and commitment are not met, feelings of isolation and of being out of the mainstream of life develop.

The early 20s are years of transition from childhood and adolescence when development was rather clear-cut and changes were made a step at a time. At about 20 years of age, the individual takes a gigantic step into the unknown of adulthood where suddenly he is expected to get about efficiently and behave according to the rules of an adult society. The family's protection and guidance are no longer present as the young adult pulls up his last roots.

Another transition the young adult ordinarily makes can be illustrated with the apocryphal story of the 18-year-old who went off to college believing that his parents knew little of life and living. When he returned home after graduation, he was astounded at how much his parents had learned in that short period. This shows part of the crunch the young adult experiences as he leaves youth and enters adulthood only to discover he has much still to learn.

The 20-year-old experiences many firsts: first marriage, first home, first child, first job. Figure 9-15 illustrates some of early adulthood's first experiences. The "firsts" are urgent but often terrifying to the young adult who feels that his choices are relatively final so that he must do it right the first time.

Today's American society has fewer traditional standards for young adults. For example, in past generations, women married, usually in their early 20s, started a family shortly, and were homemakers while the men were breadwinners. Today, traditional marriage is being challenged. Women are often expected, and find it necessary, to work in order for the couple to establish conjugal living. Some of the "firsts" of the 20s, especially that of having a family, are being delayed until the late 20s and into the 30s.

During the 30s, the time depending to an extent on when marriage occurs and children arrive, another type of strain develops. While ordinarily men are consumed with their careers and pressures to succeed and get ahead, women are busy with child-rearing and homemaking. With a "settling down" attitude at this time in life, there also appear to be problems, for at least some couples, resulting from feelings of restlessness. Women begin asking whether child-rearing and homemaking are all of life and wondering whether they are functioning at their optimum level. Men are asking whether they are doing the best they can with what they want to accomplish in life.

The glow of earlier years of marriage with the many "firsts" may seem to be fading. Divorce now becomes an important factor in life for many American families today. The difficulties of suddenly being single, rearing children in one-parent homes, and possibly entering marriage again and beginning still another family add to the strains of life during this period for many people.

Communication. Communication skills are developed further during early adulthood. Vocabulary ordinarily increases as educational and work experiences broaden

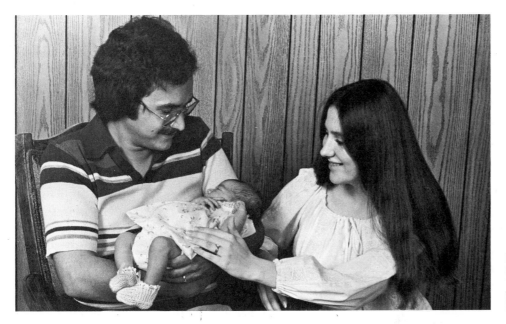

Figure 9-15 This young family has experienced many typical "firsts" in the last couple of years: marriage, home, and a baby.

the adult's horizon and semantics and subtleties in both verbal and nonverbal communications increase to a high degree. Cognitive skills are well-developed.

Self-Image. The American culture idolizes youth. Self-image during early adulthood reflects this value. Importance is placed on intactness of the body, slimness, energy, sexuality, style, sophistication, and beauty.

Sexuality. Research in adult sexuality took a big step with Alfred Kinsey's work of several decades ago. Exploration into sexual matters continues and it is commonplace to read of new findings and understandings almost daily. Standards for sexual relationships and morality had been believed to be rigid. Paradoxically, research suggests that these standards had not been observed in previous generations to the extent once thought. However, today what is considered right or wrong about sexuality has broadened and more people appear to accept the philosophy that consenting adults have the right to choose when their behavior does not hurt others. This attitude and more openness in discussing sexuality have brought about an increased general acceptance of the importance and normality of intimate sexual experiences that begin during adolescence but that can and do continue throughout the life span.

A love relationship with sexual fulfillment is ordinarily attained during early adulthood. Most persons marry during these years and decisions about types of sexual techniques used, the frequency of having intercourse, and whether to have children, become important.

With the emphasis on youth and sexuality in our culture, the young adult is much consumed with the sex act and the concepts of masculinity and femininity. There has been a marked increase in the dissemination of information concerning sexuality. There is also increased willingness and social acceptance to work toward solving sexual problems, such as frigidity, inability to reach organism, impotence, and early ejaculation.

The previous discussion has focused on *heterosexuality,* that is, having feelings for a person of the opposite sex. Some persons have other sexual orientations. *Homosexuality* is defined as having sexual feelings for a person of the same sex. The word *gay* is often used as its synonym. A *lesbian* is a female homosexual.

The sexual behaviors of the heterosexual and the homosexual are the same except for penile-vaginal penetration. Hence, the difference between a hetero-

sexual and a homosexual is primarily in the gender of the sex partner and not in a particular type of behavior. Studies have also shown that a well-adjusted homosexual could not be differentiated from a well-adjusted heterosexual on the basis of results from certain objective psychosocial examinations. As one author stated, homosexuality and heterosexuality are probably more alike than different.

Many theories have been advanced concerning the cause of a person's particular sexual orientation but none has had universal acceptance. Homosexuality has often been considered an illness or deviant behavior. In 1974, the American Psychiatric Association removed homosexuality from the category of a mental illness. While this move and certain research findings eliminated some of the stigma attached to homosexuality, society as a whole has made slow progress in accepting the gay movement that strives for equal rights and acceptance of their sexual orientation as being different from most but not deviant.

There are other sexual orientations but they occur less frequently than heterosexuality and homosexuality. Persons showing sexual feelings for others of both sexes are called *bisexual. Autosexuality* refers to behavior which focuses on the self. Masturbation can be observed in persons of any sexual orientation throughout life. The difference is that the autosexual is uninterested in sexual relations with others while this is not the case among persons who masturbate for temporary sexual gratification. The term *asexual* has been used in some literature to describe persons who apparently experience no interest in sexuality. However, the term is used more commonly to describe reproduction in plants and in some animals low in the phylogenic scale.

When sexual orientation is placed on a continuum, it becomes easier to understand that between homosexuality and heterosexuality lies considerable latitude. Normal, healthy individuals may fluctuate between these ends of the scale under certain conditions. Either heterosexual or homosexual persons may have bisexual relationships at times. A person who is heterosexual may use homosexuality under certain circumstances, such as while incarcerated in prison, while in the army, or while attending a school whose enrollment is limited to one sex. Asexuality may be experienced also by both heterosexuals and homosexuals, at least temporarily, such as following the death of the sex partner.

Many beliefs have developed concerning sexuality which research has proven wrong. Table 9-1 summarizes some of the more common myths and the facts that disprove them.

TABLE 9-1   Sexual myths and facts to refute them

MYTHS (OR COMMON MISCONCEPTIONS)	FACTS (BASED UPON RESULTS OF CURRENT RESEARCH)
The sex drive or "libido" is of primary importance in early development and behavior in infancy.	The bases for one's developing sexuality are established during the first five years of life as a result of learning, mainly through nonverbal channels. The self-gratifying behavior and pleasure-seeking activities of the infant are not "sexual" in the adult sense of the word, for sex as such, is rarely a human need prior to adolescence.
Each person is endowed with a finite amount of sexual drive which is overdrawn in youth or in young adult life leaves little reserve for the later years.	Actually the correlation between sexual activity and length of time it persists throughout life is just the opposite. The more sexually active a person is, the longer it continues into the later years of life.
The need for expressing one's sexuality becomes less important in the latter half of one's life.	Physiologically, sexual desire and ability do not decrease markedly after middle age. The expression of one's sexuality, as an integral part of development, follows the overall pattern of health and physical performance.
Sexual abstinence is necessary in training for the development of optimum physical performance in sports, dance, or other strenuous activities.	While there is great variation in sexual activity, physiologically the achievement of orgasm is rarely more demanding than most activities encountered in daily life. The desire for sleep which often follows is most commonly due to factors other than physical exhaustion from sexual activities. Orgasm may bring a relief of sexual tension with a feeling of relaxation and a readiness for sleep. A sense of weariness is more likely due to related activities resulting in improper eating, sleeping, drinking, or feelings of guilt.
Excessive sexual activity can lead to mental breakdown.	The biological significance of man's sexuality is of no greater impact on his total development than any other necessary biological function. Most behavioral scientists do not regard sex as *the* prevailing instinct in man so that his sex life must be paramount in his emotional development. There is no scientific basis for believing that one will develop a mental or physical illness unless one's sex needs are satisfied.
Nocturnal emissions (wet dreams) are indicators of sexual disorders.	Erotic dreams that culminate in orgasms are common physiological phenomena in at least 85 percent of all men. They occur at any age, beginning in the teens when the maturing sex organs exert a new primacy in masculine development. The phenomenon is also common among females, who report in clinical studies, that their sexual dreams culminated in orgasm. In women, this practice is believed to increase with advancing age.
Because of the anatomical nature of the sex organs, the female is inherently passive and the male inherently aggressive.	Physiological studies disprove this myth by showing the woman to be far from passive. Maximum gratification requires each partner to be *both* passive and aggressive in participating mutually and cooperatively.
It is "unnatural" for a woman to have as strong a desire for sex as a man—for women normally do not enjoy sex as much as men.	These myths have been reinforced by a society which has traditionally taught women that they are to suppress sexual desires to gain love, security, and society's respect—based on the assumption that it is the "basic nature" of women to be submissive, dependent, and subordinate. Physiological studies indicate that, in some respects, the woman's sex drive is not only as strong but may be even stronger than that of the male.
Women who have multiple orgasms or who readily come to climax are actually nymphomaniacs.	Physiological studies at this time suggest that we do not know women's sexual potential—but indicate that there is a wide range of intensity and duration of orgastic experience—and the potential for multiple (or frequent orgasms within a brief period of time) is not at all uncommon. Therefore, women have greater orgastic capacity than men with regard to duration and frequency of orgasm.

TABLE 9–1   (*Continued*)

There is a difference between vaginal and clitoral orgasm. The former being the more "mature" according to Freudian theory; the latter indicating signs of narcissism or inadequacy.	Physiological misunderstanding has produced the myth of separate clitoral and vaginal orgasms rather than their interrelationships. Female orgasm is normally initiated by clitoral stimulation, but since it is a total body response there are marked variations in intensity and timing. There is no reason to believe that the quantitative differences in the female response to the sex act are due to vaginal rather than a clitoral orgasm.
A mature sexual relationship requires the male and female to achieve simultaneous orgasm.	While simultaneous orgasm may be desirable it is an unrealistic goal in view of the complexity of human sexuality. Often it is possible only under the most ideal circumstances and is not a determinant of sexual achievement or of satisfaction (except to someone who accepts this as dogma).
It is dangerous to have intercourse during menstruation.	Since the source of the menstrual flow is from the uterus rather than the vagina, there is no basis for concern about tissue damage to the vagina nor is there any reason for the woman's sexual drive to diminish during the menstrual period. There is no physiological basis for abstinence during the menses.
The larger penis has greater possibilities for pleasurable stimulation or for producing orgasm in the female.	Physiologically, there is practically no relationship between the size of the penis and a man's ability to satisfy a woman sexually. Furthermore, there is very little correlation between penile size and body size and their relationship to sexual potency.
The face-to-face coital position is the proper, moral and healthy one for it is this position that distinguishes the sexual activity of man from the remainder of the animal kingdom.	Recent knowledge of human sexual practices dispel this myth with the recognition that there is no *normal* or *single most acceptable* sexual position. Whatever position offers the most pleasure and is acceptable to both partners is correct for them. Any variation is normal, healthy, and proper if it satisfies both partners.
The ability to achieve orgasm is an indicator of an individual's sexual responsiveness.	Achievement of a satisfactory sexual response is the result of the successful interaction of numerous physical, psychological, and cultural influences. Too often the physical fact of orgasm (or lack or orgasm) is taken to be symbolic of sexual responsiveness and seen out of context of the entire relationship between man and woman. Such distortions add to the tension and anxiety of those who strive to attain this singular goal—contributing to conditions of impotence and frigidity.

An important implication for nursing is that an understanding of sexuality is essential in order to participate in offering complete health care for all persons regardless of their sexual preference. If a nurse feels uncomfortable caring for a person with a sexual orientation different from her own and believes her feelings may interfere with the care she is able to give, it is best that she ask her supervisor to be assigned to the care of other persons. It would be unfair to deny someone the kind of care exemplified by a nurse who can accept other people without any regard for their sexual preferences.

As this discussion indicates, the 20s are years of being accepted in the adult world and gaining adult authenticity. The years of the 30s are settling down years and a time to deepen commitments for the self. Early adulthood is a time of building for a future by getting everything together now.

Common Health Problems During Early Adulthood

Young adulthood is relatively free from illness although unhealthful life-styles lay groundwork for many later health problems. Examples include such practices as smoking, abuse of alcohol, overeating with overweight and poor nutrition, and living with high levels of tension and strain. A malignant disease typically observed during early adulthood is Hodgkin's disease. Accidents, especially those involving motor vehicles, remain high during this age of life. Problems related to child-bearing as well as child-rearing are commonly observed now, such as concerns with infertility, contraceptions, complications of pregnancy and delivery, and child-rearing practices. Cardiovascular problems are being increasingly noted late in the period of early adulthood.

MIDDLE ADULTHOOD: APPROXIMATELY 40 TO 65 YEARS

Physiological Growth and Development

As mentioned previously, physiological processes decline beginning at about age 35 and continue until death. The height of physiological efficiency has passed by the time middle adulthood is reached. The basal metabolism rate tends to decline and hormonal levels taper. Arriving at the age of 40 is an important milestone in life, as figure 9–16 illustrates, and for at least some people, a crisis too. The results of declining physiological processes and thoughts of death become realities.

The time for leisure ordinarily increases as children leave home and careers become established. However, the physical demands of participation in leisure-time activities characteristically becomes more conservative. Life in general becomes more sedentary.

During middle adulthood, the most dramatic physiological change occurs with the *climacteric,* that is, the decline and then the cessation of reproductive ability in women. Psychological changes accompany the physiological changes; some of them will be discussed later in this section.

There is the question of whether men experience a climacteric. Certainly there is not the marked physiological changes that women experience, although the testosterone level begins to decline. Nor does the male lose the ability to produce sperm capable of fertilizing an ovum. Fatherhood has been noted in some males as late as the seventh and even the eighth decade of life. However, as is true of most females, psychological changes occur during this period. As a result, many people speak and write of the climacteric in men although from a technical standpoint, the term refers to females.

Psychosocial Growth and Development

The fourth and fifth decades of life are often called the prime of life. The 40s are important halfway years. By this time, children are reared and leave home. A career has ordinarily been well-established although some people do make career changes in these years. It is a time for taking stock, to reassess, and to enjoy fulfillment. There is now more concern with a psychosocial task of being needed by the young, to guide a new generation, to create something of lasting and worthwhile value, to receive respect, and to enjoy the dignity of having done life's work well. Society looks to people of middle years to assume social and civic responsibility which adds to prestige and fulfillment. When this task of generativity is not accomplished, the adult experiences feelings of stagnation, boredom, and personal impoverishment.

Cognitive skills are usually at a high peak during the middle adult years. Many authorities believe that the highest degree of cognition occurs during the fourth and fifth decades when persons, from the experience of living, often make their greatest contribution to society. Skills in this area have been honed to a fine degree and creativity is often at its maximum.

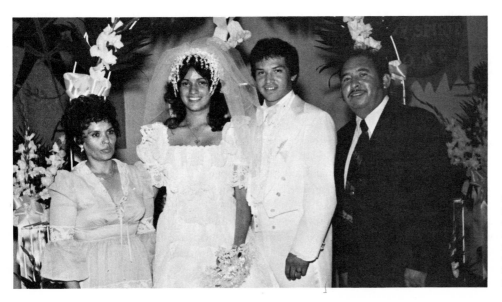

Figure 9–16 For parents, marriage of their children is often an important milestone in life. Feelings of not being needed any longer and realizing that we are mortals frequently influence behavior during middle adulthood.

Communication. There need not necessarily be a decline in communication skills as adulthood progresses. In fact, many persons who depend on the arts and skills of communication for a livelihood often experience greatest maturity and creativity during late adulthood and on into the years of the elderly.

Self-Image. When some of the chronic illnesses begin to make their appearance, adjusting to an older acting and appearing body sometimes becomes a psychological problem of sufficient magnitude to warrant counseling help. This is especially true when illness threatens intactness of the body, and particularly sexuality.

A good self-image for the older adult requires an acceptance that all dreams of a younger age may not have come true. Life may not be as beautiful as the imagination had created earlier in life. Living in an imaginary world is not possible. There must be adjustments of goals which are realistic and an acceptance of not having met some established earlier in life.

The 40s and 50s are seen as years when one becomes one's own person. Healthy middle adulthood involves a continual process of developing a maturing and blossoming self-image that accepts the realities of aging.

Interest in youth and beauty are still present during middle adulthood. Greater efforts now are needed to maintain the figure and the body of youth. Many men and women become active in a variety of programs that help keep the body in good physical condition and more youthful appearance. Both sexes become interested in the work of the plastic surgeon. Such practices as wearing wigs, having hair transplants, removing hair on the face that appears in many women after menopause, and applying a variety of cosmetics for a more youthful look become common.

Sexuality. As adulthood progresses, sexuality tends to take on a different pattern. Rather than thinking of this pattern as a decline, it is now more often described as a change. The sex act, while still important, assumes a less demanding role and becomes less intense and urgent. Proving masculinity and feminity becomes less important as problems experienced in adolescence and early adulthood have been resolved with experience and experimentation. Acts that do not necessarily include orgasm for both sexual partners are often found to be very satisfying and sexually fulfilling. Sexuality does not become less important in life but assumes a tone of maturity as life progresses. Sexual expression becomes associated more with feelings of total awareness than with meeting an urgent demand.

For some persons, the change in sexual behavior during middle adulthood may cause problems. The male may feel distress by growing old and diminishing virility. He may try to recapture the sexual prowess of youth and turn to challenges with new sex partners. The female may become more interested and aggressive in the act of sex when pregnancy cannot occur and the daily chores of rearing children have ceased. She may find it difficult to cope when her partner seems uninterested in meeting sexual needs while he struggles with a feeling of inadequacy. This is another age when inability to cope often results in divorce which adds to the strain of everyday living for both men and women. A woman especially may experience feelings of worthlessness when she interprets herself to be uninteresting as a sexual partner. Children have left home and no longer seem to need her which fuels the so-called empty nest syndrome. Self-esteem suffers and despair may result. This is a time when women are encouraged to find new interest and many return to work with resulting improved self-esteem and self-image.

Couples in middle adulthood often need help to understand maturing sexuality and to learn and explore new techniques for sexual gratification. It becomes important to teach that boredom, physical fatigue, too much food and alcohol, and preoccupation with outside matters usually stand in the way of sexual fulfillment. Changes in patterns of sexuality can be expected with a proper attitude and sexual pleasure can continue.

Middle adulthood can be said to begin with a rude awakening. Life is ebbing. There are feelings of aloneness when children are reared and leave home to marry. It is time when many wonder if they can accomplish earlier dreams. By late in this period, the satisfaction of generativity and adjusting to a self-image to fit physiological declines help prepare for the age of the elderly.

Common Health Problems During Middle Adulthood

During the middle adulthood years, the harvest of life-styles that are filled with stresses and indescretions are likely to be reaped. Gastric and duodenal ulcers and myocardial infarctions become leading causes of morbidity and mortality. Emphysema and cirrhosis of the liver are likely to appear when cigarettes and alcohol have been used indiscriminately over a period of years. Overweight is a common problem of middle adulthood. Unless dietary and exercise programs are well-planned, they contribute to health problems also.

The malignant diseases become a common cause of death during middle adulthood. Other conditions frequently seen in this age period include biliary diseases, especially in women, and arthritic diseases.

THE ELDERLY: APPROXIMATELY 65 YEARS AND OLDER

Physiological Growth and Development

The reduced efficiency of the body becomes a fact of life for the elderly. Even when an older person appears in good health, physiological functioning becomes more fragile. For example, glucose tolerance drops and the blood pressure normally rises, although increased blood pressure is also associated with certain illnesses. As a result, a situation that may be handled with relative ease in a younger person, such as a fractured bone, the pneumonias, a urinary tract infection, or surgical intervention, may become catastrophic for an elderly person.

The decline in body organ and system efficiency continues. Bones tend to lose mass as calcium escapes; the muscles have less bulk and firmness and hypertrophy from disuse occurs; there is a loss of neurons which are not replaceable; the efficiency of the gastrointestinal and cardiovascular systems decreases, and so on. Approximately 30 percent of people over 65 years of age have handicaps due to chronic diseases with which they must cope in addition to decreased physiological efficiency as shown in Figure 9–17.

Sensory decrements occur, as sight, hearing, sensations of pain, and tactile senses decrease in acuity. Reflexes and the thought process become slower as age progresses.

By the age of about 65, many persons have lost their teeth, usually because of periodontal diseases. When dentures are ill-fitting and uncomfortable, eating habits change and there is danger of malnutrition due to poorly balanced diets. There is also a decrease in the total amount of body fluids in relation to body weight which adds to the fragility of fluid balance.

Medical science has made great strides to increase life expectancy. However, the life span for the human, which is approximately 100 years, has not increased. There is a loss or malfunctioning in body cells with aging. The cause for this deterioration which finally terminates life is unknown.

The position of the aged becomes one of flexion. Several factors contribute to this bent over posture,

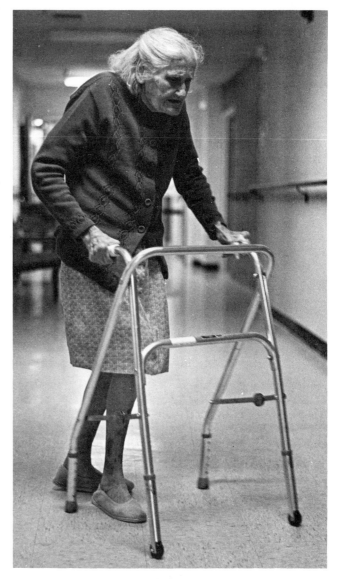

Figure 9–17 This resident in a nursing home illustrates many characteristics of the elderly: chronic disease, in this case, arthritis; the stooped body posture; grey hair; wrinkled skin; and loss of teeth. Yet, she maintains a certain amount of independence and personal integrity by wanting to walk about with the assistance of a walker.

including decreasing musculoskeletal integrity and diminishing locomotion cues from sensory organs, especially that of sight. There is also a general decrease in the perception of the body in space which threatens coordination and balance. Moving slowly and a shuffling gait while keeping the feet close to the walking surface help overcome the change in posture and perception. Tiring easily in order to cope with these changes in locomotion becomes understandable. Figure 9–18 illustrates one of the many characteristics of the elderly.

Psychosocial Growth and Development

There is a trend toward continuing to use the skills of persons after what has been the traditional age for retirement at 65 years of age. However, the age of the elderly is often thought of as the time for retirement. For many, there are rituals associated with leaving careers, the traditional retirement luncheon being one. Also moving to smaller living quarters and, for some, migrating to communities for the elderly in the sunbelt of the United States are often part of retiring. There is ordinarily a drop in income which may force a change in living standards. The loss of a mate can change life for the elderly in a profound manner too.

In some cultures, the Oriental culture being one, the elderly are held in respect for the wisdom and understandings acquired over the period of their lives. This is not particularly true in the American culture where youth is venerated. The phenomenon of lack of interest in the elderly tends to make the task of maintaining dignity and a healthy ego integrity difficult for some older persons. However, when the elderly can con-

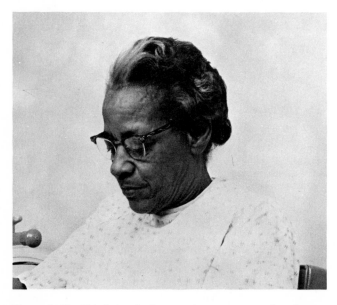

Figure 9–18 This lady who is several years younger than the one in Figure 9–17, appears to be reminiscing and she seems to be enjoying what she is recalling. Reminiscing often helps the elderly maintain ego-identity and a secure self-identity.

template life, accept it, and adapt to both the triumphs and disappointments of the past, ego integrity is maintained. When the task of developing ego integrity is insurmountable, the elderly are likely to live in despair and suffer from feelings of uselessness and of being unwanted. Time becomes too short to reorder goals. These feelings are more pronounced when younger persons appear to have no respect for the elderly and seem to have found no satisfactory way to put up with them.

In cognitive skills, there is a decreased capacity for adaptation, especially when stressors become formidable. But intellectual and reasoning capacity, the ability to think abstractly, and memory do not necessarily decline unless illness destroys vital nervous system tissues. Thinking becomes slower but the elderly can learn—it just takes a little longer than it once did.

Communication. The ability to communicate does not necessarily deteriorate with age unless a handicap interferes with speech or cognition. Speech and the thought process become slower and interest in semantics and linguistics may diminish. However, ability to use verbal and nonverbal communication skills are often as acute as they were during earlier stages in life.

Self-Image. During the years of the elderly, the individual must learn to develop a self-image that accepts a body with diminishing efficiency. Intactness is still important and there is real concern for having to change life-styles, especially when illness is present. The necessary adjustments have to be incorporated during these later years into a self-image that is quite different from that of the young and middle-aged adult. The elderly person, while shifting gears, must rethink who he is and what is expected of him. As growing older is accepted in realistic terms, so ordinarily is acceptance of a changed self-image. It has been noted that acceptance of this decline is often accompanied with great self-esteem when coping abilities triumph over the vicissitudes of aging.

A characteristic of the elderly is that they tend to reminisce. This behavior has adaptive qualities. It helps to resolve doubts and conflicts about the self and to restructure a new self-identity in terms of what is. There is a sharpening of the present when the past is examined. Reminiscing is also adaptive in helping the elderly to develop ego integrity. As can be seen, maintaining a secure self-identity and a healthy self-image are tasks throughout the life span.

Sexuality. The need for sexual gratification does not disappear with age as was once thought to be true. Research has demonstrated that there appears to be no time limit for having sexual intercourse for women. Typically, after menopause, vaginal secretions decrease, the vaginal mucosa becomes thinner, and the ability of the vagina to expand decreases. Many women in this country now use prescribed hormonal therapy so that these physiological decreases can be abated for many years. It has been demonstrated that a healthy male with an interested and interesting partner can perform sexual intercourse into the 80s and beyond.

Sexual needs persist until death. When intercourse is not possible, other expressions of intimacy, such as companionship, affection, love, and feelings of closeness are necessary in order for the elderly to enjoy a full and normal life. It is a myth that the elderly have no sexual desires or that they cannot participate in sexually satisfying relationships.

Many speak of the time after approximately 65 years of age as the golden or vintage years and they can well be. In order to avoid bleakness, just as was true during earlier periods in life, the elderly need interests, tasks that make them feel needed and wanted, friendships, and opportunities for sexual expression. They need experiences that bolster self-esteem, as Figure 9–19 illustrates. They also need encouragement to remain independent as long as it is feasible. The stereotype of the lonely and unhappy elderly concerned only with aches and pains need not necessarily be the case.

Until life ends, the elderly can experience a full life with satisfaction and happiness as he adjusts to physiological waning. This is especially true when the environment is supportive and there is interest in the person's total welfare.

Common Health Problems of the Elderly

The three most common causes of death in this country are diseases of the heart, malignant neoplasms, and cerebrovascular disorders. These three disease conditions demand much of the health personnel's time and effort, in terms of prevention, health promotion, rehabilitation, and the care of persons ill with these disorders. Infections, particularly in the respiratory and urinary systems, are conditions to which the elderly are very prone. Because of bone fragility, falls are dangerous for the elderly, especially when a fall results in a fracture of the hip. Conditions resulting in failing acuity of the eyes and ears are common. Arthritis ranks second to heart disease as the most common chronic disease in this country and is responsible for much prolonged suffering and disability among the elderly. Although diabetes mellitus is not frequently the prime cause of death, it predisposes to cardiovascular and renal complications which are frequent causes of death.

The psychosocial problems frequently encountered by the elderly are of concern to health practitioners. Typical examples include the loneliness of living when mates and friends die and children are grown and away from home; despair when life itself seems worthless; and hopelessness when chronic diseases interfere with normal living. Economic insecurity occurs at a time in life when it is usually too late to seek employment. There is loss in self-esteem when it seems that no one any longer cares. It is little wonder that suicide is becoming increasingly common among the elderly.

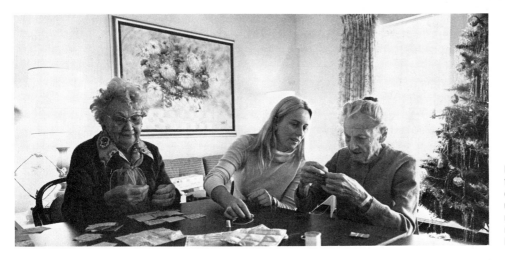

Figure 9–19 A destructive force during the years of the elderly is feeling unwanted and useless. These residents in a nursing home are helped to feel needed as they make items for holiday gift giving.

THE FAMILY

A _family_ may be defined as a small group of people who consider themselves bound by ties and who accept the responsibility for rearing children. The _nuclear family_ is the immediate family unit, that is, the father, mother, and their children. A nuclear family is illustrated in Figure 9–20. The _extended family_ includes the nuclear family as well as grandparents, uncles, aunts, and cousins.

The discussion thus far has focused on the individual and how he changes from birth to death. A significant influence in all of life is that of the family. A few current trends that are changing traditional family units in this country will be given here. Some of the far-reaching effects of these trends on the individual may not be predictable at this time. However, because of the important influences the family has on its members, at least some trends seem worth noting.

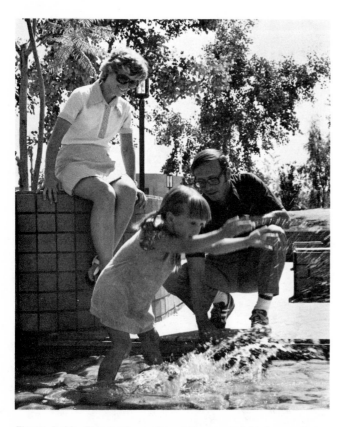

Figure 9–20   This family, mother, father, and child, is a nuclear family. As is typical of many families today in the United States, this family's extended members (grandparents, aunts, uncles, and cousins) live in other parts of the country.

- Many functions once assumed by the family have been transferred to other social institutions. For many years, the primary responsibility for the education of the young has been given to the school and meeting religious needs has been largely delegated to the church. A few more recent trends include the following: law enforcement agencies have been given many responsibilities once assumed by the family, such as the handling of delinquent children; many agencies have been providing sex education for the young when once it was considered the family's entire responsibility; the rearing of the young during early childhood is being increasingly shared by substitute care, such as day care centers and preschool nurseries; and more families are turning to governmental agencies to care for their old and poor.

- The close association among members of the extended family has almost disappeared. For example, homes are shared by members of the nuclear family and rarely are extended family members included. Close ties among extended and nuclear family members are becoming less common.

- Many children are being reared in single-parent homes. Approximately one-sixth of all children in the United States live with a single parent. With changes in divorce and child custody laws, fathers are increasingly rearing children when once it was the mother who reared children after divorce.

- The increase in the number of abortions performed in this country has resulted in fewer children available for adoption. Also, many unwed mothers are choosing to rear their children alone when they have not wished to have an abortion. Single men and women are beginning to be reported as adoptive parents who choose to rear children alone.

- One marriage in three ended in divorce in the early and middle 1970s. This is an all-time high, but there is evidence to suggest that this rate is leveling off, according to the National Center for Health Statistics.

- It has been estimated that about $1\frac{1}{4}$ million single men and women live together without being married; some of these couples have children. Yet, about 98 percent of the men and women in this country who are cohabitating are married.

- Time was when only men deserted homes and families. It is reported that women are increasingly doing so also and child runaways are no longer uncommon.

- About 40 percent of all married women work outside of the home and that percentage is on the increase. Over 50 percent of the women who work have school-age children and over one-third of working women have pre-schoolers. These statistics indicate that women in relatively large numbers are tending to move away from traditional homemaking roles.

- The traditional roles of husband and wife are being challenged. Role reversal is becoming more common with men helping to assume housekeeping and child-rearing responsibilities and women assisting with the economic support of the family. (Fig 9–21).

- The home has traditionally been accepted as the environment for sexual gratification of husband and wife. Satellite affairs and sexually open marriages are becoming more commonplace. For these people at least, monogamy is being challenged.

- The family is an extremely mobile unit. Changing work locations several times during adulthood is becoming more common in our complex, technological society. Moving creates stresses and strains in most families and requires severing relationships with relatives and friends and establishing ties in new communities.

- The size of families has been slowly decreasing for well over a century. With concern for an environment able to support increasingly larger populations and an interest in zero population growth, the trend for smaller families has become more evident in recent years.

Other changes from the traditional could be cited. The ones given here have been used by many who believe that the American family is falling apart and doomed to failure. Yet, persons observing less rigid and traditional roles and promoting more individualized behavior believe many of these changes are long overdue and are making for happier and healthier families. They believe the family remains strong and will survive. History is on the side of this latter group.

The family as a social institution has demonstrated remarkable stability throughout the ages of mankind and has shown great capabilities for adapting to change. Families may not be what they used to be but they are here and thriving nonetheless. Many alternatives have been tried in the past and a few can be seen today, such as communes, trial marriages, and kibbutzes. But the family, possibly the most flexible of all human institutions, has survived despite years of criticism. It appears to be doing well as it adapts to changes today.

Sociologists suggest several reasons for the family's existance and for predicting its continued survival. The family is particularly well-suited to socialize the young by conveying knowledge, values, and patterns of social behavior to next generations. It serves as the best source

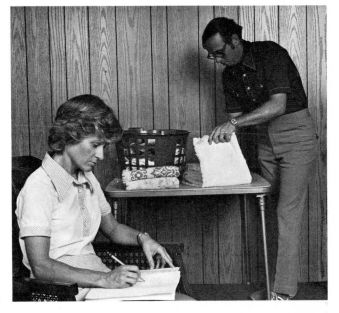

Figure 9–21 Traditionally, women were homemakers and men were breadwinners. This couple illustrates role reversal. The husband assists with household chores. His wife is completing graduate education. She has plans to continue with her career and to help in the economic support of the family.

for love and affection and for the physical care of the young. The family gives a sense of belongingness to living and of being wanted and needed. These are critical factors in the rearing of children. A cartoon caption once described the family well: it's a place where they will always take you in.

Thus, the enduring power of the family remains. It adapts to change and takes advantage of choices society allows. Family member roles may blur and formal structures change. But it still seems to be an essential institution necessary for the very survival of mankind.

IMPLICATIONS FOR NURSING

Implications for nursing in relation to the life span are numerous and can be considered from a variety of viewpoints. In terms of the nursing process, knowledge of growth and development through the life span and of the developmental tasks confronting various age groups is important for data gathering, assessment, planning nursing care, intervention, and continuous evaluation. A few examples will illustrate.

The nurse familiar with human growth and development has knowledge to guide her when she obtains a health history. Thus her interest in the typical diet of a teenager who is experiencing a growth spurt becomes important. Compare this with data-gathering the nurse will use when a mother expresses concern because her eight-year-old child who seems to eat too sparingly in the mother's opinion. Or, consider the elderly gentleman whose nutritional status appears poor. Has he been eating poorly because of ill-fitting dentures? Is he economically handicapped and unable to purchase foods that are necessary for good nutrition? Perhaps he is alone and unfamiliar with the ways of preparing an adequate diet.

In order to assess, one must have a standard with which to compare findings. This chapter is rich in such standards. The eight-year-old child who dislikes school may be tussling with feelings of inferiority when the more positive achievement of industriousness of this age is not being attained. Many parents, as well as other adults, fret when the teenager seems concerned about who he is and where he fits into the scheme of things. The nurse can help these persons when she understands that their behavior is important as they seek identity. A young couple speaks of great sexual gratification in their marriage and add that they dread the 40s and 50s when they assume their sex life will come to a natural end. It is important for the nurse to know that sexual gratification is part of all of living and need not necessarily end during middle and late adulthood.

After data have been collected and assessed, the nurse can then plan nursing care that is appropriate for each person she is serving. For instance, the nurse who understands that the cardiac sphincter is immature at birth knows that her care plan should include bubbling the baby in order to help prevent regurgitation. An elderly patient has been eating and drinking poorly. The nurse who knows that with age, physiological functioning becomes fragile, the skin becomes dry, thin, and more easily injured, and the circulatory system's efficiency has decreased, wisely plans accordingly. Care will include measures that will help promote improved fluid and food intake and that will help prevent skin breakdown. A one-year-old infant requires an injection. Since the infant is likely to be very fearful when mother is out of sight, the nurse can plan to have the mother present and assist in the infant's care.

Nursing intervention requires taking age into consideration. The elderly patient needs the respect and dignity afforded by providing proper explanations and privacy when nursing measures are being carried out, even though his mental state may not be as alert as it once was. The choice of a site for an intramuscular injection for a newborn requires special precautions since his muscles are small and underdeveloped. Special care is also indicated for the elderly whose muscular tissue has atrophied with age and whose vascular system is declining in efficiency. Knowledge that preschoolers are interested in knowing about sexual matters guides the nurse in answering the five-year-old's inquiry concerning how babies are "made." In just about all ages except the very young, surgical intervention threatens the person's self-image and helping persons cope with the threat becomes an important nursing intervention measure.

Earlier chapters have pointed out the importance of helping persons build on their potentials in order to enjoy the best possible state of well-being. This type of nursing care can be accomplished much more effectively when the nurse knows common characteristics of persons of various ages. For example, it is usually unrealistic to expect that an elderly patient with failing coordination and balance can become mobile after a hip fracture with the use of crutches. However, the patient might well be able to regain mobility and an improved sense of well-being by learning how to use a walker. A nine-year-old child who has learned he has diabetes mellitus is ordinarily a good subject for being taught how to give himself insulin. At this age he is motivated to learn and eager to continue progress toward independence. Illness is an unwelcomed intruder but when the strengths of the individual are used to help build coping behavior, the person moves from illness to health and well-being.

The nurse has important teaching responsibilities as she works for health promotion, disease prevention, and rehabilitation. It is of little value to understand the human being if the knowledge is reserved only for use when an individual is ill. This chapter contains much information which the nurse can share with persons for whom she cares. The sections on common health problems for each age group was given with the intent of alerting the nurse not only to disease conditions per se, but also to offer her clues for teaching about health promotion and disease prevention. This can be seen in the following instances.

The excesses of smoking, food, and alcohol commonly seen in early adulthood often predispose to health problems later in life. During the 20s and 30s, health promotion by helping persons adjust life-styles before it is too late is important.

Accidents and suicide are common causes of death early in life. Teaching programs, as well as being alert to psychosocial problems underlying depression, are important for helping to decrease common causes of death.

Dental science has progressed to the point that periodontal disease which is the primary cause of losing teeth late in life can be halted and prevented. Teaching the importance of proper dental care is essential when working toward health promotion during childhood and adulthood.

The nurse often serves as the patient's advocate. When the nurse judges that the patient needs help for which she is inadequately prepared, she seeks the assistance of others on behalf of the patient. For example, counselors who deal with adult sexuality problems have much more information than this chapter could appropriately present as well as special counseling skills. The nurse can plan with the patient interested in such services by contacting a counselor and paving the way for a patient-counselor relationship.

A knowledge of the life span and characteristic developmental tasks for each age teaches the nurse typical concerns of patients of various ages when illness strikes. The infant is primarily mother bound and illness with possible separation from mother creates fear and feelings of mistrust. The toddler responds by shame and feelings of doubt when his drive for autonomy is interrupted. The preschooler tends to feel guilty when he assumes he is the cause of his illness and thinks his body will be permanently mutilated. Children of middle childhood years hate the restrictions of illness which disturbs their developing industriousness. Illness causes most adolescents to feel irritated and put upon when disability immobilizes them. They are concerned about the effects illness may have on their self- and body-image. An intact body is of special concern during adulthood and threats to intactness become particularly troublesome. The elderly person tends to view illness as a threat to life itself and may find coping abilities so reduced that despair results.

Concerns or problems of sexuality can occur as the result of illness. The patient may ask the nurse for assistance. Or, the nurse may observe indications of a problem and may seek other information for validation. Some patients are reluctant to initiate a discussion on sexuality but would appreciate the opportunity to talk about it if the occasion is presented. Some may wish only to discuss sexual matters with a nurse of the same sex while others are willing to talk about the topic with any supportive, accepting nurse. In other instances, the nurse may need to refer the patient to a professional with special training in the area of sexuality.

Masturbation by children and adults may be observed by the nurse. As indicated, in young children, masturbation is merely an exploring of the body. Often, parents need help in understanding that it is normal behavior.

In the adolescent or adult who is confined to a health care agency, masturbation may be an indication of boredom or it may be a continuation of a form of sexual stimulation that the person practices routinely. Masturbation may also be used to relieve anxiety created by confinement or illness as a substitute for the person's sexual feelings while being separated from his usual sexual partner.

If the purpose of masturbation is to relieve boredom, providing activities which interest the patient can engage his attention. If masturbation is used to relieve anxiety, the nurse may assist the individual by providing another outlet, such as a relationship which allows the patient to discuss his concerns. If the individual is merely continuing his normal practices, providing privacy for him by closing the door or drawing a curtain can be appreciated. In any case, the nurse's action should not be punitive or engender feelings of guilt or shame in the patient. If the nurse views masturbation as an outlet for normal sexual feelings, she can more easily meet the patient's needs in a nonjudgmental manner.

Men and women may turn to the nurse for assistance with family planning. The nurse will need the appropriate information before she engages in teaching. Family planning is discussed in various speciality and clinical texts.

The nurse may be called upon to provide information about surgical procedures which cause sterilization. Many patients need assistance in understanding the effect of a vasectomy or tubal ligation performed for sterilization.

Women who are deciding about whether to have an abortion may turn to the nurse for information and support. The nurse may also be expected to provide nursing care for patients who have had therapeutic, criminal, and self-induced abortions. Depending on the viewpoints of the patient and the nurse, this may be an emotionally charged time which requires objectivity and skill on the part of the nurse.

Many patients experience anxiety about the effect of some types of surgery on their usual sexual activities. Women who have hysterectomies and radical mastectomies often worry about the effect of the absence of their uterus or breast on their femininity and how this will affect their sexual partner. Men frequently are concerned about the effects of prostate surgery or a vasectomy on their sexual functioning. The effect of colostomy and ileostomy surgery and of paralysis of the lower part of the body on sexual activities also cause anxiety in many patients and their partners. Teaching and emotional support are important in these instances.

Persons with chronic illnesses, such as diabetes and heart disease, frequently experience problems with sexual functioning. In some instances, impotence and sterility exist. In others, the problem may be more psychological than physiological.

Persons with pathology which affects their sexuality often need information and emotional support. The nurse frequently is in a position to provide both. In addition, the person who is unable to function sexually or experience sexual satisfaction may need encouragement to develop new ways of achieving sexual gratification with the sexual partner.

Some illicit and prescribed drugs have side effects which influence sexual functioning and interest in sex. For example, antihypertensives, antidepressives, antihistamines, sedatives, tranquilizers, and narcotics, when taken over a period of time, tend to depress sexual functioning. Patients and their sexual partners often need an explanation of this fact and an understanding that the effect generally disappears once the medication is discontinued.

Substances, such as alcohol, marihuana, LSD, and amphetamines, have been thought by some to heighten the satisfaction of sexual activity. This impression seems to result from the fact that inhibitions are lowered by these substances and the person may therefore experience new and pleasurable sensations. The substances are depressants and in sufficient quantity, will inhibit sexual drive and functioning.

Recently, since the reporting of sexual rape has become more common, nurses often come in contact with women who have been raped. This is usually an emotionally traumatic time. Acceptance of and support for the patient are of utmost importance, along with the necessary physical care.

The detection and treatment of venereal diseases can be traumatic for some patients. Many have a poor factual understanding of the cause and effect of these infections. Nonjudgmental teaching by the nurse can be of great assistance.

The nurse may also be called upon to deal with various questions and problems related to menstruation and menopause. Objectivity and sensitivity to the feelings of the patient are important.

Chapter 1 discussed the nurse's right to withdraw from caring for a patient when she feels unable to do so, for whatever reason. It is generally agreed that she has the right to withdraw when she has taken steps to see to it that care will be given by another person. This general guide to action applies also if the nurse feels incompetent or psychologically uncomfortable when caring for patients with sexual problems. The nurse will then wish to take steps to seek more knowledge or to explore her own feelings on the matter.

Persons for whom the nurse cares are members of families. Often it is assumed that the patient's family unit is traditionally structured and organized. But with changes in the family, nursing services must be planned so that they are appropriate in each situation. For example, reasonable adaptations must be made in the home care of a convalescing youngster when both parents work. It is best to look at family member roles rather than assuming they are traditional in nature when offering family health services. The pregnant runaway teenager does not want to be told to go home. She needs someone to listen to her problems in an environment free of moralizing and scolding and to help her plan for the future. The male in a home situation may not be the husband or the father of children and may not assume typical head-of-household responsibilities. Adult children may need help in selecting a nursing home for the elderly parent. The single parent may need help in learning the developmental changes of children of the opposite sex.

CONCLUSION

It seems worth a reminder to point out again that every individual is unique and that to describe nursing through the life span was not intended to suggest that everyone can be fitted into a particular pattern of behavior. Nor is the material presented here appropriate for all cultures. As stated in the introduction, many influences mold the individual. This chapter was based on findings most typical of the American middle class. This applies especially to the psychosocial development of the individual.

The purpose of this chapter will have been well met when the information presented serves as a foundation upon which deeper insights concerning the life span and the family can be built. There are many specialty texts that include information to deepen understanding and some appear in the references at the end of this unit. Commitment to caring for patients of all ages is an integral part of nursing. A knowledge of growth and development throughout the life span is necessary to fulfill that commitment.

SUPPLEMENTAL LIBRARY STUDY

1. How does the author of the following article explain that the concept of self can be divided into two parts?

   Lewis, Michael. "The Busy, Purposeful World of a Baby." *Psychology Today,* 10:53–56, February 1977.

   What are several typical behaviors of an infant that are described in this article and that are important in the baby's development of self-image? Indicate how research this author describes demonstrates that an infant's sense of gender comes with the emergence of self-identity.

2. The mother of a 16-year-old was critical of the effects of care given by nurses while her son was hospitalized. Read her letter.

   Gast, Marilyn. ". . . the effects of patronizing, overprotective behavior . . ." (Letters) *American Journal of Nursing,* 75:1439, September 1975.

   What did the mother describe as the nurses' reason for their protective behavior toward her son? How did this behavior influence her son's self-image, in the mother's opinion? How does the mother's opinion support this chapter's discussion concerning self-image in the adolescent?

3. The following article describes crises common to many persons in the middle to late adult years:

   Peplau, Hildegard E. "Mid-Life Crises." *American Journal of Nursing,* 75:1761–1765, October 1975.

   Indicate three or four role transitions the author describes to which most persons must adjust during the adult years. How does the author describe an "Acceptable Look" as a social game that presents a dilemma for most adults? Self-image and bodily reality are often incongruent. To what is this primarily attributed, according to research reported by the author?

4. Read the following article:

   Watts, Rosalyn Jones. "Sexuality and the Middle-Aged Cardiac Patient." *The Nursing Clinics of North America,* 11:349–359, June 1976.

   What advice does the author give about suitable positions and coital style when counseling the middle-aged cardiac male patient? What suggestion is offered as a therapeutic modality for the cardiac patient who has not yet recovered to the point of its being advisable to have sexual intercourse? Note the sexual activity program outlined on pages 357 and 358. Describe the criteria that are suggested to determine appropriate sexual activity as the patient with uncomplicated myocardial infarction progresses through convalescence.

5. The following article written by a pediatric nurse practitioner describes how she helped a family in need of various health services:

   Brown, Marie Scott. "The Gordons Needed All the Help They Could Get." *Nursing 77,* 7:40–43, October 1977.

   Indicate how the Gordon family resembled the traditional American family in terms of organization and structure. How did it differ from the traditional family? Describe how the nurse used the nursing process while caring for this family of three. Indicate how the nurse acted as a patient advocate for the Gordon family.

10

BEHAVIORAL OBJECTIVES

When content in this chapter has been mastered, the student will be able to

Define the terms appearing in the glossary.

Describe how man functions as an open system and why using a closed system is unsatisfactory.

Explain how physiological and psychosocial homeostasis functions as an open system.

Discuss Maslow's theory of the hierarchy of human needs and indicate the order of priority.

Explain Selye's concept of stress and list at least 12 characteristics of stress.

Summarize Selye's general and local adaptation syndromes and how they relate to each other.

Describe Cannon's fight-or-flight pattern and indicate how it resembles Selye's general adaptation syndrome.

List and describe at least five common emotional responses to stressors.

List and describe at least eight defense mechanisms commonly used by man and indicate the criterion usually used to differentiate between the pathological and nonpathological use of defense mechanisms.

Describe how the concepts of health or wellness and illness can be placed on a continuum.

Discuss the three typical stages of illness which most patients experience.

List and describe at least ten implications for nursing which are related to concepts presented in this chapter.

Human Needs; Stress and Adaptation; Health and Illness

GLOSSARY

Adaptation: Adjusting to different circumstances and conditions, the end result of which is behavior that is constructive to human integrity.

Anger: An emotional state characteristically associated with frustration and struggling with threatening or unpleasant experiences.

Anxiety: An emotional state characterized by feelings of uneasiness and apprehension of a probable danger or misfortune.

Continuum: A continuous whole.

Defense Mechanism: An unconscious process used to protect oneself from anxiety.

Denial: Refusing to acknowledge the presence of a disturbing condition; self-deception.

Displacement: Satisfying a need by substituting one type of behavior for an unacceptable type of behavior.

Distress: Harmful or unpleasant stress.

Emotion: A bodily state involving consciously or unconsciously motivated feelings.

Equilibrium: A state of balance in which opposing forces are equal.

Fantasy: Using the imagination to create a picture that exists only in the mind.

Fear: An emotional response characterized by an expectation of harm or unpleasantness.

General Adaptation Syndrome: Manifestations of stress involving the whole body that evolves in three stages: alarm reaction, stage of resistance, and stage of exhaustion. Abbreviated GAS.

Health: The state of physical, psychological, and sociological well-being that results in the wholeness of the human organism. Synonym for wellness.

Helplessness: An emotional pattern characterized by a "fear of fear" and feelings of being unable to avoid an unpleasant experience.

High-Level Wellness: A state of health or wellness in which one is functioning at one's most favorable status.

Homeostasis: The process of maintaining uniformity, stability, or constancy.

Hostility: An emotional state characterized by feelings of unfriendliness and animosity. It may be associated with aggressive action that is intended to hurt or humble others.

Illness: A state characterized by malfunctioning of the biopsychosocial organism. A loss of wholeness.

Intellectualization: Detaching oneself from an emotionally disturbing situation by dealing with it in abstract terms.

Local Adaptation Syndrome: Manifestations of stress involving a local area that evolves in stages in the same manner as the general adaptation syndrome. Abbreviated LAS.

Maladaptation: Failure to adjust to different circumstances and conditions, the end result of which is behavior that has adverse effects on the individual or society.

Need: A necessity or requirement.

Need Gratification: The satisfying of a necessity or requirement.

Overdependency: An emotional state characterized by feelings of helplessness which are beyond those considered normal.

Problem: That which stands in the way of meeting human needs.

Projection: Attributing undesirable impulses to another person or object.

Rationalization: Giving questionable behavior a logical or socially acceptable explanation.

Reaction Formation: Giving a reason for behavior which is the opposite of its true cause.

Reframing: Altering one's point of view by placing circumstances or conditions into a different perspective.

Regression: Returning to an earlier method of behavior.

Repression: Excluding an anxiety-producing event from conscious awareness.

Self-Pity: Feeling sorry for oneself.

Stress: A nonspecific response of the body to any demand made upon it.

Stressor: The factor or agent which produces stress.

Sublimation: Successful displacement behavior. Often used in relation to sexual desires.

Wellness: The state of physical, psychological, and sociological well-being that results in the wholeness of the human organism. Synonym for health.

Worry: A mild form of anxiety characterized by preoccupation with an unsolved conflict.

INTRODUCTION

Knowledge of the total functioning of the human being is still not complete despite years of study and research. However, in order to offer meaningful health care, courses of action are necessarily built on knowledge presently available. This chapter will present some current concepts concerning how the human being functions as a total, integrated organism and the implications these various concepts have for nursing during stages of health and illness.

THE HUMAN BEING AS AN OPEN SYSTEM

For many years, health care literature tended to speak of the human organism as though it were a closed system, that is, a system that seeks equilibrium when taking initial conditions only into account. It was often described as consisting of a linear relationship and can be illustrated as follows:

cause or stimulus → effect or response

By using the concept of a closed system, the person was not viewed as a whole interreacting with the world about him. Hence, a patient with pneumonia was treated for pathology in his lungs. He was reduced to physical and chemical quantities and viewed as an organism without consideration of the psychosocial factors within him and in his environment.

With increased knowledge of the biopsychosocial characteristics of man, it became clear that the concept of a closed system was unsatisfactory. The open system has become the basis for viewing how the human functions. The open system was described in Chapter 4.

How can the concept of an open system be applied to the human being? It takes the initial condition into account but adds much to that. When using an open system approach, all parts of man, the manner in which the parts interact, and man's total environmental influences are taken into consideration. The human system exchanges information both within the body and with the outer world as well. This approach can be illustrated by a circular pattern showing man interacting with his environment dynamically and continuously, as Figure 10-1 attempts to illustrate.

The word environment is used here in its broadest sense. The external environment includes everything that in some way influences what is inside the human skin—the whole of the biopsychosocial being. Some external environmental influences are microorganisms, the weather, daily news events, relationships with friends and family, work experiences, and education. The internal environment lies within the body and it also influences man's behavior. Thus, when the body's cells need nourishment and water, the person responds behaviorally by seeking food and water for ingestion. When a microorganism enters the body, the body's defense system goes to work to destroy the invader.

The concept of wholeness applies when using an open system. A popular term for the wholeness of man is holism which was defined earlier in this text. The human body has interrelated and interacting parts that form a whole. For example, the body has legs, arms, eyes, a nose, a stomach. a central nervous system, and so on. Each part has its own purpose, but each part is related to all of the other parts. Each one influences all of the others as well as the whole. The concept of wholeness of the human organism is generally accepted in nursing. It can also be said that because of the complexity of human nature, the sum of the parts is equal to even more than the total! The human body is more than the sum of its various cells, organs, and systems and more than a receiver of information from its external environment. Man also gives to his environment and is creative through such processes as perception and learning. And what he gives also returns to influence his internal environment.

HOMEOSTASIS

Homeostasis is the process of maintaining uniformity, stability, or constancy. The term was first used by Walter B. Cannon in his book *The Wisdom of the Body*. Credit for the original concept of homeostasis, though not the word, is given to the French scientist, Claude Bernard who described how the body fights disease to maintain constancy in its internal milieu.

Some persons have equated the concept of homeostasis with that of equilibrium. The dictionary defines *equilibrium* as a state of balance when opposing forces are equal to each other. For example, a scale is in a state of equilibrium when the weights on each side are equal. Hence, equilibrium does not imply a constantly changing state that is reacting in a dynamic way to influences about it. Man is never static—he continually changes to meet the challenges of influences that are forever present within his body and in his outer world.

Homeostasis functions as an open system. Thus, we are saying that man, as an open system, strives to

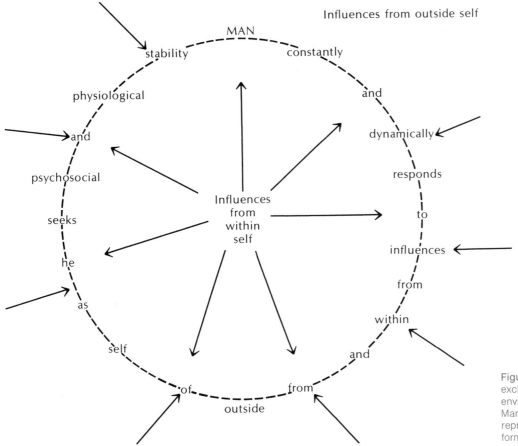

Figure 10-1 Man constantly exchanges information with his environment and within himself. Man as an open system is represented with the broken line forming the circle.

maintain stability and constancy as he is subjected to influences from everything about and within him. He is normally an integrated biopsychosocial whole.

The concept of homeostasis has been used in relation to physiological functioning of the body for some years. Cannon pointed out that the purpose of homeostasis is freedom; that is, man is free from second-by-second attention to such bodily processes as maintaining proper fluid acidity, water balance, cell nourishment, and so on. This freedom allows us to enjoy beauty, to create and work, to invent and explore, and otherwise reach for our potential as humans.

Within the last decade or so, the concept of homeostasis has been used with regard to man's psychosocial functioning as well. Just as man functions to establish physiological homeostasis, so also he seeks psychosocial stability. Psychosocial homeostasis can be illustrated when an individual first learns that he has an incurable illness. Man constantly seeks survival. Hence, psychosocial stability is ordinarily upset by knowledge of

impending death. Chapter 26 will describe the fairly typical stages through which most persons pass as death approaches, beginning with denial and anger and usually proceeding to a stage of acceptance, tranquility, and readiness for the inevitability of death.

Physiological and psychosocial homeostasis cannot be separated into two distinct entities for they are completely interrelated and constantly influencing each other. As a result, it can be seen that homeostasis may well require more than one mechanism working at any one time. For example, during an emotional crisis, an individual will use his resources to restore psychosocial stability. But he may fail to observe the need to eat properly while in an emotionally charged state. Hence, the body's reserves of glucose will be called forth through mechanisms that will help maintain physiological homeostasis.

The numerous processes of homeostasis have their limitations. The body can do only so much to maintain stability. When limits are surpassed, outside help becomes necessary. For instance, the body has normal defense mechanisms that function when microorganisms invade the body. However, when an infectious process becomes overwhelming, antibiotic therapy may need to be prescribed to give the body an assist.

The processes of homeostasis do not occur in a haphazard manner. The body is extremely well-organized. Much of its functioning is automatic, although still well-coordinated. Chapter 23, which discusses fluid balance, will demonstrate the intricacies and the beauty of mechanisms that help the body maintain physiological homeostasis within relatively narrow ranges of normality. As one example, the body normally maintains fluid acidity/alkalinity within a very narrow margin of approximately 7.35 and 7.45.

HUMAN NEEDS

What prompts the body to take whatever action is necessary in order that the processes of homeostasis can occur? It would appear that there has to be certain motivation in the human in order to bring about behavior that fosters homeostasis.

It has been demonstrated that humans have certain needs, which when met satisfactorily, help maintain physiological and psychosocial homeostasis. A _need_ is that which is necessary, useful, or desirable to maintain homeostasis and life itself. A need becomes the motivation for behavior. The motivation as well as the resulting behavior may be observable, that is, overt, or it may be imperceptable, or covert. For example, the human being needs oxygen in order to survive. The act of respiration functions to meet the body's need for oxygen. In other words, the motivation for respiration is the need for oxygen. Needs may be met consciously or unconsciously. Certain aspects of respiration can be voluntarily controlled to a certain extent—one can voluntarily hold one's breath for a length of time. However, most of the process of respiration is an involuntary, unconscious, and imperceptable act. When hunger and thirst are present, the adult consciously seeks food and fluid but the processes involved in the use of food and water by the body are involuntary, unconscious, and imperceptable behaviors.

Many philosophers, psychologists, and physiologists have described human needs and have discussed them from various points of view. Possibly the first person to describe human needs was Aristotle when he discussed man's needs for profit, pleasure, and morality. Abraham Maslow's theory of human needs, which he de-

veloped in the 1950s, has been used extensively by health care personnel and was discussed in Chapter 6.

Maslow's theory has been called by some a force-for-growth concept. Maslow believed that every person strives to become everything he is capable of becoming. He identified a hierarchy of needs, as described in Chapter 6. The base of the hierarchy consists of physiological needs which man shares with other forms of life; these include the need for nourishment, water, and oxygen. As one moves up the hierarchy, one eventually reaches for self-actualization which differentiates man from other forms of life. The central theme is that man has an urge to grow to attain his highest potential. According to Maslow, upper-level needs in the hierarchy will not be met, or be permitted to be met, unless lower-level needs are gratified, at least to some degree, first. Thus, a person who is in need of food will concentrate all of his efforts on obtaining nourishment before seeking ways to meet his need for self-esteem or love. Figure 10–2 illustrates and further explains Maslow's theory of human needs.

There are times when needs are not met entirely in accordance with the hierarchal theory. The person completely engrossed with meeting self-actualization needs may delay eating or obtaining sufficient fluid intake. The artist whose need to paint becomes more important to him than his need to eat is often given as an example. However, more commonly, persons do appear to meet needs in accordance with Maslow's theory.

Using the hierarchal concept, it can be seen that man is constantly varying. His needs continually evolve, develop, change, and grow. When the individual experiences gratification, he enjoys well-being and is free to develop to his greatest potential.

When the processes of meeting needs are frustrated, pathological conditions may develop. In the context of homeostasis, a _problem_ can be defined as that which stands in the way of meeting man's needs, and hence, threatens physiological and psychosocial homeostasis. The person with a disease of the respiratory tract may have a problem because of inadequate ventilation. His body cells are not receiving sufficient oxygen to maintain homeostasis.

It is important for the nurse to differentiate between needs and problems. Needs are requirements for the maintenance of well-being. The person unable to have his needs gratified experiences a problem. He often turns to health personnel whose role it is to help overcome the obstacles to meeting his needs. The person with a respiratory disease may require oxygen therapy in addition to other forms of therapy in order to

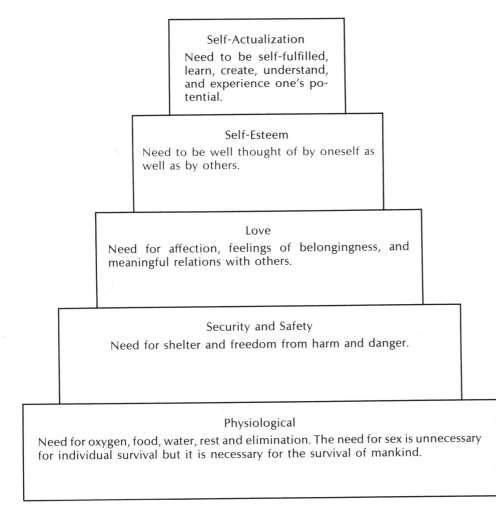

Figure 10–2 This sketch of Maslow's theory indicates that man is constantly evolving so that he can reach his highest potential. Higher needs in this scheme cannot fully grow and develop until lower ones are adequately met. When the meeting of needs at any level is frustrated, a pathological condition will eventually develop.

overcome the problem of poor ventilation and to meet his need for adequate oxygen.

How do needs and problems function when the concept of an open system is used to study the human being? A human need is input for an open system. The need for oxygen is input. If the need is being met by the normal respiratory process, the system is evaluated as performing satisfactorily when the person experiences the well-being of having oxygen needs met. If a pathological condition is present so that the respiratory process cannot function properly, the problem of oxygen deprivation becomes input in an open system. The body will try to compensate by increasing the respiratory rate and depth, increasing its production of red blood cells to improve oxygen-carrying capacity, increasing the work of the heart to carry blood more rapidly to cells, and so on. If the body's compensating behavior is successful, feedback tells the body to continue what it is doing. However, if compensating be-

havior is inadequate, the suffering from oxygen deprivation continues. This suffering in turn becomes input and asks the body to do still more to make up for the deficit. When this type of feedback continues, the body will eventually wear itself out and death will ensue unless intervention measures are used.

The same processes just described occur with other needs and problems and in the same manner. Other human needs could be substituted in the example given above, as well as the resulting problem when the need is not being met adequately.

STRESS

The human body constantly makes adjustments to promote physiological and psychosocial homeostasis. The word stress has become useful when studying such behavior.

Hans Selye, a world reknown authority on *stress,* defined it as the nonspecific response of the body to any demand made upon it. He called the factor or agent which produces stress a *stressor.* Selye was careful to explain that demands made upon the body are specific in nature: exposure to cold makes us shiver; lack of sufficient fluid makes us thirsty; a diuretic drug increases the production of urine, and so on. The specific demand causes the body to make a readjustment of some sort. However, the resulting adjustment is nonspecific, according to Selye, because it occurs without regard to, and independently of, the specific stressor. It makes no difference whether the stressor is pleasant, such as the joy of getting married, or unpleasant, such as the fear of death. Selye goes on to state that this nonspecific response to stressors is the essence of stress itself. It seems contradictory to think that two such opposite feelings as joy and fear may have the same effect on the body; that is, certain reactions within the body to very different stressors can be identical. Yet, research has shown this to be the case.

To help clarify the concept of stress, consider some characteristics of stress and some things which stress is *not.*

Stress is not nervous energy. Many persons equate stress with emotional or nervous exhaustion. Emotional reactions are common stressors, but, as Selye points out, lower animals with no nervous system—even plants!—also have stress reactions.

Stress is not always the result of some damage to the body. The stress one experiences when competing in a tennis match is not the result of damage.

Distress is the word Selye used to mean harmful or unpleasant stress. Stress does not always result in feelings of distress. The body's needs for food, water, and oxygen are normally not associated with unpleasantness unless a problem arises. Nor is the stress normally associated with such events as the birth of a child or marriage considered unpleasant. On the other hand, the distress associated with fear, anger, and sadness are usually considered unpleasant. So also is the inability to breath or eliminate wastes.

Stress is not necessarily something to be avoided. Complete freedom from stress cannot even be accomplished except in death. Stress is a necessary part of all of life and essential for growth. If stress related to thirst is not present, we will die of dehydration; if stress related to high levels of carbonic acid is absent in our body, we will die of acidosis; if stress to attain self-esteem is absent, we may not study sufficiently to succeed in school. Even when sleeping, stress is present as internal organs work to maintain homeostasis.

Because some stress is part of the fabric of all of life, if it could be measured with a pressure gauge, the pointer would never be on zero. However, problems result if stressors are either too great or too little because of the body's inability to make proper adjustments. If a person is hemorrhaging, the body responds in various ways so that the heart can pump remaining blood as efficiently as possible. But, if the blood loss is overwhelming, that is, the stressor is too great for the body to make adjustments to a sufficient degree, blood pressure falls, the pulse rate becomes rapid, and the person will eventually die as the circulatory system fails. On the other hand, if the stress related to hunger is too little, the person may suffer malnutrition and even starve to death. Selye's model showing the relationship between stress and various life experiences is shown in Figure 10–3.

An overload or underload of stress may lead to bizarre psychosocial behavior. Even though we often long for a quiet and peaceful life, depriving a person of normal sensory input can be disasterous. The opposite has also been demonstrated—an overload of sensory input can also lead to problems. There will be further discussion of sensory deprivation and overload in Chapter 13.

Both the number of stressors present at one time and the duration of stress will influence the body's ability to cope. For example, if a person has been injured in an accident, the body can cope with greater ease when the injuries are few rather than numerous. To illustrate the

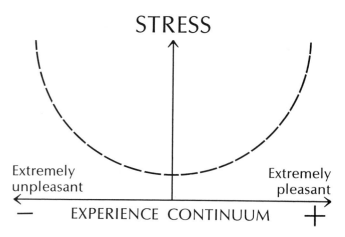

Figure 10–3 This sketch shows the relationship between stress and various types of life experiences. Note that the stress level never reaches zero in life. Either pleasant or unpleasant events may produce stress in varying degrees. Both pleasant and unpleasant emotional experiences result in increased physiological stress but not necessarily distress. (Seyle, Hans. *Stress Without Distress.* New American Library, New York, 1974, p. 20.)

effects of the duration of stress, experiencing short periods of depression are easier to handle than a state of depression that continues for a long time. Ordinarily, stress of long duration or repeated exposure to stress will take its toll, with the body falling into a state of physiological and psychosocial exhaustion.

The anticipation of a particular event can be more stressful than the event itself. A person may experience more unpleasantness while anticipating a diagnostic procedure than he experiences during the procedure itself. A child who is about to have an injection may cry in terror, and yet, indicate that the injection "didn't hurt all that much" after the injection has been completed.

The lack of anticipating a stressful situation may amplify its effects. The presence of sudden and unexpected stressors ordinarily require more coping effort on the part of the body than when stress occurs gradually or when expected. For example, the body can cope with small losses of blood over a period of time more easily than it can cope with large losses of blood occurring in an emergency situation. Also, an untimely death in a family ordinarily requires more coping ability than the expected death.

Each individual handles psychosocial stressors in his own unique way. The person's past experiences become important in relation to how he will cope with the phenomenon of stress. A situation that may be markedly stressful for one person may present little difficulty for another person. For example, some patients, especially those who have never had surgery, may find the experience more stressful than the patient who has had several surgical experiences. On the other hand, the reverse may occur; if a person has had an unpleasant experience with a surgical procedure in the past, this may add to the magnitude of the stressor. For persons desiring employment, being without work is usually stressful. Some may use the experience as a challenge and put forth great efforts to find employment while others may find the experience so upsetting that they may be immobilized and unable to put forth effort. Still others may appear to take the experience in stride with little evidence of its being distressful.

Stress involves the entire body acting as a whole and in an integrated manner. It is erroneous to view stress as being either physiological or psychosocial. A person suffering with an infection has physiological responses, such as an elevated temperature, rapid pulse and respiratory rates, and so on. He is also likely to experience psychosocial stress related to the experience of being ill, having limited physical activity, losing time at school or work, and being separated from his family when

hospitalization is necessary. The opposite also occurs. The stressor, fear, has definite physiological effects on the body, for example.

Stress provides feedback to promote homeostasis. When feedback indicates things are going well in the presence of stress, an individual continues with behavior that helps him return to a state of homeostasis. But when feedback is the opposite, pathological processes will result. Consider a person with a gastric ulcer. Feedback will motivate behavior that will eventually promote healing when the person can successfully alter a life-style that has many stressors. However, telling another person that a change in life-style is advisable and to "take it easy" may cause him to become even more distressed. In this case, feedback on the pathological process on stomach mucosa may further aggravate the situation.

There are some persons who appear to be addicted to stress and thrive on it. Many successful executives, athletes, and politicians seem to find their best personal well-being when stressors result in high levels of pressure and even danger. If these people suddenly were forced to slow their pace of life, their own personal sense of well-being might well be in jeopardy.

The age of the person often influences how he will cope with a particular stressor. Infants and elderly persons handle temperature extremes less well than young and middle-aged adults. An infection in the urinary tract that may be handled with relative ease in an adolescent may be completely devastating to an elderly person.

A person's physical condition will often influence his ability to cope with stressors in his life. For example, a person with a heart disease cannot cope with the demands of physical exertion as well as the person who is in good physical condition.

Selye is a physician and developed his theory on stress after extensive physiological research. The manner in which stress is related to physiological functioning will be discussed later in this chapter.

ADAPTATION

In the literature of the psychologists and sociologists, *adaptation* is described as adjusting to different circumstances and conditions. Adaptive behavior tends to bring man into adjustment with his environment. Adaptation is often characterized as resulting in behavior which indicates that the individual has an accurate perception of reality, is aware of his own motives and feelings, can control his behavior, experiences self-worth, enjoys good relationships with others, and so on.

Psychologists agree that all behavior is caused. Since man strives to reach his best biopsychosocial potential, it might seem that for each person, all behavior is adaptive since the cause for behavior is to meet an individual's needs. Nevertheless, the term *maladaptation* is often used, especially when speaking of persons with mental illnesses. It is described as behavior that has adverse effects on the individual or society. Maladaptive behavior is not in keeping with what is judged as normal, acceptable, or appropriate. For example, parents who abuse their children are meeting some personal need of their own, and for them, their behavior satisfies that need. However, society does not accept their behavior as appropriate, and therefore, judges it as maladaptive.

When Selye developed his concept of stress, he used adaptation somewhat differently from the manner just described. He speaks of a *general adaptation syndrome,* abbreviated GAS, which is a sequence of behavior involving the whole body. He described GAS in the following three stages:

Alarm Reaction (AR). During this stage, the body becomes aware of a stressor and either consciously or unconsciously is triggered into action. The body's defense forces are mobilized and normal levels of the body's resistance decrease. If the stressor is sufficiently severe, death may result during this stage. An example is a very severe burn.

State of Resistance (SR). This stage is characterized by adaptation to the stressor. The body fights the alarm reaction since no one can maintain a state of alarm indefinitely. The body's normal level of resistance increases above normal to resist the stressor with the hope of adaptation. In addition, the body's resistance to further stimuli rises.

Stage of Exhaustion (SE). If the body continues to be exposed to stressors, it will reach a stage of exhaustion. The symptoms of the alarm reaction reappear now but if the stressor is not removed, these signs become irreversible. Death follows unless somehow the body can regain adaptive techniques or find new ways to cope with the stressful situation.

Figure 10–4 illustrates the three stages of the general adaptation syndrome. Selye called this syndrome *general* because it is produced by situations that have a general effect on many parts of the body. He called it *adaptive* because it helps the body acquire and maintain a state of adjustment to the stressor. And he called it a syndrome because the manifestations are completely coordinated and even dependent, at least to a certain extent, on each other.

Selye also describes a *local adaptation syndrome,* abbreviated LAS. The inflammation occurring at the site of an infection represents a local adaptation syndrome. The same three stages described in the GAS occur but in a local area. The LAS and the GAS coordinate closely. The alarm reaction set up at a local site sends signals to the nervous and endocrine systems and the GAS is instigated. The GAS then turns back to influence the LAS.

According to Selye, adaptation is finite. He believes that the body has adaptation energy, the amount of which is most probably genetically acquired. He suggests that the process of aging, when adaptation energy gradually depletes itself and eventually death occurs, illustrates that each individual has just so much adaptive energy. Selye also points out that each individual can be exposed to a stressor, such as cold, for just so long before exhaustion and eventually death will occur.

When the body is failing in stages of the GAS, a crisis may occur; that is, the life of the individual is at stake. As adaptation energy becomes depleted, outside intervention is necessary to prevent death. For exam-

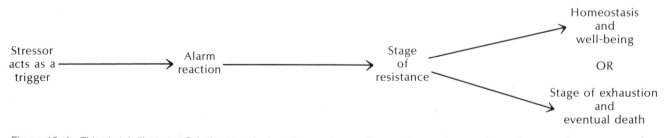

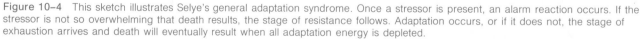

Figure 10–4 This sketch illustrates Selye's general adaptation syndrome. Once a stressor is present, an alarm reaction occurs. If the stressor is not so overwhelming that death results, the stage of resistance follows. Adaptation occurs, or if it does not, the stage of exhaustion arrives and death will eventually result when all adaptation energy is depleted.

ple, if the heart and breathing stop, for whatever reason, intervention will have to include cardiopulmonary resuscitation if life is to be sustained.

PHYSIOLOGICAL RESPONSES TO STRESSORS

When Selye was a medical student, he was struck by what he called the syndrome of being sick. He had observed that a great diversity of conditions threaten homeostasis but, no matter what the condition was, many of the signs and symptoms different patients presented were similar. He found a certain sameness, regardless of what condition brought the patient to seek medical help. He then went on in his research to look for the common underlying factors in the syndrome of being sick. His findings eventually led to his stress-GAS theory.

Cannon's work on homeostasis and on fear preceded Selye's theory. Cannon developed what became known as the fight-or-flight pattern. In order to overcome a stressful situation, the body tries to fight the stressor or tries to flee from it. Assume that a person is confronted by a vicious dog that is about to attack. The entire body will be mobilized when this trigger is present. Epinephrine will be secreted in larger than average amounts; blood pressure will rise; the pulse and respiratory rates will increase; there will be increased blood flow to skeletal muscles and to the heart, lungs, and brain; blood sugar levels will rise. All of these alarm reactions put the body in the best possible condition either to fight off the dog or to flee from it.

Selye describes physiological responses in the alarm reaction stages of the GAS in much the same way as Cannon described them in his fight-or-flight pattern. But Cannon did not study the role of the pituitary gland and the adrenal cortex which became important in Selye's theory.

In a situation involving stress, the hypothalamus is aroused and sends impulses to activate the sympathetic-adrenal medullary mechanism which prepares the body for action. It also secretes the corticotropin-releasing factor (CRF) which serves as a chemical messenger to activate the anterior pituitary-adrenocortical mechanism. The short-term changes of stress occur primarily when epinephrine (adrenalin) and norepinephine (sympathin) are secreted by the medulla of the adrenal gland. Long-term changes occur primarily when glucocorticoids are released from the adrenal cortex. Hormones from the pancreas and thyroid gland also play a role when stress is present.

The neuroendocrine responses to stressors operate through the nerve cells and fibers of the autonomic nervous system. This system consists of the sympathetic (thoracolumbar) and the parasympathetic (craniosacral) divisions. The sympathetic division carries impulses that increase heart action, inhibit salivation and gastrointestinal activity, raise blood pressure by constricting arterioles, dilate bronchioles, stimulate perspiration, and increase the secretion of epinephrine. The parasympathetic division carries impulses that tend to control normal operation of the viscera, such as facilitating smooth muscle contraction, permitting salivation, and slowing the heart rate. It brings the body back to normal. Thus, Selye theorized that the alarm reaction includes neuroendocrine responses that prepare the body for action while antagonistic impulses to bring the body back to normal occur in the stage of resistance. Figure 10–5 on page 198 illustrates the autonomic system and its inhibiting and accelerating routes.

As stated earlier, the hypothalamus plays an important part in responses to stress. So also does the cerebral cortex. Coordination of responses apparently occurs in part through activity of the hypothalamus, and the cerebral cortex appears to have a restoring or controlling effect on responses to stressors. Awareness of stressors and analyzing a stressful situation which makes use of past experiences with stress also occur in the brain.

The nature of stressors cannot be differentiated by physiological responses. For example, there is not a physiological response to joy which can be differentiated from the physiological response to anger. However, the responses are not disorganized. On the contrary, they are well-organized. Even when a stressor is strong, the body responds harmoniously. What *may* be disorganized is overt behavior that results from a stressful situation. Thus, a person experiencing extreme fear may be so consumed by his emotion that his behavior may become erratic, and, hence, less effective in eliminating or reducing the cause of the fear.

EMOTIONAL RESPONSES TO STRESSORS

The literature describing common emotional responses to stressors is voluminous. A wide variety of terms is used, some of which are defined and used in somewhat different ways. This section will describe briefly a few of the more common emotional responses to stressors.

An *emotion* is a bodily state involving feelings which

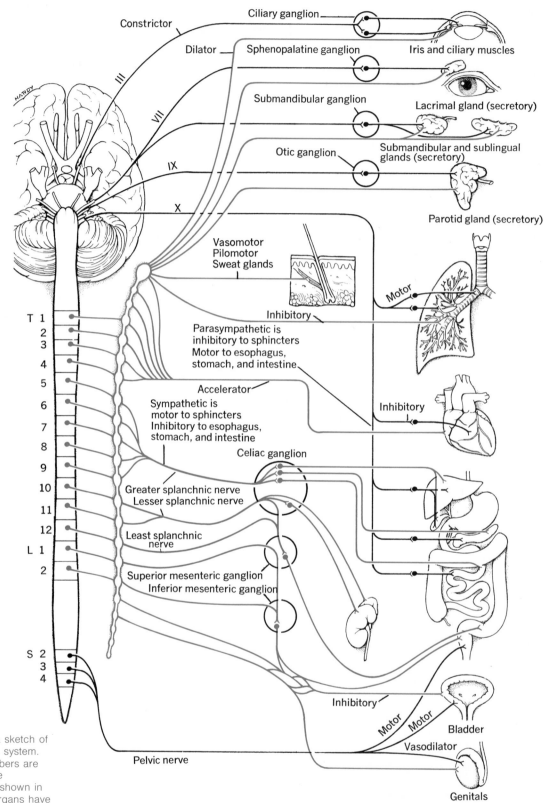

Constrictor
Ciliary ganglion
III
Dilator
Sphenopalatine ganglion
Iris and ciliary muscles
VII
Submandibular ganglion
Lacrimal gland (secretory)
IX
Otic ganglion
Submandibular and sublingual glands (secretory)
X
Parotid gland (secretory)

Vasomotor
Pilomotor
Sweat glands
Motor

Inhibitory
Parasympathetic is inhibitory to sphincters Motor to esophagus, stomach, and intestine

Accelerator
Sympathetic is motor to sphincters Inhibitory to esophagus, stomach, and intestine
Inhibitory

Celiac ganglion

Greater splanchnic nerve
Lesser splanchnic nerve

Least splanchnic nerve

Superior mesenteric ganglion
Inferior mesenteric ganglion

Inhibitory
Motor Motor
Bladder
Vasodilator
Genitals

Pelvic nerve

T 1
2
3
4
5
6
7
8
9
10
11
12
L 1
2
S 2
3
4

Figure 10–5   This is a sketch of the autonomic nervous system. The parasympathetic fibers are shown in black and the sympathetic fibers are shown in blue. Note that most organs have a double nerve supply.

may be consciously or unconsciously motivated. An emotion is a type of coping mechanism that can activate and direct behavior.

Fear

Fear is an emotional response characterized by an expectation of harm or unpleasantness. Normally the body reacts by attempting to avoid or withdraw from the threat. When we are afraid, sympathetic innervation, as described earlier, places the body in a state of readiness for action to avoid or escape harm. The person who has fear usually is aware of the danger and has insight into the reasons for his fear although he ordinarily has doubts about his ability to handle the cause of his fear. The causes in general are present and real, even though the patient may conceal his fear, as shown below.

Absence of the emotion of fear may seem ideal, but without it life would be infinitely more precarious. We have all experienced fear in our lives, and it is doubtful that we could have survived the many dangers had we not been fearful. For example, fear of accidents often results in safer automobile driving. Possibly one of the best lifesaving "devices" for the nonswimmer is his fear of being in water over his head.

Patients with fears may express them rather freely. For example, a patient said he was afraid of receiving oxygen therapy because of the danger of an explosion. A few explanations from the nurse to the patient and to his visitors alleviated the fear readily.

On the other hand, some patients may be reluctant to express fears, believing that they may appear unintelligent and a nuisance if they ask questions. One hospitalized patient eventually described having marked fear when he did not receive his breakfast when the other patients were served. Instead, a technician came to take a blood sample. The patient was sure his condition had worsened and that he was about to receive some therapy. He was both fearful of what might be happening to him and fearful of asking anyone for an explanation. When one reads in the literature what patients have described as fearful experiences, it is easy to see that many of them could have been avoided or minimized, had someone just taken the time to give some explanations to these people.

Fears may be camouflaged by other behavior. A patient, awakened postoperatively, saw that she was in a bed with siderails in place. She became very angry and told a family member that she "really told off that nurse who put up those railings." When asked why she was upset about having siderails on her bed, the patient said, most indignantly, "I came in here for a simple operation and I don't expect to be treated like someone who is insane. I've heard about how they treat insane people. They put them in beds and fix it so you can't get out. And I'm not crazy!" After the reason for the siderails was explained, the patient's anger quickly subsided, since her fear of being considered mentally ill was removed.

Anxiety

The dictionary defines *anxiety* as uneasiness of mind caused by apprehension of danger or misfortune. It is often described as a persistent, generalized fear of the unknown and is associated with some future event. *Worry* is a mild form of anxiety characterized by preoccupation with an unsolved conflict. Unlike the anxious person, the worried person usually is able to communicate the cause of the concern. Anxiety ordinarily is characterized by a lack of awareness of the cause of fear. Although pervasive, it is vaguely organized in the mind of the person; hence, he feels helpless and uncertain concerning appropriate action to take.

Anxiety is more difficult to handle than fear. Should one be afraid of a dog, he can try to get away from the situation. But when anxiety is present, the person lacking insight as to its cause feels defeated and has dread of what will happen.

The physiological reactions to anxiety result from (sympathetic innervation.) However, because of the nature of anxiety, the responses of the organs to stimulation are not usually as dramatic as when fear is present.

Because lack of insight is commonly present, an anxious person often directs his attention to the physiological symptoms of anxiety. Common ones are fatigue, insomnia, diarrhea, urgency of voiding, nausea, anorexia, and excessive perspiration. "Nervous heart" is a common lay symptom of the anxious person. Or the person may say he thinks his heart "stands still" at times. When anxiety becomes chronic and persistent, psychotherapy may be necessary.

Although anxiety can be destructive, it may also be used constructively. This is especially true when the anxiety is not overwhelming. In fact, some persons believe that without anxiety, as well as some fear, the human race might not have survived in situations that made constructive action imperative. The anxiety associated with examination periods in school stimulates many students to carry out effective study programs. The anxiety of an elected official whose neglect of slum conditions may threaten his office can serve to stimulate constructive action.

Overdependency and Feelings of Helplessness *Overdependency* is an emotional response characterized by feelings of helplessness to an extent beyond what is considered normal. *Helplessness* is a "fear of fear" and a feeling of being unable to avoid an unpleasant experience.

Human beings demonstrate dependence on others throughout life. A mother depends on health care services to help her keep her family well. The student turns to his counselor for help in planning his educational program. The employee looks to his employer for guidelines that determine what he is expected to do on his job. But characteristically during periods of illness, dependence and feelings of helplessness usually increase, unfortunately, sometimes to the point of being harmful to the patient. Usually it is the nurse who first observes overdependency in an ill person and she may be the one who must make decisions concerning whether a patient's dependency has reached an undesirable level for the patient's own good. A convalescing patient who is reluctant to assume responsibility for his personal care, for instance, may well have grown too dependent during acute illness.

It may be that a patient who has grown too dependent on others is a fearful person. A patient recovering from a myocardial infarction may be afraid that assuming graduated exercises may precipitate another heart attack. Another overdependent person may be angry because he has been permanently handicapped by an illness or injury. He may even blame health personnel for his handicap and become defiant of efforts to assist him to use remaining physical potential.

Whatever the reason for overdependency and feelings of helplessness, the nurse should observe and study possible motives for it. Simultaneously, she will want to assist a patient to surmount overdependency in a manner compatible with the patient's capabilities rather than in a manner that satisfies her own aspirations for the patient.

Anger

Anger is an emotion characteristically associated with frustration and struggling with a threatening or unpleasant situation. It is common when a goal is blocked, when respect for self has been lowered, or when a goal cannot be attained.

Anger can serve useful purposes. When it can be comfortably and safely expressed, anger may act as a relief valve in a highly charged emotional situation. Often, being able to express anger makes a person feel better, when it serves as a substitute for the uneasy, unpleasant, and powerless feelings of anxiety. The anger may be directed toward the source of the frustration or it may be aimed at someone or something else.

Like other emotions, anger may be camouflaged. This is especially true in a society such as ours that places taboos on most angry behavior. The child with a cough and sore throat who willfully destroys his toys because he cannot attend school may be angry at being ill, with his mother, and with himself. A mother may be frustrated and angered by her teenager who refuses to eat what she considers to be a balanced diet; because she is angry, she enforces a more rigid curfew policy. A person experiencing pain when no cause can be found may express his anger by being impatient and annoyed at other drivers on his way home from the clinic.

Energy is liberated by the body during periods of anger. When this energy can be directed toward constructive ends, the nurse may help an angry patient find more meaningful and useful behavior. To do so, the nurse must accept the patient's feelings of anger and not take them personally even if directed toward her. She will want to assure the patient that his feelings are not unusual and help him find the cause of his anger. Then, she and the patient can work to solve situations producing the emotion. Attempts to find the cause of the anger are helpful so that the difficulty can be dealt with realistically.

Hostility

Hostility is an unfriendliness and animosity that is sometimes associated with a desire for aggressive action. It may occur with anger and with the wish to hurt or humiliate others. Almost all adults experience at least some of it when ill, especially when confined during hospitalization.

The intensity of hostility cannot be judged safely by the intensity of the behavior overtly associated with it. Nor is it always easy to recognize the focus or cause of the hostility for there is a tendency to displace feelings of hostility onto others. For example, a quiet, almost uncommunicative patient may be extremely hostile but may present the behavior he does because expressing his hostility outwardly may be too upsetting for him. He may display his behavior to health practitioners working with him but feel hostile primarily toward relatives who, he feels, have deserted him during his illness.

Sarcasm and abusive remarks are often expressions of hostility. The overdemanding, unreasonable, aggressive, and argumentive patient may also be expressing hostility by his behavior.

Self-Pity

Self-pity is feeling sorry for oneself. The person feels sad and put upon, and lacks security and self-esteem. The person often is whiny and has many complaints.

Self-pity may have elements of both worry or anxiety and anger directed toward the self. It may be of relatively short duration, or it may continue indefinitely, especially if the person is alone and has few interests in his external environment.

Lecturing a person who feels self-pity and indicating that he can stop feeling sorry for himself if he tries are ineffectual measures. It is better to offer support by acknowledging the person's complaints, especially when they seem justified, and to be guided by knowledge that the person's feelings are valid for him.

The emotional reactions just described can increase the severity of an illness experience, the amount depending on their intensity and duration. These reactions could also lead to a state of emotional and physiological crises which add to the difficulty of coping with the situation.

Human behavior is very complex and no one is likely to be as rational and logical as he thinks he is. A particular type of behavior can rarely be understood in a simple fashion since psychological research has indicated that behavior may be motivated at either the conscious or unconscious level, or at both levels simultaneously. In addition, behavior is rarely motivated by only one determining factor. Rather, multiple influences may be at work producing a particular kind of behavior.

The danger of oversimplification when attempting to observe and analyze another's behavior is ever-present. Nonetheless, turning away from attempts to understand behavior and failing to respond with warmth and acceptance when persons are communicating via their behavior fall short of professional nursing practice.

DEFENSE MECHANISMS

A *defense mechanism* is an unconscious process used to protect oneself from anxiety. A defense mechanism does not solve a problem or alter the condition of anxiety itself. Rather, it changes the way a person thinks about whatever is disturbing him. This may relieve at least some anxiety, but rarely is a defense mechanism totally satisfying.

Denial

Denial is sometimes used as a synonym for self-deception. The individual using it refuses to acknowledge the presence of a condition that is disturbing him. An ill person uses denial when he refuses to accept a diagnosis or prognosis. The first step in the process of grieving over the death of a loved one is often denial; that is, the person refuses to acknowledge the death that has occurred in order to relieve the anxiety the situation creates for him.

Repression

Repression means that there is an exclusion of an anxiety-producing event from conscious awareness. Freud first defined it in the Oedipus complex when he said a young boy has sexual attraction toward his mother and hostility toward his father who enjoys sexual relationships with the mother. The boy represses these feelings in order to avoid distressful consequences of acting out his sexual impulses. A characteristic of repression is that because the individual ordinarily is unaware of using this defense mechanism, there will be total forgetting of a situation that is stressful. There is a tendency for humans to forget unpleasantness of the past and remember only the good times.

Projection

Projection occurs when a person's own undesirable impulses are attributed to another person or object. Consider a patient who fails to take medications as prescribed. His explanation is that his wife is responsible for reminding him and she failed to do so. He blames his wife for his own forgetfulness. As another example, a person carelessly trips over an article on the floor and blames the article rather than his own behavior for the accident.

Rationalization

Rationalization means giving questionable behavior a logical or socially acceptable explanation. It amounts to behavior justification. A person may be rationalizing when he forgets an appointment with a health practitioner and explains that the practitioner is incompetent and he does not care to continue seeing someone in whom he has no confidence. One of Aesop's fables described the fox who complained that the grapes he was unable to reach would have been sour anyway. The fox was using rationalization. Rationalization may offer a good reason but it does not describe the true cause of behavior.

Reaction Formation

Reaction formation is used when the individual gives a reason for his behavior which is opposite from its true cause. A common example is the parents of an unwanted child who overindulge the child to reassure themselves that they are good parents.

Displacement

Displacement occurs when satisfying a need becomes blocked with one type of behavior but can be satisfied by using another type of behavior. For example, the person who is angry with a co-worker displaces his anger by kicking a chair. Or, hostile impulses can be expressed in a socially acceptable manner through participation in sports. Displacement is among the most satisfying ways to handle undesirable behavior because it allows at least some gratification for an unacceptable motive.

Sublimation is a type of successful displacement since it involves substituting one type of behavior for another. The term is often used in relation to sexual desires. For example, masturbation may be used to relieve sexual tension when other means of satisfying sexual desires are absent. It is rarely, if ever, pathological behavior.

Regression

When *regression* is present, an individual returns to an earlier method of behaving. It is a turning back process. Children very often demonstrate regressive behavior when ill. For instance, the youngster who is toilet-trained and can drink from a cup begins to soil diapers and demands a nursing bottle.

Fantasy

Fantasy means using the imagination to create a picture that exists only in the mind. Daydreaming is one kind of fantasy. Unrealistic solutions to problems are usually at the heart of fantasy. Thus, an ill person may use fantasy by imagining himself well and without the need for health care.

Intellectualization

Intellectualization means becoming detached from an emotionally disturbing situation by dealing with it in abstract terms. Teenagers may intellectualize about sexual relationships and try to detach themselves from emotional experiences when facing up to their sexual impulses proves too disturbing.

Labeling a person's behavior in terms of the defense mechanism he is probably using may be one way of describing behavior but offers no reason for the behavior. One would have to explore the need a defense mechanism meets for the person using it in order to understand its use. As pointed out earlier, human behavior is complex. It becomes foolhardy to attempt to label behavior without having a good understanding of the person using it. Also, labeling tends to lead to tunnel vision with the result that one tends to turn off other avenues of exploration when studying someone's behavior.

The use of defense mechanisms is part of everyday living and when used in moderation, can be effective as a way of coping with a problem. Some persons feel that the human being may not even have the powers to survive if defense mechanisms were unavailable to temper the many stressors of daily living. Especially when a problem seems overwhelming, a defense mechanism provides time to find alternative ways to adjust. The use of defense mechanisms becomes of concern when they are used as the primary or dominant method of handling life's problems and then stand in the way of learning more mature ways of behaving.

HEALTH, ILLNESS, AND THE HEALTH-ILLNESS CONTINUUM

Professional and lay literature abounds with definitions of health, most of which in general are based on the premise that health represents physical fitness, emotional and mental stability, and social usefulness. A few examples will illustrate.

The U.S. President's Commission on the Health Needs of the Nation reported that *health* means ". . . physical, mental, and social efficiency and well-being." The Commission went on to state that the first requisite for leading a full life is health, which makes possible maximum self-expression and self-development of man.

The World Health Organization, one of the specialized agencies of the United Nations, defined health in the preamble of its constitution as ". . . a state of complete physical, mental and social well-being and not merely the absence of disease or infirmity." It also states that health is ". . . one of the fundamental rights of every human being. . ."

Health can be viewed as wholeness of the human being. It is a state that results from satisfactory interrelationships among the physical, psychological, and social components of the body. In other words, it represents biopsychosocial homeostasis.

There are some who prefer the term *wellness* rather than health since the idea of health as being only an absence of illness has become entrenched in many people's minds. Since health is the more popular term, it is used frequently in this text. However, the reader is reminded that health is used in the context as described above rather than as simply a state of not being ill.

Illness involves an event or condition that results in malfunctioning of the biopsychosocial organism so that its ability to function in a state of wholeness is restricted. In other words, there is a loss in wholeness in the presence of illness.

Most persons think of themselves as being well when they are not ill and ill when they are not well. However, neither health nor illness is a fixed quantity. For example, "efficiency and well-being" and a "state of well-being" are positive descriptions that indicate that health may not be necessarily constant in nature. Well-being fluctuates and at times so-called healthy people do not function or feel as well as they do at other times. A person considered healthy may have a headache and perform poorly in school that day. While he may not feel up to par, it is unlikely that he would consider himself sick. As long as he is able to cope with problems in his environment and maintain homeostasis, he may be considered well. A sick person also fluctuates in his state of illness. A person so ill that he cannot care for his hygienic needs may convalesce sufficiently to meet those needs and still be ill when he cannot cope with his problems sufficiently to maintain homeostasis. Everyone has a state of health, wholeness, and homeostasis. It may exist at a high level and be called *high-level wellness*. Or it may exist at a low level and be considered illness or even life-threatening.

Usually, the person is somewhere between these extremes.

The concept of high-level wellness was developed by Halbert L. Dunn whose book on the subject appears in the references at the end of this unit. He described it as the state in which one functions at one's most favorable status. It means the potential of the individual is at its maximum, integrated, and utilized with purpose and meaning within the individual's environment. Optimum health, often used synonymously with perfect health, is considered unknown or without accurate description. A better and recommended concept is that of high-level wellness.

A *continuum* is defined as a continuous whole. Fluctuations in health and illness can be illustrated on a health-illness continuum, as shown in Figure 10-6. There is no exact point at which health ends and illness begins. Both are relative in nature, and for each individual, there is considerable range and latitude in which he may be considered ill or well.

On a continuum, health and illness may be viewed as phases of coping ability. When a person copes and functions effectively, he can be considered in the health spectrum even though he may have a chronic disease, such as diabetes mellitus or arthritis. Good health and well-being involve continuous adjustment. Failing adjustment eventually results in illness. When the body fails completely and irreversible damage results, death follows.

A relationship between high-level wellness and the health-illness continuum can be observed. Consider an adult male with asthma and emphysema, two chronic conditions involving the respiratory tract. This person has permanent and irreversible damage to his respiratory tract resulting in physical limitations. He can no longer participate in sports and his exercise is limited to strolling walks; he is limited in the amount and kind of yard work he can do; and air pollution is especially troublesome to him. This man has a position demanding of his intellectual ability, but his work requires practically no physical exertion other than commuting to and from his office. His car and office are air-conditioned so that air pollution in his working environment is at a minimum. It can be observed that he is functioning at his maximum potential or at high-level wellness for him. On the health-illness continuum, he is functioning within a relatively narrow range on the continuum of illness and health. It could even be said that he is a sick man even when he is well. However, in this case, his illnesses do not necessarily prevent him from experiencing well-being and he is functioning at

Figure 10-6 This diagram illustrates the health-illness continuum.

high-level wellness for him. He is maintaining biopsychosocial homeostasis at his best potential.

STAGES OF ILLNESS

When an individual is no longer able to cope with the stressors he encounters, homeostasis is threatened. On the health–illness continuum, the person has reached an area of instability. Unless he can muster additional coping behaviors, he will fall into the illness spectrum. Now he has still another stressor with which to deal—the state of illness.

When a person becomes ill, he assumes a role that is different from the one he had when his health problem was absent. As stated earlier, behavior is purposeful in that a person acts in a manner that to him has meaning, even when he may not be able to explain the reason for his behavior. Hence, in the process of coping with illness, the person's behavior changes because it is an attempt to adjust to something new.

Some people adjust to new settings and new experiences with greater ease than others. For example, there are people who move around the country establishing new homes in markedly different surroundings with apparent ease. There are others who feel they could not live happily except in a familiar environment. So too with ill persons. Some appear to adjust with ease while others adjust with greater difficulty. This difference among patients also demonstrates the uniqueness of everyone.

The seriousness of an illness, from a health practitioner's viewpoint, may not necessarily be a useful indicator in predicting a person's attitude and reactions when illness occurs. Some persons whose illness may be considered minor in terms of complete recovery may view that illness with great alarm and concern. Other persons experiencing serious illness may appear to show little emotional reaction or concern.

Studies have shown that there appears to be a general pattern of adjustment to illness. The phrase "stages of illness" is often used when speaking of this pattern. Although investigators have described the pattern somewhat differently and used different terminology to some extent, there is commonality in general behavioral characteristics.

Denial, a defense mechanism described earlier in this chapter, is characteristically an early stage of illness. Even the suspicion of illness may be a stressor with which the individual must cope. Emotional reactions, such as anxiety, fear, irritability, and aggressiveness, often occur. The patient may avoid, refuse, or even forget needed care. As has been said, the person may appear to flee toward health in attempting to escape illness. Using denial to cope may be appropriate temporarily. However, if it occurs to any extent, or for an extended time, denial may precipitate a crisis.

When the person no longer denies being ill and is aware of what is happening to him, he tends to move toward a stage of acceptance and ordinarily turns to professional help for assistance. At first, many patients become dependent on health practitioners and also become symptom- and illness-oriented. Gradually, dependence is likely to lessen as the patient's condition changes and as he is aided to accept more responsibility in helping himself. Nonetheless, it can be expected that at least some patients will still continue to deny illness and may even appear to be challenging it. Acceptance for them may not occur, or at least not until a change in their physical condition occurs at which time they tend finally to accede to illness.

Then follows a stage of recovery, rehabilitation, or convalesence. Depending on the illness, it may be a relatively short or long period. If little adjustment is required for a patient to return to a former way of life, convalescence tends to be short. The period will be longer when patients are required to make changes in their life-style. During recovery, without regard to its length, the patient goes through a process of resolving loss or impairment of function. When the period is prolonged due to chronic illness or physical limitations, the patient may experience recurrence of illness requiring repeated efforts to cope.

IMPLICATIONS FOR NURSING

Viewing the human being as an open system offers a base upon which nursing care can be developed that takes the wholeness of man into consideration. Man is made up of many parts, the sum of which does not become the whole unless the dynamic, forever-changing interrelatedness of all behavior is also taken into account when planning nursing intervention. We are biopsychosocial beings constantly reacting to our internal and external environments.

Since environmental influences are always present, the human being must have the resources to maintain constancy and stability for life and growth. When homeostasis is upset, illness threatens. An understanding of homeostasis is important for the nurse who includes in her role helping persons to attain as well as maintain health. Homeostasis is fostered when human biopsychosocial needs are being met satisfactorily. Each person is unique and although there is commonality in the needs of man, the environments of each person are different. When meeting needs is thwarted, problems arise as homeostasis is upset. A recognition of the importance of meeting human needs and of the problems that arise when they are not met becomes a guide upon which the nurse can plan and execute nursing care.

The concept of stress becomes the basis for understanding the body's responses to stressors in the environment. A common method for describing how the body responds to stress uses the general adaptation syndrome. The three-step pattern of alarm, resistance, and exhaustion becomes a guide for the selection of appropriate nursing intervention. As long as a person experiences adaptation to a stressor during the stage of resistance, homeostasis is regained and maintained. This knowledge is essential for the nurse to plan health maintenance measures for those to whom she offers her services. When the person fails to reach adjustment and passes on to the stage of exhaustion, illness is present and unless health care measures are used, death will eventually follow. If the stage of exhaustion is not interrupted sufficiently soon, the nurse faces a crisis in which emergency care must be instigated promptly.

There are certain diseases that are considered stress-related. Some persons call them diseases of adaptation. Prolonged exposure to stressors may exhaust the body and leave it with insufficient ability to fight illness. It tends to affect skin and mucous membranes, resulting in such problems as rashes and ulcers. Another condition often associated with excessive stress is hypertension. Knowledge that excessive exposure to stressors predisposes to certain illnesses serves to alert the nurse to plan preventive care for persons exposed to numerous stressors.

On the other hand, certain amounts of stress are necessary for health. For example, muscles atrophy with disuse. Exercise that results in an appropriate amount of stress on muscles prevents atrophy. Following a myocardial infarction, many persons are taught to follow a graduated exercise program in order to help maintain muscle tone and decrease the heart's workload by promoting venous return and preventing blood stagnation.

Defense mechanisms help one cope with anxiety. When used judiciously and moderately, they can be health-promoting. Recognizing this, the nurse will wish to be alert when persons are observed using them as a primary method for handling life's problems. Nursing intervention measures then become important.

Reframing has been found helpful when judging behavior. *Reframing* is a way to alter one's point of view by placing a circumstance or condition into a different perspective. An article describing reframing appears in the references at the end of this unit. The author gives this example. A patient has been ordered to maintain bed rest but refuses to stay in bed. He could easily be labeled a problem patient whose behavior is maladaptive. By reframing, the patient's behavior can be viewed as satisfying to him since he cannot accept being sick, dependent, and helpless. While this patient may harm himself by refusing to stay in bed, he is also preserving his self-image and esteem. The technique of reframing helps health personnel avoid labeling and using tunnel vision when judging behavior.

Today's definition of health or wellness and illness are defined much more broadly than once was the case. It is helpful to think of the terms as being on a continuum since no person is in a total state of either health or illness. The continuum focuses attention on needs that may not be well met while calling attention to strengths that can be utilized for promoting homeostasis.

Man strives to use his greatest potential, even during periods of adversity. This knowledge places the nurse in the position of realizing that everyone has assets or strengths upon which the nurse can build, the end result of which will help persons in her care regain and maintain their best possible potential.

Nurses can expect that most persons will experience emotional reactions when they are ill. It has been found that bringing these emotional responses to a conscious level helps identify them and guides the nurse toward appropriate nursing intervention. For example, when a person can express his anger and be helped to identify its cause, the nurse can then better help him cope with it. It is important for the nurse to remember that people *feel* the way they do for a reason and they cannot be made to feel the way others think they should.

Observations of the person receiving care are basic to

nursing. Signs and symptoms serve as cues concerning how well or how poorly a person is meeting stressors. Using observation becomes the key for analyzing what is happening to a person, what stressors are interrupting homeostasis, what needs are not being met, and finally, what measures can best be used to restore homeostasis.

Two nurse authors have suggested questions to help the nurse gain knowledge about a person's behavior in relation to coping abilities. These questions can be used for planning health care services that are conducive to maintain and regain homeostasis. The authors explained that what may appear as duplication of some of the questions occurs in order to ensure that the patient situation is viewed from all perspectives.

A. Questions that will determine the particular structural variable profile for each person involved in the situation:
  1. What are the specific characteristics of each profile factor?
    a. What is their age and sex?
    b. What is their ethnic and cultural background?
    c. What is their religious affiliation?
    d. What is their educational and occupational background?
    e. Who are the "significant others" involved?
    f. What is their health status?
  2. What are the generalizations that might be relevant to a person with the characteristics of this profile?
  3. To what degree do the identified generalizations actually influence or govern the person's behavior in this situation?

B. Questions that identify potential problems and potential resources:
  1. What are the limitations with which the client must cope?
  2. How does the client view his situation?
    a. What priority does the client give to his human needs?
    b. Does he have only a here-and-now orientation?
    c. Is he seeing himself as a unified whole or only as his involved part?
    d. How does the individual view or evaluate his potential capacity?
  3. To what degree is he utilizing the potential of which he is capable?
  4. What are the behaviors composing the client's usual patterns of daily living?
  5. What are the disruptions in his usual behaviors caused by the illness situation?
  6. Within the limits of the medical regimen, which of the disruptions in his behavioral patterns are actually necessary?
  7. What are the external environmental resources available to him? How can they be utilized more effectively?

C. Questions that give an indication of the client's adaptation status, the appropriateness of his energy allocation, and his potential adaptive capacity:

  1. Is the client's behavioral adjustment adaptive or maladaptive?
  2. What is the client's position on the behavioral stability continuum?
    a. Are his behaviors effective and efficient, or effective but not efficient or vice versa, or neither effective nor efficient?
    b. To what degree are his behaviors consistent, coherent, and orderly?
    c. Are there any behavioral cues that may indicate intensification of the stress state in the following categories:
      (1) Accentuated use of some usual mode or pattern of behavior?
      (2) Alteration in the variety of activities usually undertaken?
      (3) Less organized behavior or a lower level of behavioral organization?
      (4) Demonstration of greater sensitivity to the environment?
      (5) Presence of behaviors reflecting alteration in his ordinary subsystem activity?
      (6) Distortion of "reality"?

D. Questions that give an indication of the client's ability to utilize his adaptive capacity constructively including the factors that affect his ability to change:
  1. Do both the nurse and the client give the same priority in the ranking of the client's basic haman needs in the specific illness situation?
  2. What is the status of the stressors for a particular situation?
    a. What is the nature of the stressor?
    b. How many stressors must be coped with simultaneously?
    c. How long has or will the client be exposed to the stressor?
    d. What has been his previous experience with a comparable stressor?
  3. How successfully can the client be motivated to change his behavior?
    a. What is the source of the stimuli?
    b. What is the intensity or number of the stimuli?
    c. What is the specific behavior or pattern of behavior involved?
    d. What importance does the client attach to the original behavior?

E. Questions that will identify nursing intervention that will be required:
  1. For whom does this particular activity have consequences?
  2. What are the consequences that can be anticipated?
  3. What is the value of those consequences for those involved?

F. Questions that will give an indication of the effectiveness of the nurse-client interactional process will have two directions:
  1. Questions of the client that may indicate stressors or potential stressors:

a. What does the person view as his rights and obligations in the client position?

b. What is his understanding of the client role behaviors and the behaviors of the nurse role?

c. Can confusion or conflict between roles attached to his other positions and that of the client role be anticipated under the prevailing circumstances?

d. Does the client understand and accept the ground rules of this nurse-client relationship?

2. Questions that nurses must ask themselves:

a. Do the client's understandings of his role and the nurse role differ from my understandings in this situation?

b. Have I clarified the ground rules of this professional relationship in my own mind?

c. Are all the stages of a relationship being fully incorporated in my interactions with a given patient?

d. Am I appropriately enacting the nurse role in this situation?

e. Do I inadvertently shift roles when the nurse position is the governing position?

f. Are there conflicting demands of other positions I occupy that influence my enactment of the nurse role?

G. Questions that nurses must continually ask of themselves so that their practice will continue to reflect the highest level of professional competence:

1. Am I fulfilling the full scope of my professional obligations in my daily practice?

2. Are my rights as a professional nurse being acknowledged in such a way that I can best fulfill my professional obligations?

3. To what degree am I depending upon external rules and regulations to govern my actions?

4. Am I using discrimination when I delegate tasks to other categories of health workers or family members?

5. Am I judicious in accepting tasks delegated to me?*

High-level wellness as a national goal involves the services of health practitioners of all types plus many other persons as well. For example, environmental experts are important, as are engineers and architects who build the structures serving society, the social scientists who are concerned with humans and their relationships with others, and the politicians who are responsible for legislating for the promotion of well-being. Certainly too, the consumers of health care are important, as Chapter 3 described. High-level wellness requires services that are broad in scope and achieving it requires team work with representation from all groups in society. Nurses must plan to work cooperatively with the consumer and many others to contribute to the health of all members of society.

---

*Byrne, Marjorie L. and Thompson, Lida F. *Key Concepts for the Study and Practice of Nursing*. Edition 2. The C. V. Mosby Company, St. Louis, 1978.

Nurses are human beings too and they have needs which must be met. The easy way out when the nurse has difficulty coping with a patient's problem is to blame the patient, avoid him, or possibly plan less than total care. When the nurse understands her own behavior, her own methods of meeting needs, and her value system, she can better accept and understand the behavior of others. Also, recognizing when the nurse may lack certain skills to deal with a particular patient satisfactorily opens up avenues for consulting those who do have those skills. For example, many nurses do not have the counseling skills required for dealing with persons with certain psychosocial problems. The nurse then is advised to turn to nurses with special counseling skills required in that particular situation rather than trying to do all things for every person she serves at all times.

CONCLUSION

This chapter presented concepts basic to an understanding of how man functions to meet his needs and to maintain homeostasis. These concepts, it is believed, provide a framework for a synthesis of knowledge necessary for the nurse to offer complete health care to those who have come to her for care.

SUPPLEMENTAL LIBRARY STUDY

1. Read the following article:

Levine, Myra E. "The Pursuit of Wholeness." *American Journal of Nursing,* 69:93–98, January 1969.

How does the author define adaptation and wholeness in relation to man's environment. On page 96, the author describes the probable results of overcrowded living. What pathophysiological changes does she theorize could very well be caused by overcrowded living that is so often found in slum and poverty-stricken areas? On page 98, the author gives an example of ill-effects that occurred when the nurse's and the patient's perceptual systems were at odds. Cite an example from your experience while caring for a patient when you believe your nursing intervention measures may have failed because you and the patient had different perceptions of a particular situation.

2. Note how a nurse was helpful when a patient's fear interfered with her recovery:

McGuire, Maggie. "Every E.R. Should Have One." *Nursing 77,* 7:80, July 1977.

What nursing observation suggested that the patient was suffering from psychosocial stress? What nursing intervention measures did the nurse use to ease the patient's tension? Discuss Maslow's human needs theory as it could be applied in order to understand the patient's behavior. What physiological findings were observed that appeared to be related to the patient's emotional stress?

3. An interview with Dr. Hans Selye is described in the following article:

"Secret of Coping With Stress." (Interview with Dr. Hans Selye) *U.S. News & World Report,* 82:51–53, March 21, 1977.

What does Dr. Selye consider to be the most frequent cause of psychological stress in man today? What suggestions does he offer to cope with psychological stress? What does he believe stands in the way of helping those people who are unable to cope with stress?

4. Note the A to Z list of characteristics the author used to describe adult wellness in the following article:

Oelbaum, Cynthia Hastings. "Hallmarks of Adult Wellness." *American Journal of Nursing,* 74:1623–1625, September 1974.

What reasons does the author give concerning why many nurses are illness- rather than health-oriented? How does she illustrate the importance of viewing man as a whole? The rights of the consumer were discussed in Chapter 3 of this text. How does the author describe the nurse's responsibilities, as related to consumer rights, in the last paragraph of this article?

5. Read the following article:

Kunzman, Lucy. "Some Factors Influencing a Young Child's Mastery of Hospitalization." *The Nursing Clinics of North America,* 7:13–26, March 1972.

The author notes that a child has fears, anxieties, and fantasies when he becomes a patient but she reminds her readers that a child is not a miniature adult. On page 15 of this article, there is a table that compares a child's situation at home with the situation that exists when hospitalization becomes necessary. Suggest ways that could be used to minimize the trauma a child faces when hospitalized. For example, describe how you believe a child could be helped to master a loss of independence when hospitalization occurs.

References For Unit III

CHAPTER 6

Angelini, Diane J. "Nonverbal Communication in Labor." *American Journal of Nursing,* 78:1220–1222, June 1978.

Belt, Linda Hagen. "Working with Dysphasic Patients." *American Journal of Nursing,* 74:1320–1322, July 1974.

Cosper, Bonnie. "How Well Do Patients Understand Hospital Jargon?" *American Journal of Nursing,* 77:1932–1934, December 1977.

Egolf, Donald B. and Chester, Sondra L. "Speechless Messages." *Nursing Digest,* 4:26–27, March/April 1976.

Fredette, Sheila. "Problem Solving with a Difficult Patient." *American Journal of Nursing,* 77:622–623, April 1977.

Gombrich, E. H. "The Visual Image." *Scientific American,* 227:82–96, September 1972.

Gordy, Helen E. "Gift Giving in the Nurse-Patient Relationship." *American Journal of Nursing,* 78:1026–1028, June 1978.

Gould, Grace Theresa, Guest Editor. "Symposium on Compassion and Communication in Nursing." *The Nursing Clinics of North America,* 4:651–729, December 1969.

Hein, Eleanor and Leavitt, Maribelle. "Providing Emotional Support to Patients." *Nursing 77,* 7:39–41, May 1977.

Herth, Kaye. "Beyond the Curtain of Silence." *American Journal of Nursing,* 74:1060–1061, June 1974.

Kalisch, Beatrice J. "What Is Empathy?" *American Journal of Nursing,* 73:1548–1552, September 1973.

Kesler, Arlene Riley. "Pitfalls To Avoid in Interviewing Outpatients." *Nursing 77,* 7:70–73, September 1977.

Kohut, Susanne A. "Guidelines for Using Interpreters." *Nursing Digest,* 4:55, January/February 1976.

Krauss, Robert M. and Glucksberg, Sam. "Social and Nonsocial Speech." *Scientific American,* 236:100–105, February 1977.

Langford, Teddy. "Establishing A Nursing Contract." *Nursing Outlook,* 26:386–388, June 1978.

McGreevy, Abigail and Van Heukelem, Judy. "Crying: The Neglected Dimension." *Nursing Digest,* 5:61–63, Spring 1977.

Maslow, Abraham H. *Motivation and Personality.* Edition 2. Harper & Row, New York, 1970, 369 p.

Mayeroff, Milton. *On Caring.* Harper & Row, New York, 1971, 106 p.

Melrose, Jay. "Audiocassettes Help Hospitals Break Language Barriers To Care." *Hospitals, Journal Of The American Hospital Association,* 51:93–94, 96, November 1, 1977.

Mitchell, Ann Chappell. "Barriers to Therapeutic Communication with Black Clients." *Nursing Outlook,* 26:109–112, February 1978.

Montagu, Ashley. *Touching: The Human Significance of the Skin.* Columbia University Press, New York, 1971, 338 p.

Mooney, Judith. "Attachment/Separation in the Nurse-Patient Relationship." *Nursing Forum,* 15:259–264, Number 3, 1976.

Munn, Harry E. Jr. "Are You a Skilled Listener?" *AORN Journal,* 25:994, 996, 998, 1000, April 1977.

Perron, Denise M. "Deprived of Sound." *American Journal of Nursing,* 74:1057–1059, June 1974.

Rogers, Carl R. *On Becoming a Person: A Therapist's View of Psychotherapy.* Houghton Mifflin Company, Boston, 1961, pp. 39–58.

Sandlan, Brenda. "Ted Can Only Blink His Eyes . . . Still We Communicate." *Nursing 75,* 5:19–21, May 1975.

Shubin, Seymour. "Familiarity: Therapeutic? Harmful? When?" *Nursing 76,* 6:18, 20, 21, 24, November 1976.

Skelly, Madge. "Aphasic Patients Talk Back." *American Journal of Nursing,* 75:1140–1142, July 1975.

Skipper, James K. Jr. and Leonard, Robert C., Editors. *Social Interaction and Patient Care.* J. B. Lippincott Company, Philadelphia, 1965, 399 p.

Stokoe, William C. Jr. "Seeing & Signing Language." *Nursing Digest,* 4:40–42, Summer 1976.

Sundeen, Sandra J., et al. *Nurse-Client Interaction: Implementing the Nursing Process.* The C. V. Mosby Company, Saint Louis, 1976, 200 p.

Walke, Mary Anne Kelly. "When a Patient Needs to Unburden His Feelings." *American Journal of Nursing,* 77:1164–1166, July 1977.

Wisser, Susan Hiscoe. "When the Walls Listened." *American Journal of Nursing,* 78:1016–1017, June 1978.

Wolf, Ellen M. "Communicating with Deaf Surgical Patients." *AORN Journal,* 26:39–47, July 1977.

CHAPTER 7

Anderson, Gwen and Tighe, Bridget. "Gypsy Culture and Health Care." *American Journal of Nursing,* 73:282–285, February 1973.

Berkowitz, Philip and Berkowitz, Nancy S. "The Jewish Patient in the Hospital." *American Journal of Nursing,* 67:2335–2337, November 1967.

Branch, Marie Foster and Paxton, Phyllis Perry, Editors. *Providing Safe Nursing Care for Ethnic People of Color.* Appleton-Century-Crofts, New York, 1976, 272 p.

Brink, Pamela J., Editor. *Transcultural Nursing: A Book of Readings.* Prentice-Hall, Inc., Englewood Cliffs, New Jersey, 1976, 289 p.

Bullough, Bonnie and Bullough, Vern L. *Poverty, Ethnic Identity, and Health Care.* Appleton-Century-Crofts, New York, 1972, 226 p.

Campbell, Teresa and Chang, Betty. "Health Care of the Chinese in America." *Nursing Outlook,* 21:245–249, April 1973.

Damsteegt, Don. "Pastoral Roles in Presurgical Visits." *American Journal of Nursing,* 75:1336–1337, August 1975.

Dickinson, Sister Corita. "The Search for Spiritual Meaning." *American Journal of Nursing,* 75:1789–1793, October 1975.

Hongladarom, Gail Chapman and Russell, Millie. "An Ethnic Difference—Lactose Intolerance." *Nursing Outlook,* 24:764–765, December 1976.

"Hospital Care: When Religious Belief Affects Therapy." *Patient Care,* 8:99–101, November 1, 1974.

Kniep-Hardy, Mary and Burkhardt, Margaret A. "Nursing the Navajo." *American Journal of Nursing,* 77:95–96, January 1977.

Leininger, Madeleine, Editor. *Health Care Dimensions: Transcultural Health Care Issues and Conditions.* F. A. Davis Company, Philadelphia, 1976, 206 p.

Leininger, Madeleine. *Nursing and Anthropology: Two Worlds to Blend.* John Wiley & Sons, Inc., New York, 1970, 181 p.

Lindstrom, Carol J. "No Shows: A Problem in Health Care." *Nursing Outlook,* 23:755–759, December 1975.

Loftus, John. "Medicine Man." *World Health,* 17–19, October 1976.

Luckraft, Dorothy, Editor. *Black Awareness: Implications for Black Patient Care.* The American Journal of Nursing Company, New York, 1976, 43 p.

McMahon, Margaret A. and Miller, Sister Patricia. "Pain Response: The Influence of Psycho-Social-Cultural Factors." *Nursing Forum,* 17:58–71, Number 1, 1978.

Primeaux, Martha. "Caring for the American Indian Patient." *American Journal of Nursing,* 77:91–94, January 1977.

Pumphrey, John B. "Recognizing Your Patients' Spiritual Needs." *Nursing 77,* 7:64–68, 70, December 1977.

Rocereto, LaVerne R. "Root Work and the Root Doctor." *Nursing Forum,* 12:414–426, Number 4, 1973.

Rosten, Leo, Editor. *Religions of America: Ferment and Faith in an Age of Crisis.* Simon & Schuster, New York, 1975, 672 p.

Scott, Clarissa S. "Health and Healing Practices Among Five Ethnic Groups in Miami, Florida." *Public Health Reports,* 89:524–532, November/December 1974.

"Symposium on Cultural and Biological Diversity and Health Care." *The Nursing Clinics of North America,* 12:1–86, March 1977.

White, Earnestine Huffman. "Health and the Black Person: An Annotated Bibliography." *American Journal of Nursing,* 74:1839–1841, October 1974.

CHAPTER 8

Ballantyne, Donna J. "CCTV for Patients." *American Journal of Nursing,* 74:263–264, February 1974.

Berni, Rosemarian and Fordyce, Wilbert E. *Behavior Modification and The Nursing Process.* Edition 2. The C. V. Mosby Company, Saint Louis, 1977, 160 p.

Carruth, Beatrice F. "Modifying Behavior Through Social Learning." *American Journal of Nursing,* 76:1804–1806, November 1976.

Engle, Veronica. "Diabetic Teaching: How To Win Your Patient's Cooperation in His Care." *Nursing 75,* 5:17–24, December 1975.

Fuhrer, Lois Mishkin and Bernstein, Ronni. "Making Patient Education a Part of Patient Care." *American Journal of Nursing,* 76:1798–1799, November 1976.

Gorman, M. Leah. "Conscious Repatterning of Human Behavior." *American Journal of Nursing,* 75:1752–1754, October 1975.

Haferkorn, Virginia. "Assessing Individual Learning Needs as a Basis for Patient Teaching." *The Nursing Clinics of North America,* 6:199–209, March 1971.

Kazdin, Alan E. "Token Economies: The Rich Rewards of Rewards." *Psychology Today,* 10:98, 101, 102, 105, 114, November 1976.

Knapp, Mary Elizabeth, et al. "Teaching Suzi to Walk by Behavior Modification of Motor Skills." *Nursing Forum,* 13:158–183, Number 2, 1974.

Kratzer, Joan B. "What Does Your Patient Need to Know?" *Nursing 77,* 7:82, 84, December 1977.

LeBow, Michael D. *Behavior Modification: A Significant Method in Nursing Practice.* Prentice-Hall, Inc., Englewood Cliffs, New Jersey, 1973, 271 p.

Loxsom, Rosalind. "Changing Obesity Patterns." *Nursing Outlook,* 23:711–713, November 1975.

Lyons, Mary Lou. "What Priority Do You Give Preop Teaching?" *Nursing 77,* 7:12, 14, January 1977.

Merkatz, Ruth, et al. "Preoperative Teaching for Gynecologic Patients." *American Journal of Nursing,* 74:1072–1074, June 1974.

Miller, Jean. "Cognitive Dissonance in Modifying Families' Perceptions." *American Journal of Nursing,* 74:1468–1470, August 1974.

Mitchell, Ellen Sullivan. "Protocol for Teaching Hypertensive Patients." *American Journal of Nursing,* 77:808–809, May 1977.

"Preoperative Teaching Found to Shorten Hospitalization." (News) *American Journal of Nursing,* 75:2078, November 1975.

Pugh, Elizabeth Jean. "Dynamics of Teaching-Learning Interaction." *Nursing Forum,* 15:47–58, Number 1, 1976.

Rottkamp, Barbara C. "An Experimental Nursing Study: A Behavior Modification Approach to Nursing Therapeutics in Body Positioning of Spinal-Cord Injured Patients." *Nursing Research,* 25:181–186, May/June 1976.

Schmidt, Mary P. W. and Duncan, Beverly A. B. "Modifying Eating Behavior in Anorexia Nervosa." *American Journal of Nursing,* 74:1646–1648, September 1974.

Shipley, Robert H. "Applying Learning Theory to Nursing Practice." *Nursing Forum,* 16:83–94, Number 1, 1977.

Tarver, Joyce and Turner, A. Jack. "Teaching Behavior Modification to Patients' Families." *American Journal of Nursing,* 74:282–283, February 1974.

Winslow, Elizabeth Hahn. "The Role of the Nurse in Patient Education. Focus: The Cardiac Patient." *The Nursing Clinics of North America,* 11:213–222, June 1976.

CHAPTER 9

Burton, Genevieve. "Families in Crisis: Knowing When and How to Help." *Nursing 75,* 5:36–43, December 1975.

"Caring for the Aged." (An AJN Feature) *American Journal of Nursing,* 73:2049–2066, December 1973.

"Denying Mastectomy." (Public Welfare) *Human Behavior,* 6:23, August 1977.

Erikson, Erik H. *Childhood and Society.* Edition 2. W. W. Norton & Company, Inc., New York, 1963, 447 p.

Gresham, Mary L. "The Infantilization of the Elderly: A Developing Concept." *Nursing Forum,* 15:195–210, Number 2, 1976.

Havighurst, Robert J. *Developmental Tasks and Education.* Edition 3. David McKay Company, Inc., New York, 1972, 119 p.

Lanahan, Colleen C. "Homosexuality: A Different Sexual Orientation." *Nursing Forum,* 15:314–319, Number 3, 1976.

Lawrence, John C. "Homosexuals, Hospitalization, and the Nurse." *Nursing Forum,* 14:304–317, Number 3, 1975.

Lee, Roberta J. "Self Images of the Elderly." *The Nursing Clinics of North America,* 11:119–124, March 1976.

Lore, Ann. "Adolescents: People, Not Problems." *American Journal of Nursing,* 73:1232–1234, July 1973.

"Nobody Home: The Erosion of the American Family." (A Conversation with Eric Bronfenbrenner) *Psychology Today,* 10:40–47, May 1977.

Sheehy, Gail. *Passages: Predictable Crises of Adult Life.* Bantam Books, New York, 1976. 560 p.

Sibille, Sister Michael. "Geriatric Care: Let's Make it More than Physical Care." (Speaking Out) *Nursing 75,* 5:54–55, July 1975.

Smith, David W. and Bierman, Edwin L., Editors. *The Biological Ages of Man From Conception Through Old Age.* W. B. Saunders Company, Philadelphia, 1973, 211 p.

"Staying Well While Growing Old." (Special Feature on the Well Elderly) *American Journal of Nursing,* 78:1334–1354, August 1978.

Sutterley, Doris Cook and Donnelly, Gloria Ferraro. *Perspectives in Human Development: Nursing Throughout the Life Cycle.* J. B. Lippincott Company, Philadelphia, 1973, 331 p.

Vaillant, George E. "The Climb to Maturity: How the Best and the Brightest Came of Age." *Psychology Today,* 11:34–41, 107, 108, 110, September 1977.

Waechter, Eugenia H. and Blake, Florence G. *Nursing Care of Children.* Edition 9. J. B. Lippincott Company, Philadelphia, 1976, 834 p.

CHAPTER 10

Andersen, Marcia DeCann and Pleticha, Jane Marie. "Emergency Unit Patients' Perceptions of Stressful Life Events." *Nursing Research.* 23:378–383, September/October 1974.

Byrne, Marjorie L. and Thompson, Lida F. *Key Concepts for the Study and Practice of Nursing.* Edition 2. The C. V. Mosby Company, Saint Louis, 1978, 160 p.

"Calling Dr. Stress." *Psychology Today,* 11:93–94, 96, 99–100, 105, September 1977.

Ciuca, Rudy, et al. "When A Disaster Happens: How Do You Meet Emotional Needs?" *American Journal of Nursing,* 77:454–456, March 1977.

Clark, Carolyn Chambers. "Reframing." *American Journal of Nursing,* 77:840–841, May 1977.

"Dealing With Rage." *Nursing 75,* 5:24–29, October 1975.

Dunn, Halbert L. "What High-Level Wellness Means," in *High-Level Wellness.* R. W. Beatty, Ltd., Arlington, Virginia, 1961, pp. 1–7.

Glass, David C. "Stress, Competition and Heart Attacks." *Psychology Today,* 10:54–57, 134, December 1976.

Graham, Lois E. and Conley, Elizabeth Myers. "Evaluation of Anxiety and Fear in Adult Surgical Patients." *Nursing Research,* 20:113–122, March/April 1971.

Kyes, Joan J. and Hofling, Charles K. *Basic Psychiatric Concepts in Nursing.* Edition 3. J. B. Lippincott Company, Philadelphia, 1974, 527 p.

Levine, Seymour. "Stress and Behavior." *Scientific American,* 224:26–31, January 1971.

Marcinek, Margaret Boyle. "Stress in the Surgical Patient." *American Journal of Nursing,* 77:1809–1811, November 1977.

Martin, Harry W. and Prange, Arthur J. "The Stages of Illness—Psychosocial Approach." *Nursing Outlook,* 10:168–171, March 1962.

Pelletier, Kenneth R. "Mind as Healer; Mind as Slayer." *Psychology Today,* 10:35–37, 40, 82–83, February 1977.

Peterson, Margaret H. "Understanding Defense Mechanisms." (Programmed Instruction) *American Journal of Nursing,* 72:1651–1674, September 1972.

Porth, Carol M. "Physiological Coping: A Model for Teaching Pathophysiology." *Nursing Outlook,* 25:781–784, December 1977.

Selye, Hans. *Stress Without Distress.* New American Library, New York, 1975, 193 p.

Selye, Hans. *The Stress of Life.* (Revised Edition) McGraw-Hill Book Company, New York, 1976, 515 p.

Selye, Hans. "The Stress Syndrome." *American Journal of Nursing,* 65:97–99, March 1965.

Sloboda, Sharon. "Understanding Patient Behavior." *Nursing 77,* 7:74–77, September 1977.

Stephenson, Carol A. "Stress in Critically Ill Patients." *American Journal of Nursing,* 77:1806–1809, November 1977.

Suinn, Richard M. "How To Break the Vicious Cycle of Stress." *Psychology Today,* 10:59–60, December 1976.

Tanner, Ogden. *Stress.* Time-Life Books, New York, 1976, 176 p.

Turnbull, Sister Joyce. "Shifting the Focus to Health." *American Journal of Nursing,* 76:1985–1987, December 1976.

Vincent, Pauline. "The Sick Role in Patient Care." *American Journal of Nursing,* 75:1172–1173, July 1975.

Wacker, Margaret S. "Analogy: Weapon Against Denial." *American Journal of Nursing,* 74:71–73, January 1974.

Weiss, Jay M. "Psychological Factors in Stress and Disease." *Scientific American,* 226:104–113, June 1972.

unit IV
Environmental Considerations in the Practice of Nursing

11

BEHAVIORAL OBJECTIVES

When content in this chapter has been mastered, the student will be able to

Define the terms appearing in the glossary.

Explain how the description of a community can apply to both a family and international groups.

Describe how the well-being of community members can be influenced by the six categories of typical community characteristics described in this chapter.

Illustrate each characteristic with at least two positive and two negative examples of its influence on the well-being of individuals.

Identify three ways the environment of a community can have implications for the nurse's practice.

Discuss the community environment, using the nursing process as a guide.

The Community Environment

GLOSSARY

Community: An aggregrate of people living in the same area and sharing common values and beliefs.
Ergonomics: The study of relationships among individuals and their work and working environment.

INTRODUCTION

Environmental influences can either interfere with or promote well-being. The nurse is often looked to for leadership in working for the kind of environment that promotes high-level wellness. This unit focuses primarily on environmental factors that may influence health and on the practitioner's interest in an environment that promotes well-being. It discusses implications for nursing action directed toward a healthful environment.

The first chapter in this unit deals with the environment of the person in his community. The last three chapters focus on practices that promote a healthful environment in the home and in health agencies.

THE COMMUNITY DESCRIBED

The dictionary defines a *community* as an aggregate of people living in the same area and sharing common values and beliefs. Communities vary in size, both in terms of number of members and of the area involved. A family is a community and is as old as mankind. A neighborhood, city or town, county, state, and country are communities. In recent times, the world has been described as an international community. In the context of this definition, it can be seen that everyone belongs to several communities that become larger beginning with the family and extending outward to the community of mankind, as Figure 11–1 illustrates.

Most authorities describe communities, (regardless of size), in a similar manner. For example, a community is generally made up of people who tend to share some personal characteristics or interests. These people live within a rather well-defined geographical area. The community has certain policies and regulations and certain institutions that serve it. There are usually activities in the community which are directed toward the general welfare of its members. And, the problems of a community often become the common concerns of its members.

The specifics of these commonalities vary among communities but they will amost always produce an environment which influences the individual's state of well-being. Some influences will be positive, or tend to promote health, while others will be negative, or be detrimental to health.

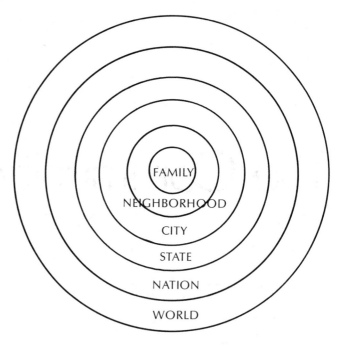

Figure 11–1 Everyone belongs to several communities and as the community continues to grow, all peoples of the world are included. Environmental concerns are the concerns of all communities, and hence, of all mankind.

TYPICAL CHARACTERISTICS OF THE COMMUNITY AND THEIR INFLUENCE ON WELL-BEING

Common characteristics observed among communities may be classified in a variety of ways. Six categories which relate to well-being have been selected for discussion here: prevailing beliefs and values; production of needed services and goods; education and recreation programs; transportation and communication facilities; protection, safety, and aesthetic concerns; and health care resources.

Communities tend to express prevailing values and beliefs. While in general, community members hold to some similar values and beliefs, they may not always be identical in nature. However, those held in common tend to be reinforced and strengthened within the community. The following examples show how values and beliefs may influence well-being.

When a community places value on recreational activities for all age groups, facilities are usually easily available and enjoy the support and interest of community members. Institutions such as churches, schools, YMCA's, and YWCA's generally support and encourage healthful activities for all. When a community places little value or interest in this type of activity, facilities and the support they need may be minimal. As a result, common leisure-time activities may be less likely to promote physical and mental well-being.

When community members tend to hold to the belief that mothers should be in the home, child care facilities are likely to be a rarity. On the other hand, communities whose members feel that mothers have the right to work if they so desire tend to support child care facilities and encourage their use.

Fear and distrust of health practitioners may result in people avoiding care except in crises. It has been observed that such attitudes tend to occur more frequently in isolated rural and poverty-stricken communities. Individuals living in higher socioeconomic communities tend to seek out preventive care from professional practitioners. Hence, they tend to have fewer preventable health-related problems than those living in lower socioeconomic areas.

Belief in assisting others in times of need can be of great value for many health-related community action programs. Churches, service organizations, and interested individuals contribute to their success. On the other hand, a general feeling that every person is responsible for helping himself can result in minimal community service to others.

As Chapter 7 pointed out, most people hold to religious and cultural beliefs, many of which have implications for health care. It is important for health practitioners to know the prevailing beliefs in a community since they may serve as important aids in the promotion of well-being.

People in the community produce services and goods to sustain livelihood. When a community's job opportunities are scarce and unemployment rates are high, the results of having limited resources to purchase the necessities for daily living become apparent. Health problems among the unemployed and unemployable are numerous and well-described in lay and professional literature. For example, when money is scarce, diets often lack sufficient nutrition, the annual physical examination is omitted, dental care is postponed, and so on. Joblessness also has many psychological implications that tend to erode mental well-being through loss of self-respect, financial independence, and control over certain decisions. The negative influence of a high unemployment rate on the welfare of a community is documented almost daily in newspapers around the world.

Job situations also are sometimes directly related to health problems as well as to the improvement of health. As a result of increased attention to the problems of people and their work, a field of study has evolved, called *ergonomics,* which deals with the relationship between individuals and their work and working environment. It is especially concerned with fitting jobs to the needs and abilities of the worker. In ergonomics, attention is focused on health-illness factors the employee brings with him to the work setting as well as the injuries and illnesses acquired as a result of his work. Extensive health programs in many industries focus on disease detection, prevention, and treatment. There are programs concerned with cardiac and respiratory diseases, alcoholism, drug addiction, mental health, and cancer detection and treatment, to name a few.

As mentioned in Chapter 2, the Occupational Safety and Health Act was passed in 1970. Its purpose is to ensure safe and healthful working conditions for employees by promoting the enforcement of standards for maintaining safe and healthful work environments, reducing work hazards, providing research in occupational safety and health, and investigating relationships between disease and illness and the working environment.

It has been observed that most industrial accidents occur at midday or near the end of the work day—the times when the body is at its lowest biological efficiency. These findings correlate with the body's biologic or circadian rhythms which will be discussed in Chapter 15. Many industries have put this knowledge to work by providing rest breaks at appropriate intervals to promote work efficiency and to reduce accidents.

Some services produced in the community, such as those related to health, generally make a direct contribution to the overall welfare of the community, as well as to the welfare of individuals. For example, home health care services make it possible for many elderly and chronically ill persons to live more healthful and active lives. Public transportation specifically designed to accommodate the handicapped makes it possible for many disabled persons to be independent and productive citizens. Day care facilities make it possible for some mentally and physically handicapped children to live part-time with their families where they tend to do better, rather than to place them in institutions. Communities in which health care services are limited or of poor quality will usually reflect a higher incidence of preventable diseases and their effects than communities in which health care services are readily available.

Communities have educational and recreational programs. Education and recreation begin in the home. In addition, most communities have a wide variety of educational programs available to their members. Basic education for children from kindergarten through twelfth grade is typical in this country. There are several trends evident in educational programs in the United States. More facilities and services are becoming available for exceptional persons, that is, those with above average and those with below average mental and physical abilities. Opportunities for learning experiences for children under five years of age are on the increase in many communities. Vocational education is on the increase, as are educational programs for adults, including programs for those with or without benefit of earlier educational opportunities. Health education for all ages is increasing in both formal and informal programs. In addition to increasing the learner's areas of knowledge, enriched educational programs tend to enhance a person's independence, opportunities for employment, and self-concept—factors that in turn tend to promote an individual's psychological well-being.

Consider the following individuals with different kinds of educational experiences, and think about the effects these experiences may have had on their well-being: the children of migrant farm workers whose parents move so frequently in order to follow the harvesting of crops that the children are unable to complete an academic year in any one school; a child with a progressive muscle-deteriorating disease but with an unimpaired intellect who has been able to graduate from high school through a homebound educational program; the teenagers in a neighborhood who are high school dropouts without vocational skills and who do not have the benefit of health teaching in the use of illicit drugs and the prevention of venereal diseases; children who live in a neighborhood where a language other than English is usually spoken but who attend schools where teaching is done in English. These examples have both positive and negative implications for mental and physical well-being.

As mentioned earlier, recreational facilities can help to promote healthful mental and physical activities for all ages. Usually too, community cohesiveness, camaraderie, and morale are increased through the social contacts afforded by the availability of recreational facilities.

Recreational facilities and activities require supervision in order to prevent accidents. For example, swimming facilities without adequate safety features often lead to tragedy. Injuries occurring when recreational equipment is improperly used or maintained is another dangerous condition. When adequate recreational facilities are lacking in a community, destructive activities tend to be more common, and delinquency and crime tend to increase.

Communities rich in opportunities for those interested in the arts, as the dance, music, literature, and art, enrich life and add to the fun and enjoyment of living for most people. These in turn help to promote the community's well-being.

Communities generally have transportation and communication. A variety of transportation facilities is available in many communities. In others, local transportation is almost entirely by automobile. Generally, increased mobility has provided ways for many persons to leave and return to their homes regularly and with ease. This means these persons are exposed to expanding communities, and as a result, often develop interests and attachments outside their immediate neighborhoods. The "bedroom" communities surrounding a metropolitan area are examples of areas where residents often have loyalties and commitments to communities in which they work as well as to those in which they live.

The marked increase in the use of the automobile for transportation in our society has created many health problems caused by pollution from auto exhausts, especially in large cities. There are times when the fumes contribute heavily to a blanket of smog around a community with harmful results. In 1952, a week's period of smog in London resulted in approximately 5,000 deaths, according to physicians who studied the disaster. The amount of respiratory damage due to auto pollution is unknown but believed to be extensive, serious, and on the increase.

Man is working to decrease pollution and thereby its related problems. Improved highway construction that moves traffic more quickly, experts say, results in less exhaust fumes than when there is much stop-and-go, slow traffic. Automobile manufacturers are faced with increasingly rigid standards designed to decrease the amount of unburned hydrocarbons and carbon monoxide in exhaust fumes. Communities are looking more and more to public transportation to ease the use of the auto. Some communities are considering banning the use of the private car in areas where traffic is particularly troublesome. It is hoped that all these efforts will decrease air pollution and the health problems resulting from it.

Availability of public transportation influences accessibility of health care services. For example, the mother without a car and with young children will seek only essential or crisis care, as a rule, if no ready means of getting to health services is available to her. In areas where there is no public transportation, the health care of many persons is poor. It has been observed in communities with limited public transportation that neighborhoods immediately surrounding a health agency, such as a hospital, generally have many elderly residents who chose the location in order to be within easy walking distance of health care facilities.

The size of the community may be said to decrease with improved communications. While the family and neighborhood members may communicate mainly by word of mouth, they are in almost constant contact with the larger communities as well through the means of mass media.

With expanded communications media, values and beliefs often change. There tends to be less solidarity in the family and neighborhood as communities exchange ideas. Also there is often less contentment with status quo and more interest in acculturation as communities view each other through the communications media.

There is little value in providing a particular health service if the community fails to inform people of its availability. Communications media have been helpful in disseminating information on health and health services. One result has been mounting consumer demands for better and more health services.

Communities are concerned with protection, safety, and aesthetics. Activities that promote the conservation of health, life, resources, and property are observed in the community in innumerable ways. Many dangers that previous generations were exposed to have disappeared. For example, the provision of safe drinking water has practically eliminated certain diseases, such as typhoid fever, in many parts of the world. However, as some dangers have been overcome, new perils have appeared. The automobile, built to serve man so that he could enjoy a better way of life, also kills more than 50,000 individuals, and maims countless others each year in the United States.

Auto research continues its attempts to make travel safer. Safety efforts in communities include signs giving traffic information, programs in driving education, the enforcement of speed limits, and the building of roads which are less hazardous.

Fire control, community health education, pet control, food handling regulations, and zoning regulations are additional community efforts to safeguard its members.

Protection from danger and the development of safety and aesthetic measures that will promote well-being require engineering, enforcement of laws, and consumer education, as the following examples show.

The disposal of wastes has brought about the development of sewage disposal plants that replace the emptying of raw wastes into our lakes and streams. It is now illegal in most places to dispose of raw wastes indiscriminately. The consumer is becoming increasingly knowledgeable about the implications of water pollution and is demanding laws and law enforcement that help to prevent it.

As in the case of water pollution, the public has been made equally aware of air pollution and its threat to health and well-being. Engineering and legislation aimed at preventing air pollution from industrial sources is also on the increase.

Indiscriminate use of our natural resources has expanded the role of the environmentalist from one of relative insignificance to one of power and persuasion in our society. Those using or destroying natural resources without consideration for the effects are often viewed as enemies of the public. Increasingly, legislation on use of natural resources reflects people's demands for considering ecological balance in the world among plants, animals, and matter.

Space, as an entity, has taken on increasing importance in recent years as the result of concern about progressive limitations on the available space in the world. Because of the vastness of this country, only within the past several decades has space even been considered a factor in healthful living. It is now an accepted concept that the amount and quality of space available to man can influence him both physically and psychologically. While there are no definitive answers as to the amount of space which is desirable, ongoing studies by social and physical scientists are bringing us new information. For example, the influence of both confinement and vast surrounding space on astronauts continues to be investigated. The effect of population density on both physiological and psychosocial well-being is also being studied. The amount and kind of space available is influenced by many factors, including climate, land usage and control, and building regulations. Communities have become more concerned with regulating the use of space. More attention will undoubtedly be focused on man's need for, and use of, space in the generations to come.

The appearance of our environment has been found to have an important effect on morale and psychological well-being. Slogans such as Keep America Beautiful

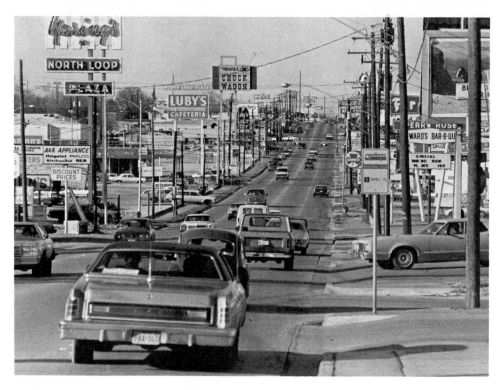

Figure 11-2 This city street, busy with traffic and lined with advertising signs, utility poles, and wires, is typical of many in our country. The clutter is indicative of the minimal concern that has been placed on the aesthetic impact of the activities and needs of large numbers of persons clustered together in recent years, some cities are becoming increasingly conscious of the need to regulate zoning and building more carefully to guard the community environment.

have caught on and assisted in efforts to improve environmental aesthetics. Concern with beauty in our environment can be seen in efforts used to eliminate littering and cluttering of our landscape with neon signs and billboards. Engineering and building of new communities and reclaiming the old are types of planning that consider both space and beauty as important factors in promoting a healthful way of life. Communities that show little interest in space and beauty tend to have disintegrating neighborhoods, citizen dissatisfaction or apathy, and little motivation to improve the quality of life.

The long-range effects of noise have been found to influence physical and psychological well-being. Noise abatement efforts have influenced the engineering and construction of jet engines and industrial equipment. The location of airports is being carefully considered in order to decrease air traffic noises in populated areas. Health practitioners often observe physical and psychological damage in people who have had prolonged exposure to loud noise.

There are various miscellaneous measures that are of community concern in efforts to eliminate environmental hazards. These efforts include the control of insects and rodents; the disposal of abandoned refrigerators and automobiles; and appropriate protection from

"attractive nuisances" such as swimming pools and wells, and cisterns not in use.

These are but a few examples that illustrate the community's concern with protection, safety, and aesthetics. When communities fall short in their efforts, physical and psychological well-being may suffer. Certainly, it appears, there is much more work to be done and there is ample opportunity for health practitioners to lead the way. As the citizens of communities have become aware of potential dangers in their environments, their general support and interest in attempts to decrease and eliminate them are evident.

Communities provide health care resources. Health care services in communities vary and may be extensive. For instance, many communities have nonofficial or voluntary agencies dedicated to serving their citizens, such as voluntary hospitals, visiting nurse service, clinics, the Red Cross, United Fund, scouting organizations, service clubs, day care centers, drug rehabilitation services, and associations concerned with specific diseases, such as heart diseases, cancer, and multiple sclerosis. The role of these voluntary agencies and the importance of their contributions in promoting physical and psychological health are well-documented. Without these agencies, needy persons would often go unattended.

Communities also have official or governmental health care agencies to serve their members with various health services, including publicly supported hospitals, clinics, and health departments. Most communities also have official social service agencies that assist individuals to supplement their own resources. These include financial assistance, psychological and legal counseling, and provisions for low-cost housing. Official and nonofficial health agencies, once devoted primarily to the care of the ill, have increasingly expanded to offer services for health promotion, health education, early disease detection, and rehabilitation. Both types of agencies have contributed heavily to health-related research as well.

Private health care resources of various types also exist in many communities. There are general and special hospitals, clinics, nursing homes and other residential facilities, emergency services, and diagnostic and treatment centers which focus on wellness care. In some communities, there are independent group practices of nurses, as well as physicians and other professional health care practitioners. Most communities have pharmacies, diagnostic laboratories, and retail stores offering health care equipment and supplies. Some communities also have exercise and fitness facilities, weight control centers, and health food stores.

As pointed out in Chapter 7, even isolated communities which may have limited professional health care services, usually have health care available from their folk medicine practitioners. Many of these communities also have herb pharmacies and other related services. However, when professional health care services and facilities are limited, the general state of well-being of members of the community is generally at a lower level than when such services are more readily available. For example, infant and maternal mortality rates are proportionately higher, the incidence of communicable diseases and their complications are greater, and malnutrition is generally more prevalent.

Figure 11-3 depicts the categories of community characteristics that have been discussed. These characteristics help to make up the community environment which in turn influences the well-being of its members.

THE COMMUNITY ENVIRONMENT AND THE NURSING PROCESS

The discussion in this chapter has offered a broad overview of environmental influences in community living. It is hoped that the reader is stimulated to think of the environment outside of the home or health agency and to be aware of the tremendous influence environmental factors have on well-being.

When the nurse initiates the nursing process and collects data, she will want to include information about environmental factors regardless of whether her patient is a community, family, or individual. The specific data she will gather will vary with the situation. However, answers to the following general questions can provide helpful information and alert the nurse to the need for certain data. What are the prevailing cultural and religious beliefs and practices in the community? What are the major means of livelihood for persons living in the community? What are the primary community resources for education and recreation, transportation, communication, protection, safety, aesthetics, and health care? What are the major health hazards in the community? Are there active programs existing to cope with existing or potential health hazards?

Standards for assessing environmental data can be found in various sources. For instance, community health, sociological, and statistical references can be useful. The nature of the specific standards which are appropriate is determined by the particular data collected.

If nursing assessment indicates the need for nursing intervention, the specific nursing diagnoses will provide guidance for nursing care planning and implementation. The following suggestions can offer more guidelines for the nurse with regard to the community environment.

- Consider the effect of the environment on the individual. Everyone is constantly reacting to environmental influences, but all persons do not necessarily react the same even to similiar environments. Therefore, the nurse must determine how the individual responds to the influences of his environment. She needs to guard against stereotyping the reactions of persons. The following are some examples of individuality. One person may be able to cope adequately with a repetitive-type occupation by participating in other satisfying activities during nonworking hours while another individual may become physically or mentally ill from such work. Some persons become intimidated and defensive if their values and practices are inconsistent with those prevailing in the community; others are not bothered by the fact that this discrepancy may exist. Some people are affected emotionally by such factors as climate and weather conditions, physical characteristics of the city, or the economic

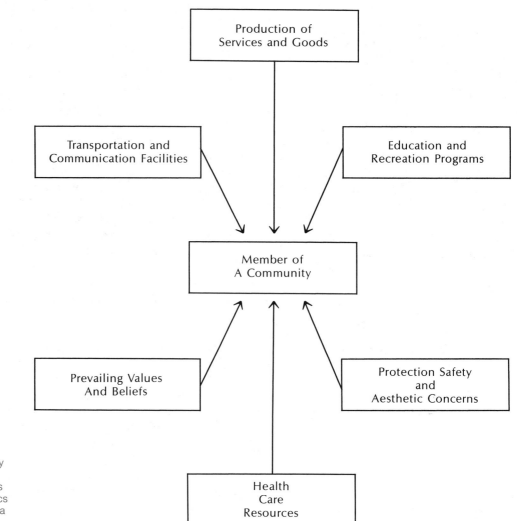

Figure 11–3 Many characteristics of a community influence the well-being of its members. This diagram shows six categories of characteristics which influence the health of a member of a community.

condition of the nation; other persons are not markedly influenced by such factors. As in other instances, the nurse needs to determine each person's responses to environmental influences on an individual basis when providing nursing care.

• Become familiar with the community environment of patients. If the nurse is to understand how the community environment influences persons with whom she comes in contact, she must first be familiar with environmental influences. In order to do this, the nurse is encouraged to make a survey of the area from which her patients come. Or, she may review the report of a recent survey conducted by someone else, if such a report is available. Such surveys usually include statistical information about the community and its members, major employers in the area, housing descriptions, public serv-

ices, formal and informal communication channels, mortality and morbidity information, and health care services. Guides for community surveys are available in many sources. A reference to one such guide is included in the Supplemental Library Study section later in this chapter.

• Use community resources to assist in meeting patients' needs. Wide varieties of community resources are often available to the nurse. Being familiar with these resources and the policies of health facilities in the community is essential if the nurse is to use them in the best interest of her patients. Mutually beneficial working relationships between health agencies can be developed with little effort. The nurse is encouraged to make contacts with other health workers to share information about available services. If this is done prior to the identification of a need for a particular patient, time can be saved when the need for the service arises. Also such preliminary personal contacts often result in greater cooperation between agencies and more satisfactory results for those receiving health care.

● Assume leadership and actively participate in supporting activities that promote the public welfare. The role of the nurse as a responsible citizen was mentioned in Chapter 1. Several examples in this chapter illustrated that health practitioners are often looked to for assistance when communities face problems related to health and well-being. The responsible nurse will assist in effecting change that promotes high-level wellness, both for her own and for her patient's health. She will initiate activities to identify environmental hazards to health, assist in helping to eliminate them, and support activities that promote well-being.

The parts of the nursing process and of the process as a whole are evaluated as described in Chapter 4.

CONCLUSION

Environmental influences are ever-present and no one exists without them. Some may tend to promote well-being; others are inimical to it. The nurse often functions as an applied ecologist and epidemiologist as she seeks data and determines clues that will help her in working with persons in the total context of their environments. The nurse can find strengths in the environment and build on them, such as the availability of agencies that may offer assistance in a particular area in which the patient has needs. She may also function as a change agent as she becomes aware of environmental influences that stand in the way of promoting health for the patients she cares for and for herself as well.

SUPPLEMENTAL LIBRARY STUDY

1. The results of a community survey can be very helpful to the nurse in understanding the community environment as she plans nursing care. Appendix B in the following book contains a community survey guide which can be useful for collecting data. Like any other data collection tool, it may need to be modified for use in a specific setting.

   Tinkham, Catherine W. and Voorhies, Eleanor F. *Community Health Nursing: Evolution and Process*. Edition 2. Appleton-Century-Crofts, New York, 1977, pp. 277–290.

   Identify the sources in your community you would use for collecting the data suggested. For example, where would you go for general descriptive information, for characteristics of the population, for morbidity and mortality statistics, and for health service information? You and your classmates may wish to conduct such a survey by dividing responsibility for acquiring the information pertaining to your community.

2. The authors of the following research report considered high-rise apartment buildings for the elderly. They conducted a community review to identify health needs resulting from the age of the residents and the characteristics of the community.

   Hain, Sister Mary Jeanne and Chen, Shu-Pi C. "Health Needs of the Elderly." *Nursing Research,* 25:433–439, November/December 1976.

   The discussion section of the report contains recommendations based on the study results. Which of the recommendations directly relate to the environment of the community? Do you believe the recommendations would be appropriate for other communities?

3. The author of the following article discusses the mental health needs of the elderly and how community resources can be utilized to meet these needs.

   Carter, Carolyn McCraw. "Community Mental Health Programs and the Elderly." *The Nursing Clinics of North America,* 11:125–133, March 1976.

   Identify the nine different community resources used to meet the needs of Mrs. M. and Mrs. T. in the case studies.

4. Most popular periodicals and many newspapers carry articles regularly on environmental issues making the news. Review several of these articles. Describe how the issues being discussed influence health and how solutions to community problems are being sought.

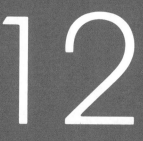

12

BEHAVIORAL OBJECTIVES

*When the content in this chapter has been mastered,
the student will be able to*

Define the terms appearing in the glossry.

Describe two ways in which space can contribute to
the well-being of persons. Indicate at least four
actions of the nurse which can promote the patient's
control over his personal space.

Discuss various ways in which safety can be
promoted in the patient's environment.

Explain the role of the three-prong plug in preventing
electrical shocks.

Describe two ways the nurse can influence the
decor, the lighting, and the noise in the patient's
immediate environment.

Identify two reasons for providing aids in the
patient's immediate environment which assist him in
accomplishing his activities of daily living. Give at
least four examples of specific aids for each.

Discuss a person's immediate environment, using the
nursing process as a guide.

The Immediate Environment
of the Patient

GLOSSARY

Ground: A conducting connection between a source of electricity and the earth.
Macroshock An electrical current passing
through a relatively large area of a person.
Microshock: An electrical current passing
through a relatively small area of a person,
generally a part of the heart.

INTRODUCTION

This chapter is concerned with the patient's immediate environment, that is, the areas in which he spends large amounts of time. The home and health care agency will be the primary focus. The work environment was discussed in the preceding chapter.

The immediate environment should be as pleasant and convenient as possible. It is relatively safe to say that there is no ideal physical environment for everyone. However, an environment that promotes well-being will take at least these factors into consideration: provisions for space, safety, comfort, and ease in accomplishing common activities of daily living.

It is expected that most persons are capable of satisfactorily maintaining their immediate environment independently. However, the nurse may need to assist in providing a healthful environment for those who lack the necessary knowledge, strength, or ability. Persons who are elderly, handicapped, ill, or inexperienced are often in need of the nurse's assistance.

PROVISIONS FOR SPACE

Each individual has a need for space in his immediate environment. These spatial needs and values vary from culture to culture. The following are a few examples of behavior in relation to space commonly observed in this country.

Siblings who share a common bed or room usually have an imaginary line that separates one child's side from the other. Classroom chairs and desks have implied ownership. It is common practice to apologize, even in crowded areas, when one person touches another unintentionally. The space one has while waiting in line at the supermarket or at the movie ticket window is considered one's own. In the home, members of a family generally have a space of their own at the dining table. In the living room, particular chairs may be designated for specific persons. In industry, the worker has his work area. A person visiting a clinic or office is usually assigned a chair or cubicle, and the hospitalized patient has a room or unit which he calls his own.

Psychologists generally recommend that all persons, including children, have a space that is designated for their own use. It is felt that the self-concept is strengthened by having some personal territory to control. The space may be one or more rooms, or a section of a room. It may be only a drawer or a box. But the individual may do as he wishes with his own

area. He should be allowed to arrange and decorate it as he prefers.

Usually, the larger the space occupied by an individual the more prestige it conveys. In industry, the larger the office the higher the status of its occupant. Research in territorial rights has demonstrated that while people tend to defend whatever space they have, the less they have the more vigorously they tend to defend it.

People need space to grow, that is, space that stimulates and permits them to develop, to change and to mature, both physically and mentally. Growth occurs in all environments and at all ages, irrespective of an individual's position on the health-illness continuum. A healthful environment is one with the space and opportunities to promote that growth. In the home, this space may be an area in which family members can read, study, or think. It may be a workshop, hobby area, or play room, or it could be a backyard area designated for baseball or a garden spot. Any space which is conducive to physical or mental activity can promote growth and health.

Health agencies are increasingly aware of the need for space as well as the facilities for growth and most now make appropriate provisions. In hospitals these include a children's play area, a library for patient use, a chapel or "quiet room" for thought and contemplation, units for recreational and occupational activities, and lounges for visiting. Often clinics and other ambulatory facilities also provide comfortable waiting areas with reading materials, as well as play areas for children.

The person who is ill, whether at home or in the hospital, often has limits put on his usual personal space. He may be restricted in his movement and/or in an unfamiliar environment. Especially if his illness is lengthy, the enforced limits in his personal space may threaten his self-concept. Therefore, special care should be taken by health care personnel to provide each ill person with some personal space and a healthful immediate environment. Figure 12-1 illustrates how a patient made her assigned space in a hospital as attractive as possible.

PROVISIONS FOR SAFETY

Safety in the Home

A safe environment is one that is free from harm and danger. It is unrealistic to think of an environment entirely free of hazards. However, there are ways in

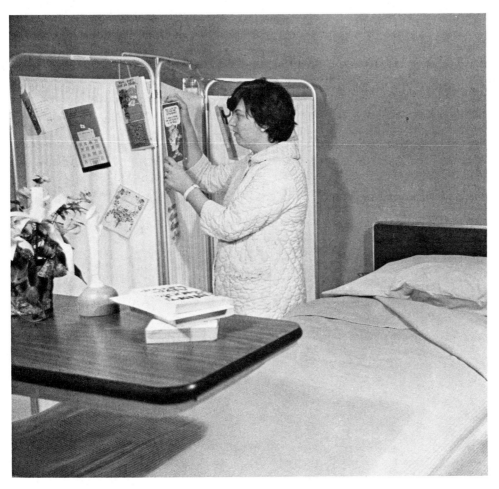

Figure 12–1   This patient has been permitted to display her get-well cards and other personal items as she prefers in the hospital space designated for her use. Encouraging patients to use the available space in a manner that suits them can contribute to strengthening of the self-concept at a time when it may be threatened by illness.

which hazardous elements in the environment can be at least minimized if not eliminated.

A modification in the design of an item can reduce a hazard. Using drug bottles with caps that are difficult to open, the "child proof" cap, has helped to reduce the incidence of young children accidentally swallowing drugs.

Hazards can be reduced when items in the environment are used with care and forethought. Acting hastily and without thinking is a common cause of accidents. For example, ceramic tile and enamel bath tubs have practical and attractive features but they tend to become slippery when wet. "I knew the tub was slippery but I was in a hurry" often explains an accident. Nonskid mats or emery strips can help prevent falls in tubs.

Using equipment for its intended purpose and maintaining equipment properly also help to minimize hazards, as will be discussed later in this chapter.

Most people tend to think of the home as a safe

place, and yet, according to the National Safety Council, it is one of the most dangerous places of all. About one-half of accidental injuries and approximately one-third of accidental deaths occur in the home.

Falls.   Falls account for nearly half of the accidental deaths that occur in the home. Major causes include slippery floors, poor lighting, worn rugs, misplaced furniture, and objects littered about. The young, the old, and the physically handicapped are especially susceptible to falls. Measures as simple as handrails in bathrooms and on stairs, good lighting, and discarding or repairing broken equipment about the home will decrease accidents.

Scalds and Burns.   Injuries caused by scalds and burns rank second to falls as the cause of accidental death occurring in the home. Common causes include carelessness in the use of matches, cigarettes, stoves, fireplaces, and barbecues.

Poisoning. Accidental poisoning causes many deaths in the home each year. It has been reported that more than half a million children under age five are poisoned annually and more than half of these accidents are caused by drugs, with aspirin being the chief cause of death. Analgesics, iron preparations, household cleaning solutions and supplies, insecticides, and paints are also commonly ingested with disastrous results.

Asphyxiation. Asphyxiation results in many accidental deaths each year. Persons die of gas inhalation from auto exhausts and gas-fueled appliances, and many choke to death on food and small objects.

Electrical Shocks. Many injuries and accidental deaths from electrical shock occur in the home. Overload of electrical circuits, faulty appliances, frayed wires, careless use of electrical tools, handling of electrical devices and cords when shoes and hands are wet are conditions which often result in injury or death.

Figure 12–2 illustrate common home hazards that often contribute to accidents.

Safety in Health Agencies

As is true of the home, it is unlikely that a health agency would be entirely free of hazards. However, as in the home, measures can be taken to help reduce common hazards.

Preventing Spread of Microorganisms. A major concern of health practitioners is the danger of spreading microorganisms from person to person and from place to place. Health agencies have policies for practices that limit the spread of microorganisms. Techniques for controlling the transmission of organisms will be discussed in Chapter 14.

Preventing Falls. The high incidence of falls occurring when patients move from place to place in health agencies is of concern to every health practitioner. The rate tends to increase in agencies caring for patients who have physical limitations and poor coordination and who are debilitated as a result of illness. Many medications also have side effects which influence the equilibrium of persons taking them. Disorientation, especially at night, is also common when persons are ill and in an unfamiliar setting. There are a variety of safety measures recommended to reduce the number of falls, including handrails, bed siderails, ramps and elevators for patient use, nonskid floor coverings, night lights in patients' rooms, beds which can be lowered to be consistent with the height of beds in homes, well-lighted corridors that are free of extra equipment and furniture, and nonskid and supportive footwear for patients.

Siderails are common equipment on agency beds. Agency policy usually guides the practitioner in their use. They are especially important for the safety of patients who are likely to be disoriented, restless, confused, or unconscious. When in doubt about the patient's mental status, it is better to err in the overuse of siderails than to contribute to a situation that results in a patient falling out of bed.

Restraining Patients. More and more, health personnel are looking for ways and means to minimize the practice of restraining patients. In the care of the mentally ill, for example, psychiatric therapy that includes the use of drugs has greatly reduced the need for the use of restraints. Nevertheless, the nurse in the course of her practice will encounter situations in which, in her judgment, restraints are required to protect patients. She may have reason to believe that the patient will crawl over siderails and fall out of bed or that he will disturb tubes leading from the body, equipment, dressings, or wounds. Figures 12–3 and 12–4 on page 230 illustrate two types of restraints. The use of restraints will be discussed further in Chapter 17.

Preventing Equipment-Related Accidents. Accidents in health agencies, as in the home, frequently result from using equipment carelessly or using malfunctioning or poorly maintained equipment. With the marked increase in the use of highly sophisticated equipment, it is especially important for health practitioners to learn to use it properly and to know how to recognize signs that indicate the equipment is not functioning correctly. For example, failure to use protective belts or siderails on carts and neglecting to lock wheelchair wheels can result in injuries to patients. Using suction devices with inadequate vacuum and rate regulators or infusion equipment that delivers erratic amounts of solution have also resulted in equipment-related accidents.

Electrical equipment can present a particular safety hazard. There have been claims, albeit unconfirmed, that as many as 1,200 persons die annually as a result of electrical shocks in hospitals. Whether or not these statistics are exaggerated, the prevalent use of electrical equipment in health agencies increases the chances of injury to both patients and health practitioners when safety measures are ignored.

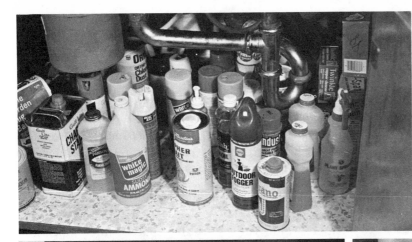
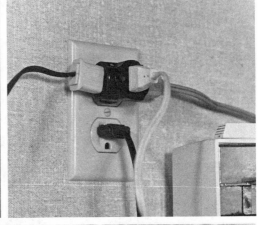
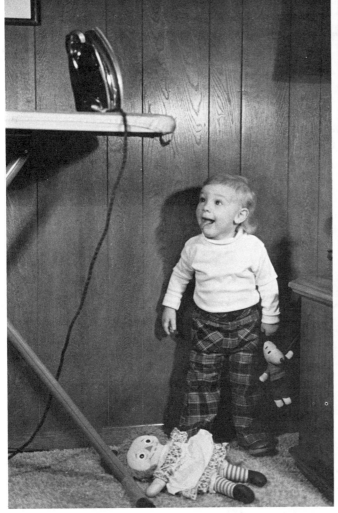
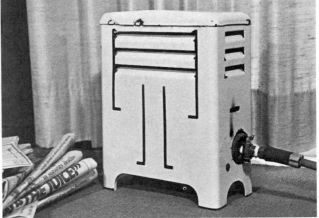
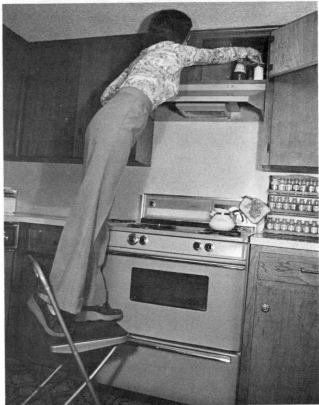

Figure 12-2 These photos illustrate some of the most common causes of accidents in the home: dangerous substances stored in an accessible area under a sink; an overloaded electrical outlet; the cord of an electrical appliance left within temptation of an unattended child; flammable items left near a space heater; and standing precariously on an unstable chair.

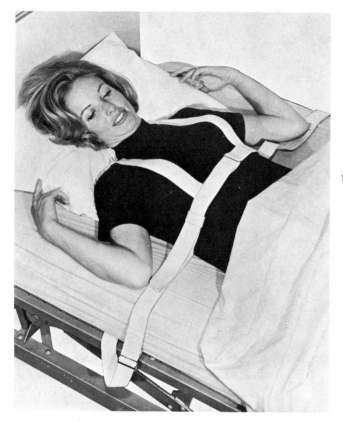

Figure 12–3 Restraints which can be adjusted to the specific activity limitation desired are more likely to be accepted by the patient and his family. For example, preventing a patient from sitting up, but allowing him to turn from side to side; permitting him to sit up and to turn from side to side, but preventing him from climbing over the siderails or from getting out of bed; or preventing a patient from turning on one side or the other. The purpose of restraints is to help to prevent the patient from harm. They should not interfere with physiological functioning, such as impairing circulation, limiting muscular activity to the point of immobilization or interfering with respiration. (J. T. Posey Company)

Most electrical equipment used in hospitals is equipped with three-prong plugs. The third prong, when inserted into a properly wired wall outlet, provides a ground for the piece of equipment. A ground is a connection from an electricity source to the earth through which electrical current leakage can be harmlessly conducted. Current leakage is not uncommon in electrical equipment, but a grounding system renders the equipment safe. Removing the third prong of a plug, using a "cheater" adapter which renders the third prong inoperative, or using an outlet which does not hold the plug securely can result in danger from the current leakage. Figure 12–5 shows a three-prong plug and an adapter.

Most persons have experienced a tingling sensation in the extremities and trunk resulting from an electrical current passing through a relatively large area of the body. This is known as _macroshock,_ and while unpleasant, it is usually not harmful. Macroshock often results from an ungrounded appliance or one in which the electrical wiring has been damaged.

Microshock is the transmission of an electrical current through a relatively small area of the body, usually directly into the heart. Because of the sensitivity of the myocardium to electrical impulses, microshock can cause serious or even fatal heart irregularities. Persons with tubes, wires, or electrodes implanted in the chest or heart are susceptible to microshock dangers, because the tubing or wire can conduct leakage electricity directly to the heart muscle. Particularly because of microshock dangers, only equipment with three-prong plugs is recommended for use in health care agencies. Suspicion of ungrounded current leakage, including

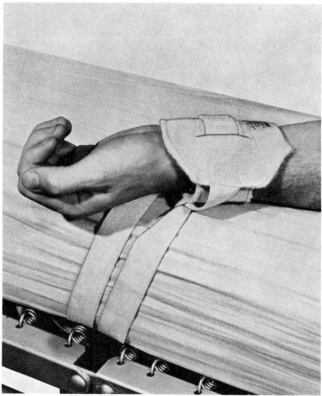

Figure 12–4 Hand restraints should not totally immobilize the person's arms. They are intended to prevent a patient from disturbing a tube, dressing, or infusion, or just to remind him to keep his arm or hand quiet. The restraint shown here controls activity while permitting the person to turn his hand and move the arm somewhat. (J. T. Posey Company)

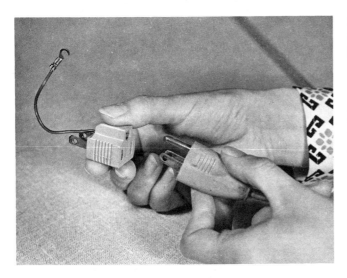

Figure 12–5 Safety experts recommend the use of the three-prong plug as illustrated on the right side of this photo. The third prong serves as a ground for the piece of equipment. The two-prong adapter, shown on the left, can be used when the electrical outlet does not accommodate the third prong of the plug. The wire on the adapter serves as the ground when it is attached to the screw holding the electrical plate in place. Then, the three-prong plug can be safely inserted into the two-prong adapter. Two-prong adapters without the ground conduction wire are called "cheaters" and should not be used. They bypass the ground and provide no safe means for the conduction of current leakage.

even a slight tingling sensation when touching a piece of equipment, or any other malfunction of electrical equipment should be reported immediately.

Means of Identifying Patients. It is extremely important that each patient receive the care and therapy intended for him. In order to avoid accidents, an accurate, easy-to-use, and reliable way of identifying patients being cared for in a health agency is essential. Even the alert patient may become temporarily confused in a strange setting; therefore, every effort should be made to assure proper identification wherever care is being given.

Most inpatient health agencies use a waterproof wrist bracelet that cannot be removed without destruction of the band. It is imprinted with the patient's name and certain other identifying information, such as the health agency's identifying number, the name of the physician caring for the patient, and the patient's unit or room number.

In delivery rooms, it is common practice to place a wrist or ankle bracelet on the newborn with information corresponding to that on the mother's bracelet. In addition, immediately after birth, infants are often

footprinted to prevent identification errors. Footprints are distinctive and easier to secure than prints of the infant's clenched fingers.

Safety Education and First Aid

Instruction in safety assumes an important place in life today. Safety education along with safety engineering and safety enforcement have helped immeasurably to reduce accidents.

Safety education begins in the home. From infancy on, children are exposed to teaching about accident prevention. Many states now require safety instruction in their school systems. For example, safety is emphasized in such courses as physical education, health education, vocational education, and driver education.

The communications media have given much assistance in teaching safety. Special educational programs are commonly offered in most communities to promote safety. These include programs in safe boating, swimming, driving, camping, and hunting. Safety education is included in curricula in schools of nursing and is a part of most continuing education programs as well. Health agencies also offer safety education, such as measures to prevent fire and practices to follow when fire occurs. Certainly, also, the nurse will include safety education in her teaching of patients.

First aid or emergency care is that given a victim of an accident. Training in first aid measures has demonstrated that effective care will be given more promptly at the time of the accident, and the person familiar with first aid care will be less likely to have accidents himself.

First aid and emergency care are an important part of the nurse's education. As a responsible member of the health team, she is expected to be able to assist effectively during emergency situations.

PROVISIONS FOR COMFORT

Comfort measures in the environment are not only desirable in themselves, but may be closely associated with such safety measures as adequate lighting. The comfort measures discussed here apply to the health agency but they are appropriate for the home also.

Decor

It is no longer considered necessary for a health agency room to be bare and "sterile-looking." White walls and white equipment are being replaced by more colorful furnishings and tastefully decorated walls. However, there is still need for careful planning in the use of color and design. It is best to use combinations that are attractive in an unobtrusive way, because unusual decor may appeal to relatively few people.

It has been found to be unsatisfactory to use wallpaper with a distinct design, such as large flowers, in rooms serving the ill. Some patients have been disturbed by designs, seeing faces and other objects in them. Pictures, bedspreads, and curtains may have the same effect if not selected carefully. Color in ceiling coverings can be pleasant for patients who are confined on their backs for long periods.

Considerable attention also is being given to floor coverings. The cold, bare look is being replaced with attractive coverings. These, too, must be selected with care since parallel lines, tiny squares, and some geometric designs cause some persons to feel dizzy when they look at them. Floor coverings should be able to withstand frequent cleaning. The floor is considered highly contaminated, and, hence, solutions with germicidal properties are commonly used for routine floor cleaning.

In recent years carpeting has become more popular in hospitals. Patients and personnel in general find it (aesthetically) pleasing and comfortable. While opinions vary, many experts tend to believe that carpeting can be cleaned sufficiently so as to eliminate the danger of it becoming a haven for microorganisms.

Lighting

Good lighting is lighting that is adequate for persons to see clearly and without strain for the task at hand. It should be without glare and produce a minimum of shadowing. Good lighting, both natural and artificial, is important for patients and workers. While it is true that the nurse cannot alter windows or some lighting fixtures, certain modifications can often be made. Light bulbs, shades, or lamps can be changed with relative ease. Simply making certain light bulbs are clean can be a help.

Adequate lighting for work and reading is essential for the preservation of sight. Lighting has also been observed to affect mood. Some lighting not only helps a person to feel cheerful, it also helps him look better. Other types of lighting, particularly "daylight" fluorescent bulbs, can do the reverse. Many architects use large, almost full-length windows that can be shaded as required for both home and health agencies. In addi-

tion to providing much more natural light, they make it more pleasant for patients who enjoy looking out-of-doors.

Usually health personnel need more light to work effectively than do the patients. The glare from overhead lights or from windows that do not have shades partially drawn and the reflection from light colored objects, such as white uniforms and bed linen, can become uncomfortable for the worker as well as the patient. Older patients are particularly disturbed by lighting irregularities. While diffuse light in the room may be easier for personnel, it still may not be appropriate for the patient if he wishes to read. The light may be coming from such an undesirable angle that it is almost impossible for the patient to see comfortably close at hand. Ideally, a light at the patient's bed should be sufficiently adjustable so that it can serve the patient and also be used by health personnel when needed for treatment of the patient.

A dim light is valuable as a comfort and a safety measure at night in both homes and health agencies. The light should be situated so that it does not shine into the patient's eyes, no matter in what position he may wish to sleep. It should give sufficient lighting to the floor around the bed so that if the patient wishes to get up, he can do so with safety. Elderly persons are in particular need of some light at night, since this helps them to orient themselves should they awaken and be confused as to their whereabouts.

Temperature, Humidity, and Ventilation

Most well people are comfortable in a temperature range of 20°C. to 23.3°C. (68°F. to 74°F.) and with a humidity range of 30 to 60 percent. When the humidity is low, the rate at which body moisture evaporates is increased, and hence, a higher environmental temperature is comfortable. Comfort is also influenced by a person's activity, age, and physical condition. For example, very young, older, sedentary, and ill persons tend to be more comfortable when environmental temperatures are in the high average range.

Most modern health agencies and many homes have air conditioning that maintains comfortable temperatures and humidity. In climates or buildings in which the humidity is very low, humidifiers are often used. Steam from boiling water will accomplish the same objective. When humidity is very high, dehumidifiers are available that remove excess moisture from the air.

Ventilation can be maintained with relative ease when the climate is temperate and when air conditioners are used. Air exchange is especially important when there are many persons in one room or when one person is in a relatively small room for prolonged periods of time. Ventilation is also important when there are odorous or toxic substances in the air. Attention to the patient's covering and clothing is necessary when ventilation creates drafts, especially to older persons who tend to be sensitive to drafts.

Furnishings

Furnishings commonly used in health agencies are often as attractive as any for the home. A trend which makes it more comfortable and safe for patients is to furnish units according to the type of care required by the patient. Self-care units for the ambulatory patient have low beds, desks, comfortable chairs and reading lamps, television sets, and other homelike items.

Nurses may be required to help arrange a functional unit for a bedfast person in the home. It may mean adjusting a bedroom or an area centrally located where the ill person can participate more fully in family life. This can be a challenge when it involves using the available furniture so as not to incur additional expenses. Homemade devices can be designed which are both useful and inexpensive. The family's activities also have to be considered in such planning.

Modern health facilities are planned with an eye for efficiency, orderliness, and cleanliness—all certainly worthwhile objectives. However, one questions whether furniture has to be firmly placed so that, as one hospitalized patient stated, "From my bed I could see only the midriff of a telephone pole through a window. I later learned that it overlooked a beautifully landscaped area." A little ingenuity at home or in a health care facility can usually result in a furniture arrangement which is both convenient and pleasant.

Bed. Design of the patient's bed is often a critical factor in his care. For the convenience of health personnel caring for the patient, health agencies have beds that are considerably higher than those found in the home. Early ambulation and encouragement of patients in self-care activities have led health agencies to purchase beds that can be lowered easily so that the patient can get in and out of bed more safely. If the height of the bed is not adjustable, a step stool should be provided for the patient's use. If a patient is to remain in bed for a long time at home, a hospital bed may be bought or rented; or a bed can be raised on solid objects such as

blocks of wood, for the convenience of those caring for him.

Mattress. There is no one type of mattress recognized as being best for all situations and circumstances. A good mattress adjusts to body contours to the degree that it permits good alignment. A "soft" mattress which permits the body to sag at points of heaviest weight is not conducive to rest; in fact, such a mattress may cause fatigue and backache.

The covering of the mattress should be a quality material that will not tear easily or separate at the seams. Mattresses with waterproof coverings are available and can be cleaned easily. It is not general practice to sterilize a mattress after each patient use. Because mattresses have filling, like horsehair, cotton, or kapok, it is best to keep the mattress protected.

Foam rubber mattresses are useful when pressure from a more rigid mattress may be harmful to the patient. Mattresses filled with water or other conforming substances are also being used in some circumstances.

Pillows. Pillows are usually filled with feathers, kapok, foam rubber, or disposable materials. In addition to the comfort that most persons derive from having a pillow under the head, pillows are extremely valuable in maintaining good posture for the bedridden patient. That is why variation in pillow sizes and type of filling is desirable.

Since pillows are used for all areas of the body for support and comfort, it is important that they be protected when there is a possibility of their becoming contaminated by secretions or drainage.

Overbed Table. An overbed table is a great convenience, especially for the bedridden patient. It enables him to eat, read, write, or work more comfortably. The overbed table also makes it possible for him to change his position by leaning forward and resting on it. It has conveniences for the nurse during the administration of care also. The type of overbed table which is supported by a wide foot piece that fits under the bed and has only one post has advantages when bed siderails are in place or when other cumbersome equipment is being used at the bedside. Most overbed tables are designed so that they can be lowered for the patient's use while he is seated in a chair and tilted to support a newspaper or a book.

Small bed tables placed directly in the bed over the patient's lap are used in some instances. They are less expensive and particularly helpful in the home. In the care of children who are in cribs, such bed tables are very practical and useful.

Bedside Stand. In most health agencies, a bedside stand for storing patient care equipment and personal items is provided. A drawer in the stand usually is used by the patient for his personal possessions; therefore, it should be placed so that it opens toward his bed. The bedridden patient at home finds a bedside stand a great convenience too. A nightstand, small table, or even a sturdy box can serve this purpose.

Lamps. Floor lamps and bed lamps are a part of most patient units. The lamps should be so arranged that the patient can control them by himself if he is able. As mentioned previously, light intensity should vary with the work or the activity of the user. A lamp that has more than one bulb or a three-way light bulb is ideal, since proper intensity is more likely to be obtained.

Chairs. Usually, a chair is an integral part of the patient's immediate environment. A straight chair with good arm and back support usually is comfortable for the majority of patients. Leg heights of a chair can be managed for the very short patient by placing some suitable object underneath his feet.

Generally, chairs with arms are more comfortable for the patient, but it is also desirable to have chairs without arms available because they are more suitable when a patient must be lifted out of a bed into a chair. An upholstered chair has disadvantages for older patients and for patients who have some limitation of movement, because more effort is required to raise oneself out of it.

Call System. A device which allows the patient to call for assistance is generally attached to the bed or located on the bedside stand. It may be an electric light or buzzer mechanism, an intercom device, or a tap-bell, but it should be accessible to the responsive patient at all times. At home, a hand bell, whistle, or other signal device can be used.

Personal Care Items

The following are basic personal care items: basin, soap dish, mouthwash cup, emesis basin, bedpan, a urinal for the male patient, and a water container and drinking glass.

Manufacturers provide wide selections of equipment

for personal care that are both attractive and safe to use. Disposable equipment is available in increasing varieties. This is an important factor in infection control. These disposable items also greatly reduce the workload of cleaning and sterilizing. If only nondisposable care items are available, sterilization between use by different patients is recommended. Both disposable and nondisposable items can be purchased or rented for home care use.

Privacy and Quiet

Anyone who is being interviewed, examined, or cared for deserves and appreciates the comfort of privacy. It is very easy for nurses and for others to feel that anything routine to them is also accepted as routine by the patient. Many patients are reluctant to protest the lack of privacy. Persons caring for patients, whether in a clinic, an office, a home, or a hospital, should try to provide as much privacy as possible. Doors should be closed, beds curtained or screened, and adequate draping provided when care is being given. Nurses will also wish to be well aware of the legal implications of invasion of privacy, as discussed in Chapter 2.

Hospitalized patients frequently complain about the following noises: careless handling of equipment in service areas and of dishes and trays on serving carts and in the kitchen; loud talking on the telephone, in the nurses' station, and during rounds; calling down the corridors; talking by visitors who gather near patients or in the corridors; loud radios, television, and the call system. Many if not all of these noises can be controlled to a great extent, but it takes constant awareness on the part of the nurse to see that they are.

There are various ways to decrease the problems associated with noise. Many buildings use acoustic materials on walls, ceilings, and floors. Carpeting, wall hangings, and draperies absorb noise. Many health agencies have found that special efforts to remind people of ways to reduce noise have been helpful. Considerable ingenuity has gone into designing posters and signs for use in health agency corridors and waiting rooms to help reduce noise.

Quiet background music has been shown to have a calming effect. Many health agencies use piped in music with good results.

The nurse should consider noise factors when planning care since environmental noise can work for or against the patient's well-being.

PROVISIONS FOR EASE IN ACCOMPLISHING COMMON ACTIVITIES OF DAILY LIVING

Using environmental resources is important to promote maximum mobility and independence—for example, for the young who are still learning how to become independent; for the elderly and handicapped who may have to learn new skills to replace those they no longer have; and for the ill who are being helped to a state of wellness. The following are some measures nurses have found helpful when patients are learning to develop, regain, or maintain independence.

For patients required to remain in bed, an overhead trapeze enables them to move about in bed with relative ease. It is a helpful device to assist in toileting, changing linen, and eating, and for providing exercise.

Most public buildings, including health agencies, are now constructed to accommodate patients who use wheelchairs, canes, crutches, and braces. Ramps and elevators have already been mentioned. Wide doorways and halls to accommodate wheelchairs are also important. For patients in the home using similar aids to mobility, it is recommended that adjustments be made to accommodate the patient to the greatest extent possible. In many instances, ramps can be built to eliminate steps. Elevator chairs can now be installed in homes for those who cannot use stairways. Any aid that keeps a patient mobile usually also helps him to remain independent.

Environmental aids to facilitate social interaction are desirable. Having the space and comfortable chairs for people to enjoy each other's company helps in meeting a patient's psychosocial needs. The bedridden patient at home may be in a living room or some area where he can more easily participate in family matters and offer his contributions as far as possible.

The nurse will wish to be aware of environmental factors that promote ease and independence in the management of personal hygiene. Devices such as shower heads that can be adjusted to various levels, tub chairs, foot basins, handrails, and supports on tubs are all helpful.

Facilities which make eating as easy and pleasant as possible are important for ill persons. The use of overbed tables and comfortable chairs has been mentioned. Some health agencies accommodate ambulatory patients in a common dining room or at least encourage several patients to eat together. The resulting social interaction often stimulates the appetite. In the home, it is generally recommended that accommodations be made for chronically ill persons to eat with other family members as frequently as possible.

Readily available facilities and space for recreational and occupational activities were discussed earlier. Using such facilities, both in health agencies and in the home, tends to promote mobility as well as offer activity that stimulates the patient mentally and physically. It has been observed that even infants respond to environmental stimulation favorably. Colored mobiles, recorded voices of mother, swings to change the baby's position in his crib, and much holding and cuddling have been found stimulating for even the tiniest patients.

Environmental factors that maintain independence in relation to elimination are recommended. For example, it is helpful to have appropriately sized toilet facilities for children or a step stool and a removable child's seat to facilitate comfort and safety. Handbars help a patient move himself from a wheelchair to a toilet.

Architectural considerations are becoming more common for persons with permanent physical handicaps. Light switches in homes are being placed at a height convenient for persons in wheelchairs. Kitchen counters, as well as bathroom sinks, are also being arranged to accommodate individuals confined to wheelchairs.

Many other ways of using the patient's physical environment to promote his independence could be cited. The reader may wish to add examples from her own experience. From the accounts of health practitioners and patients, provisions that help the patient in accomplishing activities of daily living for himself promote well-being and high-level wellness.

THE PATIENT'S IMMEDIATE ENVIRONMENT AND THE NURSING PROCESS

Some aspects of the health consumer's immediate environment are not within the nurse's control. However, the nurse can influence other aspects by her direct action and through her teaching and example. The nurse who is concerned about the well-being of people will want to be alert for opportunities to influence their immediate environment positively whenever possible.

When collecting data, the nurse should gather information about the patient's immediate environment. The type of the information will vary depending on the circumstances of the person receiving care. Consideration of the following questions will provide basic data about the immediate environment. What is the nature of the personal space available to the person? What indicators are there of his preferences about the use and arrangement of his personal space? Are safety hazards and/or precautions in evidence? That is, have common sources of injuries been safeguarded, especially when very young, the elderly, ill, or handicapped persons are involved? Is there an awareness of the need for safety precautions? Is there evidence of the presence of essential comfort items? For example, are satisfactory furnishings and personal hygiene items available and properly used? The preceding questions suggest only a general framework for collecting data about the immediate environment. Clues indicating the need for more specific information generally become apparent as the nature of the situation is examined.

Sources for appropriate standards for the assessment of data will vary and depend on the particular circumstances. Thus, personal standards which incorporate the individual's cultural and socioeconomic backgrounds and his preferences may be used to assess space and comfort data in some circumstances. In other situations, more objective standards from psychological and physiological research findings may be used. Sources, such as the National Safety Council, insurance companies, and institutional safety committees, can provide useful standards for safety. Various rehabilitation authorities produce information from which standards for assessment of activities of daily living can be derived. As indicated before, standards must be appropriate for data being judged, and, hence, the precise data collected will determine the standards which are used.

If the nursing diagnoses indicate a need for nursing intervention related to the patient's immediate environment, planning the nursing care will also vary with circumstances. A sampling of some nursing approaches which have been found to be helpful follow.

- Respect the person's need for space. The patient in the health care facility needs to be oriented to the space that is designated for his personal use. The nurse or other person admitting the patient is generally responsible for this explanation. The nurse should then respect the control an individual shows over whatever space is his. For example, she should generally knock before entering his room and seek permission before opening his bedside stand drawer, closet, or locker. She should recognize the patient's desire to express himself within his assigned space and respect his wish to have his own personal items with him. Showing interest and respect for pictures of

loved ones, a favorite piece of handicraft or art, a religious object, or a child's favorite toy, acknowledges the importance of space and its personal uses.

- Assist in arranging the personal space of the immobilized person. The area should be arranged in a way that the patient finds satisfactory, not in the manner that suits the nurse. For example, the patient may wish to have get-well cards displayed, a flower arrangement placed in a particular position, or the items on his bedside stand organized in a specific way. By allowing him to control his personal space, the nurse is acknowledging his individuality and contributing to his self-image.

- Explain the importance of space and help plan for providing it. Families caring for ill persons at home often need this assistance. Also the nurse is often in a position to teach mothers the importance of providing personal space in the home for each child. Such planning can contribute to the child's psychological growth and development.

- Assist in the identification of accident hazards in home environments. Community health nurses are frequently able to make a contribution to the well-being of individuals and families in this way. Fire dangers, improper storage of volatile and poisonous substances, slippery floors and rugs often exist because people simply have not thought about the potential for injury. The nurse can teach responsible family members how to survey their homes for potential problems and then to initiate changes that will make them more safe. Homes in which young children are exploring and learning, as well as those in which older persons with failing eyesight, hearing, and poor equilibrium live, need particular precautions. Helping families plan for alternate exit routes from each room in the house in case of fire, encouraging home fire drills, and suggesting the purchase of smoke detectors, are other ways in which the nurse can contribute to making home environments safer.

- Encourage individuals to learn first aid techniques. Proper care for injuries can often keep them from becoming serious. Other first aid measures can actually be life-saving, such as cardiopulmonary resuscitation which will be discussed in Chapter 25.

- Provide safety education. Nurses in clinics, offices, schools, industries, and other outpatient facilities can often prepare safety displays and programs for viewing by persons who are waiting for appointments. Studies have shown health education efforts can be particularly effective at this time.

- Anticipate the patient's need for protection. In the health agency, the nurse has a legal and moral responsibility for safety in the immediate environment. The nurse is expected to understand that persons who are ill, receiving medications, and in an unfamiliar environment often become disoriented or do not use the same judgment they possess when they are well. It is generally considered the responsibility of the nurse to take precautions to protect such persons from injury. For instance, the nurse is expected to see to it that night lights, siderails, crib sides, and restraints are all used properly. Equipment, footstools, extra furniture, and other items should be stored appropriately to prevent accidents. Making ill persons being cared for at home and their families aware of such hazards is also a teaching responsibility of the nurse.

- Arrange the patient's frequently used articles conveniently. For example, stretching and reaching to retrieve an item just out of reach has resulted in persons losing their balance and falling from bed. The height of the overbed table and head of the bed should be adjusted appropriately to avoid the danger of hot drinks and foods being spilled as the patient eats. The height of adjustable beds being used by ambulatory patients should remain in their lowest position except when direct care is being given. In this way, when a patient gets out of bed unassisted, his likelihood of falling is reduced.

- Demonstrate to the patient and supervise his use of unfamiliar equipment. For example, a wheelchair, walker, or remote control television can be hazardous if used improperly. Anticipate the need for assistance whenever possible, because many persons are reluctant to ask for help or are not aware of their need for it.

- Identify the patient. Check the identifying name band worn by the patient or ask him to state his name before administering care. Calling a person by name is not considered adequate identification because frightened and ill persons frequently respond even when addressed by an incorrect name. Inaccurate identification is one of the most common causes of errors in the administration of medications and treatments.

- Be familiar with the safe operation of the equipment being used. Since new devices are continually becoming available, the nurse needs to develop the habit of reading instructions, attending demonstrations, practicing, and asking for assistance as indicated. It cannot be stressed too strongly that manufacturer's instructions for use of equipment should always be followed. In addition, the following guides will help to decrease equipment-related accidents in health agencies. Use equipment for the use for which it was intended. Do not operate equipment with which you are unfamiliar. Handle all equipment with care. Three-prong electrical plugs that provide for grounding of equipment are recommended. Do not twist or sharply bend electrical cords because you may break the wires inside the cord. Report signs of trouble immediately. Be alert to signs that indicate faulty equipment, such as breaks in electrical cords, sparks, smoke, electrical shocks, loose or missing parts, and unusual noises or odors.

- Make the patient's room as satisfying to him as possible. The nurse does not ordinarily have a great deal of control over the decor or furnishings of the patient's immediate environment. However, she may exert some influence by making appropriate suggestions when redecorating is being planned or when new furnishings are being considered. In some agencies, the nurse may also be able to rearrange some furniture so that it is more suitable for the patient. In other situations, especially when persons are immobilized for long periods, the nurse may periodically be able to change pictures or other wall hangings to alter the patient's environment. Inexpensive colorful posters can be especially helpful for home use. However, she should be aware that pictures should be selected with care since they may have a soothing or disturbing effect on some persons depending on how they are interpreted.

- Alter the lighting, temperature, and ventilation as necessary. If adequate facilities are available, many persons can adjust these environmental conditions to suit themselves. However, for persons who are not able, the nurse needs to be sensitive to the need for adjusting the light, heat, cooling, and air circulation in a room. She needs to remember that it should be adjusted for the comfort of the patient, not for her personal preference. Adjusting lighting to avoid having it shine directly into the patient's eyes is one of the most frequently forgotten ways in which the nurse can make the immediate environment more comfortable for incapacitated persons.

- Avoid unnecessary noises. Because persons who are ill, frightened, and in a strange setting are often more sensitive to unfamiliar sounds, special care needs to be taken by the nurse to prevent avoidable noises. Especially at night, unaccustomed sounds can be distressing to an ill person. Often, an explanation of the nature of sounds which are not familiar will also help to allay a patient's anxiety. A radio located close to the patient and on low volume can help block out other noises and also have a calming effect on some persons.

- Explain the use of aids for activities of daily living. Even when the immediate environment has accommodations for making activities of daily living easier and safer, the nurse must explain and frequently encourage their use because they are unfamiliar to many persons. For example, taking a shower instead of a tub bath is a new experience for some persons. Showering while seated on a waterproof chair, or using a bedside commode is not familiar to many persons. Using a walker, handrails, or the back of a chair for support while ambulating generally requires initial instruction and encouragement. The nurse must be sensitive to the fact that many persons need assistance to take advantage of the facilities in the immediate environment that can promote their well-being.

The parts of the nursing process and of the process as a whole are evaluated as described in Chapter 4.

CONCLUSION

The patient's immediate environment can either promote or hinder well-being. To assist the patient most effectively, the nurse will wish to make whatever provisions she can to provide a safe and comfortable environment and one that promotes optimum independence for the patient. There will be times when ingenuity is required to overcome problems resulting from undesirable factors in the patient's environment. However, nursing care is incomplete and less than professional when environmental factors are ignored.

SUPPLEMENTAL LIBRARY STUDY

1. The following article describes how, in one long-term hospital, paralyzed patients had some control over their immediate environment by participating in the decorating of their lounge.

    "Paralyzed VA Patients Create a Mural for Their Day-room." *Hospitals, Journal of the American Hospital Association,* 51:69–71, July 1, 1977.

    What were the benefits the writer believes the participants gained from their involvement in the project?

2. The following article makes some suggestions about the proper use of lighting to avoid eyestrain.

    Linne, Andrea. "The Light Way." *Family Health,* 8:62, 64, May 1976.

    How can you incorporate the suggestions regarding the use of light in your personal life and in your nursing care?

3. The following author describes how the audit, discussed in Chapter 5, was used in one hospital to maintain the quality of the immediate environment.

    Cohn, Steven S. "Audit Enhances Patient's Environment." *Hospitals, Journal of the American Hospital Association,* 51:61–62, May 1, 1977.

4. In the following report, the authors describe a study measuring noise in the incubators of newborns, a recovery room, and acute care rooms.

    Falk, Stephen A. and Woods, Nancy F. "Hospital Noise—Levels and Potential Health Hazards." *The New England Journal of Medicine,* 289:774–781, October 11, 1973.

    The authors expressed concern because of the physiological and psychological effects of high noise levels on patients. Beside those made in this chapter, what other suggestions were made for lowering the noise levels in hospitals?

5. The reference listed below is an interview with the former chairman of the National Commission on Fire Prevention and Control.

    "Fire: How You Can Guard Against It . . . And Escape From It." *Family Health,* 8:66–67, 69, 71, 73, October 1976.

    What suggestions does the chairman make concerning the proper use of a fire extinguisher, what to do if your clothes catch on fire, and the practical values of fire detectors and sprinkler systems?

    What areas does the author indicate are included in the audit? What are the advantages of this system, as cited by the author?

13

BEHAVIORAL OBJECTIVES

When content in this chapter has been mastered, the student will be able to

Define the terms appearing in the glossary.

Describe briefly the process of sensory stimulation and perception.

List at least eight behavioral changes which can be indicative of sensory deprivation.

Identify at least three types of situations which can predispose persons to sensory deprivation.

Identify at least eight observations the nurse can make to detect persons with sensory deprivation.

Describe the nursing care of a person experiencing a problem with sensory stimulation, using the nursing process as a guide.

The Environment and Sensory Stimulation

GLOSSARY

Axon: A process that carries impulses to the central nervous system.

Dendrite: A process that carries impulses to the neuron. Synonym for dendron.

Dendron: A process that carries impulses to the neuron. Synonym for dendrite.

Gustatory: Pertaining to the sense of taste.

Kinesthesia: The perception that enables the organism to know the position of various body parts without help of vision. Synonym for proprioception.

Neuron: A nerve cell.

Olfactory: Pertaining to the sense of smell.

Perception: The awareness of a sensory stimulus.

Proprioception: The perception that enables the organism to know the position of various body parts without help of vision. Synonym for kinesthesia.

Receptor: A body structure that receives stimuli.

Sensory Deprivation: A reduction in the optimum quantity and/or quality of sensory stimulation and perception.

Sensory Overload: An excessive stimulation of the senses.

Tactile: Pertaining to the sense of touch.

INTRODUCTION

Sensory stimulation is a subject of interest to both biological and social scientists. Knowledge of the phenomenon has practical value for a variety of people, including the health practitioner.

The body receives the irritating effects of agents on muscles, nerves, or sensory end organs through the process of stimulation. Stimulation can originate from sources outside or inside the body. Stimuli are received through various senses, such as sight, hearing, touch, smell, and taste. Touch is also known as the *tactile* sense, while smell and taste are called the *olfactory* and *gustatory* senses, respectively.

Proprioception or *kinesthesia* is the sense that enables the person to know the position of various body parts without the help of vision. This sense produces an awareness of the body and its parts, movement, resistance, position, and equilibrium. There are also internal chemical stimuli to which the body responds, but they will not be discussed here.

From conception to death, the human being uses sensory organs to learn about the environment in which he lives. Stimulation of the sensory organs also promotes development of these organs and contributes to the overall well-being of the individual. Hence, development of the senses and knowledge of the world depends not only on an organism's genetic endowment, but on environmental influences as well. When an organism is deprived of stimuli from its environment, deleterious effects may result, as this chapter will explain.

THE NATURE OF SENSORY STIMULATION

The study of stimulation begins with a nerve cell, or *neuron*. The cell has a projection or process, usually one but sometimes more, called a *dendrite* or *dendron* that carries an impulse to the neuron. It also has a process called an *axon* that carries an impulse to the central nervous system. Although there is much still to be learned about an impulse, it has been determined that an electrical current is set up in a nerve when it is stimulated. Sensory nerves carry some impulses to areas of the brain where the individual becomes aware of the stimulus. *Perception* then occurs with awareness. When an impulse reaches consciousness, the individual has information about the outside world. For example, optic nerves carry messages from the eye, olfactory nerves carry information from the nose, and so on. Some impulses are transmitted to certain areas of the brain or to the spinal cord where they do not normally reach consciousness. For instance, we are not usually aware of the stimuli which produce changes in blood vessel size or which make it possible for us to remain in an upright position.

The structure that receives stimuli is called a *receptor.* The eye is the receptor of light waves and the muscle spindles are the receptors in skeletal muscles for stretch and tension. In general, the body's receptors respond best to only one type of stimulation. The exceptions are fibers that carry messages of pain. They have no special structural receptor to receive stimuli, and the nerve endings receive a variety of stimuli that are perceived as pain.

When nerve cells are studied, they do not appear very different from one another. Nor do essential differences show up when electrical currents associated with nerve cells and impulse transmission are studied. These findings pose an interesting question: how do we experience very different sensations? For example, the perception of lightning and of thunder are distinct and different sensations. We do not *hear* lightning nor *see* thunder. The quality and interpretation depends, for the most part, on the nature of the transmission of the impulse and on the particular region of the cerebral cortex where the impulse arrives. The cells in these regions interpret the impulses in a characteristic manner, accounting for differences in sensations.

A pattern for sensory perception can be seen. The receptor organs tune into specific stimuli; the impulse is carried to a particular area in the brain, depending on which receptor cells receive the impulse; and appropriate activity or a response is then initiated, depending on the nature and quality of the stimuli. From this description, it can be seen that the eye does not really *see*. Rather, it has receptor cells to receive stimuli, the impulse is transmitted to the brain, and there the impulse is interpreted as a visual sensation.

Receptors in the skeletal muscles and tendons transmit impulses to the spinal cord and cerebellum from which reflex contraction of the muscles is controlled. Impulses for the change of position of body parts are transmitted to the cord and then to the brain in order that adaptive movements can be coordinated.

There are many different receptor cells in the body. Through them we are able to receive stimuli that are perceived by the brain as shape, color, space, movement, noise, pain, cold, hot, touch, size, odor, and taste.

Our nervous system is constantly bombarded by various types of stimuli. If we were to react to all of them, we could never function in an effective manner. The overload of stimuli would result in frustration and distorted behavior. It has been estimated that as much as 99 percent of the information received by the brain is discarded or not used at the time of transmission. This phenomenon can be experienced when driving a car as the brain effectively screens out visual, auditory, and other distractions that would interfere with driving. Impulses that are not acted on when received may be used at a later date. The memory process involves the storage of that material. Thought and memory are used, for example, when a new sensory experience occurs and the organism uses a response based on previous knowledge and experience.

It has been observed that the human organism stops responding to a stimulus that is repeated many times. Thus, the repeated stimulus of a continuing noise eventually goes unnoticed. Some authorities speak of an adaptability phenomenon occurring in sensory reception. An offensive odor eventually goes undetected by a person exposed over a period of time. Adaptability to the sense of pain appears to be least likely to occur.

Man is a social animal and has constant stimulation from his physical and psychosocial environment. Current research strongly suggests that we have inborn needs for physical and psychosocial stimulation, and satisfying these needs promotes well-being.

This has been only a very brief summary of the nature of stimulation and perception. Those wishing to explore the subject further should consult texts in physiology and psychology.

SENSORY DEPRIVATION AND SENSORY OVERLOAD

It has been noted that the brain does not act upon every message it receives from the environment through the sensory receptors. To do so would destroy well-being. Furthermore, well-being is not promoted when there is a lack of variety or an insufficient amount of stimuli being received by the body. When the input is below the optimum that promotes a particular individual's well-being, sensory deprivation is present.

Optimum input varies among individuals and is largely dependent, it appears, on a person's background. Hence, optimum input for well-being can be described best on a continuum. Some individuals appear to require more input to avoid boredom and apathy while others appear to require less. *Sensory deprivation,* then, means that one is receiving less than his optimum quantity and/or quality of sensory stimulation and perception, the end result of which can effect the individual's behavior.

Sensory overload is excessive stimulation of the senses. Because the brain selectively responds to stimuli, excessive stimulation results in an ignoring or nonfocusing on the less intense stimuli and, thus, a type of sensory deprivation occurs. Researchers have found that the behavioral changes which occur as the result of excessive stimulation are similar to those found in sensory deprivation. It is theorized that in both situations, *meaningful* stimuli are absent. Hence, the effects of sensory overload are thought to result from a type of sensory deprivation.

EFFECTS OF SENSORY DEPRIVATION

Although some of the effects of sensory deprivation had been described earlier in the literature, serious observations of persons suffering from it began during World War II. Persons in submarines operating various types of monitoring equipment were found to be missing important clues for no discernible reason. The monotony of the work as well as the isolated environment in which the work was carried out were investigated as possible reasons for operator failure. When variety in the environment and rest periods were introduced at regular intervals, efficiency began to improve. Similar findings have been observed in industry also. Monotonous work environments and tasks repeated over and over again lead to inefficiency while variety with interspersed rest periods tends to promote productivity.

Since the early 1950s, there has been continued exploration into the effects of a monotonous environment on human beings. Well persons have been subjected to experimental environments in which usual and typical sensory stimulation is minimized. The exposure to an environment with no relief from identical stimuli has been observed to have deleterious effects on behavior. The subjects experience impaired thinking, illusions, hallucinations, poor visual perception, and emotional disturbances. Thought content changes, and the subjects become very irritable. The conclusion is that well-being depends on an environment that provides for continuing, as well as a variety of, sensory stimulation. Without it, behavior becomes abnormal.

The influence of sensory stimulation on behavior can also be seen in babies and young children. Children who are reared in confined environments with minimum external stimuli and hospitalized babies who are isolated in incubators and other life-saving devices for long periods have exhibited marked behavioral changes when the environment is changed. They appear unaware of objects and people, have blank expressions, cry or smile very little, and exhibit eating and sleeping disorders while in the deprived environment. When they are exposed to varying stimuli of light, color, sound, textures, human touch, and changes in position, their behavior has been observed to change quickly. They become more active, eating and sleeping improve, they become more curious and respond to things around them, and they begin to express emotion. The lack of sufficient sensory stimuli and the monotony of the environment are believed to have a negative effect on normal development.

Adults have been observed in a variety of settings when sensory deprivation existed. For example, many authorities believe that sensory deprivation plays a part in brainwashing techniques used on prisoners of war to obtain conversions in the prisoner's ideology, false confessions, or secret information. Other factors undoubtedly are involved, such as illness and lack of sleep, but a prisoner's physical and social isolation with resulting sensory deprivation has been observed to correlate with intellectual and emotional disorganization and behavioral disturbances.

In elderly people sensory deprivation may well be one cause of disturbed behavior. As age advances, sensory perception tends to become less acute, such as when hearing and vision fade. The person's earlier psychosocial environment with its variety of stimuli tends to shrink. Friends and mates die, work opportunities cease, children leave home to lead lives of their own, and problems with mobility are often present. Defects in the sensory system and a limited psychosocial environment are believed to play an important role in the disorientation and misinterpretation of environmental clues so often displayed by the elderly individual.

Even during sleep, the well-being of an individual appears to be enhanced when sensory input continues through the experience of dreaming. Some drugs are known to impede dreaming and, therefore, their extended use contributes to sensory deprivation.

Critical care units of hospitals have received much attention in recent years as environments responsible for abnormal sensory stimulation and behavioral changes in patients. For patients spending extended periods in critical care units, the environment is monotonous and sensory stimulation is unchanging. The normal stimulation from family members and other acquaintances is severely limited. Continuous artificial lighting is often used and the noise of mechanical equipment is a steady sound. Numbing around-the-clock routines are often employed. Patients frequently receive drugs which reduce the body's ability to perceive stimuli and which also prevent dreaming. Customary smells, sights, and sounds are usually absent. Sleep is often interrupted for various checks of the patient's condition and essential therapeutic procedures. While there may be no doubt that interrupted sleep plays an important role, the behavior following the experience may also be influenced by sensory deprivation and the monotony of the environment.

One study, reported by Larkin M. Wilson, observed patients in two different critical care units, one being windowless and the other having windows and a bed arrangement that permitted the patients to observe the out-of-doors. Except for the presence or absence of windows, the settings, the patients, the general nature of their surgical procedures, and the care they received were identical. Over twice as many patients in the windowless unit experienced delirium as those in the unit with windows. Depressive reactions were also more numerous among patients cared for in the windowless unit. The observer of the patients' behaviors concluded that sensory deprivation was one important cause of the differences.

The lack of privacy of patients in critical care units has also been thought to contribute to behavioral changes. The physical arrangement of the unit is usually such that the patients can be continually observed by health practitioners and others. It is believed that this constant exposure to strangers can be detrimental to one's perception of oneself.

Behavioral changes of patients in critical care units have been reduced since more attention is being paid to the use of color and sound and increased privacy and social interaction. Some units have used flexible visiting hours with good results. Dimming lights at night has been found to be helpful.

Temporary or permanent disturbances in receiving or perceiving sensory stimuli can result in sensory deprivation. For example, the person who sustains an injury or illness which results in the inability to see or who has damage to the area of the brain where the sensory impulses are interpreted, is deprived of sensory stimuli in the same way as if the stimuli were absent

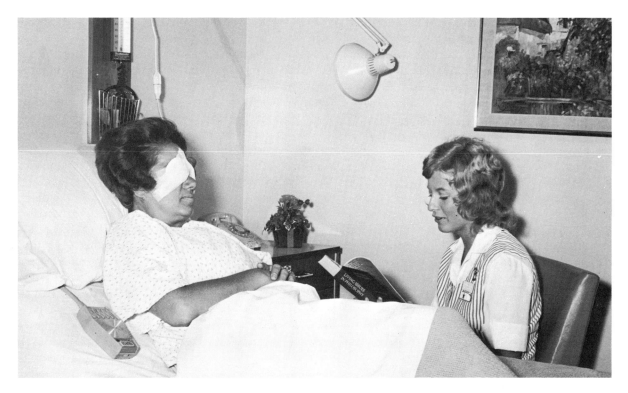

Figure 13–1   For this temporarily blind woman, the day could be long and monotonous. The volunteer reads to the patient which helps to promote sensory stimulation during the time when the patient cannot see.

from his environment. When efforts are made to increase stimulation of other functional senses, at least temporary symptoms of sensory deprivation often occur.

Excessive sensory stimulation from the same type of stimuli is also felt to be harmful because it produces the same monotony as inadequate stimulation. The patient who is experiencing continuing intense pain or itching can focus on little else other than the discomfort resulting from the stimuli. Thus, he is deprived of perceiving other stimuli that are present in his environment.

Long-term maintenance of the same position can result in sensory deprivation. For example, the pressure and/or tension in particular muscles which results from the inability to move prevents the person from experiencing variations in tactile and proprioceptor stimulation. It has been hypothesized that immobility and the resulting decreased kinesthetic sensations can have the same effect as the deprivation of other stimuli.

In summary, sensory deprivation can arise from numerous causes. Certain behavior seems to be characteristic of persons who have experienced sensory deprivation, regardless of its cause. The following typical behavioral changes have been described: visual and auditory hallucinations, illusions, paranoia, disturbances in the thought process and content, apathy, boredom, listlessness, feelings of strangeness, deterioration in ability to concentrate and fluctuations in attention span, and decreased coordination and equilibrium.

PRINCIPLES OF SENSORY STIMULATION AND SENSORY DEPRIVATION

Sensory stimulation and its perception are important for well-being. Heredity is certainly important to the development of an organism. However, the influences of the environment are essential also. Genetic and environmental influences interact and produce the individual organism. The environment providing stimuli to the organism appears to offer the setting in which an organism's potentials unfold. We do not grow in a vacuum. Hence, without adequate sensory stimulation and properly functioning sensory perception, the individual has been observed to suffer ill effects.

A changing sensory environment promotes well-being. Monotony is a curse to mankind. Curiosity and interest in the environment appear to be natural characteristics of the human organism. An environment that provides variety and opportunity for satisfying curiosity and interest appears to promote an individual's state of well-being.

When these two principles are violated, that is, when sensory stimulation is in short supply and is unchanging in nature and when perception is below par, the resulting sensory deprivation produces deleterious changes in an individual's behavior. Investigation is necessarily limited by the amount and type of hardship factors that can be introduced when research on human beings is being conducted, and it is difficult to limit human research to one variable. Nevertheless, there appears to be sufficient evidence to theorize safely that human behavior deteriorates when sensory deprivation exists.

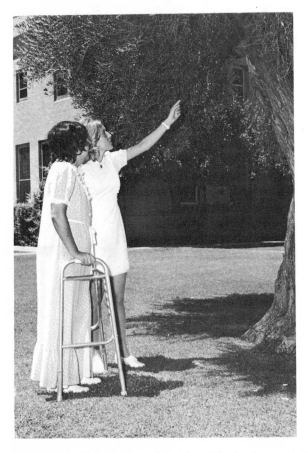

Figure 13–2 Following a period of immobilization in a cast, this patient is learning to walk again. She welcomes the walk out-of-doors with her nurse and the variety of new and different stimuli it presents after confinement in her hospital room.

Observations of persons who have suffered sensory deprivation indicate that the effects of sensory deprivation occur relatively rapidly. Also, the human organism has remarkable ability to cope with sensory deprivation and to return to normal behavior when sensory deprivation is terminated. The literature abounds with information concerning the remarkable recoveries men have made, such as after harrowing experiences with marked sensory deprivation as war prisoners. Also, many battered and isolated children have been observed to make great strides toward recovery when the abuses are discontinued. The wonder is that many of these people survive their devastating experiences at all. Also, the return to normal, especially when sensory deprivation has not been unusually long or severe, can occur in a relatively short time.

For example, patients who have spent time in critical and coronary care units and have demonstrated behavioral changes attributed to sensory deprivation have been observed to display excellent progress toward recovery within 24 hours after transfer to other environments. In addition, many persons permanently handicapped because of destruction of sensory organs demonstrate great ability to adapt to these losses. Motivation to surmount handicaps and to return to a state of well-being, and the body's inherent ability to strive for and reach homeostasis, no doubt play critical roles in the organism's remarkable ability to cope with adversity.

SENSORY STIMULATION AND THE NURSING PROCESS

The nurse who is concerned about the well-being of individuals will want to plan ways of assuring that the environment contributes to quality sensory stimulation. She will want to be alert to situations in which sensory deprivation may occur, think of ways it can be prevented, and plan for assisting persons to cope with it when it is present.

When collecting data, the nurse should gather information about sensory deprivation. She will want to pay attention to situations which are believed to predispose to sensory deprivation and be sensitive to clues that indicate that a potential or existing problem is present.

Persons who have had damage or trauma to the sense organs are candidates for the effects of sensory deprivation. For example, the individual who has lost his sight or his hearing is a likely prospect. So also are persons who have impaired perception, such as may occur following a head injury or a cerebrovascular accident. As was pointed out earlier, elderly patients whose senses are beginning to diminish and whose stimuli in their psychosocial environments are decreasing can also show at least some of the characteristic effects of sensory deprivation.

Individuals who are physically or socially isolated for any reason often display signs of sensory deprivation. An example is the person who must be isolated from others because of an infectious disease or because he is highly susceptible to acquiring infections from others. Care for these patients will be discussed in Chapter 14. Patients whose death appears imminent often are isolated from their usual environment and describe feelings of loneliness and fear. Suggestions to help these patients will be given in Chapter 26. Anyone with a chronic disease who may need long periods of care in a health agency or even at home is susceptible. Many persons in nursing homes, generally elderly to begin with and separated from their usual environment by requiring the constant care offered by these facilities, can be expected to display ill effects from sensory deprivation if steps are not taken to prevent it.

Patients who must be immobilized for extended periods will often display signs of sensory deprivation. These include patients who have had a heart attack and those placed in restrictive casts or traction following injuries. The typical surgical patient generally has limited mobility postoperatively with accompanying social isolation for a time. Mention was made of the sensory deprivation so often found in the environment of the critical and coronary care units, and patients needing these facilities may be expected to display changes in behavior. Patients using respirators and kidney dialysis machines also have limited mobility.

When collecting data, answers to the following questions should provide the nurse with helpful clues. What type of sensory stimuli are present in the person's environment? Are they varied? Does he appear to perceive stimuli accurately? For example, what is the magnitude and type of his responses to stimuli, such as changes in light, sound, odor, texture, taste, pain, and position? If he normally uses eyeglasses, contact lenses, dentures, or a hearing aid, are these devices available to him? Does he display any symptoms associated with sensory deprivation? For example, are his verbal responses consistent with reality? Is he oriented to time and place? Can he follow simple directions? Are his emotional and motor responses consistent with his verbal responses? Is he able to be aroused? Can he concentrate when aroused? Is he easily distracted?

In order to assess data collected from the patient, the nurse will find standards useful that relate to the age and physical status of the individual. Standards relating to the usual behavior of the individual can also be useful to determine if behavioral changes have occurred.

If potential or existing sensory stimulation or perception problems are identified in the nursing diagnoses, the nurse will then plan nursing care for preventing or dealing with the problems. Nursing approaches that can increase the variety and amount of sensory stimulation and/or approaches that will help maintain sensory stimulation at optimum levels may be necessary. Alternative nursing measures that can be considered in planning are numerous. The appropriate ones for implementation will depend on the circumstances in each patient situation. Some suggested approaches the nurse may find helpful follow. Most of them can be used for patients who are confined at home or in a health agency.

- Involve patients and allow them to take an active role in planning and decision-making for their care. The patient who is active mentally and physically to the extent possible is less likely to experience sensory deprivation.

- Encourage a variety of diversional activities. Most patients have television and radio at their disposal. While these are certainly helpful, their overuse can be monotonous too. Many other diversions that actively involve the person can be used in eliminating boredom resulting from nothing to do or think about. The use of lounges and dining rooms was mentioned, as one means to promote social stimulation among patients being cared for in inservice facilities. Conversations with others, playing games, or singing can be enjoyable and stimulating. Handicrafts and tending to fish or plants can also be satisfying for persons whose environments are limited. Maintenance of an active role in family affairs, even though it may be very limited, is important for the homebound person.

- Provide an immediate environment that relieves monotony. The use of interior decorating techniques to relieve the monotony of the room in which the patient spends a great deal of his time has been mentioned. Moving patients about to the extent possible from room to room when being cared for at home and moving a patient to various places in a room if he is in a health agency were suggested. One patient who had nothing but a telephone pole to look at from her hospital window expressed how much more interesting it would have been had she been placed so that she could have seen the lovely landscape and outdoor activity from her bed. Varying the lighting in a room is also helpful in providing optimum stimulation.

- Encourage visitors to the extent permitted by health agency policy and the patient's condition. The patient who is with those he knows and loves is in an environment that is as near normal as possible. Many times, this text has pointed out instances in which the patient's family members and friends can be included in his overall care, and encouraging this usually works in the patient's favor.

- Teach and explain to the patient so that he knows what is happening to him. The more knowledge the patient has about his condition and how he can cope with it, the better able he is to handle fears, frustration, and confusion of unfamiliar stimuli.

- Promote well-being by offering care that provides rest and comfort. Interrupted sleep and discomfort often lead to uncomfortable perceptions. Measures to relieve them help to provide for normal sensory perception.

- Encourage physical activity and exercises. A variety of activities and exercises, all of which help to maintain normal sensory perceptions and decrease the likelihood of sensory deprivation, will be discussed in Chapter 17.

- Provide communications avenues for the patient. The importance of communications has been described.

Paticipating with the patient in goal-directed communication can hardly be overemphasized. The interactions that occur during verbal and nonverbal communications offer innumerable sensory stimuli. Nurses who work in agencies where intercoms are available for communicating with patients are advised that overuse can be detrimental to the patient's welfare. If use of the intercom is substituted for direct social interactions extensively, the patient may be denied an important sensory stimulus. Appropriate use of the telephone can be a significant communication link both for persons confined at home or in a hospital. For those so inclined, communicating with others through correspondence can be another type of sensory stimulus.

- Stimulate as many senses as possible. Varied sights, sounds, smells, body positions, and textures can be helpful in providing a variety of sensations. Rearranging pictures on the wall or other furnishings can change the environment of an immobilized patient. Current newspapers, magazines, and other printed matter can be a source of stimulation. Using different soaps, body lotions, shaving creams, toothpastes, and other items of personal hygiene provide new stimuli. Altering the nature of the wearing apparel or bed linens of a bedfast person can provide different color and texture stimulation. It is especially important to alter the position of the person who cannot move independently. Various mechanical lifts, beds, and

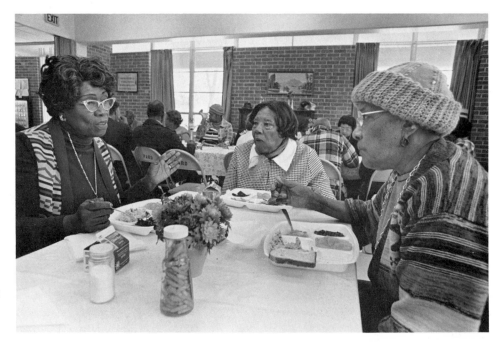

Figure 13–3 These well and retired persons who live alone enjoy the stimulation of each other's company while eating together. Many communities have centers where a daily meal is provided for elderly persons. (Photo by Michael Patrick. Austin, Texas).

tilt devices are available to assist in changing the position of such persons. For the person whose condition does not permit him to be moved, mirrors and prism glasses can be helpful in changing his visual environment.

- Offer reassurance to the patient. Reassuring a patient occurs in many ways. Sometimes just the touch of a hand will help. On other occasions, explanations and teaching are indicated. In still other situations, just being present is more important than any activity can be as a means of offering reassurance.

- Be aware of and take cultural factors into consideration when offering nursing care. This is especially important when caring for patients from cultures other than one's own. The isolation from familiar cultural behaviors and the inability to communicate with others in his native tongue, for example, can significantly decrease a patient's usual sensory perceptions.

- Provide privacy for the patient. The legal implications when the patient's privacy is violated have been discussed. This chapter also mentioned the importance of providing privacy in order to sustain the patient's self-esteem. Providing privacy is conducive to the satisfying promotion of psychosocial interactions.

- Provide a continuing means of orientation, especially for persons whose perceptive abilities are depressed due to age, illness, or drugs. The following aids assist orientation: a calender, a clock, and the opportunity to be aware of the passage of day to night.

- Provide a variety of textures, flavors, and temperatures of food. Limited diets are necessary for many ill persons but generally, some variety can be introduced. Even food that must be ground or pureed can be varied according to color and flavor. Special effort should be taken to see that food is served at the appropriate temperature.

- Be aware of the need for sensory aids and prostheses and make them available as necessary. Examples include eyeglasses, contact lenses, hearing aids, dentures, canes, walkers, and artificial limbs.

- Position mechanical devices which make a continuous noise in way to make the sound least audible to the immobilized patient. There are practical limits which restrict the positioning of humidifiers, cardiac monitors, suction devices, respirators, and other such equipment. However, sometimes turning the machine to another angle, moving it a bit, or placing it on the opposite side of the bed can move the motor sufficiently so that the sound is decreased for the patient.

- Provide the opportunity for persons experiencing perceptual and thinking distortions to acknowledge that fact. For example, it is not unusual for some persons who experience minimum sensory deprivation to have hallucinations and to be aware that the perceptions are not consistent with reality. For these individuals, the opportunity to discuss the experience and to be reassured that they are not unusual and are usually temporary generally eases their anxiety. The nurse should not minimize the patient's concern over these experiences nor should she attempt to convince the patient that they did not happen. She may also need to reconsider her measures to maintain optimum sensory stimulation.

- Control discomfort of the patient whenever possible. Pain, itching, burning, an irritating dressing, or other forms of discomfort have significant physiological implications for patients. Specific nursing measures for dealing with these discomforts will be discussed in other chapters.

- Use touch as a means of sensory stimulation. The use of touch for communication has been discussed in several chapters. There are times when wearing rubber gloves is essential for the protection of the patient or the nurse. However, it is advisable to avoid using them when possible since they provide a barrier between the patient and the nurse.

- Teach the importance of sensory stimulation. Sometimes, even well and active persons become so engrossed with their daily routines and responsibilities that they are unaware of their need for varying sensory stimulation to maintain their well-being. For example, changes in sensory input are important for the industrial worker who performs a monotonous job in an environment with a steady noise level, the parent who is confined at home caring for a baby or young active child, the secretary who types all day, the businessman who routinely schedules appointments one after the other, the college student who spends days studying alone, or the elderly person who lives alone. The nurse's explanation about the role of sensory stimulation and suggestions for simple ways of influencing the environment and its stimuli can be helpful in promoting the well-being of many individuals.

The parts of the nursing process and of the process as a whole are evaluated as described in Chapter 4.

CONCLUSION

The relationship of sensory stimulation and sensory deprivation to health care is a relatively new concern for many health practitioners. In the past, behavioral changes that appeared to be without a definite etiological basis often remained unexplained and accepted as normal in the course of events. With the blossoming of research in sensory deprivation, possibly much of this behavior can be better explained.

It would appear that once again, knowledge of sensory deprivation and sensory stimulation reemphasizes the futility of thinking of the human body as a physical entity and a psychological entity. Observations of the interrelatedness of the body's functions, the interdependence of genetic and environmental influences, and the uniqueness of each individual continue to mount and they support the use of a holistic approach when offering patient care. It is knowledge no health practitioner can afford to ignore when offering health services, including nursing that meets the patient's need for adequate sensory stimulation.

SUPPLEMENTAL LIBRARY STUDY

1. In the first article given below, the author describes her experience with sensory deprivation while she was confined in a critical care unit. In the second article, the researcher reports on the experiences of 180 healthy subjects in an experimental study on the effects of social isolation.

    Thomson, Linda Reckhow. "Sensory Deprivation: A Personal Experience." *American Journal of Nursing,* 73:266–268, February 1973.

    Downs, Florence S. "Bed Rest and Sensory Disturbances." *American Journal of Nursing,* 74:434–438, March 1974.

    In what ways were the experiences reported by the ill nurse and the healthy subjects alike? In what ways were they different? Can you think of nursing actions based on these articles that might help to decrease abnormal sensory experiences for patients?

2. The author of the following article reviews the reports of a number of research studies on sensory deprivation:

    Bolin, Rose Homan. "Sensory Deprivation: An Overview." *Nursing Forum,* 13:240–258, Number 3, 1974.

    Review the 24 terms in Table A that the author states are used synonomously with sensory deprivation. Can you identify ways in which their meanings are not synonomous? If there are any terms with which you are unfamiliar, check their meaning in a medical or psychological dictionary.

3. The following article describes care designed to provide sensory stimulation for seriously ill newborns.

    Brown, Josephine and Hepler, Ruth. "Stimulation—A Corollary to Physical Care." *American Journal of Nursing,* 76:578–581, April 1976.

    Review the general guidelines for stimulation of the infants on page 579 and the stimulation program designed specifically for Chrissie. While the circumstances surrounding critically ill infants require that special stimultion efforts be taken, normal newborns also need environmental stimuli. How would you incorporate the suggestions provided by the authors in a teaching plan for the parents of a healthy baby?

4. The following report describes the results of an investigation of a person's estimation of the passage of time while on bed rest.

    Smith, Mary Jane. "Changes in Judgment of Duration with Different Patterns of Auditory Information for Individuals Confined to Bed." *Nursing Research,* 24:93–98, March/April 1975.

    While the results were not conclusive, what major suggestion does the investigator make for possible application to the hospitalized patients? What are some specific ways you could incorporate this suggestion in your nursing care?

14

BEHAVIORAL OBJECTIVES

When content in this chapter has been mastered, the student will be able to

Define the terms appearing in the glossary.

Identify at least four factors that are considered when selecting sterilization and disinfection methods and indicate the significance of each factor.

Explain the recommended method and underlying rationale for cleaning supplies and equipment used in direct health care.

Describe advantages and disadvantages of four methods of sterilization and disinfection using heat, and two methods using radiation, and give an example of a practical use of each method.

Identify advantages and disadvantages of ethylene oxide and the two preferred chemical disinfectants and antiseptics in current use.

Explain the infection process cycle and the goal of infection control.

Describe the recommended handwashing technique.

Identify at least five examples each of practices of surgical asepsis, medical asepsis in the home, and medical asepsis in the health agency.

Compare and contrast the purposes and recommended techniques for the seven categories of isolation procedures and provide at least one example of an illness for which each category would be appropriate.

Discuss infection control practices, using the nursing process as a guide.

Infection Control

GLOSSARY

Antiseptic: A substance that inhibits the growth of bacteria.

Asepsis: The absence of disease-producing microorganisms.

Bactericide: A substance capable of killing bacteria but not necessarily their spores. Synonym for germicide.

Bacteristat: A substance that prevents the growth of bacteria.

Blood Precautions: Practices designed to prevent the transmission of pathogens by contact with blood.

Carrier: A person or animal who is without signs of illness but who has pathogens on or within his body which can be transferred to others.

Clean Technique: Practices designed to reduce the number and transfer of pathogen. Synonym for medical asepsis.

Communicable Disease Technique: Practices that prevent the transmission of specific microorganisms. Synonym for isolation technique.

Concurrent Disinfection: The ongoing practices which are observed in the care of a patient to limit or control a pathogenic organism.

Contagious Disease: A disease conveyed easily to others.

Contamination: The process by which something is rendered unclean or unsterile.

Discharge Precautions: Practices designed to prevent the transmission of pathogens by direct contact with body secretions or excretions.

Disinfectant: A substance used to destroy pathogens but generally not resistant spores.

Disinfection: The process by which pathogens but not spores are destroyed.

Enteric Precautions: Practices designed to prevent transmission of pathogens through contact with fecal matter.

Entry Portal: The entry route for microorganisms into a new host.

Exit: The point of escape for organisms from a reservoir.

Fungicide: a substance that kills fungi.

Germicide: A substance that kills bacteria. Synonym for bactericide.

Host: An animal or a person upon which or within which microorganisms live.

Infection: A disease state resulting from pathogens in or on the body.

Isolation Technique: Practices designed to prevent the transmission of specific microorganisms. Synonym for communicable disease technique.

Medical Asepsis: Practices designed to reduce the number and transfer of pathogens. Synonym for clean technique.

Nonpathogen: A microorganism which does not normally cause disease.

Nosocomial Infection: A hospital-acquired infection.

Pathogen: A disease-producing microorganism.

Portal of Entry: The point at which organisms enter a host.

Protective Isolation: Practices designed to prevent contact between potential pathogens and a highly susceptible person. Synonym for reverse isolation.

Reservoir: A natural habitat for the growth and multiplication of microorganisms.

Resident Flora or Bacteria: The microorganisms that normally live on the skin of an individual.

Respiratory Isolation: Practices designed to prevent the transmission of pathogens from the respiratory tract by direct contact or airborne droplets.

Reverse Isolation: Practices designed to prevent contact between potential pathogens and a highly susceptible person. Synonym for protective isolation.

Sterile Technique: Practices that render and keep objects and areas free from all microorganisms. Synonym for surgical asepsis.

Sterilization: The process by which all microorganisms, including spores, are destroyed.

Strict Isolation: Practices designed to prevent the transmission of highly communicable diseases spread by contact and airborne routes.

Subungual: An area beneath the nail of the finger or toe.

Surgical Asepsis: Practices that render and keep objects and areas free from microorganisms. Synonym for sterile technique.

Susceptibility: The degree of resistance of a host to a pathogen.

Terminal Disinfection: Practices used in caring for a patient's environment and belongings after his illness is no longer communicable.

Transient Flora or Bacteria: The microorganisms picked up on the skin as a result of normal activities and that can be removed readily.

Virucide: A substance that kills viruses.

Vehicle: The means for transmitting organisms.

Wound and Skin Isolation: Practices designed to prevent transmission of pathogens by direct contact wounds and articles contaminated by wound drainage.

INTRODUCTION

Microorganisms are naturally present in the environment. Some are beneficial and some are not. Some are harmless to most people and others are harmful to many persons. Still others are harmless except in certain circumstances.

The efforts of many persons are involved in maintaining a microorganism-safe environment. Governmental agencies at the international, national, state, and local levels, health personnel, citizens from every walk of life, and family members are all involved in making and keeping the environment as free from harmful organisms as possible. Such efforts include mass immunization programs; laws concerning safe sewage disposal; regulations for the control of certain communicable diseases, such as tuberculosis, hepatitis, and venereal diseases; hospital infection surveillance programs; and so on.

The Center for Disease Control of the U.S. Public Health Service in Atlanta, Georgia, has been instrumental in developing many of the infection control practices discussed in this chapter. A special committee of the American Hospital Association is also very active in infection control. In addition, a national multidisciplinary group, the Association for Practitioners in Infection Control, has been organized to focus on limiting infections in health agencies and communities.

STERILIZATION AND DISINFECTION

Definitions

Asepsis is the absence of disease-producing microorganisms, called *pathogens*. *Nonpathogens*, constantly present in the environment or on the host, are microorganisms that do not normally cause disease. The *host* is an animal or a person upon which or within which microorganisms live.

Asepsis generally is divided into two types: medical asepsis and surgical asepsis. Concepts of medical and surgical asepsis and related terms used in this text are based on the following definitions.

Medical asepsis refers to practices which help to reduce the number and hinder the transfer of disease-producing microorganisms from one person or place to another. These practices are sometimes called *clean technique*. The reason for observing medical asepsis is that there are always microorganisms in the environment

which in some individuals and under certain circumstances can cause illness. Therefore, reducing their number and hindering their transfer increase the safety of the environment. Any number of methods may be used to help achieve this aim, including dusting, vacuuming, washing, boiling, sterilizing, and disinfecting.

Generally speaking, medical asepsis is used continuously both within and outside health care agencies because it is assumed that pathogens are likely to be present, even if the exact kind is undetermined. For example, public drinking cups are considered unsanitary, because pathogens may be present on the cup after use by someone harboring the organisms. On the other hand, there are times when a specific pathogen is known to be present in the environment; for instance, the rubella or German measles virus is known to be present in and on the patient having the disease, and also in his environment. In such instances, additional precautions are taken to prevent further spread of this particular organism, a procedure generally called *isolation or communicable disease technique*. Isolation technique includes the use of specific measures related to the way the microorganism is transmitted and to ordinary medical asepsis. One specific measure is the use of a gown worn by personnel caring for the patient. Isolation technique is discussed more fully later in this chapter.

Surgical asepsis includes practices which render and keep objects and areas free from *all* microorganisms. These practices are also called *sterile technique*. Surgical asepsis is concerned with the handling of objects and areas which must be kept sterile. It is used extensively in operating and delivery rooms. The sterile gown and the sterile gloves that the surgeon wears during an operation protect the patient from being contaminated by the surgeon; the forceps used in handling sterile dressings protect the patient from contamination by the fingers.

Contamination is the process by which something is rendered unclean or unsterile. In medical asepsis, areas are considered to be contaminated if they bear, or are suspected of bearing, pathogens. In surgical asepsis, areas are considered to be contaminated if they are touched by *any* object which is not also sterile. In medical asepsis, the gown worn by the nurse or the coverall apron worn by a mother when caring for a child who has measles is to protect the nurse and the mother from contamination by the child.

Disinfection is the process by which pathogenic organisms, but generally spores, are destroyed. A *disinfectant* is a substance used to destroy pathogens. It is not usually intended to be used for destroying pathogens in or on the living person.

An *antiseptic* is a substance which inhibits the growth of bacteria. Certain antiseptics can be used safely on the living person.

A *bacteristat* is a substance that prevents the growth of bacteria. A *bactericide* is a substance that kills bacteria but not necessarily their spores. The term *germicide* is used interchangeably with bactericide. A *fungicide* kills fungi, and a *virucide* kills viruses.

Sterilization is the process by which all microorganisms, including spores, are destroyed. It usually pertains to methods involving the use of heat, such as steam under pressure and dry heat, but radiation, chemicals, and germicidal gases may be used also. Chemical methods of sterilization are not considered as reliable as physical means.

While sterilization is an integral part of surgical asepsis, there are innumerable instances when it is also an integral part of medical asepsis. When working against unknown pathogens, it is generally considered preferable to use measures which can be relied on to destroy all microorganisms in order to be safe. Thus, in the hospital, personal care items which are reused by patients are usually sterilized by steam under pressure before being offered to another patient. It is possible that the items could be made safe by washing with soap and water and rinsing well. However, since the exact nature of the contaminants is not known, it is safer to use additional precautionary measures.

One of the most important things to remember about surgical or medical asepsis is that the effectiveness of both depends on the faithfulness and the conscientiousness of those carrying them out. Failure to be exact and meticulous cannot be detected in many instances. For example, an article such as a drinking glass, a comb, a syringe, or a needle can be cleaned superficially or not even disinfected, and no one except the person responsible would really know.

Handling and Caring for Supplies and Equipment

Central Supply Units. Most larger health care facilities in the United States maintain a central supply unit where a major portion of reusable equipment used in patient care is cleaned, kept in good working order, and sterilized. Central supply units also commonly store and dispense disposable equipment which has been sterilized by the manufacturer. Safety measures for the patient have increased as hospitals have found it economically feasible to centrally purchase, care for, and distribute equipment and supplies. More nursing time is available for patient care when responsibility for cleaning and sterilizing equipment and for preparing trays for procedures, as well as purchasing and distributing supplies, has been delegated to personnel in central supply units. Also, equipment usually receives better care from persons especially taught and employed to care for it.

Disposable Equipment. Recently, health agencies have been using more disposable items that are sterile and ready for use. Certain items such as syringes, needles, instruments for changing dressings, and linens are used only once and then discarded. Other items, such as bedpans and some thermometers, may be used repeatedly, but by one patient only, and then discarded upon his discharge. Almost monthly, health care periodicals report new disposable equipment as it appears on the market.

The use of disposable equipment has not only greatly decreased the amount of time involved in cleaning, repairing, and sterilizing equipment, it has also reduced problems of cross-transmission infections. But its use has created a new problem, that is, the disposal of these supplies after use. It has been estimated that at least 10 pounds of solid wastes are produced daily for each patient in a general hospital. Many agency administrators continue to work on safe ways to dispose of the tons of contaminated solid wastes that accumulate each year.

Regardless of whether equipment has been sterilized by the agency or is sterile when purchased, the responsibility for assuring and maintaining its sterility through proper storage and appropriate checks rests with agency personnel. The nurse should develop the habit of not using a sterile item that has its outer covering damaged or removed because the sterility of the contents is no longer assured.

Trends toward the development of central supply units and the manufacturing of disposable items have changed many responsibilities once assumed by nurses. However, in some situations, such as small clinics, offices, and homes, nurses are responsible for the care, disinfection, and sterilization of equipment and supplies or for teaching others to do so. Therefore, it remains important for the nurse to have current knowledge of sterilization and disinfection techniques.

Procedures for sterilizing and disinfecting equipment and supplies are based largely on principles of microbiology. Certain of these which affect the choice of sterilization and disinfection procedures will be reviewed briefly.

The Selection of Sterilization and Disinfection Methods

Nature of Organisms Present. Some microorganisms are destroyed with considerable ease, while others are able to withstand certain commonly used sterilization and disinfection techniques. The tubercle bacillus is one organism that is relatively resistant to most disinfection processes, especially by chemical means. The gonococcus and meningococcus are very fragile organisms that are susceptible to common means of destruction. Bacterial spores are particularly resistant and can withstand many germicides that readily destroy other types of organisms.

Although not a great deal is known about transferring viruses by means of contaminated supplies and equipment, there are two notable exceptions: Types A and B viral hepatitis, also known as infectious and serum hepatitis respectively, can be spread by contaminated needles and syringes. While hepatitis A is more readily transmitted by this mode than hepatitis B, a simple prick of the skin with a contaminated needle may result in illness. Studies also indicate that the viruses causing these conditions are destroyed with certainty only by subjecting them to steam under pressure, such as in an autoclave.

Until fairly recently, it was thought that if the nature of organisms on equipment and supplies was known, the selection of a sterilization or disinfection method was relatively easy. However, such practices were based on the belief that organisms were relatively stable, and if they were determined to be nonpathogenic, they continued to be harmless in most circumstances. Over the past three decades, such thinking has proven false. A number of organisms previously considered harmless have modified to the point that they are now pathogenic. *Pseudomonas aeruginosa* and *Serratia marcescens* are two examples. For this reason, the trend in health care agencies is to treat all microorganisms as potentially pathogenic and dangerous. As noted earlier, this means that whenever possible, sterilization methods are selected over disinfection. When surgical asepsis is being practiced, the only safe method is one that is capable of destroying all organisms. When sterilization is not possible or practical, careful adherence to prescribed medical asepsis techniques for decreasing the number of microorganisms is vital, such as when human skin surfaces, walls and floors, and furniture are involved.

It is particularly important to respect the recommended time for the various sterilization and disinfection methods. It is unwise to assume that the contaminating organisms are easily destroyed or that the remaining organisms are harmless. *Time* is a key factor in sterilization and disinfection. Anyone who fails to allow sufficient time for sterilization or disinfection is guilty of gross negligence!

In the home, where the nature of contaminating organisms occasionally may be ascertained with some certainty and where the patient may have developed immunities to certain organisms commonly found in his environment, sterilization and disinfection procedures can be modified more safely than they can in a health agency.

Number of Organisms Present. The more organisms that are present on an article, the longer it takes to destroy them. Thus, an instrument that is contaminated with relatively few organisms can be rendered sterile more quickly than one contaminated with large numbers of organisms. If organisms are protected by coagulated proteins or harbor under a layer of grease or oil, it will take longer to sterilize or disinfect the article. Therefore, articles that are cleaned thoroughly prior to sterilization or disinfection will be made sterile or clean more quickly and with more certainty than an article that has not been cleaned.

Bacteriologists have found that bacteria exposed to sterilization procedures die in a uniform and consistent manner. The rate of death has been found to be governed by definite laws, so that computation of death rates of bacteria is possible. Theoretically, 90 percent of the bacteria are killed in each minute of exposure. Therefore, *absolute* sterility is probably not actually possible because only a percentage of the surviving organisms is killed during each succeeding time period. However, for practical purposes, sterility is defined as, and generally accepted to mean, the absence of all organisms, because the percentage of those remaining is very small and not generally considered to be of practical consequence. The term is so used in this text. Table 14–1 illustrates a theoretical example of the order of death of a bacterial population; the order of death is said to be logarithmic in nature.

Knowledge of bacterial death has important practical implications, and some bacteriologists maintain that this knowledge is applicable for heat sterilization, chemical disinfection, and pasteurization.

Type of Equipment. Equipment with small lumens, crevices, or joints that are difficult to clean and to

TABLE 14–1 Theoretical example of the order of death of a bacterial population

MINUTE	BACTERIA LIVING AT BEGINNING OF NEW MINUTE	BACTERIA KILLED IN MINUTE		BACTERIA SURVIVING AT END OF MINUTE
First	1,000,000	90% =	900,000	100,000
Second	100,000	=	90,000	10,000
Third	10,000	=	9,000	1,000
Fourth	1,000	=	900	100
Fifth	100	=	90	10
Sixth	10	=	9	1
Seventh	1	=	0.9	0.1
Eighth	0.1	=	0.09	0.01
Ninth	0.01	=	0.009	0.001
Tenth	0.001	=	0.0009	0.0001
Eleventh	0.0001	=	0.00009	0.00001
Twelfth	0.00001	=	0.000009	0.000001

Perkins, John J. *Principles and Methods of Sterilization in Health Sciences.* Edition 2. Charles C Thomas, Springfield, Illinois, 1969. p. 68.

expose requires special care. For example, if catheters are being placed in a chemical solution, disinfection will be ineffectual if the solution does not fill the lumen of the catheters. It also must be remembered that certain pieces of equipment are damaged by various sterilization and disinfection methods. For instance, certain chemical solutions cause the corrosion of some metals. Before using any disinfectant for such a purpose, the nurse should read the directions carefully. Most common sterilization and disinfection methods will ruin lens mountings in instruments such as cystoscopes. Such equipment requires special handling in order to keep it in good condition.

Intended Use of Equipment. If equipment and supplies are being used when medical asepsis is practiced, it is sufficiently safe for them to be free of pathogenic organisms. But when surgical asepsis is required, equipment and supplies must be sterile. Therefore, the intended use of equipment and supplies will influence the selection of a particular procedure for rendering the equipment safe.

In most health care agencies, in order to ensure safety for the patient, almost all articles used for patient care are sterilized prior to use. As noted previously, the nature of contamination is not always certain, and, even though in some instances it may be safe to use equipment that is clean, most agencies follow a policy of using, whenever possible, only sterilized equipment and supplies for patient care.

Available Means for Sterilization and Disinfection. Sterilization and disinfection may be accomplished by physical and chemical methods. Chemical sterilization is accomplished by using solutions or gases that kill organisms by chemical processes. Physical sterilization usually is accomplished by dry or moist heat or by radiation.

There is no ideal sterilization or disinfection means since each has limitations. The choice of method is made on the basis of the nature and number of organisms, the type and intended use of the equipment, and the availability and practicality of the means.

Cleaning Supplies and Equipment

Proper cleaning of items used in health care prior to their being sterilized or disinfected is essential. Organisms embedded in organic material, such as blood, mucus, pus, or fecal matter, or protected under a layer of fat or grease are difficult to destroy. Furthermore, cleaning reduces the number of organisms present, and, as has been pointed out, the fewer the organisms the easier it is to sterilize or disinfect equipment.

Persons cleaning equipment should wear waterproof gloves if the articles are contaminated with highly pathogenic materials or if they have skin abrasions on their hands. A brush with stiff bristles is an important aid for cleaning equipment.

It is generally recommended that all equipment first be rinsed in cold water to remove any organic material. The protein in organic materials is coagulated by heat and, therefore, is more difficult to remove after exposure to hot water. Then, warm water containing a detergent or soap should be used to complete cleaning the items. The brush, the gloves if used, and the sink or basin in which the equipment is cleaned should be considered contaminated and treated and cleaned accordingly. After the equipment has been cleaned thoroughly, it is ready for sterilization or disinfection.

Physical Means of Sterilization and Disinfection

Physical sterilization and disinfection usually are accomplished by using heat and radiation. Both means alter the internal functioning of the organisms. The most common methods using heat are steam under pressure, boiling water, free-flowing steam, or dry heat.

Dry heat kills organisms by an oxidation process, while moist heat coagulates protein within the cell. Sterilization and disinfection occur when heat is sufficient to destroy organisms, and, the higher the temperature, the more quickly organisms will die. Therefore, an essential factor for heat sterilization and disinfection is that equipment and supplies be exposed to the heat properly. Overloading a sterilizer or packing it in such a manner that equipment and supplies are not exposed to the heat defeats the effectiveness of the process. In the following discussion, the recommended times for sterilization and disinfection are based on the assumption that the items are prepared properly and sterilizers loaded properly so that the contents are exposed to heat adequately.

Steam Under Pressure. Moist heat in the form of saturated steam under pressure is the most dependable and practical means known for the destruction of all forms of microbial life. Steam is water vapor, and in the saturated state it can exist only at a definite pressure corresponding to a given temperature. The amount of pressure has nothing to do with the destruction of bacteria. It is the higher temperature resulting from higher pressure that destroys bacteria.

The autoclave is a pressure steam sterilizer. Most hospitals and many clinics and offices are equipped with pressure steam sterilizers today. Texts dealing with sterilization describe their operation in detail.

Many homes today have pressure cookers that operate on the same principle as pressure steam sterilizers. Foods cooked in a pressure cooker can be prepared more quickly because of the higher temperature attained by steam under pressure. Pressure cookers can be used for sterilizing equipment in the home by placing articles for sterilization on a rack or a screen above the level of water in the cooker.

The amount of time necessary to expose equipment and supplies in a pressure steam sterilizer in order to assure sterility depends on several factors: the type of equipment or supplies to be sterilized, the manner in which they are wrapped or packaged, the way in which the sterilizer is packed, and the temperature and the pressure maintained. It is generally recommended that saturated steam at 121° to 123° C. (250° to 254° F.) under 15 to 17 pounds of pressure per square inch can achieve sterilization of items in 15 to 45 minutes.

It will be recalled that the temperature and not the pressure is the factor responsible for destruction of microbes. As altitude increases, a higher pressure is needed in order to reach a specific temperature; and in mountain areas persons operating pressure steam sterilizers must take this fact into consideration in order to secure sterilization.

Steam under pressure is both efficient and economical for sterilizing items that are not damaged by high temperatures and moisture. For example, most smooth hard-surfaced objects, such as many surgical instruments, metal basins, and bedpans, can be autoclaved safely. Its primary disadvantage is that items which are sensitive to high temperatures, such as most plastics, lensed instruments, drugs, and thermometers, are damaged by steam under pressure and cannot be sterilized in this way.

Dry Heat. Dry heat is no longer recommended for general sterilization and disinfection in health agencies. There may be a few exceptions when an article must remain dry, such as some powders and laboratory supplies. Dry heat has the advantage of being harmless to objects which are damaged by moisture, such as the cutting edge of sharp instruments and the ground surfaces of glass. However, its disadvantage is that the penetration ability of dry heat is not believed sufficient to destroy all microorganisms and, therefore, its reliability is questionable for most health agency uses.

Dry heat may be used in some home situations to achieve disinfection. A hot-air or ordinary baking oven can be used for this purpose. Authorities agree that, for most articles, disinfection occurs when a temperature of 160° C. (320° F.) is maintained for two hours. For equipment and supplies that will not tolerate this temperature, a longer time at a lower temperature is required.

Boiling Water. Placing equipment in boiling water for a time has been a common method of sterilization and disinfection. The advantages of this method are that it is inexpensive and simple. However, the disadvantage is that if spores are present on equipment, boiling water is not a practical method of sterilization since the temperature of the water cannot rise about 100° C.

(212° F.). Some spores are exceedingly resistant and the time required to kill susceptible spores is too long and too unspecific. Also, some viruses are resistant to boiling. Therefore, using boiling water is no longer recommended for sterilization because its effectiveness is too uncertain.

Boiling is usually used for disinfection in homes. Although authorities differ, it is believed boiling an item for a minimum of 15 minutes can achieve disinfection.

Free-Flowing Steam. The temperature of free-flowing steam is 100° C. (212° F.). Therefore, free-flowing steam for disinfection should be used for the same period of time as boiling water. It is not recommended for sterilization for the same reasons that boiling water is considered inadequate for this purpose. Its primary advantage is that it is relatively inexpensive. The major disadvantage of the free-flowing steam method is that it has limited practical value because it is difficult to load a free-flowing steam chamber in such a way that all equipment is exposed fully to the steam. Therefore, it is no longer recommended for use in health agencies. In the home, ironing with steam is believed to achieve disinfection in five to ten minutes.

In the past, many hospitals installed bedpan flushers which flushed bedpan and urinal contents and then released free-flowing steam on the items for a period of one to two minutes. Because such mechanisms are still in use in some hospitals and were labeled as sterilizers by some manufacturers, the nurse needs to be aware of their limitations. Bedpan flushers do not render equipment sterile. Because of the short cycle of free-flowing steam, certain pathogenic viruses are not destroyed and, therefore, even disinfection of the items is highly questionable in most instances.

Radiation. Nonionizing and ionizing radiation are used for sterilization and disinfection. They cause the death of microorganisms by altering their essential metabolic processes. The most common type of nonionizing radiation is ultraviolet rays which can be used for disinfection. While it can destroy some organisms, ultraviolet radiation has the disadvantage of having limited practical use in health agencies because of its minimum penetration ability and the need for careful controls while using it. In the home natural ultraviolet rays in the form of sunlight can be used to achieve some degree of disinfection. When it is feasible to use this form of radiation, its chief advantage is that it is inexpensive.

In recent years, ionizing radiation has been developed for sterilization. This method is used for pharmaceuticals, foods, plastics, and other heat-sensitive items. Its major advantage is that it is believed to be extremely effective for many items which are otherwise difficult to sterilize. Its primary disadvantage is that the facilities and equipment for the use of ionizing radiation are complex and expensive. Therefore, it is not generally available in health care agencies but is used by commercial industries which manufacture and sterilize prepackaged health care items and other products.

Chemical Means of Sterilization and Disinfection

Chemical sterilization employs liquid solutions or gases. Objects to be sterilized are immersed in a solution or exposed to fumes in a chamber or oven for a specified time. Various studies have found serious shortcomings in the use of chemicals for sterilization. In fact, some authorities state that no chemical solution can be considered completely safe for sterilization. Hence, the use of chemicals ordinarily is limited to items that are heat-sensitive or to situations in which a more reliable method is not available.

A chemical commonly used for sterilization is ethylene oxide gas. The gas destroys microorganisms by interfering with metabolic processes in cells and it has been found to effect lethal action on spores as well as vegetative cells. Optimum action can be attained at relatively low temperatures 54.4° to 65.5° C. (130° to 150° F.) when humidity in the sterilizer is held between approximately 30 to 60 percent. Its penetrating qualities are excellent. Although steam under pressure is the preferred sterilizing method, ethylene oxide has the advantage of being useful for sterilizing heat-sensitive items, including rubber, plastic, and paper. The major disadvantage of ethylene oxide is that it is considered to be toxic to humans in high concentrations. Therefore, it is extremely important that health personnel adhere to recommendations for adequate ventilation of the sterilizer and aeration of the sterilized materials. At the time of the preparation of this manuscript, the federal Environmental Protection Agency is reported to be considering banning the use of ethylene oxide for sterilization because of its toxicity. Nurses are encouraged to follow the development of this proposal.

Chemical disinfectants on the market are numerous and new ones are added almost daily. One must be especially careful with substances sold as "all-purpose" disinfectants for home use. Before depending on advertisements, one should be certain that the solution has been adequately tested and is recommended for its safety and effectiveness by a reliable source.

In large health care agencies, the selection of chemical disinfectants is generally not made by the nurse, but in smaller facilities and in the home, she may be called upon to do so. When selecting a disinfectant, the nurse should follow the principles discussed in the previous section of this chapter.

Disinfectants are generally used for instrument and equipment disinfection and for housekeeping disinfection. While it was stated earlier that the term disinfectant described substances used on inanimate objects, because of their mildness, *some* disinfectants are also used as antiseptics on human tissue.

Disinfectants destroy organisms by disturbing their structure or their metabolic processes through coagulation and alterations of the cell membrane and cell protein. The time of exposure, concentration and temperature of the chemical, and the type of organism are key factors in achieving disinfection. Most disinfectants are also particularly susceptible to being inactivated by the presence of various substances, such as soap and organic matter. Because of the vast number of available disinfectants and their varying uses, the reader is advised to seek information on specific disinfectants in recent chemistry and microbiology texts and current periodicals. A brief description of the major classes of disinfectants used in health settings follows.

Phenolic Compounds.   Phenolic compounds are good substances for housekeeping disinfectants. Beside their bactericidal action, they have the property of stability which means they remain active even after exposure to mild heat and prolonged drying.

Chlorine Compounds.   Chlorines are useful for disinfecting water and for housekeeping disinfectants. They should not be used on metals because of their tendency to cause corrosion.

Iodine and Iodophors.   Iodine has an effective bactericidal effect but also an undesirable staining quality. This characteristic is reduced when a detergent is added to the solution. The combination is distributed as iodophors. Iodophors are one of the preferred antiseptics because of their fairly rapid germicidal effect and because they are relatively nontoxic.

Formaldehyde.   Aqueous solutions of formaldehyde are known as Formalin. They are very effective bactericides. Unfortunately, however, they also have highly irritating fumes and are toxic to human tissue. Therefore, articles disinfected in Formalin must be rinsed thoroughly before coming in contact with human tissue. Since formaldehyde is extensively inactivated by proteins, the removal of organic material is essential before disinfection can occur.

Glutaraldehyde.   This substance is a newer member of the same chemical family as formaldehyde and is an even more effective bactericidal disinfectant. It is also somewhat less irritating to human tissues and less inactivated by organic substances.

Alcohols.   Ethyl (grain) and isopropyl (rubbing) alcohols are most commonly used as antiseptics, although occasionally they are also used as disinfectants. They act rapidly as germicidals but the effectiveness of ethyl alcohol is sometimes reduced because it is not as good a fat solvent as is isopropyl alcohol. Extensive use of the alcohols is drying to the skin and can damage plastics. However, alcohol in appropriate strength is still considered to be one of the preferred chemical disinfectants available today.

Quaternary Ammonium Compounds.   The "quats" have been used extensively as both disinfectants and antiseptics. However, in recent years their effectiveness has come under close scrutiny. The "quats" have been found to harbor the growth of organisms when the solutions are contaminated and are easily inactivated by the presence of soaps, proteins, and certain fibers. Therefore, in 1972, the Center for Disease Control concluded that the hazards and misuse of these substances outweighed their potential benefits. Since these chemicals continue to be available as bactericides and are still recommended in some references, the nurse should be alert to prevent their inappropriate use. Benzalkonium chloride, or Zephiran, is one such substance.

Mercurials.   These substances have been used in the past, but because they are relatively slow-acting and bacteristatic only, they are not considered as satisfactory disinfectants.

Table 14–2 illustrates the uses of the various classes of chemicals commonly used for disinfection and antiseptic purposes.

TABLE 14-2 Classes of chemicals commonly used for disinfection and antiseptic purposes in health care settings

CLASS	DISINFECTANT	ANTISEPTIC
Phenolic compounds	X	
Chlorine compounds	X	
Iodine and iodophors	X	X
Formaldehyde	X	
Glutaraldehyde	X	
Alcohols	X	X

MEDICAL AND SURGICAL ASEPSIS

Principles Used in Practices of Medical and Surgical Asepsis

There are three basic principles underlying practices of medical and surgical asepsis.

Certain microorganisms are capable of causing illness in man.

Microorganisms harmful to man can be transmitted by means of his direct or indirect contact with them.

Illness caused by microorganisms can be prevented when there is an interruption of the infectious process cycle.

The presence of a pathogenic microorganism does not in itself ensure that a disease will occur. When a disease state, called an *infection,* does result from the presence of pathogenic microorganisms in or on the body, it occurs as the result of a cyclical process. The essential components of the process are the reservoir for the growth and reproduction of infectious agents; a means of exit from the reservoir for the infectious agent; vehicle(s) for the transmission of the agent; an entry portal for the agent into a host; and a susceptible host. The susceptible host becomes the new reservoir and the cycle continues. Figure 14-1 illustrates the infectious process cycle and a brief discussion of its components follows.

The *reservoir* for growth and multiplication of the causative microorganism is the natural habitat of the organism. Reservoirs which support organisms pathogenic to man are other humans, animals, or the soil. For example, tuberculosis bacillus, measles virus, and syphilis spirochete grow in man. Viruses suspected of causing some types of encephalitis thrive in wild birds, and the rabies virus grows in many types of animals. Bacteria that cause gas gangrene, tetanus, and anthrax grow in the soil. Man and animals can harbor patho-

gens yet not demonstrate an illness. Persons and animals who have no indications of illness but who have disease-causing organisms on or within their bodies which can be transferred to others are called *carriers.*

The *exit* is the point of escape for the microorganism from the reservoir. The organism cannot extend its influence unless it moves away from its original source. While there may be more than one means of exit, most often there is a primary exit route for each type of microorganism. Common escape routes in man are the respiratory, gastrointestinal and genitourinary tracts, and breaks in the skin.

Pathogens must have a means of mobility. Various *vehicles* act as a means of transmitting microorganisms, including water and food. For example, water can be the vehicle for the typhoid bacillus; shellfish that live in the contaminated water can also carry this microorganism. Mosquitos, ticks, and lice can transmit organisms causing malaria, encephalitis, and typhus. Air currents can serve as a vehicle, particularly for (droplet nuclei) *Sneezing* which may contain the causative organisms for tuberculosis, chicken pox, smallpox, and measles. Inanimate objects, such as books, can sometimes serve as vehicles for transmitting pathogens, though much less frequently than was once thought.

The microorganism must now find a *portal of entry*

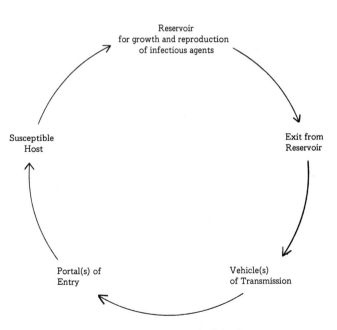

Figure 14-1 Infection process cycle. An infection occurs as a result of interrelated factors. An infection will not develop if the sequence is interrupted. Hence, efforts to control infections are directed toward interrupting the sequence.

on a new host. The entry route is often, though not exclusively, the same as the exit route. The respiratory and gastrointestinal tracts and the skin are common entry points.

For the microorganism to continue to exist, it must find a source which will accept and support it. *Susceptibility* is the degree of resistance the potential host has to the pathogen. Many factors, including nature's protections such as intact skin and mucous membrane, gastric secretions, genitourinary system pH level, phagocytes, and hormones, influence the resistance of a person to a pathogen. Such factors as age, sex, and race have been shown to be influential also, even though the reasons are not entirely clear. Fatigue, climate, general health status, presence of preexisting illnesses, previous or current treatment with ionizing radiation, and some kinds of medications may also play a part in determining the degree of susceptibility of the potential host.

Because the cyclical process just discussed must exist for infections to spread, breaking the cycle can control infections. Complete elimination of the cyclical process for all pathogens is impossible, but breaking the cycle as frequently as possible is the never-ending goal of infection control. Attempts to eliminate the pathogen reservoirs, to prevent or control the escape and transmission of microorganisms, to prevent new entry sites, and to increase resistance of potential hosts are ongoing infection control activities.

Because there is usually a large number of persons whose bodies harbor pathogens in hospitals than in other places, patients frequently come in contact with harmful microorganisms and some develop infections while hospitalized. An increased awareness of such occurrences has resulted in a recently coined term, *nosocomial infections,* to describe hospital-acquired infections. In 1969, the Center for Disease Control established a nationwide cooperative surveillance network known as the National Nosocomial Infections Study. The purpose of the group is to develop detection and prevention methods for nosocomial infections and to support research on them. Member hospitals have active surveillance systems and make monthly reports on the incidence of nosocomial infections. Other hospitals are also putting great effort into detection and prevention programs.

The role of sterilization and disinfection in asepsis has been discussed. Additional methods of preventing the transmission of pathogens in the practice of medical and surgical asepsis will be discussed in the remainder of this chapter. Attention will also be drawn to other aseptic practices, as appropriate, throughout this text.

Bacterial Flora of the Hands

In 1938, Price, a noted researcher in skin bacteriology, published a summary of studies conducted to determine the bacterial flora normally found on the hands. His research findings are still considered valid today. He pointed out two types—one called *transient* flora or bacteria, the other called *resident* flora or bacteria.

Transient bacteria are relatively few on clean and exposed areas of the skin. Usually, they are picked up by the hands in the normal activities of living and working; therefore, the type and the nature of the organisms will depend largely on the nature of work in which each individual is engaged. For example, a librarian may have many organisms on his hands that can also be found readily on books and papers. Similarly, one who has handled a dressing soaked with drainage may find organisms on her hands similar to those found in the drainage of the wound. Transient bacteria are attached loosely to the skin, usually in grease, fats, and dirt, and are found in greater numbers under the fingernails. Transient bacteria, pathogenic as well as nonpathogenic, can be removed with relative ease by washing the hands thoroughly and frequently.

Resident bacteria are relatively stable in number and type. They are found in the creases and the crevices of the skin, and it is believed that they cling to the skin by adhesion and adsorption. Resident flora cannot be removed easily from the skin by washing with soap and water unless considerable friction is also applied with a brush, and they are less susceptible to the action of antiseptics than are transient flora. Some of them are embedded so deeply in the skin that they do not appear in washings until the skin has been scrubbed for 15 minutes or longer. For practical purposes, it is not considered possible to clean the skin of all bacteria.

It was found also that transient flora may adjust to the environment of the skin if the flora are present in large numbers over a long enough time; they then become resident flora. For example, if one handles contaminated materials over a period, the organisms in the materials, although originally transient in nature, may become resident flora on the hands. If such flora contain pathogenic organisms, the hands may become carriers of the particular organisms. To prevent transient flora from becoming resident flora, it is important that the hands be cleaned promptly after each contact with contaminated materials, and especially if the materials contain pathogenic organisms. Since nurses in the course of their work often handle materials contaminated with pathogenic organisms, the importance of frequent and thorough handwashing becomes evident.

Soap and Detergents and Water as Cleaning Agents

Because soap and detergents lower the surface tension and act as emulsifying agents, they are generally good cleaning agents when used with water and friction. The resulting lather suspends the soil and organisms and allows them to be rinsed away.

When soap is used in hard water, an insoluble flaky precipitate is formed when the salts of soap react with the salts found in hard water, and the reaction of the two salts makes the soap ineffectual as a cleaning agent. However, soap used with soft water is an invaluable cleaning agent.

Detergents are popular and effective as cleaning agents because of their surface-tension-reducing power. Such representative household products as Dreft, Cheer, and Tide, and Electro-Sol for automatic dishwashers have effective cleaning and emulsifying properties. Detergents do not react unfavorably with the salts in hard water, and therefore, they lather readily in any water of any temperature. Few if any household detergents, however, are effective disinfectants.

Price used various types of soap in his studies on skin cleaning. He experimented with green soap, institutional soap, castile soap, and several popular toilet soaps. None had a germicidal agent added. His studies, and other studies also, have found that all the soaps cleaned the hands equally well, and that, although certain toilet soaps may leave a pleasing odor on the skin, their cleaning effect is enhanced neither by the perfumes added nor by their cost.

Since nosocomial infections have become a problem, it was often recommended that soaps and detergents containing a germicide or antiseptic be used in the handwashing technique. However, experience has shown that routine washing with such substances tends to cause skin dryness and irritations. These irritations defeat the purpose of decreasing the number of surface organisms because irritated skin harbors organisms and is difficult to clean adequately. Therefore, handwashing with only soap or detergent and water under routine circumstances is now recommended for health personnel. However, prior to special procedures, such as urinary catheterization and some dressing changes, and in high-risk areas, such as operating rooms, nurseries, delivery rooms, and isolation units, handwashing with other substances is recommended.

Substances containing hexachlorophene were used extensively for this purpose in health care settings and had also become very popular for home use to control microorganisms. In 1972, the Federal Drug Administration ruled that hexachlorophene products would no longer be generally available on the commercial market and recommended that such routine practices as bathing newborns, handwashing and surgical scrubbing with agents containing hexachlorophene be reconsidered. Restrictions came about as a result of experimental studies which showed potential toxic hazards through absorption of hexachlorophene. While the effectiveness of hexachlorophene against Gram-positive organisms has been well-documented, recent studies have questioned its effectiveness against Gram-negative organisms and fungi. Cleaners containing hexachlorophene are available for home use with a physician's prescription. They are also still used in the high-risk areas of some health agencies. A number of authorities recommend the iodophors, such as povidone-iodine (Betadine), as the preferred cleaning agent, however.

Tap water is as effective as sterile water for skin cleaning. The few nonpathogens in tap water are not implanted on the skin during washing, and therefore, they rinse or wipe off with ease.

Suggested Handwashing Technique

Studies on handwashing techniques have been reported in the literature since well before the end of the last century. Admonitions concerning the importance of clean hands date back even further, to the time of the ancient Hebrews as reported in the Old Testament. Despite much evidence to support the importance of careful and frequent handwashing, contaminated hands are considered by many authorities to be the prime factor in cross-infections to this day. Hands in health settings and homes are in constant use: the nurse giving an injection, the physician examining a patient, the maid folding linen, the volunteer helping a patient select reading material, the aide making a patient's bed, the engineer repairing a television control switch, children playing with toys, and mothers carrying out household tasks. Still, much handwashing appears to be more ritualistic than realistic, even though the role of hands in cross-infection is no longer debatable.

Cleaning the hands prior to performing certain procedures using surgical asepsis, such as surgery or the delivery of a baby, is taught when the nurse learns to assist with these procedures. The suggested technique described here is intended for use when *medical asepsis* is being practiced.

Many researchers have illustrated the value of certain antiseptics for cleaning the hands. However, if there is no reason to believe that the hands harbor pathogenic organisms in the resident flora of the skin, and if contact with patients in high-risk areas is not involved, there would appear to be no need to use antiseptics for medical asepsis. Avoiding antiseptics unless necessary also minimizes the associated irritating effect on the skin. Transient bacteria are removed easily by thorough washing with soap or a detergent and water. The Center for Disease Control recommends at least a 15-second hand wash before and after routine care of patients. If the hands have been contaminated with blood, purulent materials, mucus, saliva, or secretions from wounds, washing should be done for a longer period. Regardless of the type of soil, friction and a lather are essential to emulsify and mechanically remove the microorganisms. A sterile brush may be used if the hands are grossly contaminated. If used, a sterile brush should be handled with great care, because it is easy to break the skin around the nails with a stiff brush. Broken skin can serve as a reservoir or as an entry portal for organisms. The *subungual areas,* that is, the areas under the nails, should be cleaned with a sterile nail file or an orange stick, and again caution should be exercised to prevent breaking the skin. If good nail hygiene is maintained, it may not be necessary to clean the subungual areas with a stick or file with every washing, but the procedure should be followed if special circumstances warrant it.

It is preferable to wash the hands under running water at a sink with foot- or knee-controlled faucets. If the faucets are hand-controlled, a policy should be observed concerning whether they are considered to be clean or contaminated. A paper towel should be used to *open* the faucets before washing if the policy is to keep them clean; a paper towel should be used to *close* the faucets if the policy is to consider them contaminated. Basins for handwashing are not recommended because of the likelihood of contamination. When running water is not available, scrubbing with specially prepared antiseptic foam is considered preferable by some authorities. However, if it is necessary to use a basin, the water should be changed frequently while washing and after each person's use. The inside of a sink or a basin should be considered contaminated.

If bar soap is used for cleaning, the bar should be picked up at the beginning of the washing period and held in the hands during the entire period. Following washing, the bar should be rinsed and then dropped onto the soap dish. A soap dish that allows water to drain from the soap is preferable in order to keep the soap firm and dry between uses. It has been found that jellylike soap can harbor pathogens that transfer from user to user. Soap granules, leaflets, and impregnated tissues are also satisfactory. Liquid soap dispensers are convenient but some have been found to harbor organisms. If used, liquid soap dispensers should be cleaned and refilled with fresh soap solution on a regular and frequent basis.

The hands and the forearms should be held lower than the elbows during the washing in order that soiled water will not run up the arms. Following washing and rinsing, the hands should be dried on an individual linen or paper towel. Laundry problems when using linen, and disposal problems when using paper, have increased the use of forced hot air for hand drying in many agencies. It is suggested that a lotion or a cream be used following washing in order to keep the skin soft and pliable. Chapped and rough skin is difficult to keep clean and will break more easily with repeated washing. Some lotions have been found to harbor organisms, and hence, protection from contamination and frequent fresh supplies are recommended.

If at any time during the handwashing the hands accidently brush along the inside of the sink or on the soap dish, the entire washing should be repeated. It is suggested that a timer be placed near the sink or that personnel develop a habit of looking at their watch so that the washing period can be determined with accuracy. Figures 14–2 through 14–6 show a recommended handwashing technique.

It seems worth repeating that handwashing is recommended *before* and *after* patient care. Most health personnel wash their hands following contact with a patient but the practice of doing so before care is considered to be even more important. It is not necessary to repeat handwashing between two patients if little time elapses and if no possibility of contamination of the hands occurs. However, if several minutes elapse or there is the possibility of exposure to microorganisms, the hands should be washed again before caring for the second patient.

The technique just described may need to be taught to patients or family members who have infections in the home.

Keeping hands clean, regardless of the particular technique followed, is no more reliable than the individual whose conscientiousness, concern for cleaning all areas thoroughly, and respect for his own health, as

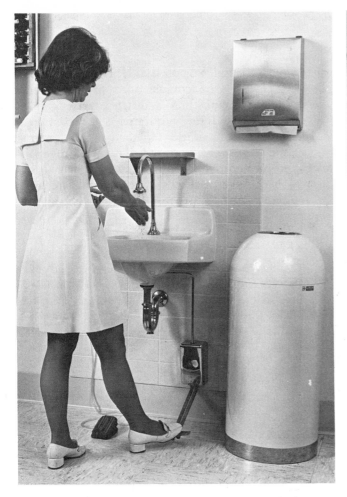

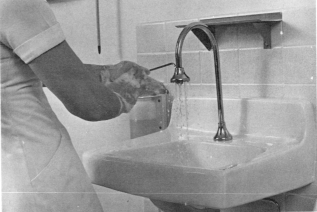

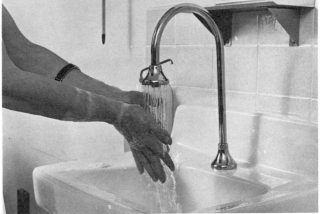

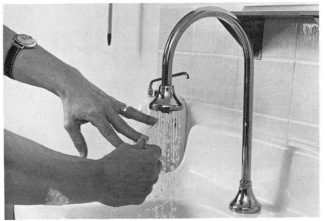

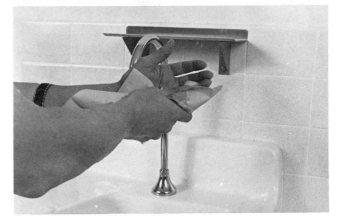

Figure 14–2 The importance of careful handwashing in the control of infection cannot be overemphasized. In this figure, the nurse is regulating the temperature and force of the running water and will wet her hands and wrists as she prepares for soaping them. In this agency, the water is regulated with foot controls. So also is the liquid soap dispenser.

Figure 14–3 The nurse uses friction on all surfaces of her hands and onto her wrists to develop a good lather. She holds her hands in a manner to prevent water from running up her arms. A minium of 15 seconds is recommended for this step in the procedure.

Figure 14–4 The nurse is rinsing the lather and suspended soil from her hands by allowing the water to run off her fingers. Note that her watch is high on her arm so that she can wash and rinse her wrists as well as her hands.

Figure 14–5 The nurse is shown cleaning the area under her nails under running water. This is an important part of handwashing and should be done at least once a day at the beginning of work and oftener as indicated.

Figure 14–6 The nurse dries her hands and wrists with paper towels. Complete drying is recommended to prevent chapping and skin irritations.

well as for the health of others, will determine to a great extent the effectiveness of handwashing. For aesthetic reasons as well, persons caring for the ill should practice good handwashing techniques.

Common Practices of Medical Asepsis

The following examples help to illustrate the fact that medical asepsis is constantly being practiced in daily living:

Paper towels are used when a large number of persons share common wash facilities; paper straws, such as those used at soda fountains, are wrapped individually so that they are not contaminated by constant handling; cafeterias frequently provide tongs for customers to use when taking rolls or bread; pillows and mattresses must be sterilized before they are sold, and they must have a label attached at the time of sale indicating that they have been sterilized; hairdressers and barbers are required to sterilize combs and other items after use on each customer.

Practices of medical asepsis in the home include the following: the homemaker washes her hands before beginning any food preparation; she roasts some meats to a higher temperature in order to ensure that they are safe to eat; she washes fruits and uncooked vegetables before serving them; she teaches the children to wash their hands before eating and after going to the toilet; she provides individual items for personal care for each member of the home, such as washcloths, towels, and toothbrushes.

Because certain diseases may be transmitted insidiously, there are many regulations enforced by law in most communities which aim to prevent their spread. Some of these regulations deal with the examination of food handlers, the management of eating establishments, the disposal of garbage, the construction of sewage systems and public building ventilation, and sanitation requirements. In every sense, these regulations constitute medical asepsis. They are defenses against the occasions when contamination may be present.

Most patients practice habits of medical asepsis which they do not recognize as such. However, these persons have an understanding of the need for protecting themselves and the means by which it can be done. Never underestimate the patient's ability to evaluate practices of asepsis in a hospital. He is as capable of doing this as he is of judging the practices he sees in a restaurant, a food store, or a motel in light of how they may affect him. Since patients have some "know-how" in this area, it is only natural that they would expect

the nurse to exemplify good health practices in all that she does. Even such activities as stripping the linen from the bed occupied by a patient, carrying linen, washing an item, visiting with a patient, or holding a child provide opportunities for good health teaching.

The following are actions which a nurse carries out, based on the fact that appropriate precautionary measures applied to daily activities and personal care aid in preventing the transmission of microorganisms and disease.

- Wash the hands frequently but especially before handling foods, before eating, after using a handkerchief, after going to the toilet, and before and after each patient contact. Clean underneath the fingernails frequently to keep the areas clean and free from contaminated materials.

- Keep soiled items and equipment from touching the clothing. Carry soiled linens or other used articles so that they do not touch the uniform. When stooping or bending, do not allow the uniform to touch the floor, a grossly contaminated area.

- Avoid having patients cough, sneeze, or breathe directly on others. Provide them with disposable wipes, and instructions as necessary, to cover their mouths when close contact is necessary, as during an examination.

- Clean away from yourself, especially when brushing, dusting, or scrubbing articles. This helps to prevent contaminant particles from settling on the hair, the face, or the uniform.

- Avoid raising dust. Use a specially treated cloth or a dampened cloth. Do not shake linens. Dust particles constitute a means by which bacteria may be transported from one area to another.

- Clean the least soiled areas first and then the more soiled ones. This helps to prevent having the cleaner areas soiled by the dirtier ones.

- Dispose of soiled or used items directly into appropriate containers or holders. Wrap items which are moist from body discharge or drainage in waterproof containers, such as plastic bags, before discarding into the refuse holder so that handlers will not come in contact with them.

- Pour liquids which are to be discarded, such as bath water, mouth rinsings, and the like, directly into the drain so as to avoid splattering in the sink. Most agencies caring for the sick have sinks or hoppers which are used primarily for disposing of contaminated liquids and washings.

The combined efforts of experts in microbiology, medicine, nursing, and sanitary engineering are necessary to study communicable diseases that are still posing problems and to arrive at flexible and workable techniques to prevent their spread. Thus, all the facts about the illness, the causative organisms, the existing facilities of the community, and the problems nursing care can be presented and evaluated. For example, some communities have sewage disposal systems which are inadequate to destroy all disease-producing organisms; therefore, action must be taken to disinfect waste materials before disposing of them in the sewage system; or if the causative agent exists only in the patient's blood, the only items that would be managed with additional care would be those that come into direct contact with the patient's blood; or, if the patient's respiratory secretions contain the causative organism, it may well be that a gown should be worn when coming in close contact with the patient and his bedding; or, if the organism is destroyed easily, the dishes may be safe if washed with hot soapy water. Knowledge of such factors is important when making the decision as to whether a person with an infectious disease can safely be cared for at home or must be hospitalized.

Psychological Implications When Using Communicable Disease Control Techniques

Regardless of the specific technique that is used and whether the patient is at home or in a health care facility, one need in his care does not change: attention to the psychological effects of the necessary restrictions. The implications of this are great whether the patient is strictly separated from others or whether he merely needs to observe simple precautions. The feeling of being undesirable to others is generally intense for the patient. He often feels frightened, lonely, "unclean," guilty, and rejected. The likelihood of the effects of sensory deprivation occurring from the isolation of persons with communicable diseases was also mentioned in Chapter 13. Because the person responds as a total being, his emotional state can influence his recovery rate and needs to be considered carefully.

Teaching and supportive measures are probably the two biggest contributions the nurse can make during this period of a patient's illness. The patient and his family need to have an accurate understanding of the pertinent epidemiological facts of the situation and of how to carry out the specific precautions necessary. The idea that it is the pathogenic organism which is un-

wanted, not the patient must be emphasized. Since misunderstanding can breed distrust, resentment, and fear, it is extremely important for the nurse to validate that the patient and his family have an accurate understanding of the situation. Their feelings often prevent them from asking for clarification or assistance. The nurse may find that she needs to extend her teaching to a patient's fellow employees or classmates. Misunderstanding on the part of a patient's aquaintances can also influence a patient's feelings of rejection, even after he has recovered.

Both the patient and his family may need support and reassurance regarding handling the isolation precautions and the feelings that may evolve. If the patient is being cared for at home, family members may need much help in understanding why the patient's behavior may change extensively and in how to cope with it. The patient who resents and ignores the precautions needs help in being accepted as a person and in constructively expressing his feelings.

Studies have been done which show that the extensive separation of persons from others can be extremely traumatic. The goal now is to minimize the extent of the precautions and the length of time they must exist as much as can safely be done. The problem of striking a balance between what is best for both the patient and for others is a delicate one. The skill and ingenuity of the nurse are often taxed extensively in caring for the patient with a communicable disease.

A well-informed nurse who understands how to protect herself and her patients and a well-informed patient who is cooperating in his care are by far the best communicable disease precautions.

Types of Isolation Practices

As stated previously, there are many variations of specific isolation techniques. In an attempt to organize communicable disease precautions, the Center for Disease Control has epidemiologically categorized isolation procedures into seven groups: strict, respiratory, enteric, wound and skin, discharge, blood, and protective. A patient's particular pathogen and its means of transmission determine which category of precautions is appropriate to institute. The specific techniques are described in the publication, *Isolation Techniques for Use in Hospitals*. The book is listed in the references at the end of this unit. A brief description of the categories follow. In each category, handwashing before and after patient care is considered mandatory for all health practitioners.

Strict Isolation. The purpose of *strict isolation* is to prevent the transmission of all highly communicable diseases spread by both contact and airborne routes. The technique requires that the patient be in a private room and that persons coming in contact with the patient wear gowns, masks, and gloves and observe rigid precautions. Strict isolation is frequently used with patients who have illnesses such as smallpox, diphtheria, or *Staphylococcus aureus* infections of extensive burns.

Respiratory Isolation. The objective of *respiratory isolation* is to prevent the transmission of pathogens from the respiratory tract by direct contact or airborne droplets. It also requires that the patient be in a private room, that masks be worn, and that particular precautions be taken with respiratory tract secretions. This method may be used for patients with diseases such as pertussis (whooping cough), measles, and active pulmonary tuberculosis.

Enteric Isolation. The goal of *enteric isolation* is to prevent diseases which can be transmitted through direct or indirect contact with infected fecal material. Persons can be safely cared for in rooms with others as long as care is taken to avoid fecal-oral cross–contamination. Gowns and gloves should be worn by those having direct contact with the patient or his excretions. It is recommended that persons with either Types A or B hepatitis have both enteric and blood isolation techniques incorporated in their care. Cholera and salmonellosis are other diseases that may require enteric precautions.

Wound and Skin Isolation. *Wound and skin isolation* is designed to prevent infection from pathogens transmitted by direct contact with wounds and articles contaminated by wound drainage. It is preferable that the patient have a private room. Persons in direct contact with the patient must wear gowns and masks. Gloves must be worn by persons in direct contact with the infection area, and special precautions should be taken when dressings are changed. A fresh pair of gloves is worn when the soiled dressing is removed and another pair is worn for applying the new dressing, with careful handwashing between glove changes. Patients with such conditions as gas gangrene, bubonic plague, and generalized wound infections may warrant these precautions.

Discharge Precautions. The purpose of *discharge precautions* is to prevent infections from pathogens transmitted by direct contact with excretions and secretions or contaminated articles when the likelihood is slight but possible. The primary precautions pertain to the handling of lesion drainage, oral secretions, and fecal excretions. Patients with minor infected wounds and burns, gonorrhea, scarlet fever, and poliomyelitis may require one of these precautions.

Blood Precautions. *Blood precautions* are designed to prevent infections from organisms transmitted by contact with blood or items contaminated with blood. Special care is taken with needles and syringes contaminated with the patient's blood. Blood specimens of the person are also prominently labeled so that adequate precautions may be observed. Hepatitis and malaria are two diseases which may require this care.

Protective Isolation. The purpose of *protective isolation* is to prevent contact between potential pathogens and a person with greatly increased susceptibility. These techniques are also known as *reverse isolation* and are discussed later in this chapter.

Regardless of the type of isolation practices being observed, the patient needs to be located in a physical environment in which it is feasible to carry out the intent of whatever precautions are necessary. Handwashing facilities in the immediate area are vital. Adjoining bathing and toilet facilities are desirable, whenever possible. Adequate space separating the person harboring the pathogen and others helps to decrease the possibility of transmission in all situations. A separate room with a door that can be kept closed is essential in circumstances where the causative organisms are airborne. Ventilation in the area should have a minimum of six air changes per hour. To prevent cross-circulation or recirculation of air between the isolation room and other areas, slight negative pressure in the room in relation to adjoining areas is desirable. Exhaust window fans can be used for this. Facilities to discard excretions, drainage, and other contaminated substances safely are important.

Facilities for diversion and sensory stimulation may be especially important for persons who are confined alone. Selection of the environment for the patient should be based on the patient's needs and availability of facilities to carry out the appropriate techniques to prevent pathogen transmission.

Personal Contact Precautions

The most common vehicles of transmission for communicable diseases are personal contacts, excretions, secretions, equipment, and supplies. Figure 14–9 depicts the commmon vehicles and the role of barriers in preventing their transmission. This section discusses methods used to develop vehicle barriers.

As indicated earlier, personal contacts between the patient with a communicable disease and others is extremely important from a psychological standpoint. Depending on the degree of illness, the patient may need personal contacts for physical assistance also. Important as the contact is, it is probably the contact that is most responsible for pathogen transmission. More specifically, inadequately cleaned hands transmit more microorganisms than any other single transmission vehicle. Handwashing technique has been discussed and its importance cannot be overemphasized.

Patients and family members need to have an explanation of the purposes for using handwashing and wearing apparel as barriers to vehicle transmission of organisms through personal contacts. As stated in Chapter 6, because touch is such an important part of communication, it may be important to the nurse-patient relationship to set up barriers to vehicle transmission so the avoidance of touch is not necessary.

Gown Technique. When gowns are worn, individual gown technique is recommended. This means gowns are worn only once and then are discarded for disinfection if they are not disposable. Disposable gowns are destroyed in an appropriate manner. Multiple gown technique, or the reuse of gowns, was practiced extensively in the past. This technique required careful re-

moval and donning of the gown to avoid contamination. Since contamination often occurs, the Center for Disease Control recommends this approach be abandoned.

Gowns that are used for isolation technique are made of washable or disposable material; most are made to be worn over the outer garments of the wearer. They are designed with the opening in the back and a tie around the waist to help to keep the gown secure and closed. Some have stockinet at the wrists; others have buttons. They may have buttons or tie strings at the neck. These minor variations do not affect the use or the value of the gown. All have the same purpose of protecting the clothing of those who come in contact with the patient from contamination.

Supplies of gowns should be available outside the immediate patient environment so the wearer can put one on before entering the patient's area. There is no special way in which a clean gown must be put on. However, it should be closed well in the back so that all parts of the wearer's clothing are covered.

When the wearer is ready to leave the unit, the gown is unfastened and removed so that the wearer turns it inside out. In other words, the wearer takes off the gown and rolls it up so that the contaminated part is inside. Then the gown is discarded in a special hamper provided for it. The wearer now washes her hands thoroughly, making certain that special precautions are taken to prevent contaminating the faucets if foot- or knee-controlled faucets are not available. Figure 14–10 on page 274 shows proper gown technique.

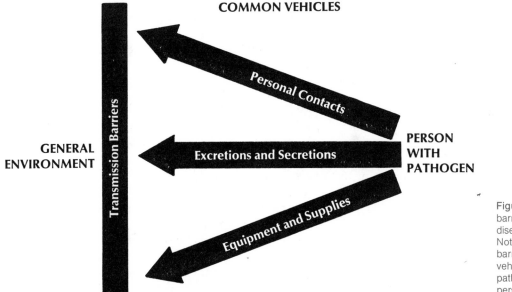

COMMON VEHICLES

Transmission Barriers

Personal Contacts

GENERAL ENVIRONMENT

Excretions and Secretions

PERSON WITH PATHOGEN

Equipment and Supplies

Figure 14–9 The transmission barriers are communicable disease or isolation techniques. Note that the transmission barriers prevent common vehicles from transporting pathogens from the infected person to the general environment.

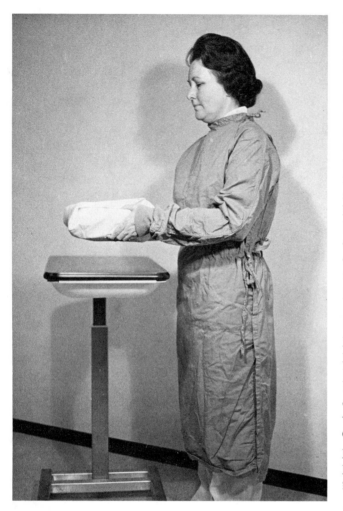

Figure 14–10 This nurse is properly gowned for working in isolation. The isolation gown will protect her uniform when she comes in close contact with the patient.

Masks. A variety of practices is observed in the use of the mask as a barrier in caring for a patient who has a communicable disease which can be transmitted via the airborne route. In some instances, all personnel and visitors to the patient wear masks; in others, personnel, visitors, and the patient wear masks.

Theoretically, the mask is intended to filter inspired and expired air in order to trap the organisms in its meshes. The purpose of the mask should be understood by the wearer; for example, if a patient has active pulmonary tuberculosis, it is recommended that he wear the mask to provide a barrier for the pathogens he may exhale. When the patient is unable to cooperate by wearing the mask, persons coming in contact with him then may need to wear masks. When used in the

newborn nursery or other areas where protective techniques are used, the purpose is to protect the infants or the patient from the air expired by the workers, and hence, personnel wear masks.

If masks are worn by persons coming in contact with the patient, they should be stored with the gowns outside the patient area and put on before entering the room. Masks should cover both the nose and mouth and be worn only once. They should never be lowered around the neck and then reused. Moisture makes masks ineffective and so they should be removed and appropriately discarded as frequently as necessary to keep them dry. The actual length of time a mask can be worn safely, which is partly determined by the type of mask, is a debatable question. Newer high-efficiency, disposable masks are more effective than reusable cotton gauze masks and are preferred for preventing airborne and droplet-spread infections.

Gloves. Gloves may be worn during certain phases of patient care. They may be used as a barrier for the person handling wound dressings or when carrying out treatments if drainage is present. Sterile gloves may also be worn to protect the patient from the introduction of organisms when caring for an open wound. Gloves are worn only once and then discarded appropriately. Gloves should be changed after direct handling of potentially contaminated drainage and before completing the patient's care. Both reusable and disposable gloves are available commercially.

Hair and Shoe Covers. Hair and shoe covers are not used generally except in the care of patients with smallpox and in some protective isolation situations. When they are worn, all hair on the head should be covered, and the shoe covers should also protect the open ends of trouser legs.

Excretion and Secretion Precautions

Organisms can escape from the host through body secretions and excretions. Urine and feces and respiratory, oral, vaginal, and wound drainage may require special precautions.

Urine and feces may need to be treated before disposal into the sewage system. As mentioned previously, this precaution is unnecessary in communities in which the sewage disposal techniques are adequate to destroy organisms. Home sewage systems may make disinfection necessary in some situations.

The problems that the disinfection of excreta brings

to any nursing service usually are numerous. The psychological implications as well as the hazards of handling several pails or bedpans of excreta make it an unpopular procedure. Therefore, efforts should be made to ascertain the absolute necessity for disinfecting excreta before it is done.

The disadvantages of the free-flowing steam bedpan flusher have been discussed. The safest practice is to empty the bedpan, rinse it thoroughly with cold water, wash it with soap or detergent and water and then sterilize it with steam under pressure before reuse.

If there is drainage, tissues and other items may be contaminated by wound, mouth, nose, or vaginal drainage, and they should be considered as pathogen vehicles and handled carefully. The usual technique is to place the contaminated materials in an impervious bag and close it tightly. This is illustrated in Figure 14–11. When the bag is removed from the patient area, it should be placed in a larger, clean disposable bag or container, keeping the outer surface uncontaminated to protect persons handling refuse. The entire container then is discarded by incineration or other methods deemed appropriate by the agency. Figure 14–12 shows nurses using the double-bag technique.

Specimens of body secretions or excretions may need to be collected for laboratory analysis. As with the dressings and other items, it is important that the outside of the container not be contaminated with the pathogens for the protection of laboratory personnel. A second larger, clean bag or container is also often used in these situations to provide a barrier between the pathogens and the persons handling the container.

Equipment and Supplies Precautions

Equipment and supplies contaminated by pathogens can become vehicles for infection transmission if effective barriers are not developed. Equipment which is reused in providing patient care, such as a sphygmomanometer, stethoscope, and other physical examination equipment, should be left in the patient's room whenever possible for his exclusive use until the illness has subsided. Disinfection of the equipment should be in the manner appropriate to the causative organisms and situation. Disposable thermometers are available and preferable. If a reusable thermometer is used, it should also be left at the patient's bedside in a container of disinfectant. Cleaning the thermometer before placing it in the disinfectant and appropriate changing of the disinfectant solution are important points to remember. It is recommended that electronic thermom-

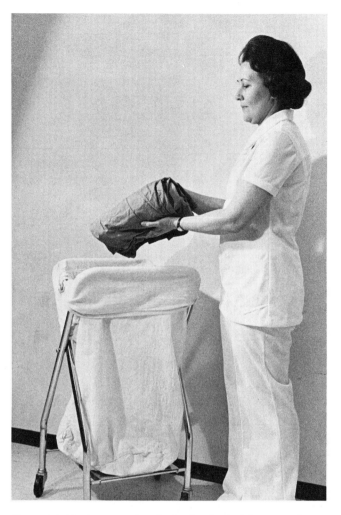

Figure 14–11   In preparation for leaving the isolation area, the nurse has removed her isolation gown and folded it with the contaminated side in before discarding it in the linen hamper. She will wash her hands carefully before leaving the area.

eters not be used for patients on isolation because of the difficulty in rendering them safe for the next patient. Needles and syringes must be handled carefully, especially if contaminated by the hepatitis virus. Nondisposable syringes and needles should be rinsed thoroughly in cold water and then disinfected before they are prepared for reuse. The extensive availability of disposable equipment today makes the safe handling of contaminated supplies much easier. Disposable thermometers, physical examination equipment, and needles and syringes can be merely prepared for destruction after use.

If linen and personal laundry are contaminated with pathogens, they should be removed from the patient's

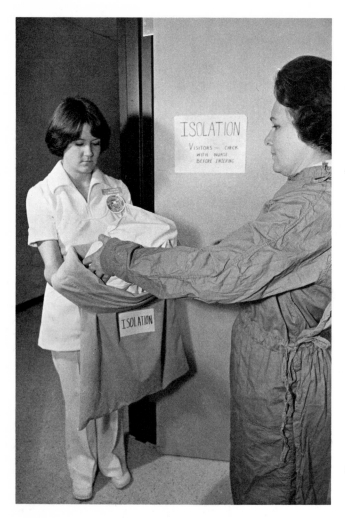

Figure 14–12 Double-bagging is used to remove contaminated items from an isolated area. This figure shows a so-called clean nurse prepared for receiving contaminated linen. She holds a specially designated laundry bag with her hands protected by a wide cuff. The gowned nurse carefully inserts the contaminated linen, which is already enclosed in a bag, into the isolation laundry bag. After the contaminated linen is inside the second bag, the clean nurse will close it so that only the inner surface will be contaminated.

diseases to be handled in the usual manner. Preferably, hot water-soluble bags are available so that linen and bags can be placed directly in the hospital washing machine. Nonsoluble bags should be opened and the linen carefully placed in the washer.

For items of clothing that are not washed easily in a machine, gas sterilizers, discussed earlier in this chapter, may be used. This would be a suitable procedure for items that are not washable, such as decorative bed jackets.

Home laundering can generally be safely accomplished with sufficient hot water or boiling the items and using an appropriate detergent and household bleach or disinfectant, such as Clorox or Lysol.

Most health agencies use mechanical dishwashers that leave dishes free of pathogens. If this is not the case, it then becomes necessary to take special precautions when a patient has a communicable disease, especially one that is transmitted via secretions from the mouth. In some agencies, the dishes are rinsed and then boiled. Other agencies use disposable dishes so that only the silverware needs boiling. The technique of placing soiled dishes in a container of water and boiling them before being washed is a questionable practice. The heat of the water often coagulates the food particles remaining on the dishes. If the organism is contained within these solids and is particularly resistant, it may survive the washing process. Therefore, the dishes should be rinsed thoroughly first before being washed and subjected to heat. Many mechanical dishwashers used in restaurants and hospitals provide for rinsing the dishes before they are washed. Rubber gloves should be worn if the dishes are rinsed by hand.

If contaminated, leftover food should be wrapped and discarded along with other wastes from the patient's room. Liquids should be poured down the drain or the toilet if a satisfactory sewage system is available. If not, they may be disinfected before discarding.

Protective (Reverse) Isolation

As noted previously, protective isolation includes those practices designed to prevent a highly susceptible person from coming in contact with pathogens. Protective isolation is also called reverse isolation, because its goal is the opposite of the usual isolation process. The purpose of protective isolation is to protect a *specific* person against encounter with *any* pathogens in contrast to the usual isolation goal of keeping a *known* microorganism away from any person. The barriers for protective

immediate environment using the double-bag technique described earlier. The outer bag's external surface should always remain clean and the bag's contents should be clearly marked to indicate that the contents are contaminated. Vigorous movements when changing bed linen should be avoided to prevent air movement and spread of microorganisms.

Modern hospital laundering processes make it possible for almost all linens of patients with communicable

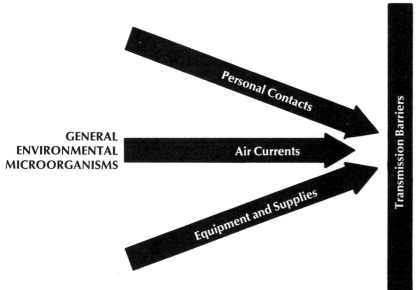

GENERAL ENVIRONMENTAL MICROORGANISMS

Personal Contacts

Air Currents

Equipment and Supplies

Transmission Barriers

SUSCEPTIBLE PERSON

Figure 14–13 This diagram illustrates protective or reverse isolation. Note that the susceptible person is protected from common vehicles transporting microorganisms from the general environment by transmission barriers.

isolation must be designed to prevent vehicles from conveying organisms to the patient. Figure 14–13 demonstrates the goal and common pathogen vehicles.

As indicated earlier, some persons are highly susceptible to infections, even from microorganisms they could normally resist. Persons with certain diseases (leukemia, agammaglobulinemia, and lymphomas) or those receiving certain treatments (total body irradiation) or certain medications (steroids, antimetabolites, or immunosuppressives) need to be protected from as many microorganisms as possible.

Specially constructed rooms or commercial devices can be used to provide an environment as free from organisms as possible. The special space should be under slight positive pressure with respect to adjacent rooms so air flow from the protected room or area moves to the adjoining spaces. Persons caring for the patient do so by wearing a sterile "space suit" type of apparel or by working through special sealed openings in the "plastic walls" of the area. All substances coming in contact with the patient are sterilized, that is, air, linen, food, medications, equipment, and supplies. This is a highly sophisticated and complex type of technique to implement.

Modifications of protective isolation may merely provide for sterilization of all supplies entering the patient's room, plus sterilization of clothing worn by health care personnel. Masks, gloves, and hair and foot covers are also worn by personnel.

INFECTION CONTROL AND THE NURSING PROCESS

The practicing nurse should be conscious of the need for infection controls at all times. During her data collection, she will want to gather information about existing or potential pathogens and infections. The following questions suggest some areas which can be helpful when collecting patient information pertinent to infection control. Does the person have a wound with drainage? Does he have a break in the skin or mucous membrane or is there a potential for such a break? Are there suspected or confirmed pathogens in his excretions or secretions? Does he exhibit indications of the presence of an infection? For example, does he have suspicious laboratory test results or symptoms? Has he had known exposure to a pathogen? For example, has he had contact with a person with a communicable disease or contact with pathogens through an injury? Are there reasons to suspect he has an increased susceptibility to infection? For example, is he very young or very old? Has he had therapy which is known to lower resistance to infections? Does he have an illness which causes an increased susceptibility to infection? What type of barriers to the transmission of pathogens exist? What is the status of his immunizations?

The nature of the data and the patient's situation will determine the type of standards which will be appropriate for assessing the data. Microbiology, public health, and various clinical texts plus federal, state, and agency infection control directives are among the sources that can provide useful standards.

Nursing care planning and intervention will depend on the nature of the nursing diagnoses and the existing circumstances. Many nursing measures for infection control have already been identified in this chapter. Nursing measures for specific pathogens and pathogenic states are discussed in various clinical texts. The following generalizations are intended to summarize the nursing implications of infection control.

- Consider the patient as your primary concern. It is easy to become so engrossed in complex laboratory studies, the patient's symptoms, and elaborate techniques for confining the organism that the patient as a person can be nearly forgotten. It is important to remember that it is the *patient* who has the existing or potential infection and that he is the focus of nursing care. The patient is not only responding physiologically if a pathogen is present, but he is responding psychologically to the care directed toward controlling the pathogen. It is important that he feels that the health practitioners are concerned about his total well-being. The techniques of infection control are employed as a means to improve the welfare of the patient and others. They should not become ends in themselves.

- Make habits of common infection control techniques. Since the nurse is in frequent contact with potential pathogens, she should perfect routine infection control techniques so that they do not require conscious thought. For example, washing before and after each patient contact, as well as using the proper handwashing technique, should become a routine that is automatic. The handling of sterile, clean, and contaminated articles and personal hygiene habits should also be performed routinely according to a recommended technique. Like all other habits, infection control techniques must first be performed consciously. With repeated performance, they can become automatic. It can be helpful for the beginner to ask a knowledgeable person to observe her techniques and provide suggestions for improvement. Periodically, the nurse would be wise to request a critique of her routine practices to make certain that she has not unconsciously allowed an improper technique to appear. Such a critique also can help to keep her current with changes in recommended infection control practices. The nurse who practices infection control routinely is protecting her patients as well as herself.

- Serve as an example of infection control practices. The typical patient and his family observe the habits of the nurse. Often they imitate her. She can serve as a good or poor model. If the nurse routinely washes her hands before changing a patient's dressing, the probability is greater that the patient also will do so as he continues the dressing changes at home. He will also probably be inclined to mimic her handling of both the soiled and fresh dressings. If the nurse fails to cover her mouth when coughing or sneezing, a patient is not likely to think such a practice is important either. Teaching by example can be very significant in influencing people's health care habits beyond the time when the nurse has contact with the patient.

- Select specific pathogen control practices according to the characteristics of known organisms. Appropriate means for disinfection and sterilization, medical and surgical asepsis, and transmission barriers should be chosen and altered according to the causative organism and its potential for causing infection. Therefore, knowledge of the particular organism and pertinent aspects of the infection process cycle are essential to sound nursing care.

- Be continually aware of changes in the recommended ways of controlling pathogens. Recently, it has become very apparent that organisms change their characteristics and new organisms are discovered. For example, some pathogens that were initially susceptible to control with various antibiotics have developed resistance to them. Nearly every year, organisms previously unknown, or unknown as pathogens, are isolated as the cause of new illnesses. Such discoveries along with the continual refinement of knowledge about organisms and their control and the development of new products and technologies, result in changes in the recommended techniques for caring for persons harboring or exposed to pathogens. The nurse must take the responsibility to keep her knowledge and skills current with these changes. The present revision of this text is believed to be current with present recommendations, but it is anticipated that changes will continue to occur.

The parts of the nursing process and of the process as a whole are evaluated as described in Chapter 4.

CONCLUSION

Disinfection, sterilization, and isolation techniques vary. They should be based on knowledge of the causative pathogen, its reservoir, exit mode, transmission vehicles, entry portals, and susceptibility of new hosts. Barriers to prevent transmission of pathogens are the most realistic means of preventing diseases caused by microorganisms. The nurse must use her knowledge judiciously in order to provide safe patient care when dealing with infections and communicable diseases.

SUPPLEMENTAL LIBRARY STUDY

1. Recommendations for immunizations change from time to time. For example, with smallpox nearly eradicated, immunizations for it are no longer routinely recommended for persons in this country. The following articles describe recommendations on immunization.

    Brown, Marie Scott. "What You Should Know About Communicable Diseases and Their Immunizations: A Guide for Nurses in Ambulatory Settings: Part I: The Three Rs." *Nursing 75,* 5:70–72, September 1975.

    Brown, Marie Scott. "What You Should Know About Communicable Diseases and Their Immunizations: A Guide for Nurses in Ambulatory Settings: Part II: Diphtheria, Pertussis, Tetanus, and Polio." *Nursing 75,* 5:56–60, October 1975.

    Brown, Marie Scott. "What You Should Know About Communicable Diseases and Their Immunizations: A Guide for Nurses in Ambulatory Settings: Part III: Mumps, Chickenpox, and Diarrhea." *Nursing 75,* 55–56, 58–60, November 1975.

    Read the articles and evaluate yourself and members of your family to determine if your immunizations are adequate.

2. As indicated in the title of the following article, the author has coined a new term in infection control.

    Beck, William C., Guest Editor. "Abridged Sterility—A Level of Disinfection." *AORN Journal,* 26:242, 244, August 1977.

    What is the definition of "abridged sterility"? How is it different from sterility and disinfection? Even though the author has suggested a new concept, what two reasons does he give for not recommending adoption of the concept in health care?

3. In the following article, a study of the handwashing practices of nursing personnel is reported.

    Fox, Marian K., et al. "How Good Are Hand Washing Practices?" *American Journal of Nursing,* 74:1676–1678, September 1974.

    The study indicates that many of the personnel observed did not follow the recommended procedure. Using the criteria and scale on page 1677, how many points would you score with your handwashing technique?

4. The author of the following article conveys that every nurse has a role in infection control.

    Jenny, Jean. "What You Should Be Doing About Infection Control." *Nursing 76,* 6:78–79, November 1976.

    How many different infection control practices can you identify in the article? Can you suggest additional ways the nurse can help control infections?

5. Characteristics of the probable or identified causative organisms and the nature of the infection can provide standards for determining nursing diagnoses and the basis for planning nursing care and selecting nursing intervention measures. Use the following examples of data to practice implementing the nursing process. Identify the standards, make the nursing diagnoses, state the nursing care objectives, and specify the nursing care measures related to infection control for each hypothetical patient situation.

   - A mother is concerned about preventing her two- and three-year-old children from acquiring German measles from their six-year-old brother who has just begun to develop the rash.

   - A young man has just entered the hospital with an infected leg injury acquired from an accident involving a piece of farm equipment. As he removes his trousers, you note that purulent drainage has soaked through his dressing.

   - A woman hospitalized for observation begins to have symptoms of diarrhea and vomiting. This occurred after her husband has been diagnosed as having salmonella food poisoning from some food they ate.

References For Unit IV

CHAPTER 11

Aase, Jon M. "Environmental Causes of Birth Defects." *Nursing Digest,* 4:12–14, Winter 1976.

Bayer, Mary. "Community Diagnosis—Through Sense, Sight, and Sound." *Nursing Outlook,* 21:712–713, November 1973.

Bertz, Edward J., et al. "Viewing the Hospital as a Working Environment." *Hospitals, Journal Of The American Hospital Association,* 50:107–112, October 16, 1976.

Burkeen, Oleta E. "Occupational Health Nursing and the Low-Wage Worker." *Occupational Health Nursing,* 23:12–14, April 1975.

Ellingson, Harold V. "Industrial Diseases and the Industrial Nurse." *Occupational Health Nursing,* 23:7–11, February 1975.

Goldmark, Peter C. "Communication and the Community." *Scientific American,* 227:143–150, September 1972.

Goldstein, David H. and Benoit, Joyce N. "Occupational Safety and Health." *American Journal of Nursing,* 75:1759, October 1975.

Gosnell, Davina J. "Know Your Community Resources." *Journal of Gerontological Nursing,* 3:65–66, May/June 1977.

"Habitat and Health." *World Health,* 4–9, May 1976.

Hackley, John A. "Full-Service Hospice Offers Home, Day, and Inpatient Care." *Hospitals, Journal Of The American Hospital Association,* 51:84–87, November 1, 1977.

Karvonen, Martti J. "Fitting the Job to the Worker." *World Health,* 30–35, July/August 1974.

Lanuza, Dorothy M. "Circadian Rhythms of Mental Efficiency and Performance." *The Nursing Clincs of North America,* 11:583–594, December 1976.

McMichael, A. J. "An Epidemiologic Perspective on the Identification of Workers at Risk." *Occupational Health Nursing,* 23:7–11, January 1975.

Milio, Nancy. *The Care of Health in Communities: Access for Outcasts.* Macmillan Publishing Co., Inc., New York, 1975, 402 p.

Philippe, Robert. "Clues in the Community." *World Health,* 14–17, May 1974.

Pierce, John R. "Communication." *Scientific American,* 227:31–41, September 1972.

Rubenstein, Reva and Bellin, Judith S. "Chemical Hazards in the Workplace." *Occupational Health Nursing,* 24:16–21, October 1976.

Rushwood, Elizabeth. "Hazards Around Us." *World Health,* 10–13, May 1974.

Ruybal, Sally E., et al. "Community Assessment: An Epidemiological Approach." *Nursing Outlook,* 23:365–368, June 1975.

Sammond, Peter H. and Davis, Samuel. "Hospital-Community Cooperation Brings Care to Senior Citizens." *Hospitals, Journal Of The American Hospital Association,* 50:117–120, May 16, 1976.

Solomon, Jeffrey R. and Lichtman, Marc. "Nursing Home Nucleus Generates Array of Outreach Services." *Hospitals, Journal Of The American Hospital Association,* 51:85–86, 88, 90, December 16, 1977.

"The Community—New Focus for Nursing." *Nursing Digest,* 4:53–55, Summer 1976.

Ward, Barbara. "'Water' The Key to Health." *World Health,* 3–7, January 1977.

Wreford, Brian M. "Prevention and Noise." *Nursing Mirror and Midwives Journal,* 141:57–59, September 11, 1975.

CHAPTER 12

"Auto Safety Myths: What You Think You Know Can Kill You." *Family Health,* 8:36–38, 64, September 1976.

Caplan, Frank. "How to Select the Right Toys for *Your* Child." *Family Health,* 8:48–50, 62, November 1976.

Emmons, Howard W. "Fire and Fire Protection." *Scientific American,* 231:21–27, July 1974.

Insel, Paul M. and Lindgren, Henry Clay. "Too Close for Comfort: Why One Person's Company is Another's Crowd." *Psychology Today,* 11:100–106, December 1977.

Kukuk, Helen M. "Safety Precautions: Protecting Your Patients & Yourself, Part One." *Nursing 76,* 6:45–51, May 1976.

Kukuk, Helen M. "Safety Precautions: Protecting Your Patients & Yourself, Part Two." *Nursing 76,* 6:49–52, June 1976.

Kukuk, Helen M. "Safety Precautions: Protecting Your Patients & Yourself, Part Three." *Nursing 76,* 6:45–49, July 1976.

Mylrea, Kenneth C. and O'Neal, L. Burke. "Electricity and Electrical Safety in the Hospital." *Nursing 76,* 6:52–59, January 1976.

Phegley, Dianne and Obst, Jerry. "Improving Fire Safety with Posted Procedures." *Nursing 76,* 6:18–19, July 1976.

Sovie, Margaret D. and Fruehan, C. Thomas. "Protecting the Patient from Electrical Hazards." *The Nursing Clinics of North America,* 7:469–480, September 1972.

Trought, Elizabeth A. "Equipment Hazards." *American Journal of Nursing,* 73:858–862, May 1973.

CHAPTER 13

Bizzi, Emilio. "The Coordination of Eye-Head Movement." *Scientific American,* 231:100–106, October 1974.

Carnevali, Doris and Brueckner, Susan. "Immobilization—Reassessment of a Concept." *American Journal of Nursing,* 70:1502–1507, July 1970.

Ellis, Rosemary. "Unusual Sensory and Thought Disturbances After Cardiac Surgery." *American Journal of Nursing,* 72:2021–2025, November 1972.

Julesz, Bela. "Experiments in the Visual Perception of Texture." *Scientific American,* 232:34–43, April 1975.

Kramer, Marlene, et al. "Extra Tactile Stimulation of the Premature Infant." *Nursing Research,* 24:324–334, September/October 1975.

Lee, Robert E. and Ball, Patricia A. "Some Thoughts on the Psychology of the Coronary Care Unit Patient." *American Journal of Nursing,* 75:1498–1501, September 1975.

Neu, Carlos. "Coping with Newly Diagnosed Blindness." *American Journal of Nursing,* 75:2161–2163, December 1975.

Perron, Denise M. "Deprived of Sound." *American Journal of Nursing,* 74:1057–1059, June 1974.

Wahl, Patricia R. "Psychosocial Implications of Disorientation in the Elderly." *The Nursing Clinics of North America,* 11:145–155, March 1976.

Wesseling, Elizabeth, Guest Editor. "Symposium on Patients with Sensory Defects." *The Nursing Clinics of North America,* 5:449–538, September 1970.

West, Norman D. "Stresses Associated With ICUs Affect Patients, Families, Staff." *Hospitals, Journal Of The American Hospital Association,* 49:62–63, December 16, 1975.

Wilson, Larkin M. "Intensive Care Delirium: The Effect of Outside Deprivation in a Windowless Unit." *Archives of Internal Medicine,* 130:225–226, August 1972.

CHAPTER 14

American Hospital Association Committee on Infections Within Hospitals. *Infection Control in the Hospital.* Edition 3. American Hospital Association, Chicago, 1974, 198 p.

Beletz, Elaine E. and Covo, Gabriel A. "The Case of the Hidden Infections in the Elderly." *Nursing 76,* 7:14–16, August 1976.

Boyle, Sister Mary T. and Kaufman, Arthur. "Strep Screening to Prevent Rheumatic Fever." *American Journal of Nursing,* 75:1487–1488, September 1975.

Castle, Mary. "Help Stamp Out Infections: Be an Infection-Control Coordinator." *Nursing 76,* 6:90, 92, 95, September 1976.

Castle, Mary. "Isolation: Precise Procedures for Better Protection." *Nursing 75,* 5:50–57, May 1975.

Center for Disease Control. *National Nosocomial Infections Study Quarterly Report.* Fourth Quarter 1972, Issued April 1974, pp. 18–25.

Center for Disease Control. *National Nosocomial Infections Study Quarterly Report.* Third and Fourth Quarters 1973, Issued March 1974, pp. 19–28.

Chavigny, Katherine Hill. "Microbial Infections in Hospitals: A Review of the Literature and Some Suggestions for Nursing Research." *International Journal of Nursing Studies,* 14:37–47, 1, 1977.

Chobin, Nancy, et al. "Strep Screening to Prevent Rheumatic Fever: From Project to Ongoing Program." *American Journal of Nursing,* 75:1489–1491, September 1975.

Cockburn, W. Charles. "Saving Young Lives." *World Health,* 8–13, February/March 1977.

Costerton, J. W., et al. "How Bacteria Stick." *Scientific American,* 238:86–95, January 1978.

Davies, Julian and Pankey, George A. "Controlling Infection: Will the Microbes Beat Us Yet?" *Nursing Digest,* 11:35–41, September 1974.

Donley, Diana L. "Nursing the Patient Who Is Immunosuppressed." *American Journal of Nursing,* 76:1619–1625, October 1976.

Henderson, Donald A. "Smallpox Shows the Way." *World Health,* 22–27, February/March 1977.

Henderson, Donald A. "The Eradication of Smallpox." *Scientific American,* 235:25–33, October 1976.

Litsky, Bertha Y. "Microbiology of Sterilization." *AORN Journal,* 26:334–350, August 1977.

MacClelland, Doris C. "Are Current Skin Preparations Valid?" *AORN Journal,* 21:55–60, January 1975.

MacClelland, Doris C. "Sterilization by Ionizing Radiation." *AORN Journal,* 26:675–684, October 1977.

Morley, David C. "Six Killers." *World Health,* 4–7, February/March 1977.

Nordmark, Madelyn T. and Rohweder, Anne W. *Scientific Foundations of Nursing.* Edition 3. J. B. Lippincott Company, Philadelphia, 1975, pp. 306–326.

Perkins, John J. *Principles and Methods of Sterilization in Health Sciences.* Edition 2. Charles C Thomas, Springfield, Illinois, 1969, 560 p.

Riemensnider, Dick K. and Richards, Ruth F. "Providing Supportive Information to the Patient in Isolation." *Hospitals, Journal Of The American Hospital Association,* 51:103–104, 106, June 1, 1977.

Robinson, Alice M. "Nurse-Epidemiologist: Key to Infection Control." *RN,* 38:63–67, October 1975.

Stamm, Walter E. "Elements of an Active, Effective Infection Control Program." *Hospitals, Journal Of The American Hospital Association,* 50:60, 62, 64, 66, December 1, 1976.

"Symposium on Infections and the Nurse." *The Nursing Clinics of North America,* 5:85–177, March 1970.

U.S. Department of Health, Education, and Welfare, Public Health Service, Center for Disease Control. *Isolation Techniques for Use in Hospitals.* Edition 2. U.S. Government Printing Office, Washington, D.C., 1975, 104 p.

Ventura, Jacqueline N. "The International Traveler's Health Guide." *American Journal of Nursing,* 77:968–974, June 1977.

unit V
Technical Skills in and Underlying Principles of the Practice of Nursing

15

BEHAVIORAL OBJECTIVES

When content in this chapter has been mastered, the student will be able to

Define the terms appearing in the glossary.

Differentiate between the four methods commonly used to collect data on the physical health status and provide several examples of the appropriate use of each method.

Describe requirements for an appropriate setting, equipment, and supplies for collecting data on the physical examination.

Explain the physiological basis of the vital signs, describe the common techniques for measuring the vital signs, and identify normal findings for well adults.

Describe the major characteristics to be observed in each anatomical area when doing a physical examination, identify the appropriate examination method(s), and give at least one normal finding for each anatomical area.

Explain how the characteristics of an electrocardiogram reflect the action of the heart.

Discuss the role of the nurse in collecting blood, urine, and secretion specimens.

Describe the preparation of a person who will have contrast radiography, ultrasound examinations, and radioisotope scanning.

Describe the nurse's responsibility in conducting a gastric analysis, lumbar puncture, thoracentesis, abdominal paracentesis, and proctosigmoidoscopy.

Discuss the physical examination, using the nursing process as a guide.

Collecting Data on the Patient's Physical Health

GLOSSARY

Accommodation: The focusing ability of the eye.

Amplitude: The size or fullness of the pulse.

Anoscopy: A visual examination of the anal canal.

Anoxia: An absence of oxygen.

Antipyretic: A fever-reducing agent.

Apical-Radial Pulse: The pulse rates counted at the apex of the heart and at the radial artery simultaneously.

Apnea: The absence of breathing.

Arrhythmia: An irregular pulse rhythm.

Ascites: The accumulation of fluid in the peritoneal cavity.

Atrioventricular or Auriculoventricular Node: The tissue at the base of the atrial septum that normally picks up the electrical current from the S-A node. Abbreviated A-V node.

Audiometer: A device used for testing hearing.

Auscultation: A method of examining by listening to sounds within the body.

Auscultory Gap: The disappearance of the sound of the blood flowing through the artery during Phase II of Korotkoff's sounds.

Barium Enema: The x-ray visualization of the large intestine.

Bigeminal Pulse: Two regular pulse contractions following by a pause.

Biopsy: The removal of a piece of tissue for microscopic examination.

Bounding Pulse: The feel of the pulse when it is difficult to obliterate the artery.

Bradycardia: A slow heartbeat.

Cardiac Output: The volume of blood forced out of the left ventricle each minute.

Cardinal Signs: Measurements of body temperature, pulse, respirations, and blood pressure. Synonym for vital signs.

Cheyne-Stokes Respirations: The gradual increase and then gradual decrease in depth of respiration followed by a period of apnea.

Circadian Rhythm: A biological or behavioral process that recurs in approximately every 24-hour cycle.

Conduction: The transfer of heat to another object by direct contact without perceptible movement.

Confusion: A condition of mental bewilderment.

Continued Fever: A temperature that remains consistently elevated and fluctuates very little.

Convection: The dissemination of heat by motion between areas of unequal density.

Core Temperature: The internal body temperature.

Crisis: A rapid drop of body temperature to normal.

Cyanosis: The bluish coloring of the skin and mucous membrane.

Dehydration: A depletion of body fluids.

Depolarize: To destroy polarity.

Diaphoresis: Excessive perspiration.

Diastole: The period when the least amount of pressure is exerted on the arterial walls during heartbeat.

Dicrotic Pulse: An exaggerated ending of the pulse wave which feels like a double pulse to touch.

Dimpling: A puckering of the skin.

Disoriented: The state of being unaware of time, place, and/or surroundings.

Dorsal Position: A position in which the patient lies flat on his back, legs together. Synonym for horizontal recumbent position.

Dorsal Recumbent Position: A position in which the patient is placed on his back close to the edge of the bed, legs separated, and knees flexed.

Dyspnea: Difficult breathing.

Ecchymosis: A collection of blood in subcutaneous tissues, causing purplish discoloration.

Ectopic Pacemaker: The areas where heart impulses may originate in the heart other than at the S-A node.

Edema: An excess amount of fluid retained in body tissue.

Electrocardiogram: A graphic record produced by the electrocardiograph. Abbreviated EKG.

Electrocardiograph: The instrument that measures and records electrical impulses of the heart.

Empyema: A collection of purulent fluid in the pleural cavity.

Endoscope: A lighted tubular instrument used to visualize the inside of organs and cavities.

Erect Position: The position in which the patient stands normally.

Essential Hypertension: An abnormally high blood pressure with no known cause. Synonym for primary hypertension.

Evaporation: The conversion of a liquid to a vapor.

Exhalation: The act of breathing out. Synonym for expiration.

Expiration: The act of breathing out. Synonym for exhalation.

External Respiration: The act of lung ventilation, oxygen absorption, and carbon dioxide elimination.

Fast: Abstinence from food and fluids.

Feeble Pulse: The feel of the pulse when blood volume is small and the artery can be easily obliterated. Also called weak or thready.

Fever: The lay term for an elevated body temperature. Synonym for pyrexia.

Fluoroscopy: The radiological visualization of motion without its being recorded on film.

Flush: A redness of the skin.

Fremitus: Vibratory tremors of the body.

Gastric Analysis: The laboratory examination of gastric contents.

Genupectoral Position: A position in which the patient rests on his knees and chest with the body flexed approximately 90° at the hips. Synonym for knee-chest position.

Hernia: The protrusion of an organ or a part of an organ through the cavity wall which normally contains it.

Homeothermal: The maintenance of the same body temperature, irrespective of environmental temperature.

Horizontal Recumbent Position: The position in which the patient lies flat on his back, legs together. Synonym for dorsal position.

Hyperpnea: An increased depth of respirations.

Hyperpyrexia: A high fever, above 41°C. (105.8° F.).

Hypertension: An abnormally high blood pressure.

Hypotension: An abnormally low blood pressure.

Hypothermia: A body temperature that is below the average normal range.

Hypoxia: Low oxygen content.

Incoherent: Pertaining to disconnected thought or speech.

Inhalation: The act of breathing in. Synonym for inspiration.

Inspiration: The act of breathing in. Synonym for inhalation.

Intermittent Fever: The alternating temperature between a period of pyrexia and a period of normal or subnormal temperature.

Intermittent Pulse: A period of normal pulse rhythm broken by periods of irregular rhythm.

Internal Respiration: The act of using oxygen by body cells. Synonym for tissue respiration.

Intravenous Pyelogram: The x-ray visualization of the kidney's ability to excrete urine. Commonly abbreviated IVP.

Jaundice: A yellowness of the skin.

Knee-Chest Position: A position in which the patient rests on his knees and chest with the body flexed approximately 90° at the hips. Synonym for genupectoral position.

Korotkoff's Sounds: The sounds that indicate systolic and diastolic pressure when determining blood pressure.

Lead: The placement pattern of electrodes used in electrocardiography.

Lesion: A circumscribed area of diseased or injured tissue.

Lithotomy Position: The same as the dorsal recumbent position except the feet are placed in stirrups and the buttocks are at the edge of the examining table.

Lumbar Puncture: The insertion of a needle into the subarachnoid space. Synonym for spinal tap.

Lysis: The gradual return of an elevated body temperature to normal.

Meniscus: The curved surface at the top of a column of liquid in a tube.

Mucus: The viscid watery-appearing secretion produced by mucous membrane.

Obesity: An excess amount of fat on the body.

Ophthalmoscope: A lighted instrument used for examining the interior of the eye.

Oriented: The state of being aware of time, place, and surroundings.

Orthopnea: A type of dyspnea in which breathing is easier when the patient sits or stands up.

Otoscope: A lighted instrument used for examining the external ear canal and the tympanic membrane.

Pallor: Paleness of the skin.

Palpation: A method of examining by feeling a part with the fingers or hand.

Palpitation: The perception of one's own heartbeat.

Paracentesis: The withdrawal of fluid from a body cavity; usually from the abdominal cavity.

Parallax: An apparent change of position of an object when seen from two different angles.

Percussion: A method of examination that helps to determine the density of a part by means of tapping the surface.

Percussion Hammer: An instrument with a rubber head used for tapping a body surface.

Poikilothermal: The maintenance of the same body temperature as environmental temperature.

Polarity: The existence of opposing attributes.

Polypnea: A respiratory rate above average normal range.

Precordium: The anterior surface of the chest wall overlying the heart and its related structures.

Premature Beat: A cardiac contraction occurring before the normal one.

Primary Hypertension: An abnormally high blood pressure with no known cause. Synonym for essential hypertension.

Proctoscopy: A visual examination of the rectum.

Proctosigmoidoscopy: A visual examination of the rectum, rectosigmoid junction, and lower sigmoid colon.

Prosthesis: An appliance or artificial part used for a natural part of the body.

Pulse: A wave set up in the walls of the artery with each beat of the heart.

Pulse Deficit: The difference between the apical and radial pulse rates.

Pulse Pressure: The difference between systolic and diastolic pressure.

Pulse Volume: The feel of the blood flow through the vessel.

Purkinje System: The interlacing network in ventricles that carry electrical currents through the ventricles.

Pyrexia: An elevation of body temperature. Synonym for fever.

Radiation: The diffusion or dissemination of heat via electromagnetic waves.

Radiography: The use of x-rays for securing data.

Radioisotope: A radioactive chemical.

Radiopaque: A substance which x-rays cannot penetrate.

Rash: An eruption of the skin.

Recrudescent Fever: Recurring pyrexia after the temperature has returned to normal.

Remittent Fever: An above normal fluctuating temperature.

Repolarization: The process of restoring polarity.

Respiration: The act of breathing and of using oxygen in body cells.

Responsive: Answering with word and/or gesture.

Retraction: A skin depression.

Roentgen Ray: A high-energy electromagnetic wave which is capable of penetrating solid matter and acting on photographic film. Synonym for x-ray.

Secondary Hypertension: An abnormally high blood pressure which is caused by known pathology.

Sims's Position, Right or Left: A position in which the patient is on his side with the top knee flexed sharply onto the abdomen and the lower knee less sharply flexed.

Sinoatrial or Sinoauricular Node: The tissue in the upper part of the right atrium where the heartbeat originates. Abbreviated S-A node. Also called the heart's pacemaker.

Sphygmomanometer: An instrument used for indirect measurement of the blood pressure.

Spinal Tap: The insertion of a needle into the subarachnoid space. Synonym for lumbar puncture.

Sputum: A substance from the respiratory tract ejected from the mouth.

Stertorous Respiration: Noisy breathing.

Stethoscope: An instrument used to amplify sounds made by the body.

Stroke Volume: The quantity of blood forced out of the left ventricle with each contraction.

Symmetry: A correspondence in relative contour, size, color, and position of parts on opposite sides of the body.

Systole: A period when maximum pressure is exerted on the arterial walls during heartbeat.

Tachycardia: A rapid heartbeat.

Thoracentesis: The entrance and aspiration of fluid from the pleural cavity.

Tidal Air: The volume of air exchanged with each respiration in a state of rest.

Tissue Respiration: The act of using oxygen by body cells. Synonym for internal respiration.

Tonometer: An instrument for measuring pressure within the eye.

Transducer: An instrument which converts energy from one form to another.

Tuning Fork: An instrument which sets up vibrations which are used for testing hearing.

Turgor: The tension of a cell determined by its hydration.

Tympany: A drumlike sound on percussion

resulting from the presence of air or gas.

Ultrasonography: The use of ultrasound to produce an image or photograph of an organ or tissue.

Ultrasound Waves: Extremely high-frequency and inaudible sound waves.

Unconscious: The lack of capacity for sensory perception.

Unresponsive: The apparent unawareness of one's surroundings.

Upper GI Series: The x-ray visualization of the esophagus, stomach, and duodenum.

Urinalysis: The laboratory examination of a urine specimen.

Vaginal Speculum: A two-bladed instrument used for opening the vagina for examination of it and the cervix.

Vasoconstriction: The condition in which arterioles are in a state of contraction to a greater than usual degree.

Vasodilation: The condition in which arterioles are in a state of enlargement to a greater than usual degree.

Vital Signs: Measurements of body temperature, pulse, respirations, and blood pressure. Synonym for cardinal signs.

Wound: A break in the continuity of the skin.

X-ray: A high-energy electromagnetic wave which is capable of penetrating solid matter and acting on photographic film. Synonym for roentgen ray.

INTRODUCTION

The collection of data and their assessment are essential before nursing care can be planned and given, as Unit II described. This chapter presents common methods used in collecting data about the state of the individual's physical health. Usual techniques for determining vital physiological functions, an introduction to conducting a physical examination, and general methods of collecting certain other information are discussed. In addition, standards in the form of normal findings which can be used in assessing data, are also included.

According to the dictionary, the word physical means the body as distinguished from the mind. As this text has stated earlier, it is almost impossible to separate the mind and body; rather, both function interdependently and as a whole. Although the primary focus of this chapter is on the physical health state, the patient's mental and emotional status are not to be ignored.

The expanded role of the nurse was discussed in Chapter 1. In many schools of nursing, students are being taught to assume more responsibility for collecting data about the person's physical status and using it to make nursing judgments than once was the case. Also, in many health agencies, graduate nurses are taking increased responsibility for the physical examination. In some settings now, the nurse is often expected to conduct the entire initial physical assessment. The reader will be expected to observe the policy in her school of nursing or in the health agency in which she practices concerning the exact responsibility she will assume for collecting physical data and using the information.

It is assumed that the nurse has a sound knowledge of anatomy and physiology before she proceeds with collecting data about the person's state of physical health. Except for the vital signs, anatomy and physiology are not discussed here, and if necessary, the reader should review appropriate texts. Details of specific techniques and the interpretation of abnormal findings of a physical examination are also not described here. These techniques and their interpretations are more appropriately discussed in clinical nursing texts.

IDENTIFYING APPROPRIATE DATA

Before the nurse collects information about the patient's physical status, decisions must be made about selecting appropriate data. The guidelines offered in Chapter 4 are applicable here. For example, three questions to assist the nurse in selecting relevant data are helpful. Who is the patient? Why is the person being considered for nursing care? What factors in the person's life are playing a part in influencing his present health status?

The particular circumstances of the person will determine which data will be appropriate for his situation. In some instances, data may be collected about only one or two physiological functions, such as cardiac and respiratory functioning. In others, a complete physical examination may be necessary. Frequently, the physical examination is conducted when the patient has his initial contact with the health agency or practitioner. Data about specific bodily functions are often repeatedly collected when there is an indication of a particular problem or when comparative information about a physiological response is desired. The nurse decides which data are appropriate, based on knowledge of the patient's situation.

The collection of physical health data may be said to begin when the person is admitted to a health agency. Certain basic information gathered on admission will be useful during the examination, such as the person's name, address, age, sex, primary complaint if any, and so on. This type of background information was discussed in Chapter 5. A health history is then obtained, generally from the individual. History-taking was discussed in Chapter 4.

There is no one correct method of organizing data. Health agencies generally have forms to help guide the nurse in selecting as well as in organizing data. The importance of recording data accurately cannot be overemphasized. The forms are used according to health agency policy.

DETERMINING SOURCES AND METHODS FOR COLLECTING DATA

This chapter will focus primarily on the use of observation for collecting data. Four methods are commonly used: inspection, palpation, percussion, and auscultation.

Inspection is purposeful and systematic observation. Most often, inspection involves the visual sense, such as looking to observe the color of the skin or wound drainage. Inspection can also involve the sense of hearing, such as listening to the nature of a cough or the quality of a voice. Inspection can utilize the olfactory sense as well, such as smelling to detect the characteristic of an odor.

Palpation involves the sense of touch as the examiner uses his hands and fingers to feel or press on the body. Palpation is used when the skin is touched to detect a change in temperature, or when the abdomen is examined to feel the various internal organs.

Percussion involves tapping a particular area of the body, either with the fingertips or with a percussion hammer, in order that the examiner may listen for sounds to determine density of the tissue. For instance, percussion is used when the examiner taps the patient's chest wall to determine the sound created. If fluid or a solid mass is present, the sound will be dull when the level of fluid or obstruction is passed, a hollow sound will be heard.

Auscultation uses the sense of hearing for interpreting sounds made by the body and usually is performed with the aid of the stethoscope. Auscultation is used when the examiner listens to the patient's heart and lung sounds with the stethoscope or when the blood pressure is measured.

In most instances, the person himself is the chief source of data. Occasionally, past records also serve as sources. When the individual has past health records available, the nurse may want to examine them. In some situations, the previous records may be current, and after validation, the nurse may decide some data on the record are satisfactory and need not be gathered again. In other instances, the collection of new information is necessary and may be used to determine changes in bodily functions which have occurred over time.

COLLECTING DATA

The discussion in this chapter, will begin with a general overall observation of the person followed by measurement of the weight and height and the vital signs. Then, a general head-to-toe order of examination will be described. In practice, only selected data may be collected in a particular patient situation.

Preparation for Collecting Data # 3

The patient should be prepared for the collection of data about his physical health by an explanation from the nurse. She should explain the purpose of the data collection, what she intends to do, and what use will be made of the information. Especially if the person has never had a physical examination, he needs to be assured that the examiner will instruct him in what to expect. A few minutes spent in explanation often helps a great deal in allaying anxiety and in securing the patient's cooperation. Relaxation and active participation by the patient can make data collection easier, more accurate, and more productive.

If a complete physical examination is to be performed, the person should be requested to undress and wear a patient gown to facilitate the examination. The individual is also asked to empty his urinary bladder before the examination because abdominal organs can be distorted by a distended bladder.

Data about the status of the person's physical health are usually collected in an examination or treatment room. The hospitalized patient's room or a room in the home may be used, but these settings are generally not as convenient. The setting should provide privacy. The room should be quiet, because excessive environmental noises may make detection of some physiological sounds difficult. The availability of adequate lighting is also an important factor in selecting a room. The examiner should be able to darken the room to facilitate some parts of the eye examination. A bright, nondistorting light for accurate inspection of skin surfaces is also necessary.

Most health agencies have a tray for storing necessary equipment. The following items should be available when a physical examination is conducted, even though they may not all be used.

An *ophthalmoscope* is a lighted instrument used for examining the interior of the eye. An *otoscope* is a lighted instrument used for examining the external ear canal and the tympanic membrane. The ophthalmoscope and otoscope heads are often interchanged on the same light source. The otoscope is usually equipped with varying sizes of funnel-shaped tips, including one which can be used for examining the nose. A *vaginal speculum* is a two-bladed instrument used for opening the vagina for examination of it and the cervix. A *percussion hammer* is an instrument with a rubber head used to tap the body surface, test reflexes, and determine tissue density. A *tuning fork* is an instrument which sets up vibrations which are used for testing hearing. These instruments are pictured in Figure 15–1. A *tonometer* is an instrument for measuring pressure within the eye.

A *stethoscope* is an instrument used to amplify sounds made by the body. A *sphygmomanometer* is an instrument used for indirect measurement of the blood pressure.

A thermometer, watch with a second hand, tongue depressors, skin pencil, pen light, tape measure, eye chart, safety pins, cotton, test tubes, specimen containers, sterile and clean gloves, and lubricant are also necessary. In addition, paper towels, a drape, disposable pad, waste container, and a soiled instrument container should be accessible.

As part of a physical examination, several laboratory tests are commonly done. Each agency has its own procedure or laboratory manual concerning the type of container in which to collect the specimen, the amount of specimen needed, preparation of the specimen, the laboratory to which the specimen is sent and so on. The nurse's responsibilities will vary, depending on the agency's procedure.

The nurse will wish to have material available for draping. Some agencies have disposable paper drapes, but the same purpose can be achieved with a bath blanket, a draw sheet, or the top bedcovers if the patient is examined in a bed. The purpose of draping is to avoid exposing the patient except for the part being examined. Sometimes, it may be necessary to provide and extra cover to prevent the patient from drafts or being chilled. This is particularly true when the patient is very ill or elderly.

The patient may need assistance in assuming and retaining proper positions for examining. While the examination is being conducted, the nurse keeps the patient draped properly, exposing areas of the body only as indicated. The legal implications when a patient is exposed unnecessarily were discussed in Chapter 2 in the section dealing with invasion of privacy.

Observing the Person's General State of Health

At the moment of her first contact with the person, the nurse begins her observation of the individual's general state of health. Her purpose is to collect information about the overall functioning of the person in contrast to specific body functions or parts, which will be examined later.

Observations which can be included are as follows: What is the person's body build and proportions? Does he appear thin or overweight? What is his general skin condition? Does he have any obvious lesions or deformities? Is his posture erect? If he walks, is his gait smooth and coordinated? Are his other motor movements purposeful and coordinated? Does his appearance indicate that personal hygiene is attended to? Is his speech clear and paced and pitched appropriately? Is there obvious evidence of a physiological problem? For example, is he having difficulty breathing, or is he grimacing in pain? Descriptive recordings of these and other physical observations help to provide an overall picture of the person's general state of health.

While observing general physical characteristics, the nurse should become aware of the individual's mental

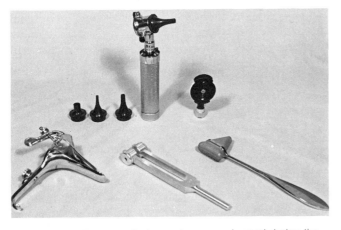

Figure 15–1 These are instruments commonly used during the physical examination. Top, left to right: various sizes of otoscope tips, otoscope, ophthalmoscope head. Bottom, left to right: vaginal speculum, tuning fork, percussion hammer.

responsiveness and orientation and of emotions he may be experiencing. The following are some common terms used to describe a person's mental state.

To be *oriented* means to be aware of time, place, and surroundings; to be *disoriented* is the opposite. The word *confusion* describes a condition of mental bewilderment. A *responsive* patient answers by word, or gesture, or both; the *unresponsive* patient appears to be unaware of his surroundings and unable to answer when spoken to. The word *incoherent* describes disconnected thought or speech. The thoughts are unrelated and the listener is unable to make sense from what is being said. The *unconscious* patient lacks the capacity for sensory perception. When using such terms, it is helpful to describe what the patient actually says or does, or does not say or do; for example: "Could not answer appropriately when asked current date and city where he was"; "Responded appropriately to all questions"; "Spoke of brother, who has been dead for years, as if he were alive"; "Speaks in phrases which have no apparent relationship to each other."

Chapter 10 described common emotions, and the nurse will wish to be alert to behavior that reflects the patient's emotional state. Terms such as anxious, accepting, pleasant, cooperative, frightened, unconcerned, resentful, and uncooperative are often difficult to define and may be interpreted differently among health and nursing team members. Therefore, it is better to record the behavior observed; for example: "Facial and extremity muscles tense, jaw set, hands clenched, perspiring heavily"; "Moves frequently about room, talking rapidly, exaggerated response to sound stimuli"; "Smiles and converses readily, initiates removal of dressing."

Measuring the Person's Height and Weight

It is common practice to measure a person's height and weight when the individual is admitted to a health agency. Even though the person may have been weighed recently, it is preferable to weigh him on admission so that subsequent weights can be taken on the same scale, thus making comparisons more accurate. The person's height is measured at the same time. He should be asked to remove his shoes or slippers for this procedure. It is good medical asepsis to place a paper towel on the scale before the person stands on it with his bare feet and to use a clean towel for each succeeding person.

Weighing the individual and measuring his height may be delayed if he is too ill, unless it is necessary to

know his weight for purposes of therapy. To make weighing easier for very ill patients, some agencies have portable or bed scales. The scale can be rolled to the patient's bedside where he can be assisted onto it.

Many factors enter into a consideration of what is normal weight, such as age, body build, height, and sex. Therefore, it is difficult to determine where abnormality begins. Most authorities accept a 10 to 15 percent variation from the norm described in weight tables as being within acceptable limits. The standard for *obesity,* which is an excess amount of fat on the body, is 20 percent over the weight norm. Table 15–1 provides a standard for assessing weight and height data. Other body measurements used in some situations include triceps size, skin-fold thicknesses, and arm circumferences. The nurse will wish to be aware of evidence that suggests the person is experiencing unusual weight losses or gains.

THE VITAL SIGNS

Alterations in body function often are reflected in the body temperature, the pulse, respirations, and the blood pressure. Physiological mechanisms governing them are very sensitive and normally keep them regulated within a narrow range. Any change from normal is considered to be a significant indication of the person's state of health. That is why they are frequently called *vital signs* or *cardinal signs.*

Palpation and auscultation are the primary methods used to measure the vital signs. The introduction of monitoring devices has made it possible to keep patients' vital signs under constant surveillance in hospital settings. This has been a lifesaving measure for many patients because it provides a far more accurate means of observing the effects of pathology and therapy.

Obtaining a person's vital signs is part of most agency admission procedures. These data provide part of the baseline information from which a plan of care is developed. It is recommended that upon the person's admission, the nurse obtain these signs whenever possible rather than assigning the task to auxilliary nursing personnel who may have less knowledge about measuring these important indicators of the health status.

Measurement of the vital signs is also routinely repeated for both hospitalized and nonhospitalized persons for comparison with previous measurements. The intervals between repeating the measurements vary

TABLE 15–1. Desirable Weights for Women and Men.

Weight in Pounds According to Frame (In Indoor Clothing)

	HEIGHT (with shoes on) 1-inch heels Feet Inches	SMALL FRAME	MEDIUM FRAME	LARGE FRAME
MEN OF AGES 25 AND OVER	5 2	112–120	118–129	126–141
	5 3	115–123	121–133	129–144
	5 4	118–126	124–136	132–148
	5 5	121–129	127–139	135–152
	5 6	124–133	130–143	138–156
	5 7	128–137	134–147	142–161
	5 8	132–141	138–152	147–166
	5 9	136–145	142–156	151–170
	5 10	140–150	146–160	155–174
	5 11	144–154	150–165	159–179
	6 0	148–158	154–170	164–184
	6 1	152–162	158–175	168–189
	6 2	156–167	162–180	173–194
	6 3	160–171	167–185	178–199
	6 4	164–175	172–190	182–204

	HEIGHT (with shoes on) 2-inch heels Feet Inches	SMALL FRAME	MEDIUM FRAME	LARGE FRAME
WOMEN OF AGES 25 AND OVER	4 10	92– 98	96–107	104–119
	4 11	94–101	98–110	106–122
	5 0	96–104	101–113	109–125
	5 1	99–107	104–116	112–128
	5 2	102–110	107–119	115–131
	5 3	105–113	110–122	118–134
	5 4	108–116	113–126	121–138
	5 5	111–119	116–130	125–142
	5 6	114–123	120–135	129–146
	5 7	118–127	124–139	133–150
	5 8	122–131	128–143	137–154
	5 9	126–135	132–147	141–158
	5 10	130–140	136–151	145–163
	5 11	134–144	140–155	149–168
	6 0	138–148	144–159	153–173

For girls between 18 and 25, subtract 1 pound for each year under 25.

Courtesy of the Metropolitan Life Insurance Company, New York.

with the individual. It can be as often as several times an hour for hospitalized patients, each visit with ambulatory persons, or much less frequently. The comparison of vital signs is considered a good gauge of changes in the person's condition.

Most adults are familiar with the procedures for obtaining body temperature, pulse and respiratory rates, and blood pressure. However, an explanation of the procedures by the nurse may help put the person at ease, especially if he is anxious about the results. Distress can cause the vital signs to increase, and hence, every effort should be made to help the person relax as much as possible. Explanations should be given to children also for the same reason.

Body Temperature

A phenomenon known as the "24-hour" or *circadian rhythm* has been observed in many animals, including man. Certain daily events in biological man appear to recur every 24 hours, and therefore, the word circadian, meaning "nearly every 24 hours," is often used to describe the rhythm. The rhythm can be observed in biological functioning that involves body temperature, sleep, and blood pressure. Body temperature, for instance, is usually 0.6 to 0.12° C. (1° to 2° F.) lower in the early morning than in late afternoon. This variation tends to be somewhat higher in infants and young children.

Man is *homeothermic;* that is, he is warm-blooded and maintains body temperature independently of his environment. Cold-blooded animals are *poikilothermic,* meaning their body temperature is the same as their environment. Fish, frogs, and reptiles are poikilothermic animals.

Temperature Regulation. There are various factors that influence body temperature regulation or control. Temperature is maintained through a balance between heat loss and heat production. This balance is influenced by physical and chemical means and through nervous system stimulation.

The body produces heat chemically through the metabolism of food. Body metabolism will increase in order to produce more heat for the body as necessary. In cold weather, a diet high in protein which stimulates metabolism aids in heat production. During hot weather, a high-protein diet will place added work upon mechanisms that produce heat dissipation. Heat production is increased also by epinephrine, norepinephrine, and thyroxin.

Physically, the body gains heat from its environment, but this is of lesser significance than heat produced chemically. For example, clothing, sun, and the ingestion of hot foods may increase body temperature.

The body "stokes its furnace" to produce heat through stimulants to metabolism. This is generally brought about by increased muscular tone. The contraction of smooth muscles when "gooseflesh" occurs is an example. Shivering is movement of skeletal muscles by involuntary nervous control which stimulates metabolism. Exercising, often found comforting when one is cold, increases muscle tone and stimulates metabolism which in turn increases heat production.

Heat is dissipated from the body primarily through physical processes. As much as 95 percent is lost through radiation and convection and through evaporation of water from the lungs and skin. *Radiation* is the diffusion or dissemination of heat via electromagnetic waves. *Convection* is the dissemination of heat by motion between areas of unequal density, such as from the body to cool moving air or to the water in a swimming pool. *Evaporation* is the conversion of a liquid to a vapor, such as occurs when water leaves the lungs and skin as vapor. Most of the remaining amount of heat is lost through urine and fecal excreta and in raising the temperature of inspired air to body temperature. A negligible amount is normally lost through conduction. *Conduction* is the transfer of heat to another object by direct contact without perceptible movement. The

body can lose heat by conduction when it is in contact with a cold surface for a prolonged time, such as when lying on a cold floor.

Temperature regulation is an example of homeostasis, which was discussed in Chapter 10. To maintain constancy of temperature, the hypothalamus in the central nervous system, located at the base of the brain, plays an important role as the body's thermostat. The hypothalamus has two parts: the anterior hypothalamus controls heat dissipation and the posterior hypothalamus governs heat conservation efforts.

What happens when body temperature is elevated? It is generally theorized that the thermostat in the temperature-regulating center is at a higher level and heat dissipation is decreased. The regulation of the temperature has not broken down; rather, the thermostat has been set at a higher degree. When fever begins, the skin is often pale and dry while metabolism is normal. Once fever reaches a certain level, balance begins again. The thermostat theory is also supported when one observes the action of *antipyretic,* or feverreducing, drugs; they are believed to reset the heatregulating center since these same drugs do not affect body temperature when the person's temperature is within normal range.

In summary, thermal balance is maintained through heat production and loss. Heat is produced primarily through metabolic activity and through exercise. Heat is lost to the environment through radiation, convection, evaporation, and conduction. Changes in the vascularity of the skin modify body temperature; when blood is directed to the skin through vasodilation, heat loss is increased, and when the skin vessels contract, heat is conserved. Perspiration protects the body from overheating because the body is cooled by evaporation. Shivering is an adaptive mechanism to conserve heat.

Normal Body Temperature. Body temperature is recorded in either degrees of Celsius or degrees of Fahrenheit, abbreviated C. or F., respectively. The Celsius designation has been official in this country since 1948 but its equivalent (centigrade) continues to be commonly used and is also abbreviated C. Table 15–2 illustrates comparable Celsius and Fahrenheit temperatures and explains how temperatures are converted from one scale to the other.

The thermometer is placed in the mouth to obtain an oral temperature, in the anal canal to obtain a rectal temperature, in the axilla to obtain an axillary temperature, or in the esophagus to obtain an esophageal temperature. The bodily organs require a fairly con-

TABLE 15–2 Equivalent Celsius and Fahrenheit temperatures and directions for converting temperatures from one scale to another.

CELSIUS	FAHRENHEIT	CELSIUS	FAHRENHEIT
34.0	93.2	38.5	101.3
35.0	95.0	39.0	102.2
36.0	96.8	40.0	104.0
36.5	97.7	41.0	105.8
37.0	98.6	42.0	107.6
37.5	99.5	43.0	109.4
38.0	100.4	44.0	111.2

To convert Celsius to Fahrenheit, multiply by 9/5 and add 32. To change Fahrenheit to Celsius, subtract 32 and multiply by 5/9.

stant internal or *core temperature* for optimum functioning. Detection of the internal temperature is complex and difficult, and hence, the body temperature is ordinarily measured rectally or orally. The axillary area is also used to obtain the body temperature because of its convenience when other sites are contraindicated, but it is generally considered to be the least reliable site. The esophagus is considered to be the site where the temperature is closest to the core temperature. However, because of difficulty in measuring in this location, it is usually used only when the most precise knowledge of the body temperature is considered necessary, such as in certain types of therapy using hypothermia. Table 15–3 shows the average normal temperature standards for well adults in the various body sites.

Variations occur in each individual and a range of 0.3° to 0.6° C. (0.5° to 1.0° F.) from the average normal temperature is considered to be within normal limits. However, wider variations from the average temperature have been found to be normal for certain individuals. Factors, such as endocrine secretions, environmental conditions, exercise, drugs, food, emotions, and age, are felt to have some effect on variations in body temperature.

The body temperature has been observed to be lowest during the early morning hours and highest during the late afternoon or early evening hours. An inversion of this cycle has been observed in persons who routinely work at night and sleep during the day. Exercise, manner of living, amount and kind of food ingested, and external cold may also influence body tempera-

ture. Newborns and young children normally have a higher body temperature than adults.

Elevated Body Temperature. *Pyrexia* is an elevation in normal body temperature. The lay term for pyrexia is fever. *Hyperpyrexia* is high fever, usually above 41° C. (105.8° F.). Pyrexia is a common symptom of illness, and there is sufficient evidence to believe that an elevation in body temperature aids the body in fighting disease. For instance, in an infectious disease, when the causative organisms are destroyed by a total body response, the elevated temperature apparently helps to destroy bacteria as well as to mobilize the body's defenses. In children, this response is often seen quickly. Sudden high fever is often the first sign of illness in a child. In the very old person, pyrexia may be one of the last signs when illness occurs and the temperature may be elevated only one or two degrees above normal.

The physiological reason for pyrexia is not understood clearly, but it is believed commonly that it is the result of a direct action on the temperature-regulating center in the hypothalamus. Heat loss is decreased or heat production is increased or both occur when body temperature rises above normal. Cells in the central nervous system may be impaired when the body temperature surpasses 41° C. (105.8° F.), and survival is rare when it reaches 43° C. (109.4° F.). When high body temperature occurs, death is usually due to failure of the respiratory center, but may be due also to inactivation of body enzymes and destruction of tissue proteins.

Pyrexia may take a variety of courses, usually depending on the pathological process occurring in the body. Several terms are used to describe the course of an elevated body temperature. The onset or invasion is the period when pyrexia begins; it may be either sudden or gradual. When the temperature alternates regularly between a period of pyrexia and a period of normal or subnormal temperature, it is called an *intermittent fever*. A *remittent fever* is one that fluctuates several degrees above normal but does not reach normal between fluctuations. A *continued fever* is one that remains consistently elevated and fluctuates very little. When pyrexia subsides suddenly, the drop to normal is called a *crisis;* a gradual return to normal temperature is called *lysis.* In certain instances, when body temperature has returned to normal following pyrexia, a patient may experience a temporary *recrudescence* or recurrence of fever. This may be due to increased activity or exertion, in which case there is usually little cause

TABLE 15–3 Average normal temperatures for well adults in various body sites.

	ORAL	RECTAL	AXILLARY	ESOPHOGEAL
C.	37°	37.5°	36.7°	37.3°
F.	98.6°	99.5°	98°	99.2°

for alarm. However, a recurring fever may also be a sign of relapse; therefore, the temperature warrants frequent checking.

When pyrexia occurs, body metabolism is elevated above normal, and the respiratory rate and the pulse rate will also increase, as a rule proportionately with increased body temperature. The patient usually experiences loss of appetite, headaches, general malaise, depression, and occasional periods of delirium. Observing for other signs as body temperature rises is important, such as decreased urinary output and dehydration of the skin and mucous membrane. Nursing measures associated with these conditions are discussed in other chapters.

Lowered Body Temperature. A body temperature below the average normal range is called *hypothermia*. Death usually occurs when the temperature falls below approximately 34° C. (93.2° F.), but exceptional cases of survival have been reported when body temperatures

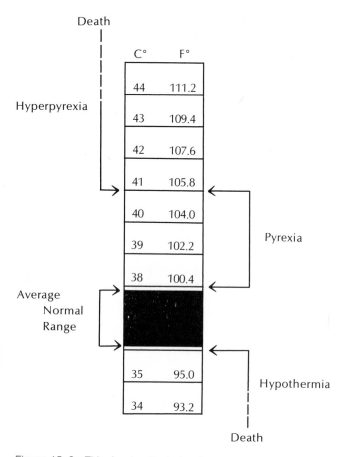

Figure 15-2 This drawing illustrates the range of human body temperature, as measured orally.

have fallen considerably lower. There are a few illnesses associated with hypothermia, especially those producing unconsciousness; therefore, it is important to observe a patient closely when body temperature falls below normal.

Just as an elevated body temperature is a protective device for the body, a lowered body temperature may be beneficial also. Rates of chemical reactions in the body are slowed, thereby decreasing the metabolic demands for oxygen. Hypothermia as a form of therapy is discussed in clinical texts. Figure 15–2 illustrates the range of human body temperature.

The Thermometer. The glass thermometer has traditionally been most commonly used to measure body temperature, but newer devices are now becoming popular. The glass thermometer has two parts, the bulb and the stem. Mercury is in the bulb and, being a metal, will expand when exposed to heat and rise in the stem. The stem is calibrated in degrees and tenths of a degree. The range is from approximately 34° C. (93° F.) to approximately 42.2° C. (108° F.). A wider range of temperature is not necessary, since human life rarely exists above or below these temperatures.

Fractions of a degree usually are recorded in tenths, such as 0.2 to 0.6 or 0.8. If the mercury appears to be a bit more or less than an even tenth, it is common practice to report the nearest tenth.

Some oral thermometers have a long slender mercury bulb, and others have a blunt bulb similar to that used on almost all rectal thermometers. The blunt bulb on the rectal thermometer helps to prevent injury when it is inserted. The long slender bulb on the oral thermometer is thought to give a larger surface area for contact. When using a thermometer in the home or in a different agency, check to see whether it is an oral or a rectal thermometer. Some thermometers have this printed on them; others do not. Rectal thermometers should not be used orally.

Most hospitals have adopted the procedure of using one thermometer for each patient. The thermometer is kept in the patient's unit and is disposed of when he is discharged or it is sent home with the patient. It has been recommended that thermometers used for patients having hepatitis be discarded when the patient is discharged.

Electronic thermometers measure body temperature in a matter of seconds. They are felt to be more accurate than glass thermometers. Most have two temperature probes, one for oral and one for rectal use, both of which are nonbreakable. They are equipped with disposable covers, a feature that minimizes chances for cross-infection and cleaning chores. There are various models available; some are hand held, others are desk models, and still others fasten to clipboards.

Disposable single-use thermometers are also available. They register within seconds, are nonbreakable, and because they are used only once, eliminate the danger of cross-infectiion.

Another device for measuring temperature is a disposable patch or tape which is applied to the abdomen. The temperature-sensitive tape changes color at different temperature ranges. It is generally recommended for use with well infants born at term. A thermometer should be used to check the infant's temperature if the color on the tape illustrates that the temperature is either above or below normal average range.

There are also devices which provide for a constant monitoring of a patient's temperature. These are generally used when the patient is critically ill. The thermometer probe can be attached to an alarm device that indicates when the patient's temperature moves beyond a specific range.

Palpation can be used for making a gross estimate of the body temperature. It is recommended that the nurse use the dorsal surface of her hand because it is more sensitive to temperature stimuli than the palm of the hand. However, using a thermometer or other heat-sensitive device is a more accurate and more precise way to determine body temperature.

Selecting a Site for Obtaining Body Temperature. Most agency policies specify the site to be used for obtaining the temperature. However, the nurse must make modifications in certain circumstances.

Oral temperatures are contraindicated for unconscious, irrational, and seizure-prone patients and for infants because of the danger of breaking the thermometer in the mouth. Oral temperatures are also contraindicated for persons who breathe through their mouths, and those with diseases of the oral cavity or surgery of the nose or the mouth. Traditionally, oral temperatures have not been taken on patients receiving nasal oxygen therapy because it was believed that the oxygen caused a false low reading. Present research is challenging this belief.

If the patient has had either hot or cold food or fluids or has been smoking or chewing gum, it is generally recommended that a period of approximately 30 minutes should elapse before an oral temperature is obtained to allow time for the oral tissues to return to normal temperature.

A rectal temperature has traditionally been considered to be more accurate than an oral temperature. However, this opinion is now being challenged by some authorities. If a patient having an oral temperature taken routinely shows a considerable change in his temperature, it is good practice to check it rectally. Some hospitals require rectal readings on patients having an elevated temperature. It is usual procedure to obtain rectal temperatures for most ill infants and for unconscious and irrational patients. Rectal temperatures are contraindicated for patients having rectal surgery, diarrhea, or diseases of the rectum. Because insertion of the thermometer can act as a cardiac stimulant, rectal temperatures are also generally not taken on persons with certain heart diseases.

An axillary temperature is generally obtained only when both oral and rectal temperatures are contraindicated or the sites are not usable or accessible. Some hospitals take routine temperatures by the axillary method on normal newborns. Unless the patient is capable of cooperating, the nurse will need to remain in attendance to hold the thermometer. The axillary method is the least accurate way of obtaining body temperature, since the axilla is easily influenced by environmental conditions and because it is often difficult to approximate skin surfaces while the bulb of the thermometer is held in place. If the axilla has just been washed, taking the temperature should be delayed, since the temperature of the water and the friction created by drying the skin will influence the temperature.

The procedures for obtaining oral, rectal, and axillary temperatures are described on pages 296–297.

Cleaning Clinical Thermometers. Making a glass clinical thermometer safe for use with another person presents a problem. Heat sufficient to kill pathogenic organisms will ruin thermometers by causing the mercury to expand beyond the column within the thermometer. Therefore, the method of choice is to disinfect thermometers in a chemical solution.

The suggested action and the underlying rationale for the procedure on page 297 apply to either oral or rectal glass thermometers. However, since a lubricant is used on a rectal thermometer, cleaning to remove the lubricant completely prior to disinfection is essential. If this is not done, organisms may harbor in a film of lubricant, and the disinfection procedure becomes ineffective. Detergents are particularly effective for emulsifying oils and fats even in cool and hard water; therefore it is preferable to use a detergent rather than soap.

Obtaining body temperature with a glass clinical thermometer

The purpose is to measure body temperature.

ORAL METHOD

SUGGESTED ACTION	RATIONALE
If the thermometer has been stored in a chemical solution, wipe it dry with a firm twisting motion, using clean soft tissue.	Chemical solutions may irritate the mucous membrane and may have an objectionable odor or taste. Soft tissue will approximate the surface, and twisting helps to contact the entire surface.
Wipe once from the bulb toward the fingers with each tissue.	Wiping from an area where there are few or no organisms to an area where organisms may be present minimizes the spread of organisms to cleaner areas.
Grasp the thermometer firmly with thumb and forefinger, and with strong wrist movements shake the thermometer until the mercury line reaches the lowest marking.	A constriction in the mercury line near the bulb of the thermometer prevents the mercury from dropping below the last temperature reading unless it is shaken down forcefully.
Read the thermometer by holding it horizontally at eye level, and rotate it between the fingers until the mercury line can be seen clearly.	Holding the thermometer at eye level facilitates reading. Rotating the thermometer will aid in placing the mercury line in a position where it can be read best.
Place the mercury bulb of the thermometer under the patient's tongue and instruct him to close his lips tightly.	When the bulb rests against the superficial blood vessels under the tongue and the mouth is closed, a measurement of body temperature can be obtained.
Leave the thermometer in place for seven to ten minutes.	Allowing sufficient time for the oral thermometer to reach its maximum temperature results in a more accurate measurement of body temperature.
Remove the thermometer and wipe it once from the fingers down to the mercury bulb, using a firm twisting motion.	Cleaning from an area where there are few organisms to an area where there are numerous organisms minimizes the spread of organisms to cleaner areas. Friction helps to loosen matter from a surface.
Read the thermometer and shake it down as described above.	
Dispose of wipe in a receptacle used for contaminated items.	Confining contaminated articles helps to reduce the spread of pathogens.

RECTAL METHOD

SUGGESTED ACTION	RATIONALE
Wipe, read, and shake the rectal thermometer as the suggested procedure for obtaining an oral temperature indicates.	
Lubricate the mercury bulb and an area approximately 2.5 cm. (1 inch) above the bulb.	Lubrication reduces friction and thereby facilitates insertion of the thermometer and minimizes irritation of the mucous membrane of the anal canal.
With the patient on his side, fold back the bed linen and separate the buttocks so that the anal sphincter is seen clearly. Insert the thermometer for approximately 3.8 cm. (1½ inches). Permit buttocks to fall in place.	If not placed directly into the anal opening the bulb of the thermometer may injure the sphincter, or hemorrhoids if present.
Leave the thermometer in place for two to three minutes. Hold the thermometer in place if the patient is irrational or is a restless child or infant.	Allowing sufficient time for the thermometer to register results in a more accurate measurement of body temperature.
Remove the thermometer and wipe it once from the fingers to the mercury bulb, using a firm twisting motion.	Cleaning from an area where there are few organisms to an area where there are numerous organisms minimizes the spread of organisms. Friction helps to loosen matter from a surface.
Read and shake the thermometer and dispose of wipe in a receptacle used for contaminated items.	

AXILLARY METHOD

SUGGESTED ACTION	RATIONALE
If the thermometer has been stored in a chemical solution, wipe it dry with a firm twisting motion, using a clean tissue.	Chemical solutions may irritate the skin. The presence of solution may alter the skin temperature. Soft tissue with the aid of friction helps in removing the solution.
Read and shake the thermometer as the suggested procedure for obtaining an oral temperature indicates.	
Place the thermometer well into the axilla with the bulb directed toward the patient's head. Bring the patient's arm down close to his body and place his forearm over his chest.	When the bulb rests against the superficial blood vessels in the axilla and the skin surfaces are brought together to reduce the amount of air surrounding the bulb, a reasonably reliable measurement of body temperature can be obtained.
Leave the thermometer in place for ten minutes or more.	Allowing sufficient time for the axillary thermometer to reach its maximum temperature results in a reasonably accurate measurement of body temperature.
Remove, read, and shake the thermometer and dispose of wipe.	

Disinfecting glass clinical thermometers

The purpose is to disinfect a glass clinical thermometer that has been used for obtaining a patient's temperature.

SUGGESTED ACTION	RATIONALE
Use a soft tissue for cleaning the thermometer.	Adhered organic matter interferes with disinfection.
Use a clean, soft tissue each time the thermometer must be wiped.	Soft tissue comes into close contact with all surfaces of the thermometer.
Hold the tissue at the end of the thermometer near the fingers.	Cleaning an area from where there are few organisms to an area where there are numerous organisms minimizes the spread of organisms to cleaner areas.
Wipe down toward the bulb, using a twisting motion.	Friction helps to loosen matter from a surface.
After the thermometer has been wiped, clean it with soap or detergent solution, again using friction.	Soap or detergent solutions loosen adhered matter.
Rinse the thermometer under cold running water.	Rinsing with water helps to remove organisms and foreign material loosened by washing. Also, certain chemical solutions are rendered ineffective in the presence of soap—for example, benzalkonium chloride (Zephiran Chloride).
Dry the thermometer after it has been rinsed.	The strength of a chemical solution is decreased when water is added to the solution.
Immerse the thermometer in the chemical solution specified.	Chemical solutions must be used in proper strength for the proper length of time in order to be effective.
Rinse the thermometer with water after disinfection and before reuse.	Chemical solutions may irritate the mucous membrane of the mouth or the rectum. Also, they may have an objectionable odor and taste.
Return the thermometer to the storage receptacle.	

In many agencies, it is common practice to have thermometers issued from a central supply unit. After being used, one thermometer for each patient, they are returned for cleaning and disinfection. The central supply unit may have a machine for shaking down the mercury in many thermometers simultaneously.

In the home, thermometers should be cleaned with soap and water and then stored for reuse by the same person. If the thermometer is to be used by more than one person or if the person has a known or suspected infection transmitted by oral secretions, it should be disinfected with an appropriate disinfectant following the cleaning.

The care and disposal of electronic and other types of thermometers vary with the manufacturer. The nurse should follow the manufacturer's recommendations.

Pulse

The stimulus for contraction of the heart starts in the sinoauricular or sinoatrial node, which is in the upper part of the right atrium. Because the node sets the pace of the beat, it is often called the pacemaker. The contraction stimulus, a type of electrical current, passes as a wave through the rest of the heart.

The heart is indeed a remarkable organ. In the average lifespan, it beats millions of times and pumps millions of gallons of blood. It rests for only part of a second between each beat and except for a malfunctioning heart, seldom is there a beat misplaced. About 5 liters of blood are estimated to be pumped from the heart every minute.

Each time the left ventricle of the heart contracts to eject blood into an already full aorta, the arterial walls in the blood system expand or distend to compensate for the increase in pressure. This expansion of the aorta sends a wave through the walls of the arterial system which, on palpation, can be felt as an impact or light tap. The sensation of the impact or tap is called the pulse.

The quantity of blood forced out of the left ventricle with each contraction is called the stroke volume. The cardiac output is the volume of blood forced out of the ventricle each minute or the stroke volume per minute. The stroke volume is multiplied by the number of contractions per minute to calculate the cardiac output. When the stroke volume decreases, such as when the blood volume is lowered because of hemorrhage, the contraction rate usually increases to maintain the same cardiac output.

Pulse Rate. On awakening in the morning, the pulse rate of the average healthy adult male is approximately 60 to 65 beats per minute. The pulse rate for women is slightly faster—about seven to eight beats per minute more than for men. Pulse varies with age, gradually diminishing from birth to adulthood and then increasing somewhat in very old age. It has been noted that body size and build of an individual may affect the pulse rate. Tall, slender persons often have a slower rate than short, stout ones. Very wide variations in pulse rates have been noted in normal healthy adults. The American Heart Association accepts as normal for adults a pulse rate of between 50 and 100 beats per minute. Table 15-4 shows the average pulse rates for well persons of various ages.

There are numerous causes for changes in the pulse rate. The rate of the heartbeat responds readily to

TABLE 15-4 Average pulse rates per minute for well persons at various ages.

AGE	PULSE RATE/MINUTE
Birth	120
1 year	110
5 years	95
10 years	85
Adolescent	80
Adult	75

impulses conducted along the sympathetic and the parasympathetic nervous systems. Stimulation of the sympathetic system increases the heart rate and, therefore, the pulse rate. This system responds quickly to emotions; consequently, the pulse rate increases when a person experiences fear, anger, surprise, or worry. The sympathetic system also receives impulses from internal organs of the body. Pain in the abdomen will cause the pulse rate to quicken, usually due to sympathetic stimulation. The rate also increases with exercise as the heart compensates for the increased need for blood circulation. Because the heart rate is influenced by activity and emotions, the pulse rate should be determined when the person is in a resting state whenever possible.

Prolonged application of heat to the skin will stimulate the heartbeat and increase the pulse rate. The pulse rate increases when blood pressure decreases as the heart attempts to increase the output of blood. When blood pressure returns to normal, the pulse rate usually will decrease. Elevated body temperature is accompanied by an increase in pulse rate—usually an increase of about seven to ten beats per minute for each 0.6° C. (1° F.) of elevation above normal.

When the pulse rate is over 100 beats per minute, the condition is called tachycardia. The word comes from two Greek words meaning quick and heart.

Stimulation of the parasympathetic system decreases pulse rate. The drug digitalis, commonly taken by patients having heart ailments, is one agent that decreases the pulse rate by stimulating the vagus nerves of the parasympathetic system.

The term used to describe the pulse rate when it falls below approximately 50 beats per minute is bradycardia. A slow pulse rate is less common during illness than a rapid pulse rate. Therefore, when bradycardia does occur, it should be reported to the physician immediately.

Rhythm of the Pulse. Normally, the pulse rhythm is regular, and the time interval between beats is equal.

The force of the normal pulse is equal with each beat. Irregular pulse rhythm is called *arrhythmia.* An *intermittent pulse* is one that has a period of normal rhythm broken by periods of irregular rhythm. An intermittent rhythm may be a serious sign, as in certain heart diseases, or it may be a temporary condition due to emotional upset or fright. If the ending of the pulse wave is exaggerated, the pulse wave feels double to touch, and the pulse is said to be a *dicrotic pulse.* A *bigeminal pulse* is two regular contractions followed by a pause.

Another form of arrhythmia is the premature contraction. A *premature beat* is a cardiac contraction occurring before the normal one. Because the contraction is early, it usually results in decreased stroke volume and thus is palpated as a weak pulsation. Sometimes persons with premature beats feel a sensation in the chest and describe their heart as "fluttering" or "skipping." Perception of one's own heartbeat is called *palpitation.*

Volume of the Pulse.   The *pulse volume* is the feel of the blood flow through the vessel. Under normal conditions, the volume of each pulse beat is equal. The pulse can be obliterated with relative ease, by exerting pressure over the artery, but it remains perceptible with moderate pressure. When blood volume makes it difficult to obliterate the artery, the pulse is called *bounding.* If the volume is small and the artery can be obliterated readily, the pulse is called *feeble,* weak, or thready. A thready pulse usually is associated with a rapid pulse rate.

The pulse is also sometimes described according to its size or fullness which is called *amplitude.* The amplitude reflects the strength of the left ventricular contraction. Amplitude is similar to volume and often recorded according to the following scale:

3+ —Bounding
2+ —Normal
1+ —Weak, Thready
0   —Absent

The Arterial Wall.   When the fingertips are placed over an artery, the sense of touch will determine certain characteristics of the arterial wall. Normally, it is elastic, straight, smooth and round. With advancing age, the arteries become less elastic and smooth, and a normally straight artery may feel tortuous to touch.

Common Sites for Palpating the Pulse.   Usually, the radial artery at the wrist is used for palpating the pulse rate, because it is easily accessible and it can be pressed against the radius. If it is not possible to palpate the pulse at the wrist, other superficial arteries of the body which overlie a bone may be used. A site should be used that does not produce exertion or discomfort for the person because this could alter the pulse rate. Alternate sites for palpating the pulse are described later.

Occasionally, a patient has a radial pulse that is difficult to count. It may be so irregular and the force of the beats so uneven that it is difficult to determine an accurate count. Using alternate sites may not provide any more accuracy. Two nurses checking the pulse may have different counts. A more accurate estimate of the heartbeats per minute should be obtained by auscultating with a stethoscope over the apex of the heart. The impulse contraction of the heart usually can be heard in the space between the fifth and sixth ribs about 8 cm. (3 inches) to the left of the median line and slightly below the nipple.

There are times when the *apical-radial pulse* rate may be taken; that is, the pulse rate is counted at the apex of the heart and at the radial artery simultaneously. This requires two persons; one listens over the apex of the heart with a stethoscope, and the other counts at the wrist. They use one watch conveniently placed between them. After listening and feeling to be sure that they can get the best possible count, they decide on a time to start counting, for example, when the second hand is at a specified place. At this time, both persons start counting for a full minute. Both the apical and radial counts are recorded. The apical-radial pulse is generally taken when the radial pulse is irregular. If a difference exists between the apical and radial pulse rates, it is called the *pulse deficit.*

Of the possible alternate sites for obtaining the pulse, the carotid, facial, and temporal arteries are the most common. The femoral and dosalis pedis arteries may be used also. They are used when information about the pulse in the lower extremities is desired. Figure 15–3 on pages 300–301 illustrates the common sites for palpating the pulse. The chart on page 302 describes how to obtain the radial pulse rate.

Respiration

Respiration, in its broadest sense, begins with the act of breathing and includes the body's use of oxygen and the elimination of carbon dioxide. *Inspiration* or *inhalation* is the act of breathing in, and *expiration* or *exhalation* is the act of breathing out. *External respiration* includes lung ventilation, the absorption of oxygen, and the

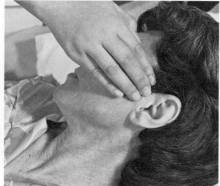

Temporal artery

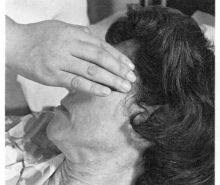

Facial artery

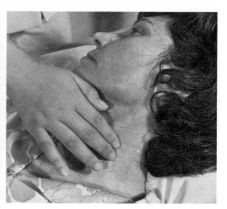

Carotid artery

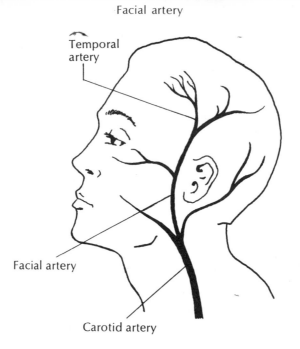

Temporal
artery

Facial artery

Carotid artery

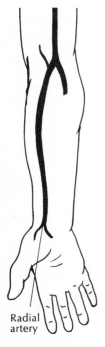

Radial
artery

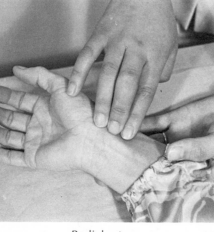

Radial artery

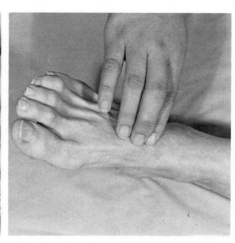

Dorsalis pedis artery

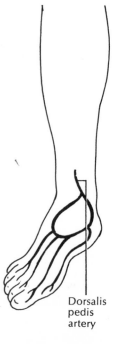

Dorsalis
pedis
artery

elimination of carbon dioxide. *Internal respiration,* sometimes called *tissue respiration,* includes the use of oxygen by body cells for the production of heat through oxidation and the liberation of energy from the food we eat.

The thorax is a closed structure. The air sacs of the lung communicate through the air passages (nose, pharynx, trachea, and bronchi) with the atmosphere. With inspiration, the thorax is enlarged, causing the pressure in the thorax to be less than atmospheric. The atmospheric pressure, being greater than the pressure in the thorax, forces air to the lungs that expand to fill the space of the enlarged thorax. The muscles involved with respiration contract to produce expiration. The diaphragm and the external intercostal muscles are the primary muscles of respiration. Other muscles of the thorax and those of the abdominal wall may also be involved; however, when breathing is difficult for any reason, they become important for assisting with respiration.

The chemical stimulation of an increased carbon dioxide tension in the blood is an important phenomenon of involuntary respiration. As carbon dioxide accumulates in the blood, the respiratory center is stimulated directly and also indirectly by the carotid and the aortic glomi, and the rate and the depth of respiration are increased. This involuntary chemical stimulation is responsible for the limitation of voluntary control of breathing. A new mother, not realizing this, may panic when her child has a temper tantrum and holds his breath.

When breathing is voluntary, impulses travel to the respiratory center in the medulla oblongata from the motor area of the cerebral cortex. Because of this arrangement, a person can automatically control his breathing when talking and singing, and voluntarily hold his breath until the carbon dioxide tension builds up excessively in the blood. Laughing from amusement or happiness and crying or sobbing from grief or sadness modify respirations by impulses from the brain that are carried to the respiratory center.

The respiratory center responds reflexly from impulses that can be carried over any sensory nerve in the body; excitement, anger, fear, pain, unusual sights and sounds will reflexly alter respiratory rates and depths. Coughing, sneezing, and hiccuping are modified acts of respirations also largely brought about reflexly. Afferent fibers or the pulmonic vagi also reflexly stimulate the respiratory center. Through this course, impulses from the lungs reflexly end each respiratory act. It is

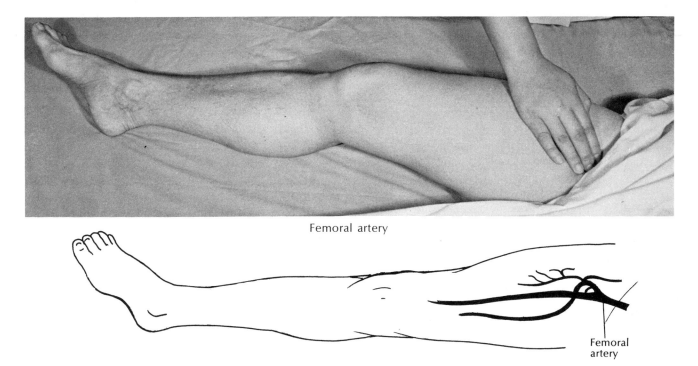

Femoral artery

Femoral artery

Figure 15–3 These photos illustrate common sites where the pulse rate can be readily obtained. The artist's sketches illustrate the location of the artery the nurse is palpating in each case.

Obtaining the radial pulse rate

The purpose is to count the number of times the heart beats per minute and to obtain an estimate of the quality of the heart's action.

SUGGESTED ACTION	RATIONALE
In the lying position, have the patient rest his arm alongside his body with the wrist extended and the palm of the hand downward. In the sitting position, have the forearm at a 90° angle to the body resting on a support and with the wrist extended and the palm of the hand downward.	These positions are ordinarily comfortable for the patient and convenient for the nurse.
Place the first, second, and third fingers along the radial artery and press gently against the radius; rest the thumb in apposition to fingers on the back of the patient's wrist.	The fingertips, sensitive to touch, will feel pulsation of patient's radial artery. If thumb is used for palpating the patient's pulse, the nurse may feel her own pulse.
Apply only enough pressure so that the patient's pulsating artery can be felt distinctly.	Moderate pressure allows the nurse to feel the superficial radial artery expand and contract with each heartbeat. Too much pressure will obliterate the pulse. If too little pressure is applied, the pulse will be imperceptible.
Using a watch with a second hand, count the number of pulsations felt on patient's artery for 30 seconds. Multiply this number by two to obtain the rate for one minute.	Sufficient time is necessary to study the rate, volume, and quality of the pulse.
If the pulse rate is abnormal in any way, count the pulse rate for a full minute or longer. Repeat counting if necessary to determine accurately the rate, quality, and volume of the pulse.	When the pulse is abnormal, full minute or longer countings are necessary to allow for the detection of irregular timing between beats.

believed that certain centers in the brain also reflexly affect respirations.

Respiratory Rate. Normally, healthy adults breathe approximately 16 to 20 times a minute. Wider variations have also been observed in healthy persons. The respiratory rate is more rapid in infants and young children. It has been noted that the relationship between the pulse rate and the respiratory rate is fairly consistent in well persons, the ratio being one respiration to approximately four heartbeats. Increased rate of respiration is called *polypnea*.

During illness, the respiratory rate may vary from normal. When body temperature is elevated, the respiratory rate increases as the body attempts to rid itself of excess heat. Any condition involving an accumulation of carbon dioxide and a decrease of oxygen in the blood also will tend to increase the rate and the depth of respirations.

There are conditions that characteristically predispose to slow breathing. An increase in intracranial pressure will depress the respiratory center, resulting in irregular and shallow, slow breathing, or both. Certain drugs will also depress the respiratory rate.

Respiratory Depth. At rest, the depth of each respiration is approximately the same. The volume of air normally exchanged in each respiration, the *tidal air,* varies greatly with individuals, but the average is about 500 ml. of air for a well adult. The depth of respirations is described as deep or shallow, depending on whether the volume of air taken in is above or below normal. Increased depth of respiration is called *hyperpnea.*

Nature of Respiration. Ordinarily, breathing is automatic, and respirations are noiseless, regular, even, and without effort. Between each respiration there is normally a short resting period.

Difficult breathing is called *dyspnea.* Dyspneic patients usually appear to be anxious, and their faces are drawn from exertion. Often, the nostrils will dilate as the patient fights for his breath. Usually, both abdominal and costal breathing are present. In abdominal breathing, the abdominal wall muscles relax and contract with respirations as they assist in making movements of the diaphragm more forceful. In costal breathing, the intercostal muscles raise the ribs to enlarge the chest cavity and thus assist respirations.

Dyspneic persons frequently find some relief if they sit in an upright or near upright position. This places the thorax in a vertical position. The condition of being able to breathe easier while in an upright position is known as *orthopnea.* The chart on page 303 describes obtaining the respiratory rate.

Cheyne-Stokes respirations refer to breathing consisting of a gradual increase in the depth of respirations followed by a gradual decrease in the depth of respirations

Obtaining the respiratory rate

The purpose is to obtain the respiratory rate per minute and an estimate of the patient's respiratory status.

SUGGESTED ACTION	RATIONALE
While the fingertips are still in place after counting the pulse rate, observe the patient's respirations.	Counting the respirations while presumably still counting the pulse helps to keep the patient from becoming conscious of his breathing and possibly altering his usual rate.
Note the rise and fall of patient's chest with each inspiration and expiration.	A complete cycle of inspiration and expiration constitutes one act of respiration.
Using a watch with a second hand, count the number of respirations for a minimum of 30 seconds. Multiply this number by two to obtain patient's respiratory rate per minute.	Sufficient time is necessary to observe the rate, depth, and other characteristics.
If respirations are abnormal in any way, count the respiratory rate for a full minute. Repeat if necessary to determine accurately the rate and characteristics of breathing.	Full minute countings allow for the detection of unequal timing between respirations.

and then a period of no breathing or *apnea*. Dyspnea is usually present. Cheyne-Stokes respirations are a serious symptom during illness and very often occur as death approaches. They also occasionally occur in well, elderly persons, especially when at high altitudes.

Breathing that is unusually noisy is called *stertorous*. A snoring sound is common.

There are still other terms that describe various types of respirations. Describing the specific character of the respirations rather than attempting to use an uncommon term that may be misinterpreted is recommended.

Frequency of Obtaining Temperature and Pulse and Respiratory Rates

As indicated earlier, obtaining the patient's temperature and pulse and respiratory rates is a part of the physical examination. At other times, agency policies govern when and how frequently they are to be obtained. It is common policy in hospitals for patients having elevated temperatures and those who are in the immediate postoperative period to have vital signs taken every four hours. Severely ill patients may have these observations made more frequently. In some self-care, chronic illness, or psychiatric units, these observations are not made routinely. When a patient does not have an elevated temperature or other vital sign disturbances, there seems to be little justification for observing these signs several times a day. When the nurse visits an individual at home, his condition determines the frequency of obtaining data about vital signs.

Although auxiliary personnel may make temperature, pulse and respiration observations, the nurse responsible for the patient is ultimately responsible for

these observations. Should a patient show untoward symptoms or change in pulse and respiratory rates, the nurse should count the pulse and the respirations, and if necessary, take the temperature. These are cardinal signs and good clues to what is happening in the body.

Monitoring devices in hospitals make it possible to have a constant measurement of a patient's vital signs. Use of such equipment enhances the nurse's ability to gather these data.

Blood Pressure

From the study of human physiology, it can be recalled that maximum pressure is exerted on the wall of the arteries when the left ventricle of the heart pushes blood through an open aortic valve into the aorta. The highest point of pressure in the arteries is called *systolic pressure*. The lowest point, or pressure which is constantly present on the arterial walls, is called the *diastolic pressure*. The difference between the two is called the *pulse pressure*. Determining systolic and diastolic pressure is an excellent way of determining the work of the heart and the resistance offered by the peripheral vessels. Blood pressure is recorded in millimeters of mercury, abbreviated mm. Hg, and recorded as a fraction. The numerator is the systolic pressure and the denominator is the diastolic pressure. For example, if the blood pressure is 120/80, 120 is the systolic pressure and 80 is the diastolic pressure. The pulse pressure is 40.

Persons whose blood pressures are above normal are in a state of hypertension. When the cause of the hypertension is due to pathology and known, it is called *secondary hypertension*. *Primary* or *essential hypertension* is hypertension without a known cause. A blood pressure below average is called *hypotension*.

Maintenance of Blood Pressure. The following five factors are responsible for maintaining blood pressure.

Peripheral resistance. The circulatory system has a high pressure system (arteries) and a low pressure system (capillaries and veins). Between the two are the arterioles, very fine muscular tubes. When the arterioles contract, their caliber becomes small and less blood flows through the capillaries. When the arterioles are in a state of overcontraction, the condition is called *vasoconstriction.* In the opposite condition, the arteriole walls are relaxed and increased amounts of blood reach the arterioles. The arterioles are then in a state of dilation, or *vasodilation.* Normally, arterioles are in a state of partial contraction—they are neither fully dilated nor fully relaxed. Constriction greater than normal results in a higher blood pressure; less constriction results in a lower blood pressure. All other factors being normal, the degree of vasoconstriction affects diastolic pressure and is its chief determinant. Persistent diastolic hypertension is the most serious and most common blood pressure disturbance in man.

The pumping action of the heart. When increased amounts of blood are pumped into the arteries (that is, when cardiac output is increased) the arteries will distend more, resulting in an increase in blood pressure. When less blood is pumped into the arteries (that is, when cardiac output is decreased) blood pressure will fall. Hence, a weak pumping action results in a lower blood pressure than a strong pumping action.

The blood volume. When blood volume is low, such as following a hemorrhage, blood pressure is low because there is decreased pressure on the arteries. Increasing the quantity of blood will increase the pressure because there will be more pressure on the arteries.

The viscosity of the blood. Viscosity is the quality of adhering, that is, having a sticky, glutinous consistency. The viscosity of the blood depends on the proportion of blood cells to plasma. The more viscid the blood, the higher the blood pressure will be; that is, the more viscous the fluid, the more force is required to move it.

The elasticity of the vessel walls. Arteries have a considerable quantity of elastic tissue that allows for their ability to stretch. When the heart rests between each beat, the walls of the arteries recoil although pressure in them does not drop to zero. The state of pressure keeps the blood entering the capillaries and veins in a continuous flow, not in spurts. Simultaneously, the arterioles, normally in a moderate state of contraction, offer certain resistance; therefore, the elasticity of the walls, in addition to the resistance at the arterioles, helps to maintain normal blood pressure. Vessels that have little elasticity offer more resistance than vessels with great elasticity. As resistance increases, such as when arteriosclerosis is present, so does the pressure.

Normal Blood Pressure. Studies of healthy persons indicate that blood pressure can be within a wide range and still be normal. Since individual differences are considerable, it is important to know what is the normal blood pressure for a particular person. If there is a rise or fall of 20 to 30 mm. Hg in that person's pressure, it is significant, even if it is well within the generally accepted range of normal.

The normal newborn infant has a systolic pressure of approximately 20 to 60 mm. Hg. Blood pressure increases gradually until puberty when a more sudden rise occurs. At 17 or 18 years of age, blood pressure reaches adult level. At 20 or so, a man's average, normal blood pressure is usually given as 120/80 mm. Hg. A steady but not great rise continues from then to old age in healthy individuals. For a young adult, a systolic pressure of 140 may be considered high, but for a person of 60 years of age, it may not arouse great concern. Having a consistently low blood pressure, for example, a systolic reading of 90 to 115 mm. Hg in an adult, appears to cause no ill effects. Rather, this is usually associated with longevity.

The average range of pulse pressure is about 30 to 50 mm. Hg for a well, middle-aged adult. It increases normally with age. The pulse pressure becomes an important factor in certain illnesses inasmuch as it varies directly with the amount of blood being pumped out during systole.

In most instances, blood pressure is measured in the brachial artery over the antecubital space. If a measurement is not designated to be taken at another site, the brachial artery is used. Occasionally, blood pressure is measured in the leg when the arms are not accessible or when pressure measured over a leg artery is significant because of existing pathology. The popliteal artery over the popliteal space on the leg is ordinarily used. Systolic pressure in the leg of the well adult is normally 10 to 40 mm. Hg higher than that in the arm. The diastolic pressure may normally be lower or the same as that in the arm. Blood pressure measured in the leg, should be recorded as having been obtained there.

It has been found that nearly all persons will show

normal fluctuations within the course of a day. The blood pressure is usually lowest upon arising in the morning before breakfast and before activity commences. The blood pressure has been noted to rise as much as 5 to 10 mm. Hg. by late afternoon, and it will gradually fall again during the sleeping hours.

There are several factors that will influence blood pressure in the average healthy person. Age has already been mentioned. The sex of the person influences blood pressure, females usually having a lower blood pressure than males at the same age. Blood pressure has been observed to rise after the ingestion of food. It will also rise during a period of exercise or strenuous activity. Emotions such as anger, fear, and excitement will generally cause a rise in blood pressure. Generally, a person who is lying down will have a lower blood pressure than he will when he is sitting or standing.

Hypertension is a prevalent health problem in this country. It is a major cause of early death and serious disability in an estimated 25 million persons annually. Although the exact reason has not yet been determined, hypertension occurs almost twice as frequently in blacks than in Caucasians.

One of the most menacing aspects of hypertension is the fact that it is undetected and untreated in many persons and, therefore, causes permanent damage before it it discovered. The brain, kidneys, heart, and retina are particularly susceptible to damage from hypertension. It has been estimated that approximately one-half of the persons with hypertension are undiagnosed. Of those who have been identified, about one-half are not being treated. For these reasons, a massive national campaign has been undertaken in recent years to identify and treat persons with hypertension.

Since blood pressure normally varies in well persons, the state of hypertension is somewhat relative in nature. However, some norms have been established to act as guidelines when assessing blood pressure. Table 15–5

TABLE 15–5 Maximum normal blood pressures over the brachial artery for persons of various ages.

AGE	BLOOD PRESSURE
Infants	90/60 mm. Hg.
3 to 6 years	110/70 mm. Hg.
7 to 10 years	120/80 mm. Hg.
11 to 15 years	130/80 mm. Hg.
15 to 20 years	130/85 mm. Hg.
20 to 40 years	140/90 mm. Hg.
40 to 60 years	160/95 mm. Hg.
60 to 75 years	170/95 mm. Hg.
75 years and older	180/100 mm. Hg.

shows the upper limits of normal blood pressures over the brachial artery, as determined by the American Heart Association. Persistent readings higher than these limits should be evaluated by a physician for treatment. Because of the many factors which influence blood pressure, the measurement of a single elevated blood pressure is not necessarily significant. Every person with a reading above normal should be reexamined several times to determine if the measurement persists.

Measuring Blood Pressure. A sphygmomanometer and a stethoscope are necessary for measuring blood pressure by the indirect method. The sphygmomanometer has a cuff which consists of an airtight, flat, rubber bladder covered with elasticized cloth. The cloth extends beyond the bladder to various lengths. There are two tubes attached to the bladder within the cuff. One is connected to a manometer. The other is attached to a bulb that is used to inflate the bladder. The bladder is inflated to the extent necessary to obstruct the flow of blood through the artery. A needle valve on the bulb allows the operator to deflate the cuff while pressure is being read.

One type of manometer is a mercury manometer which has a mercury-filled cylinder or tube calibrated in millimeters. When mercury rises in the tube, the upper or top surface of the mercury is curved convexly. The top most point on the curved surface is called the *meniscus.* It is caused by the cohesive force of the mercury molecules. When determining blood pressure on the mercury manometer, the meniscus indicates the pressure. The meniscus of the mercury is read at eye level. If the meniscus is above eye level, the pressure reading will appear higher than it really is. If the meniscus is lower than eye level, it will appear lower than it really is. The apparent change of position of an object when seen from two different angles is called *parallax.* Figure 15–4 on page 306 illustrates meniscus and how pressure readings may be incorrect when the meniscus is above or below eye level.

Another type of manometer is called the aneroid manometer. It too has a cuff but it is attached to a round calibrated dial with a pointer that indicates pressure. Figure 15–5 on page 306 shows a mercury and an aneroid manometer.

When the blood pressure is measured, the cuff is inflated to the extent necessary to occlude the blood flow through the artery. The pressure within the cuff registers on the manometer.

The width of the cuff is a factor in obtaining an accurate blood pressure reading. If the cuff is too nar-

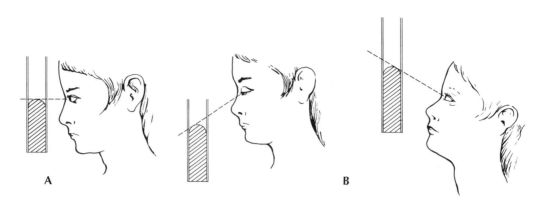

Figure 15–4   A. This sketch illustrates meniscus, the point at which a reading of pressure should be made. B. These sketches illustrate how blood pressure readings could vary when eye is at different levels in relation to the meniscus. This phenomenon is known as parallax.

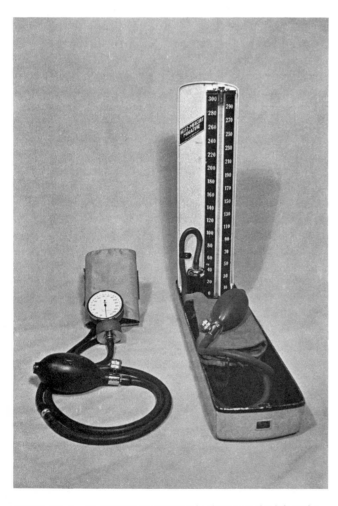

Figure 15–5   An aneroid manometer is shown on the left and a mercury manometer is shown on the right.

row, the reading could be higher than the actual pressure in the artery because the pressure is not evenly transmitted to the artery. An example would be using an averge size cuff on an obese person. If a cuff is too wide, the reading may be less than the pressure in the artery because pressure is being directed toward a proportionately larger surface area. An example would be using an adult cuff on the thin arm of a child. It is recommended that the cuff width be 20 percent wider than the diameter of the limb.

The length of the cuff bladder is also important. It should be sufficiently long to encircle the limb completely in order that pressure on the extremity is equally applied to all parts. An average adult requires a cuff width of 12 to 14 cm. or about $4\frac{1}{2}$ and $5\frac{1}{2}$ inches, and a bladder length of 23 cm. or about 9 inches. Measurement of the blood pressure in the thigh requires a proportionately larger cuff. A baby may require a cuff as narrow as 2.5 to 5 cm. or 1 to 2 inches. A school-age child generally requires a cuff width of 9 to 12 cm. or about $3\frac{1}{2}$ to 5 inches.

The stethoscope is used to auscultate the sounds directly over the artery as the pressure in the cuff is released and the blood is permitted to flow through the artery. The construction of the stethoscope magnifies the sounds in the artery and these sound waves are transmitted to the listener. By listening to the sounds and watching the manometer, the blood pressure reading is obtained.

The acoustical stethoscope, the type most commonly used, has an amplifying mechanism connected to ear pieces by tubing. The preferred amplifying mechanism has a large, flat side which is called the diaphragm. The opposite side is smaller in diameter and more upright and called the bell. The diaphragm is more useful for hearing high-frequency sounds since it is constructed to screen out low-frequency sounds. For example, the diaphragm is generally used for listening to respiratory sounds. The bell screens out high-frequency sounds and is more useful for hearing low-frequency sounds, such as those commonly made by the heart and the blood within the vessels. Figure 15–6 illustrates the bell and diaphragm of the amplifier stethoscope.

The ear tips of the stethoscope should be selected to fit the ear canals comfortably and snugly for most effective auscultation. The tips should be sufficiently large to block out extraneous environmental noises when the stethoscope is being used. The tips should be adjusted to be directed into the ear canal, not against the ear itself. The selection of an appropriate stethoscope for maximum efficiency during auscultation is an individual matter but should be considered carefully.

It is preferable to obtain the blood pressure measurement in as little time as possible in order to prevent venous congestion. The inflated cuff acts as a tourniquet. Venous congestion in the arm below the cuff will affect the reading. Also, prolonged venous congestion causes discomfort for the patient.

Sometimes it is necessary to repeat the procedure in order to be certain that an accurate blood pressure reading is obtained. Before successive measurements, the cuff is completely deflated and venous circulation in the lower arm is allowed to return to normal for 20 to 30 seconds or more if necessary. When it is difficult

to hear the blood pressure sounds, asking the person to elevate his arm before inflating the cuff and having him open and close his fist eight to ten times after the cuff is inflated will often help make the sounds more prominent. These actions lower the venous pressure and thus make the arterial sounds easier to hear.

If the patient is to have frequent blood pressure readings taken and the cuff is left in place, it is necessary to check to see that it has not rotated out of position before taking the next reading. Also it is essential to make certain that the cuff cannot be inflated accidently between readings.

The series of sounds for which the nurse listens when measuring blood pressure are called the *Korotkoff's sounds.* The first clear sound when blood initially flows through the artery is called Phase I and is recorded as the systolic pressure. This sound then normally becomes louder. At Phase II, the sound becomes muffled and may disappear. The change in the vessel size as the cuff pressure is released causes vibrations which are responsible for the muffling. The disappearance of the sound is called the *ausculatory gap.* At Phase III, the sound becomes more distinct since the lowered cuff pressure allows the artery to remain open during systole of the heart. At Phase IV, the sound changes and becomes muffled because the pressure in the cuff is falling below the pressure within the artery. The American Heart Association accepts this last distinct sound as the diastolic pressure. At Phase V, all sounds disappear because the artery remains open throughout the entire cardiac cycle. Some authorities feel Phase V more accurately represents absolute diastole. When a recording of Phase V is desired, the nurse notes both the Phase IV and Phase V sounds. A blood pressure recording then includes three numbers and is recorded, for example, as 130/92/86. Figure 15–7 on page 308 illustrates the artery occlusion and blood flow and the associated blood pressure sounds.

The chart on page 308 describes how to obtain the blood pressure with a mercury manometer. There are electronic instruments also available for measuring blood pressure. Readings are available in a matter of seconds. These instruments have a built-in microphone to detect surface vibrations which activate circuitry and audibly indicate systolic and diastolic pressures. The manufacturers point out that these devices eliminate errors due to poor hearing, interference by outside sounds, and poor visual and auditory correlation.

The direct method of obtaining blood pressure is done by placing a needle in an artery and connecting it to a manometer. This method is used when very pre-

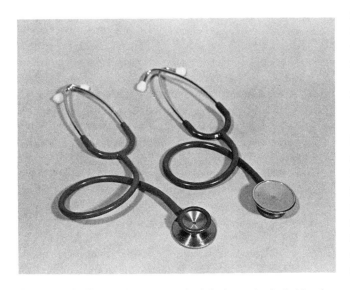

Figure 15–6 The stethoscope at the left shows the bell side of the amplifier. The diaphragm of the amplifier is shown on the stethoscope at the right.

Figure 15–7   When the cuff has been inflated sufficiently, it will occlude the flow of blood into the forearm (left). No sound will be heard through the stethoscope at this time. When pressure in the cuff is reduced sufficiently for blood to begin flowing through the brachial artery (center), the first sound is recorded as the systolic pressure. As the pressure in the cuff continues to be released, the last distinct sound heard through the stethoscope is the diastolic pressure. At this time, blood flows through the brachial artery freely (right).

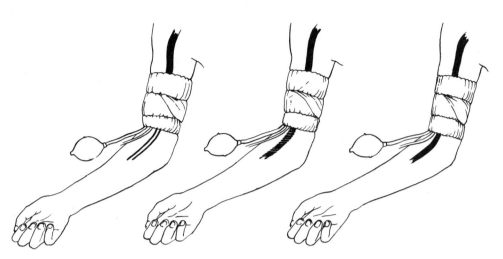

Obtaining the blood pressure with a mercury manometer

The purpose is to measure the systolic and diastolic blood pressure in the brachial artery by an indirect method.

SUGGESTED ACTION	RATIONALE
Position the person comfortably with the forearm supported at the level of the heart and the palm upward.	This position places the brachial artery in alignment with the heart for the most accurate measurement, and makes the antecubital area accessible.
Place yourself so that the meniscus of the mercury can be read at eye level, no more than 3 feet away.	If the eye level is above or below the meniscus, the reading will be inaccurate. A distance of more than 3 feet may result in an inaccurate reading.
Place the cuff so that the inflatable bladder is centered over the brachial artery, which lies midway between the anterior and the medial aspect of the arm, so that the lower edge of the cuff is approximately 2 cm. or almost 1 inch above the antecubital space.	Pressure applied directly to the artery will yield most accurate readings.
Wrap the cuff smoothly around the arm and secure the end of the cuff.	A twisted or loose cuff could produce unequal pressure and thus an inaccurate reading.
Use the fingertips to feel for a strong pulsation in the antecubital space.	Locating the artery allows the stethoscope to be placed for maximum auscultation.
Place the stethoscope firmly but lightly over the brachial artery in the antecubital space where the pulse was noted.	The transmission of sound can be distorted when the stethoscope is misplaced.
Pump the bulb of the manometer until the mercury rises to approximately 20 to 30 mm. Hg above the point at which it is anticipated that systolic pressure will be heard.	Pressure in the inflated cuff must be greater than the systolic pressure to occlude the flow of blood through the brachial artery.
Using the valve on the bulb, release air at a rate of 2 to 3 mm. Hg per heartbeat and note on the manometer the point at which the first sound is heard. Record this figure as the systolic pressure. Increase the drop by 5 to 6 mm. Hg for patients who have a known wide pulse pressure until near the expected diastolic pressure.	Systolic pressure is that point at which the blood in the brachial artery is first able to force its way through, against the pressure exerted on the vessel by the cuff of the manometer.
Continue to release the air in the cuff evenly and gradually. Sounds may become a bit muffled.	The artery is still partly occluded.
Note the point on the manometer when the last distinct loud sound is heard. Record this figure as the diastolic pressure.	Diastolic pressure is that point at which blood flows freely in the brachial artery and is equivalent to the amount of pressure normally exerted on the walls of the arteries when the heart is at rest.
When appropriate, note the point on the manometer when the sound disappears entirely. Record this figure as the second diastolic pressure.	Some authorities believe the cessation of sound indicates the diastolic pressure more accurately.
Allow the remaining air to escape quickly, remove the cuff, and clean the equipment according to agency procedure.	

cise measurements are needed. The direct method is discussed in clinical texts.

Frequency of Measuring Blood Pressure The patient's blood pressure usually is obtained on admission to a health agency and when a physical examination is done. If the patient has an illness involving the circulatory system, has had surgery, or is receiving a medication for blood pressure control, daily or more frequent readings may be necessary. As with observations of body temperature, pulse, and respirations, the nurse must exercise judgment. Very ill patients who are in need of almost constant recording of vital signs are usually hospitalized in intensive care units where this recording can be done with monitoring systems. Persons who are maintained on blood pressure medications at home are often taught to check their own blood pressure, with the health practitioner validating for accuracy at regular intervals. If a layperson is taught to take blood pressure measurements, care should be taken to be sure he understands the technique and can perform it accurately.

Care of Equipment It is important that equipment used for measuring blood pressure be in good repair and function accurately. Improperly functioning equipment is a major cause of inaccurate measurements. The nurse should check routinely to see that there are no air leaks in the rubber bladder, sphygmomanometer connectors, tubings, or valve. The mercury meniscus and the needle on the aneroid manometer should be checked to see that they are exactly on zero when the cuff is deflated in order for pressure to be measured accurately. The mercury manometer should be cleaned and checked at least annually to see that the mercury is free of foreign matter and air. The aneroid manometer must be checked for accurate calibration frequently against an accurate mercury manometer. Some authorities recommend weekly calibration for the aneroid manometer while others suggest checking it every six months. At any time that the accuracy of the equipment is questioned, it should be checked and repaired or replaced, as indicated.

THE PHYSICAL EXAMINATION

The physical examination is often conducted by the nurse as a screening device. She must know normal physical characteristics sufficiently well to recognize deviations from normal. In most instances, the human body is symmetrical. *Symmetry* means that there is a corrrespondence in relative contour, size, color, and position of parts on opposite sides of the body. The nurse observes for symmetry as well as for indications of normal functioning of body parts.

Positioning the Patient

There are several common positions used when a physical examination is done. The *erect* position is the normal standing position. The patient wears slippers, or the floor is protected. The draping is arranged so that body contours, posture, muscles, and extremities can be inspected conveniently.

In the *dorsal* or *horizontal recumbent position,* the patient lies flat on his back with his legs together, in bed or on the examining table. His head may be supported with a pillow and his legs extended or slightly flexed at the knees to relax the abdominal wall. He is covered with a drape. Parts of the drape are folded back to expose the area being examined. The dorsal position is assumed most commonly for examination of the abdomen, the chest anteriorly, and the breasts. This position may also be used for examination of the reflexes, the extremities, the head, the neck, the eyes, the ears, the nose, and the throat if the person is unable to sit.

In the *dorsal* or *horizontal recumbent position,* the patient close to the edge of the examining table while lying on his back with the legs separated and the knees flexed; the soles of the feet rest flat on the bed or table. One pillow may be placed under the head. A drape is placed diagonally over the patient with opposite corners protecting the legs and wrapped around the feet so that the drape will stay in place. The third corner of the drape covers the patient's chest, and the fourth corner is placed between the legs. A disposable pad may be placed under the patient's buttocks to avoid soiling linen. The corner of the drape between the patient's legs is raised and folded back on the abdomen to expose the part of the perineum being examined. Figure 15–8 on page 310 illustrates the dorsal recumbent position.

The *lithotomy position* is the same as the dorsal recumbent position except that the patient is usually on a table equipped with foot stirrups. The patient's buttocks are brought to the edge of the table. The knees are flexed, and the feet are supported in the stirrups. A disposable pad may be placed under the patient's buttocks, and draping is the same as for the dorsal recumbent position. The position is assumed usually for digital examination of the rectum or instrument

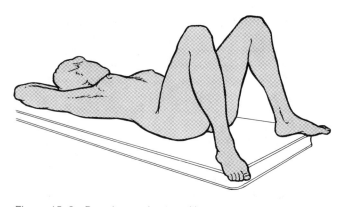

Figure 15–8   Dorsal recumbent position.

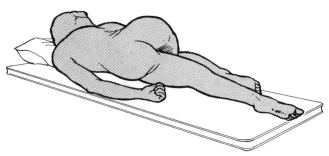

Figure 15–10   Sims's position.

examination of the vagina. Figure 15–9 illustrates the lithotomy position.

In the left *Sims's position,* the patient lies on his left side and rests his left arm behind his body. The right arm is forward with the elbow flexed and the arm resting on a pillow placed under the patient's head. The patient's body inclines slightly forward. The knees are flexed, the right one sharply. In the right Sims's position, the placement of the extremities is reversed. The position usually is assumed for a digital examination of the rectum or the vagina. A disposable pad may be used under the buttocks. One corner of the drape is folded back on the patient's hip to expose the area being examined. Figure 15–10 illustrates the Sims's position.

In the *knee-chest* or *genupectoral position,* the patient rests on his knees and chest with the body flexed approximately 90° at the hips. The head, turned to one side, rests on a small pillow. A small pillow also may be placed under the chest. The arms are above the head or they may be flexed at the elbows and rest alongside the patient's head. The lower legs are placed perpendicular

to the thighs. The knee-chest position frequently is assumed for an instrument examination of the rectum. The drape is placed so that the patient's back, buttocks, and thighs are covered. Only the area to be examined is exposed. This is a very difficult position for most patients to assume, especially the elderly patient. Therefore, the nurse should have all equipment ready and should not assist the patient into position until she is to commence. Figure 15–11 illustrates the knee-chest position.

The dorsal recumbent, lithotomy, Sims's, and knee-chest positions are used to examine areas of the body which cause embarrassment to some patients. The examinations can be made easier for the patient if the nurse takes every precaution to prevent exposure and to give explanations and directions slowly and carefully. Even when a patient is properly draped for an examination, there may be concern that someone can see into the unit or come into the room. The nurse should make every effort to see that this does not happen.

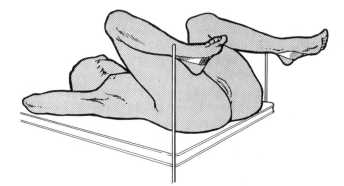

Figure 15–9   Lithotomy position.

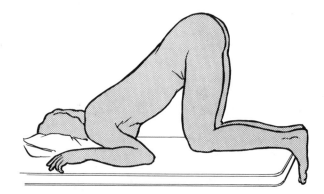

Figure 15–11   Knee-chest position.

Examining the Skin, Mucous Membrane, Nails, and Hair

The skin is a good indicator of a person's health state. The mucous membrane and nails are differentiated tissues but continuous extensions of the skin. Because hair originates in the skin, it is also considered a part of it. The nurse observes the skin of each area of the body as the examination proceeds.

The skin is observed for *turgor,* which is the tension of a cell determined by its hydration. Normal turgor results in an elasticity of the skin which allows it to be picked up in a fold and to return to its normal shape when released. Inspection and palpation are used for examining the skin.

The skin is inspected for color and abnormalities. The skin color varies among races and among individuals. Normally, skin ranges from a pinkish-white to various shades of brown depending on the person's race. The skin areas which are normally exposed, such as the face and hands, may have a somewhat different color from areas that are usually covered with clothing, but generally the color is relatively constant. Special care must be taken to detect color changes in dark-skinned persons, such as some blacks, Mexican-Americans, American Indians, individuals of Mediterranean extraction, and Caucasians who are deeply sun-tanned. Some body areas of dark-skinned persons, such as the palms of the hands and the soles of the feet, normally have less pigmentation than other areas of the body.

The following terms are used to describe the skin.

A *flush* is a redness of the skin, such as in a blush or sunburn. It is usually associated with an elevated temperature, and the face and the neck are more likely to be affected than other parts of the body. Palpation with the back surface of the fingers often reveals an increased temperature more readily than inspection for skin color in the dark-skinned person.

Cyanosis is a dusky, bluish color of the skin and can usually be observed in the lips and around the mouth, nailbeds, and earlobes. Cyanosis can be detected more readily in the conjunctiva, lips, and inside of the mouth in dark-skinned persons.

Jaundice is a yellowness of the skin. Usually, it affects the entire body and almost always, the sclera of the eyes. Jaundice in the dark-skinned person is more difficult to observe because the sclera often has a yellowish color normally.

Pallor is a paleness of the skin. It often results from an inadequate amount of circulating blood. The decrease in circulating blood results in an inadequate amount of oxygen being supplied to the tissues. This condition is called *hypoxia. Anoxia,* which means an absence of oxygen, is not technically correct when used as a synonym for hypoxia. Depending on its severity, pallor may be visible over the entire skin surface. At other times, it can be detected in the mucous membrane, lips, nailbeds, and conjunctiva. The detection of pallor may be more difficult in dark-skinned persons. The person's family may best be able to determine changes in the skin color of these individuals.

Besides color, the skin is inspected for evidence of *lesions,* circumscribed areas of diseased or injured tissue. Normally, the skin should be smooth and without breaks in its continuity. The presence of scars usually indicates skin breaks which have healed. Evidence of bruises, scratches, cuts, insect bites, and wounds should be noted.

A *wound* is a break in the continuity of the skin. Any wound should be described as to its size, shape, depth, and location. The amount and character of drainage, if present, should also be described. Wounds will be described in more detail in Chapter 22.

A *rash* is an eruption of the skin. Because the descriptive details of a rash are complex, including type of spots, size, elevation, coloring, and presence or absence of drainage or itching, they are dealt with more appropriately in a text on skin diseases. The nurse should indicate exactly where on the patient's body a rash is noticed and its general appearance.

Ecchymosis is a collection of blood in subcutaneous tissues, causing purplish discoloration. The nurse should note its location, size, and color, the last of which is an indication of how recently it occurred.

The moisture, temperature, and turgor of the skin are determined by palpation. When a person is at rest in an environmental temperature of approximately 21° to 29° C. (70° to 84° F.), his skin is normally warm and dry.

Abnormal skin temperature, moisture, or turgor can indicate illness. For example, an increase in skin temperature and in skin moisture from perspiration can signify an elevation of body temperature. An excessive amount of perspiration, such as when a person's entire skin is moist, is known as *diaphoresis.* The elevated temperature can result in *dehydration,* the depletion of body fluids and a decrease in skin turgor. Typically, the skin is loose and wrinkled and the mucous membrane cracked and dry when dehydration is present.

A below normal skin temperature can indicate circulatory impairment which can be either generalized or localized.

An increase in skin turgor may mean excessive fluid in the tissues. This condition, known as *edema,* results in swelling, and the skin is usually taut and shiny over the area. The tension within the affected tissue cells can be sufficiently great so that the skin cannot be picked up readily. If depressed with the fingers, an indentation may remain after the pressure is released. An illustration of edema appears in Chapter 23.

The nails are inspected for shape, texture, and color. The shape of the nails should normally be somewhat convex and follow the natural curve of the finger. The angle between the nail and its base in the finger should be about 160°. The texture of the nails should be smooth and the nail bases firm. Increased brittleness and angulation between the nail and nailbed and disturbances of the thicknesses or texture of the nails can indicate illness.

Hair is inspected for distribution, texture, and quantity. Hair normally covers all parts of the body except the palms of the hands and the soles of the feet. A difference in hair distribution exists in male and female adults and is usually evident by the time of adolescence.

The texture of hair normally varies among persons and on different parts of the body. Generally, a change in the texture of the individual's hair is of greater significance than the texture itself.

The quantity of hair normally varies extensively among persons. A change in hair quantity usually is more important than the amount of hair. However, excessive or inadequate quantities of hair can have psychological significance for many persons.

Examining the Head and Neck

The head and neck are generally observed with the person in a sitting position.

Skull and Face The skull is examined for size and shape by inspection and palpation. The parts of the head and face should be in proportion to each other and to other parts of the body. There is considerable variation in the shape of the normal skull, but generally, the shape is gently curved with some prominences. The scalp may be examined by parting the hair at intervals and observing for lesions.

The face is inspected for symmetry and placement of the parts, such as the eyes and the ears. Movement of the facial structures is observed. For example, do both corners of the mouth assume the same angle when the person smiles? Is the movement of the eyelids symmetrical?

Eyes The eyes are inspected for general characteristics and visual acuity, after which the internal structures are examined. The eyelids and lashes, conjunctiva, sclera, cornea, and iris are inspected for consistency of configuration and color. The eyes are inspected for pupillary reaction to light, for coordinated movements, and for *accommodation,* which is the focusing ability of the eye.

Visual acuity is usually tested by asking the person to read from the Snellen eye chart. The Snellen chart contains letters of various sizes. Each eye is tested separately with the person at a distance of 20 feet from the chart. The visual acuity is expressed as a fraction. The numerator indicates the distance the person is from the chart and the denominator the distance at which a person with normal vision can read the chart. The Snellen test standard for normal vision is expressed as 20/20.

The nurse inspects the internal structures of the eye by looking through the pupil with the ophthalmoscope. This examination is preferably conducted in a darkened room which allows the pupils to dilate. Eyedrops that dilate the pupils may also be used. The optic disc, retinal vessels, and macula are examined for size, shape, and color.

The internal eye pressure is measured with the tonometer. After anesthetizing the cornea with eyedrops, the tonometer is applied lightly to the cornea and the pressure within the eyeball registers on a gauge. Measurement of the intraocular pressure is not routinely performed as a part of all physical examinations, but it should be conducted periodically on persons over the age of 40. An increase in normal pressure is a typical sign of glaucoma which is a common cause of blindness.

Ears. The external ears are inspected for shape, size, and lesions. The external surfaces of the ear should be smooth and the shape and size symmetrical and proportionate to the head. The otoscope is used to examine the ear canal and the tympanic membrane. To achieve better visualization, the ear canal of an adult can be straightened by gently pulling the lobe up and back. The ear canal of a child is straightened by pulling the lobe back. The ear canal should be smooth and pinkish in color. The tympanic membrane is translucent, shiny, and gray in color. Anatomical landmarks should be observable.

Hearing can be tested, one ear at a time, by determining if the person can hear the nurse's whisper from 1 to 2 feet away. The nurse must be certain that the person is not lip reading, and, hence, positions herself out of the patient's vision or covers her mouth. A device called an *audiometer* is used for more precise testing of hearing. Audiometry is not generally used in a routine physical examination. When hearing loss is present, a tuning fork can be used for distinguishing between auditory nerve and bone conduction abnormalities.

Nose. The nose is inspected with an otoscope with a short, wide tip or with a nasal speculum and penlight. The mucous membrane of each nostril is examined for color and the presence of any exudate or growths. The nasal septum is observed for intactness and deviation. Normally, the nasal mucous membrane is redder than the oral mucosa and should appear moist. Any exudate, swelling, perforation, or differences between the nostrils should be noted.

Sinuses. Symmetry of the face is inspected to detect swelling of the sinuses. Palpation over the sinuses is then used to determine sensitivity. Normally, the sinus cavities are not tender or uncomfortable when palpated.

Mouth and Pharynx. Examination of the mouth and oropharynx begins with inspection of the lips, tongue, and mucous membrane. The lips should be symmetrical and smooth. The tongue and mucous membrane are normally pinkish in color and moist, and free from swelling and lesions. The tongue surface should be rough, and the mucous membrane smooth and shiny. If the person wears dentures, he is asked to remove them for inspection of the gums and roof of the mouth. The gums should be pink and smooth. With the tongue relaxed on the floor of the mouth, the mucous membrane of the oropharynx is examined when the base of the tongue is retracted with a tongue depressor. The uvula normally is centered and freely moveable. The tonsils, if present, are small, pinkish and symmetrical.

Neck. The neck should first be inspected for symmetry. Palpation for lymph nodes on each side of the neck, ears, and jaw, follows. Except in children, the nodes in most persons normally cannot be palpated. If nodes are palpated, their location, size, consistency, mobility, and tenderness should be noted.

Trachea and Thyroid. The neck is inspected for deviations of the trachea and thyroid. Observation is facilitated by asking the person to swallow. Normally, movement of the tracheal cartilages should then be observable, but the thyroid should not. Palpation is used to determine the size and shape of the thyroid. In many persons the thyroid is not normally palpable. If it can be felt, it should be smooth and symmetrical.

The neck vessels may also be observed at this time although more detailed examination is usually deferred until the patient is in the dorsal position. The jugular veins are not normally visible when the person is in a sitting position.

Examining the Chest

Lungs. With the patient in a sitting position, the chest is initially inspected for symmetry, shape, and respiratory movements. The chest should normally have a greater crosswise diameter than a front to back diameter. The respiratory movements are normally regular and smooth. Men and children tend to have proportionately more abdominal movement with respirations while women tend to have greater thoracic movement.

Palpation is used to detect areas of sensitivity, chest expansion during respirations, and fremitus. *Fremitus* means vibratory tremors.

Palpation should not detect areas of tenderness. Chest expansion is determined by placing the hands over the anterior and posterior chest wall and feeling the amount of movement during shallow and deep inhalation and exhalation.

Tactile fremitus can be detected through the chest wall. The person is asked to speak while the nurse palpates the chest wall with her fingertips. The vibrations normally vary among persons depending on the pitch and intensity of the voice. However, fremitus is greater over the larger bronchi because they are filled with larger quantities of air. Increased or decreased fremitus may be indicative of the presence of pathology.

Percussion is used to determine lung position and size and to detect the presence of air, liquids, or solids within the lungs. The shoulder area and anterior and posterior chest walls are percussed in a systematic pattern. The nurse listens for the intensity, pitch, duration, and quality of the sounds produced. When a normal air-filled lung is percussed, the sound is hollow, loud, low-pitched, and of long duration.

Auscultation is used to detect air flow within the respiratory tract. A stethoscope is used to listen to the sounds of inspiration and expiration over the chest wall in a pattern similar to that used with percussion. Normally, breath sounds result from the free movement of air into and out of all parts of the bronchial tree. The nurse listens for the duration, pitch, and intensity of the sounds which normally vary over different parts of the lung. Abnormal sounds can indicate that air flow is obstructed. The cause may be a foreign body, mucus, fluid, or a tumor.

If the patient has a cough, it is described as nonproductive if no matter or discharge from the respiratory tract is produced. If there is expectoration, it is called a productive cough, and the expectoration is described. *Mucus* or *sputum* can be viscid watery-appearing secretion of the mucous membrane or it can be of greater viscosity and color, depending on its cause and origin. It can be expectorated with or without a cough. If a patient has a cough, the nurse should determine whether the patient understands how to protect others when he coughs and how to dispose of tissues safely.

Heart and Neck Vessels.

The patient may be sitting up or lying down for this part of the examination. Inspection is used to detect pulsations over the precordium and neck vessels. The *precordium* is the anterior surface of the chest wall overlying the heart and its related structures. The neck vessels of concern here are the jugular veins and the carotid arteries.

The precordium is inspected for evidence of pulsations of the left ventricle, known as the apical impulse. The normal rhythmical movement can often be visualized when the person is in a recumbent position and the light is good.

Palpation is used with the visual observations. Systematic palpation can reveal the apical impulse, some abnormal movements and vibrations, and heart enlargement. Steady, rhythmical pulsations are generally present in the healthy person.

Percussion is not generally used in the examination of the heart except for an estimation of heart size. X-ray is felt to give a more accurate indication of size and is commonly used.

Auscultation is used to observe cardiac sounds. The sounds are studied for their pitch, intensity, duration, and timing in the cardiac cycle. In the healthy person, the closing of the mitral and aortic valves are the major heart sounds. The density of the various thoracic structures influences the transmission of the sounds. Therefore, auscultation is performed in a systematic pattern over the anterior and posterior chest wall to develop a comprehensive picture of the person's heart sounds. Abnormalities, such as extra heart sounds and murmurs, can also be detected by auscultation.

The jugular veins and carotid arteries should be examined on both sides of the neck for symmetry. They should be palpated, one side at a time, for fullness and pulse rate, rhythm, amplitude, and symmetry. Care must be taken to distinguish between the veins and arteries. Auscultation is used to detect local obstructions and some abnormal heart sounds. In the normal individual, palpation and auscultation should reveal rhythmical and steady pulsations and smooth filling and emptying of the neck vessels.

Breasts and Axillary Area.

The patient may be in a sitting or lying position. Inspection and palpation are the techniques used in the breast examination. The breasts and nipples are inspected for symmetry, contour, and skin lesions. The breasts should be relatively symmetrical although many women normally have some variation in breast symmetry. The size of the breasts varies among women. The contour of the breasts should be rounded and smooth with no skin depressions or puckering, known as *retraction* and *dimpling*. There should be no discharge from the breasts unless the woman is pregnant or has recently delivered a baby.

Palpation is used to examine the breast tissue for consistency. Breast tissue may normally vary from homogenous soft tissue to generalized nodules or small swellings within the tissue. The purpose of palpation is to detect any type of mass or lump which could be cancerous. The difference between malignant lumps and benign nodules is often hard to detect by palpation. One of the key factors is to determine whether there have been changes in the breast tissue. For this reason, the patient's cooperation and participation are important and the patient should be encouraged and taught self-examination of the breasts. If a mass is detected or suspected, its location, size, shape, consistency, and tenderness should be noted carefully and follow-up care with a physician is recommended.

The entire axillary areas should be palpated for lymph nodes. Usually, the nodes cannot be felt and they should not be tender. Detection and sensitivity of nodes may be significant and should be reported.

While breast examinations are usually the concern of women, the breasts of men should be examined also since males are subject to breast malignancies too.

The breast is the most common site for cancer in women. Caucasian women past the age of 50 have the highest incidence of breast cancer. Other risk factors include an immediate family history or personal history of breast cancer and not having borne children.

3

Lying down:

To examine your right breast, put a pillow or folded towel under your right shoulder. Place right hand behind your head — this distributes breast tissue more evenly on the chest. With left hand, fingers flat, press gently in small circular motions around an imaginary clock face. Begin at outermost top of your right breast for 12 o'clock, then move to 1 o'clock, and so on around the circle back to 12. A ridge of firm tissue in the lower curve of each breast is normal. Then move in an inch, toward the nipple, keep circling to examine *every part of your breast*, including nipple. This requires at least three more circles. Now slowly repeat procedure on your left breast with a pillow under your left shoulder and left hand behind head. Notice how your breast structure feels.

Finally, squeeze the nipple of each breast gently between thumb and index finger. Any discharge, clear or bloody, should be reported to your doctor immediately.

2

Before a mirror:

Inspect your breasts with arms at your sides. Next, raise your arms high overhead. Look for any changes in contour of each breast, a swelling, dimpling of skin or changes in the nipple.

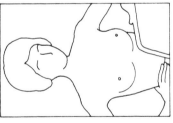

Then, rest palms on hips and press down firmly to flex your chest muscles. Left and right breast will not exactly match—few women's breasts do.

Regular inspection shows what is normal for you and will give you confidence in your examination.

1

In the shower:

Examine your breasts during bath or shower; hands glide easier over wet skin. Fingers flat, move gently over every part of each breast. Use right hand to examine left breast, left hand for right breast. Check for any lump, hard knot or thickening.

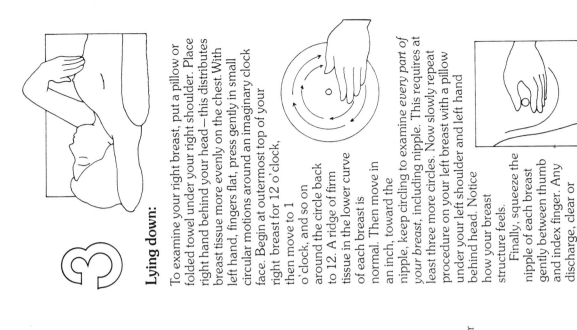

Figure 15–12   These sketches and instructions illustrate a recommended technique for self-examination of the breasts. (Reprinted by permission of the American Cancer Society)

During the physical examination, the nurse can often do health teaching. The technique of self-examination of the breasts can frequently be taught and demonstrated at this time. This examination is felt to be an effective technique for the early detection of breast cancer. Figure 15–12 on the preceding page illustrates the technique that is recommended by the American Cancer Society. It is advised that the breasts be examined on a monthly basis and after menstruation.

Examining the Abdomen and Back

The abdomen is usually examined with the person in the dorsal position. The back may be examined while the individual is seated.

Abdomen. Palpation is generally the most effective method used for examining the abdomen. In order to facilitate the description of an abdominal examination, the area has been mapped into four quadrants. A line drawn from the tip of the sternum to the pubic bone through the umbilicus and a horizontal line crossing the other at the umbilicus divides the abdominal area. The quadrants are called the right and left upper quadrants and the right and left lower quadrants. They are abbreviated RUQ, LUQ, RLQ, and LLQ, respectively. Figure 15–13 illustrates these four quadrants.

The abdomen is inspected for lesions, symmetry, distention, visible peristaltic waves, and the effect of respiratory movements. The abdomen should be free of obvious lesions. There may be evidence of old wounds indicated by scars. The abdomen is symmetrical with flat or rounded contours. Local or generalized distention or edema should not be present and may indicate the presence of pathology. While in some thin persons peristaltic waves may be visible, peristalsis is not usually seen through the abdominal wall. Abdominal movement associated with respirations are often visible with children and adult men. In adult women, abdominal repiratory movement is normally absent.

Auscultation is used in the abdominal examination to detect motility in the gastrointestinal tract and vascular sounds. The noises produced by the movement of air and fluids in the gastrointestinal tract are described as bowel sounds and are normally heard over the abdominal wall. The frequency of the sounds varies considerably and may depend on how recently the person has eaten. A decrease, the absence, or an increase of bowel sounds can have pathological significance.

Sounds produced by the flow of blood through the major abdominal vessels can be heard by auscultation.

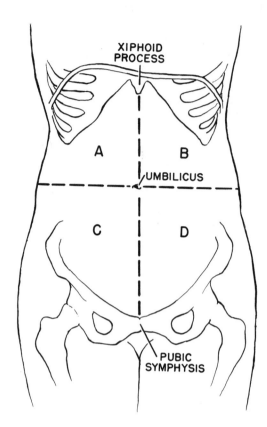

Figure 15–13   Quadrants of the abdomen: (A) the right upper quadrant—RUQ; (B) the left upper quadrant—LUQ; (C) the right lower quadrant—RLQ; (D) the left lower quadrant—LLQ.

Narrowed or dilated vessels can cause abnormal vascular sounds.

The normal presence of air or gas in the stomach and intestines produces a drumlike sound upon percussion called *tympany.* If a solid mass or fluid is present, percussion will produce a dull sound over the involved area.

Palpation is used to determine size, position, mobility, and consistency of major abdominal organs. In addition, muscular resistance, tenderness, and masses can be detected. Each quadrant of the abdomen is systematically examined. Except for the sensations caused by the nurse using deep palpation, the abdomen normally should not be tender or sensitive. The liver, gallbladder, spleen, pancreas, and often the kidneys are ordinarily not palpable if they are of normal size. If they are enlarged or tender, they may be palpable. The urinary bladder is only palpable when distended. Abnormal masses can often be detected by palpation.

Palpation of the inguinal areas for hernias and lymph nodes may be done as a part of the abdominal examination. A *hernia* is the protrusion of an organ or a part of the organ through the cavity wall which normally contains it. Lymph nodes are not normally palpable.

Back. At the conclusion of the abdominal examination, the back can be inspected for symmetry and percussed for tenderness. Swelling or tenderness over the lower back area can be indicative of kidney pathology.

Examining the Musculoskeletal and Peripheral Vascular Systems

The musculoskeletal and peripheral vascular systems are examined when the person is sitting, standing, and lying down. The extremities and back are inspected for symmetry of contours, and for mobility, size, and color.

The spine should normally have cervical, thoracic, and lumbar curves. Each joint should be examined for mobility and size. The range of joint motion may be measured for greater accuracy. The major muscles of the extremities may also be measured for size and tested for control. The skin should be smooth and relatively consistent in color except for the lighter pigmentation on the palms and soles of dark-skinned persons. The individual should be observed to see that he has sufficient muscle control to carry out normal activities of daily living. The vascular system should be inspected on the lower extremities with care. The veins may normally be visible, but they should not be visibly pulsating or greatly distended.

Palpation is used to study temperture, pulsation, muscle strength, and tenderness. In low environmental temperatures, the skin temperature of the extremities may normally be slightly cooler than the trunk of the body. However, the skin temperature of the extremities should be generally consistent. The palpation of pulses in the extremities was discussed in the section on vital signs earlier in this chapter. The strength of symmetrical muscles should normally be consistent. Except on deep palpation, the major muscles should not be tender.

Examining the Neurological System

The neurological system is usually examined while the person is in the sitting and dorsal positions.

Palpation is used to examine the neurological system to determine the sensations of pain, vibration, and touch, and to test the reflexes.

Sensory functions and reflexes are usually tested in a routine physical examination. Other more complex testing is done only when indicated. Sensory functioning is tested by applying a cotton wisp, the point of a sharp object, such as a safety pin, test tubes containing hot and cold water, and a tuning fork to various surfaces of the body. This technique helps to determine whether the person correctly perceives the stimuli. Normally a person can identify the sensations although some body surfaces, such as the back and the soles of the feet may require more intense stimulation than other areas.

Most reflexes are tested by percussion. Usually the reflexes in the biceps, triceps, knee, and Achilles tendon are tested. A normal reaction is a jerking movement. The plantar and abdominal reflexes are generally tested by moving a pointed object over the skin surface of the areas. The plantar reflex normally causes contraction of the toes. The abdominal reflex normally results in contraction of the rectus abdominis muscle.

Examining the Anus and Rectum

The patient may be in the Sims's, knee-chest, or lithotomy position, or standing but leaning over a table for examination of the anus and rectum.

Inspection is used to examine the anal area. Lesions, scars, swellings, or drainage may be evident and should be noted when present. The anal area has increased pigmentation and some hair growth.

Palpation is used to examine the rectum. The nurse wears a glove to palpate the rectal canal with the index finger. The mucosal lining should be smooth. Tissue swellings, distortions, or hard fecal material should be noted. Fecal specimens may be taken at this time for culture and examination.

In the male patient, the size, shape, and consistency of the prostate gland can be palpated through the anterior rectal wall. The gland should normally be approximately 4 cm. or about $1\frac{3}{4}$ inches in size and feel smooth and firm. In addition, it should not be tender to touch.

In the female, the cervix may be felt as a small round mass through the anterior rectal wall.

Examining the Genitalia

The genitalia of the male are usually examined with the patient in the standing position. Gloves may be worn by the nurse for this part of the examination.

Inspection and palpation are used in examining the genitalia. The penis is inspected for lesions, swelling, inflammation, and discharge, none of which should normally be present. The scrotum is inspected for symmetry, swelling, and lesions. While the sides of the scrotum may vary somewhat in size, they should be relatively symmetrical. Palpation is used to study the testes, epididymes, and spermatic cords. Their size, shape, and consistency should be similar. If a discharge is present, specimens may be taken at this time in the examination.

The genitalia of the female are examined with the patient in the lithotomy position. Gloves are worn by the nurse.

The external genitalia of the female are inspected initially. The pubic area, vulva, labia, clitoris, urinary meatus, and perineum are examined for color, size, lesions, or discharge. The vulva normally has more pigmentation than other skin areas and the mucous membrane should be dark pink and moist. The skin and mucosa should be smooth and without lesions or swelling. A small amount of clear or whitish discharge from the vagina is normal. Palpation of the external genitalia may detect abnormal swelling and tenderness.

A speculum is used to visualize the cervix and vagina. They are inspected for color, position, size, and lesions and discharge. A specimen for a cervical Papanicolaou smear is ordinarily obtained at this time.

The uterus is also palpated between the examiner's hands for size, shape, consistency, mobility, and tenderness.

Noting Physical Limitations

The presence of physical limitations will usually have been identified in the health history. However, any physical disability observed during the physical examination should be noted. Observing for limited vision or hearing has been discussed earlier. Other disabilities to note include various types of amputations, loss of function in a body part, and artificial orifices. Some persons may use a *prosthesis,* which is an artificial part of the body. Examples include an artificial eye, an artificial limb, and an artificial breast. Others may use a crutch, a cane, braces, and special girdles. Still others may use such items as a colostomy belt and bag, elastic hose, or mositer-proof undergarments. Some persons have cardiac pacemakers. A high anterior chest scar with some protrusion is a clue that a pacemaker is present. However, most individuals having a pacemaker are likely to indicate voluntarily that they have one. Any such items suggest possible limitations, and the nurse will wish to note their presence and reasons for using them.

Some persons may speak freely about items just described and warn others to be careful of them. Other persons may not feel as free to talk about their limitations and a cautious approach is then necessary. It is not a matter of ignoring the presence of such items but rather one of determining if something can be done to make it easier for the person to manage his activities of daily living.

It is important to ask the person if he has any allergies to drugs or other agents. An allergic reaction can be a serious manifestation. This information is usually secured in the health history, but if not, it should be done at the time of the physical examination. When allergy problems are present, the information should be clearly and conspicuously stated in the person's record.

Following the physical examination, the nurse assists the patient as necessary. For safety and courtesy reasons, he should be assisted off an examination table. He may also need assistance with dressing.

The nurse will follow the agency's policy on the care of equipment used during the physical examination. This includes cleaning and returning items to their proper place and discarding disposable items carefully.

The collection of data about the physical health of the patient may include various other tests and examinations. Some of the most common tests and examinations are discussed in the remaining sections of this chapter.

ELECTROCARDIOGRAPHY

The *electrocardiograph* is an instrument that measures and records electrical impulses of the heart. The findings are important for studying heart function. The graphic record produced by the electrocardiograph is called the *electrocardiogram* and is commonly abbreviated EKG.

The electrical activity in the heart can be picked up through electrodes place on the skin. These electrodes are placed in various places on the body. The placement patterns of electrodes are called *leads.* The same cardiac activity is monitored on each lead, but the waves on the electrocardiogram look somewhat different. The trained observer recognizes normal and abnormal findings for each placement of electrodes.

Heart muscle cells are electrically charged, or polarized, in a state of rest. *Polarity* is the existence of opposing attributes. In the case of the heart, polarity results from the positively and negatively charged ions in the tissue fluids separated by the cell membrane. When cells are electrically stimulated, they depolarize and contraction follows. *Depolarization* is the destruction of polarization and the positive and negative charges are changed across the cell membrane. The cells repolarize during the resting phase that follows contraction. *Repolarize* means to restore polarity. Depolarization and repolarization are electrical happenings that are recorded by the electrocardiogram.

When atrial depolarization occurs, the atria contract. Atrial repolarization occurs when the atria are at rest. When ventricular depolarization occurs, the ventricles contract. Ventricular repolarization occurs during ventricular rest.

The heartbeat originates in the *sinoatrial* or *sino-auricular node,* commonly abbreviated *S-A node,* which is located in the upper part of the right atrium. It is frequently called the heart's pacemaker. Currents radiate quickly throughout the atria from the *S-A* node and stimulate their contraction. A second node, the *atrioventricular* or *auriculoventricular node,* commonly abbreviated *A-V node,* picks up the current. The node is

situated at the base of the atrial septum. The A-V node divides into two bundle branches and each in turn, gives rise to numerous "twigs" that interlace throughout the ventricles. This interlacing system is called the *Purkinje system.* Figure 15–14, left, illustrates the structures through which electrical current travels through the heart.

Figure 15–14, right, shows a drawing of a normal EKG. The waves on the electrocardiogram are lettered, as illustrated. The P wave occurs when electrical charges, originating in the S-A node, cause the atria to depolarize and contract. The wave of Q, R, and S occurs when the electrical charges result in ventricular depolarization and contraction. Wave T represents relaxation of the ventricles during which time ventricular repolarization occurs. Repolarization of the atria occurs during the QRS segment but it is not usually as visible on the electrocardiogram as ventricular repolarization is. The sum total of P, Q, R, S, and T represents the cardiac cycle. Another way of describing the cardiac

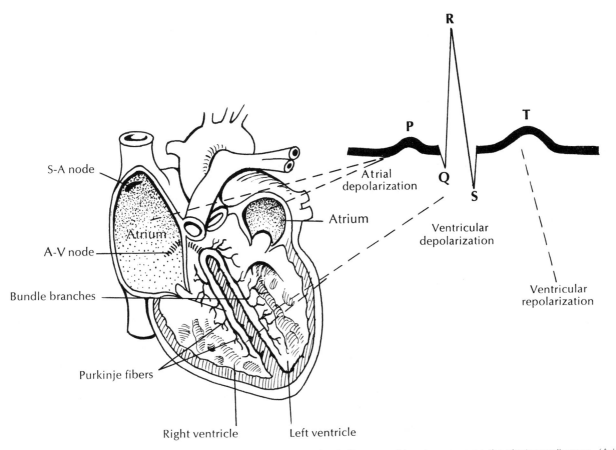

Figure 15–14 Illustration of how electrical phenomenon occurring in the normal heart appears on the electrocardiogram. (Adapted from illustration in Meehan, M.: EKG Primer. Am. J. Nurs., 71:2201, Nov. 1971)

cycle is that it consists of atrial and ventricular depolarization and repolarization.

Look again at Figure 15–14. It illustrates how each electrical phenomenon occurring in the normal heart appears on the electrocardiogram.

When the S-A node is not functioning properly as the heart's pacemaker, other areas in the heart become potential pacemakers. These pacemakers, called *ectopic pacemakers,* may be in the A-V node, atria, or ventricles. Heart block is one condition in which an ectopic pacemaker develops. There is a disruption in the passage of current between the atria and ventricles. The ventricles do not stop beating when this occurs. Rather, they beat independently from impulses of their own and usually at a slower rate than the atria.

The ruled paper use for an EKG aids immeasurably when reading the EKG. The paper is calibrated in 1 mm. squares, as Figure 15–15 illustrates. The horizontal lines represent the measurement of voltage while the vertical lines measure time. When the heart is diseased, the waves may be abnormal in size, form, or position. The time interval between waves also has diagnostic significance. The following EKG findings are commonly found when certain pathological conditions exist. An atrial flutter is characterized by rapid and identical P waves; an ectopic pacemaker has probably originated in the atria. The distance between similar waves is short in time when tachycardia is present; it is long in time when bradycardia is present. An irregular rhythm is often due to disease in the coronary artery. The drug quinidine tends to retard electrical conduction; the result is that the P waves may be notched and the QRS segment may be wider than normal.

Interpretation of an EKG requires skill and practice. When properly used, it is an invaluable tool for studying heart function. More and more, nurses are expected to have at least a basic understanding of electrocardiography. For nurses working with patients having heart diseases and with patients in intensive care and coronary care units, additional study and practice are necessary since understanding EKG readings is critical in the care of these patients.

Patients who are seriously ill frequently have constant monitoring of the heart action including the impulse transmission and myocardial response. Devices which permit the patient to move around and carry on some activity while being monitored increase the patient's comfort. Some monitoring is now possible for persons outside of health agencies and carrying out normal activities of daily living. The electronic devices extend the health personnel's ability to secure data about the patient. Their usage generally requires explanation for the patient and his family.

The person who is having an electrocardiogram for the first time needs an explanation of the purpose and technique being used. It should be explained that he will have electrodes applied to his chest and extremities with an adhesive paste, and that he will be asked to lie quietly while the tracing is being recorded. It should be clearly explained that the electrodes pick up the electrical impulses coming from his heart and they are recorded on the paper. Electricity will not be transferred to his body. Some persons misunderstand the use of the word electrical and are fearful that they will receive an electrical shock. This fear needs to be allayed. There should be no sensation of discomfort from the electrocardiograph.

SECURING CERTAIN ADDITIONAL DATA

Additional data may be secured to compile a more detailed picture of the patient's state of health. The nurse may participate by instructing and preparing the patient, by collecting specimens, and in some situations, by assisting the physician. The report of examination results often provides data useful in planning nursing

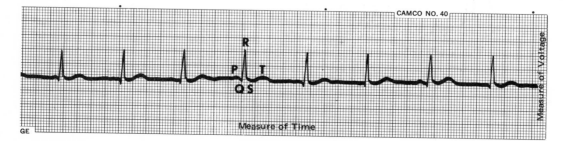

Figure 15–15 The calibrated paper used for the electrocardiogram illustrates time and voltage measures. (From Sharp, L. N., and Rabin, B.: Nursing in the Coronary Care Unit. Philadelphia, J. B. Lippincott, 1970.)

care. Most health agencies have prescribed routines and policies regarding the procedures involved in securing these additional data. The nurse is expected to comply with their routines and policies.

Specimens

The nurse often has the responsibility for instructing the patient and for securing specimens for laboratory examinations. She is also usually responsible for the correct labeling of specimens before they are transported to the laboratory. An inaccurate or unmarked specimen can be more hazardous than no specimen at all. A request for the type of examination desired should accompany the specimen.

Blood Specimens. Blood is one of the most significant body fluids that conveys information about the person's health state. The majority of physical examinations include some type of blood analysis. Multitudes of laboratory tests can be done with blood specimens. The role of the nurse is generally one of explaining to the patient what will happen and what preparation is necessary for the examination. Many blood specimens are secured while the patient is in the fasting state. *Fasting* means abstinence from food or fluid ingestion. The period of fasting will vary with the tests to be done and laboratory techniques used. Whether patients are in their homes or in a health agency, they need a careful explanation about the fast period.

Blood specimens are generally collected by laboratory personnel. Sometimes, the nurse may be responsible for deciding what laboratory tests are to be done and for taking action, depending on the results of the examinations.

In all situations, the nurse should be sufficiently familiar with the more common normal blood examination values in order to be able to recognize deviations. Blood examination results are additional data she collects about the patient in order to provide effective nursing care. Normal adult values for some of the more common laboratory blood tests are given in Table 15–6 on page 322.

Urine Specimens. A *urinalysis* is the laboratory examination of a urine specimen. Analysis of the urine is another common way of securing data about the health state of an individual. The nurse is often responsible for instructing and/or securing a sample of urine. A cooperative patient can be instructed to put the specimen into a clean or, in some instances, a sterile container.

Care should be taken that the outside of the container is not contaminated.

Most laboratories prefer a specimen of several hundred milliliters that is collected soon after arising from sleep. Special urine collection techniques will be discussed in Chapter 20.

Like common blood specimens, the nurse should be able to recognize deviations from normal in the urinalysis. Table 15–6 shows normal adult laboratory analysis values for urine.

Secretion Specimens. Specimens of body secretions are collected for microscopic examination or to introduce them into a culture medium to promote growth of microorganisms present. Body secretions from the throat, vagina, rectum, and wounds or lesions are most often collected for these purposes during the physical examination.

A sterile, long-handled applicator and sterile test tubes are generally used. Some agencies also use sterile glass slides.

The sterile cotton-tipped end of the applicator should be placed directly into the area where the specimen is desired and rotated to make certain secretions adhere to the applicator. The applicator is then carefully placed directly into the test tube or onto the slide and handled according to the laboratory policy. Precautions should be taken so that the applicator is not contaminated before or after securing the secretion specimen. Nor should the secretions be allowed to contaminate other surfaces.

Radiology

Radiology is the use of x-rays to secure data about the patient's health status. An *x-ray* or *roentgen ray* is a high-energy electromagnetic wave which is capable of penetrating solid matter and acting on photographic film. X-ray films are commonly taken to determine the size, shape, and functioning of some organs, the characteristics of bones, and the detection of masses. The role of the nurse in the diagnostic use of x-rays is generally to teach and to prepare persons as necessary.

An x-ray examination of the chest, skeleton, or abdomen generally requires no advance preparation. Several views of the area from different angles are generally taken so that the patient will usually have to change positions during the procedure.

In order to secure more detailed viewing of some organs, a radiopaque contrast substance is used. *Radiopaque* means impenetrable to x-rays. The radiopaque

TABLE 15–6 Normal laboratory values

CONSTITUENTS	NORMAL RANGE
Blood	
Bleeding time	1–3 min.
Cholesterol, total (plasma or serum)	150–250 mgm. %
Clot retraction time	begins in 1 hr.—complete in 24 hrs.
Coagulation time	6–12 min.
Erythrocytes	4,500,000–5,000,000/cu. mm.
Glucose	70–120 mgm. %
Hemoglobin (average for both sexes)	14–16 Gm./100 cc.
Hematocrit average for men	47% ± 7%
Hematocrit average for women	42% ± 5%
Icterus index (serum)	4–6 units
Leukocytes	5,000–10,000/cu. mm.
Basophils	0.25–0.5%
Eosinophils	1–3%
Lymphocytes	25–33%
Monocytes	2–6%
Polymorphonuclear neutrophils	60–70%
pH	7.35–7.45
Platelets	200,000–400,000/cu. mm.
Prothrombin time (Quick)	10–15 sec.
Reticulocytes	0.8–1.0%
Sedimentation rate (Westergren) in first hour	
Men	0–12 min.
Women	0–20 min.
Volume	7–9% body wt.
Cerebrospinal fluid	
Cell count	1–7 lymphocytes/cu. mm.
Colloidal gold	negative
Diffusible calcium	4.5–5.5 mg./100 cc.
Pressure (in resting position)	120–200 mm. water
Specific gravity	1.003–1.008
Sugar	40–70 mg./100 cc.
Total protein	20–40 mg./100 cc.
Urine	
Average amount in 24 hrs.	1,000–1,500 cc.
Chlorides (Na)	10–15 Gm./24 hrs.
Phenosulfonphthalein (P.S.P.)	60–75% in 2 hrs.
Urea clearance	54 cc. blood/min.
Urea	20–35 Gm./24 hrs.
Uric acid	0.4–1 Gm./24 hrs.

Courtesy of Becton, Dickinson and Company.

substance, often containing barium or iodine, produces a contrasting shadow on x-ray films as compared to tissues which are penetrated by the x-rays. For these examinations, the patient usually is in a fasting state.

An *upper GI series* is the x-ray visualization of the esophagus, stomach, and duodenum. The person is asked to drink a radiopaque barium preparation immediately prior to the x-ray examintion. Fluoroscopy may also be used in the upper GI series. *Fluoroscopy* is the radiological visualization of motion without its being recorded on film. Swallowing and the emptying of the stomch may be observed in this way. The examination should not be uncomfortable.

A *barium enema* is the x-ray visualization of the large intestine. A barium solution is instilled through the anus to distend the rectum and colon. In addition to fasting, preparation for the barium enema generally includes cleansing of the colon with laxatives and enemas. The technique for giving enemas will be discussed in Chapter 20. Laxatives and enemas may also be used to cleanse the intestine of residual barium following the examination. The patient should be prepared for the fact that a barium enema is rather uncomfortable and a tiring procedure. He should also be told to expect that his fecal material may be white from the barium for several days following the examination.

A gallbladder x-ray or oral cholecystogram is the x-ray visualization of the gallbladder. An iodine radiopaque substance is taken orally, absorbed by the liver, and concentrated in the gallbladder. Preparations generally include some dietary modification on the day preceding the examination, followed by taking pills containing the contrast material during the evening. The procedure should cause no discomfort although occasionally some persons may experience side effects from the contrast material. An intravenous cholangiogram uses contrast material given intravenously. The examination is similar to the oral cholecystogram.

An *intravenous pyelogram,* or IVP as it is commonly called, is the x-ray visualization of the kidney's ability to excrete urine. A radiopaque dye is injected intravenously and films are taken at timed intervals to determine the amount of dye excreted by the kidneys. Preparations for an IVP usually include a laxative or enema and having the person urinate before the examination. Normally, there should be no discomfort. However, some persons are sensitive to the dye and may have allergic reactions to it.

Ultrasonography

Ultrasonography is the use of ultrasound to produce an image or photograph of an organ or tissue. The kidneys, liver, spleen, pancreas, gallbladder, thyroid, heart, eyes, lymph nodes, aorta, and female reproductive organs can be examined in this way. *Ultrasound waves* are extremely high-frequency and inaudible sound waves. The ultrasound waves penetrate and bounce back according to the density of the tissue. A *transducer,* an instrument which converts energy from one form to another, produces the ultrasound waves and converts the reflected waves into electrical energy. The electrical energy then produces an image on a viewing screen. The person will be asked to remain quiet while the transducer, which is approximately 2.5 cm. or 1 inch in diameter, is applied to the lubricated skin and moved about over the area to be examined. Generally, no special preparations are necessary and the person experiences no discomfort with this procedure.

Radioisotope Scanning

A *radioisotope* is a radioactive chemical. When used for diagnostic examination, a substance containing a small amount of radioisotope is taken orally or by injection. The particular substance is selected according to its ability to localize in the target organ. Blocking agents are sometimes given to prevent its absorption by other organs. The heart, vessels, brain, spinal canal, lungs,

thyroid, and abdominal organs are examined in this way. The size, shape, and function of organs and the presence of abnormal masses can be determined. A mechanism called a scanner detects emission of the radioactive waves and records them on a photographic plate. Preparation for radioisotope scanning should include reassurance that the amount of radioisotope normally used is minute and produces no more radiation than that of a single x-ray. Some individuals fear that they will become dangerously radioactive. The person should also be prepared for the fact that lengthy placement in an awkward position may be necessary during the test. No discomfort should normally be experienced except for that caused by injection and the positioning.

Gastric Analysis

Gastric analysis is the laboratory examination of gastric content. The stomach contents are removed by means of aspiration through a tube which has been inserted through the mouth or nose and the esophagus into the stomach. Removal of the gastric specimens is often the responsibility of the nurse. The tube itself may be inserted by nurses in some health agencies and by physicians in others.

A gastric analysis can be done to examine the volume or constituents of stomach secretions. It is done most commonly when stomach pathology is suspected.

Since the stomach is not a sterile cavity, the equipment need not be sterile, but medical asepsis is observed. The tube is introduced through one of the nares or the mouth. It is made of rubber or plastic and is 30 to 60 cm. or 12 to 24 inches longer than the distance from the patient's mouth to his stomach. The tube commonly used is the Levin tube. Either a bulb-type syringe or a plunger-type syringe is used to aspirate the stomach contents. Usually a 50 ml. syringe is preferred.

The larger the lumen of the tube, the easier it is to remove thick stomach contents. However, the larger the tube, the more discomfort the patient experiences in swallowing it. When a small tube is used, it is passed through one of the nares; if a larger tube is used, the patient is asked to swallow it through the mouth.

Before the tube is inserted, it may be helpful, especially when using rubber, to place the tube on cracked ice for 15 to 20 minutes. This cooling of the tube makes it less flexible and therefore easier to handle. In addition, a water-soluble lubricant should be available for lubricating the tube.

The number and type of specimen containers needed will be determined by the tests to be performed and the laboratory procedure.

In most instances, the patient is placed in the sitting position so that gravity aids the passage of the tube. If the patient is unable to sit up, he may lie either on his back or on his side. The chin should be elevated. This facilitates passage of the tube by following the body's natural contours.

The approximate distance to the stomach is determined by measuring the distance from the tip of the sternum to the bridge of the nose. The length should be marked on the tube before initiating insertion. The lubricated tube is introduced through one of the nares or over the top and middle of the tongue. Asking the patient to breathe through his mouth is generally helpful. When the tip of the tube reaches the pharynx, the patient is asked to begin swallowing. As the patient swallows, the tube is inserted until the marked point is reached. Since the delicate mucous membrane can be damaged, insertion through the nasal or oropharyngeal areas should be gentle. Force should not be used. Usually, adequate lubrication and rotation of the tube with gentle pressure will aid ease of movement. Since some persons have nasal septum deviations and other pathological states of the nasopharyngeal area, if one naris cannot be entered readily, the alternate one should be used. If the tube cannot be inserted readily, another more experienced practitioner should be called on. If the patient is allowed water, permitting him to take sips while the tube is being swallowed helps to ease passage of the tube.

The gag reflex is stimulated by tube insertion in most patients. However, it should be a temporary reaction. Persistent gagging may mean the tube is being passed too slowly or too rapidly.

Sometimes, the tube may enter the trachea rather than the esophagus. Coughing, difficulty with breathing, and the inability to hum are indications of this misplacement. The tube should be immediately removed when the trachea has been entered.

Once the tube has been inserted the appropriate distance, placement within the stomach should be positively ascertained. There are a number of techniques to determine tube placement, but the only completely reliable one is the aspiration of gastric contents through the tube. However, there are situations when the tube may be properly placed and because of the viscosity of the gastric contents, they do not move readily up the tube when suction from the syringe is applied. Holding the end of the tube under water to observe for bubbles can be tried. If the tube is in the lung, air should escape through the tube in the form of bubbles. Another method is to inject air into the tube while auscultating over the upper abdomen. If the tube is properly placed, the nurse will hear air entering the stomach. If there is any doubt about the tube placement, seeking the opinion of another nurse or a physician, or repositioning the tube is essential.

When proper placement is assured, the tube should be taped securely at the nose or cheek. If the tube is not secured, swallowing, coughing, sneezing, and even talking can displace it.

Removal of stomach contents is achieved by aspirating with the syringe. The number of specimens to be taken and the time intervals between them will vary according to the procedure of the laboratories in the various agencies. However, almost all request a fasting specimen initially. Then some require the administration of a drug or a test meal to stimulate gastric secretions. At specified intervals, samples of gastric contents are taken. The specimens are labeled and handled according to the agency policy.

Following completion of the examination, the gastric tube can be removed. After the tape holdings are loosened, the tube is pinched tightly near the patient's face and quickly withdrawn. A towel or similar cloth should be available to cover and remove the tubing from the patient's view immediately. The tube's removal may stimulate the gag reflex, but this will usually only last momentarily.

The gastric analysis is usually done to determine the volume of hydrochloric acid in the stomach. A tubeless gastric analysis, involving dye ingestion and urine specimen collection, is also possible to determine the presence of free hydrochloric acid, but it does not determine how much acid is present.

Lumbar Puncture

A *lumbar puncture,* or *spinal tap,* is the insertion of a needle into the subarachnoid space in the spinal canal. The procedure is part of the physical examination for some patients. It is generally performed by a physician with the nurse assisting.

Indications for a Lumbar Puncture. Cerebrospinal fluid normally fills the ventricles of the brain, the subarachnoid space, and the central canal of the spinal cord. The fluid is clear and transparent. It may be necessary to enter the subarachnoid space for several reasons: to obtain a specimen of the fluid for analysis and for culture; to establish any alterations in the usual pressure of the cerebrospinal fluid; to relieve pressure; to inject drugs or to inject dyes for x-ray visualization. Table 15–6 on page 322 includes norms for laboratory analysis of spinal fluid.

Necessary Equipment. Because the subarachnoid space is a sterile cavity, surgical asepsis is observed. Normally, the cerebrospinal fluid pressure is greater than atmospheric pressure, and many pathogenic conditions of the central nervous system are characterized by an increase in this normal pressure. Therefore, the lumbar puncture needle contains a carefully and precisely fitted stylet so that fluid will not escape while the needle is in place, except when the physician removes the stylet.

The necessary sterile equipment includes a 20- or 22-gauge lumbar puncture needle, 7.5 to 12.5 cm. (3 to 5 inches) long; a small syringe and a 22- or 25-gauge needle for the injection of local anesthesia at the site of injection; a fenestrated drape, gauze and cotton balls, and gloves for the physician. Many sets include specimen containers and some a manometer for measuring the pressure of the fluid. If not included, they are added at the appropriate time. Commercially prepared disposable spinal tap trays are available also. If the physician wishes to inject a drug into the spinal canal, another sterile syringe of the appropriate size is necessary. The local anesthetic of the physician's choice should be available. One percent procaine hydrochloride usually is used. The physician may want a stool so he can be seated during the procedure.

Prior to the procedure, the nurse examines the skin area where the lumbar puncture will be performed. If hair is present, the physician is asked whether he wishes the area to be shaved.

Assisting the Physician. The fourth or the fifth lumbar space is the usual site of entry. The needle enters the subarachnoid space by passing between the vertebrae into the canal. In order to spread the vertebrae and to provide the widest possible space for easier insertion of the needle, the patient is positioned on his side and with his back arched. Figure 15–16 illustrates this position. He is brought near the edge of the bed or the treatment table where the physician will work. The patient is asked to flex his knees and bring his head and shoulders down as close as possible to the knees. A small pillow may be placed under the patient's head and between the knees for comfort. Some patients are unable to assume or maintain this position without assistance. This can be done by facing the patient and grasp-

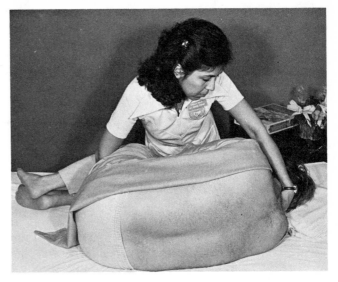

Figure 15–16   The patient is positioned for a lumbar puncture. The nurse is helping the patient maintain the desired position with one arm behind his flexed knees and the other arm behind his flexed back. In this position, the back is arched and the vertebrae are separated to facilitate introduction of the spinal needle.

ing him behind the knees with one arm and behind the neck with the other arm so that the back remains arched as much as possible. Other patients may have difficulty in understanding or be disoriented. They will need repeated assurances of what is being done. However, the head should not be pulled down or the knees pressed against the abdomen, since this increases intraspinal fluid pressure, leading to a falsely elevated pressure.

The nurse may have to help the patient to maintain the desired position. After helping the physician to get his equipment in order, the nurse returns to the opposite side of the bed to do this. It is important to explain to the patient that he must remain motionless during the procedure. Moving about makes insertion of the needle more difficult and also may cause the needle to break.

Occasionally, the physician may prefer having the patient in the sitting position during the lumbar puncture. The patient sits on the edge of a treatment table, the feet are supported on a chair and the arms are placed over the shoulders of a person who helps to support him in position, or the arms are supported on an overbed table placed in front of him.

The fourth or the fifth lumbar space is located approximately at the same level on the back as the iliac crest. After an antiseptic has been applied to the area, the physician puts the sterile fenestrated drape in place. The opening is over the area that has been cleaned and where the needle will be inserted. Care should be taken so that the drape does not slip during the procedure and thereby contaminate the working area. The area of the drape surrounding the working area is kept sterile.

The nurse prepares the bottle of anesthetic that the physician has ordered and holds it so that he can check the label and withdraw some, or the nurse may pour the drug. The physician begins the procedure by anesthetizing the skin and the subcutaneous tissue at the site of injection.

When the anesthesia is effective, the physician inserts the lumbar puncture needle. After the needle is in place, the physician may apply the manometer to the needle to determine the cerebrospinal pressure. The pressure normally is not constant and will be observed to fluctuate somewhat with each pulse beat and each respiration. The normal average range of pressure is about 6 to 12 mm. of mercury or 90 to 150 mm. of water. The physician may ask the nurse to make a notation of the pressure reading. If the lumbar puncture needle is resting freely in the subarachnoid space, pressure usually can be increased when venous compression occurs. The physician may ask the nurse to apply hand pressure to the abdomen. The pressure can also be increased by compressing the jugular vein. This is called the Queckenstedt's test and is used if intraspinal lesions are suspected. The most reliable reading can be obtained by inflating a blood pressure cuff wrapped about the neck. This provides for a more even pressure. The mercury column is elevated to 50 mm. As there is variation in this practice, the nurse should always understand the physician's procedure if she is to assist in this test.

After pressure has been determined, specimens will be collected if desired. If sterile tubes are provided in the set, the physician may collect the specimens himself and hand them to the nurse for proper labeling and handling.

If not included, the physician may ask the nurse to hold the tubes below the opening of the needle while he regulates the flow of cerebrospinal fluid with the stylet. Care should be taken to prevent touching the needle or the hands of the physician with the collecting tubes. It may also be important to note and mark the order of fluid removed on each specimen container. Table 15–6 indicates normal cerebrospinal fluid values.

During the procedure, the nurse observes the patient's reaction carefully. His color, pulse rate, and respiratory rate are noted and reported to the physician immediately if they deviate from his norm. Care should be exercised to prevent alarming the patient if any report is being given to the physician.

When the procedure is completed, the needle is removed, and compression is applied to the site for a short while. A small sterile piece of gauze may be applied to the site and fastened with adhesive.

Immediately following the procedure, the patient may be placed in the recumbent position, preferably without a pillow. Fluids usually are offered. This is intended to avoid postspinal headache. It generally is believed that the headache is due to the tear in the dura mater made by the needle, which allows for seepage of small amounts of cerebrospinal fluid. Differences of opinion do exist about the effectiveness of positioning in avoiding the occurrence of the headache. The nurse will want to follow the practice preferred in her agency. If a headache does occur, the patient usually is treated symptomatically.

The patient's general physical reaction to the procedure is observed. This is of particular importance if the procedure was carried out to relieve pressure. Any unusual reactions such as twitching, vomiting, or slow pulse are reported to the physician promptly.

Thoracentesis

A *thoracentesis* is the entering and aspirating of fluid from the pleural cavity. The pleural cavity is a potential cavity, since normally it is not distended with fluid or air. Its walls are in approximation, and normal secretions keep them from adhering. The physician generally performs the thoracentesis with the nurse assisting.

Indications for Thoracentesis. When a thoracentesis is done as a part of a physical examination, the pleural cavity is entered to determine whether fluid is present, if this cannot be established satisfactorily by other means. If fluid is present, specimens usually are obtained and analyzed to assist in diagnosis. If an accumulation of fluid in the pleural cavity causes difficult respiration and discomfort, a thoracentesis may also be done for therapeutic reasons to remove the fluid. This, in turn, relieves respiratory embarrassment.

Fluid in the pleural cavity results from inflammation caused by an infection which increases the normal secretions in the pleural cavity. If the fluid is purulent, the condition is called *empyema*. Fluid may accumulate also in the pleural cavity as a result of impaired circulation. This is common when a tumor is present. Air in the pleural cavity is almost always due to accidents when the chest wall has been punctured.

Equipment Needed. Because the cavity being entered is sterile, surgical asepsis is used. The basic equipment for entering the pleural cavity includes a small syringe and a 22- or 25-gauge needle for administering a local anesthetic at the site of injection; a blunt 15-gauge needle, 5 to 7.5 cm. (2 to 3 inches) long; gauze and cotton; sterile gloves for the physician; sterile specimen tubes; and a fenestrated drape. A skin antiseptic and a local anesthetic agent are also necessary. Commercially prepared disposable trays containing the equipment are also available.

Normally, the pressure in the pleural cavity is less than atmospheric pressure; therefore, equipment for suction is almost always necessary to remove the fluid. The physician indicates the method that he will use.

One way to remove fluid or air from the pleural cavity is to aspirate it with a syringe. A large syringe, usually 50 ml., frequently is used. When this method is employed, a sterile syringe with a three-way stopcock attached is added to the sterile equipment. The physician withdraws the fluid into the syringe and adjusts the stopcock so that he may push the fluid into the collecting container. He readjusts the stopcock and reaspirates the pleural cavity. A hand-operated large volume bellows pump can also be attached to the needle for aspiration. This device eliminates stopcock manipulation.

Another method for removing fluid from the pleural cavity is to drain the fluid into a bottle in which a partial vacuum has been created. The bottle has a stopper on it to which is attached a two-way stopcock. To one opening in the stopcock is attached rubber tubing which connects with the needle in the pleural cavity. Air is removed from the bottle through the other opening in the stopcock with either a motor-driven or a hand-operated suction pump. When this method is used, the tubing which connects the needle and the bottle should be sterile. It is convenient to use a calibrated bottle for the drainage in order to determine readily the amount of fluid that has been removed.

To enhance the safety and the effectiveness of the procedure, a sterile plastic catheter to thread through the needle after it is in the site can be used. Then the needle can be withdrawn. The catheter reduces the possibility of puncturing the lung or doing other damage; also, its flexibility makes it possible to feed it into a pocket of fluid which the needle may not have

reached accurately. The catheter is also more comfortable for the patient.

Prior to the procedure, the nurse examines the skin area where the physician will be working. If hair is present, the physician is asked whether he wants the area shaved.

Assisting the Physician. Usually, this procedure is carried out when the patient is in a sitting position on a chair or on the edge of a treatment table or bed with the feet supported on a chair. Figure 15–17 illustrates this position. If the patient cannot sit up, he may lie on his side. Usually, he is placed on the affected side with the hand of that side resting on the opposite shoulder.

The skin is prepared over the area where the physician indicates that he will insert the needle. The exact location will depend on the area where fluid is present and where the physician can best aspirate it. The needle will be inserted between the ribs through the intercostal muscles, the intercostal fascia and into the pleura. After the skin is prepared, the physician places the drape. The nurse may need to help anchor it in front of the patient's shoulders to prevent its slipping about on the field of work. The nurse prepares the bottle of anesthetic drug and holds it so that the physician can read the label before he withdraws some or she pours some.

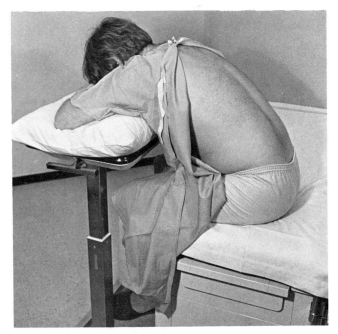

Figure 15–17 This patient is properly positioned for a thoracentesis.

The physician begins by anesthetizing the area where the needle is to be inserted. When anesthesia is effective, the physician inserts the needle. The nurse usually is asked to assist with the collection of specimens. The nurse is responsible for having the container ready for the physician to empty the syringe if the syringe method is being used. If a bottle is being used to collect the drainage, the nurse assists by operating either the hand- or the motor-driven pump that creates the partial vacuum in the bottle.

During the procedure, the nurse observes the patient for reactions. The patient's color, pulse rate, and respiratory rate are observed, and any deviation from his norm is reported to the physician immediately. Fainting, nausea, and vomiting may occur.

When the procedure is completed, the needle (or plastic catheter) is removed. The nurse assists with placing a small sterile dressing over the site of entry.

Following the procedure, the patient should be observed for changes in his respirations. If a large amount of fluid is removed, respirations usually will be eased. If the lung has been punctured inadvertently (the use of a blunt needle aids in preventing this accident), respiratory embarrassment becomes acute. If present, sputum should be observed, and if blood appears or if the patient has severe coughing, the physician should be notified promptly.

Abdominal Paracentesis

The withdrawal of fluid from the peritoneal cavity is called an abdominal paracentesis. The word *paracentesis* means the withdrawal of fluid from any body cavity, but it is common practice to use the term when referring to the removal of fluid from the peritoneal cavity. The technique is used to secure abdominal fluid for analysis or for the therapeutic value of removing excess fluid. This procedure also is normally performed by a physician with the nurse assisting.

The accumulation of fluid in the peritoneal cavity is called *ascites* and often occurs with certain liver, cardiac, and renal diseases.

Indications for a Paracentesis. When used for diagnostic purposes, specimens of the fluid are taken for examination in order to identify certain organisms or cells. The fluid may be analyzed to determine whether or not cells of a malignant tumor are present. A paracentesis will help to relieve symptoms caused by the accumulation of fluid in the peritoneal cavity. The symptoms are caused by the pressure of the fluid. For example, respi-

rations may be embarrassed if the fluid causes pressure on the diaphragm, or frequency of voiding may be increased, since the fluid may make it difficult for the urinary bladder to fill to normal capacity.

Equipment Needed. Since the peritoneal cavity is normally a sterile cavity, surgical asepsis is observed for the procedure. Normally, the pressure in the peritoneal cavity is no greater than atmospheric pressure, but, when fluid is present, pressure is greater than atmospheric. Gravity will aid in the removal of fluid; therefore, the fluid will drain of its own accord until pressure is equalized.

A sterile trocar and cannula are used to enter the peritoneal cavity. This instrument is usually 10 to 12.5 cm. (4 to 5 inches) in length with a bore of approximately one-eighth of an inch. In order to introduce the trocar easily, a very small incision is made in the skin which is sutured following the procedure. The sterile items needed include a small syringe and a 22- or 25-gauge needle for anesthetizing the skin prior to making the incision; a scalpel for making the incision; suture material, small clamps or forceps, a suture needle, and scissors for closing the incision; tubing to be attached directly to the trocar for drainage; a fenestrated drape or towels; gauze and cotton balls, and gloves. Skin antiseptic and an anesthetic usually will be needed. Disposable paracentesis trays are also available.

A clean container for drainage, preferably a calibrated bottle, is necessary. The use of a plastic catheter threaded through the trocar once it is in place is a method used by some physicians. It provides for greater safety and comfort to the patient. In addition, its small caliber reduces the rate of flow of the fluid. When the plastic catheter is used, both the physician and the nurse may need to consider available equipment for connecting the catheter to drainage tubing. A large-gauge needle inserted into the plastic tubing and then attached to suitable-sized drainage tubing is one means used.

Prior to the procedure, the nurse examines the patient's abdomen. If hair is present, the physician is asked whether or not he wants the area to be shaved.

Assisting the Physician. The patient is weighed prior to and after the treatment. The patient should be encouraged to void before the procedure is begun. This is of particular importance when a paracentesis is to be performed because, if the urinary bladder is full, there is danger of puncturing it with the trocar. If the patient is unable to void, the physician should be notified; then he may order the patient to be catheterized.

Since gravity will be used to assist the drainage, the patient is placed in a sitting position. The patient may be supported in the sitting position in bed; he may be placed at the side of the bed or the treatment table with his feet supported on a chair; or he may sit on a chair during the procedure. A chair is most comfortable because it offers good back and arm support. This is important, since the procedure may take an extended period of time if a large amount of fluid is to be withdrawn. After the patient is in position, with legs slightly separated so that the site of entry is readily accessible, he should be covered adequately for warmth and to prevent unnecessary exposure. A pair of pajama pants helps to keep the patient's legs covered and also to prevent exposure. The trocar will be passed through the abdominal wall into the peritoneal cavity near the midline of the abdomen approximately halfway between the umbilicus and the pubis. The skin over this area is cleaned, and the physician places the sterile drape in position. The nurse may need to secure it to prevent its slipping.

The physician then anesthetizes the site of entry, incises the skin, and introduces the trocar and the cannula. When the trocar is in place, the physician will pull back on the cannula to see if fluid will drain; if it does, the drainage tube is attached. The specimens will be obtained and should be carefully labeled. If a plastic catheter is used it is threaded through at this time. The nurse places the distal end of the tubing in the container for drainage. The greater the vertical distance between the trocar and the container for drainage, the greater will be the pull of gravity. If fluid is draining too rapidly, the container should be elevated on a stool. Rapid drainage may produce symptoms of shock.

During the treatment and after, the nurse observes the patient for untoward reactions associated with electrolyte imbalance. His color and respiratory and pulse rates are noted. Signs of fainting are watched for. The patient may begin to experience relief from the pressure of the fluid, and these signs are observed by the nurse also.

The nurse notes the type and the amount of drainage present. After the needle has been withdrawn and the incision sutured, the nurse should place a sterile heavy dressing over the site of incision, since leakage usually occurs. The dressing is changed as necessary. The patient often is more comfortable if an abdominal binder is used for support following the procedure.

Proctosigmoidoscopy

A *proctosigmoidoscopy* is a visual examination of the rectum, rectosigmoid junction, and lower sigmoid colon. A *proctoscopy* is a visual examination of the rectum, and an *anoscopy* is a visual examination of the anal canal. A lighted tubular instrument called an *endoscope* is used for examining the inside of these and similar organs or cavities. The length of the instrument and the portion of the intestine which is viewed vary with each examination. The physician usually performs the examinations with assistance from the nurse.

Indications for Proctosigmoidoscopy. When a proctosigmoidoscopy, proctoscopy, or anoscopy is performed as a part of a physical examination, it is generally to detect the presence of a malignancy. When suspicious tissue is found, a biopsy is usually done. A *biopsy* is the removal of a piece of tissue for microscopic examination. Because of the prevalence of cancer of the lower intestinal tract, it is recommended that an endoscopic examination be done routinely each year on persons past age 45. It should also be performed on anyone with such symptoms as changes in bowel habits or blood in the stool. The examination is also used to detect the presence of other intestinal abnormalities.

Equipment Needed. Because the area being examined is not sterile, medical asepsis is sufficient. However, surgical asepsis is often used as an added safety precaution, particularly if a biopsy is anticipated. The required equipment includes an endoscope of appropriate size and length for the intended purpose, mechanical suction, an air insufflator for forcing air into the colon in order to separate the mucosal folds, and a biopsy forceps. Gloves, lubricant, a specimen container, and a drape should be available. The physician may also wish a stool so that he can be seated during the examination.

Assisting the Physician. The lower colon should be emptied of fecal material in preparation for the endoscopic examination. Enemas, laxatives, or suppositories, or a combination may be used.

The patient is assisted into the knee-chest position for the examination. Some examining tables can be adjusted to make the position easier to assume and maintain. Adequate draping of the patient is important to minimize exposure and discomfort for the patient. A large fenestrated drape or two draw sheets are used.

The physician generally initially performs a digital rectal examination to dilate the anal sphincter and to determine that no obvious obstructions are present. The lubricated endoscope is then gradually inserted its full length unless the patient cannot tolerate it. As it is slowly withdrawn, all areas of the intestinal mucosa are inspected. Air from the insufflator may be introduced and suction is used to remove fecal matter and other secretions as necessary to achieve maximum visualization. Suspicious tissue can be biopsied at any site.

Usually, the patient will experience the urge to defecate during the digital examination and when the endoscope is introduced. Encouraging him to breathe deeply and slowly through his mouth generally relieves this sensation. The head-down position, the deep breathing, and the discomfort may cause the patient to become dizzy. The nurse should also observe the patient for pulse and color changes and notify the physician of the patient's reactions.

The physical and psychological discomfort makes the intestinal endoscopic examination unpopular among patients. The nurse should make every effort to assure the patient's privacy, assist him in positioning, and help him to relax.

Following the examination, the patient may need to rest in a horizontal position for a few minutes to regain his equilibrium before sitting or standing. He should be observed for abdominal pain or rectal bleeding. If they occur, the physician should be notified. Abdominal and anal tenderness and a small amount of rectal bleeding are not unusual.

THE PHYSICAL EXAMINATION AND THE NURSING PROCESS

This chapter is concerned primarily with the collection of data about the patient's state of physical health. As Chapter 4 indicated, validation of data is important but it is neither necessary nor practical to validate every bit of information collected.

When there are discrepancies in data, validation is advisable. For example, if there are discrepancies when the patient's blood pressure is taken by different people, the measurement should be validated.

Doubt about the accuracy of data calls for validation. For example, a patient's temperature, taken orally, falls within normal range; yet, the patient feels warm to touch and complains of a headache and nausea. The nurse will wish to recheck the patient's temperature since she realizes that an elevated temperature is commonly found with the symptoms presented.

Data are evaluated to determine appropriateness and accuracy. These questions, offered in Chapter 4 will aid the nurse to evaluate data: Do the findings accurately reflect the patient's present state of health? Have all relevant factors in the patient's situation been considered? Are the relationships between factors in the patient's situation appropriate and accurate? The reader is encouraged to review Chapter 4 for a more detailed discussion of the entire data-gathering process.

Many standards were given in this chapter that will help the nurse assess data. For example, the tables in this chapter, except for Table 15–2, give valuable norms for assessment.

When nursing diagnoses related to the patient's physical health are determined, a nursing care plan is developed with the patient. Using the assessed data increases the probability of planning comprehensive and individualized patient care.

The particular nursing measures selected for intervention will depend on the patient's situation. The following are some general guidelines the nurse will wish to keep in mind when collecting information about the patient's physical health.

- Use and abuse will damage any equipment eventually. Many different nursing and other health personnel use the equipment ordinarily provided by health agencies and offices for collecting data. Before using equipment for gathering information, be sure the equipment is in good working order and serves its intended purpose accurately.

- Use and care for equipment utilized for the collection of data properly and carefully. Much of the equipment is very expensive, and if not properly used, will not provide accurate data.

- Collect data from the patient in a thoughtful manner. Gathering data automatically and without thought while observing a particular routine often results in care that does not meet the patient's individual needs. For example, obtaining vital signs is often done on a routine basis without much consideration for what the signs mean and in what way they reflect the patient's health status.

- Assume the ultimate responsibility for accuracy of data you are expected to collect. Auxiliary nursing personnel are often assigned to carry out such procedures as obtaining vital signs and weighing patients. While many are capable of doing so, they do not have the theoretical background of the nurse and cannot be assumed able to make the kinds of judgments expected of the nurse.

- Note the patient's psychological responses to the collection of data. Many procedures discussed in this chapter are frightening to most patients. The patient has the right to explanations so that he will know what to expect and why particular procedures are being done. Before, during and after data collection, the nurse should offer emotional support and care as indicated.

- Take advantage of teaching opportunities while carrying out the various parts of a physical examination. As the nurse examines and interviews the patient, she will note when there is need to share health information and will proceed to do so as indicated.

The parts of the nursing process and of the process as a whole are evaluated as described in Chapter 4.

CONCLUSION

The health state profile, developed from collected data, is an important tool for assessing and planning nursing care and for nursing intervention. This chapter has described the gathering of certain data that are important to have in order to prepare an objective and accurate profile. Some norms used in assessing have also been presented. This text will describe data gathering in remaining chapters also. However, basic data necessary in nearly every situation have been presented here.

SUPPLEMENTAL LIBRARY STUDY

1. The increasing popularity of nurses learning skills to conduct physical examinations has not been without controversy. The following authors identify several erroneous assumptions they believe are common.

    Lynaugh, Joan E. and Bates, Barbara. "Physical Diagnosis: A Skill for All Nurses?" *American Journal of Nursing*, 74:58–59. January 1974.

    What assumptions did these authors describe? What are the risks associated with the assumptions? Do you agree with their recommendations for developing a balance between competence and confidence in the practitioner?

2. Laboratory test results make up an important part of data used to study a patient's physical health. A four-part series about common hematological studies is included in the following issues of a nursing periodical.

    Byrne, Judith. "Hematologic Studies: Part 1. A Review of the CBC: The Quantitative Test." *Nursing 76*, 6:11–12, October 1976.

    Byrne, Judith. "Hematologic Studies: Part 2. A Review of the CBC: The Differential White Cell Count." *Nursing 76*, 6:15–17, November 1976.

    Byrne, Judith. "Hematologic Studies: Part 3. A Review of the CBC: Stained Red Cell Examination." *Nursing 76*, 6:15, December 1976.

    Byrne, Judith. "Hematologic Studies: Part 4. Tips for Interpreting the Sedimentation Rate and Reticulocyte Count." *Nursing 77*, 7:9–10, January 1977.

    How are laboratory test results useful in planning nursing care? For instance, what significance could an elevated white blood count have for nursing care?

3. Comprehensive observations of a person's physical health is often difficult and sometimes complex. These authors suggest a practical tool for making the collecting and assessing of physical data easier.

    Wolff, Helen and Erickson, Roberta. "The Assessment Man." *Nursing Outlook,* 25:103–107, February 1977.

    Use the authors' tool in your clinical practice and evaluate to determine if it helps to make your data collection more organized and logical.

4. The *American Journal of Nursing* has published a series of programmed instructions on the physical examination. Each part of the series focuses on a different part of the body. Some examples of the programs are given below.

    "Patient Assessment: Examination of the Chest and Lungs." (Programmed Instruction) *American Journal of Nursing,* 76:1453–1475, 1516, September 1976.

    "Patient Assessment: Examination of the Eye. Part 1." (Programmed Instruction) *American Journal of Nursing,* 74:2039–2063, November 1974.

    "Patient Assessment: Examination of the Head and Neck." (Programmed Instruction) *American Journal of Nursing,* 75:839–862, May 1975.

    Review the programs to acquire an understanding of the knowledge and skills which are considered necessary for conducting a physical examination. These programmed instructions can be helpful resources to acquire and improve your skills.

16

BEHAVIORAL OBJECTIVES

When content in this chapter has been mastered, the student will be able to

Define the terms appearing in the glossary.

State four basic principles which guide the nurse when she cares for the skin and mucous membrane.

Describe skin cleaning agents, grooming aids, and cosmetics and indicate problems that may be associated with the use of each of them.

Indicate the primary purposes of the bath and back rub and briefly describe the procedure for each, including the shower bath, tub bath, bath taken in bed, bath given in bed, and the towel bath.

Discuss the care of the hair, including grooming Caucasian and non-Caucasian persons; care of the mouth and teeth, including dentures; care of the nails, feet, and eyes, including eyeglasses, contact lenses, and an artificial eye; care of the ears and nose; and perineal care. Describe modifications in care when the person is ill.

Summarize the manner in which a decubitus ulcer develops, factors which predispose to the development of decubitus ulcers, and how decubitus ulcers can be prevented and treated.

Describe the nursing care of a patient requiring assistance with personal hygiene, using the nursing process as a guide.

injury. Very thin and very obese people tend to be more subject to skin irritation and injury.

Body cells adequately nourished and hydrated are more resistant to injury. Chapter 19 discusses the importance of nutrition to good body functioning. Cells in the skin and the mucous membrane need adequate nourishment and hydration. The better nourished the cell, the better its ability to resist injury and disease.

Adequate circulation is necessary in order to maintain cell life. When circulation is impaired for any reason, the cells involved are nourished inadequately; hence, they are more subject to injury. The importance of this principle will be illustrated more clearly in the discussion on the prevention of bedsores, later in this chapter.

CARE OF THE SKIN

The skin consists of two distinct layers. The superficial portion is called the *epidermis* and is made up of layers of stratified squamous epithelium. It contains pores of sweat glands and shafts of hair in most parts of the body. The deeper layer is called the *dermis* and consists of smooth muscular tissue, nerves, fat, hair follicles, certain glands and their ducts, arteries, veins and capillaries, and fibrous elastic tissue. The skin covers the entire body and is continuous with the mucous membrane at normal body orifices. Figure 16–1 on page 336 illustrates a cross-section of normal skin.

The skin serves to protect underlying body tissue and organs from injury; it prevents microorganisms from invading the body; water, including nitrogenous wastes, is excreted through the skin; and the skin houses sense organs of touch, pain, heat, cold, and pressure. The skin also plays an important part in the regulation of body temperature. Heat is lost from the body through vasodilation and evaporation of perspiration. Heat is retained through vasoconstriction, and the phenomenon known as "goose pimples," which are formed by the contraction of muscular tissue in the dermis, makes the hair stand on end.

The cutaneous glands include the sebaceous, the sweat, and the ceruminous glands. The *sebaceous glands* secrete an oily substance called *sebum* which lubricates the skin and hair and keeps the skin and scalp pliant. The sweat glands secrete perspiration. The *cerumen* in the external ear canals, consisting of a heavy oil and brown pigment, is secreted by the *ceruminous glands*.

Age is a factor in caring for the skin. Because an infant's skin is injured easily and subject to infection he should be handled and bathed gently to prevent injury. Young children's skin becomes more resistant to injury and infection but requires frequent cleaning because of toilet and play habits.

During adolescence, the skin should be kept immaculately clean and free from irritation to aid in the control of acne. This condition is common during these years and is discussed later in this chapter. During adolescence and up to approximately 50 years of age, secretions from skin glands are at their maximum. Hence, more frequent bathing is necessary to prevent body odors and the accumulation of secretions and dirt.

As age advances, the skin becomes thinner and less elastic and supple. Subcutaneous fat that normally helps to absorb injury to the skin decreases. Wrinkles appear, most of which are deep in the dermis. Since less oil is secreted from sebaceous glands, the skin becomes dry, often scaly, and rough in appearance. Brown freckle-like spots often appear on the hands, arms, neck, and face. They may begin appearing as early as 35 years of age and tend to become more numerous and larger with aging. These spots are often called old-age freckles or liver spots. Liver diseases do not cause these spots; rather, they are due to exposure to the wind and the sun. If they become thickened or develop crusts, it is wise to seek medical advice to determine whether any are precancerous lesions. Changes that occur in the skin with aging are irreversible.

Illness very often alters the condition of the skin and makes special care necessary. Severe fluid loss through fever, vomiting, or diarrhea reduces the fluid volume of the body. This condition makes the skin appear loose and very often flabby. The skin can be lifted easily, and it may not spring back as it does when the patient is well. Also, excessive perspiration may present a problem during illness. Some illnesses are accompanied by a change in pigmentation of the skin. The most commonly seen change in the skin color is that of jaundice. This symptom of several pathological conditions is a light to deep yellow pigmentation of the skin. Other diseases may produce tiny hemorrhagic spots on the skin or mottled areas, and the skin appears as though the underlying blood vessels are barely covered.

Soaps, Detergents, and Creams

A great variety of soaps and detergents is available on the market today. However, there is very little difference in their quality, despite advertising claims. The expensive ones, with their color, perfume, and en-

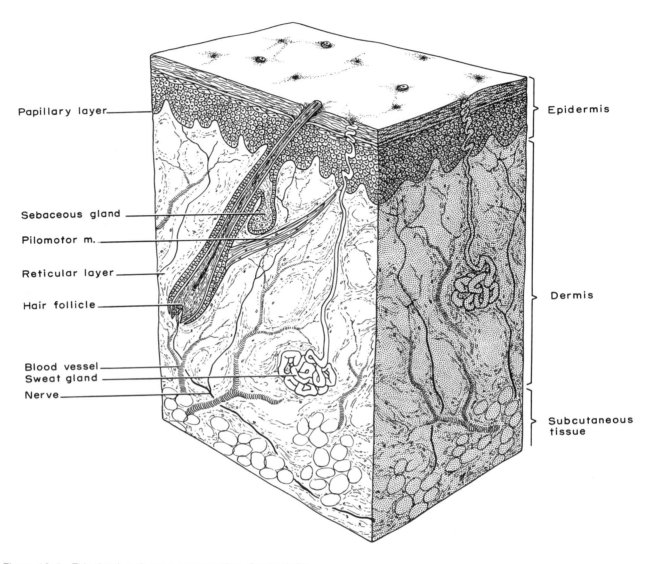

Figure 16–1   This drawing shows a cross-section of normal skin.

dorsements, have not been found to be superior to the less expensive ones as cleaning agents.

Although the skin may be cleaned in various ways, for most people, the best way is with soap or detergent and water. The choice of soap is largely a matter of personal preference. Some contain more oils or fats than others; some contain (abrasive) substances; still others contain detergents. Nearly all are scented.

Soaps are made from vegetable and animal fats. Most detergents are made from petroleum derivatives. Detergents are especially satisfactory when the water is hard, cold, or salty. Persons who are sensitive to soap often find that they can use detergents without difficulty. Detergent bars are available, but there is no

contraindication for using the mild granulated or liquid detergents on the skin as long as they do not irritate or dry the skin. Laundry detergents may cause burning and irritation of the skin. Youngsters and elderly people require special help in selecting an appropriate soap or detergent, since their skin is more subject to injury and to irritation. If the skin at any age is very dry, creams may be used. Bath oils help to control the symptoms of dry skin. Alcohol or any other defatting agent should be avoided on dry skin.

To prevent drying of the skin, when the outdoor temperature and humidity are low, less frequent bathing and using creams more often are recommended. Soaps and detergents should be rinsed off well after bathing. Since wool often acts as an irritant to dry skin, other types of fabric usually are preferable. Some of the chemicals used to produce wrinkle-resistant fabrics are irritating, especially to dry skin. It is recommended that clothing made of these fabrics be washed one or two times before wearing. Adding moisture to the air with a humidifier and increasing fluid intake help to relieve dry skin.

Bath oils are often used when the skin is dry, although most appear to be removed when rubbing the skin dry. These oils make bath tubs slippery, and care must be exercised when oils are used, especially for the elderly, to prevent mishaps. They may help an itchy skin, provided the itching is not due to systemic diseases. Most bath preparations contain chemicals that help to soften water, and a fragrance; some have bubble ingredients. Bubble bath preparations should be mixed well in the bath water before the person sits in the tub. Urinary tract infections have been reported in children when there was direct contact with concentrated solutions.

For those who are sensitive to both soap and detergents, creams may be used. Cold creams consist of an oil or wax, water, and perfume. The cream feels cold because the water evaporates, producing a feeling of coolness. The oil and wax liquifies on the skin and loosens or suspends dirt, oily secretions, perspiration, bacteria, makeup, dead cells, and other foreign material on the skin surface. They are then removed with tissue or a soft cloth. The oil in cold cream is a nonvegetable oil that will not become rancid.

Cleansing creams are similar to cold creams except they contain little or no water. Cleansing lotions and foams are essentially cleansing creams prepared in fluid or foam form. A washing cream is also a cleansing cream but so prepared that it can be removed by rinsing it off with water.

Emollient creams are a type of cold cream. They are intended to remain on the skin and to prevent dryness and, therefore, usually are less greasy than cold creams. If the oil base has a high melting point, it does not feel greasy and seems to disappear into the skin; hence, creams made of this type of base are often called vanishing creams. Emollient or moisturizing creams do not add moisture to the skin. Rather, the oily film they leave on the skin retards normal moisture evaporation, and the film helps to hold down the scaly skin surfaces. Cocoa butter, petroleum jelly, and lanolin are effective emollients and are used in many cosmetic emollient creams.

Soap and detergents and water are more effective than creams for cleaning the skin. Personal preference, sensitivities, and the amount of moisture in the skin will serve as guides for determining whether to use soap or a detergent and water, or creams, or both.

Deodorants and Antiperspirants

Perspiration, commonly associated with body odor, is essentially odorless, although it contains some waste products, such as uric acid and ammonia. The odor occurs when bacteria, normally present on everyone's skin, act on the skin's normal secretions. When one perspires from a warm environment or from nervous tension, the body is attempting to rid itself of excess heat through evaporation of the perspiration. Hence, perspiring is a compensatory response of the body to rid itself of excess heat. Perspiration is normally acid and helps keep some of the microorganisms on the skin at a minimum.

Keeping the body and clothing clean is the prime requisite for preventing body odors. Deodorants and antiperspirants may be used *after* the skin is clean. Boric acid or zinc stearate and a fragrance usually are used in deodorants to mask or diminish body odors. Antiperspirants are intended to reduce the amount of perspiration. They act as astringents and tend to close the exits of the sweat glands. Most often, they contain aluminum chloride, tannic acid, or zinc sulfate. Chlorophyll has been advertised as being able to control body odors. However, studies do not support the claim.

Body odor is not often a problem with children and the elderly. Hormones that stimulate the growth of sweat glands begin during adolescence and gradually decrease with age.

Antiperspirants and deodorants should be used with care in order to prevent irritation of the skin. There are toilet soaps that, according to manufacturers' claims, kill skin bacteria and therefore eliminate body odors. However, deodorants, medicated soaps, toilet waters, and powder cannot substitute for bathing.

Deodorants to control odor in the vaginal area have become widely marketed. They may be applied directly to the area or they may be placed on sanitary napkins. Although these deodorants do not contain aluminum salts which are irritating to the mucous membrane, they are intended for external use only. They should not be used on tampons. Some have been reported as possibly harmful when sprayed into the vagina. Repeated use is not generally recommended because of reported irritation and rashes, nor should they be used on broken skin areas. No therapeutic benefits from their use have been proven to date. As was true of other deodorants, these special deodorants cannot replace cleanliness of the area.

Vaginal Hygiene

In normal healthy women, regular daily internal douching is believed to be both unnecessary and unwise. The practice tends to remove normal bacterial flora from the vagina, and if the solution is high in acid content, it may irritate or injure normal cells. Many women use douches for personal hygiene reasons after intercourse. The practice is satisfactory when the solution is nonirritating. There are many products on the market that can be used in douching solutions. Personal preference will guide the woman in her selection. Many gynecologists apparently feel that a mild white vinegar solution, using a tablespoon or two in a quart of warm water, or normal saline, is just as satisfactory. Douching oftener than twice a week is not recommended for normal personal hygiene purposes.

The preferred method for douching is to use a bag with tubing and a douche tip or a rubber catheter. While lying in the bathtub, the woman gently inserts the catheter or tip; the bag is held 2 or 3 feet above the level of the hips. Contracting the muscles around the vaginal orifice or holding the vulva to close the orifice allows the solution to collect and to distend the vagina, making a thorough cleansing more possible. The solution is allowed to escape, and filling and emptying the vagina continues until all the solution is used. Using undo force during douching with an appliance, such as a bulb syringe, is contraindicated because of the danger of introducing microorganisms into the cervix.

Medical assistance is recommended when a discharge or irritation and itching about the vaginal orifice persists. Frequent douching to relieve the symptoms may only tend to aggravate the cause of the problem. Before a vaginal examination, a douche is contraindicated because it will remove secretions and any discharge—specimens which are necessary for a diagnostic procedures. Most authorities recommend not douching for 24 to 48 hours before a vaginal examination.

Cosmetics

Cosmetics frequently enhance the appearance of a clean and healthy skin, although certain cultural and religious groups would not agree with this opinion. For older people, makeup used judiciously helps to disguise blemishes, improves skin coloring, and makes wrinkles appear less obvious. Creams and lotions made by reputable concerns are safe to use, but it has not been demonstrated that their cost is commensurate with their quality. The choice is one of personal preference.

The skin has absorbent ability but to a very limited degree. Nourishment is transported to the skin through the blood; absorption by skin tissue cells is negligible. Claims for creams that nourish and rejuvenate the skin tend to be misleading. Most contain estrogens, but the primary benefit of the creams is their emollient effect. Various exotic ingredients such as mink and turtle oil have been added to creams, but there is still a lack of scientific evidence to support manufacturers' claims for their rejuvenating effects. At present, there is no way in which results of aging on the skin can be reversed.

For persons sensitive to one type of cosmetic, the variety is large enough so that often another brand with a different type of base, dye, or perfume can be found. However, from time to time, cosmetics containing harmful ingredients have appeared on the market, various dyes used to color cosmetics being an example. The nurse should be alert to such agents and help consumers avoid their use. The Food and Drug Administration of the United States Department of Health, Education, and Welfare enforces federal laws on the purity of foods, drugs, and cosmetics and the advertising claims of their manufacturers. The agency is a good source of information about these products.

It has been found that cosmetics often become contaminated with bacteria and fungus. It is better to discard cosmetics after they are approximately four months old, especially those applied near the eyes. Makeup applicators and puffs should be kept immaculately clean.

Medicated Soaps and Cosmetics

Various antiseptics have been incorporated in soaps and cosmetics, but they have not been proven to be as beneficial as most advertisements claim. A danger is that users may develop sensitivities not only to the particular antiseptic, but also to chemically related products. Hexachlorophene was one antibacterial agent commonly used in soaps and powders. As mentioned in Chapter 14, the Food and Drug Administration has banned its use except by prescription.

Shaving Methods and Cosmetics for Men

There does not appear to be evidence that one shaving method is better than another. Individual preferences are based on such factors as type of skin, quality of beard, the frequency with which one shaves, the presence of skin problems, and convenience. Blade razors tend to give a closer shave than electric razors, but many men find electric razors convenient and practical. They are especially convenient for the ill and bedridden patient.

Preparations used prior to shaving are intended to soften the beard for easier shaving. After-shave preparations consist primarily of alcohol, water, and perfume. They tend to make the freshly shaven face feel good and have a cosmetic rather than a therapeutic effect.

An ingrown hair is one that curves back into the skin. The cause is not clearly known, although shaving with the grain of the beard and with a sharp blade and shaving more frequently but less closely help to reduce the problem for many men. Black men are more prone to ingrown hairs than men from other racial backgrounds.

Permanently removing ingrowing hairs may be required in severe and persistent cases.

It is recommended that warts that are in the way of shaving be removed to prevent injuring them and to prevent their spread.

Men are tending to use more cosmetics, deodorants, and antiperspirants than previously. They should exercise the same care in their selections and use as do women.

Hirsutism

Hirsutism is the excessive growth of body hair. Custom dictates what hair on the body is (superfluous.) In American culture, axillary hair is considered superfluous for women, but it is not so considered in some European and Oriental countries. Hence, superfluous hair has more important psychological implications than physical.

Superfluous hair can be removed by tweezers, waxing, chemical depilation, shaving, or electrolysis. Waxing is usually done by a beautician. A warm wax which imbeds the hair is applied to the skin, allowed to harden, and then removed quickly, plucking the hair in the process.

The safest and the most economical way to remove unwanted hair is to use a razor. It has not been proven that repeated shaving causes excessive growth and coarseness of hair. Depilatories which either destroy hair shafts or mechanically remove hair often irritate the skin and cause infection, although many persons find them safe to use.

The only way to remove hair permanently is by electrolysis, a process by which the hair follicle is destroyed with a mild electric current. This is an expensive and tedious process and requires an experienced operator. A hair remover that is advertised to destroy the hair root permanently is available.

Older people tend to have softer and finer hair. Superfluous hair on the face is common in women after the menopause and the nurse can give advice on its removal if the person finds that it is a problem.

A 6 percent solution of hydrogen peroxide (20 volume peroxide with 20 drops of ammonia added to 1 ounce of peroxide) may be used as a bleach for superfluous hair, especially on the face. The bleached hair is hardly noticeable and often solves the problem easily and inexpensively.

Excessive body hair is thought to be an inherited characteristic. Hirsutism has been observed to occur at the time of menopause; authorities do not agree on its cause. However, it is a misconception that it results from the overuse of creams. Excessive body hair is commonly associated with the use of certain pharmaceutical agents, such as corticotropin (ACTH) and vitamin A in large doses.

Acne

Acne is an eruption of the skin due to inflammation and infection of the sebaceous glands. Medically speaking, acne is not a serious condition, although it can lead to permanent scarring. It occurs most commonly during the teen years when its appearance is especially disturbing from a psychological viewpoint. Acne usually appears on the face, neck, shoulders, and back.

During adolescence, endocrine gland activity increases, and among other things, the hormones cause enlargement of the sebaceous glands and increased glandular secretions. When these secretions become dammed up in the sebaceous ducts and inflammation with infection occurs, blackheads and (pustules) appear.

There are various ways to control acne and minimize scarring. The infected areas should not be squeezed and picked. Because of oiliness of the skin and hair, typical during adolescence, frequent washing with soap and hot water is recommended. Cosmetics, especially oily ones, should be used sparingly. Some persons find that the sun or ultraviolet exposure helps, but caution to prevent burning is important. If certain foods, usually chocolate and cola beverages, appear to make the condition worse, they should be eliminated from the diet. Using dietary restrictions indiscriminately usually is of no avail and may endanger the general health of the person.

In severe cases, the services of a physician are recommended. Drugs are sometimes necessary but are prescribed with great care because of the danger of sensitizing the person to the drug and of developing a strain of microorganisms that become drug resistant. Cold quartz lamps and liquid nitrogen are often used to dry the skin. These therapeutic measures are not curative, but they help to prevent scarring of the skin. There are surgical procedures that help to eliminate scarring, should this become a psychological problem.

BATHING THE PATIENT

An important purpose of the bath is to clean the skin. Some persons may require daily or even more frequent bathing while others may bathe less frequently and still be clean. The condition of the skin, the type of work, the place of work, the type of activities, and the weather conditions are all guiding factors in establishing bathing habits.

In addition to its cleaning purpose, a bath can be very refreshing for many patients when they are feeling restless and uncomfortable. Depending on the situation and the temperature of the water used for the bath, the patient may feel stimulated and ambitious following it, or he may relax to the point that sleep follows soon after. To those who enjoy a bath, the feeling of cleanliness and relaxation that accompanies it is satisfying. Hence, warm water usually is used for bathing, since the warmth tends to relax muscles. The cooling effects of the bath, even when warm water is used, result from evaporation of water from the body surface.

The cleansing bath also affects physiological activities. Massaging the skin will affect the (peripheral nerve) endings and the peripheral circulation. If firm movements are used in stroking the various areas, muscles will be stimulated, and circulation will be aided. This action on the circulation often results in increased kidney function. It is not uncommon for a patient who has been given a bath to void immediately following it.

The activity involved in bathing also can be of great value to the musculoskeletal system as a form of exercise for an ill person. If the bath is taken or given with this advantage in mind, it is possible to exercise all of the major muscle groups and place almost all joints through full range of joint motion. Chapter 17 will describe exercises to accomplish this. As the muscle groups contract, blood within the veins is assisted to return to the heart. The activity of the muscle groups helps to maintain muscle tone.

If, during the bathing process, there is a definite attempt to include some planned exercise, stimulation of respirations also will be involved. Increasing the rate and the depth of respirations has physiological advantages, such as increasing the oxygen intake and preventing congestion within the lung tissue.

Whether given by the nurse or taken by the patient, a bath can be so managed that it functions effectively as a conditioning activity for the body. Middle-aged and elderly patients often will say that they are too stiff to reach down and wash their legs while in bed, to get into a bathtub, to brush their hair, to button or tie a bed gown in the back. They may very well be correct, but investigation often will show that there is no pathological basis for this limitation. Possibly their knees are stiff, and they cannot reach in back because they have not attempted to do so for a long time. If limited activity continues, the patient may develop _ankylosis_ which is an abnormal immobility and fixation of a joint. Laypersons frequently call this condition a "frozen joint." Many of these patients can be helped to increased activity by nurses who can explain the values of good body mechanics.

Bathing the patient offers the nurse one of her greatest opportunities for getting to know the patient, for observing his physical and emotional status, and for identifying possible health-related problems. It offers an excellent opportunity for health teaching at a time when the patient often demonstrates readiness for learning. The importance of _caring_ in nursing was discussed in Chapter 1. Many patients have expressed the feeling that sincere interest and caring about the patient's welfare are best shown by those who give personal care. While it is possible to have numerous contacts with the patient during the course of the day, few are as prolonged as the time spent in preparation for and assistance with the bath. Therefore, the nurse will consider carefully before delegating the bath to others when the opportunity to use this time with the patient is available to her.

Some people prefer a shower to a tub bath, and vice versa. Some bathe in the morning on arising and others in the evening before retiring. Some bathe daily, others every other day, and still others once a week, or even less frequently. It may be difficult to satisfy all these habits in hospital situations, but, when practical, most patients appreciate having their home bathing habits observed. It is helpful to indicate changes in health agency bathing routines for a particular patient on the patient's nursing care plan.

No matter where or when the patient is to be bathed, the nurse still has the responsibility for assisting the patient as needed, seeing that he has his necessary articles and checking to see that safety and privacy measures have been considered. Protecting the patient from possible sources of injury or harm include avoiding drafts; making certain that the water is a safe, comfortable temperature; and providing means for preventing slipping in the tub or the shower. The patient should never be left out of easy calling distance of the nurse, the doors of bathrooms should not be locked, and a calling device should be within easy reach. These precautions help to avoid serious problems should the patient suddenly feel faint or fall and apply to adults of all ages. Children should never be left alone in bathrooms!

The Shower Bath

Even if the patient can manage by himself, the nurse should make certain that supplies are available and the facility is in order before permitting him to use the shower. If the patient is weak, he should be watched closely and every precaution taken to avoid an accident. Health agencies generally have guide rails on the wall both inside and outside the shower stall for safety purposes. These rails are available and relatively easy to install in home showers. It is best if there are two levels of rails in the stall; one placed low enough so that if a patient prefers to sit on a stool while in the shower, he can assist himself to stand. Sitting in the shower is much safer for the older patient or the patient who is still weak. Also, sitting on a chair or a stool makes it easier for the patient to wash his legs with less likelihood of slipping. Some nurses have reported that portable commodes with the pan removed have been used effectively as shower chairs. They offer the patient more support than a stool.

Portable showers are available on the market. The patient remains in the back-lying position during the shower. They are especially helpful for bathing immobile, chronically ill patients.

Figure 16–2 illustrates several features that add to the safety of a shower bath for the hospitalized patient.

The Tub Bath

For the physically limited person, the advantages of the tub bath are often defeated by the disadvantages of the tub itself. It is not a particularly easy device to get in and out of. In some instances, the addition of an attachment to the tub or a rail on the wall will make it easier to enter and leave. Another arrangement that has helped many patients is the use of a chair alongside the tub. The patient sits on the chair and eases to the edge

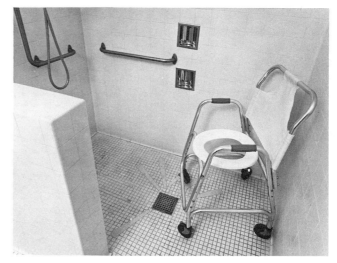

Figure 16–2 This shower can be used by the ambulatory patient or by one who can be transported by and remain in the shower chair. Note the bars for the patient to grasp and the emery strips on the floor to help prevent falling from slipping on a wet floor. Out of the camera's view was a bell cord to summon help; it was located at the head of the room divider. In order to prevent accidents with electrical appliances, this room had no electrical outlets.

of the tub. After putting both feet into the tub, it is then easier for him to reach the opposite side of the tub and ease down into the tub. Occasionally, it is easier if the patient has a towel or a mat in the tub and then, instead of easing down directly, to kneel first and then to sit down. Sometimes, it is best for the bath water to be run after the patient is seated and then drained before the patient attempts to get out of the tub. Some health agencies have hydraulic lifts which can also be installed in home tubs. The person sits on a seat, swings over the tub, and then lowers himself into the tub. The reverse is done for getting out of the tub. Tubs are available that can be lowered in order to make it easier for persons to get into them and then raised for the convenience of the nurse. Also available are walk-in tubs. A watertight door makes it possible for a person to walk into and out of the tub. Figure 16–3 on page 342 illustrates several features that add to the safety of a tub bath for the hospitalized patient.

The Bath Taken in Bed

Some patients must remain in bed as a part of their regimen, even if they are permitted to care for themselves, feed themselves, read, and possibly do some prescribed exercises. If they have not had a bed bath previously, they may need some suggestions on how to bathe themselves.

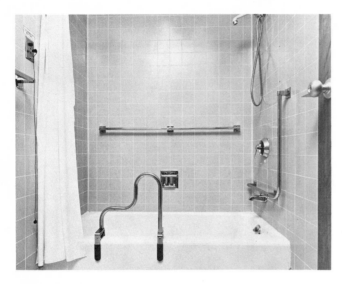

Figure 16-3   Note the hand support on the tub, and bars at different angles and heights for the patient to grasp, as necessary. This tub can be used for showering also; emery strips in the bottom of the tub to help prevent slipping are out of the camera's view. A bell cord, within reach to summon help, is near the shower curtain. This room has no electrical outlets to prevent accidents with electrical appliances.

In addition to providing the patient with all of the necessary articles for oral hygiene and for washing, the nurse prepares the unit so that it is more convenient for the patient. This includes removing the top bed linen and replacing it with a bath blanket so that the patient does not get the bedding wet. The necessary articles should be placed conveniently, usually on the bedside or overbed table. Clean clothing should be placed within easy reach. Makeup items for the woman patient should be left where she can obtain them after she has finished her bath. Male patients may wish to shave either before or after they have bathed. A mirror and good light are necessary and clean hot water also if a blade razor is used.

Patients in bed will have varying degrees of physical ability to bathe themselves. Some patients will be able to wash only the upper parts of their bodies. The rest of the bath is then completed by nursing personnel. Other patients will be able to wash all but their backs. Some patients are able and are encouraged, as a part of their bed exercises, to wash their backs as well. Washing every area of the body while in bed requires considerable manipulation and exercise. This activity in itself is a good conditioner for someone who is not up and about. With good teaching the nurse can help the patient to understand its values.

The Bath Given in Bed

For patients who are restricted in their activity and for those who are unable to move, the bath is refreshing and physiologically stimulating. For the very ill and inactive patient, bathing with modifications of water temperature and types of strokes used can bring considerable relief from discomfort and serve as a sensory stimulus.

Before starting the bath, it is best to offer the patient the bedpan.

The following description of a bed bath assumes that the patient is able to be raised or lowered in bed and that, while there is limitation of movement, it is possible for the nurse to manage the patient alone. It also assumes that only routine hygienic care is needed. Bathing procedures vary. The suggested actions on page 343 are given as guides.

The Towel Bath

An in-bed towel bath, or lotion bath as it is sometimes called, was devised by Gus Totman, a nurse employed by the Veterans' Administration. The bath uses a

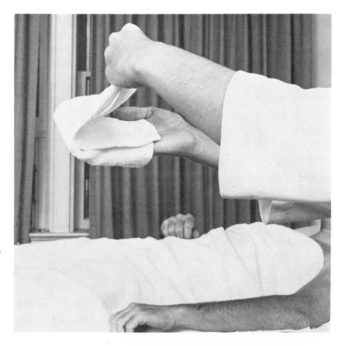

Figure 16-4   To form a thumbless mitten, fold a washcloth in thirds, slip the hand into the pocket, flip the remainder of the washcloth over the fingers and palm, and place the extra length of washcloth between the palm and the folded washcloth, as this nurse demonstrates.

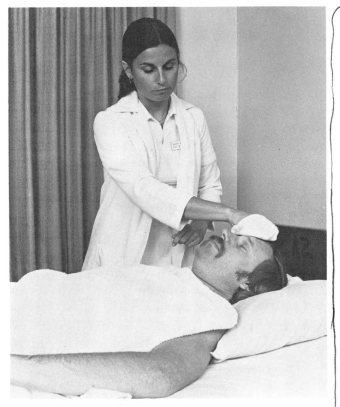

Figure 16-5 The nurse has the patient draped with a bath blanket. She starts the bath by washing his face. There is a bath towel over the patient's chest for drying after she washes and rinses the face.

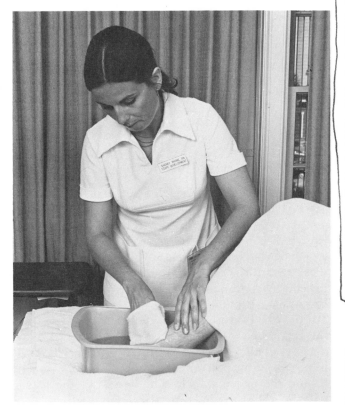

Figure 16-6 An important part of the bed bath is washing the patient's feet. Patients enjoy being able to place their feet in a basin of water when bedridden. They also enjoy placing their hands in a basin of water; the hands are washed earlier in the bath after the arms and axillae have been done.

Suggested procedure for bathing a patient in bed

Obtain all articles needed for hygiene and bed-making. For the patient's psychological comfort, provide for privacy. The bath water should be between approximately 43.3 and 46.1° C. (110° and 115° F.).

Arrange the articles in order of use for convenience in working.

Remove the top bedding and fold linen to be replaced on the bed so it is ready when needed without being rearranged. Place the bath blanket over the patient to avoid exposure and to provide warmth.

Assist the patient to the side of the bed for convenience and ease in working.

Elevate the head of the bed slightly while oral hygiene is being done, to avoid having the patient aspirate liquids.

Lower the head of the bed and remove either all pillows or all but one. Assist the patient to raise the head and the shoulders in order to remove the pillows.

Arrange the washcloth to form a thumbless mitten with all corners tucked in. Figure 16–4 on page 342 illustrates.

Wash the patient's face, as illustrated in Figure 16-5, ears, and neck. When washing the eyes, wipe from the inner canthus outward and use a separate portion of the washcloth for each eye. The *inner canthus* of the eye is at the medial angle of the eye where the upper and lower lids meet, and the *outer canthus* is at the lateral angle where the upper and lower lids meet.

Wash the patient's face, ears, and neck. When washing the eyes, wipe from the inner canthus outward and use a separate portion of the washcloth for each eye.

Wash and dry the patient's arms, axillae, and hands. Wash and dry the patient's chest. Then wash and dry the abdomen, including the area of the thighs near the groin.

Drape the bath blanket around the upper thigh to prevent exposure of the patient while washing the leg.

Lift the patient's leg at the bony prominence at the ankle and the heel and then support the leg on your arm until you can place the foot carefully into the basin of water. Wash each leg and foot separately. Wash the foot as illustrated in Figure 16-6.

Change the water.

Roll the patient to the side-lying position and bring him close to the edge of the bed.

Place the towel along the back and turn the bath blanket back to expose the patient's back. Wash the back of the neck, the shoulders, the back, the buttocks, and the posterior upper thighs. Use firm, long strokes.

Roll the patient back to the back-lying position.

Wash the genital area. If the patient is able to do this, provide water, soap, and towel within easy reach and leave the unit. Remove equipment which can be cleaned while the patient is busy. Perineal care given by the nurse is discussed later in this chapter.

Give the patient a back rub, as described later in this section.

Comb the patient's hair after the bed is made. The old pillow case or towel can beused to protect the bed from combings. The bed-making procedure and the care of hair are described later in this chapter.

quick-drying solution containing a cleaning agent, a disinfectant, and a softening agent mixed with water of 43.3° to 48.9° C. (110° to 120° F.). A commonly used solution developed cooperatively by Totman and Vestal Laboratories is called Septi-Soft.

A large terry cloth towel of about 3 feet wide by 7 feet long is saturated in a plastic bag containing the cleaning agent mixed with water. It is then wrung out until it is nearly dry. This towel is unrolled over the patient as the upper sheet is removed simultaneously. An extra amount of towel is folded under the patient's chin for later use.

The bathing begins with the feet. The nurse moves up the patient's body using a massaging motion. The towel is folded upward as the bathing proceeds while a clean top sheet is unfolded over the patient. The face, neck, and ears are cleaned with that part of the towel folded under the chin. The towel is then folded in quarters, soiled side turned in, the patient is turned on his side, and the folded towel is then used to wash the back and buttocks. When the bath is completed, the towel is removed, clean linen is placed on the bed, and the patient is dressed and positioned. The patient need not be dried since the cleaning solution dries in a matter of two or three seconds. The entire bathing procedure and linen change takes approximately ten minutes, once the technique is learned.

Totman reports that most patients for whom he has cared prefer the towel bath to the traditional in-bed bath using a basin of water. He states that the towel bath can be accomplished with less fatigue to the patient; the towel remains warm during the short procedure; patients report feeling clean and refreshed; and the oil in the bathing solution eliminates dry and itchy skin.

According to Totman, the brevity of the towel bath may well also be a disadvantage. The nurse has more time with her patients when giving the traditional bath in bed which is especially important for developing helping relationships, at least with certain patients. Some patients and nurses also reportedly have questioned the effectiveness of cleaning a person in the short time required for a towel bath.

The Back Rub

Following the bath, it is recommended that the patient be given a back rub. A back rub acts as a general body conditioner and promotes peripheral circulation. It takes approximately four to six minutes to give an effective back rub. A lotion or powder is usually used although alcohol is sometimes recommended when the skin is oily. For the comfort of the patient, the lotion or alcohol should be warmed before applying it to his back.

A back rub to promote relaxation uses a long, slow, rhythmic stroke along the length of the back, across the deltoid muscles, up the neck and along the top of the shoulders. The hands with the fingers together should be kept on the skin at all times and follow the muscle groups while moving up the back. The strokes should be firm but gradually become somewhat lighter as the back rub is ending. Sufficient pressure should be used to prevent a tickling sensation for the patient.

If stimulation is desired, the strokes of the back rub should be rapid and firm and the hands should move in a circular pattern. This produces friction between the skin and the underlying tissues. However, friction should not be great enough to cause trauma to the skin. The back may be lightly struck with the side of the hands and areas of the skin may be picked up between the fingers for stimulation. This latter type of stroke is especially effective as one moves up on either side of the spine, along the top of the shoulders and up to the nape of the neck. It is sometimes called the kneading movement. Figures 16–7 through 16–10 illustrate various techniques used during a back rub.

A back rub is a nursing measure that dates back many years. Its prestige has increased with recent studies that illustrate the communicative and psychological value of touch and the "laying on of the hands." The time with the patient offers the nurse a good opportunity to learn to know him better and it is the rare patient who does not enjoy, appreciate, and remember a good back rub.

Making an Occupied Bed

It is usual procedure to change linens at the time that the bed bath is given, since the top bedding will be already off. The occupied bed is made by rolling the patient over to the far side of the bed and tucking the soiled bottom linens and the rubber or plastic draw sheet toward the center of the bed and well under the patient. The clean linens are then placed so that one-half of the bottom of the bed can be made. The patient can then be rolled over onto the freshly made part of the bed. The soiled linens are removed, and the clean linens are pulled through tightly. A smoother bed will be possible if the pull on the clean linen is done directly behind the patient's back. The weight of the patient will then hold the linen in place. The bottom of the

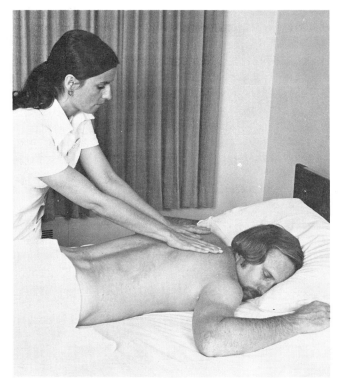

Figure 16-7 The nurse uses long, firm strokes for the length of the back when giving a back rub. Note that she places her entire hand flat on the patient's skin. The back rub should begin and end with this type of stroke.

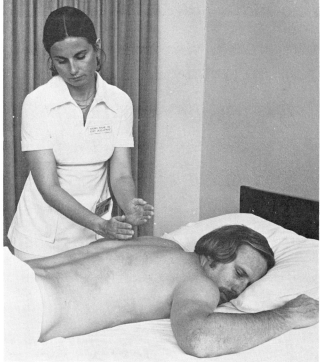

Figure 16-8 For extra stimulation, the nurse strikes the back lightly with the sides of her hands.

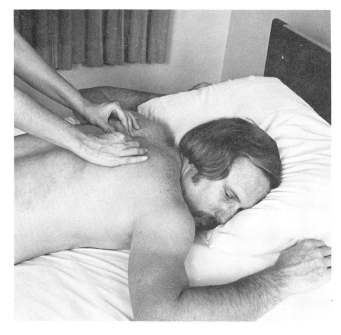

Figure 16-9 Picking up the skin between the fingers is effective for stimulation along the length of the spinal cord.

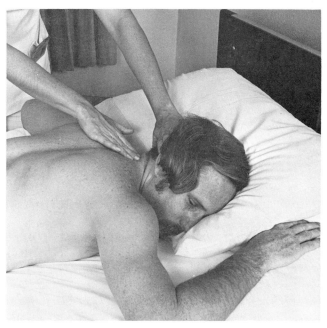

Figure 16-10 The area at the back of the neck and along the hair line often feels tense. Including this area in the back rub promotes comfort and relaxation.

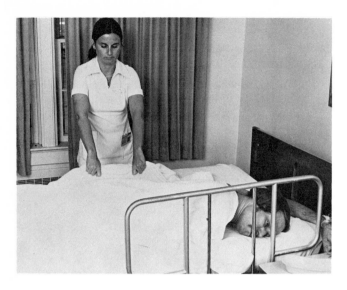

Figure 16–11   When pulling the bottom sheet for tight foundation linen, the patient might easily roll out of bed. Note that the nurse has the siderail in place to prevent an accident.

bed is then completed. The patient is usually turned back toward the center of the bed, and the top of the bed is made. The use of (contour) bottom sheets has greatly reduced the amount of time needed to tighten sheets. While placing the bottom bed linen as the patient lies on the far side of the bed from the nurse, special care is necessary to keep the patient from rolling out of bed. Raising the bed siderails is recommended, as illustrated in Figure 16–11.

There are variations in the procedure for making the occupied bed. However, these small differences have no real effect on the patient's comfort. In some instances, it is necessary for nurses to devise unique ways to change the linens on a patient's bed because of the nature of the patient's condition, orthopedic appliances on the bed, or treatments that may be in progress.

CARE OF THE HAIR

The hair is one of the accessory structures of the skin. It is normally shiny and is neither excessively oily, dry, nor brittle. As illustrated in Figure 16–1 each hair consists of the shaft, which projects through the dermis beyond the surface of the skin, and the hair follicle, which lies in the dermis. Hair grows in the follicle and receives its nourishment from the blood which circulates through each follicle. It has been found that hair can carry bacteria. This is of special importance to

health workers caring for debilitated patients with open wounds and those working in operating and delivery rooms. Short hair, frequent shampooing, and hair coverings are recommended for these health workers.

There are many cultural overtones associated with hair, and its care and styling are often influenced by one's values. Styles change within a culture. Note, for example, the change from a short-cut style for men to a longer hair style in this country. Black people have favored the "Afro" or "natural" style. Women tend to change hair styles and color more often than men in this country.

Good general health is essential for attractive hair, and like the skin, cleanliness aids in keeping it attractive. Illness affects the hair, especially when endocrine abnormalities, increased body temperature, poor nutrition, or anxiety and worry are present.

The hair is exposed to the same dirt and oil as the skin. It should be washed as often as necessary to keep it clean. For most persons, a weekly shampoo is sufficient, but more often or less frequent shampooing may be indicated for others. Daily brushing of the hair aids in keeping it clean and in distributing oil along the shaft of each hair. Brushing also stimulates the circulation of blood in the scalp.

A comb used for arranging the hair does not replace brushing. Personal preference dictates the selection of a comb, but sharp and irregular teeth which may scratch the scalp should be avoided. A large-tooth comb is recommended for very curly hair. The comb and the brush should be washed each time the hair is washed and as frequently as necessary between shampoos.

If the hair is dry, oils may be used. Pure castor oil, olive oil, or mineral oil is satisfactory, but perfumed preparations may be used with safety if sensitivity of the skin is no problem. If the hair is oily, more frequent washing is necessary.

The care of short hair rarely presents problems. However, time and attention to an important part of grooming may be necessary when the hair is long. During the acute phase of illness, the patient may ask to have the hair left undisturbed. To do so, especially if the hair is long, may prove to be disastrous. Hair which becomes entangled is difficult to undo. Hours of careful combing of tiny sections of hair may be necessary if a patient's hair is not combed for even one day. The best way to protect long hair from matting and tangling is to ask the patient for permission to braid it (some patients may not wish to have their hair arranged in braids). Patients usually will consent to such a procedure if it provides them with more comfort during a time when they are unable to manage the arranging of their own hair. Parting the hair in the middle on the back of the head and making two braids, one on either side, prevents the discomfort of lying on one heavy braid on the back of the head.

Occasionally, a patient's hair is almost hopelessly matted, and cutting the hair may be necessary. Before a patient's hair is cut, it is usual procedure to have the patient sign a written consent. It is also recommended that the nurse discuss the necessity for cutting the hair with an immediate member of the patient's family.

Nurses should be aware of the fact that most patients have a hair style that is most satisfying to them. If it is necessary to comb and arrange a patient's hair, the nurse should ask the patient how it is to be arranged. Doing so in the fashion the patient considers best is often a big boost to morale.

The care of the black person's hair usually requires special attention. The hair is normally dry, very curly, and becomes easily matted and tangled. The comb used for arranging hair should have widely spaced teeth. Oil should be used and white petrolatum or mineral oil are often recommended. However, a skin lotion has been used effectively also. Braiding the hair of a black person is usually the best way to prevent matting and tangling. References in the Supplemental Library Study section of this chapter describe ways of combing and braiding the hair of a black person for those unfamiliar with the procedure.

Hair Loss

A certain number of hairs are lost and some start growing each day. Some permanent thinning of hair normally accompanies aging. Hair loss from plaiting, excessive back combing and "teasing," or the use of hair rollers is usually temporary, and hair returns when the tension on the hair shaft is halted. Some people experience hair loss due to illness with high fever, certain medications, x-ray therapy of the head, childbirth, and general anesthesia. There appears to be no evidence that hair loss occurs as a result of wearing wigs or excessive shampooing. It is believed by some that an excessive intake of vitamin A may play a role in hair loss.

Baldness is called *alopecia.* It is rare in women and common in men. There is no known cure for baldness despite the promises of many advertisements. Alopecia is believed to be hereditary and no amount of external treatment is likely to help. Hairpieces, frequently worn by persons who are bald, require the same care as normal hair, but less frequent washing is necessary since they are not lubricated with oil from the sebaceous glands.

A surgical procedure for baldness is the hair transplant. Hair is taken from donor sites, usually from the back or sides of the scalp, and transplanted to areas with no hair. It is a long and expensive procedure but reportedly has decided benefits for persons who find baldness especially disturbing.

Dandruff

Dandruff is a condition characterized by itching and flaking of the scalp. Nearly everyone experiences dandruff at some time. Persistent severe cases usually require medical attention. Although microorganisms play a role in infections often associated with severe dandruff, they apparently are not the cause of it. Proprietary products have not been found to be effective for "curing" dandruff although some help to suppress it temporarily. Daily brushing and shampooing as necessary in most cases will aid in keeping the scalp free of dandruff.

Shampoos and Rinses

A large variety of shampoo products are marketed, many of which are advertised to care for special hair problems. Personal preference guides purchasing, but shampoos that dry the hair excessively or irritate the scalp should be avoided. Certain shampoos on the market, recommended for dry hair, are designed to remove all substances except the natural oils. However, if the hair is dry and unmanageable after washing, a few drops of oil rubbed into the hair produce satisfactory results. Detergents are more effective than soap when used with hard water. Liquid and cream shampoos rinse from the hair with greater ease than does bar soap.

Various rinses may be used following a shampoo, such as antistatic creme rinses, protein rinses, beer rinses, and lemon juice or vinegar rinses. In each case, a film remains on the hair shaft that helps to give the hair body and a glossy appearance. Rinses tend to make freshly shampooed hair more manageable; however, there is no scientific evidence to indicate that they penetrate the hair shaft.

A variety of waterless or dry shampoos are available. They usually consist of an alkali and an absorbent powder. Or, a fine, white body powder can be used as a dry shampoo. The dry shampoo or powder is applied and then combed or brushed from the hair. The teeth of a comb can be placed through gauze which will help remove and capture the powder. Dry shampoos cannot replace the cleaning benefits of regular shampoos, but they are helpful in removing at least some of the dirt, oils, and odors from the hair. They have been especially helpful for patients too ill or incapacitated to have a water shampoo. Dry shampoos or powder are not recommended for black persons because of their normally dry hair and scalp.

Permanent Waves

Home permanent waves have become very popular with women who have learned how to use them, and they often mean additional comfort for patients confined for long periods. In some situations, as in a chronic illness unit or geriatric center, the nurse may be asked to assist a patient with a home permanent wave. If the nurse feels that she has the necessary competence, the procedure could result in considerable satisfaction for the patient.

Pediculosis

Infestation with lice is called *pediculosis*. There are three common types of lice: *Pediculus humanus,* var. *capitis,* which infests hair and scalp; *Pediculus humanus,* var. *corporis,* which infests the body; and *Phthirus pubis,* which infests the shorter hairs on the body, usually the pubic and the axillary hair. Lice lay eggs, called *nits,* on the hair shafts. Nits are white or light gray and look like dandruff, but they cannot be brushed or shaken off the hair. Frequent scratching and scratch marks on the body and the scalp suggest the presence of pediculosis. Although anyone may become infested with lice, the continued presence of pediculosis is usually a result of uncleanliness.

Pediculosis can be spread directly by contact with infested areas or indirectly through clothing, bed linen, brushes, and combs. The linen and the personal care items of patients with pediculosis require separate and careful handling to prevent spreading from person to person.

There are any number of preparations, called *pediculicides,* for the treatment of pediculosis, some of which will destroy the nits as well as the lice. Several treatments are usually necessary before all the nits are destroyed. The procedures and the medications used for the treatment of pediculosis vary from health agency to health agency. Shaving off the infested hair is frequently done, especially when pubic and axillary hair are infested. Although shaving is a relatively simple way of handling pediculosis, shaving the scalp is rarely done.

Giving a Shampoo

Many health agencies have beauticians and barbers to assist with the care of the patient's hair, including shampooing it. However, this convenience does not relieve the nurse of her responsibility to see that the patient's hair is cared for properly.

If a beautician is not available, shampooing a patient's hair may become a nursing responsibility. If the patient is ambulatory, there is no real problem. The procedure should begin with a thorough brushing and combing to stimulate the scalp and remove tangles of hair. The hair can be shampooed while the patient is showering or at a large sink. If the patient is confined to bed but is able to be moved onto a stretcher, he can be transported to a convenient sink for a shampoo. The hair is washed and rinsed over the sink while the patient remains lying on the stretcher.

For patients who must remain in bed for a shampoo, the patient's head and shoulders are moved to the edge of the bed. A protective device is placed under the head. This may be a Kelly pad or an improvised trough made from a large rubber sheet which has been built up on both sides by rolling a towel into each side. To prevent the bed from getting wet and to ensure a thorough cleaning and rinsing of the hair, it is necessary that the patient and the trough or pad be so placed that the water constantly drains. Many new devices for shampooing hair in bed are now available. Special trays with rigid frames reduce the likelihood of water flowing into the bed. Portable sinks that can be moved to the patient's bedside are available. So also are automatic shampooers, a device into which the patient's head is placed while he sits back in a wheelchair. Procedures for shampooing a patient's hair depend on the equipment and the facilities available in the agency or the home. Following a shampoo, the patient's hair is dried as quickly as possible to prevent him from becoming chilled.

ORAL HYGIENE

The mouth is the first part of the alimentary canal and an adjunct of the respiratory system. The ducts of the salivary glands open into the vestibule of the mouth. The teeth and the tongue are accessory organs in the mouth and play an important role in beginning digestion by breaking up food particles and mixing them with saliva. Saliva is also important as a mechanical cleaner of the mouth. It is estimated that healthy adults secrete between 1-and-1½ liters of saliva in each 24-hour period. The mucous membrane which lines the mouth is not as sturdy as skin; therefore, care is needed while cleaning the mouth to prevent injury.

General good health is as essential as cleanliness for maintaining a healthy mouth and teeth. The relationship, for example, between good teeth and a diet sufficient in calcium and phosphorus along with vitamin D, which is necessary for the body to utilize these minerals, is well-established.

Dental disease is considered epidemic in the United States. The American Dental Association has estimated that there are about a billion untreated cavities, with the average American having five. The following are some additional findings of interest:

- The cost of repairing tooth cavities in this country amounts to several million dollars each year.

- In one study of patients admitted to a hospital, approximately 80 percent had some form of oral disease.

- Blacks tend to have fewer tooth cavities than do Caucasians. The theory is that whites tend to have a diet higher in carbohydrates, especially sugar, than do blacks.

- Millions of people have teeth removed each year which could have been saved with good dental care.

- Research continues, but to date, the use of tooth implants, that is, replacing a tooth with another, is in the experimental stage and is not being used on a large scale. For most persons, the loss of a permanent tooth represents a lifetime loss which can only be temporized with artificial teeth.

The benefits of good oral hygiene and dental care are numerous. There is aesthetic value in having a clean and healthy mouth. Having one's own teeth contributes to an intact body image. When the mouth and teeth are in good condition, gustatory pleasure and the beginning of the digestive process are enhanced. The nurse's role is to teach the benefits of good oral and dental hygiene, offer instructions on how oral hygiene is maintained, and give nursing care that includes oral hygiene to persons who cannot manage on their own.

The decay of the teeth with the formation of cavities is called *caries*. A rather well-defined chain of events appears to foster dental caries. An accumulation of mucin, carbohydrates, and lactic acid bacilli in saliva normally found in the mouth form a coating on the teeth that is called *plaque*. Plaque is transparent and colorless and very adhesive to the teeth. Carbohydrates are acted upon by bacilli of saliva to form lactic acid. The plaque prevents acid dilution and neutralization and prevents colonies of bacteria from being dispersed. The acid eventually destroys the enamel of the teeth through decalcification, and caries result.

To prevent decay, the chain must be broken somewhere. Cutting down on carbohydrate intake helps. Sweets are the worst offenders. It is impractical to remove sweets from the diet, but dentists highly recommend that sweet snacks between meals, such as soft drinks, candy, gum, jams, and jellies, be eliminated as much as possible. The mouth cannot be cleaned of all bacteria, but dispersing the bacteria with careful cleaning is helpful. This can best be done by brushing and flossing the teeth.

The major cause of tooth loss in adults over approximately 35 years of age is gum disease. *Gingivitis* is an inflammation of the *gingiva*, which is tissue that surrounds the teeth. Gingivae (pleural) are often called the gums of the mouth. A common cause of gingivitis is Vincent's angina or trench mouth. *Periodontitis* is a more marked inflammation of the gums and involves the alveolar tissues also; it is commonly called *pyorrhea*. Symptoms include bleeding gums, swollen tissues, receding gum lines with the formation of pockets between the teeth and gums, and loose teeth. If unchecked, plaque builds up and, along with dead bacteria, forms hard deposits called *tartar* at the gum lines. The tartar attacks the fibers that fasten teeth to the gums and eventually attacks bone tissue also. The teeth then loosen and fall out. Regular dental care, limiting sugar intake, and good oral hygiene are the best preventive measures for periodontal disease.

The old saying, "an ounce of prevention is worth a pound of cure," can be applied very aptly to the care of the teeth. Most dentists recommend a dental examination every six months and preferably every three months, but frequent dental examinations are not a substitute for good oral hygiene.

Water Fluoridation

The addition of fluoride compounds to drinking water that is fluoride-deficient, for the prevention of dental caries, has been under study for several decades. In general, studies have indicated that fluoridation has aided in reducing dental caries and that it is a safe community health measure. Still, in certain areas public opposition has been sufficient to prevent its use.

Some dentists apply a fluoride compound directly to the teeth at regular intervals. Studies indicate that this procedure has reduced tooth decay among children by as much as 40 percent. Fluorine mouth rinses are also recommended by some dentists. The rinse is swished about the mouth for about 30 seconds and then expectorated. There is fluoride normally present in tooth enamel. The fluoride appears to increase the enamel's resistance to caries, and it also helps lower the bacteria level in the mouth.

Toothbrushing and Flossing

The brush should be small enough to reach all teeth. The bristles should be sufficiently firm to clean but not so firm that they are likely to injure tooth enamel and gum tissue. Many dentists recommend a soft-textured multitufted toothbrush with a flat brushing surface. Others recommend brushes with widely spaced tufts because the brush is somewhat easier to keep clean and dry. Several brushes are recommended for each person so that they can dry well between uses.

There is a difference of opinion concerning the best way to brush one's teeth. Many dentists are recommending that the brush be placed at a 45° angle at the junction between the teeth and the gums with the tufts facing in the direction of the gums. This method is illustrated in Figure 16–12. Other dentists recommend that the brush be placed at the same angle but with the tufts facing in a direction away from the gum line. When assisting and teaching patients, the nurse will wish to follow the preference of the patient's dentist.

Food clearance time helps to determine frequency of brushing. It takes about 15 minutes for decay-producing foods and liquids to be cleared from the teeth after their ingestion. Sticky foods such as candy will adhere longer. It is during this time, directly after eating, that most damage is done by bacteria. Therefore, it is ideal practice to brush one's teeth immediately after eating and drinking. Most children eat frequently between meals, and it is particularly important for them to be taught to brush their teeth and rinse their mouth often. The tongue also should be cleaned with the brush. Many persons are unaware of the need for frequent cleaning, and the nurse often finds herself in an excellent position to teach patients and members of their families of its importance.

Automatic toothbrushes, electric or battery-operated, have been found to be simple to use and as good as hand brushes in removing debris and plaque. Water spray units are available to assist with oral hygiene. These units spray pulsating water under pressure on areas to which directed. If an undue amount of water pressure is used, damage to gum tissue and forcing particles of debris into tissue pockets may occur. Therefore, it is recommended that their use be discussed with a dentist.

Many bacteria in the mouth become lodged between the teeth. The toothbrush cannot effectively reach these areas, and hence, flossing several times a day is highly recommended. The practice not only removes what the brush cannot, but helps to break up colonies of bacteria. Some dentists prefer dental tape or unwaxed floss to waxed floss. Figure 16–13 illustrates a recommended way to floss teeth, and below are flossing suggestions.

Suggestions for flossing

1. The fingers controlling the floss should not be more than 1.3 cm. or ½ inch apart.

2. Do not force the floss between the teeth. Insert it gently by sawing it back and forth at the point where the teeth contact each other. Let it slide gently into place.

3. With **both** fingers move the floss up and down six times on the side of one tooth, and then repeat on the side of the other tooth until the surfaces are "squeaky" clean.

4. Go to the gum tissue with the floss, but not into the gum so as to cause discomfort, soreness, or bleeding.

5. When the floss becomes frayed or soiled, a turn from one middle finger to the other brings up a fresh section.

6. At first flossing may be awkward and slow, but continued practice will increase skill and effectiveness.

RINSING

Rinse vigorously with water after flossing to remove food particles and plaque that you have cut loose. Also rinse with water after eating when you are unable to floss or brush. Rinsing alone will not remove the bacterial plaque. Water spraying devices alone will not remove the bacterial plaque because of the fatlike material in the plaque.

From Effective Oral Hygiene. Developed by USAF School of Aerospace Medicine, Brooks Air Force Base, Texas. Published by The Academy of Periodontology, Chicago.

A disclosing dye, commonly dispensed in tablets which are chewed after brushing the teeth, reveals areas where plaque and debris remain on the teeth. Using a disclosing dye points out quickly where brushing has been inadequate. Most people find that their usual brushing habits do not clean all areas of the teeth particularly well.

Toothpastes and powders aid the brushing process, usually have a pleasant taste, and often encourage brushing, especially among children. Most dentrifices are safe to use, but those containing harsh abrasives

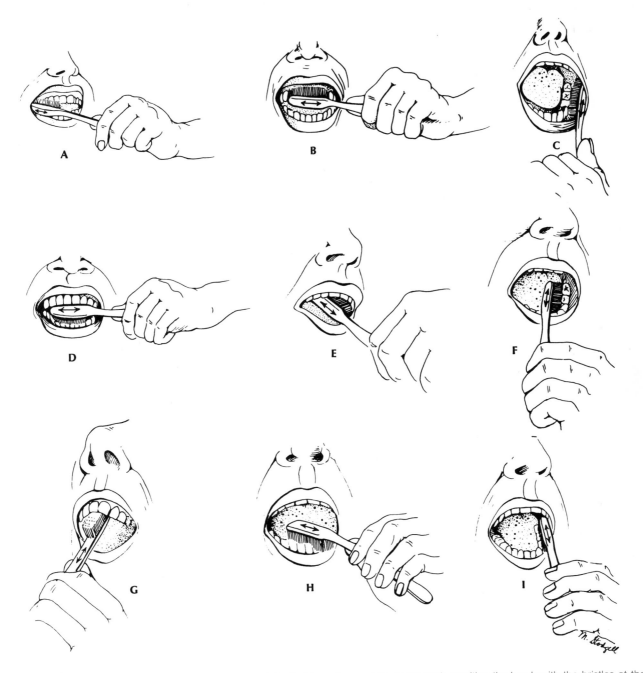

Figure 16–12 For the outside surfaces of all teeth and the inside surfaces of the back teeth, position the brush with the bristles at the junction between the teeth and gums, as in A; note the exact position of the brush. Then move the brush back and forth with short strokes several times as in Figs. B through F. Study each figure carefully. For the inside surfaces of the upper and lower front teeth, hold the brush vertically, as in Figs. G and H, and make several gentle back and forth strokes over the gum tissue and teeth. To clean the biting surfaces brush back and forth as in Fig. I. (From Effective Oral Hygiene. Developed by USAF School of Aerospace Medicine, Brooks Air Force Base, Texas. Published by The Academy of Periodontology, Chicago.)

may scratch the enamel of the teeth, and therefore, are not recommended. Salt, sodium bicarbonate, or pre-cipitated chalk are just as effective for cleaning the mouth and the teeth and are far less expensive than proprietary products on the market. Dentifrices containing stannous fluoride have proven to be effective in helping to decrease dental caries, and, hence, are rec-ommended by many dentists.

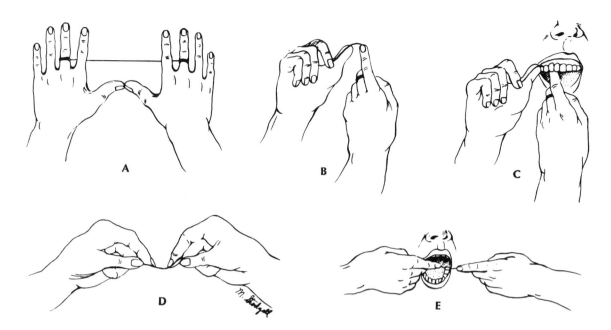

Figure 16–13   Flossing technique, A. Wrap floss on middle fingers. B. Thumb to the outside for upper teeth. C. Flossing between upper back teeth. D. Holding floss for lower teeth. E. Flossing between lower back teeth. (From Effective Oral Hygiene. Developed by USAF School of Aerospace Medicine, Brooks Air Force Base, Texas. Published by The Academy of Periodontology, Chicago.)

An offensive breath or *halitosis* is often systemic in nature. For example, the odor of onions and garlic on the breath comes from the lungs where the oils are being removed from the bloodstream and eliminated with respiration. When halitosis results from a systemic cause, oral treatment can only mask the odor temporarily at best. Mouthwashes may be pleasant to use, and some persons prefer a mildly flavored mouthwash to a salt or a sodium bicarbonate solution, but they cannot remove halitosis when odors are being eliminated by respiration.

If the cause of halitosis is poor oral hygiene, cleaning will reduce the odor. Certain mouthwashes claim antiseptic value which supposedly decreases the bacteria in the mouth. However, such claims are not well-founded; mouthwashes have little more, if any, value than plain water. If they are used in a concentrated form, they may injure oral tissue, and infection and additional odor may result.

Oral hygiene is equally important for persons with dentures. They should be cleaned as often as hygiene indicates. The removable type are removed and cleaned with a brush. There are brushes designed for dentures which are helpful in cleaning small areas and crevices. Any nonabrasive paste or powder may be used for cleaning dentures. There are also preparations in which to soak dentures to help in removing hardened particles.

When dentures are kept clean, the person is more likely to keep them in his mouth. However, if permitted to become coated with mucus, they will annoy the patient and he will wish to have them removed. When the patient is unable to clean his own dentures, it becomes a nursing responsibility to do so.

When dentures are cleaned, they should be held over a basin of water or over a soft towel so that should they slip from the nurse's grasp, they will not drop onto a hard surface and possibly break. Warm water should be used since hot water may warp the plastic material from which most dentures are made.

Keeping dentures out for long periods permits the gum line to change, thus affecting the fit of the dentures. If the patient has been instructed to remove his dentures while sleeping, a disposable denture cup is convenient and easy to use. From an aesthetic point of view, dentures should not be placed in cups, glasses, or other dishes used for eating purposes. It is recommended that dentures by stored in water to prevent drying and warping of plastic materials. A deodorant solution of water and a few drops of ammonia or white vinegar can be used. A few drops of essence of peppermint may be added also. Dentures made of vulcanite which is a porous material are especially prone to develop unpleasant odors.

Extreme care should be taken when managing a patient's dentures. They represent a considerable financial investment and damage or loss is not only expensive but embarrassing for all concerned.

Giving Oral Hygiene

While the care of the mouth described earlier is still applicable during illness, there are numerous occasions when it must be modified to meet changes in the mouth. If the patient is able to assist with his own mouth care, it may very well be a matter of providing him with the materials necessary to clean his mouth more frequently. If the patient is helpless, the nurse will help make certain that special attention is given to the patient's mouth as often as necessary to keep it clean and moist. It is not unusual to provide special mouth care as often as every hour, especially for patients who are unable to take fluids or are not permitted fluids by mouth.

Medicated mouthwashes may be used for special mouth care, especially if the patient likes the taste of an aromatic solution. An accumulation of mucus and crust formation on the teeth and around the lips is called *sordes*. When the condition is present or when the mucus in the mouth is very tenacious and the tongue is coated, a solution of half water and half hydrogen peroxide is effective for cleaning. Hydrogen peroxide solution should not be used regularly and frequently without approval by the dentist. Repeated exposure to hydrogen peroxide is likely to damage tooth enamel.

It may be necessary for the nurse to open the patient's mouth for cleaning if the patient is unconscious. A tongue blade usually works satisfactorily. Several methods are possible for cleaning the mucous membrane after the mouth is opened, but each has certain limitations. If gauze is wrapped about a tongue blade and secured with adhesive so that it does not come off, the resulting applicator is usually too large to clean all surfaces of the mouth well. If small gauze squares are held with a clamp, it is easier to reach all surfaces, but there is a danger of damaging the membrane with the clamp. Large cotton applicators, prepared so that the cotton will not come off the stick, seem to be effective. The cotton is less irritating than gauze, and the size can be varied easily, depending on the situation. A disadvantage is that the cotton becomes smooth and slippery, thus making it difficult to remove more than superficial debris from the teeth and the mucous membrane. The patient's toothbrush is perhaps the best, but care must be exercised not to injure the mucous membrane. If the brush is stiff and hard, running hot water over it softens the bristles and there is less tendency to injure gum tissue.

Whenever placing an object, such as a toothbrush or an applicator, into a patient's mouth, a mouth gag should be used to hold it open if the patient tends to close his mouth. One should not use the fingers to hold a patient's mouth open. The mouth constantly harbors organisms, and a human bite is a potentially dangerous wound.

When introducing fluid into the mouth of an unresponsive patient, keep the head in such a position that even a small amount will not be aspirated by the patient. For example, turn the patient's head to the side over the edge of a pillow. Using suctioning equipment is recommended to remove excess fluid so that the patient does not aspirate. A bulb syringe can be used but it is not as effective as suctioning equipment. When dipping the applicator or toothbrush into a solution to be used for cleaning the mouth, make certain that it is moist but not so wet that solution will pool in the mouth. Figure 16–14 illustrates oral hygiene.

After cleaning the surfaces of the mouth, clean the teeth, using the patient's toothbrush, and then clean the tongue, using gauze held on a clamp or wrapped over a tongue blade or the patient's toothbrush. The tongue is not as subject to injury as the mucous membrane of the mouth. After the entire mouth has been cleaned and wiped or rinsed with water or normal saline solution, moisten the mucous membrane with water. An emollient may be applied to the lips to help prevent cracking. The skin on the lips is very thin, and evaporation of moisture from the lips takes place rapidly, especially when the patient has an elevated temperature. White petrolatum, lanolin, and cocoa butter are suitable agents. Oil *may* be used, but sparingly and with extreme care to prevent its being aspirated.

If the patient is able to take fluids by mouth, an excellent aid to oral hygiene and comfort is frequent moistening of the lips and mouth with water.

A glycerin and lemon juice mixture has been used extensively to protect the mucous membrane of the mouth. Cotton swabs moistened in the mixture are ordinarily used. Glycerin is *hydrolytic,* that is, it is a substance that takes up water. Hence, glycerin used regularly for several days is likely to dry the mucous membrane. The lemon juice helps overcome this drying effect by stimulating salivation, but usually not to a

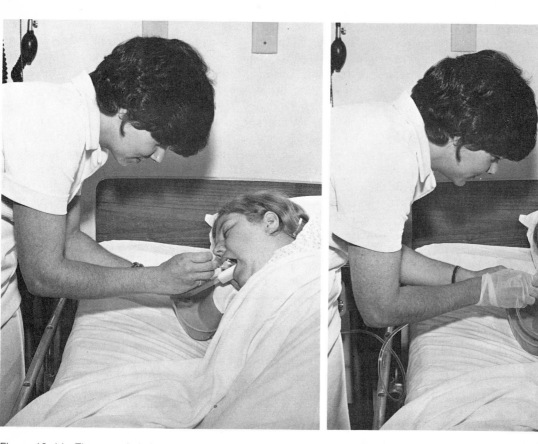

Figure 16–14 The nurse is holding the patient's mouth open with a protected tongue blade while brushing the patient's teeth and mouth. On the right, suction is used to remove secretions pooling in the patient's mouth. The nurse is wearing a glove as she suctions but this may not be necessary for many patients. Note that the patient's head is turned to the side and resting on the edge of a pillow in order to facilitate drainage from the patient's mouth while oral hygiene is given.

sufficient degree to prevent drying when glycerin is used for any length of time.

To care for the mouth of the acutely ill patient is a well-recognized responsibility of the nurse. While a variety of solutions and moisturizers have been used to clean and moisten oral tissue, studies suggest that the procedure appears to be more important than the agent that is used. This finding supports the personal experience of many well persons, that is, that no mouthwash, breath freshener, ointment, or paste replaces a thorough mechanical cleaning of the oral cavity.

CARE OF THE NAILS

Like the hair, the nails are an accessory structure of the skin. They are composed of epithelial tissue. The body of the nail is the exposed portion; the root lies in the skin in the nail groove where the nail grows and is nourished. Healthy nails have a pink color and are convex and evenly curved. With certain pathological conditions, and to some extent with aging also, the nails become ridged and saucered and areas become concave.

The fingernails may be trimmed by filing or cutting in an oval fashion. Trimming the nails too far down on the sides is contraindicated because of possible injury to the cuticle and the skin around the nail. Great care must be exercised if a nail scissors is used to prevent injuring tissue surrounding the nail. Hangnails are broken pieces of cuticle; they should be removed by cutting. Hangnails can be prevented by pushing the cuticle back gently with a blunt instrument or with a towel after washing the hands when the cuticle is soft and pliable. Using emollients helps to prevent hangnails. Cleaning under the nails is best accomplished by using a blunt instrument, being careful to prevent injuring the area where the nail is attached to the underlying tissue.

Splitting and peeling of the nails is usually due to

dryness. To decrease the condition, it is helpful to avoid contact with soap and water as much as possible, use a good hand cream frequently, and avoid the use of nail polish and polish remover, both of which have a tendency to dry the nails.

There are preparations on the market that are advertised as helping to reduce splitting and peeling of nails. Some of them contain formaldehyde, a chemical that easily irritates skin tissue. The manufacturer's instructions should be followed carefully when using these preparations.

CARE OF THE FEET

Proper foot care is important at any age; however, with aging and especially when illness is present, it becomes even more so. In her teaching role, the nurse will wish to assist patients to appreciate the importance of foot care.

Proper care starts with cleanliness. This includes bathing the feet, rinsing off the soap or detergent thoroughly, and drying the feet well, being careful to include the interdigital areas. It is best to place the feet in a basin of water when caring for a bedridden patient during the bath procedure. If the feet tend to perspire freely, frequent bathing and using foot powders with deodorant ingredients are helpful. These powders are more absorbent than are regular after-bath powders and often contain menthol which makes the skin feel cool.

The nails are trimmed, but in a manner that avoids digging into or cutting away nail at the lateral corners of the nail and toe. Patients with ingrown nails, especially older people and patients with circulatory disorders or diabetes mellitus, may require the services of a physician or podiatrist. A *podiatrist* is one who treats foot disorders. A synonym is *chiropodist*. *Podiatry* is a health discipline that deals with the treatment of foot disorders. A synonym is *chiropody*.

For older patients whose nails can be expected to be brittle and striated, it is recommended that the feet be soaked first to soften the nails for easier trimming. The feet may be placed in a basin of water. Or, they may be wrapped in damp cloths and placed in plastic bags if this procedure is more convenient than soaking in water. Adding an alkali such as Epsom salt or soda bicarbonate to the water helps soften dry scaly skin.

Improperly fitting shoes are a major cause of foot problems and can lead to corns, calluses, bunions, and blisters. The back of the shoe, or the counter, should fit snugly but not tightly. A heel offering safe support is recommended. There should be about $3/4$ inch of space in the shoe beyond the great toe when standing and the widest part of the shoe. In a good fitting shoe, the arch of the foot will lie comfortably over the arch in the shoes. The soles should be flexible and nonslippery. Shoes with rough ridges, wrinkles, or tears in the linings should be discarded or repaired.

Improperly fitting, worn, or soiled hosiery contribute to foot problems. For some persons with allergies or skin infections, nylon hosiery is contraindicated.

For most people, especially the elderly and persons with diabetes mellitus, going barefoot is not recommended. The practice is likely to result in injuries to the skin. Going barefoot in public rest rooms is especially dangerous because of the likelihood of contracting athlete's foot, a common fungus infection that is easily transmitted in showers and tubs. The causative fungi of athlete's foot are species of *Trichophyton* or *Epidermophyton floccosum* and are capable of attacking the hair and nails as well as the skin.

The nurse will wish to be alert to any symptoms of foot problems, including infections, inflammations, ingrown nails, breaks in the skin in the interdigital area, fissures or cracks, corns, calluses, bunions, and pressure areas that may result in ulcerations.

CARE OF THE EYES

The eyes very frequently reflect the state of health. Normally they are clear and kept clean with lachrymal secretions which contain lysozyme, an enzyme that protects the eye from certain microorganisms. The nurse will observe that, during illness, the eyes may water more freely and appear glasslike. As health returns, the eyes regain their normal appearance. Secretions from the eyes may adhere to the lashes, dry, and become crusty, or there may be slight discharge from the mucous membrane. If discharge is present, it may accumulate in the corners of the eyes, especially during sleep. Water or normal saline should be used to wipe the eyes clean. Boric acid solution, once popular for cleaning the eyes, is no longer recommended because of its toxicity when absorbed from injured body surfaces. Wipe from the inner canthus to the outer canthus. This is to minimize the possibility of forcing the discharge into the area drained by the nasolacrimal duct. Use a clean portion of the patient's washcloth each time the eye is wiped. Soft, disposable tissue may also be used, especially if there is any question about the cleanliness of the washcloth. If a patient is unable to close his eyelid for any reason, the eye becomes dry and its surface is subject to injury. A sterile lubricant should be applied to the eye and if necessary, an eye patch may be used to keep the eye closed and protected.

Eyeglasses

Most problems with glasses result from losing or misplacing them. Glasses are essential for many persons and represent a considerable financial investment. Hence, the nurse should take precautions to prevent breakage and loss. She should also encourage patients needing glasses to wear them in order to avoid eyestrain.

In recognition of the need for safety, the Food and Drug Administration now requires that all eyeglass lenses and sunglass lenses be impact-resistant. Lenses are most often made impact-resistant by heat treatment, chemical treatment, or by making the lenses thicker. Plastic lenses are more impact-resistant than glass lenses.

Plastic lenses have become popular because they are considerably lighter in weight than glass lenses. A refraction or correction for eye faults is as accurate when using plastic as when using glass. The one decided disadvantage of using plastic is that the material scratches very easily. The nurse will wish to be aware of this when handling and cleaning a patient's glasses.

Eyeglasses should be cleaned with water. Soap is used as necessary and a thorough rinsing should follow. The frames, which often become soiled with perspiration, hair preparations, dust, and dirt, should be washed also. Glasses are washed in warm water. Hot water is likely to damage and warp plastic that is commonly used in frames and lenses. The glasses are dried with clean, soft, paper wipes. Glasses should be cleaned over an area protected with a soft towel to avoid damage should they accidently slip from the hands. Scratching is very likely to occur when glasses are cleaned with a dry paper wipe or cloth, especially if the lenses are made of plastic.

Contact Lenses

A contact lens is a small disc worn directly on the eyeball. It stays in place by surface tension of the eye's tears. The so-called hard lenses are made of a nonpliable and nonabsorbent plastic material. Soft lenses are of a plastic material that absorbs water to become soft and pliable. They are brittle when dehydrated and absorb water when placed in solution, usually normal saline, or when in contact with tears.

Contact lenses offer several advantages over glasses. Some eye defects, such as a misshapen cornea, sometimes cannot be corrected as well with ordinary lenses. Contacts cannot be seen when worn which for many people, especially entertainers, is important for cosmetic reasons. Many athletes have found them safer to use than eyeglasses when participating in contact sports.

It is recommended that persons contemplating the use of contacts consult a physician and study their care and use under the supervision of one who specializes in the fitting and dispensing of contact lenses. Improperly fitted contact lenses can cause abrasions on the cornea. Persons wearing contact lenses need to take special precautions to keep them free of microorganisms that may lead to eye infections and to use them in a manner that will not injure or scratch the surface of the eye. They are to be removed before sleeping or swimming and when the person is in the presence of irritating vapors and smoke. The lenses should not be in contact with cosmetics, soaps, and hair sprays since eye irritation may result. It is recommended that any adverse reaction to their use be reported to the prescribing physician immediately.

The cornea which consists of dense connective tissue does not have its own blood supply. It is nourished primarily by oxygen from the atmosphere and from tears. When wearing contact lenses, the cornea requires more than its normal supply of oxygen since its metabolic rate increases. For this reason, it is recommended that contact lenses not be worn continuously for more than 10 to 16 hours in order to allow the cornea to again receive a maximum supply of oxygen. This also explains why contact lenses should be removed before sleep.

The nurse should determine whether or not her patient is wearing contact lenses. There may be times when she may be required to remove them if a patient cannot do so. To leave them in place for long periods could result in permanent eye damage. This may occur, for example, when the nurse is attending a patient who is unconscious following an accident or sudden illness. Figure 16–15 illustrates and describes how to remove contact lenses when the person is unable to do so himself.

Artificial Eyes

Most patients who wear an artificial eye will prefer to take care of it themselves, and they should be encour-

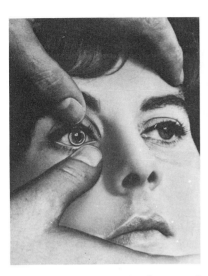

Directly over the cornea: This normal wearing position of a corneal contact lens is also the correct position for removing it. If the lens cannot be removed, however, slide it onto the sclera.

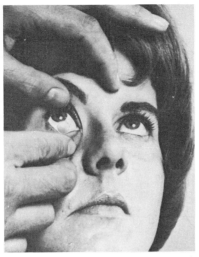

On the sclera only: Here the lens can remain with relative safety until experienced help is available; other white areas of the eye to the side or above the cornea might also be used. If the lens is to be removed, however, slide it to a position directly over the cornea.

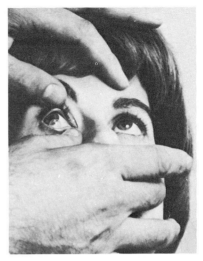

On both the cornea and sclera: A lens in this position—or a similar one anywhere around the periphery of the cornea—should be moved as soon as possible. If the lens is to be removed, slide it to a position directly over the cornea; if the lens cannot be removed immediately, slide it onto the sclera.

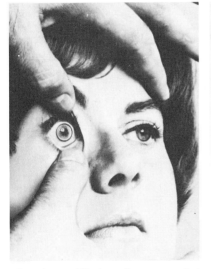

After the eyelids have been separated and the corneal contact lens has been correctly positioned over the cornea, you widen the eyelid margins beyond the top and bottom edges of lens (as shown).

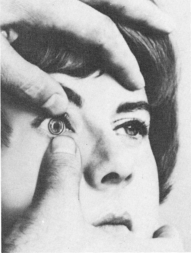

After the lower eyelid margin has been moved near the bottom lens edge and then the upper eyelid margin has been moved near the top lens edge, you are ready (as shown) to move under the bottom edge of the lens by pressing slightly harder on the lower eyelid while moving it upward.

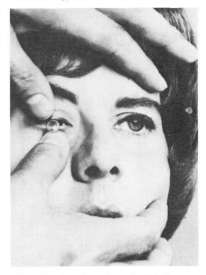

After the lens has tipped slightly, you move the eyelids toward one another and thereby cause the lens to slide out between the eyelids (as shown).

Figure 16–15   These photos illustrate how to remove contact lenses. After removing lenses, they should be stored so that lenses for the right and left eye are clearly identified. (From Contact Lens Emergency Care Information & Instruction Packet. Published by American Optometric Association Committee on Contact Lenses.)

aged to do so when possible. However, the nurse should provide the necessary equipment, which usually includes a small basin, soap and water for washing, and solution for rinsing the prosthesis. Normal saline or tap water can be used for rinsing. Most persons have their own method for cleaning the eye socket and the area around it. The nurse should ask the patient how he does this and make it possible for him to continue with his usual practice.

If the patient needs assistance, an artificial eye may be removed by placing suction on the artificial eye itself. A simple method is to use the rubber bulb of an eyedropper. The bulb is compressed to expel the air and placed near the center of the eye. When pressure on the bulb is released, the bulb will cling to the eye and it then can be removed by gently lifting. Figure 16–16 illustrates another method for removing an artificial eye and also illustrates how to replace it. The socket is ordinarily flushed with normal saline before replacing the artificial eye. Care should be taken to avoid scratching an artificial eye.

Practices differ concerning the frequency of removing and cleaning an artificial eye and irrigating the socket. It may be as often as daily or as infrequent as biweekly. There are some artificial eyes now being used that are never removed. The nurse should observe practices recommended by the patient's physician.

CARE OF THE EARS AND NOSE

Cleaning the Ears

Other than cleaning the outer ears, little more is needed for routine hygiene of the ear. After the ears are washed, they should be dried carefully with a soft towel so that water and wax are removed by capillary action. Forcing the towel into the ear for drying may aid in the formation of wax plugs.

If a wax plug is present in the auditory canal, it is removed by gentle syringing of the ear. An ear syringe is used. Some persons use a water-pik appliance, such as the one used for cleaning the teeth, for removing a wax plug in the external canal. Whatever appliance is used, great care must be taken to prevent damage caused by excessive pressure by the water spray. The stream of water should be directed against the sides of the ear canal rather than directly toward the eardrum. Using items, such as bobby pins or a hairpin, to remove wax is extremely dangerous since the eardrum may be punctured.

Cleaning the Nose

The best way to clean the nose is to blow it gently. Both nostrils should be open while blowing the nose. Closing one nostril adds to the danger of forcing debris into the eustachian tubes. Irrigations are usually contraindicated because of the possible danger of forcing material into the sinuses. Small objects should be kept away from the nose to prevent aspiration and to prevent injuring the mucous membrane of the nose.

If the external nares are crusted, applying mineral or cotton seed oil helps to soften and remove the crusts. Disposable paper tissues are recommended for nasal secretions. A cotton applicator may be used to clean the nares but with great care to avoid injury. The applicator should never be introduced into the nares.

PERINEAL CARE

An important part of personal hygiene is perineal care. The patient unable to clean the perineal area will need the nurse's assistance. To neglect this important part of care may result in physical and psychological discomfort for the patient, a breakdown in the skin, and offensive odors. The perineal area is a dark, warm, and often a moist area which favors bacterial growth. Especially in patients with indwelling catheters, organisms from the area may reach the bladder, a possibility that increases when microorganisms are numerous in an unclean perineal area.

When practical, the patient is placed on a bedpan. The perineal area is flushed with a warm, mild soap or detergent and water solution. Rinsing well with plain water follows. When flushing is insufficient for cleaning, scrubbing becomes necessary. Using cotton balls or other disposable material for scrubbing is psychologically preferable to using a washcloth. The area is then dried and emollients or powder are used on the skin areas as indicated. If it is not possible to place the patient on a bedpan, the patient is placed on a towel or pad, and the area is cleaned and then wiped free of soap or detergent solution with disposable material.

In the female, the labia are separated carefully and the exposed areas then cleaned. Special care is needed to remove the thick secretion of *smegma* found under the labia minora and clitoris. Smegma allowed to collect in the area becomes foul-smelling very quickly.

In the uncircumcised male, the foreskin or prepuce is retracted, and the exposed glans penis and prepuce are carefully cleaned. Smegma also collects in this area and

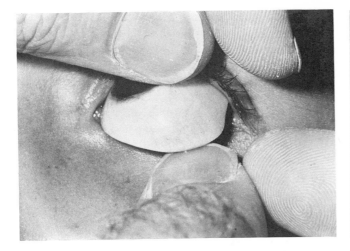

Depressing lower lid allows prosthesis to slide out and down.

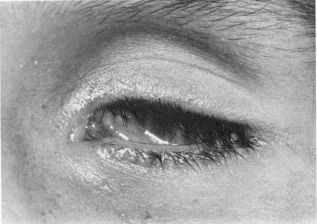

Socket after removal; wash off external matter and encrustations.

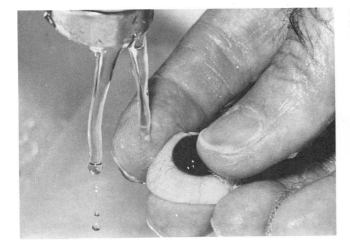

Wash prosthesis with soap and water; scrub with thumb and finger.

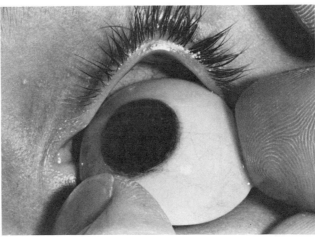

Lift upper lid, depress lower lid, and slip artificial eye in place.

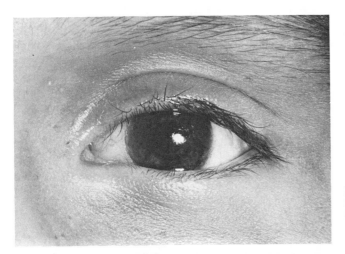

Once prosthesis is in place, eye should be wiped toward the nose.

Figure 16–16 This figure illustrates how to remove, clean and replace an artificial eye. (Zucnick, Martha. "Care of an Artificial Eye." *American Journal of Nursing,* 75:835, May 1975. Photographs by John Bishop and William Cox, Eye Foundation Hospital, Birmingham, Alabama.)

should be well washed and rinsed away. It is important to pull the prepuce back into place over the glans penis to prevent constriction of the penis which may result in serious edema and tissue injury. The penis and scrotum are washed, including the posterior and lateral aspects. The scrotum houses the testicles. They are very tender and should be handled with great care to prevent discomfort to the patient.

The crotch area in both the male and female should be carefully washed, rinsed, and dried. The area may be powdered.

The stroke used while cleaning the perineal area and the genitals in both the male and female should be long and sufficiently firm to avoid discomfort or a tickling sensation for the patient. In the female, the cleaning stroke should move from the pubic area down toward the anal area. This helps prevent carrying organisms from the anal area back over the genitals. In the male, the cleaning stroke begins at the tip of the penis and moves toward the pubic area.

The patient is turned on his or her side in order to clean the anal area. Soap and water for cleaning should be rinsed away thoroughly to prevent skin irritation. The area is then dried and powder may be applied.

It is not always possible for male nurses to attend to male patients and female nurses to attend to female patients. When the perineal cleaning is carried out in a matter-of-fact and dignified manner, patients generally do not find care by a person of the opposite sex to be offensive or embarrassing. Some persons suggest that the male penis be handled with a gloved hand or with a towel if erotic stimulation occurs during the cleaning procedure.

The bidet has long been used for perineal hygiene, especially in Europe and South America. A stream of water is directed over the perineal and anal area as one sits on the bidet. The water leaves the bidet with a flushing-type action or, in the case of the portable bidets, by draining into a toilet or tub. Persons using them report satisfactory results although they are not intended to replace the bath or shower. A sitz tub has also been used for helping to clean the perineal and anal area. The portable type is especially handy when it is cumbersome to move a patient to a stationary sitz tub.

THE DECUBITUS ULCER

A *decubitus ulcer* is an area of cellular necrosis which is caused by a lack of blood circulation to the involved area. *Necrosis* means that there is death of cells. The terms *decubitus ulcer, pressure sore, and bedsore* are used synonomously. Decubitus derives from a Latin word meaning lying down. Lying down is not necessarily the cause of a decubitus ulcer and one need not be bedridden to develop one. Therefore, some persons prefer the term pressure sore since pressure is the most prominent underlying cause of a decubitus ulcer.

Pathological changes at the site of a decubitus ulcer are caused by a collapse of blood vessels, especially the arterioles and capillaries, in the area of the ulcer. The damage to vessels is due to pressure, usually from body weight. When the blood supply is occluded because of the pressure on vessels, cells are not adequately nourished and cell wastes accumulate. Death of cells eventually occurs, leading to the characteristic ulcer of a pressure sore.

The first sign that a pressure sore may be developing is a blanching of the skin over the area under pressure. Instead of a healthy pink color, the skin becomes pale and white. In the non-Caucasian, this blanching is more difficult to see. However, insufficient blood circulation in the capillaries makes the skin appear pale when compared with areas where circulation is good. Local anemia due to poor circulation in the area is called *ischemia,* which means containing little blood.

When pressure is relieved, ischemia is rapidly followed by *hyperemia;* that is, an unusually large amount of blood is present in the area. The area now appears red and feels warm. In the non-Caucasian, hyeremia may best be detected by touch. The skin will feel warm. Hyperemia is a compensatory mechanism. The body literally floods the area with blood in order to nourish and remove wastes from the cells. This phenomenon is called *reactive hyperemia.* If pressure is not relieved, the area remains red but circulation cannot occur to the extent necessary for cell survival and the tissue cells eventually will die. The skin breaks and a shallow crater or ulcer develops. The pressure sore then is often called superficial and with proper care, ordinarily will heal with relative ease.

The skin can tolerate considerable pressure without cell death but for short periods only. Duration is more important than amount of pressure in the formation of a decubitus ulcer. One to two hours of pressure will result in ischemia, and if the pressure is sustained, a pressure sore is in the making.

A decubitus ulcer is usually described as deep when a superficial pressure sore extends and involves underlying tissues. Shearing forces are often responsible for deep decubitus ulcers. A *shearing force* results when layers of tissue move on each other. Small blood vessels and capillaries are stretched and may even tear, thus resulting in poor circulation to tissue cells under the skin. The area of skin over an area damaged by a shearing force usually appears bluish in color and sometimes a lump can be felt under the skin. A small break in the skin which leads to (necrotic) tissue in the underlying area eventually appears. Situations causing shearing force are described later in this section.

Common Sites for Decubitus Ulcers

Decubitus ulcers usually occur over bony prominences since body weight is distributed over a small area that has little subcutaneous tissues to cushion damage to the skin. Common sites for decubitus ulcers are illustrated in Figure 16–17. Of the susceptible areas, most pressure sores occur over the sacrum and coccyx. Decubitus ulcers have even been seen on the sternum and ribs of persons who lie on their abdomens for a long time.

Factors that Predispose to the Development of Decubitus Ulcers

internal + external

There are numerous factors which predispose to pressure sores. Usually a combination is responsible.

The most formidable predisposing factor for a decubitus ulcer is pressure over an area to an extent and of a duration that blood capillaries are occluded and blood circulation to tissues in the area is poor. Immobility is usually involved. The person who sits or lies most of the time and moves about little is a candidate for a pressure sore. The up-and-about person does not develop decubitus ulcers since no part of his body suffers from prolonged pressure. Even during sleep, the well person tends to move about in bed freely.

As mentioned earlier, shearing forces can cause decubitus ulcers. Patients who are moved about in bed or from bed to stretchers or chairs carelessly often will suffer from shearing forces as skin and underlying tissues are pulled over each other. A patient who is partially sitting up in bed is also susceptible. His skin may stick to the sheet while underlying tissues move downward with his body, thus creating shearing forces, usually in the sacral area. This may occur also with the patient who sits in a chair but slides down while his skin sticks to his clothing and the back of the chair.

Friction may cause skin damage and lead to decubitus ulcers. The patient who lies on wrinkled sheets is likely to suffer tissue damage due to friction. The skin over the elbows and heels often suffer from friction when the patient lifts and helps himself move in bed with the use of his arms and feet. Friction burns occur on the back also when patients are pulled or slid over sheets in bed.

Various kinds of debris in bed or on a chair produce damage to skin that can lead to pressure sores. Such debris includes crumbs, hair pins and clips, buttons, pencils and pens, and pieces of silverware.

Prolonged moisture of the skin reduces its resistance to trauma. Warmth increases the cells' demand for oxygen. Hence, an area that is moist and warm will soon lead to cell destruction and especially when pressure is present. If personal hygiene is poor, the skin will contain many organisms that will thrive in the warm, moist, environment, adding to the danger of developing a decubitus ulcer that will become infected.

Persons who suffer from malnutrition and anemia are prone to develop decubitus ulcers. Vitamin C deficiency causes capillaries to become more fragile and, hence, more subject to breaks, causing poor circulation to the area. Older persons whose skin is wrinkled because of loss of subcutaneous fat are good candidates for developing pressure sores. Their skin forms folds and becomes irritated easily. Bony prominences are better protected by persons with considerable fat tissue. Pressure sores tend to occur more readily in men than in women, for reasons that are not usually clear. Persons who have debilitating diseases with decreased mobility are likely candidates. If an elevated temperature is present or if the normal functioning of the cells is altered in any way, destruction of tissues becomes relatively easy.

The unconscious patient is especially subject to the development of pressure sores when preventive measures are not taken. So also are paralyzed patients, emotionally depressed persons who ordinarily tend to be immobile, and patients with skin abrasions. Patients whose skin is very dry and those whose skin has been irritated with adhesive tape are likely candidates for pressure sores.

The Prevention and Treatment of Decubitus Ulcers

Of utmost importance in the prevention of decubitus ulcers is the elimination of continuous pressure that restricts blood flow to an area. This can best be accomplished by changing the patient's position frequently, as often as every hour or two for those who are especially susceptible to decubitus ulcers. The position in bed that is most likely to cause the greatest amount of pressure to the largest number of areas is the back-lying posi-

362

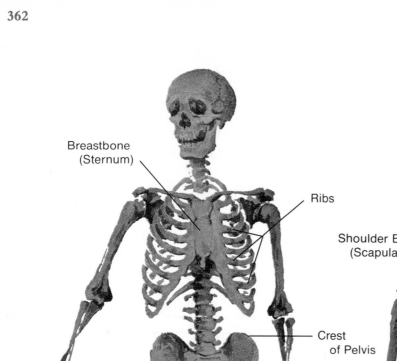

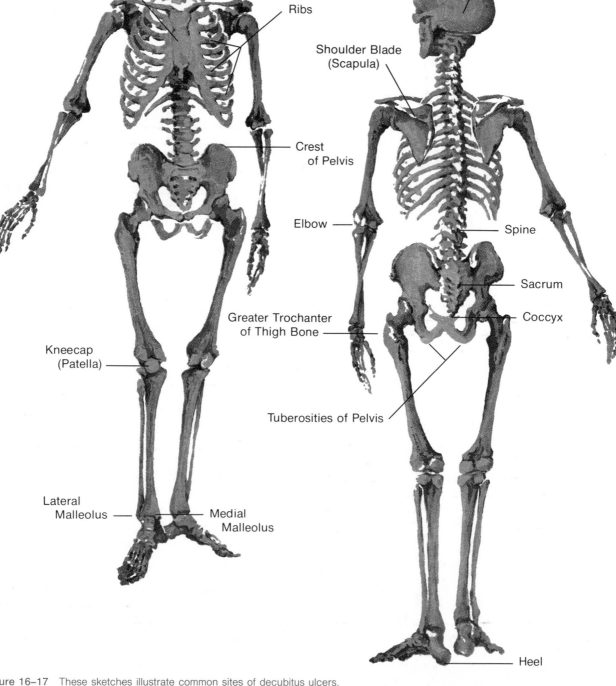

Breastbone
(Sternum)

Ribs

Crest
of Pelvis

Greater Trochanter
of Thigh Bone

Kneecap
(Patella)

Lateral
Malleolus

Medial
Malleolus

Tuberosities of Pelvis

Occipital Bone

Shoulder Blade
(Scapula)

Elbow

Spine

Sacrum

Coccyx

Heel

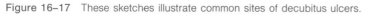

Figure 16–17   These sketches illustrate common sites of decubitus ulcers.

tion. The details of a plan to change the patient's position should be indicated on the patient's plan of care.

Keeping the patient clean and free from irritation is of extreme importance in the prevention of decubitus ulcers. Dressings may need to be changed more frequently and arranged to keep drainage from irritated areas. Patients who are unable to control urinary or bowel functions require special consideration. As a precautionary measure, an indwelling catheter may be inserted into the patient's urinary bladder if the patient is in constant danger of urinating and seems to be a likely candidate for a decubitus ulcer. Patients should be washed locally following each bowel elimination.

The skin always has microorganisms on it. While the skin manages well with its own flora, the presence of organisms from infected wounds or from feces is potentially dangerous if the skin is irritated. As mentioned earlier, if the skin is moist and warm, and the area dark, conditions become ideal for the growth of transient bacteria. Infection of the skin may occur, and, once the area is broken, the problem of healing it complicates the patient's plan of care and his illness.

Patients who must lie on sheets over plastic or other protective materials perspire, and evaporation of the moisture is difficult. The constant presence of the moisture, along with continuous pressure, presents an ideal situation for decubitus ulcer formation. Good results have been reported from placing patients especially prone to bedsores on a piece of sheepskin. The air spaces in the tufts allow air circulation and help keep the patient's skin dry. The material also eases pressure on the area and helps to distribute weight. Most sheepskins are made of synthetic materials and can be laundered. A disadvantage of real sheepskin is that it cannot be cleaned sufficiently well with washing.

In addition to keeping the skin surfaces clean and dry and changing the patient's position often, a light rubbing of the areas which receive a great deal of pressure is helpful. These areas should be examined often and massaged with a lotion. The lotion reduces friction to make massaging easier and more comfortable. The massaging stimulates circulation to the area. Lanolin is frequently recommended for dry skin areas but other emollients may also be used.

While mattresses should be firm to help maintain good alignment of the body, their firmness also may be cause for concern. The alternating pressure mattress pad, also called ripple-celled mattress, has been designed to help reduce this constant pressure. The principle on which it operates is that sections of the pad distend with air or fluid while other sections remain flat. Then those that remained flat distend, and the other sections deflate. In this way, no one area of the body is receiving constant pressure. These pads are placed over the regular bed mattress. Caution is necessary with such a pad because puncture by sharp instruments and pins can cause a leak of the fluid or the air.

The alternating pressure pad is not disturbing to the patient. The fact that it produces occasional tickling sensations which cause muscular contractions is considered to be beneficial. For the most part, however, patients become adjusted to them and do not seem to realize that they are on the pad.

The use of the water bed has caught the consumer's attention in recent years, and many are now used in hotels, motels, and homes. They had been in use for years for patients with decubitus ulcers or for those most prone to develop them on a limited basis. In recent years, the materials and designs have made them cheaper, lighter in weight because less water is used than once was the case, and easier to handle and maintain. As a result, they are becoming more commonplace in health agencies, especially those where there are many patients who are likely to develop or who have decubitus ulcers. Their effectiveness in the treatment and prevention of decubitus ulcers is based on the following physics principle. An increase in pressure on an enclosed liquid will be distributed uniformly and undiminished to all parts of the liquid. Hence, a water-filled mattress distributes pressure evenly over the body surface in contact with it. This results in better delivery of oxygen to areas of the body where ordinarily, pressure from a firm mattress is sufficient to decrease blood supply. To avoid chilliness when lying on the water mattress if there is no heating device on the mattress, extra bed covering may be necessary. Water-filled pads that can be made at home with plastic bags for the protection of parts of the body from pressure can also be used.

Sources of irritation and friction should be eliminated. Contour sheets are helpful to prevent lying on wrinkles; flat sheets should be securely anchored. Top linen so applied that it restricts freedom of movement, and pressure and irritation from casts, adhesive, tubing, arm boards, and the like, should be guarded against. For persons completely immobilized, Foster and Stryker frames and CircOlectric beds are used to make turning patients easy. These frames and beds will be discussed in Chapter 17.

Good results have been reported with the use of polystyrene foam blocks to protect ankles and heels.

The blocks, one for each ankle, are cut in half, hollowed to fit the ankle, padded (preferably with sheepskin), and gripped together around the patient's ankles. The device keeps the foot above the mattress level, thus preventing pressure and irritation. Hyperextension of the knees can be eliminated by placing a pillow under them.

A special plastic foam developed by the National Aeronautics and Space Administration has been used with effectiveness in the prevention of decubitus ulcers. The material conforms to the body when it is warmed by normal body temperature and relieves sustained pressure. Packs filled with gelatinous material can be used to relieve pressure and are available in various sizes and shapes to fit different parts of the body.

Several preparations have been used to protect the skin from irritation in areas especially susceptible to pressure sores. A silicone and zinc oxide mixture dispensed in aerosal has been used and tincture of benzoin can be swabbed on the skin as a protective measure.

Various air-inflated rings, doughnuts as they are often called, have been used to relieve pressure over an area susceptible to pressure sores. However, their use is questionable. The ring itself often causes pressure around the area involved, and, thus, it creates more problems than it solves.

A decubitus ulcer is not confined necessarily to those persons who are in bed. Some patients who are able to be out of bed but remain in a chair for a good portion of the day are also likely to develop decubitus ulcers if not cared for properly. Old as well as young patients are vulnerable.

Many topical agents have been used for the treatment of decubitus ulcers. The following agents have been reported in the literature within the last few years: tannic acid, gelatin sponges, karaya powder, sugar and sugar paste, gelfoam, gold leaf, oxygen under-pressure, whipped egg whites, antacids, proteolytic enzymes, and insulin. The ulcerated area is thoroughly cleaned first and then the topical agent is applied. According to reports, success with certain patients is reported with each agent. But, as can be seen by the number of agents being tried, an effective treatment appears more illusive than real. One person who expressed pessimism about a sure treatment for decubitus ulcers wrote that one can put anything on a pressure sore except the patient! According to some authorities, most of the time it is perhaps best to put nothing on a pressure sore.

The presence of a decubitus ulcer adds to the patient's morbidity, often complicates recovery from other pathological conditions, and can even threaten the life of a debilitated or paralyzed patient. The best treatment is *prevention* and prevention is a nursing responsibility. The best preventive measures include avoiding pressure sores by turning and moving the patient regularly, frequently, and carefully while keeping the patient clean, dry, and well-nourished and -hydrated.

PERSONAL HYGIENE AND THE NURSING PROCESS

The collection of data concerning a person's habits and the status of his personal hygiene will seek answers to such questions as the following. What habits of personal hygiene does the person ordinarily observe? Are the habits generally considered conducive to well-being? Is the person knowledgeable about sound practices of personal hygiene? Is there evidence that the person's present health status is influenced adversely by certain habits of personal hygiene? For example, has neglect of oral hygiene resulted in a person's having teeth and gum diseases? Is the person with contact lenses observing habits of hygiene that are conducive to good eye health?

As she collects data, the nurse will be interested in the person's reason for seeking health care and whether his present health status and therapeutic regimen may require that the nurse assist the patient with personal hygiene measures. For example, is the patient a likely candidate for developing a decubitus ulcer? Or, what type of bathing procedure is indicated in a particular situation?

In general, there is wide variation in habits of personal hygiene which promote well-being. While recognizing and respecting each person's individuality, there are general standards for assessment purposes. For example, when a pathological condition is not the cause, is the person exhibiting skin, hair, or scalp problems from lack of cleanliness or is the problem perhaps due to misuse of personal grooming aids? Is body odor due to poor bathing habits? From her assessment, the nurse's diagnoses form a basis for developing a plan of care.

Ordinarily, nursing care planning for personal hygiene includes encouraging the patient to take responsibility for his own personal hygiene when his habits promote well-being and when he has the ability to do so; and assisting the patient with measures he cannot manage on his own. If the nurse notes lack of knowledge about sound habits of personal hygiene, teaching becomes important. The patient and his family, as indicated, are included with planning appropriate nursing care.

The following general guidelines will assist the nurse as she implements the patient's plan of care for personal hygiene:

- Use the time when assisting the patient with personal hygiene measures to learn to know the patient better. Many times, auxiliary personnel are assigned to assist patients needing help with various personal hygiene measures. Even when these persons are capable of carrying out a particular procedure efficiently, to delegate all such care to others robs the nurse of many excellent opportunities to develop helping relationships with patients. In addition, she has lost a time to demonstrate that she personally cares and is interested in the patient's overall well-being. The importance of touch in nursing care has been discussed in this text. Many personal hygiene measures include touch that can be used therapeutically for both psychosocial and physiological purposes. Typical examples of personal care involving touch include the bath, a back rub, hair grooming, and nail care.

- Numerous opportunities for teaching become available while assisting patients with personal hygiene measures. The nurse is present and with the patient, sometimes for fairly long periods, and the time can be utilized effectively for teaching about personal hygiene as well as about whatever illness condition may be present. What better time is there for teaching a patient with diabetes mellitus the importance of proper foot care than when the nurse cares for his feet during the bathing procedure?

- Demonstrate good personal habits of personal hygiene. The nurse can set a good example when she observes good habits herself. Furthermore, it is offensive to others, especially during illness, to be cared for by persons who are careless about such things as body odor, halitosis, nail and hair grooming, and so on.

- Remember that although the skin and the mucous membrane have considerable ability to cope with many microorganisms and normal wear and tear, this ability tends to be lower during most illnesses and in the young and the elderly. When time seems consumed with therapeutic regimens that often include highly technical and complicated procedures, it may be easy to overlook such measures as oral hygiene and techniques to prevent decubitus ulcers. Nevertheless, these measures are important nursing responsibilities and the presence of poor oral hygiene and decubitus ulcers very often are the result of low standards of nursing care.

- Personal hygiene includes perineal care. It has been observed in many instances that patients are asked to finish the bath when they are unable to do so sufficiently well. Unfortunately, these patients are often unwilling or too embarrassed to ask for assistance. The nurse interested in her patient's well-being will not overlook this important aspect of personal hygiene.

- Chapter 3 stated that people unable to care for themselves expect the nurse to assist them with personal hygiene. One of the hallmarks of nursing since its inception has included assisting patients to meet hygienic needs when they are unable to do so on their own. Nursing has changed, but this important aspect of care still should command the nurse's attention and concern.

The parts of the nursing process and of the process as a whole are evaluated as described in Chapter 4.

CONCLUSION

Personal hygiene habits differ rather substantially. As the nurse remains loyal to the principle that each individual is a unique being, she will demonstrate respect for patients with personal hygiene habits that may differ from her own.

If one follows advertising in our communications media, it would seem that we are all either very clean from using the many personal care products available to us, or very dirty for needing so many different products. Certainly, personal cleanliness is an important aspect of health and grooming. It is also an important part of nursing care as nurses assist patients to meet personal hygiene needs. But in addition to meeting personal care needs, the nurse plays an important role as a health teacher in helping to differentiate fads and fallacies from facts while still being supportive of a wide variety of perfectly acceptable personal hygiene habits.

SUPPLEMENTAL LIBRARY STUDY

1. The following article presents a guide for assessment of the mouth:

    Bruya, Margaret Auld and Madeira, Nancy Powell. "Stomatitis After Chemotherapy." *American Journal of Nursing,* 75:1349–1352, August 1975.

    Discuss briefly how the guide to assess the mouth on page 1350 might be used for patients other than those having stomatitis and receiving chemotherapy. List at least five standards of mouth care the authors discuss. What cleaning agent do the authors recommend for mouth care?

2. The author of the following article describes how a back rub is a carrier of messages:

Temple, Kathleen D. "The Back Rub." *American Journal of Nursing,* 67:2102–2103, October 1967.

What purposes does the author give for a back rub? What does the author mean when she states that a back rub opens channels of communication between the patient and the nurse?

Now read the following article:

Krieger, Dolores. "Therapeutic Touch: The Imprimatur of Nursing." *American Journal of Nursing,* 75:784–787, May 1975.

What does the author describe as an essential in order for a person to help or heal by touch? What objective observation did the author use to measure the effects of therapeutic touch? Describe what relationship you see between therapeutic touch and a back rub.

3. Test your understanding in the use of contact lenses:

   "Contact Lenses." (Test Yourself) *American Journal of Nursing,* 77:267, February 1977.

4. The following two articles discuss and illustrate the care of hair for the black person:

   Grier, Marian E. "Hair Care for the Black Patient." *American Journal of Nursing,* 76:1781, November 1976.

   Davis, Mardell. "Getting to the Root of the Problem: Hair-Grooming Techniques for Black Patients." *Nursing 77,* 7:60–65, April 1977.

   Describe the mixture which Ms. Grier uses to clean the hair of a black patient. According to Ms. Grier, how does hair care meet psychosocial as well as physiological needs? Describe Ms. Davis's explanation concerning why black persons are proud of curly and thick hair. How does Ms. Davis suggest that tangles be removed from the hair?

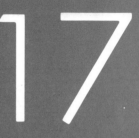

17

BEHAVIORAL OBJECTIVES

*When content in this chapter has been mastered the
student will be able to*

Define the terms appearing in the glossary.

Explain the role activity plays in maintaining well-
being and describe harmful effects of prolonged bed
rest.

Identify at least seven guidelines to use when
applying principles of physics to body mechanics.

Describe two types of conditioning exercises which
help to prepare the patient for ambulation.

Describe the proper techniques for helping persons
who have impairment of mobility; include assisting a
patient to get out of bed, walk, and use crutches,
and moving, lifting, and carrying a helpless person.

Discuss at least six general principles of nursing care
for the patient confined to bed and illustrate each
principle with several examples of appropriate safety,
comfort, and self-help devices.

Explain two principles related to leisure-time activities
and illustrate each principle with examples of
pertinent nursing approaches.

Describe the nursing care of a person experiencing a
problem with activity or exercise, using the nursing
process as a guide.

Promoting Exercise and Activity

GLOSSARY

Abduction: The lateral movement of a body part away from the midline of the body.

Active Exercise: A joint movement activated by the person.

Adduction: The movement of a body part toward the midline of the body.

Ankylosis: The fixation or immobilization of a joint.

Anterior: The front.

Atony: The absence of muscle tone.

Atrophy: A decrease in the size of a body structure.

Body Mechanics: The efficient use of the body as a machine and as a means of locomotion.

Center of Gravity: The point at which the mass of an object is centered.

Cervical Curve: The concave curve of the vertebral column at the neck.

Circumduction: The circular movement of a body part.

Contracture: The permanent contraction state of a muscle.

Dangling: The position in which the person sits on the edge of the bed with his legs and feet hanging over the side of the bed.

Extension: The state of being in a straight line.

External Rotation: A body part turning on its axis away from the midline.

Flexion: The state of being bent.

Footdrop: A complication resulting from extended plantar flexion.

Fowler's Position: A semisitting position.

Friction: The rubbing of one surface against another.

Hyperextenion: A state of exaggerated extension.

Hypotonia: A decrease in muscle tone.

Insertion: The more movable attachment of the muscle to the bone.

Internal Rotation: A body part turning on its axis toward the midline.

Isometric Exercises: Exercises in which muscle tension occurs without a significant change in muscle length.

Lateral: The side.

Line of gravity: A vertical line which passes through the center of gravity.

Lumbar Curve: The concave curve of the vertebral column at the lower back.

Medial: The middle or midline.

Origin: The less movable attachment of a skeletal muscle to a bone.

Orthopedics: The correction or prevention of disorders of the locomotion of the body.

Orthostatic hypotension: A decrease in blood pressure associated with assuming an upright position.

Passive Exercise: The manual or mechanical means of moving the joints.

Posterior: The back.

Prone: A face down recumbent position or the position in which the hands are held with the palms down or backward.

Range of Motion: The complete extent of movement of which a joint is normally capable.

Resistive Exercise: An active exercise using an external resistive force.

Rolling Friction: The rubbing caused by a circular object being moved over another surface.

Rotation: The turning on an axis.

Sacral Curve: The convex curve of the vertebral column at the end of the spine.

Sliding Friction: The rubbing of two flat surfaces over each other.

Supine: A back-lying recumbent position or the position in which the palms of the hands are facing upward or forward.

Thoracic Curve: The convex curve of the vertebral column at the chest.

Tonus: The partial steady state of muscle contraction.

Trapeze Bar: A handgrip suspended from a frame near the head of a bed.

INTRODUCTION

Research has demonstrated that an inactive body suffers both physically and psychologically. Therefore, exercise and activity, including leisure-time activity, are of concern to the nurse who has physical and psychological well-being as her goal when offering care to her patients. This chapter will focus on exercise and activity as important considerations in high-quality nursing care.

The concept of rehabilitation becomes important when promoting exercise and activity for patients. In the past it has usually meant the restoration of health or function to a handicapped person. This is still true, but the dimension of prevention has been added to the concept. The purpose of rehabilitation is to prevent loss of function and to restore as many functions as possible. Both physical and psychological functions are included.

Because the process of rehabilitation is so broad, many specially prepared persons are usually involved, and many special facilities are utilized: physicians with advanced preparation in physical as well as psychic functioning; physical, occupational, speech, and recreational therapists; mental health workers of many kinds; and vocational workers and employers join nurses in promoting rehabilitation. Teamwork among these persons is important for promoting reinforcement of efforts and goal achievement. Facilities such as special units or hospitals; social, educational, and recreational agencies; employment services; residential treatment centers; day care centers; and halfway houses are among the many agencies designed to promote rehabilitation.

There are extensive variations in patients' needs and their potential for rehabilitation. Nurses play important roles in both prevention and restoration of function loss in health agencies and in homes. They very often work with family members almost as much as with the patient to provide necessary teaching, assistance, and support.

Since a major goal of rehabilitation is prevention of disability, this chapter stresses preventive measures. There is some discussion of function restoration, but that aspect can be found in greater detail in more advanced texts. Because physical rehabilitation of a helpless patient often involves much physical exertion for the nurse or family members providing the care, measures to protect those responsible for the patient are discussed also. Several references at the end of this unit deal with safety precautions.

THE NEED FOR BODY ACTIVITY TO MAINTAIN HEALTH

The values of exercise and good posture have long been recognized. From past experience, we know that sitting in a chair in a class for an hour or more with the shoulders and the head brought forward may cause fatigue and altered breathing. If, in addition, the muscles of the legs have not contracted during that time, there may be a certain amount of swelling of the feet. The reason for this is that skeletal muscles serve many functions in addition to movement, heat production, and maintenance of posture. When the muscles contract they squeeze veins. This squeezing action helps to move the blood back to the heart. Together with breathing which changes the pressure within the closed chest cavity and the tiny valves located along the inner surface of the veins, venous circulation is maintained even against the pull of gravity. If inactivity eliminates most of this squeezing action and if poor posture prevents normal breathing, venous circulation is slowed down. Persons confined to their seats during long air flights often experience decreased venous circulation in their lower extremities. Fatigue can develop as a result of too much waste material accumulating and too little nourishment going to the muscles. Muscle fatigue usually is attributed to the accumulation of too much lactic acid in the muscles.

We have already seen that the workload of the heart and blood vessels is influenced by body activity. Many persons are not readily aware of some of its other influences on the body. Because the movement of gases and fluids in the lungs is related to position and activity, the acid-base balance determined partially by the blood's carbon dioxide content, can be altered by activity. The ease or difficulty of ingestion and movement of food in the gastrointestinal tract, as well as intestinal elimination, are related to body movement. Activity also influences calcium moving into and out of the bone tissue, the production and excretion of urine, and the metabolic activities of cells. If the reader has observed a person whose activity has been limited for an extended period, he is also aware of the influence movement has on the self-concept and psychological functioning. Body activity, then, has a widespread effect on the total well-being of an individual.

Persons with sedentary occupations need to plan for making physical activity a part of their daily lives in order to help maintain well-being. Besides being physically healthful, active diversionary activities provide a different type of sensory stimulation and can be fun.

The dependency on the automobile and labor-saving devices requires conscious planning for many people to assure that they get adequate exercise. For example, parking the car and walking several blocks to one's destination can be appropriate. Developing an interest in yardwork or do-it-yourself projects at home can provide exercise. The type of activity can vary, but the point is that it should involve physical activity, be satisfying to the person, and be performed on a regular basis.

Many persons reduce their physical activity at the time of retirement. The routines of their daily work may have incorporated the use of many muscles. When they no longer perform these routines, if substitute activities or exercises are not undertaken, evidence of muscle disuse often occurs. Even elderly persons who experience chronic health problems or merely the effects of aging can perform some physical activities within the limits of their health state.

The nurse must be physically fit also. A regular routine of conditioning exercises will help her to strengthen and maintain muscle tone. Exercises which develop the knee and hip extensors and the abdominal wall are especially helpful for many activities in her work.

By being physically fit the nurse can serve as an example to others. She is often in a position to discuss, encourage, and demonstrate the role of appropriate daily exercises. It is felt that the lack of adequate physical activity is a major factor in the suboptimum health state of many persons of all ages in this country today. Therefore, the encouragement of adequate exercise can be an important contribution of the nurse to health promotion. Physical activity does not necessarily prevent illness, but it makes the human body less susceptible and better able to respond to illness when it does occur.

Every person initiating an exercise regimen needs to be cautioned about selecting appropriate exercises and building the program gradually. Too strenuous exercises or overzealousness can cause harm to a person's body. Patients with health problems should consult a physician before starting an exercise program.

There are many lay and professional sources available which describe exercises for maintaining well-being. Several are included in the references at the end of this unit.

PRINCIPLES OF BODY MECHANICS

No one would question the relationship of rest to health or of good nutrition to health. Also, there is a direct relationship of body mechanics to the effective functioning of the body. *Body mechanics* has been described as the efficient use of the body as a machine and as a means of locomotion. Good health depends not only on how expertly we choose our foods, but also on how carefully and efficiently we utilize our body parts in relation to internal and external forces. For example, a truck driver may eat adequately nutritious meals; but if he does not understand how to use his body properly to lift a heavy object onto his truck, he may injure himself. Or the homemaker may be well aware of the essentials of proper menu planning, and she may have many modern conveniences to assist her. But improper use of the body in activities performed throughout a good part of her day, such as reaching, bending, stooping, or standing, may tire her.

The importance of understanding body mechanics is universal, regardless of health-illness status. The basic principles of body mechanics should be evident in every activity and even during periods of rest. Because correct use of the body is another phase of prevention of illness and the promotion of health, the nurse has a major responsibility to teach, both directly and indirectly, by example.

To remember to use the correct muscle groups for every activity can be a chore when one already has developed a life pattern of using muscle groups in another way. As with all habits, it takes time to learn a new pattern, especially when the process involves breaking down an established one. However, in the final analysis, good body mechanics will pay dividends in good health and appearance and body function, which in turn produces happiness and comfort for the person using them. Good body mechanics is not accomplished by following a set procedure; it is achieved through knowledge which guides actions in every activity performed and is a fundamental concept of nursing.

To be able to evaluate the patient's musculoskeletal needs and to teach by example, the nurse must understand and utilize the principles of body mechanics. Every activity in which she engages will require understanding and use of these principles, from as simple a thing as moving a chair to lifting a patient out of bed.

Terms and Concepts of Body Mechanics

All that is involved in body mechanics is sometimes called basic *orthopedic principles in nursing care*. *Orthopedics* means the correction or the prevention of disorders of the body's structures for locomotion. Since body mechanics is concerned with preventing injury to or limitation of the musculoskeletal system, these terms could understandably be interchangeable.

Nurses have long recognized that basic orthopedic principles are applicable to all areas of nursing, not just to the patient who has a bone fracture or some other pathological skeletal change. For example, the person who has a sedentary occupation and little physical activity may have poorly developed muscles. The patient who is on complete bed rest is in danger of losing muscle tonus. Should the bed rest be prolonged, the patient is in danger also of developing contractures if he does not have exercise and joint motion and if provision is not made for maintaining good posture. Functioning of various internal body processes is also influenced by position and movement or their absence.

Tonus, a normal quality of healthy muscle, is a partial, but steady state of contraction present except during sleep. Muscles usually contract by shortening their fibers, but in some types of muscle contraction the length of the muscle fibers remains the same while the tension within the muscle increases.

A contracture is a permanent contraction state of a muscle. It usually results from prolonged contraction and is observed in flexor muscles rather than in extensors because flexors are generally stronger. Flexor muscles, when they contract, decrease the angle of a joint formed by two adjacent bones. Extensors increase the angle. Knee and elbow contractures are common complications when bedridden patients have not had proper preventive exercises.

While the plight of the bedridden patient might be easy to comprehend, everyone who is up and about also faces problems. A person who is hyperactive may very well exhaust himself and become fatigued. Or, when patients are depressed or for some reason become quite inactive, they may have diminished (muscle tonus) because of inactivity. This is due to the fact that the use of muscles is essential for maintaining muscle tone. Inactivity leads to hypotonia or atony, decrease or absence of tone, respectively. Continued inactivity also leads to atrophy, which is a decrease in size of the body structure, in this case, a muscle.

The woman who is going to have a baby, if taught how to adapt to her weight changes, is able to continue her routine activities more easily. If she understands how to use her muscles effectively during pregnancy, she also helps prepare herself for an easier labor and delivery.

A person who uses specific muscles routinely can plan exercises to involve other major muscles. Thus, the executive would generally find golf, tennis, or gardening helpful for maintaining leg and back muscle tone.

The nurse who understands how to help maintain musculoskeletal functioning is able to care for patients in such a way that their recovery may be speeded, their limitation from inactivity reduced to a minimum, and their convalescence shortened.

A first step in understanding body mechanics is to consider posture.

Good posture or good body alignment is that alignment of body parts which permits optimum musculoskeletal balance and operation and promotes good physiological functioning. Good posture is essential in all positions: standing, sitting, or lying down. M. C. Winters describes the body as being in good functional alignment when:

. . . the feet are at a right angle to the lower legs and face forward in the same direction as the patellae; the weight-bearing line passes through the center of the knee and in front of the ankle joints; the knees are extended but are not tense or hyperextended; the thighs are extended on the pelvis; the spine is elongated, and the physiologic curves are within normal limits; the chest is upward and forward and the head is erect.*

Figure 17–1 illustrates good posture. The term anterior means the front, while the back is called posterior. Lateral means to the side and medial means close to the middle or midline.

Posture in itself is a key point in body mechanics and should not be considered as merely the simple procedure of holding oneself erect. Good standing posture involves maintaining balance, which constitutes an effort even though we are not consciously aware of it. To balance the body and maintain good alignment in the standing position, and to engage in various activities such as lifting, stooping, pushing, and pulling, require more effort on the part of the body than sitting or lying. This everyone knows from experience, but probably few persons stop to analyze the reasons. There are forces which are present constantly and must be overcome. There are laws of physics which, if utilized properly, will help to reduce the effort expended in maintaining good posture and balance, and in lifting and moving.

Concepts most helpful to the understanding of body mechanics are those concerned with the effect of gravity on balance. Figure 17–2 illustrates balance.

The center of gravity of an object is the point at which

---

* Winters, Margaret Campbell. *Protective Body Mechanics in Daily Life and in Nursing: A Manual for Nurses and Their Co-workers.* W. B. Saunders Company, Philadelphia, 1952, 150p.

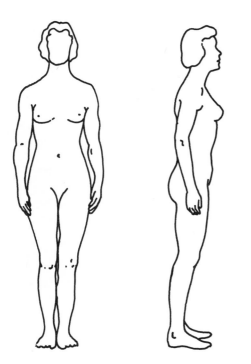

Figure 17-1 (Left) Anterior view of the body in good alignment. (Right) Lateral view of the body in good alignment.

its mass is centered. In humans, when standing, the center of gravity is located in the center of the pelvis approximately midway between the umbilicus and the symphysis pubis.

The *line of gravity* is a vertical line which passes through the center of gravity.

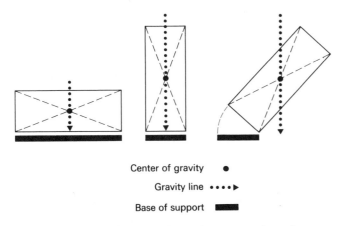

Center of gravity   ●

Gravity line   ● ● ● ▶

Base of support   ▬▬

Figure 17-2 The effect of the base of support and gravity on balance is shown. Left, the line of gravity passes through the wide base of support. This object is the most stable of the three. Center, the line of gravity also passes through the base of support, although the base is narrower. This object is less stable than the one on the left. Right, the line of gravity does not pass through the base of support. This object is unstable.

To understand further what is involved in the struggle to maintain balance and good posture, it is also necessary to know that there is an accelerating tendency of all bodies toward the center of the earth, called gravity (equal to the earth's attraction minus the centrifugal force arising from the rotation of the earth on its axis; equal to about 32.16 feet per second). This constant pull toward the earth's center is a phenomenon which nurses should understand, because it is a factor in innumerable nursing activities, such as the flow of fluids, drainage of body areas, and the stability of objects.

From the diagrams in Figure 17-2, three basic points can be made. An object is more stable if its center of gravity is close to its base of support, if the line of gravity goes through the base of support, and if the object has a wide base of support.

While these points are important when considering inanimate objects, they are equally important to humans. To demonstrate that these points have a direct relationship to stability, try standing with the feet close together and then begin to lean forward. As soon as the line of gravity is outside the base of support, you will place one foot forward in order to avoid falling. When standing, a person provides a base of support wide enough so that the line of gravity goes through the base, and he thereby stabilizes himself.

But the act of standing is not merely one of providing a base of support. Synergistic or cooperative muscle groups contract sufficiently to steady the joints, such as those formed by the head of the femur in the acetabulum of the hip and the knee joints, formed by the lower end of the femur and the upper end of the tibia. Usually, muscles work in groups, and synergistic action produces a smooth coordinated action.

An additional point developed from the three basic ones is that the stability of an object also depends on the height of the center of gravity and the size of the base of support. The wider the base of support and the lower the center of gravity, the greater is the stability of the object. For example, a can of evaporated milk requires little manipulation in order to stabilize it on a table; however, a candle, perhaps, could be made to balance itself, but in order to ensure its remaining erect it is necessary to provide a base of support for it.

In humans, as was mentioned, muscular effort is necessary to maintain the erect position. Therefore, the amount of effort required by the muscles is related directly to the height of the center of gravity and the size of the base of support. Thus, the ballet dancer, while on her toes, utilizes more effort to maintain herself erect than when she has her feet directly on the floor.

Posture when standing and lying, as well as exercise and maintenance of balance, are only initial phases of body mechanics. While there is concern if the body is not kept in good alignment and active, there is equal concern when the body is put to use. When motion of the body is extended to include activities, such as moving and lifting, there are additional factors which should be considered, since efficient use of the muscles will conserve energy and reduce the possibility of strain.

How to Use Muscles Effectively

One of the primary factors in efficient musculoskeletal activity is that the longest and the strongest appropriate muscles should be used to provide the energy needed. When muscles which cannot provide the best strength and support are forced into exertion, strain, injury, and fatigue frequently result. *Origin* is the name given to the less movable attachment of a skeletal muscle to a bone. *Insertion* is the name given to the more movable attachment of the muscle to the bone, in other words, the attachment to the bone that is being moved.

In addition to using the longest and the strongest muscles of the arms and legs properly, the muscles in the pelvic area must also be prepared for any vigorous activity. This preparation of the muscles to stabilize the pelvis, to support the abdomen, and to protect the body from strain is comprised of two activities: putting on the internal girdle and making a long midriff.

The internal girdle is made by contracting the (gluteal muscles) (buttocks) downward and the abdominal muscles upward. The internal girdle is helped further by making a long midriff. This is done by stretching the muscles in the waist. One has the feeling of standing up tall, and of trying to increase the length of the waistline. Figure 17–3 shows this posture. It is especially important that the muscles involved in the internal girdle and the long midriff assist the long strong muscles of the arms and the legs in activities such as lifting, moving, and carrying heavy objects. When lifting or carrying objects, the object should be held as close to the body as possible. If stretching or leaning causes the line of gravity to fall outside the base of support, more exertion is required to maintain one's balance. If the object is heavy, the added exertion can cause muscle injury. Figure 17–4 illustrates the proper and improper way to pick up an object.

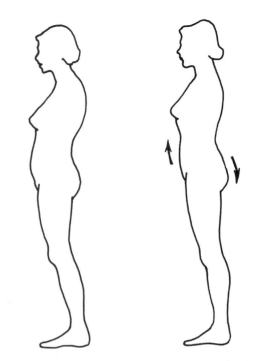

Figure 17–3   (Left) Slouch position, showing abdominal muscles relaxed and body out of good alignment. (Right) Internal girdle ''on.'' Abdominal muscles contracted, giving feeling of upward pull and gluteal muscles contracted, giving a downward pull.

Another factor in musculoskeletal physiology is that persistent exertion without adequate rest is harmful. Muscles must have alternate periods of rest and work. Therefore, activities should be conducted accordingly, especially if the task is a strenuous one.

Using the combination of the longest and strong-

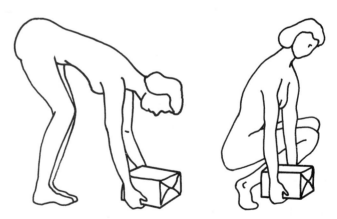

Figure 17–4   The figure on the left illustrates poor position for lifting since pull is exerted on the back muscles and leaning causes the line of gravity to fall outside the base of support. Good position for lifting is illustrated on the right, using the long and strong muscles of the arms and legs and holding the object so that the line of gravity falls within the base of support.

est muscles of the arms and the legs, the internal girdle, and the long midriff in lifting or moving heavy objects is as much a protective measure as it is an efficient use of muscles. Both the back and the abdominal wall are susceptible to injury. It will be recalled that the spinal column is composed of a series of irregularly shaped bones called vertebrae. These are separated from each other by cushions of cartilage or discs and held together by strong bands of connective tissue called ligaments. Viewed from the side, the vertebral column looks somewhat like a double S. It has a concave curve at the neck called the *cervical curve,* and a convex one at the chest, called the *thoracic curve.* Another concave curve, the *lumbar curve,* is located at the lower back. Then a convex curve, called the *sacral curve,* is located at the end of the spinal column. Muscles are attached to the vertebrae and permit flexion and extension as well as some lateral movement in certain areas.

When severe strain is placed on the muscles attached to the vertebrae and the force is transmitted to any one of the curves in the spinal column, injury can result. Many low-back or lumbar injuries are caused by such strain as lifting heavy objects incorrectly. The so-called whiplash injury occurring in the cervical area is a frequent result of an automobile accident in which the car is hit from the rear and the person's head is thrown backward suddenly and forcefully. Even in the course of everyday activities, strain and fatigue can be felt in the thoracic or the cervical regions if we sit with the head flexed forward for long periods when reading or writing. If our backs were absolutely straight many of these injuries would not occur, but then neither could we enjoy the degree of mobility that we have.

While the back is susceptible to injury because of its general structure and muscle groups, the abdominal wall also can be injured by improper use of muscle groups. Weakened musculature of the abdominal wall from decreased tone or from cutting muscle fibers as in surgery can contribute to making the back more susceptible to injury. Because the organs in the abdomen are not protected by any anterior or lateral bony cage, they rely on strong and supportive abdominal muscles. If they are not protected, the organs can cause a protrusion of the abdominal wall which in turn can result in an exaggeration of the lumbar curve (sometimes called swayback). Exaggerated back curves are sufficiently serious that they can cause some individuals to be excluded from occupations where lifting is required. Such people may also be prevented from engaging in some sports or other activities.

The abdominal wall has its own areas of inherent weakness which are subject to hernias. These areas are at the umbilicus and the inguinal canals which transmit the spermatic cords in the male and the round ligaments in the female, and at the femoral rings which transmit the femoral vessels to the legs. A hernia can occur in any of these areas if a strain imposed on the abdominal muscles exceeds the capability of the muscles at these points. Some persons having had abdominal surgery have suffered incisional hernias because of weak musculature and improper use of the muscles when lifting or moving heavy objects. Those who have hernias often describe the discomfort they experience when sneezing or coughing and their need to protect the area on such occasions by pressing their hands against it.

When practiced consistently, using the longest and the strongest muscles of the extremities and putting on the internal girdle and the long midriff can become almost an automatic act. Many nurses have saved themselves from injury by just such actions. It is not an infrequent occurrence in nursing to have a patient or a visitor feel faint and start to slide to the floor or to have a patient almost fall out of bed while reaching for something. The nurse must act instantly and put herself in the best protective position in order to avoid injury to herself as well. It could be disastrous for the nurse to attempt to hold someone up or for that matter to ease him down when in a position that is putting strain on her back or abdomen.

The nurse will need to teach many patients how activities can be done with greater ease and less fatigue. There is an efficient and safe way and a wrong way of performing such taken-for-granted acts as picking up a baby from a play pen, shoveling snow, raking leaves, skiing, dancing, lifting a turkey out of the oven, or unloading heavy objects from the trunk of a car.

Principles of Physics Which Guide Body Mechanics

Correct application of some basic laws of physics is essential for good body mechanics. If applied effectively, they will conserve energy, reduce the amount of effort exerted, and prevent injury. A few guidelines based on these laws are as follows:

- Use the longest and the strongest muscles of the arms and the legs to help provide the power needed in strenuous activities.

- Use the internal girdle and a long midriff to stabilize the pelvis and to protect the abdominal viscera when stooping, reaching, lifting, or pulling.

- Work as close as possible to an object which is to be lifted or moved. This brings the center of gravity of the body close to the center of gravity of the object being moved, thereby permitting most of the burden to be borne by the large muscles.
- Use the weight of the body as a force for pulling or pushing by rocking on the feet or leaning forward or backward. This reduces the amount of strain placed on the arms and the back.
- Slide, roll, push, or pull an object rather than lift it in order to reduce the energy needed to lift the weight against the pull of gravity.
- Use the weight of the body both to push an object by falling or rocking forward and to pull an object by falling or rocking backward.
- Place the feet apart in order to provide a wide base of support when increased stability of the body is necessary.
- Flex the knees, put on the internal girdle, and come down close to an object which is to be lifted.

Figure 17–5 shows how these guidelines can be used in sliding a patient to the edge of a bed.

The nurse can protect herself as well as demonstrate to others the proper way of using the musculoskeletal system if she consciously develops good habits of movement. The remainder of this chapter discusses additional ways of providing therapeutic physical activities for patients.

HELPING THE PATIENT TO MAINTAIN OR ATTAIN AN AMBULATORY STATUS

Fortunately for most patients, prolonged periods of bed rest are no longer considered necessary in most illnesses. The benefits of keeping persons up and about as much as possible are evident. A regular exercise routine in health, especially for the elderly whose activities have decreased, is important to maintain body functioning. Activity, even as mild as a stroll around the room, down the hall, from the bedroom to the living room, or out into the yard, is a protective measure for all body systems. It improves circulation and respiration, helps maintain muscle tonus, and promotes elimination from the urinary bladder and intestines. One only has to have a mild case of an upper respiratory infection and rest in bed for a day or two to emerge with "sea legs." Decreased activity because of age or disinterest can result in physiological as well as mental dysfunctions.

Most persons do not wish to stay in bed and so, no problem is presented. But many times, keeping some persons in bed does present a problem. Occasionally, some persons, especially elderly ones, will decrease their ambulatory activities. Many factors contribute to this, such as arthritis, aches, and stiffness. Some of their problems are in a sense self-induced by lack of exercise of certain joints and muscles over a long period. Since these persons are frequently at home, they and family

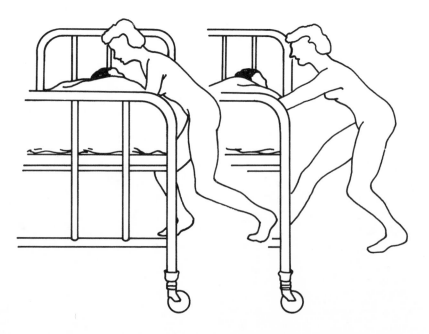

Figure 17–5 The figure on the left shows good position prior to sliding a patient to the edge of the bed: there is a wide base of support with one knee under the edge of the bed and both knees flexed; and arms are under the patient as far as possible while the person is close to the patient and leaning over him. On the right, the person is about to rock backward to use her own body weight to assist in moving the patient toward her.

members need to be encouraged to move about, take walks, climb stairs, do toe-heel exercises, and perform any other activity that helps keep them in condition to be on the move.

Patients who have surgery may need some encouragement to take that first walk the day of or following their surgery. Incisional discomfort, a running intravenous infusion, or fear of harming themselves act as deterrents. However, most patients understand that it is to their benefit to do so. Assistance in moving them and supporting them in their first efforts will make the process easier.

Physical Conditioning in Preparation for Ambulation

Patients who are not confined to bed for long periods and have good nights of sleep and possibly short periods of rest during the day may not require special considerations for increased physical activity. However, there are other patients who will have to be prepared for the day when ambulation is resumed. They may need to do conditioning exercises to maintain their muscle tone during extended periods of enforced inactivity, or they may need to strengthen weakened muscles before activity can be resumed. Even if they are active in bed, preparation for walking will have to be made for some persons who have not ambulated for a long time. Certain exercises that strengthen the overall efficiency of the musculoskeletal system can be done in bed.

Quadriceps Drills (Sets). One of the most important muscle groups used in walking is the quadriceps femoris. This muscle group helps to extend the leg on the thigh and flexes the thigh. In addition, it helps lift the legs as in stair climbing. The "sea legs" following even short periods of bed rest result from disuse of these muscles. To help to reduce weakness and make first attempts at walking easier, bed patients should be encouraged to contract this muscle group frequently. It is done by asking the patient to contract the muscles which pull the kneecap up toward the hips, during which the patient has the feeling that he is pushing the knee downward into the mattress and pulling the foot upward. This should be held to the count of four: 1-and-2-and-3-and-4. The exercise should not be done so that fatigue of the muscle group results. It is a very simple exercise that can be done two or three times hourly. Exercises like this, in which muscle tension occurs without a significant change in muscle length, are called *isometric exercises.*

Push-Ups or Sit-Ups. In preparation for getting out of bed, the muscle strength of the arms and the shoulders also may need to be improved. Exercises improve the strength needed to hold on to or get into a chair and to move about better. They are part of the preparation for all patients who must learn to walk on crutches.

A trapeze attached to the bed of a patient who has limited use of the lower part of his body helps him to move about in bed. However, this does not strengthen the triceps, which is the muscle group necessary for crutch-walking or moving from bed to chair. More suitable exercises are sit-ups or push-ups, frequently considered by some physical therapists to be two different types of exercises.

The exercise may be done by having the patient sit up in bed without support and then lift the hips up off the bed by pushing the hands down into the mattress. If the mattress is soft, it may be necessary to use blocks or books under the hands. The other form of the exercise is to have the patient lie face down on the bed. The arms are brought up so that the patient pushes his head and chest up off the bed by completely extending his elbows. This is repeated several times each time the exercise is done, and the exercise is repeated several times a day. Some patients find the latter method more difficult to do.

Daily Activities for Purposeful Exercise. In addition to specific exercises, many other activities can be carried out with benefit to the patient. These include placing the bedside stand so that the patient must use shoulder and arm muscles to reach what he needs instead of placing it so as to require little effort to take things from it; placing the signal cord so that the patient must engage in either arm or shoulder action in order to reach it; encouraging the patient to sit up and reach for the overbed table, to pull it close to him, and then to push it back in place; encouraging a patient to try to wash his back; and having him put on his socks while still in bed. There are innumerable ways in which patients can be helped to exercise, and when they understand the purpose, they very often adopt other exercises for themselves.

Preparing the Patient to Get Out of Bed

In addition to the attention given to the patient's physical state, the nurse is concerned with the necessary items needed, such as a chair or a wheelchair when the patient first gets out of bed. If the patient is going to stand or to walk about, a walker or crutches may be necessary. Positioning of the chair may be important to conserve the patient's energy. If the patient is to move from the bed to the chair without walking, the chair should be positioned parallel to the bed. If the patient is to ambulate, the chair can be positioned an appropriate distance from the bed. The type of chair varies with the patient, but generally patients who are having difficulty moving find a supportive straight chair easier to get into and out of than a soft upholstered chair.

If the patient is going to walk, it is best for him to wear shoes or supportive slippers. Having to walk with loose slippers or with shoes that have little support adds to the difficulty of ambulation if there is any physical limitation. This applies to all patients, whether young or old and whether sick for a long or a short time.

While it is not possible to set the exact manner in which any one patient should be dressed when out of bed, several points should be mentioned. The amount and the type of clothing worn by the patient will depend on the temperature and the air movement in the environment. It is the nurse's responsibility to protect the patient from discomfort due to overdressing and against the danger of becoming chilled because of insufficient clothing. Changes in the physical state as a result of illness usually make patients more susceptible to environmental factors such as drafts. Patients who may be permitted to sit outdoors on porches or patios may need to be given some sort of head covering. For most patients, it is usually better for their morale if they can be dressed in street clothes. Agencies for the chronically ill make every effort to reduce the association with illness by having their patients dress in clothing other than that which is worn in bed. The same should be true at home and in hospitals when possible.

Assisting the Patient Out of Bed

If a patient has sufficient strength to stand and to support his own weight, getting him out of bed is a relatively simple matter. However, during the time that the patient is being assisted out of bed, he should be observed for signs of faintness and difficulty in breathing. It is not uncommon for patients to become faint due to a fall in blood pressure. A decrease in blood pressure associated with assuming an upright position is called *orthostatic hypotension*. It is best to assist the patient to the sitting position slowly and to provide a short period of rest between each movement. Taking the pulse is a good way to determine the patient's reaction to the activity. His usual pulse rate and its quality are used as

norms. If the pulse rate is more rapid or irregular than usual, proceed with caution.

If the patient is too weak to walk, the preparation of the chair should precede the preparation of the patient. If a wheelchair is used, the wheels should be locked. If this is not possible, it should be placed against the wall or held in place by another person.

The patient is brought to the side of the bed and assisted to the sitting position. The head of the bed should be elevated to help support him in this position. As soon as the patient feels comfortable, the nurse supports his shoulders and legs and pivots him around so that his legs and feet are over the side of the bed. If the bed is not low enough so that his feet rest on the floor, the feet can be placed on a chair or footstool so that he can support his body and so that pressure against the posterior thigh is reduced. If the feet are not supported, the patient may not feel comfortable, and there is always danger of his sliding off the bed. This position is frequently used preparatory to ambulation and is called *dangling*.

While the patient is sitting on the edge of the bed, it is easy to dress him in his robe and to put on his shoes. A footstool should be provided for stepping down if the patient's feet do not touch the floor.

When helping the patient out of bed, the nurse stands directly in front of the patient. The patient places his hand on the nurse's shoulders. The nurse places her hands in the patient's axillary region with thumbs pointing upward. In this position, she is able to support the patient's shoulders should he begin to fall. If the nurse's hands are held against the chest instead of up in the axillary region as described, she would need to press the patient's chest tightly if he were to fall. This would be extremely uncomfortable for the patient. As the patient pushes himself to a standing position with his legs, the nurse assists by lifting the upper part of his body.

The patient is permitted to stand for a few seconds to make certain that he is not feeling faint. The nurse continues to face the patient and pivots him around so that his back is toward the chair. Then she lowers the patient to the edge of the chair first. While doing this, the nurse should have one foot forward and the knees flexed and again come down with the patient. She may even wish to brace her knees against the patient's knees for added leverage as she lowers him into the chair. Next she assists the patient to sit well back in the chair and adjusts the foot rests if it is a wheelchair. Figure 17–6 illustrates assisting a patient out of bed.

If a high-low bed is used, the nurse may wish to

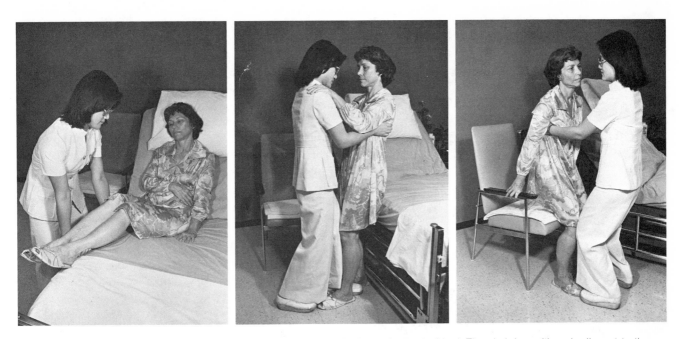

Figure 17–6   In the photo on the left, the nurse is preparing to assist the patient out of bed. The chair is positioned adjacent to the bed, the head of the bed has been elevated, and the patient's feet and legs are being moved over the edge of the bed. In the photo in the middle, the nurse has helped the patient to stand. She has positioned her hands under the axillary area for support in case the patient should become weak. Her feet are positioned to prevent the patient's feet from slipping. The nurse is now ready to pivot the patient to the chair. In the photo on the right, the nurse is easing the patient down into the chair. Note that the nurse's knees are bent and her back is straight to prevent strain on her back. Her feet are positioned to prevent the patient's feet from slipping.

prepare the patient and permit him to dangle his legs while the bed is in the high position. This creates less strain on her arms, and she is in a better position to support the patient. When the patient is ready to stand, the low position would eliminate the need of a footstool. However, if the patient is very weak, the nurse is in a better position to support him and to use her long and strong arm and leg muscles, if she does not lower the bed and follows the procedure described above.

Assisting the Patient to Walk

Many patients who have been confined to bed for a long time find that they must almost learn to walk all over again. An activity which needed no special teaching or encouragement in childhood now becomes a real challenge. Often, it is the nurse who plays a major role in the patient's recovery and mental outlook, his hope and faith, especially when he must stick to a rigid and often difficult schedule of reeducating muscle groups. Physicians have said that a patient able to raise his leg only 2.5 cm. or 1 inch from the bed possesses sufficient power to permit walking.

When a major problem of muscle reeducation pre-

sents itself, the patient will need the assistance of experts in physical medicine. However, nurses assist patients out of bed and help them to walk when a physical therapist is not present. There are several aspects to this problem of ambulation with which the nurse should be familiar.

Walking.   The normal pattern of walking is to move alternate arms and legs. For example, the right arm and the left leg move forward, and then the left arm and the right leg move forward. If a patient is able to be supported from the rear at the waist while he practices these movements and has no real limitations to the muscle groups of the hips, the legs, and the feet, he will soon be walking well again. A walking belt with handles for the assistant's hands is often worn by the patient for this purpose.

If the patient is quite weak and is reluctant to try to stand with support only at the waist, it may be necessary to support him under the arm until he feels that he is able to try the other method. A patient who seems to be very weak can be assisted to regain a sense of balance and stability by supporting himself with a walker or the backs of two chairs. Figure 17–7 shows a patient

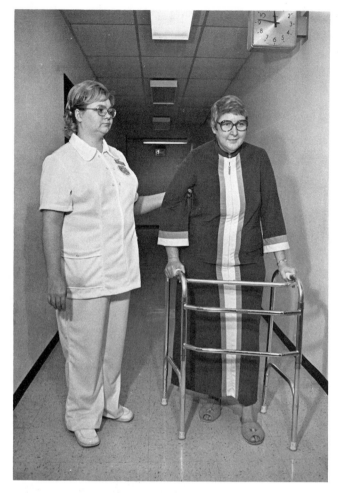

Figure 17–7   The nurse is encouraging this patient in learning to use a walker for support.

using a walker. Then when the patient walks, if he needs some additional support for a while, the nurse should walk alongside him, keeping her arm which is near the patient under his arm in an arm-in-arm position. The advantage of this position is that, if the patient begins to feel faint, the nurse's arm is in a position to slide up into the patient's axilla. The nurse throws one foot out to the side to make a wide base of support and rests the patient on her hip. Figure 17–8 shows a nurse helping a patient to walk.

To assist patients in the retraining process of walking, there are a number of supportive measures available. Patients may use canes, walkers, or crutches, or the supportive bars often found on health agency corridor walls. Some persons find pushing a straight-backed chair in front of them provides good support and a place to rest if they tire.

Crutch-Walking

Sometimes, it is necessary for patients to use crutches for a time in order to avoid using one leg or to help strengthen one or both legs. This procedure is taught best by a physical therapist; however, there are numerous instances when the nurse is called on to measure patients for crutches and to teach them to use the crutches. Even if a patient is being taught to crutch-walk by a physical therapist, it is necessary for the nurse to understand the patient's progress and the gait he is being taught. The nurse must often guide the patient at home or in the hospital after the initial teaching is completed.

There are several ways by which axillary crutches can be measured, but the two methods described here are considered satisfactory. These are done when the pa-

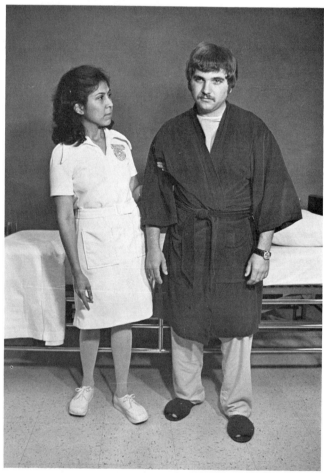

Figure 17–8   This nurse is supporting the patient during his first attempt to walk after surgery.

tient is in bed. One way is to measure from the anterior fold of the axilla straight down to the heel and then add 5 cm. (2 inches). The other way is to measure from the anterior fold of the axilla diagonally out to a point 15 cm. or 6 inches away from the heel. The patient should be measured in the shoes he will be wearing as he learns to walk. The measurement to the crutches includes the axillary pads and the crutch tips at the bottom. Then the crutches will need to be adjusted for the location of the handgrip according to the height of the patient. This may be done when the patient is in the upright position. The handgrip should be placed so that the elbows are slightly flexed while the patient is using them. The elbows should not be extended and the wrists should be hyperextended. *Flexion* is the state of being bent. *Extension* is the state of being in a straight line. *Hyperextension* is a state of exaggerated extension. It often results in an angle greater than 180°. A correct length of crutches and proper placement of the handgrips is important to prevent damage to the radial nerve in the axilla and to provide well-balanced support.

Gaits. Essentially, there are three gaits: four-point, three-point, and two-point. There is also a swing-through gait which is used by some patients when they become more accustomed to the crutches and wish to get about quickly and by patients who have had a leg amputated. The swing-through gait, however, does not simulate normal walking and extended use will lead to atrophy of the muscles of the lower extremities.

Four-Point Gait. Weight-bearing is permitted on both feet, and the pattern is as follows: right crutch, left foot, left crutch, right foot. It is the normal reciprocal walking pattern.

Two-Point Gait. Weight-bearing is permitted on both feet and the pattern is a speedup of the four-point gait: right crutch and left foot forward at the same time, left crutch and right foot forward at the same time.

Three-Point Gait. Weight-bearing is permitted on only one foot. The other leg cannot support, but it acts as a balance in the process. It is used also when partial weight-bearing is allowed on the affected extremity. The pattern is as follows: both crutches and the nonsupportive leg go forward, and then the good leg comes through. The crutches are brought forward immediately, and the pattern is repeated. Figures 17–9

through 17–11 on pages 382–383 show a patient crutch-walking while using various gaits.

Exercises Preparatory to Crutch-Walking. Before the patient is asked to use the crutches, several exercise drills will help him to be more confident and skillful. The patient must begin by strengthening the arm and the shoulder muscles. The sit-up exercise described earlier is most helpful. The muscles of the hand must also be strengthened. Squeezing a rubber ball 50 times a day by flexing and extending the fingers helps to do this.

The patient should be assisted into a chair which is close to the wall. Then he should be helped to stand against the wall and the crutches placed in his hands. Next, standing slightly away from the wall, he should sway on the crutches from side to side. This accustoms the hands and the arms to weight-bearing.

After this, he should be asked to lean against the wall and pick one crutch up about 15 cm. (6 inches) from the floor and then place it down. This should be repeated with the other crutch and the whole exercise done six to eight times. Then, still leaning against the wall, he should be asked to pick up both crutches from the floor and place them down. This too should be repeated several times.

After these exercises, it will be possible to judge the patient's ability to hold and manage the crutches without the added concern for movement. If the patient is judged capable, he proceeds to the practice of a gait. If possible, it is recommended that he begin with the four-point gait.

The patient's posture with the crutches should be guided by the physics principles described previously. The line of gravity should go through the base of support, and the base of support should be wide. The crutches should be placed about 10 cm. or 4 inches in front and about the same distance at the sides of the feet for best balance.

Patients using crutches with the axillary support should be cautioned about exerting pressure against the axillae. When patients begin to use crutches, they should be taught that the support should come primarily from the arms and the hands. The crutches should not be forced into the axillae each time the body is moved forward.

There are crutches available which have no axillary support. A supportive frame extends beyond the handgrip for the lower arm to help guide the crutch. Such crutches are more likely to be used by patients who have permanent limitations and will always need crutch assistance for ambulation.

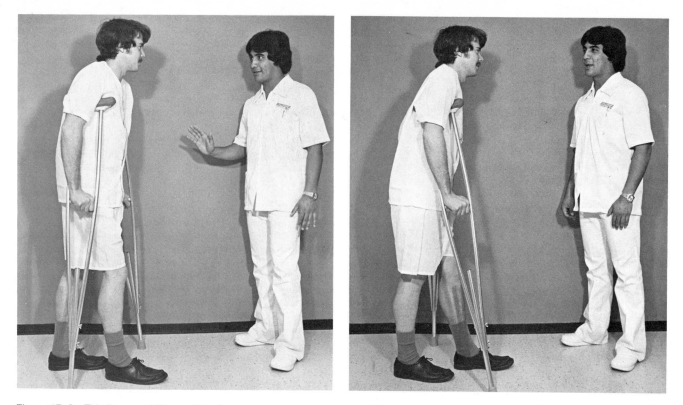

Figure 17–9 This figure and Figures 17–10 and 17–11 demonstrate crutch-walking gaits. Note that the patient wears sturdy, nonskid shoes for practicing with crutches. This figure demonstrates the four-point gait when some weight-bearing is permitted on both feet. In the photo on the left, the right foot and the left crutch are moved forward together and then, the left foot and right crutch are moved forward together, as shown in the photo on the right.

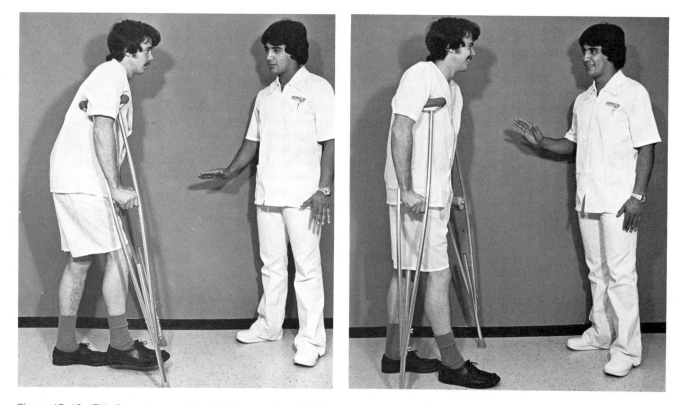

Figure 17–10 This figure demonstrates the three-point gait. Weight-bearing is permitted on one foot only. On the left, the right foot, which cannot bear weight, and both crutches are moved forward while the weight is borne by the left foot. Then, as shown in the photo on the right, the left foot is moved forward while weight is borne on the crutches with the right foot providing balance only.

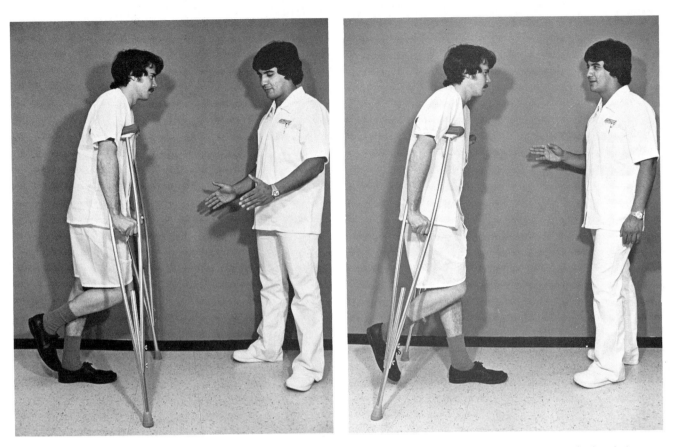

Figure 17–11 These photos demonstrate the swing-through gait. In this instance, the right foot can bear no weight. In the photo on the left, weight is borne by the left foot while the crutches are moved forward. Then, both legs are swung between the crutches and, as the photo on the right shows, the left foot again takes over weight-bearing.

GENERAL PRINCIPLES OF AND INTERVENTION MEASURES FOR THE PATIENT CONFINED TO BED

One of the greatest challenges in nursing is the care of the patient confined to bed, especially when the patient's illness renders him immobile also. He is dependent on others to do for him what he cannot do for himself and to help keep him in the best possible physiological and psychological state. It is essential that persons caring for helpless patients be aware of and use principles of body mechanics to protect themselves. One person can generally manage a helpless patient safely and easily if knowledge of body mechanics is put to use.

The Dangers of Bed Rest

Prolonged bed rest can have detrimental effects on well-being. As was mentioned earlier, keeping the patient as active as his physical condition allows is a goal in the care of any patient. Being able to walk about is of great psychological value. Therefore, when a person must be confined to bed, it can be expected that this will affect his behavior. Immobility usually restricts the patient's variety of sensory stimuli and may expose him to new and unpleasant stimuli. Being confined to bed also generally means a role change for the patient and may also have a detrimental effect on his self-concept and body image.

The physiological damage that can result from prolonged bed rest is also significant. Some effects on the musculoskeletal system have already been mentioned. For example, loss of muscle tone and resulting muscle weakness, difficulty in walking, and contractures that limit joint motion are common. In addition, bone demineralization can occur which results in discomfort and brittleness of the bones with consequent ease of fracturing.

Circulatory dysfunction often occurs following long

confinement in bed. The circulation becomes sluggish since blood tends to pool, especially in the lower part of the body. Thrombi, or blood clots, form more easily and the heart is placed under strain. Decubitus ulcers may result from impaired circulation and pressure from maintaining the same position.

Pulmonary secretions tend to pool in the lungs of the person whose activities are limited. The respiratory movements are generally decreased also. These two conditions tend to result in a disturbance of gas exchanges in the lung and in tissue cells. The pooled secretions also predispose the patient to pulmonary infections.

Prolonged bed rest influences elimination from the urinary and intestinal tracts. The retention of urine is common. Urinary tract infections and stones occur with frequency in these patients. Constipation is common in bedfast patients because their appetite and food intake are ordinarily decreased and bowel elimination is difficult while lying in bed.

Electrolyte disturbances can also occur in the immobilized patient since bone demineralization, cellular metabolic changes, and alterations in hormone productions can cause fluid imbalances. Fluid balance will be discussed in Chapter 23.

These are some of the physiological effects of prolonged bed rest. Clinical texts describe them and their treatment in more detail. The preferred treatment is to prevent them. For this reason, every effort should be made to limit the amount of time a patient is confined to bed. When bed rest is necessary, nursing care is initiated to help keep the patient as active as possible.

Even persons who are not confined to bed for long periods can lose muscle tone and coordination so that simple activities of dressing, bathing, eating, and moving are difficult. While the limitations may be temporary, they frequently need not occur if the nurse or family members take adequate precautions. The nurse needs to initiate preventive measures from the beginning of bed confinement.

Nurses need to encourage the patient to engage in routine activities of daily living (sometimes abbreviated ADL) to the extent he is capable. For the bedfast patient, these include such activities as sitting up in bed without assistance, rolling over from side to side while in bed, brushing the teeth, combing the hair, cutting meat into small pieces, lifting a cupful of liquid, buttoning a shirt button, and so on.

Bed rest can have many different interpretations. It is important that the degree of limitation be clearly understood by the nurse as well as by the patient and his family. The term bed rest may mean absolute inactivity, which means feeding, bathing, toileting, and turning the patient. It may mean that the patient is restricted to bed but he may feed and bathe himself. Or, it may mean that he is to remain in bed at all times except for elimination when he may use the bathroom. An exact understanding of the patient's activity limitations is needed to plan nursing care.

Terms Related to Body Positions

Some terms have been defined earlier. The following additional ones are commonly used when describing body positions.

Abduction is lateral movement of a body part away from the midline of the body, such as when the arm is lifted perpendicularly from the trunk. *Adduction* is the movement of a body part toward the midline of the body, such as when lowering the outstretched arm to a resting position alongside of the body.

Prone is the face downward recumbent position or the position in which the hands are held with the palms downward or backward. *Supine* means a back-lying recumbent position or the position in which the palms of the hands are held upward or forward.

Rotation is the turning on an axis, in this case, the turning of a body part on the axis provided by its joint. *Internal rotation* is a body part turning on its axis toward the midline. Internal rotation occurs when the leg turns inward at the hip joint, resulting in the foot being pointed across the body instead of aligned with the midline. *External rotation* is a body part turning on its axis away from the midline. The leg turned outward at the hip joint so that the foot points away from the body is an example of external rotation. Figure 17–12 shows internal and external rotation of the leg.

Devices for the Safety and Comfort of the Patient

Resting in bed usually is comfortable if the body is held or supported in a restful position. Merely being in a horizontal position does not ensure rest. It is as important to be in good alignment and posture when lying down as it is when standing or sitting. To sit with the knees crossed may be comfortable for a short while, but it soon becomes uncomfortable and fatiguing. Having the knees crossed while sitting is not too different from having one leg adducted and rotated inward while lying on the side. It is only when the body is supported properly and the position changed frequently enough to rest certain muscle groups and utilize others that rest in bed can serve its best purpose.

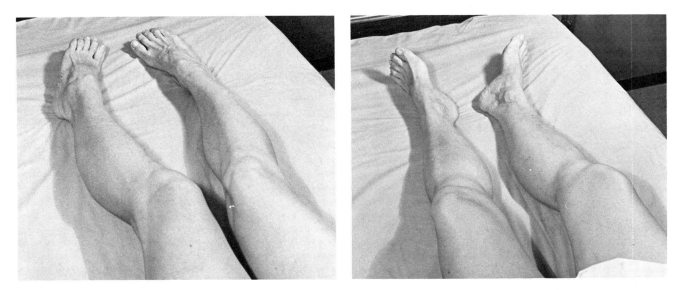

Figure 17-12   Leg rotation occurs as a result of gravity when the legs are not adequately supported. For patients who are bedfast for long periods of time, uncorrected rotation can result in serious complications. The photo on the left demonstrates internal rotation of the legs. The photo on the right demonstrates external rotation of the legs.

Modern adjustable beds used in homes and in health agencies make it possible to adjust the patient's position and still provide adequate support. Both electric and manually operated beds facilitate positioning and movement.

There are many devices which help to maintain good body alignment and muscle tonus in bed and to alleviate discomfort or pressure on various parts of the body.

Pillows.   Pillows are used primarily to provide support or to provide elevation of a part. Variety in sizes of pillows increases their usefulness. Pillows intended for the head are usually full- or large-sized pillows. Small pillows are ideal for support or elevation of the extremities, shoulders, or incisional wounds. Specially designed heavy pillows are useful to elevate the upper part of the body when an adjustable bed is not available, as in a home situation.

Mattress.   For a mattress to be comfortable and supportive, it must be firm but have sufficient "give" to permit good body alignment. Figure 17-13 on page 386 shows the effect of a supportive and a nonsupportive mattress on body alignment. If a patient were to remain in a bed, such as the one shown at the bottom of Figure 17-13, he might very well complain of backache and other discomforts.

A well-made and well-supported foam-rubber mattress retains a uniform firmness and therefore helps to protect the patient. These mattresses are made of natural or synthetic rubber, or both in combination. A large volume of air is incorporated. The foam-rubber mattress conforms to the contours of the body and supplies support at all points. Its greatest advantage is that it does not form slopes and valleys as the innerspring mattresses are likely to do. Nor does the foam rubber mattress create as much pressure against bony prominences, such as the ankles, the elbows, the scapulae, and the coccyx.

Bed Board.   If the mattress does not provide sufficient support, a bed board may help to keep the patient in better alignment. Bed boards usually are made of plywood or some other firm composition. The size varies with the needs of the situation. If sections of the bed can be raised, such as the head and the foot of a hospital bed, it may be necessary to have the board divided and held together with hinges. For home use, full bed boards are available commercially or can easily be made at home from available materials.

High-Low Tilt Bed.   Another useful device is the bed which can have its height as well as total angle adjusted. The value of having an adjustable-height bed has been discussed earlier. These beds also permit the angle to be changed so that the head is higher than the feet, or vice versa. Such beds are extremely helpful for patients forced to lie flat. They have several advantages, one of which is the fact that when the head is up the

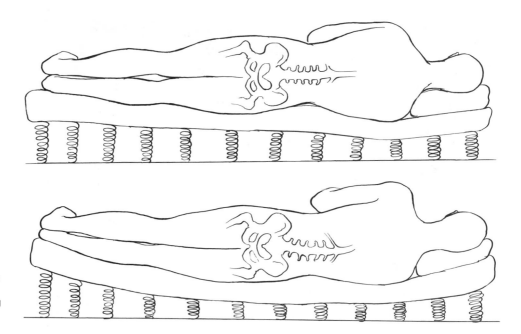

Figure 17-13 These sketches illustrate the effects of a good and a poor mattress and spring on body alignment.

patient is able to see about him without flexion of the neck. Also, the patient is assisted to a more nearly vertical position without the effort of standing. The shift in the position of the abdominal organs and the alteration in the circulation in the extremities and other body areas help to prevent complications and prepare for the day when weight-bearing and standing will begin. The upright position also provides proprioceptor stimulation when weight is borne against the feet.

Rocking Bed.   The rocking bed, while used primarily in the care of patients with vascular or respiratory diseases, is also of great value in the care of other immobile patients. This bed is mounted on a frame rather than the usual bedstead. By means of a motor, the bed can be made to rock rhythmically up and down in seesaw fashion. There is a foot rest on the bed to help keep the patient from sliding and also to help to keep the feet in good alignment. If the patient is in a moderate sitting position there is little danger of his sliding. The bed is adjusted to rock at the frequency of the patient's respirations. The rocking aids respiration by shifting the abdominal viscera, which in turn helps to move the diaphragm up and down helping air to be forced out and into the lungs.

Also, the constant changing of position aids the flow of blood. The rocking bed operates on the same principle as does the tilt bed. In some vascular diseases, it is helpful if venous circulation is assisted during the time the patient must be confined to bed.

Other patients, because of their inactive state, also need some measure to assist or improve circulation. It will be recalled that venous blood is assisted in its return to the heart by the contraction of muscle groups in the legs. Pressure against the veins helps to move the blood along its course. If activity is at a minimum, elevation of the extremities is helpful in that the position aids the blood in its return flow.

Chair Bed.   Another type of bed used in the care of patients requiring bed rest is one that can be placed into a chair position. These beds were designed primarily for the patient who has a heart ailment. In some instances, they are called cardiac beds. They permit the patient to be in a semisitting position which may aid the patient's cardiac output.

Circular Bed.   The electric circular bed is a 6 or 7 foot metal frame with a diameter support for the patient. The direction of the support can be changed so the patient can be placed in a variety of positions, including supine, prone, and vertical. This bed is especially useful for the patient who will be completely helpless for an extended period.

Stryker Frame.   The Stryker frame is a narrow support for a patient which can be turned 360°. The patient can be alternated between the supine and prone positions without changing his alignment. This bed also is particularly useful for the totally immobilized patient.

Rubber Air Rings, Cushion Rings, and Doughnuts. Inflated rubber rings, cushion rings, and handmade doughnuts for relieving pressure on bony prominences by lifting them from the mattress surface, have been used extensively in the past. Their disadvantage lies in the fact that, in protecting one area, they create pressure in immediately surrounding areas. This pressure, in turn, impairs circulation to the area of most concern and thus reduces the supply of oxygen and nutrients.

There are more effective means of relieving pressure on bony prominences and protecting the patient from developing pressure sores. A piece of sponge rubber large enough to be supportive placed adjacent to the pressure point so that it fills the space and thus reduces some of the pressure is effective. Small pillows are also helpful in elevating an area such as the heels, so that the pressure is reduced. Pieces of synthetic sheepskin are useful and protective.

Rubber or plastic air rings have some value for patients who are having sitz baths following rectal and perineal surgery. In such instances, they provide comfort for the brief period when the patient must sit in the tub. They are not recommended as a device for the prevention of a bedsore on a patient's coccygeal area.

Footboards. The footboard place at the foot of the mattress and perpendicular to it is used to keep the patient's feet in the position of dorsal flexion. In the normal anatomical position, the feet are at right angles to the legs. The footboard also provides a firm surface against which the feet of the bedfast patient can be placed for proprioceptor stimulation. In addition, if the footboard is of sufficient height, it can keep the upper bed linen from pressing on the toes and forcing the foot into a dropped position.

Commercial footboards, such as the one pictured in Figure 17–14, are available. They are generally adjustable for patients of different heights.

Footboards can be made easily from a sturdy box, carton, or wooden block. If a footboard that cannot be adjusted is used, care must be taken to see to it that it is the proper size for the patient. The footboard must come far enough up from the foot of the bed so that the patient's feet rest firmly against it without his sliding down in bed. Also, the footboard should not be so far from the foot of the bed that the patient's knees are flexed when his feet are against the footboard. Figure 17–15 shows a footboard being used in a home setting.

If a footboard is not readily available or if it is not suitable for the patient, an improvised foot support can

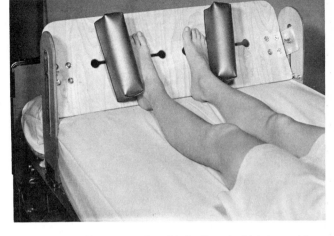

Figure 17–14 This is an adjustable footboard which is used to keep the patient's feet in dorsal flexion. (J. T. Posey Company, Arcadia, California)

be made from a pillow and a large sheet. The pillow is rolled in the sheet, and the ends of the sheet are twisted before being tucked under the mattress. The ends should be tucked under the mattress at an angle toward the head of the bed to help to keep the pillow in place. A pillow foot support does not provide the firmness of a carton, a box, or the foot block, nor does it assist in

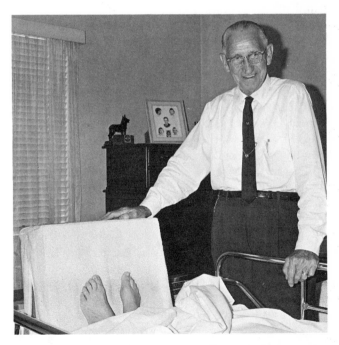

Figure 17–15 This man prepared a footboard for his wife and is obviously very pleased with the results, since they met with the approval of the visiting nurse.

stimulating proprioceptor senses, muscle contractions, and circulation; but it will suffice for a short while until a better support can be obtained.

If the patient is in a sitting position while in bed, the footboard must be placed at an angle. This is to prevent hyperextension of the knees which would result if the feet were kept in dorsiflexion while the trunk was flexed forward.

Cradle. If pressure of the top bedding is a problem, or if the top bedding must be kept off the patient's lower extremities, a device called a cradle is used. A cradle is usually a metal frame which supports the bed linens away from the patient while providing him with privacy and warmth. Some cradles are equipped with light bulbs which provide extra heat. There are any number of sizes and shapes of cradles. If used, the cradle should be fastened securely to the bed so that it does not slide or fall on the patient.

Sandbags. Some patients need to have an area of the body held in position by a firm supportive device. For example, the patient may have a tendency to rotate his leg outward. In order to prevent his lying in this position for extended periods of time, the leg can be held in good alignment by placing sandbags alongside the outer surface of the leg from the hip to the knee. Sandbags have numerous uses and their value is enhanced if they are available in various sizes. When properly filled, they are not hard or firmly packed. They should be pliable enough to be shaped to body contours and to give support. They should be placed so they do not create pressure on a bony prominence.

Trochanter Rolls. If sandbags are not available to help prevent a patient's legs from external rotation, it is possible to improvise a support that will serve the same purpose. Fold a sheet lengthwise and place the narrow dimension under the patient so that it extends from his waist to his knees. A large, bulky piece of linen should not be used because of the discomfort it will cause to the patient's back. Under each end of the sheet, which extends on either side of the patient, place a rolled bath blanket or two bath towels. Roll the sheet around the blanket so that the roll is under. In this way, it cannot unroll itself, and the weight of the patient helps to hold it secure. When the trochanter roll is in place properly, the patient will be lying on a piece of linen which has a large roll on either side of it. Fix these rolls close to the patient and tightly against the hip and the thigh so that the femur does not rotate outward. If the roll is not sufficiently long, very little support can be expected. Pillows properly placed can also serve as trochanter rolls.

Hand Rolls. If patients are paralyzed or unconscious, it may be necessary to provide a means for keeping the thumb in the correct position, namely, slightly adducted and in apposition to the fingers. To do this for short periods, any number of improvisations can be made. A rubber ball of the appropriate size, sponge rubber, or a folded washcloth may be used. However, if the hands are going to need protective support for many days or weeks, securing a commercial plastic or aluminum splint may be considered. In this way, the thumb is held in place no matter what position the hand is in. Patients who are not moving their fingers should be encouraged to do finger exercises with special attention to having the thumb touch the tips of each finger.

Bed Siderails. One of the greatest safety concerns of nursing personnel is to prevent patients from falling out of bed. Health agency accident reports show a high proportion of such events; hence, in many agencies, it is routine to use extra protection on the beds of unconscious and disoriented patients and on the beds of elderly patients. The term "bedrails" and "siderails" are synonyms for the term "bed siderails."

There is no question that the presence of siderails often has an unfortunate psychological effect on rational and oriented patients and on their families. Therefore, the use of them requires explanation beyond passing it off as "routine." The patient should be helped to understand how the siderails offer protection if he is weak, or receiving certain drugs and cannot prevent himself from falling, should he roll to the edge of the bed. They also help to remind him that he is not in his usual environment, should he awaken during the night and wish to get out of bed.

Bed siderails, even if they are the full length of the mattress, may not deter some patients from getting out of bed. Many a patient has crawled over the foot of the bed. In fact, some authorities recommend siderails that are not the length of the mattress. Then, if the patient does attempt to get out of bed, he does not have to climb over the siderail or the foot of the bed and further increase the danger of falling.

As mentioned in Chapter 12, bed siderails are used for the patient's safety, but they also have value for many weakened patients. For example, siderails make it possible for the patient to roll himself from one side to the other or even to sit up without calling for assistance. This in itself is a very good activity which helps the patient to retain or regain muscle efficiency.

The adjustable-height bed seems to be one answer for certain types of patients such as the ambulatory elderly patient. The bed can remain at the lowest height so that when the patient brings his feet over the side of the bed, he is able to place them directly on the floor. He is then safer and more stable. If, on the other hand, his feet must dangle from a higher height as from an older hospital bed, he may slide off the edge, lose his balance, and fall to the floor. Many nurses note that the incidence of hospital falls when the bed is lowered to the usual height of the home bed is greatly decreased.

Trapeze Bar. A *trapeze bar* is a handgrip suspended from a frame near the head of the bed. The patient can grasp the bar with one or both hands and then raise his trunk from the bed. The trapeze makes moving and turning considerably easier for many patients. It can also be used to perform exercises which strengthen some muscles of the upper extremities. The patient in Figures 17–34, 17–35, and 17–36 on page 404 is using a trapeze bar to help the nurse get her out of bed.

Restraints. Restraints are physical devices used to limit bodily movement. They can be used to restrict the movement of an extremity when an infusion is running. They also are helpful to prevent patients who are not voluntarily able to cooperate from pulling at wound dressings and tubings leading from the body and to prevent patients who are unsteady and in danger of falling when trying to get out of bed or up from a chair. There are numerous types of restraints available commercially. They can also be fashioned from a sufficient length of any sturdy cloth. Figures 12–3 and 12–4 illustrate on page 230 two types of restraints.

When using restraints, it is important to remember that care should be taken when limiting a patient's movements to prevent impediment of circulation or respirations and irritation to the skin. Confining movement to a safe area may be necessary, but restriction of all movement can be detrimental.

It is also important to convey to the patient and his family the reason for the application of the restraint by explaining that it is a protective device for the patient and not a punishment measure. Some patients find it helpful to consider the restraint as a reminder to limit their movements. There are some patients who become so fearful and agitated by the use of restraints that the stress induced by their presence is felt to be more detrimental than the movement. The frightened patient will often relax and become more comfortable if someone stays and calms him. Quiet talking to even the patient who appears to be unaware of his surroundings will generally have a soothing effect. Under no circumstance should the use of restraints be looked upon as alleviating the nurse's responsibility to observe the patient. Frequent observation of the restrained patient is important to ensure that the restraints are properly positioned.

Protective Positions for the Patient

Varying positioning helps to stimulate physiological functioning and provides rest. The dangers of bed rest which were discussed earlier may be prevented by frequent and careful changes in position.

Positioning which maintains body alignment and facilitates physiological functioning contributes to physical well-being. The protective side-lying, back-lying or supine, and face-lying or prone positions are intended to help maintain good body alignment. The Fowler's or semisitting position can provide variety for the patient. These positions also promote normal physiological functions. To place the patient in any of these positions, it is essential to understand the position of body parts when in good posture. For a person in the standing position, the feet are perpendicular to the legs; the knees are in a slight degree of flexion of 5° to 10°; the patellae face forward; the hips are straight; the arms are alongside of the body with the forearms slightly adducted toward the body; the hands are pronated; the thumbs are adducted into the hands; the fingers are in the grasp position; and the head is held erect on the shoulders so that vision is horizontal with the floor. For the person in a recumbent position, necessary variations are made.

The force of gravity pulls parts of the body out of alignment unless the patient consciously resists the force or unless adequate support is provided. The continued muscle tension which results from poorly aligned body parts contributes to fatigue and loss of tone in the involved muscles. Adequate support counterbalances the pull of gravity. Pillows, sandbags, footboards, and other devices can be used to counteract the force of gravity. It is especially important to provide sufficient support for the extremities of immobilized patients. By providing adequate support, many complications can be prevented and the patient's comfort can be enhanced.

The Protective Supine Position. In the supine position, two areas of the body are in need of particular attention. They are the feet and the neck. However, if the patient is unable to move, all areas of the body require attention.

The greatest danger to the feet occurs when they are not supported in the dorsal flexion position. The toes drop downward, and the feet are in plantar flexion. Because of the pull of gravity, this position of the feet occurs naturally when the body is at rest. If maintained for extended periods of time, plantar flexion can cause an alteration in the length of muscles, and the patient may develop a complication called *footdrop.* In this position, the foot is unable to maintain itself in the perpendicular position, heel-toe gait is impossible, and the patient will experience extreme difficulty in walking. If it is severe enough, the patient will not be able to walk at all. Intensive physical therapy over a long period may be required, and sometimes, surgery has been necessary to help to lengthen the shortened muscle group. The use of a foot support, such as the footboard, helps to avoid this complication.

During the time that a patient is in bed, pillows almost always are used to support the head. It will be noted that the patient frequently uses the pillows to tilt the head forward in order to improve his field of vision. This produces flexion of the cervical spine. Often one may see patients who are out of bed continue to walk about with this same flexion of the cervical spine. Since the supine position is the one in which the patient often spends the greatest length of time, the thorax, the neck, and the head should be supported properly.

If the patient is active in bed and able to move his arms, use his hands, and roll from side to side, these activities are protective in themselves and reduce the need for some supporting devices. However, if the patient is unable to move, supportive measures are necessary. Preventive measures for keeping the patient in good alignment while on his back are included in the chart on page 391 and Figures 17–16, 17–17, and 17–18 illustrate this position. The decision as to whether one, more, or all measures are necessary depends on the condition of the patient, his illness limitations, his activity status, and his body build.

The Protective Side-Lying Position. Lying on the side is a welcome relief from prolonged periods of lying on the back. Patients who have difficulty turning themselves from side to side appreciate a frequent change of position, which is also essential for alternate rest and activity of muscle groups. The protective side-lying position removes pressure from the prominent areas of the back.

While on the side, the feet are usually in a lesser degree of plantar flexion because the toes are not being pulled downward by gravity. The neck is also held in a more erect position. The primary concern for the patient in this position is the degree of inward rotation of the upper thigh and the upper arm. The pull created by both of these extremities can become very fatiguing. If, in addition, the upper arm pulls the shoulder girdle forward and compresses the thorax, respiration is impaired.

Preventive measures for keeping the patient in good alignment while in the protective side-lying position are included in the chart on page 392. Again, the decision as to whether one, several, or all measures are necessary depends on the condition of the patient, his illness limitations, his activity status, and his body build.

Pillows are arranged to support the patient's extremities, while a heavier pillow is tucked at his back to prevent him from rolling backwards. Figures 17–19, 17–20, and 17–21 on page 392 show this position.

The Protective Prone Position. The patient lies on his abdomen in the prone position. His head is turned to one side or the other. Because it is unfamiliar to many patients, they are often reluctant to be placed in this position. They may need teaching, encouragement, and a demonstration to accept what can be a relaxing position. However, there may be patients whose health state makes it impossible for them to lie in this position.

From the standpoint of alignment, the protective prone position offers the fewest sources of concern. If the patient is comfortable in the position and enjoys it, the feet are the only area of real concern. Unless supported or allowed to go over the end of the mattress, they are forced into plantar flexion, and the legs rotate inward or outward. Because the position is helpful, nurses should encourage patients to assume it on their own if they have complete freedom of activity. If the patient needs assistance, the time of the bath is often a good one for placing the patient in the prone position as when washing the back. In some instances, patients may be placed prone for specified periods of time each day to relieve pressure on the back or on the hips.

The advantages of the protective prone position are as follows: the shoulders, the head, and the neck are placed in the erect position; the arms are held in good alignment with the shoulder girdle; the hips are extended; the knees can be prevented from marked flex-

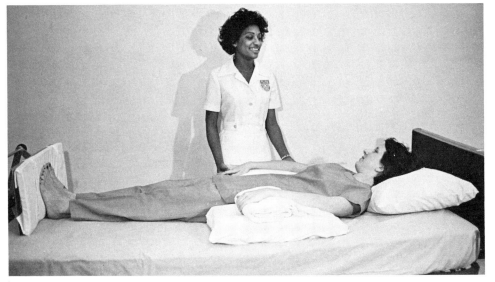

Figure 17–16 The nurse has arranged pillows to support the patient in the supine position.

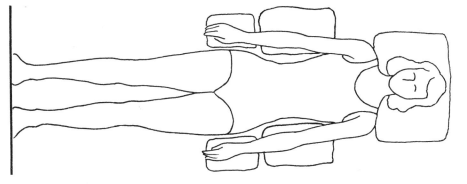

Figure 17–17 This diagram illustrates the patient in a protective supine postion as viewed from above. Note support of the head, neck, arms, hands, and feet.

Figure 17–18 This diagram illustrates the patient in a protective supine position as viewed from the side.

The protective supine position

COMPLICATION TO BE PREVENTED	SUGGESTED PREVENTIVE MEASURE
Exaggerated curvature of the spine and flexion of the hips.	Provide a firm supportive mattress. Use a bed board if necessary.
Flexion contracture of the neck.	Place pillow(s) under the upper shoulders, the neck, and the head so that the head and the neck are held in the correct position.
Internal rotation of the shoulders and extension of the elbows (hunch-shoulders).	Place pillows or arm supports under the forearms so that the upper arms are alongside the body and the forearms are pronated slightly.
Extension of the fingers and abduction of the thumbs (clawhand deformities).	Use hand rolls or small rolled towels for the hands to grasp. If the patient is paralyzed, use thumb guides to hold the thumbs in the adducted position.
External rotation of the femurs.	Place sandbags or a trochanter roll alongside the hips and the upper half of the thighs.
Hyperextension of the knees.	Place a small soft roll or sponge rubber under the knees, sufficient to fill the popliteal space but not to create pressure and not to exceed 5° of flexion.
Footdrop.	Use a footboard or make an improvised firm foot support to hold the feet in dorsal flexion.

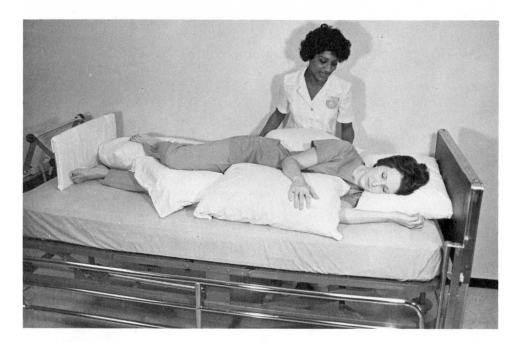

Figure 17-19   The nurse is placing a pillow at the patient's back to keep the patient from rolling back while in the protective side-lying position.

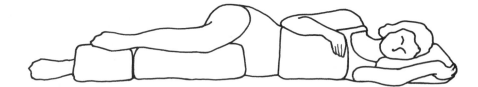

Figure 17-20   This diagram illustrates the patient in the protective side-lying position.

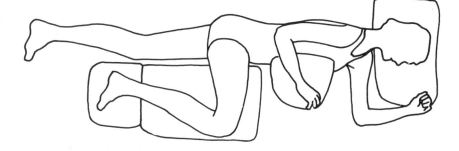

Figure 17-21   This diagram illustrates the patient in the protective side-lying position as viewed anteriorly.

The protective side-lying position

COMPLICATION TO BE PREVENTED	SUGGESTED PREVENTIVE MEASURE
Lateral flexion of the neck.	Place a pillow under the head and the neck.
Inward rotation of the arm and interference with respiration.	Place a pillow under the upper arm.
Extension of the fingers and abduction of the thumbs.	Provide a hand roll for the fingers and the thumbs.
Internal rotation and adduction of the femur.	Use one or two pillows as needed to support the leg from the groin to the foot.

ion or hyperextension; and the arms can be abducted and flexed. In a sense, it can be said that the body can be "straightened out" when placed in the protective prone position. Preventive measures for maintaining good alignment are discussed in the chart below. Figures 17–22, 17–23, and 17–24 illustrate this position.

Fowler's Position. *Fowler's position* is a semisitting position. The position is often used to promote cardiac output, respiratory movement, urinary elimination, and intestinal elimination. It also provides for ease of eating, conversing, and vision. The completely helpless person should be well-supported. The head of the adjustable bed can be elevated to the desired degree.

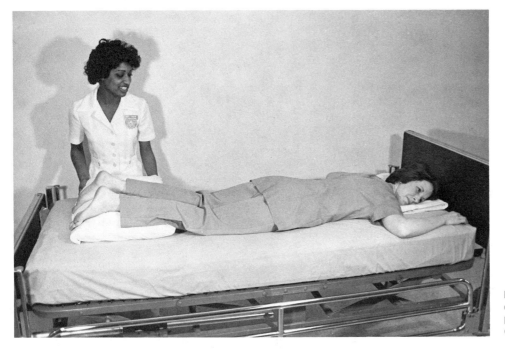

Figure 17–22 The nurse checks the placement of the patient's feet while she is in the corrective prone position.

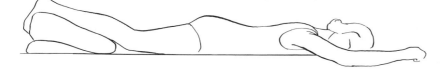

Figure 17–23 This diagram illustrates the patient in the correct protective prone position.

Figure 17–24 The diagram illustrates the patient improperly placed in a corrective prone position. The head is elevated too high which causes hyperextension of the neck, and the feet are not supported to prevent footdrop.

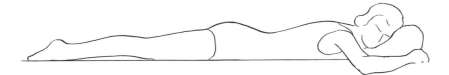

The protective prone position

COMPLICATION TO BE PREVENTED	SUGGESTED PREVENTIVE MEASURE
Footdrop.	Move the patient down in bed so that his feet are over the mattress; or support his lower legs on a pillow just high enough to keep the toes from touching the bed.
Flexion of the cervical spine.	Place a small pillow under the head.
Hyperextension of the spine. Impaired respirations.	Place some suitable support under the patient between the end of the rib cage and the upper abdomen if this facilitates breathing and there is space there.

Usually a 45° to 60° angle is used. A wedge-type, firm support can be used to elevate the patient's body from the hips up if an adjustable bed is not available. The patient should be positioned so the spine is straight and supported.

In this position, the head can be supported with a small pillow if desired. Support of the arms, especially if paralysis exists, is important because the weight of the arms and the force of gravity causes a downward pull on the shoulders and can affect shoulder joint motion in the future. Wrist and finger supports of paralyzed hands also prevent contractures and loss of joint motion. The knees can be slightly elevated with pillows or the bed knee-rest for brief periods, but they should not be in this position for a prolonged time. Impairment of circulation and knee contractures can occur from continued flexion of the knee. Foot supports may be necessary to promote dorsal flexion. Measures for promoting Fowler's position are included in the chart on page 395. Figures 17–25 and 17–26 illustrate the position.

Protective Exercises and Activities for the Patient

As indicated earlier, as little as several days in bed is sufficient time to produce temporary muscular weakness and difficulty in walking. Long-term confinement in bed can have serious effects on the muscles and joints unless they are properly cared for. The muscles can atrophy, contractures can develop, and joints can ankylose. *Anklyosis* is the fixation or immobilization of a joint. Using body parts facilitates normal functioning. By making a conscious effort to continue to use various muscles and joints, the detrimental effects of bed rest on them can generally be avoided.

Efforts to assist patients to maintain good muscle tone should begin with the first day of confinement to bed. When this is not possible, carefully planned exercises must be started and increased gradually in frequency and endurance on a day-to-day basis. Some patients may require the services of a physical therapist.

The goal of the activities discussed here is to keep the patient in the best possible physical state while bed rest is enforced. This, in turn, should help to prevent physical limitations and to reduce the length of the convalescing period. Patients can be taught the exercises and helped to develop a routine plan for their performance. Nurses and family members can carry out therapeutic regimens. When the following exercises are not considered as routine measures, the patient's physician must be consulted first.

Full Range of Joint Motion. The framework of the body is the skeleton. The bones of the skeleton are of various sizes and shapes and are held together by ligaments. These points of approximation are the joints. It is by means of the muscles and the joints that body motion is possible. The type of movement possible at the various joints of the body depends on the shape of the terminal portion of the bones and the number of bones forming the joint. It will be recalled that there are six classifications of movable joints: gliding, saddle, hinge, pivot, ball-and-socket, and condyloid. Knowing the classification and the structure of a joint is essential to understanding the type of movement it is capable of performing. *Range of motion* or full range of motion is the complete extent of movement of which the joint is normally capable. It is sometimes abbreviated ROM.

As mentioned previously, if muscle groups are altered, as in the formation of a contracture, movement of the joint is altered, and physical limitation occurs. It is essential that the nurse understand the full range of normal motion of the various joints so that preventive measures can be instituted, especially for the patient who is unable to assist in his own care to any great extent. Engaging in routine tasks, such as bathing, eating, dressing, and writing, helps to utilize muscle groups which keep many joints in effective range of motion. When all or some of these activities are impossible for various reasons, attention should be given to the joints not being used at all or to their fullest extent.

If a patient is incapable of moving himself, it may be necessary for his joints to be placed through full range of motion several times a day. This can be done during the bath or while changing the patient's position. However, the mere procedure of the bath does not ensure that all joints will have been put through range of motion. It is possible to wash the extremities without fully abducting, extending, flexing, and circumducting the joints. *Circumduction* is the circular movement of a body part, such as normally possible with the head, wrists, and thumbs. Therefore, purposeful planning for full range of joint motion is necessary. Figures 17–27 and 17–28 on pages 296 and 297 show a nurse incorporating range of motion exercises during the bathing procedure. Figure 17–29 on page 298 shows examples of range of motion exercises. This activity is necessary several times a day. In the regimen for some patients who have suffered strokes, full range of motion for specific joints, as the shoulders, the hips, and the thumbs four times a day may be required. The extent

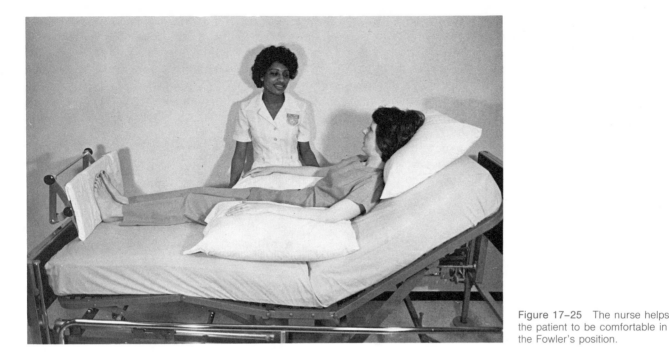

Figure 17–25 The nurse helps the patient to be comfortable in the Fowler's position.

Figure 17–26 This diagram illustrates the patient in the Fowler's position. Note how the elbow and wrist joints are supported as the shoulder is flexed.

The fowler's position

COMPLICATION TO BE PREVENTED	SUGGESTED PREVENTIVE MEASURE
Flexion contracture of the neck.	Allow the head to rest against the mattress or be supported by a small pillow only.
Exaggerated curvature of the spine.	Use a firm support for back. Position the patient so the angle of elevation starts at the hips.
Dislocation of the shoulder.	Support the forearms on pillows in order to elevate them sufficiently so that no pull is exerted on the shoulders.
Flexion contracture of the wrist.	Support the hand on pillows so it is in natural alignment with the forearm.
Edema of the hand.	Support the hand so it is slightly elevated in relation to the elbow.
Flexion contractures of the fingers and abduction of the thumbs.	Provide hand rolls for grasping and thumb supports if necessary.
Impaired lower extremity circulation and knee contracture.	Elevate the knees for only brief periods of time. Avoid pressure on the popliteal vessels.
Footdrop.	Support the feet in dorsal flexion.

to which such exercise is necessary depends on the patient's illness, physical state, and potential for recovery.

Some patients are unable to perform any joint movements themselves. When this is true, another person must move the joints through their range of motion. Manual or mechanical means of moving the joints and related tissue is called *passive exercise*. The patient is a passive recipient of the movement. *Active exercises* are self-activated range of joint movements. The patient is active in the process. *Resistive exercises* are active exercises performed by the patient using an external resistive force. The resistive force can be manual exertion applied by another person or by a mechanical device. Passive and active exercises generally can be initiated by nurses. Resistive exercises are most often used by physical therapists.

Occasionally, it is necessary to teach a patient to observe a daily routine of range of motion. In such instances, emphasis may be placed on moving the joints in directions least likely to be used by the patient. The following suggestions could be included:

While sitting up in bed without support:
move the head backward so that the cervical spine is hyperextended.
flex the trunk laterally from side to side.
rotate the trunk.
flex the arms up over the head.
extend the arms to the side of the body and then swing them in circular fashion.
While lying prone on the bed:
hyperextend the spine by lifting the head and the chest off the bed without the aid of the arms.
hyperextend the arms by lifting them off the bed toward the ceiling.
hyperextend the legs by lifting them up off the bed toward the ceiling.
While lying on the back:
flex the knees by drawing the legs up against the abdomen.
rotate the ankles inward and outward.
flex and extend the toes.
While standing and holding onto a chair back:

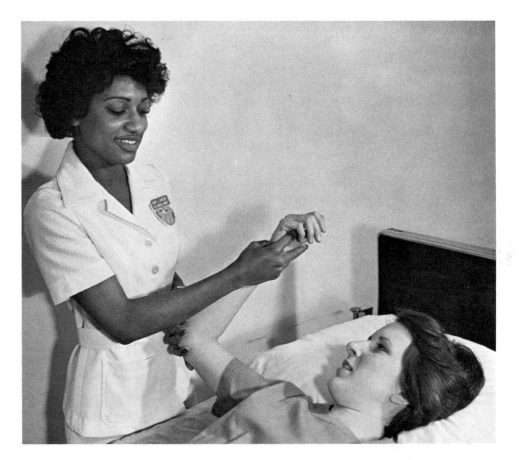

Figure 17–27 The nurse is putting the patient's shoulder joint through range of motion. Note how the elbow and wrist joints are supported as the shoulder is flexed.

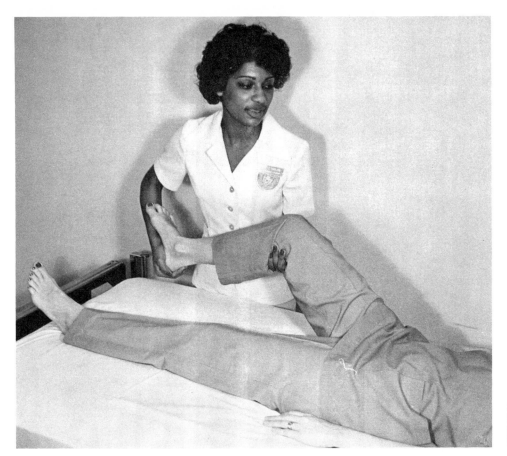

Figure 17–28 The ankle and knee are supported as the hip joint is flexed and put through range of motion.

swing each leg forward and backward and in a circular fashion.

raise the body on the toes coming down on the heels.

Attention to the thumb is of special importance. If the thumb is abducted permanently so that it cannot be brought into contact with each one of the fingers, the patient will be limited seriously. Without the full use of the thumb, it is difficult to put buttons through a buttonhole, turn a doorknob, and hold various everyday devices securely. Flexion and extension of all of the fingers and the thumb, and rotation of the thumb should be a part of the exercises.

Whenever any of the protective positions, exercises, or devices are used to help to prevent physical limitations or to restore functions, directives should be included on the nursing care plan. The nursing orders should explain what, how, and when, so that all who care for the patient observe the same routine. The Supplemental Library Study at the end of this chapter contains material on range of motion exercises.

Means by Which to Move, Lift, or Carry a Helpless Patient

Frequently, it is necessary to move a helpless patient either in the bed or from the bed to a stretcher or a chair, or vice versa. In addition to keeping him in good alignment while being moved, it is necessary that he be protected from injury.

Reducing friction makes movements easier and decreases the likelihood of tissue trauma. _Friction is the rubbing of one surface against another._ It is generally caused by the adhesion between two surfaces or the interlocking of small irregularities on the opposing surfaces. In physics, sliding and rolling types of friction have been identified. _Sliding friction is the rubbing of two flat surfaces over each other._ _Rolling friction is the rubbing caused by a circular object being moved over another surface._ Sliding friction causes more destruction than rolling friction.

In order to move a patient, friction must be reduced. It can be when sufficient energy is used to exceed resistance or when steps are taken to reduce friction.

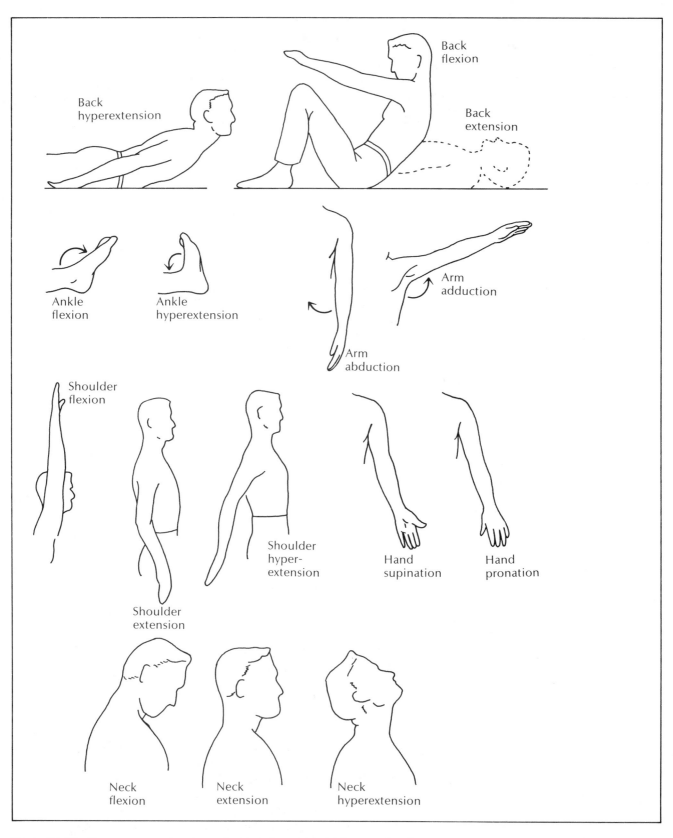

Figure 17-29 These are examples of exercises to help maintain joint range of motion.

The energy used to overcome resistance is often wasted energy. More important, the amount of energy necessary produces heat which often causes skin abrasions, sometimes called friction burns. Skin abrasions damage the protective layer of the body and increase the dangers of infections and decubitus ulcers, as described in Chapter 16. Use rolling rather than sliding movements when practical. In addition, use substances to reduce the surface adhesion and irregularities whenever possible.

Protection of the patient's skin from abrasion caused by friction is important because the skin of a helpless patient is usually very fragile and susceptible to injury. Friction burns can occur from pulling a patient across the bed or by pulling his bed linens or a bedpan from underneath him. Reducing friction by using powder or cornstarch sprinkled on the patient's dry skin and/or the linen can be helpful. Rolling, turning, and having adequate assistance are also important. Lift sheets are also useful. Mechanical devices are usually available in health agencies for moving heavy patients, and many persons have these aids in their homes. Care should be taken to make certain the operator understands how to use the device, that the patient is properly secured, and that he is instructed as to what will occur. The fears of patients who do not understand or are afraid of the devices can result in their refusal to cooperate and possible injuries.

Protection also involves understanding how to support muscles and joints which the patient cannot control voluntarily. When moving a patient, care should be taken to avoid grabbing and holding an extremity by a muscle group. The caution, "avoid grabbing the muscle bellies," is quoted frequently. An extremity should be held at the location of the insertion of the muscle tendons. For example, support at the knee or elbow rather than the midupper arm or midlower leg is preferred.

When a patient is to be moved or lifted, his comfort and safety and that of the persons involved should be considered equally important. First of all, those who lift patients must be realistic about the effort involved. two small-statured, 100-pound nurses must realize immediately that they are physically incapable of lifting a 250-pound patient. He may be rolled, pushed, pulled, or slid in bed, but lifting him from one area to another is another matter.

By using good body mechanics and the principles of mechanical laws, moving and lifting helpless patients can be made relatively easy. It is essential that the nurse understand such procedures so that she is not entirely dependent on assistance from others. Waiting for assistance which may not be necessary often means that patients cannot be moved as often as they should or when they would like to be. This is also true of helpless patients in the home. If the family is taught how to move the patient easily, home care is provided more easily.

Using Two Persons to Move a Helpless Patient Up in Bed. Children and light-weight adults are relatively easy to slide toward the head of the bed without the assistance of a second person. Average-weight adults of about 140 to 150 pounds begin to pose a problem. Many nurses have devised ways of moving heavy patients up in bed without assistance, but these methods are usually at great risk to the nurse. When moving a heavy, helpless patient up in bed, two persons should be available. Applying powder or cornstarch to the patient's back or bottom sheet will ease the move by reducing friction.

If the patient is able to push with his feet, the procedure is simple and easy. The wheels of the bed are locked first. One nurse stands on one side of the bed and the other nurse on the other side, near the patient's chest and head. Both nurses face the head of the bed. The patient is asked to flex his knees. Each nurse places the arm nearest the patient under the patient's axilla. One nurse assumes responsibility for supporting the patient's head. The other nurse places the pillow up against the head of the bed so that the patient does not hit the bed frame. Both nurses flex their knees, place one foot forward, come down close to the patient and upon a signal given by one of the nurses, the patient pushes with his feet, and the nurses rock forward, thus moving the patient up in bed.

If a patient is unable to assist by pushing with his feet, the nurses will need to hold him so that the heaviest part of his body is moved by them and not by the patient. The wheels of the bed are locked. It may be easier when the patient's knees are flexed and held in position if necessary by a third person or a pillow. A pillow is placed against the head of the bed. The nurses standing at either side of the bed face each other at a point between the patient's waist and hips. Both nurses give themselves a wide base of support, flex their knees, and lean close to the patient. They join hands under the widest part of the patient's hips and under his shoulders. At a given signal, both rock toward the head of the bed and slide the patient on the bed. The procedure may need to be repeated if he is heavy and is far down in bed. Care should be taken to avoid injury to the patient's neck and head.

Using a Sheet Pull to Move a Helpless Patient Up in Bed. While the method described previously may be necessary or convenient, the amount of effort expended by the nurses can be reduced. A draw sheet or a large sheet may be placed under the patient so that it extends from his head to below the buttocks, and can be used to lift him. When using the lift sheet, the friction that must be overcome is between the lift sheet and the bed linen. Therefore, the patient's skin is spared the effects of abrasion from friction. The sides of the lift sheet are rolled close to the patient so that they may be grasped easily. The wheels of the bed are locked. The patient's knees are flexed. The nurses stand at opposite sides of the bed at a point near the patient's shoulder and chest

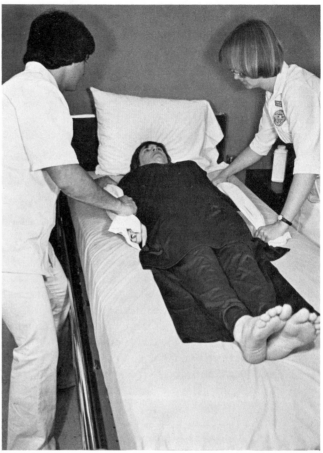

Figure 17–31 The nurses are in position following moving a patient in bed with a lift sheet.

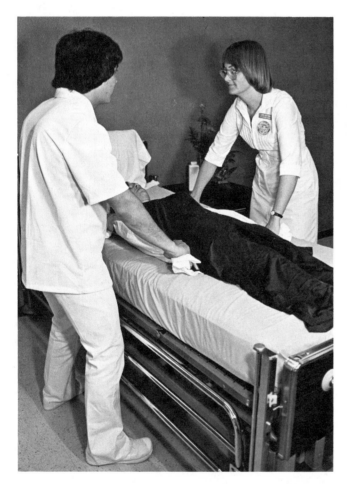

Figure 17–30 Two nurses are in position to move a patient in bed with a lift sheet. Both nurses have assumed a wide base of support, their knees are bent, and they have grasped the lift sheet close to the patient. When one of the nurses gives the signal, they are prepared to rock toward the head of the bed, sliding the lift sheet and patient as they move. Note that the pillow has been positioned to protect the patient's head.

and face the foot of the bed. They have a wide base of support with the leg nearest the bed behind them and the other leg in front. Holding the sheet securely at a point near the patient's neck and the lumbar region, they first lean forward and then rock backward. As they rock backward, the weight of their bodies helps to slide the lift sheet and the patient. At the completion of the rocking motion, each nurse usually has the elbow nearest the patient on the mattress.

The procedure can be done with the nurses facing the head of the bed. It seems easier when the backward rock is used. In the forward rock there seems to be a certain amount of upward pull necessary. Figures 17–30 and 17–31 illustrate the lift sheet pull.

Moving a Patient From the Bed to a Stretcher. Considerable care must be taken, when moving a patient from the bed to a stretcher, or vice versa, to prevent injury to the patient. If he is unconscious or helpless, the extremities and the head must be supported. The height of the bed and stretcher should be as similar as possible. Mechanical devices are available to move such patients. In the absence of such an aid, the most convenient way to move the patient is to use a lift sheet underneath him and then carefully pull on the sheet to slide the patient from one surface to the other. However, there are instances when patients must be lifted and carried. This can be done by means of a three-carrier lift. If it is done properly, the patient will feel secure, and those lifting will not suffer strain. The three-carrier lift is detailed in the chart on page 403, and illustrated in Figures 17–32 and 17–33.

When returning the patient to the bed from the stretcher, the same principles are observed. However, the carriers should first move the patient onto the bed, leaving him at the edge. Then, one member of the team supports the patient on the edge of the bed to prevent his falling off while the other two members of the team go around to the opposite side of the bed and place their arms underneath the patient in preparation for sliding him to the center of the bed. Once the two persons on the opposite side of the bed have a good grip on the patient, the third person is able to join them and assist in sliding the patient to the center of the bed. With their arms under the patient, the carriers protect his skin from some of the effects of the friction which results from the sliding. Powder would also help to reduce the friction. Sliding the patient requires much less effort than attempting to place him directly in the center of the bed. If this is attempted, the group usually is unable to hold the patient, and he is dropped onto the bed.

The three-carrier lift is used in various other situations, such as lifting a patient who has fallen to the floor and is unable to get up by himself, or lifting a patient out of a chair into the bed. Once the principles of such a lift are mastered, it becomes relatively easy to analyze situations in which it may be used.

For patients who present special problems because of their excessive weight or a cast, the three-carrier lift may not be sufficient. It may be necessary to have an additional person who is used to help support the

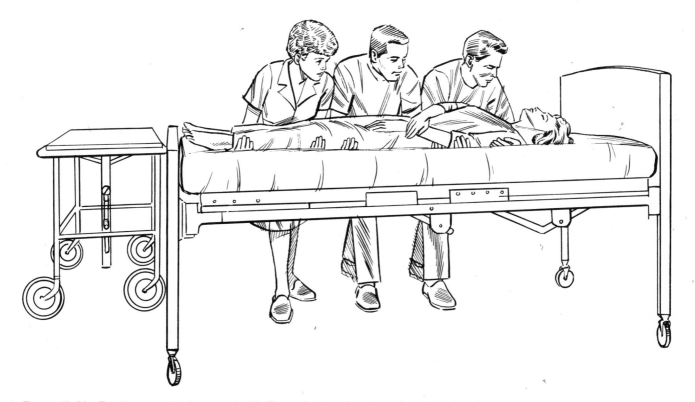

Figure 17–32 This illustrates the three-carrier lift. The patient has been brought to the edge of the bed, the stretcher is at a right angle to the foot of the bed and the three persons preparing to lift the patient have their arms well under the patient with the greatest support being given to the heaviest part of the patient. Each has a wide base of support and each is leaning over close to the patient in preparation for the lift.

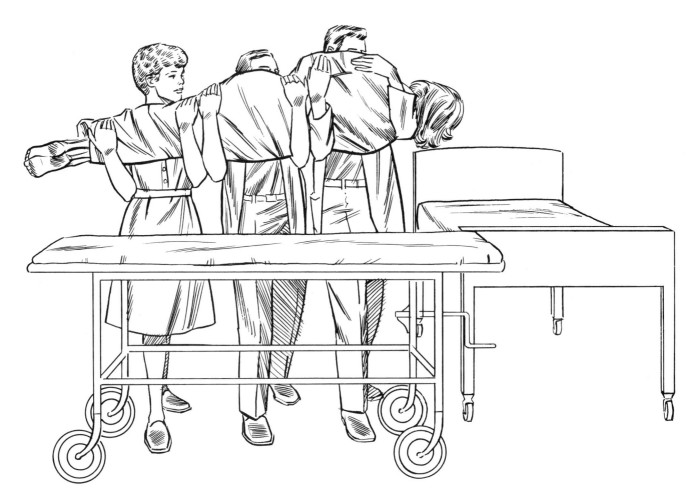

Figure 17–33 On a given signal, the three persons rock back and simultaneously lift the patient and logroll her onto their chests. They then pivot and place the patient on the stretcher. As the patient is being lowered onto the stretcher, all three carriers maintain a wide base of support and flex their knees.

heaviest or most cumbersome part of the patient. The persons distribute their arms while carrying so that the heaviest part is well-supported.

Moving a Helpless Patient From Bed to Chair. There are occasions when a patient is permitted to be out of bed but loss of various body functions makes it impossible for him to assist in the process. If the patient is able to help by using his arms for support, the problem is reduced considerably. However, some patients cannot use their arms, and nurses must be prepared to face this problem. In the health agency several persons usually are available to lift the patient from the bed to the chair. Whenever possible, lifting is preferred to prevent friction-induced skin injury. To a great extent the technique depends on the size and the weight of the

patient and the style of chair that the patient is to use. Chairs often complicate the procedure because the backrest and the arms get in the way of the persons lowering the patient.

It is possible for only one person to get a helpless patient into a chair, although two people simplify matters. The one-person technique is a valuable procedure for nurses to know for the home care of invalids and for emergency use. Often, only one family member is available to assist the patient out of bed and to return him to it. More than one person should be available if the bed and chair seat are not the same height. The technique by which one person moves a patient from a bed to a chair and to return him to the bed is shown in Figures 17–34, 17–35, and 17–36 on page 404 and included in the chart on page 405.

The three-carrier lift

The purpose is to move a patient from one place to another while maintaining his horizontal position. (From bed to stretcher is described.)

SUGGESTED ACTION	RELATED BODY MECHANICS FOR THE NURSE
Place the stretcher at a right angle to the foot of the bed so that it will be in position for the carriers after they pivot away from the bed. Lock the wheels of the bed and the wheels of the stretcher.	
Arrange the persons lifting the patient according to height, with the tallest person at the patient's head.	The tallest person usually has the longest arm grasp, making it easier for him to support the patient's head and shoulders.
Stand facing the patient and prepare to slide the arms under him. The person in the middle places the arms directly under the patient's buttocks; the person at the head has one arm under the patient's head, neck, and shoulder area and the other arm directly against the middle person's arm; the person at the patient's feet has one arm also against the middle person's arm and the other arm under the patient's ankles.	The greatest weight is in the area of the buttocks. Having the middle person's armspread smaller than that of the other two persons helps to prevent strain on this person. Having the arms of the first and the third persons touch the arms of the middle person provides additional support in the heaviest area.
Slide the arms under the patient as far as possible and get in a position to slide the patient to the edge of the bed.	Place one leg forward, the thigh resting against the bed and the knees flexed, and put on the internal girdle.
Lean over the patient and on signal simultaneously rock back and slide the patient to the edge of the bed.	Movement is accomplished by rocking backward and attempting to "sit down"; the weight of the nurses and the power of their arms, hips, and knees move the patient.
Place the arms farther underneath the patient. Prepare to "logroll" the patient onto the chests of all three at the same time the patient is being lifted from the bed.	Place one leg forward, flex the knees, and put on the internal girdle. "Logrolling" the patient onto the carriers brings the centers of gravity of all objects closer, thereby increasing the stability of the group and reducing strain on the carriers.
Pivot around to the stretcher and, on signal, lower the patient onto the stretcher.	Flex the knees, have one foot forward, and bring your own body down with the patient, thus letting the large leg and arm muscles do the work of lowering the patient.

Self-help Devices for Patients Having Activity Limitations

While it is recognized that abilities totally lost cannot be recreated, those abilities which remain should be developed to their fullest capacities. Patients who have lost the full use of a muscle group can be helped to learn new ways in which to continue their activities of daily living when they are no longer confined to bed. Of considerable help to such patients are the numerous self-help devices which are being designed and manufactured. The use of such items often helps the patient to maintain or regain independence. Independence to the degree possible enhances the self-concept. The impact of the self-concept on well-being has been discussed previously in this text.

Some self-help items are available through mail-order houses and department stores. Others are sold by medical supply companies. Items such as walkers, canes, bed trapezes, and wheelchairs are all available for home use. Some patients find that braces and prosthetic devices give them added support.

Examples of self-help items used in personal care include elastic shoe laces which eliminate the need for tying laces, long-handled shoehorns which eliminate the need for bending down to put on shoes, handbrushes and toothbrushes which need not be grasped, and a nail clipper which can be worked by a foot pedal.

For the handicapped homemaker there are numerous items which facilitate activities associated with cooking and cleaning, such as a one-handed eggbeater, a safety cutting board which holds food in place while it is being pared or cut, a long-handled dustpan, a one-handed food chopper, an automatic pressure saucepan, mixing bowls with a suction base, and an interchangeable grater, slicer, and shredder held securely on a frame. Many of these items are of value to anyone. They reduce the amount of energy expended and therefore lessen fatigue.

Self-help items for the handicapped are varied in number and complexity. They can range from homemade devices to specially designed automobiles. The purpose of all of them is to promote the independence and individuality of the patient.

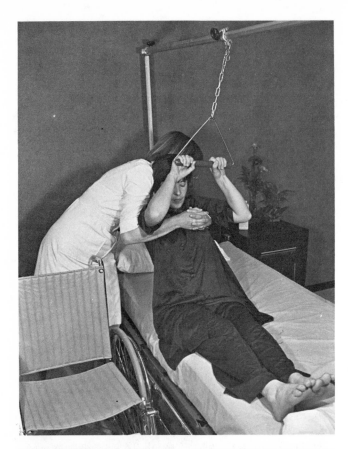

Figure 17–34   The nurse is assisting a patient who does not have use of her legs, to a chair. The nurse has prepared the wheelchair by removing the arm and positioning it adjacent to the bed. The patient is close to the edge of the bed and ready to assist by using the overhead trapeze to lift her upper body. The nurse positions herself behind the patient with her hands firmly clasped under the patient's axillary area to prevent slipping. They are ready for the nurse to slide the patient to the chair.

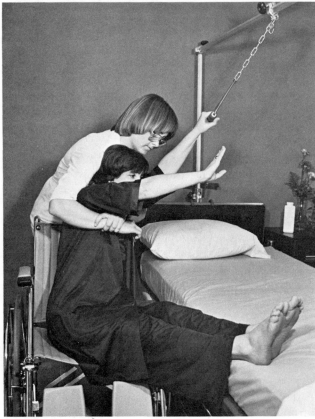

Figure 17–35   When returning the patient to bed, the nurse places the patient's feet and legs on the bed and lifts the patient to reach for the trapeze.

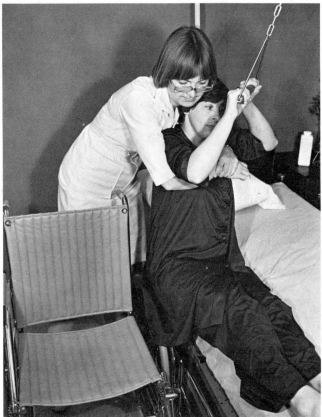

Figure 17–36   With the patient on the edge of the bed, she can use the trapeze to assist the nurse to move to the center of the bed.

One person moving a helpless patient from bed to chair

The purpose is to move a helpless patient out of bed when his weight makes it impossible for the only available person to lift him.

SUGGESTED ACTION	RELATED BODY MECHANICS FOR THE NURSE
Place the chair facing and against the bed at a point near the patient's buttocks to receive the patient and to use as a brace.	
Slide the upper portion of the patient's body to the edge of the bed. (This makes the patient lie diagonally on the bed.)	Place the arms under the patient's head and shoulders. Place one foot forward and rock backward.
Place the arms well under the patient's axillae from the rear. (The patient's head and shoulders will be resting on the nurse.)	Support the upper portion of the patient's body on yourself to reduce the weight of the patient to be moved.
Move around to the back of the chair, pulling the patient into the chair while so doing.	Lean against the back of the chair to keep it from moving and to brace yourself. Rock back and pull the patient into the chair.
Pull the chair away from the bed until the patient's feet are on the edge of the bed, being careful not to pull the chair out from under the patient.	Flex the knees, grasp the chair near the seat, and rock back.
Support the patient's legs while lowering the feet to the floor.	Flex the knees while lowering the patient's feet to the floor.

One person moving a helpless patient from chair to bed

The purpose is to move a helpless patient from a chair into a bed when his weight makes it impossible for the only available person to lift him.

SUGGESTED ACTION	RELATED BODY MECHANICS FOR THE NURSE
Bring the chair directly alongside the bed with the patient facing the foot of the bed. Place a pillow on the arm of the chair.	Slide the chair rather than lifting one side at a time. If the floor has a polished surface, slide the chair on a small rug or rags.
Lift the patient's legs onto the edge of the bed.	Flex the knees and lower the body and support both the patient's legs when coming to an erect position.
Go behind the chair, grasp the patient under the axillae from the rear and roll him onto the bed.	Face the back of the chair and the bed at an angle. Have a wide base of support and rock to move the patient onto the bed.
Move the chair and help the patient into the desired position.	Slide the chair with your foot and brace yourself against the bed to prevent the patient from falling off.

LEISURE-TIME ACTIVITIES

It was stated earlier in this chapter that the concept of rehabilitation involved prevention as well as restoration and physical as well as psychological functioning. Thus far, primarily physical measures have been discussed. While it is true that the physical body cannot truly be separated from the psychosocial, the remainder of the chapter will focus on nonphysical aspects of rehabilitation.

The concept of rehabilitation implies active involvement of the patient. Since the intention, desire, or inner drive must be present in order to be involved, the patient must possess some motivation. Motivation is usually a response to a felt need. One person cannot create or provide motivation for another, but it is possible for an individual to stimulate, support, and foster motivation in someone else. This responsibility is often part of the nurse's role. There are various types of motivational techniques that are described in other texts. The discussion here will be a brief general introduction.

Well and ill persons often can be motivated to initiate the exercises and activities mentioned earlier. They can also be motivated to use their leisure time in a meaningful fashion. Leisure time can be planned and desired, or it can be unexpectedly enforced. Diversion or recreation are terms that are frequently associated with leisure-time activities. Activities that fill this time in a meaningful way can be productive for the individual's self-concept, his learning of new ideas and skills, and his enjoyment and satisfaction. They can be a means to develop muscles, to be involved in therapeutic social interaction, to learn new skills, to retain or gain independence and dignity, or to express emotions. Or, activities can help the time to pass more quickly or to provide pleasure. The motivation that a person has for an activity depends on his felt needs.

There is a wide variety of types of leisure-time activities that may be helpful to a patient, but like all other aspects of care, the nurse must consider the individuality of the patient in order to be helpful to him. Some patients and families develop their own activities while others need the support and assistance of the nurse.

The nurse has to consider the patient's needs and his strengths, the specific purposes activities are to achieve, the patient's interests and limitations, and available facilities and resources.

Probably the most important single factor in helping a patient with planning diversional activities is his participation in decision-making. For the activity to have some positive value for him, it must be something he wishes to do. Some patients will want to pursue previous interests. Others can often be assisted to develop interests they did not have previously. Regardless of the nature of the activity or the type of assistance needed, the person should participate in determining the leisure-time activities with which he will be involved. If this principle is ignored, involvement in the activities will usually be short-lived or have limited value.

Diversional activities are seen as so important in daily living that extensive investigations of the concept of leisure time and ways it can be used are being conducted in this country. Many different community and private groups organize efforts to provide leisure-time activities. There are recreational facilities with specially prepared persons who supervise activities that appeal to all age groups and a wide variety of interests and abilities. Health institutions, especially those dealing with the chronically ill patient, often have both recreational therapists and occupational therapists, and extensive programs for both children and adults.

Helping to Select Diversional Activities

Diversional activities can serve a variety of purposes. Whether a particular diversional activity is selected to promote relaxation or interaction with others, to make time seem as though it passes more quickly, to enhance physical capacities, to substitute for past activities, or to provide an outlet for emotions, it should be purposeful. In turn, achieving the purpose or goal should result in a feeling of satisfaction and accomplishment for the individual.

It is possible to purchase or to select games or projects on the basis of age, size of group, and degree of difficulty of the activity, in relation to the desired

purpose. For example, it is possible to assist quiet and withdrawn individuals to participate comfortably in a group situation or to select a diversion which will help to quiet and relax the more active individual.

When illness or incapacity is prolonged or chronic, recreation that a person enjoyed before his illness may not interest him, or certain activities may no longer be appropriate. Recreation then may be planned to find new and suitable means of spending leisure time. For example, a person with partial permanent paralysis following a cerebrovascular accident may have to give up certain sports and find substitutes. He may lose all interest or become a passive participant.

Recreation is often a good way to keep a child contented in bed and relatively quiet during illness and convalescence. Although activity is restricted, imagination can travel far and wide through toys and games, making confinement seem less bridling. Robert Louis Stevenson's poem, "The Land of Counterpane," illustrates poignantly how toys can help the ill child roam far from his confining bed:

> When I was sick and lay a-bed,
> I had two pillows at my head,
> And all my toys beside me lay
> To keep me happy all the day.
>
> And sometimes for an hour or so
> I watched my leaden soldiers go
> With different uniforms and drills,
> Among the bed-clothes, through the hills.
>
> And sometimes sent my ships in fleets
> All up and down among the sheets;
> Or brought my trees and houses out,
> And planted cities all about.
>
> I was the giant great and still
> That sits upon the pillow-hill,
> And sees before him, dale and plain,
> The pleasant land of counterpane.

For older children, group games offer both companionship and challenge for the participants. Play can also promote learning and provide an emotional outlet.

Children's play often serves a useful purpose in evaluating physical and mental development. The observant nurse can include play when planning not only a youngster's recreation, but many other aspects of his care as well. In short, play can be used to strengthen particular muscles, to express emotions, and to teach.

Diversional activities are often used in occupational therapy. Occupational therapy is a prescribed and supervised rehabilitation procedure involving manual and/or creative activities. For instance, a patient may

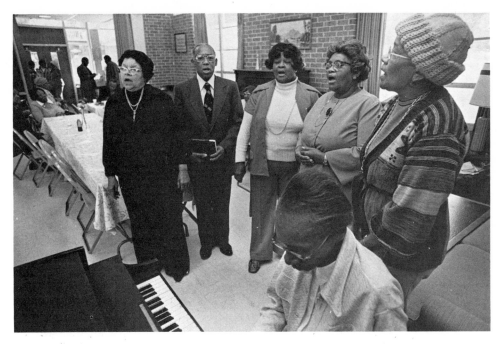

Figure 17–37 These retired persons enjoy singing together at a community center as one way of spending some of their leisure time.

be referred to the occupational therapy department for an activity which will exercise certain muscle groups in the hand and the arm. There the patient may be introduced to something that he never has done before, but in all instances the therapist will try to offer a choice of suitable activities so that the patient may enjoy doing it. Some patients may be referred to the occupational therapy department to learn a new vocation so that they may seek employment after they have recovered. Typical would be an amputee who previously was a bus driver. Or, some patients may be referred to the occupational therapy department to engage in an activity in which they already have some skill. For such a patient the immediate interest in a constructive activity is therapeutic because it gives him self-confidence from the beginning and occupies his time constructively. In still other situations, patients may wish to engage in activities which merely help to pass the time.

The diversional needs of acutely ill patients may be little other than perhaps visits with family and friends and receiving and reading mail. When convalescence is short, patients may require very little assistance in finding diversional activities, since they quickly begin to assume their usual way of life. Their ordinary interests appear, and these are pursued with little effort needed on the part of the nurse.

The person with a long-term illness or disability may require assistance. Very often, the diversion is akin to a person's occupation, but it can also be the opposite.

For example, it is not uncommon to see a person with excellent manual dexterity, such as a surgeon, paint or sculpt as a diversion, or a highway engineer building a model railroad layout at home. On the other hand, one with a confining occupation, such as a research chemist, may like gardening or golf or other outdoor hobbies. Helping a patient to feel more comfortable while ill very often requires the nurse's display of interest in his usual hobbies or diversions. It may be that he had not thought of them because he was confined. If it is not possible for him to enjoy the identical diversions, close substitutes perhaps can be found. Any diversion that can be provided which makes the patient more at ease contributes to a therapeutic climate.

The well, elderly person may need assistance from the nurse to find productive ways to use his leisure time. This is often especially true for persons who are newly retired and making adjustments to many aspects of daily living. They may need to be introduced to community senior citizen activities, volunteer programs, or part-time employment possibilities.

Like adults, children are unsatisfied with activities that are of no interest to them. The diversion selected will have to be considered carefully from the standpoint of the child's interest in it, the amount of physical activity involved, and the possible emotional reactions to it.

In certain instances, the patient may prefer group activity to solitary diversion, but here again his condition must be taken into account. Obviously, a patient in a full body cast cannot join in a game of Ping-Pong, but probably he can play cards; a game of solitaire may suffice during times when other persons cannot come to join him in a group game.

Wherever group activities are concerned, like interests are involved. When organizing such events or encouraging persons to join them, it should be remembered that recreation for one individual may not be such for another and that points of difference can cause stress and conflict for a patient. For example, if a nurse were to say to a group of patients on a sun porch, "I'll turn the television on so you can all watch the baseball game this afternoon," she may annoy those who have no interest in the game. In other words, the nurse should avoid making patients feel compelled to join in.

For persons confined for long periods, group activities usually are enjoyable. Just being in a group may be satisfying in itself. Some agencies have parties on patients' birthdays and on certain holidays, as well as planned events for other special occasions. If given the opportunity, some patients enjoy the challenge of organizing, decorating, and planning for group recreation such as a party, a skit, or a game.

When helping to select diversions, remember that most people need variety. Few care to pursue a single thing all day or day after day. Children and young adults are especially likely to succumb to boredom.

Common Diversions

Reading and Writing.   Many persons enjoy at least some reading during their leisure time. Books, magazines, and newspapers are usually available in most health agencies and many homes. For those unable to visit the library, volunteers in many agencies bring reading materials to the patients. Many recordings are available for persons whose vision makes reading impossible.

Some persons also enjoy writing while hospitalized. This is especially true with those who have long-term illness or are not acutely ill. Chronically ill persons often enjoy pen pals. New mothers usually write birth announcements while hospitalized.

The arrival of mail generally is a pleasant experience for confined patients. It is a way to keep in touch with family and friends, and many patients derive great pleasure in displaying the cards that they receive. Very ill patients, or those unable to open their mail, may appreciate help with this. The person bringing the patient his mail should offer to open the envelope and read the card or message to the patient if he so desires. It may be a comforting message from someone who is unable to visit.

Television and Radio.   Most health agencies and homes have provisions for patients to use television and radio sets. The sets may be located in the patient's room or in

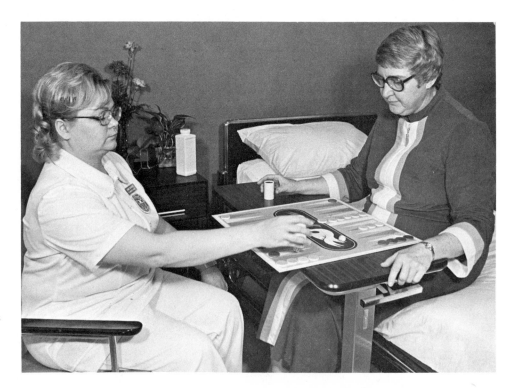

Figure 17–38   This nurse helps the hospitalized patient pass the time more quickly by engaging her in a game of backgammon.

areas shared with others. Many people enjoy watching television or listening to a radio for at least part of every day; and except for the very ill and the very young, this usually is appropriate. It should be remembered that television and radio programs may be a source of annoyance for other persons in a health agency setting; therefore, the volume should be kept at a moderate level.

Arts and Crafts. Recreation involving any of the arts and the crafts can be especially rewarding in that something is created, and the end products are useful and decorative. Frequently, arts and crafts are suggested to patients if the activity involved is also beneficial for a specific physical limitation.

Toys. Toys can be the source of much pleasure for the ill child. They should be carefully selected on the basis of factors discussed earlier in this chapter. In addition, safety must be kept in mind when selecting toys. Those with small removable parts should be avoided because of the danger of swallowing them. Also to be avoided are toys with sharp edges or points. Interesting and inexpensive toys can be made from common objects found in the home. Toys that stimulate the imagination can provide diversion for older children.

Eating and Socializing. Eating with others is a symbol of family life and is taken for granted in many cultures. Almost no one likes to eat alone, and efforts to bring an ill person to the family table or into a dining area with other patients usually are rewarding. Many of the chronic-illness hospitals have patient dining rooms, and often ambulatory patients may go to the dining room or cafeteria for meals.

Many pediatric services arrange to have children eat together. Often, children eat more willingly when with others, and the handicapped are stimulated to do their best to be more like their peers.

Patient lounges are seen commonly in hospitals and other health agencies. Here, patients can enjoy games together, meet for chatting, watch television, and so on. For persons who do not socialize readily, a patients' lounge with opportunities to meet or be near others often can make the difference between loneliness and the satisfaction of being part of a group.

Visitors. Most patients enjoy visits with family members and friends. At one time most health agencies observed very limited visiting privileges, the reason being that visitors often were thought to upset patients

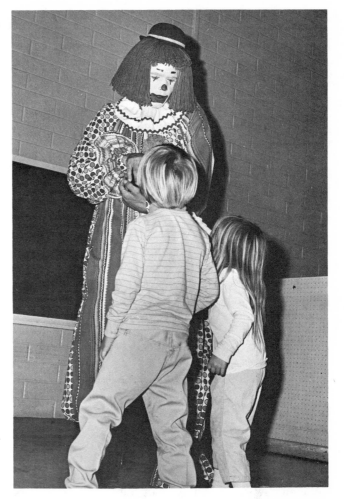

Figure 17–39 Memories are likely to be pleasant for these young patients who enjoy a visit from Mr. Clown in the health clinic's playroom.

as well as the hospital routines. However, most hospitals have become increasingly lenient in the provision of visiting privileges, as health personnel have observed the therapeutic value for patients. On pediatric services, visiting privileges in the past often were extremely limited. But in agencies where most barriers for visiting have been removed, the children have demonstrated a marked increase in morale, resulting in definite therapeutic benefit.

Visitors in the home as well as the health agency can be therapeutic for the person. In addition to the pleasure the patient has when a relative or friend visits, sometimes the visitor can assist in the patient's care by assisting the patient with eating, with walking, and with caring for the nails and hair. Under some circumstances, it may even be helpful to the patient if a family member can aid in administering medication or other treatments.

Visiting can be overdone, and health personnel generally agree that some limitations still must be observed. For the very ill, a limitation on the length of time visitors may stay or on the number of visitors present at one time may be necessary. While visiting policies are necessary, good judgment still must be used on the basis of the individual situation. In certain instances, because of the danger of infection, such as following organ transplants, no visitors may be allowed for some hospitalized patients.

Patients as Helpers.   There was a time when patients were expected to help each other and to assist with work in health agencies when such work did not interfere with their recovery. However, using patients as helpers is uncommon today in acute care facilities. In some chronic disease hospitals and nursing homes where this system is used judiciously, the results have been impressive. For some patients, being able to help is gratifying and gives a feeling of personal accomplishment, besides relieving boredom. A few things that patients can do to help are acting as interpreter when language barriers occur, reading to patients who are unable to do so, making telephone calls for bedridden patients, writing letters for patients who are incapacitated, making beds, and assisting with landscaping care.

Other Miscellaneous Diversions.   Some agencies have facilities for swimming, movies, operating a radio station, canteens, auditoriums for social events, and the like. In general, it seems that as facilities and opportunities for diversion increase, patients' attitudes toward health agencies should improve. Long-term confinement agencies need not be as dreary and impersonal as was often the case in previous years.

Community recreational facilities promote activities such as singing, dancing, group exercises, game playing, and craftwork for patients of all ages. Special activities for the handicapped and chronically ill in their homes or in community centers are available in some areas.

PROMOTING EXERCISE AND ACTIVITY AND THE NURSING PROCESS

Specific data to be collected about an individual's exercise and activity needs will vary with his circumstances. Answers to the following questions suggest data which

may be useful. Does the patient have obvious difficulty with any movements? If active, what type of body mechanics does he use when stooping, bending, and lifting? What major muscle groups and joints are not involved? What type of mattress does he use? If he spends many hours sitting each day, is the chair proportionate to his stature? Does it provide adequate support? Can and does he independently alter his position at intervals? Does he normally have or need assistance in moving? Does he use any type of device for assisting mobility? If he is confined to bed, does he understand the undesirable implications of bed rest? How does he usually spend his leisure time? What type of diversional activities interest him? These and other questions can uncover data which are useful for providing nursing care.

Assessment of collected data will determine the nursing diagnoses. The specific assessment standards to be used will depend on particular data. Some standards which can be used in assessing, such as the characteristics of normal posture and joint range of motion, and the risk factors of prolonged bed rest, have been discussed in this chapter. Other norms can be found in clinical texts.

Planning to meet the nursing care requirements of a particular person's exercise and activity needs will depend on the nature of the nursing diagnoses. Selecting the specific measures to be implemented should involve consideration of the preferences and circumstances of the patient.

Measures selected for inclusion in the patient's plan of care are implemented in nursing intervention. Many types of nursing interventions have been discussed in this chapter. The following statements summarize the nursing measures used for activity and exercise.

- Provide a positive example of the role of activity and exercise in maintaining well-being. Before saying a word to a patient, the movements and appearance of the nurse can support or undermine her attempts to promote physical activity. The health care consumer has a right to expect the nurse to serve as a model in this regard.

- Teach both ill and well persons about the importance of physical activity and safe ways of practicing it. By developing a habit of providing a simple explanation whenever related nursing care is provided, the nurse can teach and help patients to maintain or establish healthful physical activity routines.

- Include exercise as an integral part of nursing care at the earliest opportunity for every patient. This form of preventive care can contribute a significant amount to a patient's well-being.

- Change a helpless patient's position frequently. The well person shifts some aspect of his body weight every few minutes. The nurse needs to provide for meeting this need in the incapacitated, both for the sake of his comfort and for optimum physiological functioning.

- Identify the physics and physiological principles involved in common nursing measures related to moving and positioning patients. By focusing on the underlying rationales and techniques, good habits of body mechanics and protective positioning are more likely to be developed.

- Include patients in planning for activities which involve exercises and diversional activities whenever possible. Participation in planning enhances involvement and commitment. In addition, many patients come up with creative and ingenious ideas which are often very useful.

- Make the patient's self-help devices accessible to him. The person who falls because his walker or crutches are out of reach often has had a thoughtless nurse. The self-help devices should be conveniently placed and the patient should be instructed to call for assistance whenever necessary.

- Evaluate the goals of diversional activities periodically to determine if they are being met. It cannot be assumed that because a patient is participating in an activity, it is serving the intended purpose. Or, even if an activity is satsifactory for a period, alternatives may be necessary from time to time.

The parts of the nursing process and of the process as a whole are evaluated as described in Chapter 4.

CONCLUSION

Maintenance or restoration of body function is strongly influenced by posture, movement, and activity. Well persons and ill persons and family members frequently need assistance from the nurse in the form of instruction and explanation, demonstration, and support. The nurse can protect herself and promote the most effective learning of others by developing good habits in her own personal life.

SUPPLEMENTAL LIBRARY STUDY

1. A study showed that as many as 80 percent of nurses have experienced low back pain. It is hypothesized that the cause is physical inactivity and poor physical conditioning. This author suggests some conditioning exercises for the back and abdominal muscles.

   Drapeau, Janine. "Getting Back Into Good Posture: "How to Erase Your Lumbar Aches." *Nursing 75,* 5:63–65, September 1975.

   How does your posture compare with the figures on page 63? If you do not have a regular exercise routine, try those illustrated and consider incorporating them into your daily activities.

2. Before exercise is included in a nursing care plan, data must be collected and an assessment made. The following article suggests various physiological factors to consider when planning for activity needs of an individual.

   Gordon, Marjory. "Assessing Activity Tolerance." *American Journal of Nursing,* 76:72–75, January 1976.

   The writer suggests factors related to the activities which should be weighed when choosing between alternatives. Using two different types of activities, answer the questions posed on page 72 and compare the results. Would this information also help you in planning nursing care?

3. Like many other activities, the use of a cane or crutches is difficult to teach someone else if you have never had the experience of using the device yourself. Diagrams in the following book show the correct techniques.

   Dison, Norma. *Clinical Nursing Techniques.* The C. V. Mosby Company, St. Louis, 1975, pp. 53–55.

   Practice each of them until you feel comfortable and secure. If possible, use crutches for a day for your usual activities. Note how your life is influenced because of the change in your mobility. Note the amount of coordination and arm strength that is necessary for crutch-walking. Such an experience can be helpful for increasing insight into the feelings and concerns of patients.

4. Range of motion was discussed in this chapter primarily in the context of the ill person. The pictures in this article show elderly well persons performing various range of motion exercises.

   Frankel, Lawrence J. and Richard, Betty Byrd. "Exercises to Help the Elderly—To Live Longer, Stay Healthier, and Be Happier." *Nursing 77,* 7:58–63, December 1977.

   Can you identify the motion depicted in each picture, using the terms presented in this chapter? While all of the persons pictured are elderly, these exercises can be therapeutic for persons of all ages. Note how much these individuals seem to be enjoying what they are doing. Try the exercises yourself for promoting relaxation and relieving fatigue.

18

BEHAVIORAL OBJECTIVES

When content in this chapter has been mastered, the student will be able to

Define the terms appearing in the glossary.

Describe the transmission and perception of painful stimuli and how stimuli for pain may be inhibited, according to the gate control theory.

Indicate common stimuli for pain and voluntary, involuntary, and emotional responses to pain.

List six principles of pain and indicate common intervention measures that are guided by an understanding of each of these principles.

Describe the nursing care of a person experiencing pain, using the nursing process as a guide.

Discuss common characteristics of sleep, including REM and NREM sleep.

Describe the reticular system and how it functions to influence sleep and wakefulness.

List and discuss at least three factors influencing the amount of sleep an individual needs for well-being and describe common signs and symptoms of sleep deprivation.

List five sleeping disorders and common measures to control them.

List four principles of sleep and indicate common nursing measures that are guided by an understanding of these principles.

Describe the nursing care of a person experiencing sleep problems, using the nursing process as a guide.

Promoting Comfort, Rest, and Sleep

GLOSSARY

Acupuncture: A technique that uses long thin needles to prick specific parts of the body to produce insensitivity to pain.

Addictive: A substance to which an individual develops a psychological and physiological dependency.

Agrypnotic Drug: A pharmaceutical agent that causes wakefulness.

Analgesic Drug: A pharmaceutical agent that is used to relieve pain.

Autohypnosis: Self-induced hypnosis.

Biofeedback: A training program that helps an individual control certain aspects of his autonomic nervous system.

Delta Sleep: Deep sleep, occurring during Stage III and especially Stage IV in NREM sleep.

Diffuse Pain: Discomfort that covers a large area.

Diurnal Enuresis: Involuntary urination that occurs during wakefulness.

Dull Pain: Gnawing discomfort that is less intense and acute than sharp pain.

Electroencephalograph: An instrument which receives and records electrical currents in the brain.

Enuresis: Involuntary urination.

Euphoria: An unrealistic sense of well-being.

Gate Control Theory: A theory which explains that excitatory pain stimuli, carried by small diameter nerve fibers, can be blocked by inhibiting signals carried by large diameter nerve fibers, in the substantia gelatinosa cells in the dorsal horn of the spinal cord.

Hypnosis: A technique that produces a subconscious condition accomplished by suggestions made by the hypnotist.

Hypnotic Drug: A pharmaceutical agent used to induce sleep.

Insomnia: Difficulty in falling asleep, intermittent sleep, and/or early awakening from sleep.

Intermittent Pain: Discomfort that comes and goes.

Narcolepsy: A condition characterized by an uncontrollable desire to sleep.

Nocturnal Enuresis: Involuntary urination that occurs while sleeping.

NREM or Non-REM: Nonrapid eye movement that characterizes four stages of sleep.

Pain: A sensation of physical and/or mental suffering or hurt that usually causes distress or agony to the one experiencing it.

Phantom Pain: The sensation of pain without demonstrable physiological or pathological substance.

Placebo: A Latin word meaning ''I shall please.'' It consists of an inactive substance that gives satisfaction to the person using it.

Referred Pain: Pain in an area removed from that in which stimulation has its origin.

Relax: To become less rigid, to slacken effort, and to decrease tension.

REM: Rapid eye movement that characterizes the dream state of sleep.

Rest: A condition in which the body is in a decreased state of activity with consequent feeling of being refreshed.

Sharp Pain: Quick, sticking, and intense discomfort.

Shifting Pain: Discomfort that moves from one area to another.

Sleep: A state of relative unconsiousness.

Sleep Apnea: Periods of no breathing between snoring intervals.

Somatic: Pertaining to structures in the body's external wall.

Somnambulism: Sleepwalking.

Tranquilizer: A pharmaceutical agent used primarily to reduce anxiety.

Visceral: Pertaining to the body's internal organs.

INTRODUCTION

Chapter 17 pointed out the dangers of bed rest and discussed patients' needs for activity even when confined to bed. Without negating the importance of exercise and diversional activities, provisions for comfort and rest are also essential patient needs. In addition, when patients are comfortable and are meeting needs for rest and sleep, encouraging necessary activity often becomes an easier task, both for the patient and for the nurse. This chapter discusses some basic theories of pain and sleep and measures that help to promote comfort and rest.

DESCRIPTION AND CHARACTERISTICS OF PAIN

Pain is one of the body's cutaneous senses. It has intrigued the curiosity of science and has led to a huge array of pain-relieving techniques since time immemorial. Yet despite its universality and eternal presence among mankind, the nature of pain remains an enigma.

Pain has been defined, and occasionally still is, on a philosophical and religious basis as punishment for wrongdoing. Aristotle defined pain as well as anyone when he wrote that it is the "antithesis of pleasure . . . the epitome of unpleasantness." A typical dictionary definition states that *pain* is a sensation of physical and/or mental suffering or hurting that usually causes distress or agony to the one experiencing it.

There is still another aspect of pain.

> Human pain is that condition which occurs when the human being is hurt . . . it is the spirit which is affected. The greatest hurts are the loss of loved ones or the loss of their love, but pain may be felt whenever there is abuse of person . . .*

Another approach to defining pain focuses on the person who experiences the pain. The nurse, along with the physician and other health practitioners, cannot see or feel the pain to which they will attend. They function in this area of care through experiences only the patient senses and describes. Therefore, one can say that pain ". . . is whatever the experiencing person says it is and exists whenever he says it does."* The

patient may well describe pain verbally; that is, he may state that he has a throbbing pain in the foot he has injured. Or, he may communicate nonverbally; that is, he may say nothing, but he refuses to walk on the affected foot and is reluctant to let the examiner touch it.

Pain is interpreted as a threat to the organism's integrity. It is an imperative sensation and involves the whole biopsychosocial being. Its preoccupying characteristic tends to make us negate other sensations in its presence. Although the primary purpose of pain is to warn of tissue injury or disease, the degree of pain is not necessarily in direct proportion to the amount of tissue damage, nor is tissue damage always present when pain occurs.

In summary, pain is present whenever an individual states it is, even when perhaps no specific cause for the pain can be discerned. Pain is a personal and realistic experience and involves the whole human organism. A person suffering with pain ordinarily describes it in verbal or nonverbal ways or both.

The Perception of Pain

The perception of pain is concerned with the sensory process when a stimulus for pain is present. It includes the individual's interpretation of his pain. The threshold of perception is the lowest intensity of a stimulus that causes the subject to recognize pain. This threshold is remarkably similar for everyone. Still, it is theorized by some authorities that a phenomenon of adaptation does occur; that is, the threshold for pain can be changed within certain ranges. This phenomenon has been studied, for example, when prisoners of war reported that the pain of repeated torture was not as acute as it would have been under different circumstances. Many factors might well have played a role, but at least some adaptation appeared likely.

Adaptation occurs also when a person's hand is immersed in warm water. A sensation of pain eventually occurs as the water is heated. However, the person can tolerate a higher temperature as water is gradually heated to the pain level than he could have, had he plunged his hand into hot water without any preparation. This observation has practical implications, as when hot applications are applied to the body over an extended period. Even though tissues are damaged, the patient may not necessarily complain of pain when increasingly hot applications are made as he becomes accustomed to the heat.

---

*Sobel, David. "Love and Pain." *American Journal of Nursing,* 72:910, May 1972.
*McCaffery, Margo. *Nursing Management of the Patient with Pain.* J. B. Lippincott Company, Philadelphia, 1972, page 8.

The Transmission of Pain Stimuli

Pain sensations are conducted along pathways which have been rather clearly defined in certain areas, although it is still somewhat questionable in others. There are no specific pain organs or cells in the body. Rather, an interlacing network of undifferentiated free nerve endings receive painful stimuli. It is estimated that there are several million of these nerve endings in the body. They are numerous in the layers of the skin and in some internal tissues, such as the joint surfaces. In the deeper tissues of the body, the pain receptors are diffusely but unevenly spread.

Somatic pertains to structures in the body's wall. *Visceral* pertains to the internal organs in the body's various cavities. Somatic sensation is carried to the dorsal gray horn cells of the spinal cord, then to the spinothalamic tract, and eventually to the cerebral cortex. Although the autonomic nervous system is an efferent system—that is, it carries impulses *from* the central nervous system—pain sensations from the viscera apparently course along the autonomic system. Through that system, these sensations from deep-lying structures reach the spinal cord by way of the dorsal roots and then continue along the same pathways as sensations from the skin and superficial body structures. Pain impulses are also carried by the cranial nerves to the central nervous system. There is integration of the sensory impulses of pain along its entire central nervous system route, but the highest level of integration occurs in the cortex.

The phenomenon of *referred pain,* that is, pain in an area removed from that in which stimulation has its origin, has been well-described as follows:

> The afferent neurons that conduct such (pain) impulses from receptors in the viscera to the sinal cord come in contact with central neurons in the spinal cord whose axons form the lateral spinothalamic tracts. Some of these impulses, such as those from serous membranes, have a private pathway to the brain, somewhat like a private telephone line. Other impulses are not so fortunate; being on a party telephone line, they must share the central neurons with impulses from cutaneous areas. Thus, the axons of the central neurons do double duty by conducting impulses from visceral pain receptors and from cutaneous pain receptors to the same areas in the thalamus and the cerebral cortex. This arrangement is called convergence, and sometimes it can lead to confusion as you will see.
>
> In the first case, in which there is a private wire to the cerebral cortex, the pain can be localized accurately as it is projected to the point of stimulation with ease. As an example of this, the patient with pleurisy can point to a certain spot where he experiences a sensation of pain on the chest, and the physician will hear a friction rub over this area, which means that the pleural membrane is inflamed in this particular spot.
>
> In the second case, in which there is a party line, the sensation of pain is aroused in the brain as usual. However, it is projected to the cutaneous area from which impulses come to the same area in the brain. This happens since cutaneous pain is of more frequent occurrence than visceral pain, and the brain projects over the well-trod path. This phenomenon is called *referred pain,* which means that pain from a viscus is referred to a related cutaneous area.
>
> The cutaneous areas to which visceral pains are referred are of great diagnostic importance. In angina pectoris (due to lack of oxygen in the heart muscle), the pain is referred to the left shoulder and down the left arm, instead of to the heart, where the difficulty really lies. In pneumonia the pain often is referred to the abdomen, and in some cases may be confused with appendicitis.*

Figure 18–1 illustrates the cutaneous areas to which pain from various organs is usually referred.

The interpretation of pain is of a highly personal nature. An individual learns to know what causes unpleasantness for him and what he interprets as pain. His interpretation is influenced by his background, such as how he has experienced and dealt with pain in the past and what cultural factors have taught him about pain. Through past experiences, he also learns to differentiate among the various types of pain and to attach certain words to describe it, such as the pain of burning, pinching, and stretching, and pain that for him is severe, slight, dull, intense, and so on.

The *gate control theory* of pain is related to the conduction of painful stimuli. The theory suggests that certain nerve fibers, those of small diameter, conduct excitatory pain stimuli toward the brain, but nerve fibers of a large diameter appear to inhibit the transmission of pain impulses from the spinal cord to the brain. There is a gating mechanism which is considered to be located in substantia gelatinosa cells in the dorsal horn of the spinal cord. The exciting and inhibiting signals at the gate in the spinal cord determine the impulses that eventually reach the brain. The brain also appears to influence the gating mechanism. Past experiences and learned behaviors, which are interpreted by the brain, have the effect of regulating or adjusting the eventual behavioral responses to pain. This helps to explain why similar painful stimuli are interpreted differently by different people. While not everyone

---

*Chaffee, Ellen E. and Greisheimer, Esther M. *Basic Physiology and Anatomy.* J. B. Lippincott Company, Philadelphia. Edition 3. 1974. pp. 234–235.

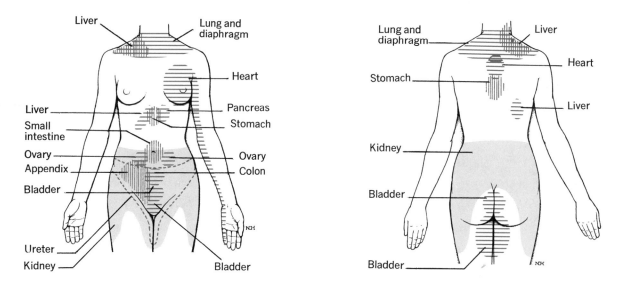

Figure 18–1 These figures, representing the anterior (left) and posterior (right) views of the body, illustrate areas to which various organs refer pain. (Chaffee, Ellen E. and Greisheimer, Esther M. *Basic Physiology and Anatomy*. Edition 3. J. B. Lippincott Company, Philadelphia, 1974. p. 234.)

accepts the gate control theory, it has been widely discussed in nursing, and specific nursing measures presented later in this chapter are believed to be effective because of this gating mechanism.

Stimuli for Pain

When the threshold of perception for pain has been reached and when there is injured tissue, it is believed that the injured tissue releases chemicals that excite nerve endings. A damaged cell releases histamine which excites nerve endings. Lactic acid accumulates in tissues injured by lack of blood supply and is believed to excite nerve endings and cause pain. Receptors in the skin and superficial organs, although incapable of responding selectively, are stimulated by mechanical, thermal, chemical, and electrical agents. Friction from bed linens and pressure from a cast are mechanical stimulants. Sunburn and cold water on a tooth with caries are thermal stimulants. An acid burn is the result of a chemical stimulant. The jolt of a static charge is an electrical stimulant.

Stretching of the hollow viscera, pulling on the omentum, and muscle spasms result in pain. Some investigators believe that at least some of the deep-lying organs have their own individual pain receptors, the uterus being an example. Some organs, such as the lungs, are insensitive to pain.

There are essentially three responses the body makes to pain: voluntary, involuntary, and emotional or psychic.

Voluntary Responses to Pain

Voluntary responses are muscle reactions that trigger efforts to remove the painful stimulus. It is a kind of fight-or-flight reaction that spells protection or defense. One kind of reaction is removing the hand hurriedly from a hot object. Grimacing and pacing the floor are also voluntary responses. Another kind of reaction is placing the injured part in a position that tends to relieve pain and by keeping the muscles rigid to maintain that position in efforts to avoid further injury. An example is to pull the knees up to the abdomen when abdominal pain is severe. These voluntary responses are protective in nature; also, through cognizance of pain, one remembers its causes and makes voluntary and purposeful attempts to avoid them in the future.

Involuntary Responses to Pain

Involuntary responses, often called autonomic responses, also are protective in nature, in that they increase the body's alertness to pain and promote organic homeostasis. In other words, the body prepares for emergency action, as described in the fight-or-flight phenomenon. Involuntary responses include increases in perspiration, blood pressure, pulse and respiratory rates, pupil dilation, muscular tension, and an increase in the output of adrenalin. The physiology of these involuntary responses teaches how each person prepares the body for necessary action when a threat to its integrity exists.

Emotional Responses to Pain

The emotional responses to pain have a wide and varying threshold among individuals. A person's previous experience with pain and his racial, cultural, and religious backgrounds all play a part. For example, in certain cultures weeping, crying loudly, and other overt expressions of distress are part of the pain phenomenon. In other cultures, this behavior may be considered unacceptable. Personality characteristics also influence pain responses. Highstrung, neurotic persons in general have a low threshold of reaction, while stoic individuals appear to have a high threshold.

Pain is almost always accompanied by anxiety and fear, and sometimes anger. Many persons are anxious and fearful of having illness that may be fatal or that may cause handicaps, when pain is present. These emotional responses tend to intensify the reactions to pain. Under these conditions, a vicious cycle forms that may be difficult to break. Increased irritability, depression, feelings of loneliness, fatigue due to poor resting, and anorexia often add to the problem of relieving pain. Anxiety and apprehension which almost always accompany pain are forms of action to escape threat when they are interpreted as the body's call for help.

Emotional reactions also help explain why some persons experience pain that appears to be without physiological cause or why some tend to complain of pain more than others when circumstances are similar. While still recognizing that the pain is indeed real as reported by the patient, can pain help to relieve a person's feelings of guilt or serve as a way to gain attention and relieve loneliness?

GENERAL PRINCIPLES OF PAIN AND ITS CONTROL

Some general principles of pain can be used to guide various intervention measures when the patient complains of pain.

Pain is a subjective and a personal experience, more often unpleasant and associated with anxiety but occasionally giving rise to ultimate pleasure for some persons. One human being cannot accurately assess the type and intensity of pain that another human being is experiencing. The nurse can only observe a patient and deduce and acknowledge that pain is present from the patient's verbal and nonverbal behavior. Thus, the nurse can assume a patient is in pain when he moans and flexes his legs sharply on his abdomen. Pain can also be detected by the body's involuntry reactions to pain, such as increased pulse and respiratory rates, perspiration, and dilated pupils. Whether signs and symptoms are present or not, when the patient states he has pain, the nurse acknowledges that he is experiencing the pain he describes.

While most pain is unpleasant and is associated with misery and stress, some individuals appear to experience pleasure and use pain to meet certain psychosocial needs. As was suggested earlier, pain may bring the attention a lonely person craves. Many times, the nurse can help meet the patient's needs in other ways so that pain becomes unnecessary. For example, visiting and staying with a patient who is lonely may be sufficient to overcome the discomfort of which he complains. In certain instances, behavior modification may be used when pain is being used to meet psychosocial needs, as will be described later in this chapter.

Cultural influences may teach some persons that to display signs of pain is to display personal weakness. Stoicism and self-control are virtues in such instances. On the other hand, outward behavioral displays when pain is present are accepted in other cultures.

Anxiety is almost always present when pain is anticipated or being experienced. The threat of an unknown is ordinarily more devastating and anxiety-producing than a threat for which one has been prepared. Studies have indicated that patients who had teaching preoperatively about what to expect postoperatively did not require as much medication for pain as did patients having similar operative procedures but who were not taught preoperatively. Admittedly, some preoperative teaching includes measures to minimize pain, such as learning how to splint an abdominal incision when the patient is coughing. This type of teaching notwithstanding general postoperative pain appeared to be less in the patient prepared for what to expect.

Anxiety tends to increase the perceived intensity of the pain. In such instances, nursing care is directed toward helping reduce anxiety. For example, anxiety generally decreases when the patient feels the nurse cares about him and is available to help and support him. Experience has demonstrated that patients who feel confident in health personnel caring for them do not require as much therapy for the relief of pain as those who are less confident. Without confidence, nothing seems to work. With it, often amazing results have been obtained using measures that ordinarily are only modestly effective.

An article given in the references at the end of this unit, written by Moss and Meyer, describes that reduction of a patient's pain occurred following certain nurse-patient interactions. After introductions to initiate the interaction, the process included discussing pain with the patient, suggesting various pain-relieving measures other than medications, and allowing the patient to decide on the method of relief. In the experimental group of adult patients with moderate pain, most of them experienced relief with this type of nursing care. In another article, written by McCaffery and Moss, the authors describe discussing pain with the patient, remaining with the patient, and providing touch as important tools for obtaining comfort.

Pain is not a pure but a mixed sensation and occurs in varying degrees. It is associated with other sensations, such as the sensation of stretching, pulling, pressure, squeezing, heat, or cold. The following are some commonly used terms to describe the quality of pain:

Sharp: Quick, sticking, and intense.

Dull: Not as intense or acute as a sharp pain, possibly more annoying than painful.

Diffuse: Covering a large area. Usually, the patient is unable to point to a specific area without moving his hand over a large surface, such as the entire abdomen.

Shifting: Moving from one area to another, such as from the lower abdomen to the epigastric region.

Intermittent: Coming and going. It may or may not be regular.

Others are sore, stinging, pinching, cramping, aching, stabbing, gnawing, and cutting.

Words used to describe the intensity of pain usually include severe, moderate, and slight or mild. The intensity is, of course, described by the patient although nonverbal and involuntary physiological signs help the nurse assess intensity.

Generally speaking, pain correlates with the intensity of the stimulation. Usually, the more intense the stimulation, the more likely it will produce pain and the more likely the pain will be severe. For example, there normally is pressure from a cast on the body part where it has been applied. The sensation of the pressure is not painful until it increases to the threshold of pain perception. Generally, it will increase sharply when injury to the tissue due to pressure of the cast occurs.

There are various ways in which pain stimuli can be altered. Removing the cause of pain is ideal and sometimes possible. Ways of doing this include removing or loosening a tight binder if permissible; seeing to it that a distended bladder is emptied; taking steps to relieve constipation and/or flatus; changing the patient's position in bed, and giving him a back rub if muscles have become tense and sore; and changing soiled linen that may be irritating the skin. It is often the nurse who identifies a source of pain that can be remedied with relative ease.

There are other factors that may contribute to discomfort and removing the source often promotes comfort. The hungry or thirsty patient may need a snack or a drink to feel more comfortable. Fatigue tends to increase sensitivity to pain, and promoting rest with measures as discussed later in this chapter is helpful. If the source of pain is an exuding wound, a soiled wet dressing may be the source of trouble and changing it will promote comfort. For the patient uncomfortable with a cast after the fracture of an extremity, elevating the extremity may relieve pressure sufficiently to promote comfort. The patient in pain usually feels more comfortable when the environment is quiet and restful. Taking steps to eliminate unnecessary noise and glaring lights is helpful. Sometimes the nurse may want to speak with visitors who may be tiring the patient in pain. These measures are also useful when caring for patients in their homes. Many other chapters in this text offer still other suggestions for decreasing or removing pain stimuli and thereby alleviating discomfort.

Certain drugs are useful to reduce the intensity of painful stimuli. Drugs that decrease smooth muscle spasms in the gastrointestinal tract and those that decrease contractions of skeletal muscles reduce discomfort. Atropine sulfate is an antispasmotic and is often used for spasms associated with spastic colitis. An example of a skeletal drug relaxant is methocarbamol (Robaxin).

It has been observed that pain may be present without injury and may not be present with injury. Therefore, tissue injury does not necessarily accompany pain in all instances. For example, tissue injury is present when the patient experiences pain due to a first- or second-degree burn. On the other hand, while physiological changes occur, tissue injury or destruction is not necessarily present when the patient has a headache due to psychological tension. In addition, intensity of pain may not accurately relate to the seriousness of a particular condition giving rise to the pain. Thus, the patient may not experience pain until the ravages of a malignancy are beyond control, while the severe pain that usually accompanies a bunion is not generally in keeping with the degree of pathology involved.

Stimulation of sensory receptors and intactness of their nerve supply are neither necessary nor sufficient conditions for pain. It would seem that a receptor for pain and a nerve route that eventually carries the impulse to the brain is necessary when pain is present. Yet, it is well-known that this is not always necessary. The pain that is often referred to an amputated leg where receptors and nerves are clearly absent is a very real experience for the patient. This type of pain is called *phantom pain* and is without demonstrated physiological or pathological substance. The person who is hypnotized can describe pain when there has been no stimulation to produce pain.

Consciousness and attention are necessary to experience pain. The unconscious patient does not perceive pain even though a painful stimulus may be present. Conscious attention appears to be necessary in order to experience pain and preoccupation with other things has been observed to distract from pain. For example, soldiers severely wounded while under fire often indicate that they felt little pain until the excitement of battle subsided. Players injured during the exciting moments in a competitive game may be unaware of an injury and pain until the game is completed. Making a loud noise, gripping an object, such as the dentist's chair, clenching the jaws, or experiencing pain elsewhere in the body are distracting and can alter perception of pain.

Numerous techniques are available to the nurse that help distract the person from his pain. The techniques themselves do not necessarily alter the painful stimulus, but they act to distract attention that tends to focus on the self and the pain. The following are some ways of distracting persons:

- A child is given his favorite toy to distract attention during a procedure ordinarily associated with pain.

- A patient in pain is engaged in a conversation on a subject of particular interest to him.

- Watching television or listening to the radio can divert attention from discomfort.

- Music has been found to be a distraction from pain for the music lover.

- Reading often distracts from pain.

- Playing a game, such as cards or checkers, takes attention away from pain.

- Using the words, discomfort and uncomfortable, when speaking to the patient takes his mind off such words as pain and painful.

- Busying oneself with a hobby tends to take the mind off discomfort.

The ingenious nurse can find many other distractors that will assist those suffering with pain. In general, one needs many more distractors and a greater variety when helping those who are suffering from chronic pain than with those experiencing pain that is of a short duration.

Biofeedback consists of a training program that helps an individual control certain aspects of his autonomic nervous system. The technique is based on the theory that man has the capacity to accept an active role in helping to solve health problems when he can learn how to achieve some control over what are ordinarily considered involuntary responses of the body. Several types of instruments are used to monitor various physiological functions, such as brain wave activity, respiratory rates, blood pressure, muscular tension, and blood flow. The person learns to reproduce changes in these functions while monitoring his own body activities.

For instance, migraine headaches have been effectively controlled by many persons who have been taught techniques of biofeedback. The pathophysiology of migraine is not clearly understood; however, when the person has learned through biofeedback to alter the blood flow from the head to the hands, the headache is relieved in many instances. The principles of pain control utilized in biofeedback include distracting the person's attention from the pain by concentrating on something else and helping the person to relax. Another beneficial aspect appears to be the sense of self-control which the person develops over his pain.

The gate control theory of pain was discussed earlier in this chapter. It is known that cutaneous nerve fibers are large diameter fibers carrying impulses to the central nervous system. When stimulated, pain is believed to be controlled by closing the gating mechanism in the spinal cord. Hence, touch using such practices as rubbing the patient's back and holding his hand often relieve pain. According to the gate control theory, the relief from discomfort occurs because many pain impulses do not reach the brain when the gating mechanism is closed, and therefore, cannot reach the brain for perception.

Acupuncture is a technique that utilizes long thin needles to prick specific parts of the body to produce insensitivity to pain. After they are inserted into the body, the needles are twirled or used to conduct a mild electrical current. The technique was developed in China and has been used for centuries in many Oriental countries. It has not been widely accepted in the Western world but is being investigated as a possible tool to help control discomfort. The relief of pain by acupuncture is generally explained on the basis of the gate control theory. The needles are believed to stimulate large diameter nerve fibers and, thereby, the gating mechanism is closed and pain impulses do not reach the brain for perception.

The Lamaze method to prepare women for childbirth is used to ease the pain associated with labor and delivery. In addition to their relaxing effect, breathing techniques which the mother is taught to use during labor are distracting. Also, the mother is taught to focus and concentrate on an object in the room during a uterine contraction. The object, ordinarily brought from home, may be a mobile, a picture, or any other object that the mother may choose. Women report less discomfort using the Lamaze method which uses the technique of distraction from the self and pain than most women who have not been taught this technique.

Hypnosis is a technique that produces a subconscious condition accomplished by suggestions made by the hypnotist. It has been used successfully in many instances for the control of pain. The person's state of consciousness is altered by suggestion so that he does not perceive pain as he normally would. It also alters the physical signs seen when pain is present, according to many hypnotists. Many persons can be taught *autohypnosis,* that is, self-induced hypnosis, for the control of pain.

Biofeedback, acupuncture, and hypnosis are used by specially prepared persons. They are not recommended when administered by amateurs since there are certain dangers associated with each technique. However, the nurse will wish to be aware of these various techniques for controlling pain in order to answer persons who inquire about their use. The Lamaze method for the control of pain is more fully described in clinical texts that deal with the care of women during pregnancy, labor, and delivery.

An *analgesic* is a pharmaceutical agent that relieves pain. The agent relieves pain in doses that do not necessarily place the patient in a state of unconsciousness although sleep often follows the administration of an analgesic when discomfort is relieved. Analgesics function to reduce the person's perception of pain primarily by their action on the central nervous system. They also change the person's responses to discomfort.

The public in general is oriented to pain relief by the use of pharmaceutical agents. Any number of analgesics are available without prescription and the news media carry innumerable messages concerning drugs to relieve pain. Many people are not even aware that there are many other measures to relieve pain and view drugs as the only measure for relief.

When drugs are required and are used judiciously for the relief of pain, their administration is indeed indicated and desirable. However, using drugs as a substitute for good nursing care that includes other measures to relieve discomfort is an indefensible act for nurses who hold to high standards of care.

When pharmaceutical agents become necessary, they are usually used with greatest effect when administered before pain occurs or becomes severe. For example, changing the dressings on patients who have been severely burned is usually a very painful procedure. It is recommended that an analgesic be administered prior to the dressing change rather than waiting until the patient complains of pain. This same guide is used for helping the terminally ill patient who is experiencing pain, as will be described in Chapter 26.

There are certain analgesics which are *addictive.* When addiction occurs, the person develops a psychological and physiological dependency on a substance and has a need to increase the intake to obtain desired effects. Many narcotic-type drugs are addictive, such as morphine, codeine, and meperidine hydrochloride (Demerol).

Drug abuse with addiction is a major public health problem in society today. However, it does not usually occur when narcotics are used for a relatively short time, such as for a week or two, for the relief of acute pain and when the patient seeks pain relief and not the euphoric effects that narcotics produce. *Euphoria* is an unrealistic sense of well-being. When used judiciously, narcotics are an important adjunct in the relief of pain. Since drugs for pain are often ordered by the physician to be administered every three to four hours at the nurse's discretion, the nurse must be aware of the possibility of addiction. But avoiding their use because of fear does not represent good nursing care.

Among the first signs that addiction may be occurring is the need for ever-increasing dosages in order to relieve pain. A second sign that should alert the nurse to the possibility of addiction is that the patient appears to seek euphoria rather than the relief of pain. It is recommended that texts dealing with pharmaceutical agents and drug addiction be consulted for detailed information.

The term *placebo* is a Latin word meaning "I shall

please." It consists of an inactive substance that is often given to satisfy a person's demand for a drug. The person, unaware of the placebo's properties, will find it to be effective for the relief of pain because he perceives it will help make him comfortable and believes in the person administering it. It is an injustice to judge a person experiencing relief from pain after the use of a placebo as neurotic. Whatever its effect on the person, he wanted pain relief and had confidence in the person giving it to him.

The placebo has its place in health care. It is often helpful in preventing an addiction problem; offering relief from discomfort when an analgesic is contraindicated, such as during certain examinations that test brain functioning; and substituting an innocuous agent when a person seems completely dependent psychologically on drug therapies which may not be deemed necessary.

The use of any pharmaceutical agent for the relief of pain does not replace good nursing care. While they have their rightful place in the control of discomfort, the nurse should also incorporate other measures when caring for patients suffering with pain.

The severity of pain and its duration affect responses to pain. Mild pain experienced briefly may produce little or no behavioral responses while intense pain experienced briefly usually brings forth reflex action to escape the cause. Pain that continues for a relatively short time, such as for a few days or a week, is very often accepted by the patient without its being all-consuming. He expects relief and believes the cause is self-limiting. However, anxiety is ordinarily present. On the other hand, chronic pain tends to consume the entire person. It demands the patient's total attention so that he has limited resources to take care of other matters in daily living. It is physically and emotionally exhausting and tends to result in depression and irritability. Chronic fatigue usually accompanies chronic pain.

Pain is ordinarily aggravated when muscular tension and fatigue are present. A vicious cycle can easily develop when pain interferes with rest and relaxation since tension and fatigue will almost always aggravate discomfort. The rested and relaxed person can often cope with great discomfort which might be completely unbearable under circumstances of fatigue and tension. Nursing measures to promote relaxation, rest, and sleep are discussed later in this chapter.

The well-informed person is often better able to cope with distressing situations, such as pain. The nurse should share knowledge with the patient experiencing pain to the extent possible as an aid in promoting comfort. Involving the patient in a pain control program, as mentioned earlier, is recommended. Teaching about pain that can be anticipated, the nature of the pain to be expected, and the usual duration are indicated. Many persons fear pain from procedures that are not uncomfortable and explanations should be included in a teaching program for these people. Such procedures include the electrocardiogram examination, ultrasound for imaging soft tissues, and electroencephalography.

Sometimes, assisting the patient to understand the cause of his pain and its function is helpful in reducing it. Or, helping the patient to know that it is usual to have pain and acceptable to express it may be important. Often these measures are also effective for reducing anxiety associated with pain. In many situations, teaching about pain should include family members in order that they understand and may help the person in pain too.

Behavior modification techniques may be used, especially when the patient's history suggests that psychosocial influences are present when pain is experienced. Thus, the person who has learned that he receives attention when he complains of pain may suffer until his psychosocial needs for attention, love, and affection are met. Pain can also be used to escape unpleasant situations. The person who dislikes a class at school may conveniently avoid the class with the socially acceptable excuse that he suffers from a severe headache. In such situations, undesirable behavior is ignored while desirable behavior that is not associated with discomfort is rewarded. Behavior modification was discussed in Chapter 8, and the reader is encouraged to review that chapter for further guides to its use.

PAIN AND THE NURSING PROCESS

Inasmuch as a patient's background is an important influence on the pain he describes, the nurse learns about her patient by using the process of data gathering. Here are some typical questions to which the nurse will wish to find answers. What cultural factors may be playing a role in the patient's experience of pain? How much does the patient know about his present illness and of the pain he is experiencing? What was the pain's mode of onset and its duration? What types of pain has the patient experienced in the past? How did he react then? What environmental and personality factors may be influencing his reactions to pain? Can the family assist in attempting to understand the patient's reaction to pain? Answers to such questions will help the nurse to select measures that are likely to promote the patient's comfort.

In addition, the nurse will want to familiarize herself with the patient's health history, his diagnosis, and the physician's plan of therapy.

Various responses to pain have been given earlier. The nurse will study the voluntary, involuntary, and emotional responses the patient exhibits when assessing in order to determine the nature of the patient's pain and how it is influencing the activities of daily living.

The nurse next proceeds to planning care that is likely to offer the patient relief from the physical and emotional ravages of pain. She selects measures she feels will be most acceptable and effective for the patient from among the wide variety of nursing measures available to her. Frequently planning should include discussing the measures with the patient, as well as with family members.

Measures to relieve pain that are included in the patient's plan of care are implemented. A variety of measures are available and many have been discussed in this chapter. Here is a summary of important aspects when using nursing measures to relieve the patient's discomfort:

- Establish a helping relationship with the patient. An important element is that the nurse be with the patient and available to offer support and comfort.

- Provide sensory input in various ways. Measures include distracting the patient from himself and his pain and providing cutaneous input with touch. While sensory restrictions by eliminating unnecessary noise, bright lights, and so on are usually indicated, it is rarely helpful to leave the patient alone in an environment with little sensory input since he will then be more likely to focus on himself and his discomfort.

- Promote rest and relaxation, using measures described later in this chapter.

- Decrease or eliminate painful stimuli to the greatest extent possible.

- Teach the patient and his family about pain, including explanations concerning how measures being used will help to relieve discomfort. Teaching techniques should be varied and, in certain instances, may include techniques of behavior modification.

- Use pharmaceutical agents as necessary. These agents may include analgesics as well as placebos.

- Use the assistance of other personnel on the health team as necessary, and the patient's family members as well.

The parts of the nursing process and of the process as a whole are evaluated as described in Chapter 4.

DESCRIPTION AND CHARACTERISTICS OF SLEEP

The word rest has a very broad meaning: refreshing ease or inactivity after exertion; relief from anything that wearies, troubles, or disturbs. In this chapter, *rest* connotes a condition in which the body is in a decreased state of activity with the consequent feeling of being refreshed. For some, rest occurs while leisurely enjoying a break in the day's activities. For others, rest may not come until sleep.

There is no concise definition of *sleep*. This text will use the word to mean a state of relative unconsciousness. The scientist recognizes that sleep, contrary to most layperson's beliefs, is not a quiescent and passive state but rather a progression of repeated cycles, each representing different phases of body and brain activity. These cycles have been studied and analyzed with the help of the *electroencephalograph* which receives and records electrical currents from the brain. The depth of unconsciousness during sleep is not uniform. Rather, it fluctuates during the different stages of sleep. This is demonstrated when it is observed that varying degrees of stimuli produce wakefulness.

The depth of unconsciousness for the sensory organs also varies. It is greatest for the sense of smell, which may explain why home fires gain headway unbeknown to the sleeping occupants, who do not smell the smoke. The depth is least for pain and for hearing. This explains why ill persons often are wakeful, because pain frequently accompanies illness.

It is frequently said that sleep is required for the body's cells to restore themselves. However, there is no scientific evidence to indicate that sleep is necessary for physiological repair. Some authorities have suggested that possibly sleep became part of man's daily living when he was a cave dweller. Man sought the safety of the cave at night to protect himself from his environmental enemies. He foraged for his food during the day when he could better escape his natural predators. The purpose of sleep was one of survival. Or, did the habit of sleeping develop when man had nothing better to do after he had found the food he needed during the day? It has been noted that animals that sleep a great deal require only a few hours to gather their food while those that sleep little need more time to find enough food to meet their needs. While the exact purpose of sleep is not clear, we know that sleep is required for well-being and that sleep deprivation is accompanied by conditions that can be devastating to the person experiencing it. Hence, no matter what its purpose, sleep is an important part of any healthful regimen to promote well-being.

REM Sleep and NREM Sleep

Research illustrates that there are two major states of sleep: rapid eye movement, called *REM* or Stage I-*REM;* and nonrapid eye movement, called *non-REM* or *NREM.*

During the REM state, it has been observed that the eyes tend to dart back and forth, respirations increase, the hearbeat becomes more rapid, and blood pressure increases or fluctuates. Body temperature and the basal metabolism rate increase and muscle twitchings are common. If persons are awakened during this state, they almost invariably report that they have been dreaming. In fact, many researchers now state that everyone dreams; those who state they do not simply are unable to recall dreams they had.

The REM state of sleep is sometimes called paradoxical sleep because it seems as though the sleeping person is close to wakefulness. Yet, it is more difficult to arouse a person during REM sleep than during NREM sleep. In normal adults, the REM state consumes 20 to 25 percent of a person's nightly sleep.

NREM sleep consists of four stages, I through IV. Stages I and II, consuming approximately 5 and 50 percent respectively of a person's sleep, is light sleep and the person can be aroused with relative ease. Stage III

sleep and Stage IV, or *delta,* sleep are deep sleep states during which time blood pressure, pulse and respiratory rates, and oxygen consumption fall to low average values.

During a person's nightly sleep, it has been demonstrated that he normally goes through the four NREM stages and the REM Stage in a circular order but with some cyclic variations. An individual usually has four or five REM periods, and these periods tend to become longer as morning approaches. Also, ordinarily more sleep occurs in the delta stage in the first half of the night, especially if one is tired or has lost sleep. These findings confirm the old saying that sleep before midnight is the best sleep since proportionately more is spent in deep sleep early in the night than toward morning when more REM sleep occurs.

Figure 18–2 illustrates a normal sleep pattern for young adults, as just described. Variations in the sleep cycle are observed according to age, as Figure 18–3 on page 424 illustrates and as its caption explains.

The hypothalamus has control centers for several involuntary activities of the body, one of which is concerned with sleeping and waking. Injury to the hypothalamus may cause a person to sleep for abnormally long periods.

The reticular formation is found in the brain stem. It extends upward through the medulla, the pons, the midbrain, and thence into the hypothalamus. It is composed of many nerve cells and fibers. The fibers have connections that relay impulses into the cerebral cortex and into the spinal cord. The reticular formation facilitates reflex and voluntary movements, as well as cortical activities related to a state of alertness. During sleep, the reticular system experiences few stimuli from the cerebral cortex and the periphery of the body. Wakefulness occurs when the reticular system is activated with stimuli from the cerebral cortex and

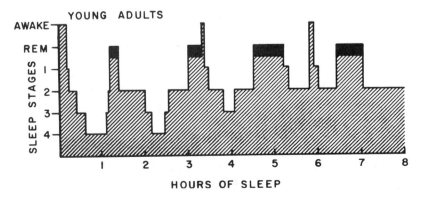

Figure 18–2 Nocturnal sleep pattern in young adults. Note the absence of Stage IV and the decreased length of NREM periods during the latter part of the night, and the short first REM period. (From Kales, A., ed.: Sleep: Physiology and Pathology. p. 20. Philadelphia, J. B. Lippincott, 1969.)

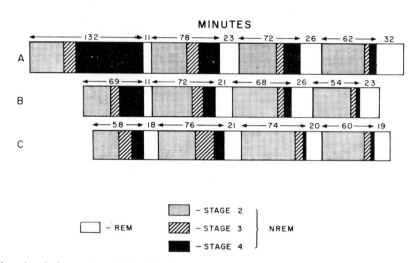

Figure 18–3   NREM-REM cycles during nocturnal sleep for three age groups (first four cycles). A, 8 children, mean age 8.4 years; B, 15 young adults, mean age 26.6 years; C, 15 normal elderly, mean age 77 years. The figure is arranged so that the onset of the first REM period coincides for the three groups. Differences in amount of Stage IV sleep apparently account for these striking differences in the length of the first NREM period. The decline in Stage IV sleep in the normal elderly may also permit the relatively long first REM period found in this group. In general, age exerts considerable effects on the durations of the sleep cycle components without greatly affecting the number of cycles. (From Kales, A., ed.: Sleep: Physiology and Pathology. p. 45. Philadelphia, J. B. Lippincott, 1969)

from periphery sensory organs and cells. For example, an alarm clock wakens us from sleep to a state of consciousness when we realize that we must prepare for work. Sensations of pain, pressure, noise, and so on, will produce wakefulness via periphery organs and cells. Wakefulness, then, is activated by the cerebral cortex and body sensations; during sleep, stimuli are minimal.

Factors Influencing Sleep and Well-Being

For no known reason, eight hours of sleep every night has been the accepted standard, despite obvious variances shown in the general population. There is no rigid formula concerning normal periodicity and duration of sleep. It is important, however, that each person follow a pattern of rest that will maintain well-being.

Despite variations, some generalities can be stated. On the average, infants sleep from 14 to 20 hours each day. Growing children require from 10 to 14 hours of sleep. Adults average seven to nine hours although a four-hour range has been observed in many normal adults. Those who are able to relax and rest easily, even while awake, often find that less sleep is needed, while others may find that more sleep is required in order to overcome fatigue. The sleep patterns of older persons vary as much as those of younger persons. However, the sleep of the elderly is less dependable; their sleeping system is fragile and they are less capable of coping with changes in their usual sleep patterns.

Evidence indicates that there are "larks" and "owls" among our population. "Larks" experience their greatest peaks of energy early in the morning and prefer an early bedtime hour. The opposite is true of "owls." "Larks" are often noted to be physical and the outdoor type while "owls" tend to lean toward nonphysical activity and greater social involvement. There is no generally accepted theory concerning why some people are "larks" and others are "owls." However, there is no indication that either of these patterns is better than the other. But studies show that there are often extra strains on marriages when the mates are out-of-phase with each other, and better than average coping abilities seem necessary for compatibility.

Certain diseases increase sleep needs, such as many of the infectious diseases. Persons with infectious hepatitis require more hours of sleep to overcome fatigue than they would ordinarily. Persons who are exposed to many emotional and physical stressors in their environment, do heavy physical work, or exercise strenuously tend to require more than average amounts of sleep for well-being. This is especially true if these activities are unusual, the person is overfatigued, or he suffers muscular discomforts from the activity.

Motivation influences sleep. A desire to be wakeful and alert overcomes sleepiness and sleep. For example, a tired person may be wakeful and alert when at a party or when attending an interesting play or concert. The opposite is also true—when there is minimum motivation to be awake, sleep generally follows.

Patterns of sleep are learned. For example, most people learn to sleep at night and to be awake and work during the day. However, many night workers learn to sleep equally well during the day once they develop the habit.

Fatigue can be considered a protective mechanism of the body and nature's warning that sleep is necessary. Fatigue is normal. However, chronic fatigue is abnormal and is often a symptom of illness. A person who complains of chronic fatigue should be advised to seek health care.

SLEEP DEPRIVATION

Symptoms of total sleep loss occur in a relatively slow but predictable pattern, mounting as time goes on. As weariness begins, normal performance fades off with lapses in attention and concentration. Unpleasant sensations, such as blurred vision, glazed and itching eyes, nausea, and headache are common symptoms of fatigue. Hallucinations and illusions eventually become vivid, and mental confusion and inability to determine reality occur. There may be a lack of memory, a decrease in intellectual effort, and an attitude of not caring what happens. The signs and symptoms of sleep deprivation indicate sleep is necessary for well-being even though we are unsure of its mechanism and purpose.

It appears that loss of sleep changes brain function and causes alterations in biochemical processes in the body. It is not known whether irreversible damage to body tissue results from prolonged or chronic sleep deprivation although animal experimentations suggest that the possibility may exist. Occasionally shortchanging one's sleep rarely produces dramatic changes in personality. However, a tired person is often irritable and depressed and may experience some hallucinating, such as seeing a fog around a light. Also, a tired person is often observed to perform less well on his job.

When dream deprivation occurs experimentally, that is, when persons are awakened and denied REM sleep, the subjects become irritable, insecure, and anxious. Inability to concentrate, often leading to poor judgment, usually can be observed with REM sleep

deprivation. Relationships with other people also suffer. Depression is a common mental symptom, and in extreme cases, a person's ethical standards have been known to deteriorate. Symptoms of psychoses have appeared in rational people after prolonged REM sleep deprivation. These same subjects, when allowed to sleep uninterrupted, experience more frequent REM periods, as if the body were trying to make up for losses.

Stage IV sleep can be said to be the sleep of the weary. If delta sleep is denied, we try to catch up on it, just as deprivation of REM sleep is followed by what appears to be an effort to catch up with it. It is not clearly known why delta sleep is important, but it is known to promote well-being when present in normal amounts.

COMMON DISORDERS OF SLEEP

Insomnia

Difficulty in falling asleep, intermittent sleep, and/or early awakening from sleep describe *insomnia*. Usually, persons complaining of insomnia have been observed to sleep more than they report. But the condition can lead to such distress as to cause further wakefulness. It is the most common of all sleep disorders and persons suffering from it are in need of help. Although there are some physical conditions that lead to wakefulness, it is believed that insomnia usually results from anxiety and stress.

Research has indicated that insomniacs tend to get more sleep and fall asleep faster than they think. However, this finding does not help the person with insomnia who suffers with what he believes is poor and inadequate sleep.

The following measures have been used with success by at least some insomniacs:

- Taking high-protein food before bedtime, such as cheese or milk. It is thought that tryptophan which is an amino acid from digested protein may help to induce sleep.
- Observing a regular bedtime hour and avoiding naps during the day or evening.
- Leaving the bed and bedroom when awake.
- Trying to sleep only when sleepy and not when wakeful.
- Avoiding stimulating activity before bedtime.
- Including exercise in each day but not before bedtime.
- Using relaxation and meditation techniques before attempting sleep.

The use of drugs has not proven to be a satisfactory solution for insomnia and may even make matters worse should dependency on drugs develop. In severe cases, skilled psychological management may be necessary.

Somnambulism

Somnambulism, or sleepwalking, is seen more commonly in children than in adults. Most children outgrow sleepwalking. It has been observed that somnambulism does not occur during REM sleep but during Stages III and IV of NREM sleep. It will be recalled that it is easier to waken a person in deep sleep than one in the dream state of sleep. Therefore, it is generally relatively easy to waken a sleepwalker. The danger for the somnambulist is that he may suffer injury, and measures to provide a safe environment are essential, such as using secure locks on doors. In at least some instances, drugs that suppress Stage IV sleep have been found effective in decreasing sleepwalking episodes; one such drug is diazepam (Valium). If a patient with a history of sleepwalking is admitted to an inservice health agency, a record should be made of this, and proper precautions to prevent injury should be taken.

Enuresis

Enuresis is involuntary urination. *Nocturnal enuresis* is involuntary urination that occurs while sleeping and *diurnal enuresis* is involuntary urination during wakefulness. Since nocturnal enuresis occurs during sleep, it is frequently called a disorder of sleep. It usually occurs during NREM sleep. The cause is unknown although some authorities now believe that it may not be only of psychological origin as was once thought. Most texts dealing with the care of children describe common measures to assist in preventing bed wetting, such as limiting fluid intake for several hours before bedtime, being sure that the bladder is empty prior to bedtime, and wakening the youngster during the night for voiding. Certain drugs have been found helpful. Those used are believed to increase bladder capacity.

Sleep Apnea and Snoring

Other than disturbing persons sharing the same bedroom, snoring is ordinarily not considered to be a sleeping disorder. However, snoring accompanied by apnea can present a problem.

Snoring is caused by an obstruction to the air flow through the nose and mouth. Enlarged tonsils and adenoids may be a contributing factor. The muscles in the back of the mouth relax and vibrate when air of respirations moves in and out. *Sleep apnea* refers to periods of no breathing between snoring intervals. The person may not breathe for periods of 15 seconds to as long as two minutes. During long periods of apnea, there will be a drop in the oxygen level of the blood and the pulse usually becomes irregular. The blood pressure often increases. The condition is most commonly seen in middle-aged men although women can also experience it, as do persons of other ages. It is often noted in persons with insomnia.

There is no known way to treat the problem of sleep apnea at present except for removing enlarged tonsils and adenoids when they appear to be aggravating the condition. Stimulating the person to a state of wakefulness is advised, especially in children and infants. In severe cases, a tracheotomy, which can be closed during the day and open during sleeping hours, may be necessary.

Fortunately, sleep apnea is not particularly common. Some investigators have theorized that possibly sleep apnea may explain certain unknown causes of death that occur during sleep.

Narcolepsy

Narcolepsy is a condition characterized by an uncontrollable desire to sleep. The person with narcolepsy can literally fall asleep standing up, while driving a car, in the middle of a conversation, or while swimming. It is considered to be a neurological disorder. The condition usually begins in susceptible persons during adolescence or early adulthood and continues through life.

Narcolepsy is sometimes confused with epilepsy, but there is no relationship between the two conditions. The brain waves of a person with narcolepsy are the same as for a normal sleeping person. There are also no blood gas or endocrine disturbances found in persons with narcolepsy.

Agrypnotic drugs are used to control narcolepsy. An *agrypnotic drug* is one that causes wakefulness. Such drugs include methylphenidate hydrochloride (Ritalin), amphetamines, such as dextroamphetamine sulfate (Dexedrine), and caffeine. Persons using drugs for narcolepsy are advised to take them faithfully because, if they are discontinued, the uncontrollable desire to sleep returns.

Sleep Talking

From observations, it appears that almost everyone talks in his sleep at some time. It occurs prior to REM sleep and rarely presents a problem unless the talking interferes with the rest of persons sharing the same room.

Sleep and Disease States

Investigations have demonstrated that sleep correlates with certain disease states. The pain frequently associated with diseases of the coronary arteries is often associated with REM sleep. Normally, gastric secretions are at a low level during the night, but they have been demonstrated to increase considerably during REM sleep in the patient with duodenal ulcers. Some research, especially when children were studied, has demonstrated that asthma attacks appear to occur less frequently during Stage IV sleep, and hence, efforts to increase Stage IV sleep is advisable. One method is to increase exercise of the nature the patient tolerates in order to assist in promoting extended periods of deep sleep.

GENERAL PRINCIPLES OF SLEEP AND SLEEPLESSNESS

The body requires periods of decreased activity in order to refresh itself. This principle, which recognizes rest as essential to well-being, becomes the basic guide to nursing practice in relation to rest.

Exactly why prolonged sleeplessness leads to ill effects is not known; however, the fact remains that sleep deprivation does produce changes that can markedly alter physical and mental functioning. When in doubt, it is best that the nurse err on the side of safety and employ efforts to promote rest as a need essential to well-being.

Rest and sleep are more likely to occur under conditions of relaxation. This principle can be stated in another way: stress and anxiety-producing situations tend to interfere with a person's ability to relax and to obtain sufficient rest for well-being. Illness and hospitalization are stress- and anxiety-producing situations for nearly everyone. Hence, nursing measures should be directed toward relieving them as much as possible. Such measures were described earlier in this chapter when anxiety related to pain was discussed, and in Chapter 10.

To *relax* means to become less rigid, to slacken effort, and to decrease tensions. One can relax without sleeping, but sleep rarely occurs until one is relaxed.

Relaxation is an individual matter. For some, purposeful effort may help. For example, a patient can be assisted to relax by having him take several deep breaths; on the last breath, encourage him to try to feel as limp as possible. Then, while the patient is in a comfortable position, instruct him to contract the muscles in his leg and then purposely allow the leg to go limp. Have him repeat this for the other leg, the gluteal muscles, each arm and shoulder, and the face, each time stressing that he must first purposely contract the muscles and then allow them to go limp. Gentle massage helps muscles to relax; therefore, massage of the back is often helpful in producing sleep.

Relieving monotony is in itself frequently relaxing. This is especially helpful to remember when caring for patients undergoing long convalescence. Suggestions for diversion may assist the nurse in promoting her patient's relaxation.

Some people have a bedtime ritual that tends to aid relaxation and promote sleep. For some, having something to eat is a *must*. A cup of coffee may relax one person despite the presence of caffeine, a central nervous system stimulant. Other persons may prefer milk or tea. Reading, listening to the radio, or watching television are common before-sleep activities. Children display similar idiosyncracies. A favorite stuffed animal or blanket, or bed-rocking are examples. Readiness for sleep is preceded by a personal hygiene routine for many persons, such as brushing the teeth, washing the hands and face, voiding, or taking a bath or shower.

There are no scientific explanations for bedtime rituals. The important thing is that they work for the persons using them. The wise nurse will be alert to the patient's bedtime rituals and make every effort to observe them as far as possible to aid in promoting relaxation and sleep. These rituals should appear in the patient's plan of care so that all health personnel can observe them.

Important for relaxation is a comfortable position in a comfortable bed. The bottom linen should be tight and clean. Upper linen, while secure, should allow freedom of movement and not exert pressure, especially over the legs and feet. Having the body in good alignment, as discussed in Chapter 17, is conducive to relaxation. For patients who must assume unusual positions because of their illness, ingenuity and skill are necessary in order to keep muscle strain and discomfort at a minimum. For example, the patient who must remain in the orthopneic position to aid breathing should be supported in a manner that relieves muscle strain, as with the use of a foot support, an arm rest, and possibly some support in the lumbar curve. Although most individuals relax best while lying down, other positions are not contraindicated.

A quiet and darkened room, with privacy, is relaxing for nearly everyone. In a strange environment, unfamiliar noises such as people walking or entering and leaving the room, and the closing of elevator doors bring complaints from most hospitalized patients. Although some of these sources are difficult for the nurse to control, every effort should be made toward reducing disturbances to promote relaxation and sleep.

Undue stimulation of the temperature receptors also interferes with rest. The temperature of the room, the amount of ventilation, and the quantity of bed covering are matters of individual choice, and the patient's wishes should be met whenever it is at all possible.

One of the greatest detriments to relaxation and sleep is pain and it is often a realistic complaint when illness is present. Nursing measures to promote relief from pain were discussed earlier.

The measures just described also apply to children. Approximately the same things interfere with rest in children as in adults. Emotional reactions are somewhat different to handle because most youngsters have not learned how to express fears and anxieties. Rather, they demonstrate these reactions by wakefulness, crying, irritability, and so on.

Picking up children, holding them securely, rocking them, and being readily available are measures that often appear to relieve their reactions to a strange environment and separation from parents. Also, leaving a night light near a frightened child is helpful. A child's fears are very real to him, and respecting them will aid in helping to promote relaxation and sleep.

The accusation often is made that a hospital is a poor place to rest. It may well be. Many patients already anxious and fearful because of illness suffer with added problems when they are surrounded by complicated and noisy equipment in a monotonous environment, are interrupted frequently with nursing and medical measures, and are bombarded with the noise of loudspeaker systems, talking, and housekeeping chores. Some patients who have presented symptoms that include hallucinations and illusions following a few days in sophisticated and complex care units where monitoring is often constant, experienced no such symptoms after a night or two of uninterrupted sleep in a private room. Common patient complaints are that they are awakened to take sleeping pills and are aroused at early morning hours to prepare for breakfast long before it is served.

The importance of sleep for physiological and psychological well-being is well-known even though possibly not as well-understood. Sleep loss can result in errors and tragedy as judgment fails. Today's living, requiring many split-second decisions, depends to a great extent on the rested person. It behooves the nurse to use measures wherever and whenever possible to promote rest and sleep for her patients. Also, the nurse will wish to observe sensible sleep habits for herself so that she can function effectively and safely.

Just as was true in helping persons in pain, developing a good nurse-patient relationship to promote relaxation and sleep is essential. Of special importance is that the patient feels the nurse cares and is readily available for extra help to promote relaxation and sleep.

Periodicity and duration of rest and sleep vary among individuals. As was true with pain, rest and sleep are individual matters. Some people require more than others; there are "good" sleepers and "poor" sleepers; and there are the restless and the quiet sleepers. Habits also apparently play a role in sleep patterns, and, as described earlier, rest and sleep are promoted when they can be observed. The sleeping person is just as much a whole and integrated person with a unique personality as is the awake person.

Just as quantity of sleep is important, the quality of sleep is also important to well-being. As discussion on the sleep cycle indicated, sleep that disallows for completing the circle of both NREM and REM sleep has been observed to decrease well-being. Some sleeping medications influence the length of both the NREM and REM states; for example, it has been found that most *hypnotic drugs,* that is, drugs used to induce sleep, suppress REM sleep. When these drugs are withheld after regular use, REM sleep increases in order to make up for the loss. The increased dreaming, often associated with nightmares, can be so distressing that persons are reluctant to give up the drugs once they have become accustomed to their use. Drugs that do not suppress REM sleep are preferred; one such drug is chloral hydrate, according to research. Some of the mild *tranquilizers,* which are drugs used primarily to reduce anxiety, promote sleep and reportedly do not interfere with REM sleep. An example is chlordiaze-poxide hydrochloride (Librium).

Because no one enjoys restless, interrupted sleep, and long periods of wakefulness, most patients accept a medication readily if they are anxious about how well they will sleep. Accepting a drug without a real need often starts patients off on habits that last long after an illness episode. Therefore, the nurse should attempt to promote sleep without the use of drugs whenever possible. If the patient is still unable to sleep, a medication may be offered. When the patient knows he can have a medication if necessary, he will often fall asleep naturally.

Hypnotics and tranquilizers are as subject to abuse as are pain-relieving drugs, and this misuse causes a community health problem also. There are certainly times when they are indicated. However, the nurse will wish to administer them judiciously and only when other measures to promote rest and sleep have not sufficed. It is recommended that texts dealing with pharmaceutical agents and drug abuse be consulted for more detailed information.

A well-informed person is often better able to cope with distressing situations, such as sleeplessness. The nurse should remember to include content on rest and sleep in her teaching programs. For both the ill and well person, rest and sleep have been found to be equally important to well-being. There have been many jokes and amusing anecdotes told about sleep, and much folklore, mystery, and magic have been associated with it. Helping patients and their families understand the nature of rest and sleep and their importance to well-being through teaching is an important nursing function.

Teaching should include such aspects as normal variations in sleep patterns and common measures to promote relaxation and sleep. When sleep disorders become a problem and common nursing measures are inadequate, the nurse can assist and teach by recommending the services of health professionals specially prepared to deal with them.

SLEEPLESSNESS AND THE NURSING PROCESS

Realizing that there are differences in rest patterns, the nurse begins data gathering by determining the patient's usual routines. It can be helpful also to inquire about the patient's activities that have tended to promote sleep in the past. For the acutely ill, for children, and for the elderly, conferring with family members is often helpful.

By observing a sleeping person carefully, one can determine when REM sleep is in progress by looking for the rapid eye movements. If the nurse finds it necessary to waken a patient for some reason, it is best not to waken him during the dream state if possible, since the importance of REM sleep has been demonstrated clearly.

A knowledge of signs and symptoms of sleeplessness and restfulness becomes the basis upon which the nurse assesses rest and sleep. These have been described earlier in this chapter.

The nurse proceeds to plan care that is likely to offer the person relief from sleeplessness. She selects measures which she believes will be most acceptable to the patient. Planning should include discussing measures with the patient, as well as with family members as indicated.

Measures to promote rest and sleep that are included in the patient's plan of care are implemented. A variety of measures are available and many have been discussed in this chapter. The following is a summary of important aspects when using nursing measures to promote rest and sleep:

- As was true when caring for the patient in pain, establish a helping relationship with the patient. Of special importance is that the nurse cares, is interested in the patient, and is available to offer support.

- Promote relaxation which is almost always necessary before sleep. Measures, such as using breathing exercises, purposely relaxing groups of muscles, relieving monotony, following the individual's personal bedtime rituals, helping the patient to be comfortable, providing a relaxing environment, and relieving pain, were described.

- Recognize that each individual is unique and measures to promote relaxation and sleep must be geared to the person and his habits.

- Teach the patient and his family concerning sleep, its importance to well-being, and the variations in sleep patterns that exist but fall within normal ranges.

- Use pharmaceutical agents as necessary to promote relaxation and sleep. These agents may include hypnotics as well as tranquilizers and placebos.

The parts of the nursing process and of the process as a whole are evaluated as described in Chapter 4.

CONCLUSION

Among the most common problems patients present are those related to the relief of pain and the promotion of sleep. While certain drug therapy may be indicated at times, the use of drugs does not eliminate the need for high-quality nursing care, including nursing measures to promote comfort and rest.

The number of over-the-counter remedies for relieving pain and promoting sleep are countless. Many have proven to be ineffective; others have been shown to be dangerous. Using them indiscriminately may delay medical attention the patient needs. Due caution and good judgment are important before using many of these products and the nurse will wish to assist patients when they are observed to be using them without discrimination.

SUPPLEMENTAL LIBRARY STUDY

1. Read the following article:

    Zelechowski, Gina Pugliese. "Helping Your Patient Sleep: Planning Instead of Pills." *Nursing 77,* 7:62–65, May 1977.

    What does the author consider as the vital first step in managing patients who have trouble sleeping? What complications did Linda develop as a result of four weeks of using hypnotics for sleep? List at least ten of the basic rules this author recommends to help patients get more sleep.

2. A study showed that nurses of different cultures vary in their perception of patients' pain, according to the following article:

    Davitz, Lois J., et al. "Suffering as Viewed in Six Different Cultures." *American Journal of Nursing,* 76:1296–1297, August 1976.

    What findings on stoicism of Orientals experiencing pain did this study reveal? Describe three similarities that cut across national groups which this study revealed related to pain. What basic proposition of the investigators was supported by this study's findings?

3. This chapter mentioned the dangers of drug abuse. Read the following article:

    Morgan, Arthur James. "Minor Tranquilizers, Hypnotics, and Sedatives." *American Journal of Nursing,* 73:1220–1222, July 1973.

    What are two attitudes the author describes that he feels are not conducive to the judicious use of medications to promote rest and reduce anxiety? What nursing measures does the author suggest the nurse use before administering pharmaceutical agents to control anxiety, stress, and sleeplessness?

4. Take the examination in the reference given below to evaluate your general understanding of pain:

    "Pain and Its Treatment." (Test Yourself) *American Journal of Nursing,* 77:983, June 1977.

19

BEHAVIORAL OBJECTIVES

When content in this chapter has been mastered, the student will be able to

Define the terms appearing in the glossary.

Describe five nutrients essential for health and their primary function in the body; indicate dietary sources for these various nutrients.

Discuss how food and fluid intake is normally regulated by the body.

List at least five cultural factors that frequently influence eating habits.

Summarize present opinion on the use of food additives and supplements.

Describe nursing responsibilities for serving food in health agencies and to patients at home.

List at least ten nursing measures that help to improve a patient's appetite.

List at least five measures that help the patient who is required to increase or limit his fluid intake.

Summarize how a patient is fed by gavage and discuss the nursing responsibilities for gastric gavage.

List at least five nursing measures to assist persons who have anorexia, nausea, and vomiting.

Summarize the nursing care of patients who have gastric and duodenal suction.

Describe how intake and output of various fluids are properly measured.

Outline essentials in a teaching program on nutrition.

Discuss teaching and helping the patient meet nutritional and fluid needs, using the nursing process as a guide.

Meeting Nutritional and Fluid Needs

GLOSSARY

Adipose Tissue: Body tissue containing masses of fat cells.

Anorexia: A loss of appetite or a lack of desire for food.

Antiemetic: A drug used to allay vomiting.

Appetite: The pleasant anticipation of food.

Basal Metabolism Rate: Heat production of the body at its lowest level of cell chemistry and of body activity.

Calorie: The amount of heat necessary to raise the temperature of 1 kilogram of water 1° C.

Coffee Ground Emesis: Vomitus containing dark brown particles that have the appearance of coffee grounds. It is a characteristic symptom of the patient with a bleeding peptic ulcer.

Emaciation: A condition characterized by leanness or thinness.

Emesis: The act of vomiting.

Eructation: A discharge of gas from the stomach through the mouth.

Feculent Vomitus: Vomitus containing contents from the small intestines. It is a characteristic symptom of the patient with a severe intestinal obstruction.

Food Additive: An ingredient added to food to improve color, flavor, consistency, or stability.

Food Supplement: A preparation added to the diet that adds nourishment to what is eaten.

Gastric Gavage: The introduction of nourishment into the stomach by mechanical means.

Hematemesis: Vomitus containing fresh blood.

Hunger: The unpleasant sensation associated with food deprivation.

Kwashiorkor: A state of extreme malnutrition due to severe protein insufficiency; caloric intake ordinarily falls within average normal ranges. *African*

Lumen: The inner open space of a tube.

Malnutrition: A condition characterized by a lack of necessary or proper food substances or improper absorption and distribution of food substances in the body.

Marasmus: A state of extreme malnutrition due to severe protein and caloric insufficiency.

Nausea: A feeling of sickness with a desire to vomit.

Nutrition: The total of processes involved in the taking in and utilization of food substances.

Pernicious Vomiting: Persistent and intractable vomiting.

Projectile Vomiting: The expulsion of vomitus with great force.

Regurgitation: Bringing stomach contents to the throat and mouth without vomiting effort.

Retching: Unproductive muscle movements that ordinarily produce vomiting.

Satiety: The feeling of having had enough to eat.

Thirst: The unpleasant sensation associated with water deprivation.

Vomiting: The forceful expulsion of gastric contents through the mouth.

Vomitus: Vomited matter.

INTRODUCTION

Food and its effects on the body have interested mankind for thousands of years. Only during the early decades of the twentieth century did nutrition become a science. Biochemistry and microchemical analysis have become useful tools in the study of food, its digestion and absorption, and metabolism.

Problems related to nutrition vary widely and usually have interrelated causes. Insufficient caloric and protein intake are major problems in many parts of the world, and usually, anyplace where poverty exists. Where people have the means to consume too many calories, as is true in many places in the United States, the problem is one of maintaining a balanced diet. Having too much food is in itself a problem for many people. Eating has many psychosocial implications also. To look only at an individual's diet without regard for his environment and his whole person and personality results in a distorted picture.

MAN'S NUTRITIONAL NEEDS

All body cells require adequate nutrition. Food is basic to life, and there are food substances essential to health. In other words, probably we could eat only what we like and remain alive, but if these foods did not contain the variety of nutrients needed by the cells of the body, physiological functioning would be impaired.

Nutrition is the total of processes involved in the taking in and utilization of food substances. The utilization of food involves the way nutrients are used by such processes in the body as growth, repair of tissue, and the maintenance of activities in the body as a whole.

The nutrients essential to health are carbohydrates, proteins, fats, vitamins, and minerals. Water is essential for maintaining fluid balance in the body. All of these are required to build and repair tissue, to furnish energy, and to make essential substances, such as enzymes and hormones. They are made available to the body by the process of digestion. The digestive process breaks them down mechanically by chewing and intestinal movements, and chemically, by oral and gastrointestinal secretions, so that they can be absorbed into the blood and the lymph.

Many nutritional needs have been fairly well-defined. We need a certain number of calories to meet energy requirements. We need specific constituents found in food to maintain health: water, protein, carbohydrates, fats, vitamins, and minerals. Of these needs water is the most urgent. We should also consider needs of palatability, availability, and the cost of food when trying to meet dietary requirements. For example, a person may be observed to need a higher protein intake than he has been getting. There is little benefit in suggesting that he eat more meat if he cannot afford to buy it or if meat is not readily available where he lives.

The constituents described below are necessary in a well-balanced diet. This can usually be accomplished with relative ease when the daily diet consists of servings of food selected from each of the four major food groups: milk and milk products, two servings; meat, including fish, poultry, eggs, and cheese, two servings; vegetables and fruit, four servings; and bread and cereals, four servings.

Calories

Heat is produced by the oxidation of food. It is a form of energy. Other forms of energy (mechanical, chemical, electrical) can also be expressed in terms of heat. If we measure the body's heat production, we can then ascertain the amount of food needed to produce that amount of heat or energy. Hence, food energy can be expressed in terms of heat.

The measurement for heat is called a calorie. A calorie is the amount of heat necessary to raise the temperature of 1 kilogram of water 1° C. We speak of food as having certain caloric value, meaning the food is capable of furnishing a specific amount of heat or energy to the body.

The heat production of an individual at the lowest level of cell chemistry and of body activity is called the basal metabolism rate. For an average adult male, the required calories to meet a basal metabolism rate is roughly 1,700; for a female, about 1,400. For many hours in every individual's day, metabolism does not go on at a basal or minimum rate because of normal activities in everyday living. Hence, intake of calories must be greater than the basal rate to produce sufficient energy to carry out these activities.

Food and caloric requirements vary among individuals. From birth to old age nutritional requirements continually vary. They are dependent on the demands of the body for growth and tissue repair and also are affected by various other factors, including the ones that follow.

The height, weight, and the sex of the individual influence caloric needs. All other things being equal, a husky 6-foot male weighing 190 pounds will need more calories than a 5-foot woman weighing 105 pounds. On the average, an adult male requires approximately 2,800 to 3,000 calories daily; a female, 1,800 to 2,100 calories daily. These requirements decrease with age.

Age is an important factor when considering caloric needs. At birth, the basal metabolism is approximately twice that of an adult. The rate gradually decreases with age. Hence, infants and young children require more calories proportionately than adults and the elderly. Infants of about six months of age need roughly 115 calories per kilogram of body weight. An infant of 5 kilograms, or about 11 pounds, would need 575 calories each day. If this need for calories existed for an adult weighing 60 kilograms, or 132 pounds, his daily caloric need would be over 7,000 calories! During the middle childhood years, caloric needs taper since growth and activity slow after about five or six years of age. During adolescence, when growth and activity spurt forward, more calories are required for health.

An individual's physical activity influences caloric requirements. Both the amount and the kind of activity must be taken into consideration. A person employed in heavy outdoor labor will require more calories than the sedentary office worker; the tennis player will need more than the chess player; and so on.

Climate influences caloric needs. Persons living in cold climates use up more calories than those living in hot climates. Various disease conditions cause the body to need more calories. The basal metabolism rate is greater in a person with an elevated body temperature, and hence, he will require more calories than one with normal body temperature. So also will the person who has suffered extensive tissue damage due to burns. Persons requiring prolonged bed rest and inactivity can suffer a loss of protein from their body and may require higher than average protein intake.

During pregnancy and lactation, there is approximately a 20 percent increase in the need for calories and a 50 percent increase in the need for calcium in the mother's daily diet. The iron requirement for women is higher than the iron requirement for men, especially during the child-bearing years.

Requirements also differ among individuals who would seem to have the same nutritional needs. There are differences in the way their foods are digested, assimilated, and used by the body.

Protein Requirements

Protein is especially important in maintaining and repairing body tissues. It is also required for the composition of many compounds in the body, such as hemo-globin, hormones, enzymes, and the plasma proteins of albumin, globulin, and fibrinogen. As will be described in Chapter 23, protein plays a vital role in one of the body's buffering systems. It breaks down into amino acids during digestion and then becomes human protein in the body. This nutrient provides the body with four calories per Gram.

Protein has great practical importance because it is generally the most expensive nutrient, except for legumes such as peas and beans. Protein is observed to be in shortest supply in most instances when malnutrition is present. It is found in both animal and vegetable foods. The presence of nitrogen, sulfur, and usually phosphorus in the chemical structure of proteins distinguishes them from carbohydrates and fats.

Meat is an important source of protein in the diet of most Americans. There is evidence that a low meat intake is conducive to health. For example, it has been found that malignant tumors of the colon occur more frequently in high meat-consuming countries, such as the United States and Canada, and less frequently in low meat-consuming countries, such as Japan and Chile. However, there are some who believe that it is the fat, not the meat, which may be related to malignancies of the colon. There also appears to be some evidence of a relationship between breast cancer and fat, or meat, intake. Research to date is hardly conclusive, but nurses will wish to keep up-to-date on additional findings of this nature.

Fat Requirements

Fats are the body's most concentrated source of energy. Nine calories are provided for each Gram of fat. Fat is an important food requirement as a source of essential fatty acids, as a vehicle for fat-soluble vitamins, and as an important contributor to the palatability of the diet. It is stored as *adipose tissue* which is tissue containing masses of fat cells. Adipose tissue acts as an insulator for the body and cushions and protects internal organs.

Cholesterol is derived from fat that is widely distributed in animal tissues and egg yolks. It has an important function in the skin by helping protect it from many chemicals and from abnormal evaporation and absorption of water. Cholesterol is also important in the formation of several steroid hormones, such as the adrenal corticoids, and of bile salts.

Fats are generally more expensive than foods high in carbohydrate content but cheaper than foods high in protein content. They provide a more concentrated form of energy than proteins or carbohydrates, but their high-caloric content is a disadvantage for persons wishing to lose weight.

Carbohydrate Requirements

Carbohydrates are the most readily available source of energy and the primary source of calories in most diets. They are also the least expensive source of food for most people. The body derives 4 calories from each Gram of carbohydrate.

Contrary to what many think, carbohydrates are important for other reasons than calories. For example, cellulose, which makes up much of the stems, leaves, and woody portion of plants, provides necessary bulk that helps digestion and elimination. Carbohydrates are essential for fat metabolism. When they are in short supply, the byproducts of fat metabolism accumulate in the body. Lactose, the milk sugar carbohydrate, promotes bacterial growth in the intestines which helps both elimination and digestion.

Most plants are primarily carbohydrates. Granulated sugar is pure carbohydrate. Extra carbohydrate in the diet can be stored and used when the body needs it. The liver stores excess in the form of glycogen; if there is still more excess, it can be changed into body fat in adipose tissue.

Minerals

In general, minerals are normally present in food in sufficient quantities; thus, a well-balanced, normal diet is rarely deficient of minerals. However, some create problems in certain circumstances. Salt may need to be limited when there is water imbalance. Calcium is necessary to build and maintain the skeletal system, especially during childhood, pregnancy, and lactation. When the body is short of calcium, the skeletal system will give up this mineral when required by other tissues. For example, the mother's skeletal system will give up calcium for fetal development and milk production if her diet is deficient in calcium during pregnancy and lactation.

Milk and milk products are a common source of calcium for persons in this country. In recent years, it has been found that a large number of individuals have symptoms of abdominal distention, flatulence, diarrhea, and pain caused by milk and milk products. As many as two-thirds of blacks, American Indians, Mexican-Americans, Orientals, and persons of Mediterranean extraction have been estimated to have various forms of lactose intolerance. Taking milk and milk products causes the symptoms described and they subside when milk is avoided. For persons with lactose intolerance, substitution of foods, such as green vegetables, to supply calcium requirements needs to be encouraged.

Iron deficiency can be serious because iron is essential for the formation of hemoglobin. Important trace minerals in the diet include phosphorus and iodine. When iodine is in short supply in the diet, the use of iodized salt is recommended.

Table 19–1 lists common minerals required by the body, their primary functions, and chief dietary sources.

TABLE 19–1 Common minerals needed by the body, their chief functions, and common dietary sources

MINERAL	CHIEF FUNCTIONS	COMMON DIETARY SOURCES
Calcium	Formation of teeth and bones Neuromuscular activity Blood coagulation Cell wall permeability	Milk products
Phosphorus	Buffering action Formation of bones and teeth	Eggs Meat Milk
Iodine	Regulation of body metabolism Promotes normal growth	Seafoods Iodized salt
Iron	Component of hemoglobin Assists cellular oxidation	Liver Eggs Meat
Magnesium	Neuromuscular activity Activation of enzymes Formation of teeth and bones	Whole grains Milk Meat
Zinc	Constituent of enzymes and insulin	Seafoods Liver

Vitamins

Vitamins are essential accessory food substances. They do not provide calories in any significant amount, but they play an indispensable role in a number of different processes necessary for health. They are organic in nature; they cannot be manufactured by the body; and they are important in maintaining normal tissue functioning.

Vitamins are either fat-soluble—A, D, E, and K—or they are water-soluble—C and the B-complex vitamins. The number of identifiable vitamins continues to grow as research becomes more sophisticated.

The exact daily requirement for some vitamins is not known. However, certain diseases that occur when vitamin intake is inadequate are well-described. Also, it is known that some disorders result from consuming too large quantities; for example, too much intake of vitamin D has been observed to be toxic to the body.

Within recent years, there has been much interest in the assertion that daily doses of vitamin C in much larger than the adult daily requirement of 60 mg. will help to prevent upper respiratory infections and strengthen arteries. Although some well-known scientists have supported the claims, proof following rigorous scientific investigation is lacking. Also, the safety of taking large doses of vitamin C over a prolonged period has not been established.

Table 19–2 on page 438 lists common vitamins, their primary functions, and chief dietary sources.

Water

From 75 to 80 percent of animal tissue is water. The water content of the body must be maintained at a fairly constant level in order to preserve health. It is important for the absorption of nutrients in the body and is the chief ingredient of extracellular fluids. It is an important constituent of body secretions and excretions. The role of water in the body will be discussed more fully in Chapter 23.

THE REGULATION OF FOOD AND FLUID INTAKE

The mechanism which makes one eat and drink the amount and kind of food and fluid required by the body is not clearly understood. Certain factors are known to play a part in the regulation of intake, but there may possibly be many more than the three usually identified: hunger, thirst, and satiety. *Hunger* and *thirst* are unpleasant sensations associated with food and water deprivation. *Satiety* is the feeling of having had enough to eat. Certainly, the influence of these factors varies too among individuals. The young and the active feel hungry often while the sedentary may rarely feel hunger pangs. It has been observed that any one or any combination of these three factors may be influenced by illness.

It is theorized that there are centers in the hypothalamus that regulate food intake. Experiments have shown that injury to one part of the hypothalamus results in overeating while injury to another part results in undereating.

It has been estimated that 15 to 25 percent of the population in the United States is above desirable body weight because of overeating. Overeating has been observed to relieve anxiety while those who are at average or below average weight tend to eat simply to satisfy hunger. Also, obese as well as underweight persons tend to eat more in the presence of boredom. In such instances, eating gives people something to do. While endocrine and genetic factors may often play a role, psychosocial factors certainly are important in determining one's weight also.

A great variety of diets to lose or gain weight are described in the layperson's literature. Many are eccentric and nutritionally unsound, especially those for persons who wish to lose weight. Weight loss after crash dieting is very often temporary since the person usually returns to the same eating habits that brought obesity in the first place. There are no reducing or weight-gaining foods but only different caloric content in various foods. For many people, the problem of obesity or thinness might well be mostly a problem of arithmetic and lack of knowledge concerning the body's caloric needs. This can be validated with relative ease by totaling the number of calories consumed each day by the obese person who states that he eats little but "it all goes to fat," or the thin person who states that he eats "well but cannot gain weight."

Obesity is no simple matter for overweight persons. It has been demonstrated rather conclusively that obesity plays an important part in premature death. In addition, it may be undesirable from the point of view of comfort and appearance.

The nurse counseling the obese person must begin by demonstrating acceptance of the individual and by recognizing that excess caloric intake can rarely be controlled without consideration of psychological as well as physical factors that contribute to the condition. The most efficient way to control obesity is through dietary discretion, exercise, and the change of eating

TABLE 19–2 Common vitamins needed by the body, their chief functions, and common dietary sources

VITAMIN	CHIEF FUNCTIONS	COMMON DIETARY SOURCES
A Fat-soluble Not destroyed by ordinary cooking temperatures	Growth of body cells Vision, healthy hair and skin, and integrity of epithelial membranes Prevents xerophthalmia, a condition characterized by chronic conjunctivitis	Animal fats: butter, cheese, cream, egg yolk, whole milk Fish liver oil and liver Green leafy and yellow fruits and vegetables
B_1 (Thiamine) Water-soluble Not readily destroyed by ordinary cooking temperatures	Carbohydrate metabolism Functioning of nervous system Normal digestion Prevents beriberi, a condition characterized by neuritis	Fish Lean meat and poultry Glandular organs Milk Whole grain cereals Peas, beans, and peanuts
B_2 (Riboflavin) Water-soluble Not destroyed by heat except in presence of alkali	Formation of certain enzymes Normal growth Light adaptation in the eyes	Eggs Green leafy vegetables Lean meat Milk Whole grain Dried yeast
B_3 (Niacin) Water-soluble	Carbohydrate, fat, and protein metabolism Enzyme component Prevents appetite loss Prevents pellagra, a condition characterized by cutaneous, gastrointestinal, neurological, and mental symptoms	Lean meat and liver Fish Peas, beans Whole grain cereals Peanuts Yeast Eggs Liver
B_6 (Pyridoxine) Water-soluble Destroyed by heat, sunlight, and air	Healthy gums and teeth Red blood cell formation Carbohydrate, fat and protein metabolism	Whole grain cereals and wheat germ Vegetables Yeast Meat Bananas Black strap molasses
B_{12} (Cyanocobalamin) Water-soluble	Protein metabolism Red blood cell formation Healthy nervous system tissues Prevents pernicious anemia, a condition characterized by decreased red blood cells	Liver and kidney Dairy products Lean meat Milk Salt water fish and oysters
B_c (Folic acid)	Protein metabolism Red blood cell formation Normal intestinal tract functioning	Green leafy vegetables Glandular organs Yeast
C (Ascorbic acid) Water-soluble Readily destroyed by cooking temperatures	Healthy bones, teeth, and gums Formation of blood vessels and capillary walls Proper tissue and bone healing Facilitates iron and folic acid absorption Prevents scurvy, a condition characterized by hemorrhagic condition and abnormal bone and teeth formation	Citrus fruits and juices Tomato Berries Cabbage Green vegetables Potatoes
D Fat-soluble Relatively stable with refrigeration	Absorption of calcium and phosphorus Prevents rickets, a condition characterized by weak bones	Fish liver oils, salmon, tuna Milk Egg yolk Butter Liver Oysters Formed in the skin by exposure to sunlight
E (Alpha tocopherol) Fat-soluble Heat stable in absence of oxygen	Red blood cell formation Protects essential fatty acids Important for normal reproduction in experimental animals, i.e., rats	Green leafy vegetables Wheat germ oil Margarine Rice
H (Biotin) Water-soluble Heat-sensitive	Enzyme activity Metabolism of carbohydrates, fats, and proteins	Egg yolk Green vegetables Milk Liver and kidney Yeast
K Fat-soluble	Production of prothrombin	Liver Eggs Green leafy vegetables Synthesized in the gastrointestinal tract by bacteria

habits. The diet should be well-balanced but limited in the amount of calories eaten. It is recommended that no person wishing to lose weight consume fewer than 1,200 calories daily without professional supervision. For many people, the will power to follow a reducing diet appears to be strengthened when people work together toward weight loss in groups. Techniques of behavior modification, as described in Chapter 8, have been used effectively for helping some overweight persons.

From a health and appearance point of view, being underweight is not as great a problem as is being overweight. Nevertheless, for the underweight person who is trying to gain weight, which may be important to him for the sake of appearance if for no other reason, the problem may be as irritating and difficult as the problem of losing weight for the obese. Behavior modification can also be used effectively for these persons.

Table 15–1 on page 291 described desirable weights for men and women of different ages. Some persons use this standard for assessing weight: a person's weight at about age 25 is an ideal weight for that person throughout adulthood. This standard may offer a very general guide but has little value when the person is either obese or very thin in his mid 20s.

Alcohol is a fairly common dietary item and when its intake cannot be regulated, drinking excessive amounts leads to many health problems. In wine-producing countries, it has been estimated that up to 10 percent of the total caloric supply comes from wine. Most of the alcohol is oxidized by the body although some is lost via the respiratory and urinary tract. Because of the caloric content of alcohol, the heavy drinker tends to gain or maintain his weight while eating less. Usually, vitamin and protein intake is insufficient in the diet of heavy drinkers. This in turn leads to some of the common problems of chronic alcoholism.

When nutritional needs are appropriately met, the person will demonstrate typical characteristics of health. He will fall within the normal range of weight for his height, sex, and build. His skin and mucous membrane will have a good color and the condition and his hair and teeth will be healthy. He will be able to carry out activities of daily living that are appropriate for him and will enjoy a good appetite.

When nutritional needs are not being met, the person will become malnourished. *Malnutrition* is a condition characterized by a lack of necessary or proper food substances or improper absorption and distribution of food substances in the body. *Emaciation* is a condition

characterized by extreme thinness or leanness. It may be the result of malnutrition or of pathological conditions, such as many of those afflicting the gastrointestinal tract. *Marasmus* is a condition of extreme emaciation due to severe protein and caloric insufficiency. The term is most commonly used with reference to infants and young children, as is the term kwashiorkor. *Kwashiorkor* is similar to marasmus except that in this condition, the infant or child has insufficient protein in his diet even when his caloric intake may be sufficient.

CULTURAL ASPECTS OF EATING

We learn to like and dislike certain foods and we learn our eating habits. The rituals associated with eating are deeply ingrained in patterns of social behavior and are learned from early childhood. Food is often associated with special occasions such as weddings, funerals, and certain religious ceremonies. Eating fads sometimes carry strong emotional overtones. The following are cultural factors related to food and eating.

- Religious practices often dictate eating patterns. The Buddhist eats no meat and Moslems and many Jews avoid pork. Fasting plays a role in some religions, and bread and wine are used in the sacraments of communion.

- Vegetarians who eat very little or no meat may be observing religious or personal convictions.

- Cultural factors influence eating habits. In western countries, plates, knives, forks, and spoons are used for eating. Arabs use bread and fingers to obtain food from common serving dishes. In the Orient, chopsticks are favored eating utensils. It is customary in the United States to have coffee, fruit, bacon, and eggs for breakfast while the English often serve meat or fish such as kidneys and kippers.

- Certain foods are associated with certain nationalities. Americans favor hamburgers, hot dogs, and apple pie. The Armenians prefer shish kebab while the Italians favor spaghetti.

- Eating is a time for family and friends to gather in most cultures. It is the rare hostess who does not offer her guests food during their visit.

- For the anxious person, food often appears to relieve anxieties.

- Food is used to show love, candy being a typical example. The denial of food is often used to punish: consider the child who is sent to bed without dinner or the prisoner who is served bread and water.

Many more examples could be cited. The observant nurse will wish to consider cultural factors associated with eating in order to be of the most assistance in helping individuals meet nutritional needs.

FOOD ADDITIVES AND SUPPLEMENTS

People in the United States seem especially obsessed with what, when, and how to eat. While there are those who have inadequate amounts of food to eat, a large majority eat too much and the wrong kind of food. In one way, food may be considered inexpensive since Americans spend less of the disposable dollar on food than do people in many other countries. However, cost in terms of human life is another matter since it is generally agreed that dietary habits account for many illnesses and premature deaths in the United States.

A relatively recent surge in writing on diet and nutrition sometimes appears to threaten the pleasures of eating. Food additives and supplements appear to be at war with the so-called natural or organic foods and the safety of using many food additives is being questioned. Myth sometimes shrouds the facts. For example, contrary to some claims, there has been no good evidence to illustrate that organically grown foods are any more nutritious than food grown in the conventional manner.

Food supplements are preparations containing vitamins, minerals, or proteins, or combinations of these and other nutrients. Their purpose is to add nutrition to the diet. Vitamins are a commonly used dietary supplement.

Certain foods such as cereals and breads may be nutritionally enriched or fortified by adding supplements to replace or restore vitamins and minerals removed by food processing. Commonly fortified products include milk to which vitamin D has been added and salt to which iodine has been added. These ingredients are food supplements.

Food additives are ingredients added to food to improve the color, flavor, consistency, and stability of the food. Use of additives is not new. Man has used salt for many centuries as a food additive to preserve foods. If additives were not used, much of the food we buy today would be uncolored and bland and would have a short shelf life. Rather than this, manufacturers have used additives as a trade-off.

The following types of additives are commonly used in food processing today.

- Preservatives to prevent spoilage in butter, margarine, soft drinks, and beer.
- Antioxidants to retard rancidity in butter, cream, shortening, and processed meats.
- Surfactants to produce stable mixtures of liquids that would otherwise separate, such as ice cream, peanut butter, and gelatin.
- Thickeners in cheese, ice cream, jellies, and jams.
- Coloring agents in ice cream, gelatin, and cake mixes.
- Artificial sweeteners in soft drinks, cakes, jellies, and jams.
- Bleaches in bread and cake.

Some of the food additives came under scrutiny when it was demonstrated that they were capable of producing pathology in animals. For example, certain food colorings appeared to be pathogenic. It had been believed that the additives, ingested more sparingly by man than by experimental animals, were harmless. However, it has been shown that many may be stored in the body and eventually build up to dangerous levels. The use of at least some additives has been linked to behavioral abnormalities in children, although evidence to date has been insufficient to convince all authorities of the relationship.

The Federal Drug Administration is the agency responsible for enforcing laws on food processing. The Delaney clause in the Food Additive Amendment of 1958 prohibits the use of food additives of any that ". . . is found after tests which are appropriate . . . to induce cancer in man or animals." The burden of proof is with the manufacturer. While the Delaney clause seems sufficiently clear, the problems are complex because the variety and number of additives are numerous, and many have been in use for years without ever having been submitted to rigorous testing. Such additives include the commonly used spices and numerous food flavorings. Saccharin, an artificial sweetener, was partially removed from the market when it was found that large quantities were carcinogenic in experimental animals.

Final or definitive answers to the controversy surrounding food additives and supplements are as yet unknown. Most authorities believe that there is a safe middle ground. While the numerous problems are being resolved, the best advice for the average consumer is to alert to news as it develops in this field.

Also, due caution is advised in judging assertions that are made by persons holding to excessive claims on either side of the controversy.

SERVING FOOD IN HEALTH AGENCIES AND TO SHUT-INS AT HOME

Nurses employed in health agencies that serve food will need to acquaint themselves with the details of nursing responsibilities such as forms to use to order diets, time limits for ordering, and ways of changing diets or canceling diets.

Patients on regular or relatively minor restrictive diets often are given menus from which they may select the foods they prefer for the next day's meals. While the type of tray, tray cover, dishes, and silver used are not within the nurse's realm of control, the general appearance of the tray should be as attractive as possible when it is served. Some agencies increase the attractiveness of the tray by using name cards and holiday favors. In the home care of patients, the nurse can do much to please the patient, such as adding a flower, using different colored cloths and napkins, serving one course at a time, and adding treats like cookies or candy if the patient is permitted to have them.

Some health agencies having self-care units permit patients to be served in a cafeteria or dining room. A dietitian may be present to help patients on special diets to make a selection from the foods available. Even if dining rooms are not available, provisions for groups of patients to eat together, as in a solarium, is a thoughtful gesture. This is true especially for holidays and special occasions. It is the rare person who prefers eating alone.

Some health agencies provide special menus for children and teenagers. The agencies attempt to offer foods these young folks like and in forms commonly served at home. Youngsters may not care for many vegetables, for example, but may relish vegetable soup. Providing youth-oriented food, these agencies report, has solved at least some dietary problems among the young.

Eligible senior citizens, unable to pick up allotments of donated foods because of poor health or no transportation, can have foods home-delivered through local volunteer efforts in parts of this country.

The federal and local governments sponsor a nutrition program for elderly persons in some communities. A hot meal is provided daily in a central location where eligible elderly persons eat together. In addition to the nutritional value of a well-balanced meal, the psychological value of eating together is conducive to the well-being of many older persons. The nurse will wish to be aware of programs for at home patients who need extra assistance in order to obtain a well-balanced diet.

Whenever it seems that modifications of the usual dietary routine or of the diet itself would make the patient feel better, the nurse should consider how this might be accomplished. Thus, if it is noted that an elderly patient leaves the meat untouched, investigation might show that he has loose-fitting dentures and cannot chew meat. He may be served ground meat instead. Or when cultural patterns affect food preferences to the extent that the patient is not getting an adequate diet, it may be necessary to consult with a dietitian so that substitutes can be made.

Some hospitalized patients find the time span between meals unsatisfactory. Three meals served within an eight- to nine-hour period and then a 15-hour wait for the next meal is not usual routine at home. They may want a snack at bedtime. Some agencies provide this, but many do not. Having the patient save some item, such as a piece of cake or fruit, from one of his trays may be an answer. Hunger is distressing, and everything possible should be done to avoid it.

Occasionally, hospitalized patients wish a substitute for something served on the trays, and this often can be managed through the kitchen on the unit. For example, the patient may have a jar of powdered coffee and may need only hot water. Or, he may have a favorite canned item, and all that is required is that it be opened and served.

Size of the food portions may also be a source of discomfort to some patients. For those who eat little and leave a part of the food served, there is no problem. But patients who are accustomed to eating larger portions will feel dissatisfied with the meal. Extra portions can be arranged with the dietary department of the health agency.

Sometimes, patients' wishes cannot be granted because of agency policies or because it would mean doing for one what cannot be done for all. For example, there are patients who would like meals brought from home. Some of the implications can be readily imagined: family members coming in at times other than visiting hours to leave the food; requests being made to heat foods; dishes being left in rooms until family members take them home; food stored in bedside stands where spoilage becomes a problem; and conflicts with the patient's regular diet. However, an occasional item of food which can be eaten immediately or shortly afterward, such as a sandwich, a piece of homemade pie or cake, or a jar of cooked fruit might please the patient very much. If hospital policy does not allow food to be brought from home, the nurse is obliged to comply. Also, even when it seems safe, many hospitals do not allow any food left at the patient's bedside except during scheduled meal and snack times. Such policies result from the danger of patients eating food that may be spoiled due to improper storage.

Not all likes and dislikes can be acted upon, but when a patient shows obvious distress, some effort should be made in his behalf.

HELPING TO MAINTAIN OR IMPROVE THE PATIENT'S APPETITE

For most people eating is a pleasure. When we recall how much a part of our life and leisure time is associated with food, we can readily see why this is so. Family celebrations, holiday meals, parties, picnics, coffee breaks, informal visits, and watching sports events, movies, and television usually include food in one form or another. We even tend to associate certain foods with particular events, such as hot dogs at baseball games, champagne at weddings, and the like.

Appetite is the pleasant anticipation of food. It is affected by many factors. Disturbances of appetite can interfere with gastrointestinal secretions, and hence, digestion. Persons who have been upset while eating or directly afterward have been known to vomit completely undigested food hours later. Not only may his physical condition affect his appetite, but what the patient can see, hear, smell, or taste may influence it as well.

Below are some suggestions nurses will want to consider for maintaining and/or stimulating the patient's appetite.

- See that the patient is in a comfortable position for eating.
- Be sure that the patient is clean and free from damp or soiled garments. Help him wash his hands if necessary.
- Alleviate pain or discomfort, as far as possible.
- Correct such annoyances as a loose or a tight dressing.

- Give the patient an opportunity to void if he desires.
- Avoid treatments such as enemas, dressings, and injections immediately before or directly after mealtimes if possible.
- See that the room is comfortable from the standpoint of temperature and ventilation.
- See that the patient is dressed adequately and comfortably.
- Remove or keep out of sight objects which would be unpleasant to look at while eating, such as urinals, bedpans, dressing trays or carts, drainage containers, suction machines, and the like.
- Screen patients who are very ill, in pain, or receiving therapy and will not be served a meal. Many patients receiving such therapy as infusions or transfusions are served meals and should not be screened.
- Make certain that the immediate environment itself is in order by removing soiled linen, treatment trays that have been used, dead flowers, and seeing that the furniture is orderly. Many persons who must remain in bed prefer not to have their baths before breakfast if it means having the bed disarranged and bathing items left about the unit.
- Make certain that the person serving the meal is pleasant and courteous and that care has been taken to avoid spilling liquids or disarranging dishes.
- Cooperate with dietary personnel in health agencies so that the meals can be served as quickly as possible. This helps to keep hot foods hot, and cold foods from wilting or melting.
- Color has been found to affect the appetite. Blues, greens, and other dark colors tend to subdue the appetite, while hot oranges, yellows, and reds have the opposite effect. Using brightly colored napkins, tray covers, and china and being sure that there is some red, orange, or yellow food as part of each meal will help overcome drabness.

The following conditions tend to decrease appetite, and the nurse will wish to control or avoid them if possible.

- Certain emotional states, such as fear and depression, decrease a person's interest in food.
- Poor oral hygiene and the inability to chew because of teeth or mouth diseases decrease the appetite.
- The person who has lost his sense of taste and smell usually finds eating uninteresting. Sometimes the loss is temporary and can be corrected, such as persons whose nasal passages are blocked or who have been smoking or

drinking alcoholic beverages in excess. In other instances, the cause may be pathological and more difficult to correct or control.

ASSISTING PATIENTS WITH SPECIAL PROBLEMS OF FOOD AND FLUID INTAKE

Some patients will need assistance with eating and drinking because of physical limitations and the need to conserve strength. For some patients, such as those in casts or in traction or those with loss of hand or arm strength, assistance may be a matter of preparing foods and placing them conveniently. It would include such things as opening the shell of a cooked egg, buttering bread, cutting meat, and preparing other foods so they can be eaten easily.

If it is difficult for a patient to drink from a cup or glass, a drinking tube should be provided. Disposable rather than reusable drinking tubes are preferred because considerable care is needed to keep the nondisposable tubes clean. Accumulated food particles in a drinking tube at room temperature make a good growth medium for microorganisms.

Some patients are unable or not permitted to feed themselves and must be fed by someone else. The patients should be positioned and supported adequately to facilitate ease of swallowing. When permissible, having the patient in as near an upright position as possible is desirable. Great care must be taken when feeding patients who are in a prone or near prone position. Having liquids and food enter the trachea rather than the esophagus can happen to anyone, but the reclining person is particularly susceptible.

When feeding a patient, a nurse or an assistant should be relaxed and in a comfortable position, so that the patient does not feel rushed. The person feeding should inquire if the patient is accustomed to saying grace. If so, permit him to do so and remain respectfully silent. A comment on his nursing care plan which indicates that the patient says grace helps to individualize his care.

Ask the patient which foods he would like to eat first and other preferences he might have. He might like his coffee with his meal or after it, a piece of bread after each piece of meat or some potato and meat together. Serve the food at the rate the patient wishes it.

If the patient is permitted slight activity and has some hand and arm functioning, permit him to hold a

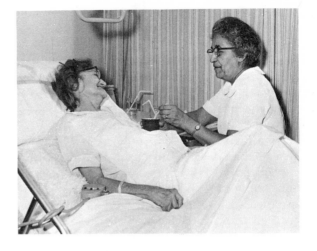

Figure 19–1 This photo illustrates the various suggestions made in this chapter in relation to assisting a patient with eating. In addition to assisting the patient, the nurse can use the opportunity to learn to know her patient better, to help in establishing a helping nurse-patient relationship, and to teach the patient as indicated.

piece of toast or a roll or to hold the drinking tube in the beverage while he sips it. If there is a beverage that he would like at the end of a meal and it can be placed so that he need only hold the drinking tube, consider doing this. It will prolong the pleasure of the meal and give the patient some feeling of independence. Avoid having to leave a patient after starting to feed him. If you must, use diplomacy so that he does not feel abandoned.

If a patient being fed is blind or if his eyes are bandaged, it is best to use some method of signaling when the next mouthful of food is ready or when it is wanted. Touching the patient's arm when the food is ready or having the patient move his hand when he wants more can make the situation much easier for both.

For certain patients, an above average intake of oral fluids is desired. Having a specific fluid intake goal is a very useful aid for many patients, their families, and nursing personnel. It is very difficult to maintain strong motivation and initiate action when the goal is simply "increase fluid intake." For some patients, the setting of short-term or interim goals is most helpful. For example, "a glass every hour," or "by the time your TV program is finished," or "a pitcher of water by lunchtime," can be good objecives.

If the reader has ever tried to increase his fluid intake when he did not feel thirsty, he realizes how important are the encouragement and support of others. These boosters can come from the nurse or the patient's family. Because normally during the night fluid intake is limited, the patient is usually able to consume a proportionately greater amount during the early hours of his waking day. It is also wise for the patient to avoid a large intake of fluid just before retiring in order to prevent sleep disturbances caused by having to void.

Having fluid available for the person whose goal is an increased intake is so obvious that it seems unnecessary to mention. However, it is amazing how many persons in homes and hospitals who are unable to secure their own fluids are left with an unfilled water pitcher, an empty glass and a full pitcher out of reach, or with a pitcher that is too heavy to lift.

The person who is unable to help himself often will be able to take only small quantities of fluids at a time. Therefore, the frequent offering of sips and single swallows is essential. Such measures as making sure certain fluids are the temperature the patient prefers are also important. If the patient wants and is permitted iced liquids, they should not be at room temperature. If he wants his coffee, tea, or water piping hot, it should be steaming. Attractive, clean, and easily handled cups and glasses can also be an encouragement.

Some persons find that the use of a drinking tube requires less effort, while others may have to have the fluids spoon fed. Increasing the fluid intake of patients is probably the single most common nursing care objective. Often, creativity and considerable patience on the part of the nurse are necessary to reach desired goals.

Having the patient decrease his intake of fluids below normal amounts is sometimes necessary. Examples of patients drinking bath water, water from flower containers, and even urine indicate how strong the desire to drink can be when thirsty. Spacing of the allowable fluids should be planned with the patient whenever possible. Since food will also provide relief through gastric distention, it is generally preferable to plan the time of maximum fluid intake for periods between meals. Setting short-term goals for hourly or two-hourly intervals may also be helpful.

Because these persons usually experience intense thirst, measures to minimize it are important. Rinsing the mouth with fluid or holding water in the mouth will moisten the mucous membrane and provide short-term relief. The effect does not ordinarily exceed 15 minutes, however. Providing oral hygiene at regular intervals can be helpful. Dry and salty foods should be avoided by the patient whose fluid intake is re-stricted, because they will tend to increase thirst. Hard candy and gum, often thought to relieve thirst by stimulating saliva, may provide temporary relief. However, their use is generally not encouraged because the high-sugar content increases the oral cavity tonicity and temporarily draws fluid to the mucous membrane. After a period of 15 to 30 minutes, the mucous membrane is even more dry than before. Diverting the person's attention by involving him in other activities to the degree he is able is often helpful in decreasing discomfort. Such measures as the use of small glasses and serving of ice which when melted is approximately one-half of its apparent volume may also be helpful. Since limiting intake for the person who is experiencing extreme thirst is very uncomfortable, the nurse needs to provide understanding and support of his feelings and encouragement for his efforts.

GASTRIC GAVAGE

When the patient is unable to take food and fluids by mouth, other methods to give nourishment are used. The patient may be given nourishment intravenously, as will be discussed in Chapter 24. Another alternative is to use gastric gavage. A gavage is used most frequently when the swallowing reflex is absent or when there is pathology present in the mouth, throat, or esophagus.

Gastric gavage is the introduction of nourishment into the stomach by mechanical means. A gavage usually is indicated when the patient is unable to take nourishment orally but when no stomach or duodenal pathological changes are present to interfere with normal digestive processes. The procedure is used often when a patient has an obstruction or a stricture in the esophagus or the throat. A tumor may be the cause of an obstruction. A stricture may be congenital or may be caused by scar tissue that has developed following injury to the esophagus. Persons with brain dysfunction sometimes lose the ability to swallow and need to be fed by gastric gavage.

Gastric gavages are used also for patients who are too weak to take nourishment by mouth. They frequently are used for feeding premature infants for whom the physical effort of sucking is too great.

Chapter 15 discussed the introduction of a tube into the stomach to obtain a specimen. The procedure for introducing a gavage tube is similar and the reader is referred to Chapter 15 for review. Extreme caution should be taken to be certain the gastric tube is positioned correctly in the stomach each time a feeding is introduced. If the tube is located in the trachea or lung, the instillation of water or liquid nourishment could have serious consequences for the patient. Even when initially positioned correctly, a tube which is left in place can become dislodged between feedings. Therefore, the location must be checked prior to each feeding.

The nourishment given by gavage is prepared in liquid form, usually with a blender. Drugs that ordinarily are administered orally may be added to the nourishment. Prepared complete liquid diets are available on the market. These liquids contain essential nutritional ingredients and may be purchased with the tube feeding delivery system also.

When a large amount of nourishment is given at regular intervals, the food is warmed to room temperature so that the patient does not become chilled. Food which is given continuously is not warmed, since it will approximate room temperature while it passes through the tubing to the patient's stomach. In addition, warmed milk and cream will sour more quickly during the time it takes for a container of nourishment to enter the patient's stomach.

After the feeding is instilled, a small amount of water should be introduced into the tube. This washes the feeding remaining in the tube into the stomach. It also prevents adhered feeding from souring.

The tube is clamped off after the food is instilled. This prevents it from draining back into the tube and escaping.

When a patient is fed by gavage on an intermittent basis, some authorities recommend removing all stomach content before adding additional nutrient. If some of a previous feeding is still in the stomach, adding still more may result in gastric distention, vomiting, and possibly aspiration of the material. The content removed by aspiration from the stomach is ordinarily refed so that the patient will not lose important electrolytes. Additional nutrient is then added in an amount small enough to avoid stomach distention. Figure 19–2 shows a patient, whose stomach tube remains in place, receiving continuous nourishment by gastric gavage.

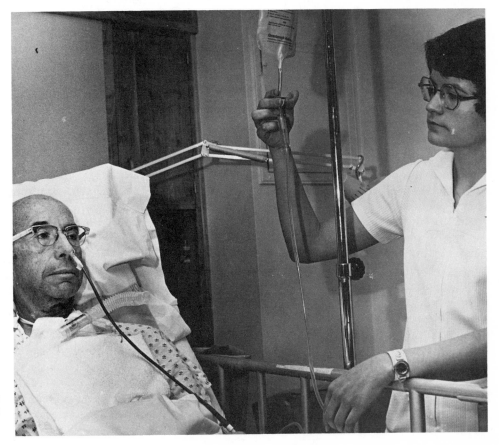

Figure 19–2 This patient is receiving nourishment by gastric gavage. The nourishment has been placed in a container that is suspended on a standard. The nurse regulates the rate at which nourishment is given with a clamp and drip meter.

THE CARE OF PATIENTS WITH ANOREXIA, NAUSEA, AND VOMITING

Anorexia

Anorexia is a loss of appetite or a lack of desire for food. The cause may be physiological, such as gastric irritation, or psychic, such as any factor that makes eating distasteful, or both. Some medications and various other therapies often cause loss of appetite. Anorexia is common when drug addiction and chronic alcoholism are present.

There does not appear to be a physiological mechanism in the body for anorexia, as is the case for vomiting. Techniques to improve the appetite were discussed earlier. Certain pharmaceutical agents also help to stimulate the appetite. In some instances, persistence of the symptom may require supplying necessary nutrients by ways other than normal eating and drinking.

Anorexia is commonly associated with nausea and vomiting. One has only to recall a personal experience or two with nausea and vomiting to remember the accompanying distress of anorexia.

Anorexia nervosa is a loss of appetite for food that cannot be explained by pathology. It is often associated with mental illness. Anorexia nervosa is most common among females between the ages of 12 and 21, but it can occur in both sexes and at any age. Unless measures are taken, persons with anorexia nervosa will literally starve to death. The person's self-perception has been found important in the cause and treatment of anorexia nervosa.

Anorexia is a common problem with hospitalized preschoolers. For example, the typical toddler responds to eating with an emphatic "No!" Various techniques have been found helpful to overcome anorexia in young children. It is important to avoid unpleasant procedures before or after meals. Children tend to eat better in groups and respond well to praise and encouragement. The attention of punishment can act as a reward for not eating. Children also respond positively to finger foods, small portions, and foods they enjoy at home, such as peanut butter sandwiches. The use of play dishes and cups often work effectively as an inducement to eat.

Nausea and Vomiting

Nausea is a feeling of sickness with a desire to vomit. "Nausea" is a noun. "Nauseous" is an adjective, and to describe a patient as being nauseous is to say that he is sickening or disgusting. The proper wording is to say that a patient has nausea, the patient is nauseated, or nausea is present.

Nausea is felt in the back of the throat and in the stomach, or both. Nausea can be accompanied by vasomotor and autonomic disturbances that result in feelings of faintness and weakness, salivation, pallor, perspiration, and tachycardia. Anorexia, dizziness, and headache commonly are associated with nausea. Retching, which is the unproductive movements of muscles that ordinarily produce vomiting, also is often present.

It is believed that increased tension, stretching, and pressure on the walls of the stomach and duodenum are responsible for the sensation of nausea. Also, distention of the lower portion of the esophagus produces nausea. If for any reason the stomach descends, tension on this general area of the gastrointestinal tract is present and nausea follows. This last phenomenon is believed responsible when such things as offensive odors and rapid changes in the speed of an elevator bring on waves of nausea. The nausea associated with motion sickness seems to result from semicircular canal stimulation. Some drugs and severe pain also may cause nausea.

Vomiting is the forceful expulsion of gastric contents through the mouth. It is also called emesis. Vomiting is a common symptom associated with numerous clinical entities. It is a reflex act that relieves the upper gastrointestinal tract of its contents. The contents are called vomitus. Vomiting is a protective mechanism that enables the body to rid itself of irritating contents. It is usually preceded by nausea.

Projectile vomiting is the expulsion of vomitus with great force, without the presence of nausea. Persistent and intractable vomiting is called pernicious vomiting. Bringing stomach contents to the throat and mouth without vomiting effort is regurgitation. It occurs commonly among infants when, it is believed, the infant spits up excess food. Eructation or belching is a discharge of gas from the stomach through the mouth.

The part of the gastrointestinal tract most sensitive to stimulants producing vomiting is the first part of the duodenum. However, sufficient stimulus in almost any section of the tract can produce vomiting. Mechanical irritation of the pharynx and fauces produces vomiting in most people. The irritation of an obstruction anywhere along the intestinal tract often produces violent vomiting. When abnormal stimulation of other organs in the body exists, vomiting is often present also. This can be observed when injury or disease affects the uterus, kidneys, heart, semicircular canals, or the brain. Cranial pressure generally produces projectile vomiting. It is a significant sign of deterioration and should be reported when it occurs.

It has been demonstrated that a vomiting center is located in the medulla oblongata. Near the center is a trigger zone that apparently collects impulses of chemical irritants, such as drugs, that in turn produce the vomiting. Other impulses eventually reach the center from the cortex and from other areas in the body, the exact pathways being largely undetermined. Some authorities believe that the vomiting center is not stimulated directly except by chemical irritants. Efferent pathways from the central nervous system carry impulses that influence the mechanical act of vomiting. Stimulants that cause vomiting include gastrointestinal irritations; intense sensations, such as pain and anger; a disturbance in equilibrium; and pressure on the vomiting center. Psychic stimuli for vomiting include nauseating odors, sights, tastes, thoughts, and so on.

The mechanism of vomiting usually begins with a few deep inspirations. The glottis is closed and the nasopharynx is isolated by elevation of the soft palate. Abdominal and diaphragmatic muscular contractions begin and aid in forcing contents from the tract. Breathing ceases temporarily and the glottis closes, both mechanisms helping to prevent the aspiration of vomitus into the respiratory tract. In the unconscious patient, the glottis may not close, thus adding to the vomiting problem the danger of respiratory aspiration of vomitus.

When nausea and vomiting are present, nursing measures are directed toward eliminating causes as much as possible, in order to avoid placing the body in jeopardy from lack of food and fluids.

When the cause can be identified and removed, the problem may be largely solved. For example, when a patient is experiencing nausea and vomiting from unsightly odors and sights, removing them may be an easy solution. When the cause is pathological, nausea and vomiting may be present until therapy begins to make amends. When cranial pressure is relieved, vomiting usually ceases. When gastritis is relieved, so also is nausea.

In some instances, drugs called *antiemetics,* which act to allay vomiting, may be prescribed. Also there are drugs that aid in reducing the nausea and vomiting associated with motion sickness. Some of them have been used effectively with other conditions as well, such as the nausea and vomiting of early pregnancy.

The patient who is vomiting needs protection and comfort. The danger of aspirating vomitus is often present and is a serious hazard, especially with the semiconscious and unconscious patient, or with infants and small children. Suctioning may become necessary for these patients to clear the upper gastrointestinal and respiratory tracts. Turning the patient's head to one side helps to rid the mouth of its contents. Gravity helps if the patient's head can safely be lowered *slightly.* Marked Trendelenburg's positions are to be avoided as gravity may then be strong enough to produce more vomiting.

For patients with abdominal wounds, supporting the area with binders, a pillow splint, or with the nurse's hand is helpful. These procedures offer comfort to the patient and help to prevent opening of a wound, although this is an uncommon complication.

Comforting the patient includes special mouth care. This should be instituted as soon as possible after vomiting ceases, because the taste and odor of vomitus often is sufficient to produce more. Soiled linen and clothes are changed and emesis basins are emptied promptly.

The tension often associated with vomiting may be relieved by giving the patient a back rub. A clean, quiet, and comfortable environment also helps.

Additional measures that assist the patient who is nauseated and vomiting include limiting the patient's activities as much as possible, especially if motion has brought on the symptoms; assisting the patient to assume a comfortable position; taking steps to alleviate pain if present; and limiting the patient's intake until the symptoms subside. Then offer fluids and food separately; offer bland and nonfatty foods; assist infants to bring up air bubbles by burping them; be prepared to offer emotional support when emotional components are present.

Notations are made on the patient's record when vomiting is present—the time it occurred, the nature of the emesis and vomitus, and the amount. The amount is recorded on the patient's record of output.

Hematemesis is vomitus containing blood. *Coffee ground vomitus* is vomitus that looks like ground coffee. It is a characteristic sign of the patient with bleeding peptic ulcers when the blood is partially digested. *Feculent vomitus* contains content from the small intestine. It is a characteristic sign of the person with a severe intestinal obstruction. An unusual odor, such as alcohol, should also be noted. When indicated, a specimen is sent to a laboratory for analysis.

THE CARE OF PATIENTS WITH GASTRIC AND DUODENAL SUCTION

Gastric and duodenal suction is used to remove contents from the stomach or duodenum or both by use of a partial vacuum. The care of patients having gastric and duodenal suction presents the problem of meeting nutritional needs because these patients cannot take fluids or food orally or by gastric gavage. Intravenous infusions are most frequently used to meet fluid and at least some nutritional needs. Hyperalimentation may be indicated in some instances. These two procedures to supply fluids and nutrients intravenously will be discussed in Chapter 24.

Suction is used when it becomes necessary to keep the stomach and the duodenum empty and at rest. For example, prior to gastric surgery, the surgeon usually wishes to have this area free of gas and undigested food; following surgery on the gastrointestinal tract, the stomach and duodenum are kept empty and at rest until healing at the site of the surgery has begun. Suctioning is effective for removing secretions and air or gas that often accumulate in the gastrointestinal tract following abdominal surgery. This helps to prevent distention. Suctioning is indicated also when there is a paralysis in the gastrointestinal tract and the normal movement of the products of digestion is interrupted, such as by a paralysis of the ileus. Suctioning then is used to prevent distention, discomfort, and the dangers associated with paralysis. Suctioning may also be used when the patient is nauseated and the prevention of vomiting is desired. Whatever the reason for removing the gastrointestinal contents, the potential for fluid and nutritional disturbances is high.

A variety of tubes is available for use in suctioning gastric and duodenal contents. If simple decompression of the stomach is desired, a single-lumen tube, such as the Levin tube, is used. The *lumen* of a tube is its inner open space. The disposable tubes are very satisfactory since they seem to be comfortable for the patient, are less objectionable when secured to the face, and eliminate the difficult problem of thorough cleaning between uses.

Another type of tube used for gastric suction has two lumens. One lumen empties the stomach while the second lumen provides for a continuous flow of atmospheric air. The air flow lumen controls suction by preventing the drainage lumen from pulling stomach mucosa into the drainage eyes, and thus, irritating the mucosa. When this tube is used, suction can be continuous rather than intermittent as is the case with a single-lumen tube. Tubes used to remove stomach contents are frequently called short gastrointestinal tubes.

If suctioning of the duodenum is desired, a long gastrointestinal tube is used. A single-lumen tube, such as the Harris or Cantor tube, or a double-lumen tube, such as the Miller-Abbott or Johnston tube, can be used. The single-lumen tubes are similar to those used for suctioning the stomach, as described above, except they are longer. Intestinal suction tubes have a balloon or bag at the end. Depending on the type, the bag is inflated with fluid, air, or mercury, usually about 5 ml. The fluid, air, and mercury bags aid the forward movement of the tube from the stomach into the duodenum. These bags also keep the tube in place by preventing the tube from moving from the intestine into the stomach.

Triple-lumen tubes with two balloons are used for specific purposes, perhaps the most common being to help control hemorrhaging from esophageal and stomach varices. There is an esophageal and a gastric balloon for two lumens and the third lumen is used to remove stomach contents. A serious complication in the use of this type of tube is erosion of the esophagus and gastric mucosa. These tubes are rarely left in place for more than 48 hours and the pressure in the balloons is released frequently, as often as every 15 to 20 minutes, to minimize mucosal irritation.

Tubes and balloons should be checked for intactness before insertion. The tube is inserted as was described in Chapter 15. If it is desired that the tube enter the duodenum, peristalsis aids in moving it through the pyloric valve. Usually, it is helpful to have the patient lie on his right side so that gravity will aid the tube in dropping into the duodenum. As a rule every 20 or 30 minutes, a few more inches of the tube are passed until the desired length has entered the gastrointestinal tract. Suctioning is started as soon as the tube has reached the stomach or is delayed until the tube is in the duodenum, depending on the physician's wishes.

Fluids and gases move from an area of greater pressure to one of lesser pressure. To remove liquids and gases from the gastrointestinal tract, it is necessary to decrease the pressure in the collection container and tubing to below atmospheric pressure to create a partial vacuum. Then the greater pressure within the gastrointestinal system will force the contents from the stomach and/or duodenum to move into the tubing and collection container.

The manner in which suction is provided on the drainage tube will depend on each agency's equipment.

Many agencies have electric pumps while others have wall suction available.

The nurse is responsible for seeing that the apparatus for gastric and duodenal suction is functioning properly at all times. The patient's tube may be irrigated at regular intervals to maintain patency. Normal saline is preferred for irrigation, usually about 30 ml. Figure 19–3 shows a nurse about to irrigate a gastric tube. When irrigating is done, it is easy to determine whether or not the tube is patent. After the solution has been injected, the suction is started again, and the irrigating fluid should return quickly. If drainage is not occurring, the suction apparatus should be checked. Open the tube at its connection and place the end of the tube removed from the suction apparatus into a glass of water. The water will be removed from the glass if the suction equipment is working properly. The following signs indicate that proper suctioning is not occurring: the stomach or duodenal contents are not returning to the drainage container; the patient's abdomen is distended; and/or the patient vomits around the tube. Vomiting carries with it the danger of aspiration of material into the lower respiratory tract.

The patient with gastric or duodenal suctioning often becomes uncomfortable from thirst and from the dryness of his oral mucous membrane. He may be allowed to have ice chips or liquids in limited quantities. Large amounts of water given by mouth are contraindicated because they would cause electrolytes to leave the body quickly by flushing out the stomach. Frequent oral hygiene is necessary to increase the patient's comfort. Oral hygiene should include lubricating the lips with cream or pomade. A common complication when oral hygiene measures are neglected is parotitis, which is an infection of the parotid glands. Signs and symptoms include pain and swelling at the angle of the jaw, little or no salivation, and an exudate from ducts of the glands in the mouth.

The nares require special care while the drainage tube is in place. Regular cleaning and the application of a small amount of lubrication help to keep the mucous membrane in good condition.

Irritation from the tube in the throat can cause considerable local discomfort. Various measures may be used to ease this discomfort: analgesic throat lozenges, local anesthetic sprayed onto the area, and lidocaine miscuous applied to the area.

When duodenal tubes are in place, the regular use of an antiseptic mouthwash is often recommended since bacteria from the duodenum can move up the tube and into the mouth. When these tubes are removed, the nurse should be prepared to give thorough oral hygiene since the odor of fecal material from the tube is common.

Reflux of stomach contents into the esophagus occurs relatively easily when the patient is flat in bed. It is recommended that the head of the bed be somewhat elevated to prevent symptoms due to reflux. The patient most often describes his symptoms as "heartburn."

The nurse is responsible for noting the type and amount of drainage present, as illustrated in Figure 19–4 on page 450. Most agencies provide a routine for measuring, emptying, and cleaning the drainage bottle every 24 hours. The amounts of solution used for irrigations, as well as any fluids the patient has taken orally, are also noted and recorded as intake. The amount of drainage, including the irrigation return, is recorded as output.

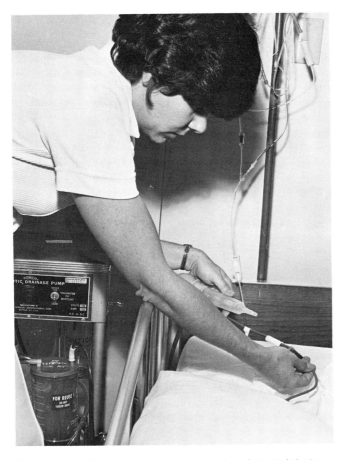

Figure 19–3 The nurse is using a bulb syringe here to irrigate the patient's gastric tube. The tube can be disconnected for irrigating purposes near where she is holding the tube in her right hand.

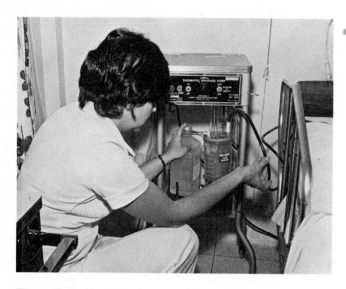

Figure 19–4　The nurse is responsible for checking the return when gastric suction is used and for measuring and recording the return as output.

THE MEASUREMENT OF INTAKE AND OUTPUT

Measuring the patient's intake and output of nourishment and fluid is an important nursing responsibility. Accuracy of the total intake and output from all sources is essential for the planning of the patient's nursing and medical care.

The measurement of urinary and fecal output will be discussed in Chapter 20. Measurement of total output should also include the amount of vomitus and drainage via suction tubes. Calibrated containers are used for measuring vomitus. Drainage bottles ordinarily are calibrated for easy measurement of output for patients having gastric and duodenal suction.

The procedure for measuring oral fluid intake varies among health agencies. Most agencies have standard-sized drinking utensils and bowls and provide the nurse with a list of these items and their liquid capacity so that determining fluid intake is relatively easy. They also ordinarily have policies concerning what foods are included with fluid intake. For example, gelatin, ice cream, and sherbet are frequently included in a fluid intake record.

The liquid nourishment given by gastric gavage is recorded as intake. As explained earlier, if the solution used to irrigate a gastric or duodenal tube is allowed to return to the drainage container, it becomes part of the patient's output while the irrigating solution is then recorded as input.

Ordinarily, the intake of solid foods is not measured. However, the nurse is expected to note how well a patient is eating and describe this on the patient's record. This is especially important when the patient is on a special diet, such as the patient with diabetes mellitus, or when he is eating poorly.

When the patient at home must maintain an intake and output measurement, the nurse can assist him by determining the capacity of several frequently used drinking containers with a household measuring cup and marking them. A household container of sufficient capacity can also be marked for measuring output.

The patient and his family should be helped to understand the purpose, importance, and technique of intake and output measurement. Their cooperation is important for accuracy. Involving the patient in this aspect of his care is also a means of promoting his independence. Maintaining his own record can be an especially helpful motivating force for the patient whose oral intake is being increased.

Various types of forms are used in health agencies to maintain fluid balance records. In most situations the patient's fluid intake and output are totaled on his record at 8- and 24-hour intervals. Figure 19–5 illustrates one type of form used for an 8-hour period. The patient at home can be assisted to adapt this type of form to his needs.

TEACHING ABOUT NUTRITION

Because the nurse is often the central person who teaches patients needing help with nutritional problems, it behooves her to share general nutrition principles when teaching and to keep abreast of knowledge in the nutritional sciences. When problems arise, a dietitian will gladly assist the nurse, and she should be consulted freely.

Health teaching should be concerned with promoting proper nutrition throughout life. This chapter included some basic information about proper nutrition, including special needs of certain persons, such as the pregnant and lactating woman. References dealing with nutrition and diet therapy and clinical texts are important sources of more detailed information.

Prescribed special diets should be followed carefully. This is more likely to occur when patients have been properly instructed on why the diet is important, what modifications may be allowed, how the diet is best prepared, and so on.

Very often, patients who are on special diets claim to have lost their appetites; what they are permitted to eat

INTAKE & OUTPUT RECORD

Name *John L. Lorre*   Room *201*

Date *6-19-'79*   Shift *7AM - 3PM*

| TIME | FLUID INTAKE | | FLUID OUTPUT | | IRRIGATION SOLUTION |
	ORAL	OTHER	URINE	DRAINAGE	
8:00 AM	240				
10:00 AM	120				
12:30 PM	300				
2:30 PM	200				
3:00 PM	120				
Total	980				

Iced Tea - 6 oz. (180 cc)
Water Glass - 6 oz. (180 cc)
Milk (carton) - 8 oz. (240 cc)
Fruit Juice - 4 oz. (120 cc)
Soup - 7 oz. (210 cc)
Ice Cream - 3 oz. (90 cc)
Jello - 3½ oz. (105 cc)

Cup of Coffee or Tea - 7 oz. (210 cc)
Styrofoam Cup - 150 cc
Paper Cup - 150 cc
Coffee Creamer - ½ oz. (15 cc)
Cereal Creamer - 2 oz. (60 cc)
Coca Cola and Seven Up - (200 cc)
H_2O Pitcher - (600 cc)

00-0550 REV. 1/76

Figure 19–5 This is an example of an intake and output record. The patient's fluid intake is given to illustrate. The form is used for an 8-hour period. At the end of a 24-hour period, the patient's total intake is recorded on his record.

does not give them any pleasure. It is difficult to be denied foods and seasonings we like, and more difficult still for a person to deny himself these pleasures when he no longer feels ill. To have an appetite for foods and to keep reminding yourself that you cannot have them takes considerable self-control. That is why many persons do not adhere to their diets after discharge from the hospital. The nurse has a responsibility to try to help make the special diet as appealing to the patient as possible. If a patient is to be on a special diet, arrangements should be made to teach and to plan with him. This teaching and planning should also include family members as indicated. When possible, having a dieti-

tian meet with the patient can often do much to help.

It is important to support patients by at least indicating an awareness and an understanding of their feelings, in addition to teaching, when special diets do not appeal to them. Reprimanding is not nursing. The patient needs the nurse's help and support. Nursing care plans for such patients should provide a consistent approach.

Persons who live alone may have a problem with adequate nutrition. This is particularly true with the older age group. Often they do not wish to cook for one person since they find it no fun to eat alone and maintain that they have no appetite anyway. Meals with friends and relatives are possible suggestions. As mentioned earlier, in some areas food service to the home has been instituted for the ill, the handicapped, or the incapacitated.

Cultural and religious factors must be considered in teaching programs. When a cultural or religious practice related to nourishment results in the patient's having a diet lacking in essential nutrients, the nurse has an opportunity for teaching how adjustments can be made without violating the person's beliefs. For example, the vegetarian may need help on how to supplement his diet with nonmeat proteins. Such foods as peas, beans, cheese, and eggs contain essential protein and can be used as meat substitutes.

The affluent society notwithstanding, an abundant food supply is not available to all in the United States. It is disheartening to know that many children and adults are chronically hungry and suffering from severe malnutrition. Sometimes teaching better food selection and using nutritious but inexpensive foods is helpful. In other situations, social agencies may need to be called upon to assist.

As a health teacher, the nurse has a responsibility to assist patients to separate fads from facts in relation to nutrition. The list of claims and facts on page 452 was prepared by the Food and Drug Administration, U.S. Department of Health, Education, and Welfare, Public Health Service. Below are suggestions offered by the Federal Drug Administration to help protect the public from nutritional fads. These suggestions were also published by the Department of Health, Education, and Welfare. Although this material was published in the early 1970s, it is still valid today.

- Don't buy a product or alter your eating habits on impulse or from fear. Take enough time to ask yourself the following questions:

  Does the promoter belittle normal foods? This is the first sign of nutritional quackery.

CLAIM	FACT
1. You are what you eat.	In one sense, yes. You are also what heredity and environment have contributed.
2. Our soil has lots its vitamins and minerals; our food crops have little nutritional value.	In the commercial production of food crops fertilizers are applied in order to produce satisfactory yields. The nutrients which promote good plant growth are added to the soil in these fertilizers, and the food crops produced contain the expected nutritional value.
3. Chemical fertilizers are poisoning our soil.	Chemical fertilizers are not poisoning our soil. Modern fertilizers are needed to produce enough food for our population. Our increasing population further increases the need for these fertilizers.
4. Natural, organic fertilizers are not only safer than chemical fertilizers, but produce healthier crops.	Organic fertilizers cannot be absorbed, as such, by plants. They must be broken down by bacteria in the soil until they finally become the same chemical elements—potassium, phosphorus and nitrogen—that are supplied directly and more quickly by modern chemical fertilizers. Their use may also contribute to the spread of certain infectious diseases.
5. Pesticides are poisoning our nation.	When pesticides on food crops leave a residue, FDA and the Environmental Protection Agency (EPA) make sure the amount will be safe for consumers. The amount allowed, if any, is set at the lowest level that will accomplish the desired purpose, even though a larger amount might still be safe.
6. Modern processing removes most of the vitamins and minerals in foods.	This is not true. While any type of processing, including simple cooking, tends to reduce to some extent the nutrient content or quality of foods, modern processing methods are designed to keep such losses as low as possible. In many instances, nutrients are restored by enrichment after processing.
7. Aluminum cooking utensils are dangerous to health.	Aluminum is the second most abundant mineral element in the soil, and it, therefore, occurs naturally in many foods. Cooking in aluminum utensils is harmless.
8. Cooking with Teflon-coated utensils is dangerous.	Careful testing of this commercial product has proved that there is no danger from normal kitchen use, or the overheating which might occur in the kitchen.
9. If you have an ache or pain, or are just feeling tired, you are probably suffering from a subclinical deficiency.	Feeling poorly, lacking pep, or experiencing an ache or pain occurs in most persons at some time or another. These are symptoms which may be caused by overwork, emotional stress, disease, lack of sleep as well as by poor nutrition. If such symptoms persist, a person should see his physician. It is extremely difficult for the average person to accurately diagnose the cause of these symptoms.
10. You have to eat special foods if you want to correct overweight.	Your physician should prescribe any special diet you may need. Personal experimenting and fad diets can be highly dangerous to your health. Successful weight control depends primarily on self-control of one's total food intake while maintaining a reasonable level of physical activity.
11. Synthetic vitamins are dead and ineffective; vitamins from natural sources are much better.	Vitamins are specific chemical compounds, and the human body can use them equally well whether they are synthesized by a chemist or by nature.
12. Everyone should take vitamins, just to be sure.	Very few of us eat exactly the same foods as our neighbors eat. There is some variation that makes our diet different from everyone else's. It is variety that helps to assure adequate nutrition for most of us. Most healthy individuals whose diet regularly includes even modest amounts of meat and eggs, milk products, fruits and vegetables, bread, and other cereal products need not resort to dietary supplements. Some persons under a doctor's care or in institutions need dietary supplements because of special conditions which greatly restrict their ability to eat a well-balanced diet. Modest supplementation with certain vitamins is generally recommended during infancy, pregnancy, and while breast feeding.

Does the product, or the person, promise or imply a quick correction for a condition you think you may have?

Is the product sold in homes by people who tell you they are interested only in helping people in need. They will agree with any ailment you may say you have, and they have a product to treat your condition. They are not doctors—they are not experts on nutrition—they are salesmen.

• When you see a testimonial, remember that legitimate practitioners do not use them. Testimonials are commonly bought and sold; some are sincere—but essentially worthless, due to the individual's lack of nutritional and medical knowledge.

• Ask known, competent authorities for all information concerning your health. You will receive honest, dependable facts.

After years of staff studies and hearings, the Select Committee on Nutrition and Human Needs of the

United States Senate issued a report in 1977 entitled *Dietary Goals for the United States.* Although the report has been both praised and condemned, it has implications for nursing in terms of nutrition and public education.

The report recommended that the American diet should include increased amounts of fruits, vegetables, whole grains, poultry, fish, and nonfat milk. It recommended decreased amounts of fat, meat, sugar, and salt. To justify these recommendations, the Select Committee associated diet with these leading causes of death: heart disease, cancer, cerebrovascular accidents (strokes), diabetes mellitus, arteriosclerosis (hardening of the arteries), and cirrhosis of the liver.

The Select Committee reported that approximately 20 percent of adults in the United States are estimated to be overweight to a sufficient degree to interfere with health and longevity. Yet, malnutrition often exists since the diets of many obese people are high in sugar and fats and low in vitamins and minerals. Here are additional items of interest to health personnel:

- Fruits, vegetables, and whole grains, the so-called complex carbohydrates, have lost a great deal of their prominence in the typical American diet. Yet, there is evidence that these carbohydrates reduce the risk of heart disease. Also, they are high in vitamins, minerals, and fibers. Low-fiber intake has been cited as a possible contributor to intestinal malignancies.

- Although to date research on food value of frozen versus fresh produce is far from complete, it was recommended that the diet consist of an even balance of each.

- Highly refined products, such as potato chips, should not be considered as nutritionally equal to the fresh produce from which they are made.

- Fortification of food with vitamins and minerals is common, but it appears doubtful that the number and balance of these nutrients in fresh form can be duplicated.

- The consumption of bread, a relatively good source of protein and calories, is on the decline, possibly because it is incorrectly viewed as fattening by many people.

- High-cholesterol intake is discouraged by many professional and governmental bodies because of its link with certain heart diseases. Americans are heavy consumers of red meat which has a high-cholesterol value. It is recommended that more protein needs be satisfied with fish, and poultry which are low in cholesterol, and vegetable proteins which contain no cholesterol.

- The average adult requirement for salt is probably about 0.5 Gm. per day. It is estimated that the average American consumes anywhere from 6 to 18 Gms. per day. There has been some research which links high-salt intake with high blood pressure.

Despite considerable controversy surrounding the Select Committee's report and a remaining lack of knowledge of many nutrients, there is no lack of interest in diet and its relationship to health. In 1977, one public poll indicated that almost 90 percent of the adults canvased stated they wanted to know more about diets and another poll found only 14 percent of those asked believed Americans had nutritious diets. Nurses have a responsibility as members of the health team to keep abreast of new findings on health and diet and to educate consumers to be more judicious in food shopping and meal planning than they have been in the past.

MEETING THE PATIENT'S NUTRITIONAL AND FLUID NEEDS AND THE NURSING PROCESS

Data gathering on how well the patient's nutritional and fluid needs are being met begins with knowing the patient. Who is he? Why is he being considered for nursing care? What factors in his life are influencing his present health status? These are typical questions to which the nurse will wish to find answers.

A nutrition history is done in order to learn more specifically how well the patient has been meeting his nutritional needs. The patient or a member of his family can be interviewed. In some agencies, a questionnaire that the patient or a family member completes has been used effectively. Examples of necessary information for a nutrition history include the number of meals eaten each day, typical foods eaten with each meal, how much and what kind of beverages are ordinarily consumed each day, food idiosyncrasies and allergies, eating habits, and so on. It may also be helpful in certain instances to ask when the patient last had something to eat or drink and what it was he ate or drank. Taking a medication history will be discussed in Chapter 24. Knowing what medications the patient is taking is important when studying a patient since some drugs influence food and fluid intake and fluid output. Laboratory data should be examined. For example, a low red blood cell count may be diet related. Additional types of data may be indicated, depending on the nature of a patient's particular illness.

Standards for assessment are the nutritional and fluid

needs of the human organism. They will reflect the person's age, sex, occupation, physical activities, and so on.

A nursing care plan is then built upon nursing diagnoses that developed as a result of data gathering and assessment and upon whatever strengths the person has for meeting nutritional and fluid needs appropriately.

The plan of care is implemented. Numerous intervention measures can be used and many were discussed in this chapter. The following are some general reminders that the nurse will wish to keep in mind when she is helping the person meet his nutritional and fluid needs.

- Hunger, thirst, and satiety play an important role in the regulation of food and fluid intake but any one or all three of these mechanisms may be faulty during states of illness. This chapter offered suggestions concerning measures to improve the appetite and to help persons to limit or increase oral fluid intake. Even though a measure may be indicated on the nursing care plan, no measure will work unless it is used. There has been some evidence to suggest that many nurses give the responsibility of helping persons meet nutritional and fluid needs low priority in nursing care. Yet, life cannot be sustained without food and water; the quality of life can be compromised when nutritional and fluid needs are not met; many illnesses have been found to be related to poor dietary habits; and recovery from illness can be delayed when nutrition and fluid needs are not properly met.

- Both this chapter and Chapter 7 discussed cultural and religious factors that influence eating. Nursing care will often be ineffectual and the patient will suffer when these factors are ignored. With ingenuity, it is the rare time when dietary modifications cannot be safely made. Some persons may be reluctant to describe eating habits resulting from cultural and religious beliefs. However, cooperation can almost always be gained when the nurse takes the time and shows sincere interest in wanting to help the patient without violating his beliefs.

- The science of nutrition is still relatively young and it may be that knowledge in this field remains limited. However, research is constantly ongoing. The nurse has a responsibility to keep up-to-date on research findings and adjust care as indicated in order to help the patient meet nutritional and fluid needs. The nurse must be alert too to the many fads and myths related to nutrition and be ready to refute them when facts prove them to be incorrect.

- Patients who cannot take food and fluid normally by mouth require special attention. Eating is ordinarily a pleasureable experience and to be denied this privilege can be most unpleasant. The physical care of these patients is not enough—they require understanding and support even when normal eating is denied them for relatively short periods.

- The importance of accuracy when a patient's intake and output are to be measured can hardly be overstressed. Unfortunately, in far too many instances, it appears as though this responsibility is handled with casualness and carelessness. Recording intake and output is often assigned to auxiliary nursing personnel but the nurse is ultimately responsible and should teach these persons the need for accuracy and also supervise their work.

- There is evidence to indicate that the public is interested in proper nutrition and wants to learn more about it. Nursing has an important responsibility for teaching patients as well as the public at large. Nurses also teach by observing sound personal habits of nutrition and fluid intake.

- Nurses are members of the health team and other members of the team very often can be called upon to assist the nurse. For example, nutritionists, dietitians, and diet therapists can be of invaluable assistance and will often share teaching responsibilities with the nurse for helping persons who need extra assistance in meeting their nutritional and fluid needs.

The parts of the nursing process and of the process as a whole are evaluated as described in Chapter 4.

CONCLUSION

During health, we tend to take eating and drinking for granted. Yet, we know that many people follow habits of nutrition that are not conducive to health. During illness, meeting nutritional needs of the patient takes on special significance. High-quality nursing care includes careful and conscientious consideration of the importance of promoting and maintaining health by helping the consumer to meet nutritional and fluid needs appropriately.

SUPPLEMENTAL LIBRARY STUDY

1. Here are nutritional tips for helping home-bound patients with a special need for high-protein intake:
   Nelson, Jane J. "Nutritional Tips for Cancer Patients." (Consultation) *Nursing 75,* 5:14–15, December 1975.
   What suggestions does the author give for stepping up

protein content in soup? How does she suggest making "double strength" milk? Describe several snacks she recommends that are high in protein content.

2. Here is a suggestion when a person's fluid intake must be limited:

Christgau, Chris. "Spray Thirst Away." (Tips & Timesavers) *Nursing 76,* 6:80, January 1976.

Could a plastic spray container used for dampening clothes be used for this suggestion? Are there other household items that could be used?

3. The following article describes a teaching tool that may be used for hard-to-teach patients:

Dwyer, Lois S. and Fralin, Florence G. "Simplified Meal Planning for Hard-To-Teach Patients." *American Journal of Nursing,* 74:664–665, April 1974.

Describe several disadvantages of oral and written insructions that the chart presented in this article helped overcome. How did the nurses and dietitians evaluate the patient's understanding of how to meet his nutrition needs? What research did the authors recommend for the use of the chart?

4. Read the following article:

McConnell, Edwina A. "All About Gastrointestinal Intubation." *Nursing 75,* 5:30–37, September 1975.

Describe three methods the author described to determine whether a tube is in the patient's stomach. Why should a tube not be taped to a patient's nose and then to his forehead? When a long gastrointestinal tube has passed the ileocecal valve, the tube can be allowed to exit the body via the rectum and anus. Describe precautions that are necessary when this procedure is used.

5. The following article describes *bulimia* and the syndrome of *bulimarexia:*

Boskind-Lodahl and Sirlin, Joyce. "The Gorging-Purging Syndrome." *Psychology Today,* 10:50–52, 82, 85, March 1977.

What do bulimia and bulimarexia mean? What usually led to the syndrome among persons studied by these authors? What basic psychological problem was commonly noted in the women they studied? What therapy was used?

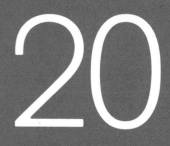

BEHAVIORAL OBJECTIVES

When the content in this chapter has been mastered, the student will be able to

Define the terms appearing in the glossary.

Identify three general principles of urinary and intestinal elimination and give examples that illustrate how failing to observe these principles stands in the way of or promotes well-being.

Describe briefly the normal production and excretion of urine and feces.

Discuss the nurse's role in promoting normal urination and defecation while including such aspects as timing, positioning of the patient, food and fluid intake, and activity.

Explain the techniques and related rationale for nursing measures commonly used for persons with problems of urinary and intestinal elimination, including urethral catheterization, indwelling catheter irrigation, changing of a stomal appliance, rectal suppository insertion, the cleansing enema, and a colostomy irrigation.

Describe the methods of securing and handling clean catch midstream urine specimens and feces specimens.

Differentiate between the action of common types of cathartics and laxatives, including chemical stimulants, bulk-formers, and fecal softeners.

List at least five measures the nurse can use to reduce the danger of nosocomial urinary infections in persons with indwelling catheters.

Discuss factors involved in bladder and bowel training, including feasibility, participation by the patient, scheduling, dietary intake, and positioning of the patient.

Describe the nursing care of a person experiencing a problem with urinary or intestinal elimination, using the nursing process as a guide.

Promoting Urinary and Intestinal Elimination

GLOSSARY

Albuminuria: The presence of albumin in the urine. Synonym for proteinuria.

Alimentary Glycosuria: The presence of sugar in the urine due to an unusually large intake of sugar or due to emotional stress.

Anal Fissures: A small linear ulcer in the anal area.

Anal Incontinence: An inability of the anal sphincter to control the discharge of fecal and gaseous material.

Anuria: The suppression or lack of production of urine.

Atonic Constipation: Dry, hardened fecal material due to sluggishness of the colon.

Bowel Movement: The emptying of the intestinal tract. Synonym for defecation.

Call: A sensation which precedes the act of micturition. Synonym for stimulus.

Cathartic: A drug used to induce emptying of the intestinal tract. Synonym for laxative.

Catheter: A tube used for injecting or removing fluids.

Colostomy: An artificially created opening from the colon to the abdominal surface for the elimination of wastes.

Constipation: The passage of dry, hard fecal material.

Cystoscope: A tubular instrument with a light in it that is used for a cystoscopy.

Cystoscopy: The visualization of the bladder, urethra, and distal ends of the ureters.

Defecation: The emptying of the intestinal tract. Synonym for bowel movement.

Diarrhea: The passage of liquid and unformed stools.

Diuresis: The excessive production and elimination of urine. Synonym for polyuria.

Dysuria: Difficult or painful urination.

Enema: The introduction of solution into the lower intestinal tract.

Excoriation: A breakdown of the epidermis.

Fecal Impaction: A hardened mass of feces in the rectum.

Feces: Intestinal waste products.

Flatulence: The excessive formation of gases in the gastrointestinal tract.

Flatus: Intestinal gas.

Foley Catheter: A type of tube inserted through the urethra into the bladder which provides for constant urinary drainage. Synonym for indwelling and retention catheters.

Frequency: Urinating at frequent intervals.

Glycosuria: The presence of sugar in the urine.

Hematuria: The presence of blood in the urine.

Hemorrhoids: Abnormally distended rectal veins.

Hydrometer: An instrument used to determine the specific gravity of urine. Synonym for urinometer.

Hypertonic Constipation: Dry, hardened fecal material due to intestinal spasms. Synonym for spastic constipation.

Ileal Conduit: A surgical connection of the ureter to the ileum with an abdominal opening for urinary excretion.

Ileostomy: An artificially created opening from the ileum to the abdominal surface for the elimination of wastes.

Incontinence: An inability to retain urine, feces, or semen.

Indwelling Urethral Catheter: A tube inserted through the urethra into the bladder which provides for constant urinary drainage. Synonym for retention and Foley catheters.

Intestinal Distention: An accumulation of excessive gas in the intestinal tract. Synonym for tympanites.

Irrigation: The flushing of a tube, canal, or area with solution.

Laxative: A drug used to induce emptying of the intestinal tract. Synonym for cathartic.

Micturition: The process of emptying the urinary bladder. Synonym for voiding and urination.

Nocturia: Excessive urination during the night. May be spelled nycturia.

Obstipation: The accumulation of hardened feces causing intestinal obstruction.

Oliguria: The scanty production of urine by the kidneys.

Orthostatic albuminuria: The presence of albumin in the urine due to physical activity or positioning.

Ostomy: An artificially created opening for waste excretion.

Overflow Incontinence: An involuntary escape of some urine from the bladder due to increased pressure. Synonym for paradoxical incontinence.

Paradoxical Incontinence: An involuntary escape of some urine from the bladder due to increased pressure. Synonym for overflow incontinence.

Peristalsis: A progressive wavelike movement of the musculature of the gastrointestinal tract.

Polyuria: The excessive production and elimination of urine. Synonym for diuresis.

Proteinuria: The presence of albumin in the urine. Synonym for albuminuria.

Pyuria: The presence of pus in the urine.

Reagent: A substance used in a chemical reaction to detect another substance.

Residual Urine: The urine retained in the bladder after voiding.

Retention: An excessive storage of urine in the bladder.

Retention Catheter: A tube inserted through the urethra into the bladder which provides for constant urinary drainage. Synonym for indwelling and Foley catheters.

Retrograde Pyelogram: The injection of contrast media through ureteral catheters into the kidneys for study of the upper urinary tract by fluoroscopy and x-ray filming.

Spastic Constipation: Dry, hardened fecal material due to intestinal spasms. Synonym for hypertonic constipation.

Stimulus: A sensation which precedes the act of micturition. Synonym for call.

Stoma: An artificial opening for waste excretion located on the body surface.

Stool: Excreted feces.

Stress Incontinence: An involuntary escape of urine from the bladder due to straining.

Suppository: A substance shaped as an oval or a cone which is inserted into a body cavity and which melts at body temperature.

Suprapubic Catheter: A type of catheter used for continuous drainage which is inserted through a small incision above the pubic area into the bladder.

Total Incontinence: An inability of the bladder to store urine.

Tympanites: An accumulation of excessive gas in the intestinal tract. Synonym for intestinal distention.

Urinary Catheterization: The introduction of a catheter through the urethra into the urinary bladder to remove urine.

Urination: The process of emptying the urinary bladder. Synonym for micturition and voiding.

Urine: The waste product excreted by the kidneys.

Urinometer: An instrument used to determine the specific gravity of urine. Synonym for hydrometer.

Voiding: The process of emptying the urinary bladder. Synonym for micturition and urination.

INTRODUCTION

Elimination from the urinary and intestinal tracts rids the body of materials in excess of bodily needs and waste products. Effective elimination is necessary to maintain well-being as well as life itself.

Because in our society it is not generally considered acceptable to discuss elimination, intestinal and bladder functions sometimes tend to be neglected in nursing care. The nurse needs to realize that these processes are essential to body functioning and handle them in a direct, objective manner. Most persons take elimination for granted unless a problem arises. However, preventive measures may be important in promoting normal patterns of elimination. In some instances, nursing intervention is necessary to facilitate elimination when malfunctioning occurs.

GENERAL PRINCIPLES OF URINARY AND INTESTINAL ELIMINATION

Efficient physiological functioning requires that waste substances be eliminated from the body. Elimination is essential to life itself. Mechanisms of elimination include not only bowel and bladder, but other organs, namely the lungs and the sweat glands.

Patterns of eliminations from the large intestine and the urinary bladder vary among individuals. Despite individual differences, as long as the intestines and the urinary bladder are eliminating wastes efficiently, there is no great need for concern.

Stress-producing situations and illness may interfere with normal habits of elimination. Persons under stress often encounter problems in elimination. For example, a patient confined to bed may find it so difficult to use a bedpan or a urinal that he may be unable to have a bowel movement or to urinate normally. Or, a person experiencing emotional stress may have difficulty maintaining normal intestinal elimination.

In addition to stress, normal elimination, especially from the large intestine, often is affected by change in diet, fluid intake, certain medications, therapeutic and diagnostic measures, and reduction in the person's normal activities.

Patterns of elimination from the urinary bladder do not vary among individuals as markedly as bowel habits. Most people urinate just before bedtime, upon arising, and several times during the day, depending on their diet, fluid intake, activity, and health state.

ELIMINATION FROM THE URINARY TRACT

The efficiency of the urinary system is vital for the maintenance of good physiological functioning. Especially during illness, considerable emphasis is placed on the patient's ability to excrete urine normally. Close observation is essential if deviations are to be detected early.

The urinary tract is one of the routes by which wastes are excreted. Certain inorganic salts, nitrogenous waste products, and water are removed from the bloodstream, accumulated, and excreted through the proper functioning of the urinary tract.

Kidneys and Ureters

The kidneys are located on either side of the vertebral column behind the peritoneum and in the posterior portion of the abdominal cavity. As one part of their overall function, they carry a major responsibility for maintaining the composition and the volume of body fluids. The kidneys function in a selective manner; that is, they single out constituents of the blood for excretion for which the body has no need and retain those substances for which the body has need. It is estimated that total blood volume passes through the kidneys for waste removal approximately every half hour. Despite varying kinds and amounts of food and fluids ingested, body fluids remain relatively stable if there is proper kidney function. The waste product containing organic and inorganic wastes which the kidneys excrete is called *urine*.

The nephron is the unit of kidney structure. There are approximately one million nephrons in each kidney. Urine from the nephrons empties into the pelvis of each kidney. From each kidney, urine is transported by rhythmic peristalsis through the ureter to the urinary bladder. The ureters enter the bladder obliquely, and a fold of membrane in the bladder closes the entrance to the ureters so that urine is not forced up the ureters to the kidneys when pressure exists in the bladder.

Urinary Bladder

The urinary bladder is a smooth muscle sac which serves as a reservoir for varying amounts of urine. There are three layers of muscular tissue in the bladder: the inner longitudinal, the middle circular, and the outer longitudinal. The three layers are called the detrusor muscle. At the base of the bladder, the middle circular layer of muscle tissue forms the internal or involuntary sphincter. This sphincter guards the opening between the urinary bladder and the urethra. The urethra conveys urine from the bladder to the exterior of the body.

Urinary bladder muscle is innervated by the autonomic nervous system. The sympathetic system carries inhibitory impulses to the bladder and motor impulses to the internal sphincter. These impulses result in relaxation of the detrusor muscle and constriction of the internal sphincter, causing urine to be retained in the bladder. The parasympathetic system carries motor impulses to the bladder and inhibitory impulses to the internal sphincter. These impulses result in contraction of the detrusor muscle and relaxation of the sphincter.

The bladder normally contains urine under very little pressure, and, as volume of urine increases, the pressure increases only slightly. This adaptability of the bladder wall to pressure is believed to be due to the characteristics of muscle tissue in the bladder and makes it possible for urine to continue to enter the bladder from the ureters against low pressure. When the pressure becomes sufficient to stimulate stretch receptors located in the bladder wall, the desire to empty the bladder becomes apparent.

Urethra

The urethra differs in men and women. In men, the urethra is common to both the excretory system and the reproductive system. It is approximately 13.7 to 16.2 cm. or $5\frac{1}{2}$ to $6\frac{1}{2}$ inches in length and consists of three parts: the prostatic, the membranous, and the cavernous portions. The external urethral sphincter consists of striated muscle and is located just beyond the prostatic portion of the urethra. The external sphincter is under voluntary control.

The female urethra is 3.7 to 6.2 cm. or $1\frac{1}{2}$ to $2\frac{1}{2}$ inches in length. Its function is to convey urine from the bladder to the exterior. The external or voluntary sphincter is located approximately midurethra. No portion of the female urethra is external to the body as is true in the male. Most literature refers to muscle at the meatus in the female as the external sphincter. Figure 20–1 on page 460 illustrates the major parts of the urinary tract.

The Act of Micturition

The process of emptying the urinary bladder is known as *micturition;* it is also called *voiding* or *urination*. Nerve centers for micturition are situated in the brain and the spinal cord. Voiding is largely an involuntary reflex act, but its control can be learned.

Following stimulation of the stretch receptors in the bladder, as the urine collects, the desire to void is experienced. Usually this occurs when about 100 ml. to 200 ml. for the child and 200 ml. to 300 ml. for the adult has collected. If the process of micturition is initiated, the detrusor muscle contracts, the internal sphincter relaxes, and urine enters the posterior urethra. The muscles of the perineum and the external sphincter relax, and micturition occurs. The act consists of relaxation of the internal sphincter, contraction of the detrusor muscle, slight contraction of the muscle of the abdominal wall, and a lowering of the diaphragm. The act of micturition is normally painless. During micturition, the pressure within the bladder is many times greater than it is during the time the bladder is filling. The voluntary control of voiding is limited to initiating, restraining, and interrupting the act.

Restraint of voiding is believed to be subconscious when the volume of urine in the bladder is small. But

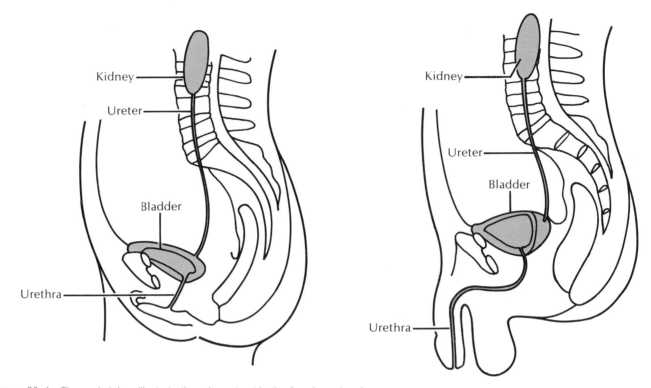

Figure 20-1   These sketches illustrate the urinary tract in the female and male.

when voiding is delayed, the bladder continues to fill. Discomfort may then be felt when undue distention occurs and the urgency to void becomes paramount.

Increased abdominal pressure, as occurs with coughing and sneezing, sometimes forces the escape of urine involuntarily, especially in the female since the urethra is shorter. Strong psychic factors, such as marked fear, may also result in involuntary urination. Under certain conditions, it may be difficult to relax the restraining muscles sufficiently to void, as when a urine specimen is requested from a shy or embarrassed person.

When the higher nerve centers develop after infancy, the voluntary control of micturition develops also. Until that time, voiding is purely reflex. Persons whose bladders are isolated from control of the brain because of injury or disease also void by reflex only.

Normal Urine

Healthy adults excrete approximately 1,000 ml. to 1,500 ml. of urine in each 24-hour period. However, this amount may vary, depending on several factors. If large amounts of fluids are being excreted by the skin,

the lungs, or the intestine, the amount excreted by the kidneys will decrease. The amount of urine will depend on the amount of fluid ingested: the greater the fluid intake, the larger will be the amount of urine produced and vice versa. Diet and age influence the amount of urine. Persons on high-protein diets will produce more urine than those on a regular diet. Children and infants excrete more urine in proportion to their weight than adults do.

The word *diuresis* is used most often to mean an excessive production and elimination of urine. *Polyuria* is a synonym. Certain fluids, such as coffee, tea, and cocoa, act as diuretics and can cause an increase in the production of urine. Certain drugs also produce diuresis.

The color of normal urine is light yellow to amber. If the urine is scant in amount and concentrated, the color will be darker; if it is dilute, the color will be lighter. Urine has a characteristic odor. Some foods and drugs will alter the odor.

Normal urine is clear. On standing and cooling, cloudiness and a sediment may occur which are due to the presence of urates and phosphates that precipitate as the reaction of urine changes from acidity to alkalinity.

Normal urine will clear again rapidly if acid is added and the urine is heated to body temperature.

Laboratory examination reveals that the specific gravity of normal urine varies on the average between approximately 1.010 and 1.025, bu it has been observed to vary between 1.002 and 1.040 in healthy persons. The inorganic constituents of normal urine include ammonia, sodium chloride, and traces of iron, and phosphorus, sulfur, sodium, potassium, calcium, and magnesium in combination with oxygen. Organic constituents include urea, uric acid, creatinine, hippuric acid, indican, urine pigments, and undetermined nitrogen. Traces of urobilin, sugar, fatty acids, carbonates, mucin, and cystine may be present.

The urine of persons on a normal diet is slightly acid. Vegetarians excrete a slightly alkaline urine. Normally, the urinary tract is sterile; therefore urine is free of bacteria. Bacteria are found at the end of the urethra, and if they are washed into a urine specimen, usually they will be identified by laboratory examination. Normal urine values were shown in Table 15–6 on page 322. The presence of casts, acetone, gross bacteria, bile, glucose, or protein in urine should be considered abnormal and reported promptly.

Frequency of Urination

The frequency of voiding depends on the amount of urine being produced. The more urine that is being produced, the more often voiding is necessary and vice versa. Unless the fluid intake is very large, most healthy persons do not void during normal sleeping hours. The first voided urine of the day is usually more concentrated than urine excreted during the remainder of the day. The nurse should remember that since the first voiding of the day is not "fresh" but rather an accumulation of a number of hours of kidney output, this urine may or may not be used as a specimen for certain tests.

Some persons normally void small amounts at frequent intervals because they habitually respond to the first early urge to void. This habit is insignificant and is not necessarily an indication of disease. Conversely, if this pattern is not a habit but a change in urination routine, it can be an indication of illness.

Other persons have habits which result in infrequent voiding. For example, some individuals go from 8 to 12 waking hours or longer without urinating. Factors, such as a habitual low-fluid intake due to environmental conditions or age, may be the reason. The inaccessi-bility of toilet facilities due to travel, work circumstances, or illness, and limitations of mobility can also be the cause of infrequent urination. Persons who habitually urinate infrequently have been found to develop more urinary tract infections and kidney disorders than those who urinate at least every three to four hours. The reason is believed to be stagnation of urine in the bladder which serves as a good medium for bacterial growth. Infrequent voiding which is a change in one's urination pattern can also be indicative of a decreased production of urine due to kidney or circulatory disorders.

NURSING RESPONSIBILITIES RELATED TO URINARY ELIMINATION

Nursing personnel are responsible for observing a person's urine. The color, odor, amount, appearance, and frequency with which voiding occurs are noted. Anything unusual should be reported. Difficulty or pain associated with the act of micturition should also be noted and reported promptly.

Adequate fluid intake is a prime factor in maintaining normal urinary elimination. If the urine is concentrated, an inadequate fluid intake is a common cause. Having an accessible supply of fresh fluids of the appropriate temperature is especially important for an immobilized patient.

Some patients find it difficult to void while confined to bed. Even Fowler's position may not be adequate. They may need to have their legs over the side of the bed while sitting on the bedpan. Some male patients on bed rest may need permission from the physician to be able to stand to use the urinal.

Female patients often need to be taught the proper technique for perineal care after urination. Drying or washing of the perineal area should be from the front to the back, or from the urethra toward the rectum. A reverse cleaning motion can result in fecal organisms being introduced into the urethra or vagina. This type of contamination is a common cause of urinary tract and vaginal infections.

Providing the Bedpan and Urinal

Men patients confined to bed usually use the urinal for voiding and the bedpan for defecation; women use the bedpan for both. When a woman patient is unable to sit up in bed—for example, when she is in a body cast—a female urinal may be used. Having to use the bedpan and the urinal is considered embarrassing by most patients. In addition, the bedpan is often difficult to use. It "fits" no one. Privacy is important to almost all patients when they use a bedpan or urinal.

Some bedpans are made of metal which takes on the environmental temperature. This is important to remember when the room is cold. The bedpan may be warmed by running warm water inside it and then rotating the water around the sides of the pan.

Bedpans of nylon resin are also available. They feel warm to touch and can be asepticized by conventional methods. Also, these bedpans eliminate the problem of noise associated with handling of metal bedpans.

A special bedpan, sometimes called a "fracture" bedpan, is frequently used by persons with fractures of the femur or lower spine. It is smaller and flatter than the ordinary bedpan but is often useful for any patient who cannot raise himself easily to use the regular-sized bedpan.

Unless contraindicated, the head of the bed should be raised slightly before placing the patient on the bedpan. This makes it easier for the patient to lift himself onto the pan. If an overhead trapeze is permitted, the patient can also move himself with less strain. If he is flat in bed, it is necessary for him to hyperextend his back in order to lift himself up onto the bedpan.

After providing privacy, the nurse folds a corner of the top bed linen over onto the patient so that it is easy to slip the bedpan under him as he lifts his hips. It is not necessary to expose a patient for this procedure. When the patient is correctly positioned and comfortable, the nurse leaves the toilet tissue within easy reach, checks to see that the signal bell is convenient, and leaves the patient alone if his condition permits. The patient should be instructed to signal when finished.

If the patient is very weak, it may be necessary for the nurse to place one hand under his buttocks and assist him to raise himself as she slides the pan under him with the other hand. If the patient cannot help to lift himself, the nurse raises the head of the bed slightly, turns the patient over on one side, places the bedpan against his buttocks, and holds it in place while the patient is rolled back onto the bedpan.

Care should be taken to avoid injuring the skin from friction by pushing the bedpan under the patient or by pulling it out. If the patient is unable to assist and rolling him is not possible, sufficient assistance should be secured to lift the patient. Powdering the surfaces of the bedpan which come in contact with the patient will also reduce friction and facilitate movement of the bedpan.

Before the bedpan is emptied, the contents should be noted and measured carefully. The excretory products are a vital clue to the patient's physiological state. Any abnormalities in the nature of the urine or in the act of elimination should be reported promptly and recorded on the patient's chart.

After a patient has used the bedpan, he should be offered a basin of water or a washcloth which has been moistened with water and soap, and a towel for cleaning the hands and/or perineal area.

Commodes can be used for patients able to be out of bed but unable to use the bathroom toilet. Commodes are chairs, straight back or wheelchairs, with open seats and a shelf or a holder under the seat on which a bedpan is placed. The commode can be placed adjacent to the bed and the patient assisted to it with minimal exertion.

If the patient is able to use the bathroom toilet, the nurse still is responsible for noting any abnormalities of elimination. In some instances, patients may need to be taught to report abnormalities to the nurse and instructed not to flush the toilet until the nurse has seen the urine. In others, the patient may go to the bathroom for voiding, but if the urine volume is to be calculated, he may need to urinate in a bedpan or some other receptacle placed on the toilet so the urine can be measured before it is discarded. Although many patients can easily be taught to measure their urinary output, the nurse should observe the urine at least once during a work shift and more frequently if warranted. Measurement of urinary output is discussed later in this chapter.

A weak patient should be assisted to the bathroom. Someone should remain in attendance if there is any danger of the patient's falling. Bathrooms should not be locked, and, especially in hospitals, a signal bell should be within easy reach of the patient so that help can be summoned easily if the patient feels weak and in need of assistance. A handrail near the toilet is helpful. So also are special raised seats on the toilet for patients who find it difficult to sit or raise themselves from the seat. Figure 20–2 illustrates.

Many a dangerous situation has been created in the absence of a signal bell or bedpan. Patients confined to bed have gotten out to go to the bathroom to void. Some climbed over or around bed siderails, and others removed oxygen masks or drainage or infusion tubings. For example, an elderly woman was admitted to

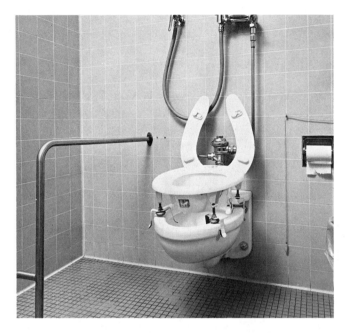

Figure 20-2 This photo illustrates several features for safety and convenience in a patient's bathroom. The handrail at the side of the toilet gives the patient something to grasp as he lowers or raises himself from the seat. A bell cord near the toilet is handy should the patient need to call for assistance. Toilet tissue is within easy reach. The elevator seat on the toilet is convenient for the patient and the nurse when the patient has difficulty bending at the hips to sit down or when the patient needs help to lift himself from the seat.

the hospital in a comatose state. The physician ordered her on *absolute* rest and oxygen as well as other medications. Several hours later when a nurse went in for one of the frequent checks on the patient, the latter was nowhere in sight. She was found in the bathroom. Asked how she got out of bed she said she had crawled around the bottom of the bed siderails. Asked why she did it, she said simply, "I had to go." It was recognized that this patient was beginning to have lucid moments; henceforth, she was offered a bedpan frequently.

Offering a bedpan or urinal frequently can save patients from a fractured hip, a dislodged infusion, or the embarrassment of soiled linen. If a patient appears very ill or is sedated, he may not think to ask in time. As a precaution, family members of patients at home may need to be made aware of this. Remember, the nurse is responsible for the patient's safety.

Securing and Testing Urine Specimens

Nurses are frequently responsible for securing urine specimens for laboratory analysis, called a urinalysis.

Urination into a clean receptacle is considered adequate in many routine situations. Other situations may require a clean catch specimen. This is especially true if a urinary tract infection is suspected and a urine culture is desired. Culture media are inoculated with the urine to allow any organisms present to grow so that they can be examined.

In the clean catch technique, the external meatus is cleaned thoroughly with sterile gauze or cotton balls and soap and water or an antiseptic solution, such as the iodophors. In the uncircumsized male, the foreskin should be retracted to expose the glans penis before cleaning. In the female, the labia are well separated before cleaning and kept apart until the specimen is collected. If the female has a vaginal discharge, she may be instructed to insert a tampon before collecting the specimen. In many agencies, it is recommended that a sterile glove be worn during the cleaning and collection. The patient voids into a sterile container.

Most agencies prefer catching the specimen in midstream. It is expected that any additional organisms harboring at the meatus will have been flushed out by the initial urine in the bladder. The specimen collected after urination has been initiated will be as near the constituency of the urine in the bladder as possible. A patient who can be adequately instructed and expected to carry out the aseptic precautions may collect his own clean catch or midstream specimens and often prefers to do so. Following the collection of urine, the foreskin of the male should be returned to its normal position. Urine specimens for culture should reach the laboratory as quickly as possible if they are not refrigerated. Most authorities feel they may be safely refrigerated for a few hours.

Twenty-four hour specimens are required for some types of laboratory studies. Instruction of the patient regarding the importance of collecting *all* urine for a period of 24 hours is important. The collection is initiated at a specified time by having the patient empty his bladder. This specimen is discarded. All urine for the next 24 hours is saved. Depending on the type of examination, the urine from each voiding may be kept in a separately marked container, indicating the time of urination, or all voidings may be put into a common receptacle. The specimens should be refrigerated and sometimes a preservative is added to retard decomposition.

Children who are too young to cooperate in urine specimen collection often require use of special techniques and apparatus. They are described in detail in texts dealing with the care of children.

In some situations, the nurse may perform tests on urine specimens, especially when specimens are being tested repeatedly for known abnormalities, when screening tests are being used, or when laboratory facilities are not readily available. For example, a nurse may test urine for the presence of glucose, protein, bilirubin, and blood, and to determine its specific gravity. The results of the test are recorded on the patient's record. Many types of commercially prepared diagnostic kits are available for determining the presence of abnormal substances in the urine. While the performance of these tests is economical and fast, laboratory analysis is generally recommended when more precise results are needed.

The diagnostic kits generally contain needed equipment and the appropriate reagent. A *reagent* is a substance used in a chemical reaction to detect another substance. Reagents are prepared in the form of tablets, fluids, impregnated paper, and plastic strips with a special coating. When the reagent is brought in contact with urine, a chemical reaction occurs which causes a color change. The reaction is then compared with an accompanying chart which describes the significance of the color.

The precise directions as to amount of specimen, time allowance for the chemical reaction, and the significance of the colors vary with the manufacturer. Therefore, it is important to read the directions accompanying the diagnostic kit carefully and to follow them exactly. Not to do so can result in erroneous and misleading results.

Since interpretation of the test results depends on the practitioner's judgment on the comparison of the chemical reaction and the color chart, the reading should be performed in a good light and by persons with good visual acuity. It is also important that a clear, nonfaded color chart be used. It is estimated that as many as 10 percent of the readings are inaccurate because of human error.

Determining the specific gravity of urine requires an instrument called a *urinometer* or a *hydrometer*. The urinometer has a calibrated scale for measurement. After a test tube is filled two-thirds full of urine, the urinometer is inserted in a circular motion without touching the bottom or sides of the test tube. The density of the urine supports the urinometer. If the urine is concentrated, as the motion of the urinometer stops, it will be buoyed up high in the test tube and will register high on the measurement scale. If the urine is dilute, the urinometer will be supported low in the urine and a low specific gravity reading will result.

Some persons with chronic illnesses are taught to perform urine tests and maintain records of the results at home. The nurse may be expected to teach the patient or his family members. After explaining the test and demonstrating the technique, having the patient or family member perform the test while the nurse observes is a useful way of identifying any problems or misunderstandings.

Preparing for Diagnostic Tests

Often the nurse prepares the patient for various examinations and tests. When the patient is taught the nature of the procedure and what to expect, any associated anxiety he may be experiencing tends to be reduced.

Visualization of the bladder, urethra, and distal ends of the ureters is called a *cystoscopy*. It is accomplished by the insertion of a lighted tubular instrument, called a *cystoscope,* through the urethra into the bladder. Preparation for a cystoscopy generally includes fasting. Sedation or anesthesia may be used depending on the patient. The preferred position for a cystoscopy is the lithotomy position. Following the procedure, the patient should be encouraged to take fluids as soon as he is able. Tissue swelling, difficult urination, and hematuria may occur because of trauma from the procedure. Therefore, the patient's voiding should be observed and measured for 24 hours or longer after the cystoscopy. The patient should be observed for signs of urinary infection after cystoscopy since it is a common cause of nosocomial infections.

The intravenous pyelogram is a common diagnostic test. A radiopaque contrast substance is injected into the circulatory system and allowed to outline the urinary tract. This test was described in Chapter 15.

When the individual has a known allergy to the contrast substance or if kidney malfunction exists, a retrograde pyelogram is often used. A *retrograde pyelogram* uses contrast material injected through ureteral catheters into the kidneys. Fluoroscopy and x-ray filming are used to visualize the urinary tract. In this way, the contrast material avoids the vascular system. With the patient in lithotomy position, a cystoscopy is performed. Ureteral catheters are inserted through the cystoscope and the contrast material injected. Preparation for the examination usually includes fasting and intestinal evacuation. Following the procedure, one or more ureteral catheters may be left in place and connected to a drainage receptacle. The amount and character of drainage from each catheter should be noted and recorded. Great care should be taken to avoid dislodging the catheters. Following a retrograde pyelogram, nursing measures and observations, such as those used following a cystoscopy, should be employed.

Other renal function tests may require that urine and blood specimens be collected at precise times. The nurse follows the procedure designated by the agency to determine her responsibility.

COMMON NURSING MEASURES FOR DEALING WITH PROBLEMS OF URINARY ELIMINATION

Before describing common nursing measures for dealing with elimination problems, it is necessary to define terms associated with urine and voiding with which the nurse will wish to be familiar. *Anuria* is suppression of urine production. When total anuria occurs, the kidneys produce no urine; therefore, the bladder remains empty. When the kidneys produce only scanty amounts of urine, the term *oliguria* is used. Anuria and oliguria are usually serious signs. *Polyuria* or *diuresis* is an excessive output of urine.

At times urine is produced by the kidneys and enters the bladder but is not eliminated. Excessive storage of urine in the bladder is called *retention*. The term incontinence is often used as a synonym for enuresis. Technically, *incontinence* is the inability to retain urine, feces, or semen. The term enuresis is used most often when referring to the child who involuntarily urinates mostly during the night, as described in Chapter 18.

Hematuria refers to urine that contains blood. If present in large enough quantities, the urine may be bright red or reddish brown in color. Pus in the urine is called *pyuria*. The urine appears cloudy. Pyuria should not be confused with the cloudiness which may occur when normal urine stands and cools. Albumin in the urine is called *albuminuria* or *proteinuria*. It is often an indication of kidney disease. Albumin is sometimes present in urine that is voided following periods of standing, walking, and running. This is called orthostatic albuminuria and is a phenomenon of the circulatory system and not necessarily a symptom of kidney disorders. *Glycosuria* is the presence of sugar in the urine. If glycosuria is due to an unusually large intake of sugar or to marked emotional disturbances and is temporary, there is little cause for alarm. This condition is called *alimentary glycosuria.*

Dysuria is difficulty in voiding. It may or may not be associated with pain. A feeling of warm local irritation occurring during voiding is called burning. *Frequency* refers to voiding at very frequent intervals. Excessive voiding during the night especially when not associated with large fluid intake is called *nocturia* or *nycturia.*

Urinary Incontinence

Incontinence may be partial or complete. If the bladder is unable to store any urine and urine dribbles almost constantly, the condition is called *total incontinence*. If the bladder cannot be emptied normally, urine continues to accumulate, and, when there is sufficient pressure in the bladder, small amounts of urine may be forced out. The dribble of urine ends when the pressure has been reduced somewhat, but the bladder is not empty. This is called *overflow* or *paradoxical incontinence*. This type sometimes accompanies retention. Total or overflow incontinence may be either permanent or temporary, depending on the cause. It is a problem faced by many elderly persons. Because it is so common, family members often need to be helped to deal with it in the home.

Stress incontinence is the involuntary escape of urine which occurs with straining, such as heavy lifting, sneezing, coughing, or laughing. It occurs most frequently in women and is thought to be due to their shorter urethras. Such incontinence may occur as early as middle-age in otherwise well females. It appears to be more prevalent in women who have had a number of pregnancies.

Nursing Measures for Incontinence. As soon as a medical evaluation of the patient's problem has been made, nursing measures should be directed toward helping to restore normal function if there is a possibility of success. Incontinence generally carries with it a significant change in self-image and loss of self-respect for the alert adult. As with fecal incontinence, urinary incontinence should not be a condition to which everyone becomes resigned.

Because of the social and psychological significance of incontinence, most persons are willing to exert a great deal of effort to regain urinary control. The psychological value of the person knowing that he is not rejected and that effort is being made to assist him should not be underestimated. A cautionary note must also be interjected. The regaining of urinary control can be an extremely difficult and lengthy process for some persons and even impossible for others. It requires the effort and complete cooperation of the individual involved. Acceptance, support, and explanation by the nurse are also important. Care should be taken to see that inappropriate goals are not established lest the person become discouraged. With realistic and progressive goals and persistent effort, most persons can be helped to some degree with urinary incontinence.

Sometimes, simple and carefully planned measures may be adequate. For example, increasing the fluid intake may be all that is necessary. Some persons do not think about the relationship between fluid intake and urination. Others deliberately decrease their daily fluid intake because of their concerns about incontinence. Such an action predisposes them to urinary tract infections and a greater likelihood of incontinence.

Conscious efforts to control or induce voiding may be sufficiently stimulating to help restore control for some persons. Especially for the elderly chronically ill, it may be as simple as taking them to the bathroom or offering a bedpan or urinal every two to three hours.

Perineal exercises, such as those used by women in childbirth preparation, can also be helpful for women experiencing stress incontinence. Alternately contracting and relaxing perineal muscles three to four times several times each day can aid in strengthening the urinary sphincter. Using muscle contraction and relaxation to stop and start the flow of urine voluntarily while voiding can also be helpful for both males and females in improving sphincter control.

In addition to efforts to help the individual regain control of urination, other measures also must be considered, such as keeping the person dry, clean, and comfortable. The nurse should provide a situation in which the individual's self-respect is nurtured. Often great skill and ingenuity are required to prevent odors and discomfort from wet clothing and linens. The ammonia resulting from decomposing urine and lying on wet linen can quickly irritate the skin and predispose the person to ammonia dermatitis and to excoriation. *Excoriation* is a breakdown of the epidermis. Such conditions also predispose to decubitus ulcers and, therefore, skin care must be meticulous.

Various types of external urinary collection appliances are available for male patients. The devices fit directly over the penis and are secured by adhesives or straps. A collection bag is usually attached to the patient's leg to permit ambulation. These devices must be applied carefully to prevent skin irritation and skin breakdown, cleaned regularly to avoid odor, and emptied at appropriate intervals to prevent accidental spillage. Since a man's trousers can cover the entire appliance, his independence and activity can be readily maintained with no embarrassment. Unfortunately, because of the anatomical structure of the female, no such device is available for women. Women with stress incontinence often wear perineal pads to absorb the urine and protect their clothing.

A quick course of action for controlling incontinence is to have an indwelling catheter inserted. An *indwelling catheter* is a tube into the bladder which provides for constant urine drainage. This will be discussed later in this chapter. The cost in terms of physical discomfort and change in body image for the person with an indwelling catheter can be exceedingly high. Infection from indwelling catheters is very common. For some patients it will require months after the catheter is removed before the infection is cured.

Patients with incontinence usually are embarrassed and insecure. The nurse can help by demonstrating tact and understanding while carrying out her nursing responsibilities. Offering emotional support, encouraging the patient to talk of his problem, and allowing him to assist with decision-making about his care also are helpful. Whenever possible, it is preferable from a psychological standpoint to consult with him about measures to collect and absorb urine, such as absorbent pads, urinary appliances, and waterproof undergarments.

In certain disease conditions, voluntary control of voiding may be impaired, but the reflex act of micturition is intact. These patients may be helped with bladder training. Drugs also are used to assist these patients.

Bladder Training. Bladder training should be instituted in consultation with the physician, since a complete evaluation of the patient's physical condition is essential. To start a patient on such a program when there is little or no possibility of his achieving results could be psychologically disastrous for him. Even if a patient is considered eligible for bladder training, he must be helped to understand that it will be a slow process and that the gains may be slight and very gradual. As in any situation, it is poor policy to permit a patient to set unrealistic goals for himself.

A primary factor in bladder training is the management of the patient's fluid intake. An intake of from 2,000 to 3,000 ml. per 24-hour period is generally considered necessary. In addition to liquids, such as milk, tea, broth, water, and soup, foods of high-liquid content may also be helpful. Because of the time relationship between drinking and the occurrence of urine in the bladder, it is best to plan a drinking schedule that will permit convenient occasions for attempting to empty the bladder. For example, most persons urinate shortly after awakening, and this is usually the first and the best time for the patient to attempt to empty the bladder. Having some water immediately on waking is usually helpful. Other liquids can be spaced throughout the day according to the patient's wishes. Liquids should be limited in the late evening hours, thus decreasing the risk of being incontinent during the night.

Position of the Patient: When the patient attempts to start bladder training, it is essential that conditions conducive to urinating be provided. The patient should be comfortable and relaxed, privacy should be provided, and adjustments should be made so that a normal position may be maintained. If the patient is not able to get out of bed and is going to use the bedpan or urinal, the head of the bed should be raised and the patient well-supported by pillows. It is also best if the patient's knees are flexed during the time that an attempt to void is being made.

The position found to be most helpful is the normal sitting or standing position. This position can be simulated by some patients if they are permitted to have their legs dangling over the edge of the bed while sitting on a bedpan. In addition, they should have a foot support and a chair or overbed table on which to lean. Men may stand by the side of the bed. A toilet or a commode is best if the patient is able to be out of bed.

Time: A regular schedule is also essential for helping the patient to establish a pattern. His usual times for voiding should be considered. If there has been any regularity to the patient's incontinence of urine, these times should be considered in the scheduling. For example, if the patient notes that incontinence often occurs near 10:30 A.M., provision for attempting to void should be made at 10:00 A.M.

The times selected for attempting to empty the bladder need not be spaced regularly, such as every four hours. However, they should be at the same time each day. The intervals between each voiding will depend on the patient's fluid intake and his bladder capacity.

The Stimulus or Call: Any sensation which precedes the act of micturition is called the *stimulus* or *call*. The patient should be informed that this may not be the usual kind of stimulus produced by a full bladder, but it may include other reactions, such as sensations in the abdomen, chilliness, sweating, muscular twitching, restlessness, and so on. It is important that the patient understand these signs to become sensitive to the clues of a need to empty the bladder.

Methods for Assisting the Process: While the patient is in the sitting position, it is helpful if he bends forward in a slow, rhythmic fashion. This creates pressure on the bladder. It also helps if the patient applies light pressure with the hands over the bladder. The pressure should be directed toward the urethra.

Other measures, such as those which are used to help patients void, also should be used if necessary. These include drinking fluids to the extent allowed or listening to running water.

It is possible for the patient to void without awareness of it or without any specific stimulus or control. This is still considered as involuntary voiding. Not until the patient is able to use a specific method to stimulate and empty the bladder is the bladder-training program considered successful.

For those patients with severe neuromuscular involvement, the best method for inducing the stimulus and emptying the bladder may require considerable exploration; 15 to 20 minutes for each attempt is sufficient. Unsuccessful attempts are discouraging, and the patient should be helped to maintain a positive and hopeful attitude toward the process. Weeks or even months of consistent effort may be necessary before results are achieved and the person should be prepared for this likelihood.

As a means of gauging the success of the attempts, examination for residual urine may be included as a part of the process. Percussion directly over the symphysis is one method. In some programs of rehabilitation, tests for residual urine are made by inserting a catheter. As the amount of residual urine diminishes and the success of emptying the entire bladder increases, the frequency of examination is reduced.

Some practitioners have used behavior modification as described in Chapter 8 to assist in bladder training. A source included in the references at the end of this unit describes the application of this approach.

Urinary Retention

Retention occurs when urine is being produced normally but is not being excreted from the bladder. The bladder continues to fill and may distend until it reaches the level of the umbilicus. The abdomen swells as the bladder rises above the level of the symphysis pubis. The height of the bladder can be determined by palpating with light pressure on the abdomen.

Retention is often temporary. It is common following abdominal surgery, especially if ambulation is delayed or fluid intake is minimal. Any mechanical obstruction, such as swelling at the meatus, which often occurs following childbirth or an enlarged prostate in the male, may cause retention. The cause also may be psychic or due to certain disease conditions.

While urine that is retained in the bladder can be removed by introducing a catheter, every effort should be made to help the patient void. Nursing measures should be instituted as soon as a patient feels that he cannot urinate even if the interval since the last voiding was only a few hours. This is particularly true if the patient has been having a normal fluid intake. Urine retained in the bladder increases the likelihood of urinary tract infection.

There are several measures that often aid in initiating normal micturition if there is no mechanical obstruction or disease condition causing retention. Placing the patient in the normal position for voiding, that is, the sitting position for females and standing position for males, is usually helpful if sitting or standing is not contraindicated. Sometimes, voiding will begin if the patient sits at the edge of the bed on a bedpan and supports his feet on a chair. If the patient is allowed out of bed, the patient can sit on a bedpan placed on a chair, or a commode can be used. The male patient often can induce voiding if he is permitted to stand. A toilet is best if the patient can walk or be moved to one. The supine position has been found to be least successful in helping to initiate voiding. If the patient's condition permits, he should be provided privacy while he attempts to void. In many instances the patient may need to wait several minutes for the urge to void to appear or reappear.

Additional measures which often assist in the voiding process include offering the patient fluids, especially warm drinks; warming the bedpan before use; allowing water to run from a tap within hearing distance of the patient; or placing the patient's hands in warm water or pouring warm water over the perineum (if no specimen is desired).

Retention is painful. The patient often becomes anxious and tense, which usually further interferes with normal voiding. A sedated or semiconscious patient may become restless because of retention even though he may not be aware of the cause of the discomfort.

Occasionally, a patient will void, but the quantity will be insufficient by comparison with the fluid intake. Or, the patient may say that he feels as though he still needs to void. Urine retained in the bladder after voiding is called *residual urine*. Normally, all but approximately 1 to 3 ml. of urine is excreted from the bladder in voiding.

Catheterization

Urinary catheterization is the introduction of a catheter through the urethra into the bladder for the purpose of withdrawing urine. A *catheter* is a tube for injecting or removing fluids. In recent years, the value of catheterization, formerly questioned, has become increasingly suspect in view of the hazards involved. It is now considered the most prominent cause of nosocomial infections. Therefore, whenever possible, it is recommended that catheterization be avoided. When deemed necessary, it should be performed with careful technique.

Several physiological facts should be recalled. The bladder is normally a sterile cavity. The external opening to the urethra can never be sterilized. The bladder has defense mechanisms, namely, the emptying of urine and intravesical antibacterial activity. These help to maintain a sterile bladder under normal circumstances and also aid in clearing an infection if it occurs. Pathogens introduced into the bladder can ascend the ureters and lead to kidney infection. A normal bladder is not as susceptible to infection as a damaged one. A patient's lowered resistance, present in many diseases and stress situations, predisposes him to urinary infection. Therefore, patients should only be catheterized when absolutely necessary because of the danger of acquiring an infection.

The hazards of introducing an instrument or a catheter into the bladder are sepsis and trauma; the possibility of the latter to the male urethra, because of its length, is obvious. An object forced through a stricture or irregularity from the wrong angle can cause serious damage to the urethra. While the urethra in the female is shorter than that in the male, it is also susceptible to damage if a catheter is forced through it. The mucous membrane lining the urethra is delicate and easily damaged by the friction resulting from the insertion of a catheter. Bacteria can enter the bladder by being pushed in as the catheter is being inserted. When the catheter is left in place, the organisms may also move up the catheter lumen or the space between the catheter and the urethral wall.

Purposes of Catheterization. It was formerly considered essential to catheterize for a routine urine specimen free of contamination, but this practice has been abandoned in most situations. The clean catch technique has been substituted. Catheterization may be used before surgery to empty the patient's bladder completely since tension and preoperative sedatives can result in incomplete emptying of the bladder. When this is necessary, it is recommended that the catheterization be performed in the aseptic conditions of the operating room. Catheterization is used postoperatively to prevent bladder distention and when patients are unable to urinate after all nursing measures to induce voiding have failed. It is used before and after delivery for the same reasons. Catheterization also may be used when the patient is incontinent or when the specimen would be otherwise contaminated, such as when a female patient is menstruating.

Catheterization also may be used to remove urine from a greatly distended bladder. Gradual decompression of the distended bladder has generally been considered to be a safer procedure than rapid removal of all urine, although there is little research evidence to support this practice. Rapid emptying of the bladder was thought to cause severe systemic reactions, such as chills, fever, and shock. Gradual decompression has been credited with preventing engorgement of the vessels as well as helping to improve the tone of the bladder wall by adjusting the pressure within the bladder in stages.

In health agencies where gradual decompression is preferred, the following practices are often used. For patients who have severe retention, for example, if as much as 2,000 ml. is suspected, a special apparatus may be used to decompress the bladder over a period of 24 hours or more. When the nurse needs to exercise judgment as to the amount of urine to withdraw at a single catheterization, no more than 750 ml. of urine is removed from a patient at any one time.

Equipment. Commonly used urinary catheters are made of rubber or plastic material. For male patients, there also are silk woven catheters that are firm, yet flexible, and following the contour of the urethra with ease.

Catheters, like rectal tubes, are graded on the French scale according to the size of the lumen. For the female adult, sizes No. 14 and No. 16, Fr., catheters usually are used. Smaller catheters are generally not necessary, and the size of the lumen is so small that it increases the length of time necessary for emptying the bladder. Larger catheters distend the urethra and tend to increase the discomfort of the procedure. For the male

adult, sizes No. 18 and No. 20, Fr., catheters usually are used, but if this appears to be too large, a smaller caliber should be tried. Sizes No. 8 and No. 10, Fr., are commonly used for children.

In addition to the catheter, a receptacle for collecting urine, a fenestrated drape, lubricant, materials to clean the meatus and area around it, and sterile gloves are necessary.

The equipment used during a catheterization should be sterile and handled with strict surgical asepsis. Sterilization with steam under pressure is recommended for reusable equipment. The trend is toward the use of presterilized disposable equipment. The equipment is used only once, thereby decreasing the possibility of introducing infection. These sets are easy to use and economical as well. When catheterization is done in the home, a disposable set is the first choice because it eliminates sterilization problems. Clean or medical asepsis is being recommended for self-catheterization for some persons with permanent incontinence problems. The technique will be discussed later in this chapter.

Preparation of the Patient. It is assumed that the patient will have had an adequate explanation of the procedure and the reason for it beforehand. A catheter being inserted produces a sensation of pressure in the area rather than one of pain. This should be explained to the patient. In addition, the patient should be assured that every measure to avoid exposure and embarrassment will be taken. The more relaxed the patient can be, the easier it will be to insert the catheter.

The most frequent position for the patient is the dorsal recumbent, preferably on a solid surface, such as a firm mattress or a treatment table. Catheterization in the bed with a soft mattress, especially for the female patient, is not as satisfactory because the patient's pelvic surfaces are not supported firmly, and visualization of the meatus is difficult. Also, sinking into the bed may cause the patient's bladder to be lower than the outlet of the catheter. If the patient is in bed, supporting the buttocks on a firm cushion is helpful.

The Sims's or lateral position can be an alternate for the female patient. It may provide better visualization for the nurse if her stature is short, and it may be more comfortable for the patient, especially one who finds hip and knee movements difficult. Reduced area of exposure also can result in less psychic discomfort for the patient. The patient may lie on either side depending on which position is easiest for the nurse and best in terms of the patient's comfort. The patient's buttocks are placed near the edge of the bed with her shoulders at the opposite edge and her knees drawn toward her chest. The nurse lifts the upper buttock and labia to expose the urinary meatus.

For the female patient, good positioning and lighting are essential to locating the meatus quickly and easily. Artificial light is almost always necessary for this procedure. The patient should be protected adequately from unnecessary exposure of the perineal area and from drafts by proper and adequate draping. Figure 20–3 illustrates alternate positions of the female patient for catheterization.

Positioning of the patient should allow sufficient space for the nurse to prepare and maintain a sterile area adjacent to the perineal area to place the necessary equipment. If the dorsal recumbent position is used, the sterile area is generally between the patient's legs near the perineum. If the Sims's position is used, the sterile area is immediately adjacent to the lower buttock. In addition, sterile drapes are usually used to extend the work area beyond the immediate perineal area.

Procedure for Catheterizaton of the Patient: As indicated earlier, bacteria can be introduced into the urinary bladder by passing a catheter through the external meatus and the urethra into the bladder. The area around the meatus should be made as clean as possible in order to minimize contamination of the catheter. In addition, the nurse should wash her hands thoroughly before the procedure. The Center for Disease Control recommends that an antiseptic agent, such as an iodophor- or hexachlorophene-containing substance, be used for handwashing prior to urinary catheterization.

The best preparation of the glans penis or the labia and the introitus prior to introducing a catheter is to clean the area thoroughly. Some agencies specify a thorough washing of the local area with soap and water immediately before the procedure, and then cleaning with an antiseptic solution on cotton balls prior to the insertion of the catheter. The Center for Disease Control recommends an iodophor solution.

The nurse wears sterile gloves for performing a catheterization. The technique for putting on sterile gloves was presented in Figure 14–7 on page 268. If at any time during the procedure the nurse suspects her gloves have been contaminated, she should change them immediately.

To catheterize the female patient, good visualization of the meatus facilitates the procedure and reduces the chance of contaminating the tip of the catheter. When the patient is in the dorsal recumbent position, this can be accomplished by inserting the thumb and the first or second finger well into the labia minora, spreading it apart and then pulling upward toward the symphysis pubis. Stretching the tissue in either position "irons out" the area and makes the meatus visible. In many women, it is rather difficult to find the meatus and it may appear as a small dimple in the area. Once the meatus has been cleaned, do not allow the labia to close over it. This risks the chance of contaminating it.

The foreskin of the penis in the uncircumcised male is retracted for cleaning and the catheter is then inserted. The urethral meatus should be visible at the tip of the penis. The penis should be held upward or near perpendicular to the body to straighten the long urethra and facilitate catheter insertion.

The catheter should be well-lubricated with a sterile, water-soluble jelly to minimize friction and to ease insertion. Slight resistance will often be met as the catheter encounters the external sphincter. Pausing briefly and asking the patient to breathe deeply will

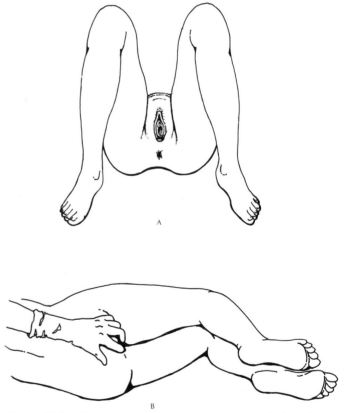

Figure 20–3 Alternate positions for female urinary catheterization. A shows the patient in the dorsal recumbent position and B shows the patient in the lateral position. Drapes are omitted in the sketches to more clearly show positioning of the patient.

generally result in sufficient relaxation for the catheter to be passed readily. Rotating the catheter gently may also be helpful. Under no circumstance should force be used. The catheter will need to be inserted approximately 5 to 7.5 cm. or 2 to 3 inches in the female patient and 18 to 23 cm. or 7 to 9 inches in the male. As the bladder is entered, urine will escape through the catheter. Following catheterization, the foreskin of the male patient should be replaced over the glans penis. Leaving the foreskin in a retracted position can cause edema and inability to void.

The insertion of the catheter normally does not produce severe pain. If the patient seems to be experiencing unusual discomfort, discontinue the procedure and notify the physician. Some patients have strictures of the urethra and urethral dilation by a physician may be necessary before a catheter can be inserted.

Immediately following the insertion of the catheter, some patients react by tightening the muscles in the area, and the flow of urine may be delayed for a few seconds until the patient is able to relax. If the nurse will merely wait a brief time after she believes the bladder has been entered, she may save herself and the patient the necessity of repeating the procedure. The chart below describes the procedure of urinary catheterization.

If a urine specimen is needed, it should be collected while the bladder is being emptied. During catheterization, there are observations which the nurse makes and later records. These include color and the transparency of the urine and the amount obtained. Occasionally, urine has an unusual odor and this should be recorded. Any unusual discomfort experienced by the patient should also be noted. A specimen is handled according to agency policy.

Self-catheterization

After World War II, many persons with bladder dysfunction due to neurological pathology, such as muscular dystrophy, paraplegia, and congenital spinal defects, were taught to perform intermittent sterile self-catheterization. Being able to care for their needs for urinary elimination at home has enhanced the independence and self-concepts of these persons.

Since 1972, persons with neurogenic bladder disorders using a clean technique for self-catheterization have been under study and the results have been promising. The individuals are taught to catheterize themselves, generally while in a sitting position in the bathroom. A clean catheter and lubricant are used rather than sterile equipment. The clean technique is far less cumbersome and more convenient than the sterile technique. Reports show no higher incidence of urinary tract infections with a clean self-catheterization technique than with the sterile technique. It is hypothesized that the cause of urinary tract infections in persons with neurological bladder dysfunction is impaired

Catheterization of the urinary bladder

The purpose is to remove urine from the bladder.

SUGGESTED ACTION	RATIONALE
Collect and prepare all necessary equipment before entering the patient's room.	Preparation of equipment where the patient can observe it may be disturbing and frightening.
After providing privacy, place the patient in the desired position.	Comfort of the patient will facilitate relaxation. Positioning should promote good visualization.
Drape the patient to provide minimum exposure. Use sufficient covering, depending on patient's age, condition, and environmental factors.	Embarrassment and chilliness can cause the patient to become tense. Tension can interfere with easy introduction of the catheter.
Arrange the lighting for maximum visualization.	Good visualization of the meatus, especially in the female, is essential for sterile insertion of the catheter.
Place the sterile tray containing equipment near the meatal area. Open it using sterile technique.	Placement of equipment near the work site increases efficiency. Inside covering of the sterile tray can be used as the sterile field.
After putting on sterile gloves, arrange sterile equipment for convenience and to avoid contamination. Place materials for cleaning the perineum so that reaching over the sterile field is avoided.	Placement of equipment in the order of use increases the speed of performance. Reaching over sterile items increases the risk of contamination.
Place the sterile drapes adjacent to the meatal area. Use the drape corners to wrap around the gloved hands.	The drapes increase the size of the sterile work area and reduce the danger of contamination. Covering the gloved hands will help keep the gloves sterile while placing the drapes.

Catheterization of the urinary bladder (continued)

The purpose is to remove urine from the bladder.

SUGGESTED ACTION	RATIONALE
Lubricate the catheter for about 3.7 cm. or 1½ inches, being careful not to plug the eye of the catheter. Lubricating the catheter is illustrated in Figure 20–4.	Lubrication reduces friction and facilitates catheter insertion.
For the female patient, place the thumb and one finger between the labia minora and identify the meatus, as illustrated in Figures 20–5 and 20–6. Maintain the separation of the labia until the catheter is in the bladder. For the male patient retract the foreskin as necessary and lift the penis perpendicular to the body.	Smoothing the area immediately surrounding the meatus helps to make it visible. Microorganisms may be harbored under the foreskin. Lifting the penis straightens the urethra.
Clean the area using as many cotton balls as necessary to assure absolute cleanliness. Use one cotton ball for each stroke, moving it from above the meatus down toward the rectum for the female, as illustrated in Figure 20–7, and in a proximal direction for the male, as illustrated in Figure 20–8. Keep the labia separated for the female and the penis elevated for the male.	Thorough cleaning of the meatus and the area surrounding it reduces possible introduction of microorganisms into the bladder. Contamination from the rectal area can result by stroking from this area toward the meatus. Permitting the labia to close over the meatus or lowering the penis may contaminate the area just cleaned.
Taking care not to contaminate it, pick up the catheter and place its distal end in the collection receptacle.	The catheter must remain sterile to avoid the introduction of organisms into the bladder. The collection receptacle must be in readiness for the urine flow to avoid soiling.
Insert the catheter into the meatus until urine begins to flow. This is usually 5 to 7.5 cm. or 2 to 3 inches for the female and 18 to 23 cm. or 6 to 7 inches for the male. Figure 20–9 illustrates the nurse about to insert a catheter into the male patient.	The female urethra is approximately 3.7 to 6 cm. or 1½ to 2½ inches long. The male urethra is approximately 13.7 to 16 cm. or 5½ to 6½ inches in length.
Hold the catheter securely in place and avoid pulling and pushing the catheter in the urethra. Obtain a specimen if indicated, as illustrated in Figures 20–10 and 20–11.	Withdrawing the catheter and then pushing it back into the bladder increases the possibility of contamination.
When the flow of urine begins to diminish, withdraw the catheter slowly, about 1 cm. or ½ inch at a time until urine barely drips.	The tip of the' catheter passes through urine remaining in the bladder.
Clean all equipment thoroughly immediately after use, if not disposable.	Secretions, lubricant, and other substances are removed more easily when they are not coagulated.

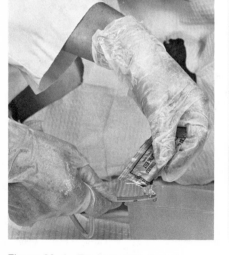

Figure 20–4   The patient is properly draped and the nurse's hands are gloved. She expresses lubricant from the package and allows it to drip onto the catheter.

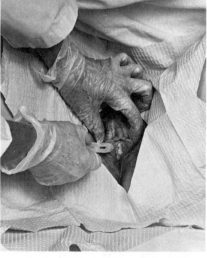

Figure 20–5   The nurse has spread the labia well. In this photo, she is pointing at the meatus with the instrument in her right hand. Note that it looks like a small dimple.

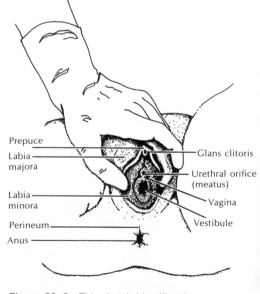

Prepuce
Labia majora
Labia minora
Perineum
Anus
Glans clitoris
Urethral orifice (meatus)
Vagina
Vestibule

Figure 20–6   This sketch identifies the various structures in the perineal area.

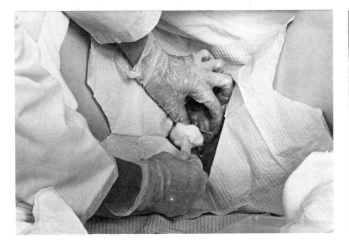

Figure 20-7   The nurse is cleaning the area at and around the meatus with a cotton ball moistened with an antiseptic. She holds the cotton ball with a pair of sterile forceps.

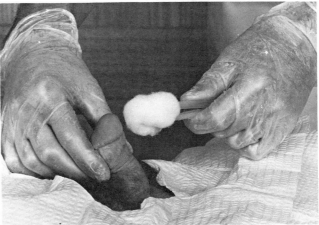

Figure 20-8   The nurse is about to clean the area at the meatus with a cotton ball moistened with an antiseptic. He holds the cotton ball with a pair of sterile forceps and will move from the area of the meatus down the penis toward the patient's body. The penis is held in position almost perpendicular to the patient's body in order to help straighten the urethra.

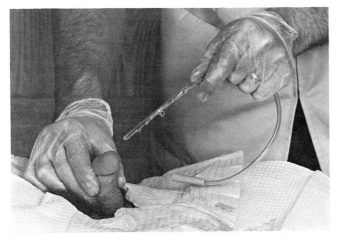

Figure 20-9   Note that the nurse has lubricated the catheter well before inserting it into the patient. Since the male urethra is tortuous, generous lubrication is recommended.

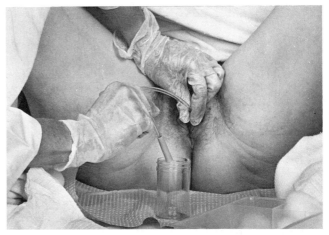

Figure 20-10   While emptying the bladder and obtaining a specimen, the nurse allows the labia to fall in place but holds the catheter securely in place with one hand. With her other hand, she holds the end of the catheter in the specimen container.

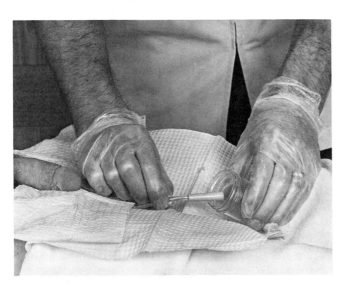

Figure 20-11   The penis is allowed to fall onto the sterile drape while the nurse holds the catheter securely with one hand. With his other hand, he holds the container to collect a specimen.

circulation to the bladder tissue resulting from frequent overdistention of the bladder. The decreased blood circulation is thought to lower the body's resistance to bacterial invasion. Frequent catheterization which keeps the bladder volume limited to 200 to 300 ml. increases resistance to the organisms and keeps the urinary tract free of infection. The ease of using the clean technique makes frequent catheterization more practical. While the procedure is too new to have long-term data, the results thus far have been encouraging. Several reports of the investigations are included in the references at the end of this unit.

Indwelling Catheters

If a catheter is to remain in place for continued drainage, an *indwelling urethral catheter* is usually used. Indwelling urethral catheters are also called *retention* and *Foley* catheters.

Occasionally, a *suprapubic catheter* is used for continuous drainage. A catheter is inserted through a small incision above the pubic area. Care of the patient with a suprapubic catheter is discussed in clinical texts.

The indwelling catheter is so designed that it does not slip out of the bladder. Such catheters are used for gradual decompression of an overdistended bladder, for intermittent bladder drainage and irrigation, and for continuous drainage of the bladder.

An indwelling catheter has a portion which can be inflated after the catheter is inserted into the bladder. Because the inflated balloon is larger than the opening to the urethra, the catheter is retained in the bladder. There are several types of indwelling catheters available, but the principles on which they operate are similar. The indwelling catheter has more than one lumen. In a double-lumen catheter, one lumen is connected directly with the balloon which may be distended with either solution or air, and the other is the portion through which the urine drains. The triple-lumen catheter provides an additional lumen for the instillation of irrigating solution. Figure 20–12 shows double- and triple-lumen indwelling catheters.

The basic procedure for inserting an indwelling catheter is the same as that for the catheter which is removed immediately. The only difference is that equipment for inflating the balloon must be available. As soon as the bladder has been emptied of urine, the balloon of the indwelling catheter is distended with air or solution, usually sterile normal saline or sterile water. The balloons are designed to hold from 5 to 30 ml. Each catheter indicates the amount to be in-

jected into the balloon. The means of injecting varies with the make of catheter. Some balloons must be distended by means of a syringe with an adaptor, and then the inlet is clamped off. Other balloons are distended with a syringe and a No. 20 needle because the inlet is self-sealing. If the patient complains of pain or discomfort while the balloon is being filled, empty the balloon and insert the catheter farther, for it may be that the balloon is in the urethra.

After the balloon has been distended, it is best to test the catheter to see that it is in place. Slight tension on it will indicate whether or not it is secure in the bladder. For patients with pathological changes of the bladder and/or the urethra, it may be necessary to irrigate the catheter after the balloon is distended. This will help to determine whether the catheter is inserted properly.

Drainage with the Indwelling Catheter. It is general practice for an indwelling catheter to be attached to a collection receptacle by tubing so that drainage occurs by gravity. This arrangement is also called straight drainage. The drainage tubing should be of sufficient length to reach the collecting container and still give the patient freedom to move about. If the drainage tubing is too long, urine pools in the tubing and may interrupt the drainage from the bladder. If it is too short, movement will be restricted.

Most urinary drainage tubing is transparent which makes it possible to examine drainage from the catheter. The drainage tube should be secured by a means which permits movement of the tubing and prevents tension and pull on the catheter and urethra. The catheter is generally taped to the patient's leg, and, in addition, the tubing may be secured to his clothing or the bed. It is essential that the tubing be placed so that it cannot be compressed by the weight of the patient's buttocks or thigh.

To place the drainage tubing over the patient's thigh has a disadvantage in that urine may pool in the bladder until there is a sufficient amount of pressure to force it up the tubing. Drainage will not occur until the urine forces its way over the thigh, and then gravity will empty the bladder. The distance between the bladder and the container will determine the rate of drainage. The drainage tube should be so arranged that accumulation of urine in the bladder or backflow into the bladder will not occur.

The drainage container should be placed so that suction on the bladder is minimized in the event that occasional siphonage should occur. Placement should also be such that the collection container is lower than

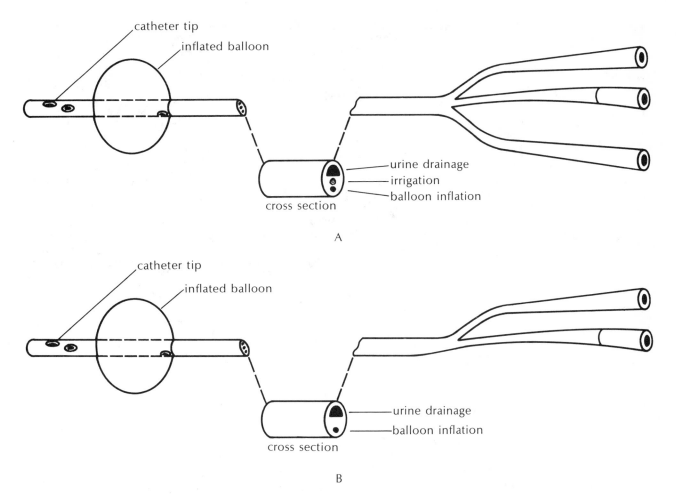

Figure 20-12 These sketches illustrate double- and triple-lumen indwelling catheters.

the catheter's entry into the bladder to prevent urine from reentering the bladder. This is especially important when the patient ambulates. Attaching the container to the bed frame is common practice when the patient is in bed. In addition, it should be inconspicuous in order to avoid embarrassment to the patient, yet be easy to examine. Figure 20–13 shows the position of the collection container. Calibrated drainage containers have several advantages. Amounts of drainage can be determined readily, and measuring when emptying the container is eliminated. In most agencies, the amount of urine in the drainage container is noted before it is emptied every eight hours.

The closed drainage system has been shown to be superior in preventing urinary tract infections. In the closed system, a continuous sterile passageway leads from the bladder to the drainage receptacle. A special air filter permits air to escape from the collection con-

tainer without bacteria entrance. An outlet valve also permits the receptacle to be emptied without contamination. The catheter, tubing, and receptacle are never disconnected from each other in order to prevent the introduction of microorganisms. Various types of commercial closed drainage systems are available.

The open system, in which catheter, tubing, and collection container may be disconnected from each other and the receptacle may even have an open top, are still occasionally used in the home. While the risk is still great, economy and elimination of cross-infection from other patients may be felt by some persons to be ample justification for its use in homes.

Chronically ill patients at home may have indwelling catheters that are cared for by the patient or family members. If nondisposable equipment is used, the nurse may need to teach the patient and/or family how to care for it. It is recommended that the collection re-

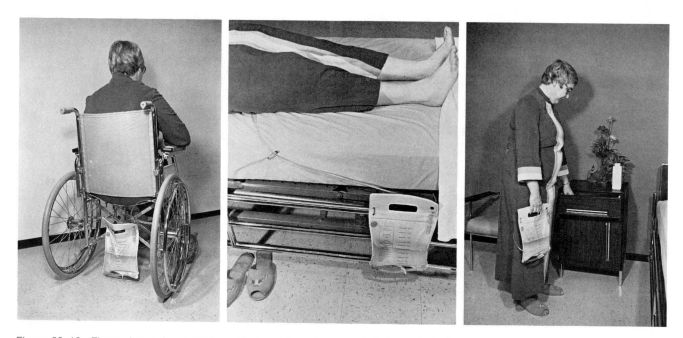

Figure 20–13 These photos demonstrate positioning of the urine receptacle for an indwelling catheter. The receptacle should be below the bladder whether the patient is seated, lying, or standing. Note that the tube is free of kinks and as straight as possible.

ceptacle and tubing be washed daily with soap and water and soaked in a vinegar solution. The tubing should be boiled approximately twice a week.

Indwelling catheters have increased the comfort of the ambulatory patient with bladder disturbances, whether he is in a health agency or at home. There are soft rubber or plastic collection receptacles available, so designed that the catheter fits into the top. The receptacle is then attached to the leg and held in place by small, soft straps. These receptacles make it possible for the patient to be completely dressed without any evidence of the attachment. However, the patient should be taught that pressure on the container could force urine back into the bladder and should be avoided because of the danger of infection. Some patients are taught to use a clamp on the catheter and to release it to empty the bladder at specified intervals, such as every two or three hours. This procedure has been questioned in recent years because of the increased incidence of infections.

Irrigation of the Indwelling Catheter.   An *irrigation* is the flushing of a tube, canal, or area with solution. The purpose of a catheter irrigation is to restore or maintain its patency. The physician occasionally orders an irrigation when blood clots or other debris threaten to block the catheter. The procedure was done routinely

for almost all indwelling catheters in the past, but because this is another means of introducing pathogens, the current recommendation is that an irrigation should be done only when there is a demonstrated need. "Natural" irrigation of the catheter through an increased fluid intake by the patient is felt to be preferable.

When irrigation is done, strict sterile technique must be followed. Sterile equipment consisting of a syringe, a basin and solution, and a clean collecting basin is necessary for irrigating at intervals. Preferably, the patient who requires catheter irrigation will have a triple-lumen retention catheter in place. This precludes the necessity of opening the closed drainage system. Otherwise, if the patient has a double-lumen retention catheter, the catheter is temporarily separated from the drainage tubing so that the solution is injected directly into the catheter. The ends of both the catheter and the tubing must be handled carefully to prevent contamination. Sterile drainage tube protectors and catheter plugs are commercially available. When it is necessary to use these items, they should be discarded after each use. It is recommended that when catheter irrigations are done at home using nondisposable equipment, the syringe should be boiled for 10 minutes before it is used.

Varying amounts of sterile solution may be specified

for irrigation, but 50 to 60 ml. per irrigation usually is sufficient. A syringe large enough to instill the entire amount at one time is preferred because it reduces the potential for introducing contaminants. The solution should be instilled and allowed to return by gravity. "Milking," or squeezing sequential sections of the drainage tubing with the fingers, may be necessary if it is obstructed. This "milking" should be done by moving from the patient toward the drainage receptacle. Pressure or suction should not be used because the mucous membrane lining of the bladder can be injured. Any irrigation solution that is unused may be refrigerated and used within a 24-hour period. After 24 hours, it should be discarded.

Preferably, the patient who needs frequent irrigation in order that the catheter and tubing remain patent will have a triple-lumen catheter with continuous irrigation. A container of sterile solution suspended above the patient is attached by tubing to the irrigation outlet of the catheter. The flow of the solution is regulated to enter the bladder slowly. It leaves via the urine drainage outlet in the catheter. Such an arrangement allows for the continuous irrigation of the catheter within the sterile system.

When it is necessary to collect a urine specimen from a patient with an indwelling catheter, it should be done from the catheter itself. A specimen from the collecting receptacle may not be fresh urine and could result in inaccurate analysis. Sterile technique must be observed.

A sterile needle, a syringe, and a pledget soaked with an antiseptic are needed to collect a urine specimen from an indwelling catheter. Most catheters have a self-sealing area which tolerates a needle puncture. After locating the area, clean it carefully with the antiseptic solution. The Center for Disease Control recommends that alcohol or iodine be used. Carefully insert a sterile 21-gauge needle into the catheter and aspirate. Care must be taken not to puncture the balloon lumen or both sides of the catheter. The specimen is then handled according to agency policy.

Nursing Implications. Great care must be taken by the nurse to prevent introducing a urinary tract infection into the patient with an indwelling catheter. Studies have demonstrated that the hands of nursing personnel are one of the primary modes of transmission of such infections. Careful handwashing between care of patients cannot be emphasized too strongly. Careful body hygiene is urged for all patients with indwelling catheters as still another effort to reduce the possibility of infection. Complete and at least twice-a-day cleaning

of the area around the meatus is recommended for both female and male patients, because organisms allowed to accumulate in this area can ascend and cause infection. Some physicians order a topical antibacterial cream to be applied to the meatus after each cleaning or at specified intervals, such as twice or three times a day. Provisions and reminders for patients to wash their hands, especially following intestinal elimination, are also important, because urinary infections from the intestinal tract can easily be acquired.

The importance of using strict sterile technique when dealing with any of the urinary drainage equipment has been indicated. If there is any doubt that any piece of equipment is sterile, it should be replaced.

There is evidence to support the theory that urinary infections are the result of cross-contamination between patients. Therefore, the Center for Disease Control recommends that patients with indwelling catheters be spatially separated whenever possible. The Center encourages avoiding placing persons with indwelling catheters in adjacent beds or in the same room. The cross-contamination again emphasizes the need for careful handwashing by the nurse both before and after handling catheter and drainage equipment.

Patients who have indwelling catheters should have the benefit of full explanation on how the system functions and on how they can assist. Teaching points include keeping the tubing free from kinks, maintaining constant downward flow of the urine, maintaining an adequate fluid intake, keeping a record of the output, and preventing contamination and the prompt reporting of bladder pain, an elevated temperature, or changes in urine characteristics.

When an indwelling catheter is in place, any comments that the patient may make about it, such as irritation, burning sensations, or annoyances with it should be noted, as well as the volume and character of the drainage. Any signs of infection should be reported. After an indwelling catheter has been removed, it should be noted on the patient's nursing care plan. There is still need for observation. Frequency, burning on voiding, interference with the urinary stream, such as inability to start it, and cloudy urine may be some of the aftermath of an indwelling catheter. Too often, patients endure the discomfort because they believe that it is to be expected. Emphasis should be placed on high-fluid intake unless otherwise contraindicated.

Removal of the indwelling catheter requires deflation of the balloon by emptying it of its solution or air. This may be done by using a syringe or by cutting the catheter section which services the balloon. The patient should be aware of the procedure being performed and should be asked to take several deep breaths while the nurse gently removes the catheter. The external genitalia should be cleaned following removal of the catheter. The patient should be provided with extra fluids and observed for urination. The nurse observes the amount and characteristics of the first several voidings and records any discomfort expressed by the patient, bleeding, elevated temperature and so on. Fluids are especially encouraged for several days after removal of the indwelling catheter.

While indwelling catheters are sometimes necessary, every effort should be made by the nurse to avoid their use or to minimize the length of time they are used. Studies have shown the incidence of urinary tract infections increases in direct proportion to the length of time the catheter is in place.

Urinary Diversions

Obstructions of the urinary tract may require that some persons have surgical diversions of the urinary flow. They may have an abdominal opening for urinary excretion, such as the *ileal conduit,* a connection of the ureters to the ileum with a stoma on the abdominal wall. A *stoma* is an artificial opening for waste excretion located on the body surface. Other types of surgery for urinary diversion are also performed, but, except for the location of the stoma, the nursing care is similar. Such diversions are generally permanent and the person wears an external appliance to collect the urine since voluntary control over elimination of the urine from the stoma is not possible.

The person who has an ileal conduit must adapt to an altered body image. The stoma will be obvious when his abdomen is exposed and using an external appliance is necessary. Therefore, the individual generally needs assistance in coping with a change in his body and new needs. The time required for adaptation varies and the adjustment can often be promoted by numerous sources of support, such as the family, friends, nurses, physicians, and persons with a similar health problem. Most of all, the person needs to understand that an active, useful life is compatible with a urinary diversion.

One problem with which most persons with a urinary diversion must deal and which often causes initial stress is the external appliance. The device consists of a soft rubber or plastic pouch, either reusable or disposable. The upper part of the pouch generally has a firm face plate several inches in diameter, which has an opening the size of the stoma. Some face plates are detachable from the pouch. Others are not. The plate surface is firmly secured around the stoma opening with a moisture-proof adherent so that no urine leakage can occur. Many persons also use an elastisized belt worn around the waist for added support. The lower end of the pouch has a drainage valve which is used for emptying the pouch.

Since it is important that every effort be made to maintain the appliance seal on the skin, the pouch should be emptied before it becomes heavy with the weight of urine and causes the seal to loosen. This means emptying the appliance several times a day for most persons. It may be necessary to measure the urine before it is discarded.

Urine collection receptacles which are designed to be placed under the bed are available for attachment to the appliance at night. In this way, the person does not have to be concerned about movements during sleep which might dislodge the partially filled pouch or disturbance of his sleep to empty the pouch.

The frequency of changing the pouch varies with the type being used. Some are changed daily while others are changed only every five to seven days. Changing the appliance should be done at a time following low-fluid intake, such as early morning. Urine excretion will be less at this time which makes changing the appliance easier. Extreme care should be used when removing the face plate from the skin surface so as not to damage the skin. In some instances, a commercial adhesive remover may be used to dissolve the adherent substance. The skin surface around the stoma must be kept immaculately clean to prevent skin irritation. A skin protectant, such as tincture of benzoin, can be used to help protect the skin. Karaya washers are also used for this purpose. With some appliances, an adhesive substance may need to be applied to the face plate of the fresh appliance. In others, the adherent is already present. In either case, a tight seal which will prevent urine leakage is necessary.

Care should be taken to make certain the opening of the face plate is appropriate for the size of the stoma. The opening in the appliance should fit snugly around the stoma. The opening is small enough so that no more than $\frac{1}{16}$ to $\frac{1}{8}$ inch of skin is visible around the opening It should be large enough so that the face plate does not adhere to the stoma itself. Too large an opening will allow excretions to irritate the exposed skin while too small an opening and adherence of the face plate to the delicate stoma mucous membrane will cause tissue trauma.

Reusable appliances may be cleaned in soap and water or commercial antiseptics. Some practitioners also recommend a white vinegar rinse to control the development of alkaline urine salts and odor. The clean appliance should be dried and allowed to air between uses. The technique for changing a stomal appliance is described in the chart below.

Many authorities believe that the urine of the person with urinary diversion should be acidified to control infection and odor. Acidification of urine may be accomplished by diet, administration of oral ascorbic acid, and/or with white vinegar placed in the external appliance.

The nurse observes the condition of the skin, stoma, and characteristics of the urine as she handles the external urinary appliance. As the patient assumes responsibility for his own care, he should be taught to make the same observations and to be aware of indications of problems and when to seek assistance. Detailed discussion of other aspects of the care of the person with a urinary diversion can be found in clinical texts.

In recent years, a new technique is being used for some persons who in the past were candidates for an ileal conduit. An internal reservoir for urine collection is created. These persons then insert a catheter at intervals to drain the reservoir. This procedure eliminates the need for an external appliance to collect urine.

ELIMINATION FROM THE INTESTINAL TRACT

Food is digested in the alimentary tract. The products of digestion which the tissue cells of the body assimilate are absorbed through the mucous membrane of the alimentary tract. Part of the residue that the body does not select for utilization becomes waste products and is excreted by the intestines. This process of excretion of wastes is essential for life and must continue during illness as in health.

Large Intestine

The large intestine is the lower or distal part of the alimentary tract. It extends from the ileocecal valve to

Changing stomal appliances

The purpose is to provide skin care and a fresh receptacle for excretions.

SUGGESTED ACTION	RATIONALE
Empty the pouch being worn.	Having the pouch empty before handling it reduces the likelihood of spilling the excretions.
Remove the pouch face plate from the skin very gently.	The seal between the surface of the face plate and the skin must be broken before the face plate can be removed. Harsh handling of the appliance can cause damage to the skin and impair the development of a secure seal in the future.
Clean the skin around the stoma with soap and water, or a commercial cleaner, and gently pat dry.	Cleaning the skin removes any excretions and traces of old adhesive and skin protectant. Excretions or a buildup of other substances can cause irritation and damage to the skin.
Place absorbent material, such as gauze, over the stoma opening.	Continuous excretions must be absorbed in order to keep the skin dry during the appliance change.
Apply skin protectant and allow it to dry completely.	The skin needs protection from the excoriating effect of the excretions and appliance adhesive. Allowing the protectant to dry completely enhances its effectiveness.
If necessary, enlarge the size of the face plate opening.	The appliance should fit snugly around the stoma. A face plate opening which is too small can cause trauma to the stoma.
Apply adhesive to the face plate and/or remove protective covering from the disposable face plate, carefully position appliance, and press in place. (Remove gauze or other covering from the stoma opening immediately prior to placing the appliance). A deodorant may be added to the pouch before adherence if desired.	The appliance is effective only if it is properly positioned and securely adhered. Commercial deodorants may be used if odor is a problem.
Secure the optional belt to the appliance and around the patient.	An elasticized belt helps to support the appliance for some persons.
Wash the reusable appliance with soap and water, or a commercial cleaner. Dry and air before reuse. Discard disposable appliance appropriately.	Thorough cleaning and airing of the appliance reduces deterioration and odor. For aesthetic and infection control reasons, used appliances should be discarded carefully.

the anus. Waste products of digestion are received by the large intestine from the small intestine.

The length of the large intestine in adults is approximately 1.5 meters or 50 to 60 inches, but variations have been observed in normal persons. The width of the colon varies in different parts. At the narrowest point, the colon is approximately 2.5 cm. or 1 inch wide; at the widest point, about 7.5 cm. or 3 inches. Its diameter decreases from the cecum to the anus.

The barrier between the large intestine and the ileum of the small intestine is the ileocecal or ileocolic valve. This valve normally prevents contents from entering the large intestine prematurely and prevents waste products from returning to the small intestine.

The waste contents pass through the ileocecal valve and enter the cecum, which is the first part of the large intestine. It is situated on the right side of the body, and to it is attached the vermiform process or appendix. When waste products enter the large intestine, the contents are liquid or watery in nature. While they pass through the large intestine, water is absorbed. Approximately 800 ml. to 1,000 ml. of liquid is absorbed daily by the intestinal tract. This absorption of water accounts for the formed, semisolid consistency of the normal stool. When absorption does not occur properly, as when the waste products pass through the large intestine at a very rapid rate, the stool is soft and watery. If the stool remains in the colon too long and/or too much water is absorbed, the stool becomes dry and hardened.

From the cecum, the contents enter the colon, which is divided into several parts. The ascending colon extends from the cecum up toward the liver, where it turns to cross the abdomen. This turn is the hepatic flexure. The transverse colon crosses the abdomen from right to left. The turn from the transverse colon to form the descending colon is the splenic flexure. The descending colon passes down the left side of the body from the splenic flexure to the sigmoid or pelvic colon. When the waste products reach the distal end of the colon they are called *feces,* and, when excreted, feces are usually called the *stool.*

The sigmoid colon contains feces ready for excretion and empties into the rectum, which is the last part of the large intestine. The rectum is approximately 12 cm. or 5 inches long, 2.5 cm. or 1 inch being the anal canal. Normally, three transverse folds of tissue are present in the rectum.

The three transverse folds may help to hold the fecal material in the rectum temporarily. In addition, there are vertical folds. Each vertical fold contains an artery and a vein. Abnormally distended veins are called *hemorrhoids.* If hemorrhoids are present, caution must be exercised when a rectal thermometer or tube is inserted. Objects introduced into the anus or rectum should always be lubricated to reduce friction. If force is applied, injury to the mucous membrane may occur. The rectum is usually empty except during and immediately prior to defecation. Feces are excreted from the rectum through the anal canal and the anus, which is about 2.5 to 3.8 cm. or 1 to 1½ inches long.

The muscular layer of the large intestine plays an important part in excretion. The internal circular muscles are thicker than they are in other parts of the gastrointestinal tract. The outer longitudinal fibers are also thicker and are arranged in three muscle bands called taeniae coli. When muscles of the large intestine contract, they are capable of producing strong peristaltic action to propel fecal matter forward. Peristalsis is a kind of wormlike contraction of the musculature.

The contents of the large intestine act as the chief stimulant for the contraction of intestinal musculature. The pressure of the contents against the walls of the colon causes muscle stretch. This in turn causes stimulation of the nerve receptors, which in turn is followed by contraction of the walls of the colon, peristalsis, and haustral churning.

Stimulation occurs by both mechanical and chemical means. The bulk of the contents acts as a mechanical stimulant; as bulk increases, the pressure in the intestine increases, causing the muscles of the large intestine to contract. Bacterial action in the intestinal tract is responsible for chemical stimulation. Certain bacteria act on carbohydrates, causing fermentation, while other bacteria are responsible for the putrefaction of proteins. The end products of fermentation and putrefaction are organic acids, amines and ammonia, which stimulate muscular contraction chemically. Various gases formed by bacterial action also stimulate muscle contraction by increasing pressure within the colon. Emotional disturbances also have been observed to produce muscle contraction in the large intestine. Such contraction occurs by reflex action.

Waste products in the large intestine are propelled by mass peristaltic sweeps one to four times each 24-hour period in most individuals. The fecal mass is moved during these sweeps. This movement is unlike the frequent peristaltic rushes that occur in the small intestine. Mass peristalsis often occurs after food has been ingested. This accounts for the urge to defecate that frequently is observed following meals. One-third to one-half of ingested food waste products is normally excreted in the stool within 24 hours and the remainder within the next 24 to 48 hours.

Anal Canal and Anus

The internal sphincter in the anal canal and the external sphincter at the anus control the discharge of feces and intestinal gas, or *flatus*.

The internal sphincter consists of smooth muscle tissue and is involuntary. The innervation of the internal sphincter occurs through the autonomic nervous system. Motor impulses are carried by the sympathetic system (thoracolumbar) and inhibitory impulses by the parasympathetic system (craniosacral). It will be recalled that these two divisions of the autonomic nervous system function antagonistically to each other in a dynamic equilibrium.

The external sphincter at the anus has striated muscle tissue and is therefore under voluntary control. The levator ani reinforces the action of the external sphincter and also is controlled voluntarily. Interference with the normal functioning of elimination from the intestines can occur in health as it can during illness. It can be affected by amount and quality of fluid or food intake, degree of activity, and emotional states. Figure 20–14 shows the parts of the large intestine.

Figure 20–14 This sketch illustrates the various parts of the large intestine.

The Act of Defecation

Defecation is the emptying of the intestines and is often called a *bowel movement*. There are two centers governing the reflex to defecate. One is situated in the medulla, and a subsidiary one is in the spinal cord. When parasympathetic stimulation occurs, the internal anal sphincter relaxes, and the colon contracts. The defecation reflex is stimulated chiefly by the fecal mass in the rectum. When the rectum is distended, the intrarectal pressure rises, the defecation reflex is stimulated by the muscle stretch, and the desire to eliminate results. The external anal sphincter, controlled voluntarily, is constricted or relaxed at will. If the desire to defecate is ignored, defecation can often be delayed voluntarily.

During the act of defecation, several additional muscles aid the process. Voluntary contraction of the muscles of the abdominal wall, fixing of the diaphragm, and closing of the glottis aid in increasing intraabdominal pressure up to four or five times normal pressure that aids in expelling feces. Simultaneously, the muscles on the pelvic floor contract and aid in drawing the anus over the fecal mass.

Normal Defecation

Normally, the act of defecation is painless. Normality is associated with the regularity and type of stool. If the bowels move at regular intervals and the stools are normal, functional problems of frequency of elimination occur infrequently. However, nurses find that many persons show concern if they do not have a daily bowel movement. The normal frequency of bowel movements cannot be stated arbitrarily. Although many adults pass one stool each day, healthy persons have been observed to have more frequent or less frequent bowel movements. Some persons have a bowel movement two or three times a week; others as often as two or three times a day.

Normally, the stool consists principally of food residues as cellulose which is not digested and other foodstuffs which the body has not utilized completely, microorganisms of various kinds, secretions from intestinal glands, biliary pigments, water, and body cells. Unless the diet is high in roughage content, little of the total amount of feces is food residue. The normal stool is a semisolid mass. The amount of stool varies and depends to a large extent on the amount and the kind of food ingested. The color of the normal stool is brown, due chiefly to urobilin, which is a result of the reduction of bile pigments in the small intestine. A change in color is significant, since it frequently indicates impaired physiological functioning. The stool has a characteristic odor due chiefly to skatole and indole produced by bacterial action on tryptophan. The diet may influence odor and color, as will certain drugs.

Normally, the stool assumes the shape of the rectum. Change in the shape of the stool is significant if such change persists. For example, pencillike stools frequently indicate a change in the lumen of the colon and may be due to a growth.

NURSING RESPONSIBILITIES RELATED TO INTESTINAL ELIMINATION

Nursing personnel are frequently responsible for observing the patient's stools or teaching him or a family member what to observe for. Color, odor, consistency, shape, and amount are noted, and anything unusual such as the presence of blood, pus, parasites, and mucus, should be reported promptly.

It is important for the nurse to know the patient's normal patterns of elimination in order to recognize any abnormality. Such information should be collected in the health history. The frequency with which stools are passed should be noted. It will be recalled that frequency varies among individuals. Therefore, the individual's own norm should be taken into account when making assessments of the frequency of bowel movements.

Passing little or no gas or unusual amounts of flatus are often important symptoms. Difficulty with passing a stool or pain during defecation also may be of pathological significance.

The nurse should understand that the establishment of bowel habits begins in childhood. Bowel habits have many psychological implications, depending on accepted practices in various cultural groups. These practices are concerned with consideration for privacy, cleanliness, frequency, and other factors. Having a bowel movement is usually easier when the person is relaxed both physically and mentally. Stress or being away from his usual environment and routine may disturb his defecation habits. Individual patterns of living will guide the selection of a convenient time. The urge to defecate often occurs following a meal; after breakfast is a common time for persons who are awake during the usual daylight hours. Responding to the urge to defecate is important in establishing and maintaining an elimination pattern. Sometimes patients are not aware of the implications of not taking the time to defecate promptly when they experience the stimuli. The nurse may need to consider all of these factors when assisting a person to establish a satisfactory defecation routine.

A person's food and fluid intakes are probably the largest influential factor in intestinal elimination. Balanced food content with varied bulk is important to the production of fecal matter and its movement along the intestinal tract. The residue after food is absorbed provides bulk which stimulates peristalsis. The food residue must therefore provide this necessary bulk. Some persons find certain foods are acted upon by their intestinal tract bacteria to cause sufficient flatus formation to result in discomfort or distress. Since the offending foods vary with individuals, eliminating their intake becomes a selective personal matter.

Fluid intake has a relationship to stool consistency. Making sure that an adequate amount of liquid is taken in daily to provide for the body's physiological needs and to maintain a soft consistency to the stool is frequently a factor that busy and older persons do not always consider. Some persons find that hot liquids on arising or prune juice helps to stimulate defecation. Teaching about the importance of these factors and providing fluids may be the nurse's responsibility.

Activity influences intestinal elimination by promoting the development of muscle tone as well as by stimulating appetite and peristalsis. The person who has minimum daily activity will generally find his intestinal elimination patterns will be irregular. Encouraging daily activity also may be an important teaching function of the nurse.

Minor rectal or anal problems, such as hemorrhoids or small linear ulcers called *anal fissures* can affect elimination patterns. They generally cause painful or uncomfortable defecation. The discomfort tends to result in the individual ignoring the stimulus and avoiding defecation as long as possible which often causes constipation. The resulting dry, hardened stool causes even more discomfort on defecation. The unpleasant and potentially serious effects of rectal fissures and hemorrhoids should alert the nurse to the need for encouraging the person to seek the services of a physician.

From the above discussion, it can be seen that certain persons are at a high risk for developing intestinal elimination problems. Such persons habitually ignore the defecation stimulus, have an inadequate fluid intake, eat an improper diet, have poor abdominal muscle tone, get minimum exercise, and have already developed minor elimination problems.

Positioning during a bowel movement influences ease of emptying the rectum. The nurse may need to assist patients or instruct family members in relation to the best position, especially for elderly, handicapped, and debilitated persons. The normal physiological semisquatting position permits the most usage of the abdominal muscles for elimination. This means a person should be in as near a sitting position as possible with the feet resting on a solid surface. A person of small stature may need a footstool or box as he sits on the toilet. Whenever possible, a person who must remain in bed will find positioning the bedpan so his legs can hang over the edge with his feet resting on the floor or a chair will make defecation easier. A person who cannot be helped to the edge of the bed will find it easier to use the bedpan if the head of the bed and his knees are elevated as much as possible. Hospitalized children may need a potty chair, small bedpans, or foot supports if they are using the commode when defecating.

As with urination, the proper technique for perineal care following defecation must frequently be taught to female patients. Children especially are often careless, but patients of any age may need reminding. After defecating the area should be cleaned with toilet tissue or a cloth in a front to back direction. Moving from the anus toward the urethra can result in fecal contamination of the urethra or vagina.

Stool specimens are sometimes analyzed for diagnostic purposes. The fecal material may be examined for blood, bile, urobilin, parasites, and ova. The nurse usually instructs the patient in the collection of the specimen or she carries out the technique.

Whenever possible, it is preferable that the fecal specimen be uncontaminated with urine, other body excretions, barium, or laxatives, or enema solutions. A clean or sterile bedpan can be used for intestinal elimination when a specimen is desired. The specimen can then be transferred to the appropriate laboratory container with two clean or sterile tongue depressors or a similar disposable instrument. Care should be taken to see that the outside of the container remains uncontaminated by the stool.

Specimens for stool cultures may be obtained by rotating a sterile applicator stick over fresh stool and placing the applicator stick in a sterile tube, preferably one containing culture medium. Occasionally, when there is difficulty obtaining a stool specimen for culture, a rectal swab may be inserted in the anus and gently rotated. If a stool is present on the swab, it can be sent for culture studies in the same manner that the applicator stick is sent.

Specimens for pinworms may be collected by pressing the sticky side of a piece of clear cellophane tape over the perianal area, removing it immediately, and placing it on a laboratory slide. The specimen should be collected after the person has been quiet for an extended period, generally in the morning before arising.

Depending on the examination to be performed, the stool specimen may be refrigerated, frozen, kept at room temperature, or transferred to a special medium. In the past, it was generally thought necessary to keep specimens warm when they were to be examined for ova and parasites in order that the organisms would survive. Recent studies have shown that artificial heat can alter the life stages of the organisms and thus make diagnosis more difficult. The agency's laboratory directives should be followed closely. Accurate and complete labeling of the specimen container is important.

Occasionally, the nurse will be responsible for "on-the-spot" testing of stool for blood or pH values. Commercial tapes, dip sticks, and solutions containing reagents are available for these tests. Directives accompanying the diagnostic kits should be followed carefully for accurate results.

COMMON NURSING MEASURES FOR DEALING WITH PROBLEMS OF INTESTINAL ELIMINATION

Constipation

Constipation is the passage of unduly dry, hard stools. This definition, it will be noted, makes no mention of frequency. Some persons may be constipated and yet have a daily bowel movement, while others who regularly defecate no more than three times a week are not constipated. The habits of elimination vary greatly among healthy persons. Therefore, defining constipation on the basis of frequency of elimination is meaningless until careful comparisons are made with the person's usual habits.

Constipation is among the commonest and oldest of all medical complaints. It is found in all cultural, economic, and age groups. There are references to laxatives in the Bible and anthropological investigations suggest the use of enemas even before recorded time. Interestingly enough, many ancient methods for treating constipation are very similar to those used today.

Common Causes of Constipation. Certain organic diseases cause constipation. Other factors causing it require attention once the physician has ruled out organic disease.

When no pathological changes are involved, a common cause of constipation is the result of poor elimination habits. If the desire for defecation is ignored repeatedly, feces become hard and dry because of increased water absorption. In addition, the colon becomes insensitive to normal chemical and mechanical stimulation, and eventually the feces in the rectum are no longer sufficient to stimulate the defecation reflex. Neglecting to observe the normal desire for defecation may result from carelessness, occupational demands, the stress of modern life, and, in children, the reluctance to interrupt play.

Certain types of diets predispose to constipation. A diet that is low in roughage often leaves so little residue that the fecal mass is small in amount and becomes dry before sufficient quantity is present to stimulate the defecation reflex. When possible, increasing the bulk of the diet with foods, such as fresh fruits and vegetables, and bran, is often sufficient for relief. Heavy-residue foods will pass through the large intestine quickly, while low-residue foods such as lean meats, rice, eggs, and sugar are moved more slowly. Since water increases the rate of movement of residue, an increase in fluids is usually helpful to the person who must consume a low-residue diet.

Investigations indicate that the colon in some individuals absorbs an unusually high percentage of water from the feces, and constipation results. For these persons, increased fluid intake often is the answer. If a bland diet is prescribed for medical reasons, the physician may recommend a medication for the patient to counteract constipation. Certain drugs, such as iron preparations, may be constipating for some persons.

Emotions, such as tension, may cause the gastrointestinal tract to become spastic, and fecal content is not moved along the large intestine sufficiently well. The importance of relaxation to aid defecation has been mentioned, and relief is often obtained as the person learns to assume a way of life that allows time for relaxation. Constipation due to spasticity usually is called *hypertonic* or *spastic constipation*.

Authorities differ in opinion concerning *atonic constipation* or constipation that is due to an abnormally sluggish and "lazy" colon. Some state that the condition is doubtful, since the colon and the rectum do not become too weak to propel feces. Others believe that the colon does become too weak to function, especially when debilitating chronic illness, emaciation, or prolonged habitual use of laxatives is present.

In addition to the hard, dry stool, the nurse will observe that some persons who are constipated complain of headache, malaise, anorexia, foul breath, furred tongue, and lethargy. It generally is agreed that these symptoms probably are reflex in nature and are due to the increased pressure in the lower colon. Relief is usually rapid following a bowel movement. These symptoms of constipation have also been produced experimentally by packing the rectum with cotton. Therefore, the general belief that the symptoms are the result of poisons being absorbed when constipation is present is unfounded.

When constipation is not due to pathological changes, the nurse can help the person to understand some of the ways in which the situation can be corrected, as by establishing habit patterns of elimination, increasing fluid intake, eating high-roughage foods, and increasing physical activity. Also, the nurse can assist by teaching the importance of establishing an elimination habit. One suggestion is that the person go to the bathroom regularly, an hour or so after a meal, and remain there for a while until the defecation urge appears. Distractions, such as reading, are helpful during this period to aid in reducing anxiety. It takes time to develop an elimination habit just as it takes time to overcome the one that was present originally. But success has been observed among persons who consistently practice a new habit pattern.

Cathartics and Suppositories

Cathartics or *laxatives* are drugs which induce emptying of the intestinal tract. Some of these drugs act chemically by stimulating peristalsis, such as castor oil, cascara, senna, phenolphthalein, and bisacodyl (Ducolax). Others act by increasing the intestinal bulk which promotes additional mechanical stimulation on the intestine, such as magnesium sulfate and psyllium hydrophilic muciloid (Metamucil). Still others act on the fecal material itself by softening it, such as mineral oil and dioctyl sodium sulfosuccinate (Colace). Another frequently used laxative is milk of magnesia. It has antacid properties in small dosages and laxative properties when taken in larger doses.

Nurses are often in a position to help patients understand the appropriate use and dangers of laxatives. Because many cathartics are available as over-the-counter drugs and because modern advertising promotes their use, many persons take laxatives frequently on their own initiative.

Most persons are aware that, because laxatives have a chemical action, they should not be taken when there is abdominal pain because of the danger of intestinal pathology and subsequent harm from increased peristalsis. While many individuals take laxatives because they believe they are constipated, most are unaware that habitual use of laxatives is the most common cause of chronic constipation. Often the person is upset or concerned when he does not have a bowel movement, so he takes a cathartic. The drug's action will stimulate peristalsis enough to empty the entire intestinal tract. Since the colon may not fill for several days and no stimulation of the defecation reflex occurs, he often repeats taking his laxative and continues the pattern. The habitual use of cathartics very soon makes it difficult for him to have a normal bowel movement.

Breaking this habit, from both a physical and psychological viewpoint, is not easy for a person who has come to depend on laxatives. It often requires a great deal of patience, support, and teaching by the nurse. The person also frequently needs to be helped with diet, fluid intake, activity, and regularity of habits.

Laxatives are necessary at times for persons whose activity is limited, or whose food intake is poor. They are also used for emptying the intestinal tract in preparation for surgical or diagnostic exploration. Their occasional use is generally not harmful for most persons, but all efforts should be taken to prevent the person from becoming dependent on this means of stimulating defecation.

A *suppository* is a conical or oval solid substance shaped for easy insertion into a body cavity and designed to melt at body temperature. Since a certain amount of absorption can take place in the large colon, some medications for systemic effect can be given by a suppository. However, the most frequent use of the rectal suppository is to aid in stimulating peristalsis and defecation. When effective, results are obtained usually within 15 to 30 minutes, but it could take as long as an hour.

A variety of rectal suppositories is available. Some act as fecal softeners, others have direct action on the nerve endings in the mucosa, and some liberate carbon dioxide when moistened.

Fecal softeners are useful when the stool is very hard, while substances that stimulate the rectum are helpful for persons with weak muscle tone or poor innervation. The carbon dioxide suppositories liberate about 200 ml. of the gas which causes distention, thus producing stimulation and elimination impulses.

Rectal suppositories can be helpful in a program to aid a person in regaining good elimination habits. An approach which has been found to be satisfactory is to insert one or two suppositories one-half hour before a meal. Since the intake of food and fluids usually results in increased peristaltic action, it is more common to have the urge to defecate after meals. In effect, the suppository reinforces the natural stimulus.

To be most effective, the suppository should be inserted beyond the internal sphincter of the anal canal. A finger cot or glove is used to protect the finger when inserting the suppository. The suppository and gloved index finger are lubricated before insertion in order to reduce friction. If the patient breathes through the mouth while the suppository is being inserted, the anal sphincter usually will relax. Often, if the nurse compresses the buttocks together for a minute or so following insertion of the suppository, the patient's urge to expel the suppository will be overcome.

Some patients are able to insert suppositories for themselves. In other situations, family members can be taught. The nurse should establish whether the patient has an understanding of the correct procedure since incorrect insertion will not produce the desired results.

Enemas

An *enema* is an introduction of solution into the large intestine, generally for the purpose of removing feces. Cleansing enemas are given for three common purposes: to relieve constipation; to prevent involuntary escape of fecal material during surgical procedures and during delivery; and to promote visualization of the intestinal tract by x-ray or instrument examination. There is some variation in the types of solutions used. Those most frequently used are tap water, normal saline, soap solution, hypertonic solutions, and oil.

Tap water, saline, and soap solutions are usually given in quantities of 500 ml. to 1,000 ml. for the average adult patient. Not more than 300 ml. of saline solution should be given to a child and much less to the very young. The quantity of solution distends the rectum and colon and usually stimulates peristalsis and defecation within 15 minutes of administration.

Tap water and saline solution appear to have approximately the same degree of effectiveness in causing bowel elimination. However, because the colon does absorb solution to some degree, their repeated use for some patients can result in fluid and electrolyte imbalances. Tap water must be administered cautiously to infants or to adults who have altered kidney or cardiac reserve. If a large quantity of hypotonic solution is absorbed through repeated enemas, the blood volume may be increased. This reaction is usually called water intoxication, and symptoms include weakness, sweating, pallor, vomiting, cough, or dizziness. The colon can conserve sodium quite effectively, so persons with abnormal sodium retention, as in congestive heart failure, may absorb sufficient sodium from repeated saline enemas to cause further electrolyte disturbance.

Soap suds solutions stimulate peristalsis by chemical irritation of the mucous membrane, as well as by intestinal distention. Too much or too strong soap can produce hyperirritation or actual colon membrane damage. Concentrated soap solutions designed for enemas are commercially available and should not be used in quantities of more than 5 ml. per 1,000 ml. of water.

Soap solutions can be made by dissolving a bland white soap or castile soap in water. However, estimates of the concentration are very difficult to determine. Bar soap that has been used previously is not recommended because it has been found that these bars can harbor organisms. Household detergents are too strong for the delicate mucosa. Many proctologists discourage the use of soap for enemas, particularly for patients having known or suspected rectal pathology or for patients being prepared for rectal examinations because of the effect on the mucosa of the intestine.

Hypertonic solutions are available in prepared, disposable enema units. An example is the Fleets enema. The amount of solution given is usually 4 ounces, or 120 ml. The action of the solution seems to be a combination of distention and irritation. The hypertonic solution draws fluid from the body into the bowel by osmosis, thus creating fluid bulk in the colon. In addition, the hypertonicity of the solution acts as a mild irritant on the mucosa The administration of this type of enema is simple, results are obtained readily within two to seven minutes, and evacuation of the colon is generally good. In many agencies, it has become the method of choice for preparation for examination of the rectum with a proctoscope or for x-ray visualization of the rectum by the barium enema. It is less fatiguing and distressing to the patient. Disposable units of hypertonic solution have been very successful for patients unable to retain large quantity enemas. Repeating hypertonic enemas within a short time should be avoided in the elderly, very young, or debilitated person.

Oils such as mineral oil, cottonseed oil, or olive oil, are used for enemas. Their primary action is as a lubricant, although they may also help to soften the fecal material somewhat. Usually, 150 ml. to 200 ml. of oil is given slowly and the patient is requested to retain the oil for as long a period as he is able, at least 30 minutes. Oil enemas vary widely in the length of time in which they are effective, since usually they are administered to severely constipated patients. It is not uncommon for an oil enema to be followed by a soap solution, tap water, or saline enema after several hours if elimination does not result from the oil enema.

Enema Equipment. The commercially prepared enema is self-contained. It is a flexible bottle containing the solution with an attached prelubricated firm tip of approximately 5 to 7.5 cm. or 2 to 3 inches in length. Its ease of use makes it particularly convenient for home situations. Patients can readily administer their own in many instances.

For the tap water, saline, or soap solutions, a container for the solution, rubber or plastic tubing with side openings near its distal end, tubing clamp, lubricant, and the solution are necessary. The solution container varies. Metal cans or plastic bags attached to the tubing are most often used. The plastic containers are usually disposable and used for one patient only, while the metal containers are sterilized for reuse. Pitchers as solution containers may be used occasionally with a funnel attached to the tubing for introduction of the solution. While the commercially produced equipment is sterile, and the reusable equipment is sterilized between patients in the health agency, the enema is an aseptic or clean technique, not a sterile one.

The larger the lumen of the rectal tube, the greater the stimulation of the anal sphincters. This is to be desired if the purpose in giving the enema is to aid in emptying the colon. If the purpose is to introduce a solution which is to be retained, a smaller sized rectal tube should be used.

If an enema is to be expelled immediately, the most commonly used rectal tubes are between No. 26 and No. 32, Fr., and for enemas to be retained, No. 14 to No. 20, Fr. The size of the tube used for retention enemas depends on the viscosity of the solution to be administered. The larger sized tubes should be used for solutions of high viscosity because of their resistance to flow.

Enema Preparation. The maximum amount of solution should generally be prepared even though it may not all be used. If the primary purpose of giving the enema is to stimulate the defecation impulse and to aid in emptying the lower colon, and if this goal is achieved with a lesser amount, it may not be necessary to use the total amount. Quantities less than the maximum are sufficient for some persons and for others, the total amount may be necessary.

The temperature of the solution should generally be slightly higher than internal body temperature, that is, 40.5° to 46.1° C (105° to 115° F.) Disposable enemas are frequently given at room temperature, but some authorities feel they are more effective and comfortable for the patient if warmed in a basin of water or under the hot water tap. Solutions that are too hot can injure the mucosa, while those that are too cold can cause cramping and difficulty for the patient to retain the enema.

After the solution is prepared and before administering the enema, the solution should be allowed to fill the tubing and displace the air. While introducing air into the colon is not harmful, it may serve to impede the inflow of solution if there is no escape and the intestinal pressure is great enough. Running a small amount of solution through the tubing before introducing it into the colon also warms the tubing.

Preparation of the Patient. Since the enema is a common procedure, many patients understand its use and how it is administered. Other patients who have not experienced an enema before will need an explanation of its purpose, what they can expect, and how they can participate. The procedure offers an excellent opportunity for health teaching, since many persons are not familiar with the functioning of the intestinal tract. Failure to observe one or more of these principles may be responsible for their considering the procedure a disagreeable one.

Most patients believe that solutions introduced into the colon are to be expelled as soon as possible. When a solution is to be retained, care should be taken to have the patient understand this. If the procedure is explained as a small enema, the patient still may believe that it is to be expelled quickly. It is best if the patient is helped to understand that it is an instillation which is to be retained. An additional precaution is to keep the bedpan out of sight.

Traditionally, the enema has been administered with the patient in the left lateral recumbent position. It was thought that the solution would flow into the colon with less resistance if the patient were to lie on his left side. It now appears that the left lateral is no more effective than the right. For some commercially prepared enemas, it is recommended that the patient be in the knee-chest position. This position helps the solution to flow further into the colon and ensures the distribution of the small amount of solution over as wide a surface area of the lower colon as possible. In this way, more fluid is drawn into the colon. Figure 20–15 shows a patient in the knee-chest position receiving an enema. The knee-chest position is difficult for some patients to assume and impossible for others. In this event, it is best if the patient is as flat as possible. In addition, it is preferable if the patient is kept in a recumbent position for a few minutes following the administration if possible. If the patient is permitted to sit up, the solution may pool in the lower portion of the colon and this would reduce its effectiveness.

A common misunderstanding about enemas is that the solution can be administered effectively while the patient is in the sitting position. The amount of pressure needed to force the solution up into the colon while sitting is far greater than that needed while lying down. In addition, solution will tend to pool and distend the lower colon since it must go against gravity in order to ascend the colon. This will cause the desire to empty the colon sooner than may be desirable for effective results.

Before the enema is administered, plan with the patient where he will eliminate the solution. If possible, most patients prefer to use the bathroom toilet. If this is not feasible, a bedside commode or the bedpan can be used. Arranging the patient's robe and slippers conveniently, making certain the bathroom is vacant or making the bedpan accessible are all important parts of helping the patient to relax.

Administering the Enema.   The enema tube should be lubricated before insertion to reduce friction and to facilitate its entry. The tip is inserted through the anus approximately 5 to 7.5 cm. or 2 to 3 inches at an angle pointing toward the umbilicus. See Figure 20–16.

Possible injury to the rectal wall is increased with further insertion. Occasionally, the tube seems to meet with some resistance as it is being inserted. In such instances, it is best to permit a small amount of solution to enter, withdraw the rectal tube slightly, rotate it, and then continue to insert. The resistance may be due to spasm of the colon or failure of the internal sphincter to open. The solution will help to reduce the spasms and relax the sphincter, and the tube may be inserted safely to the desired distance.

The disposable enema solution is forced into the rectum by applying gentle, steady pressure to the solution container. The large volume enema solution container should be elevated approximately 45 to 50 cm.

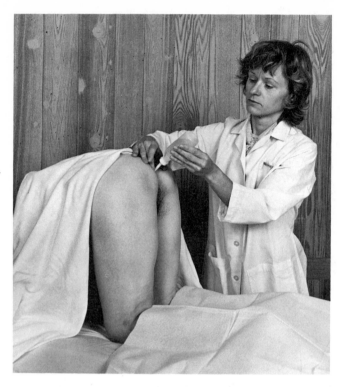

Figure 20–15   The nurse is preparing to administer a hypertonic solution enema to the patient. The patient is in the knee-chest position. Note that the patient's body is bent at approximately a 90° angle at the hips. This patient's arms are resting alongside of her head.

or 18 to 20 inches above the anus and the solution introduced slowly, that is over a five-to-ten-minute period. Faster introduction or greater elevation of the solution container and a higher pressure can result in cramping and difficulty for the patient to retain the solution. Encouraging the patient to mouth breathe during the administration usually results in muscle relaxation and ease of solution retention.

The patient should be encouraged to retain the solution as long as he is able in order to achieve maximum effects. The average time is five to ten minutes.

Occasionally it is not possible for a patient voluntarily to contract the external sphincter and assist in retaining the solution being given. Such a patient may need to have the rectal tube inserted and then be placed on the bedpan while the solution is administered. The nurse wears a glove to hold the tube in place. The head of the bed should be elevated slightly so that the patient's back is not arched. A pillow support to the lumbar region may be necessary. If the head of the bed

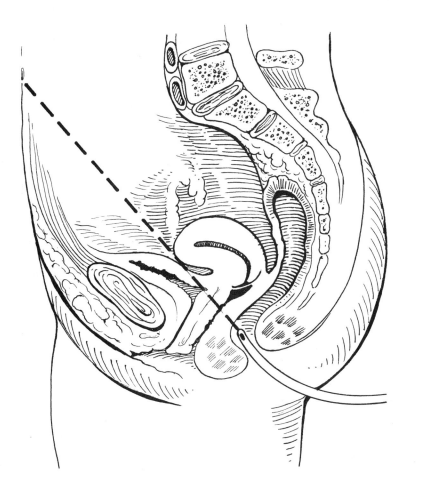

Figure 20-16   The rectal tube is inserted so that the tip of the tube is directed toward the umbilicus. The tube is inserted 5 to 7.5 cm. or 2 to 3 inches.

is elevated beyond a 30° angle, there is less likelihood of the solution entering the colon freely. Most of the solution will drain back out, and evacuation of feces in the colon may not be accomplished.

For patients who are unable to retain large quantities of fluid, the commercially prepared hypertonic solution enemas are often more satisfactory. The quantity is small enough so that usually there is no difficulty in retaining that amount. However, as a precaution, the nurse should place a pad under the patient's hips and should be sure that the patient's clothing is not soiled. These measures prevent embarrassment and discomfort. The chart on page 490 describes the procedure for administering a cleansing enema.

The results of the enema, character of the stool, and the volume and type of solution are recorded on the patient's chart. The nurse also records any unusual effects of the enema that the patient has experienced.

Fecal Impaction

A *fecal impaction* is a prolonged retention or an accumulation of fecal material which forms a hardened mass in the rectum. It may be of sufficient size to prevent the passage of normal stools.

The medical literature describes a condition called *obstipation,* which is the accumulation of hardened feces extending well up into the colon causing an intestinal obstruction. While it is common for a fecal impaction to prevent the passage of normal stools, the situation may be misleading, because the patient can have liquid fecal seepage. Small amounts of fluid present in the colon are able to go around the impacted mass. As a matter of fact, liquid fecal seepage and no passage of normal feces are symptomatic of the existence of an impaction.

Fecal impactions frequently are due to constipation and poor habits of defecation. They may result when

Administering a cleansing enema

The purpose is to introduce solution into the colon to aid in stimulating peristalsis and removing feces.

SUGGESTED ACTION	RATIONALE
Secure the commercially prepared enema or prepare the desired enema solution. The temperature of the solution should range from 40.5° to 49° C. (105° to 110° F.)	For maximum stimulation, comfort, and safety, the solution should enter the colon at a slightly higher than internal body temperature. The adult colon is estimated to hold about 750 ml. to 1,000 ml.
Place a moisture-proof pad under the patient's buttocks. Position the patient in the lateral recumbent, recumbent, or knee-chest (for commercially prepared enema) position, as dictated by the patient's comfort. Drape the patient as illustrated in Figure 20–17.	A moisture-proof pad protects the linen from possible soiling. Gravity aids the flow of fluids into the colon. The patient's comfort will help him relax.
Lubricate the end of the rectal tube for 5 to 7.5 cm. or 2 to 3 inches, as illustrated in Figure 20–18.	Friction is reduced when a surface is lubricated.
Slowly insert the rectal tube for 5 to 7.5 cm.or 2 to 3 inches at an angle pointing toward the umbilicus, as illustrated in Figure 20–19.	The anal canal is approximately 2.5 to 5 cm. or 1 to 2 inches in length. The tube should be inserted through the internal anal sphincter, but further insertion may damage the intestinal wall. The suggested angle follows the normal intestinal contour. Slow insertion of a lubricated rectal tube minimizes spasms of the intestinal wall.
Gently and steadily collapse the flexible commercial enema container with hand pressure, or elevate the reservoir to the point where the solution begins to flow *slowly* into the colon. Usually the reservoir is 45 to 50 cm. or 18 to 20 inches above the anus, as illustrated in Figure 20–20.	Pressure on the liquid forces the solution into the colon. Force on the container wall or gravity provide the pressure. The amount of pressure exerted on the solution will determine the rate of flow into the colon and the pressure exerted on the colon.
Stop the flow of fluid and remove the rectal tube when the patient has a strong desire to defecate.	Distention and irritation of the intestinal wall, which produce strong peristalic action, should be sufficient to empty the lower intestinal tract.
Place the patient in a sitting position on the bedpan, or assist him to the bathroom or to a commode if permissible.	Contraction of the abdominal and the perineal muscles which aid in emptying the colon is easier when the patient is in the sitting position.
Wash all equipment thoroughly and sterilize it before reuse, if disposable equipment is not used.	Normally, there is an abundant growth of bacteria in the large intestine.

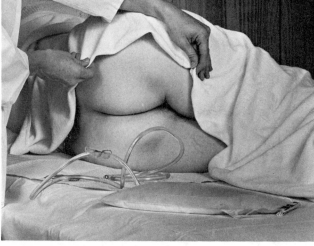

Figure 20–17 The patient is properly draped and positioned for administering a cleansing enema.

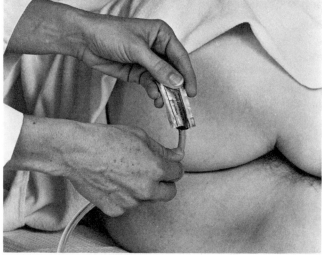

Figure 20–18 The nurse is lubricating the rectal tube by placing the end of the tube into the package of lubricant. The lubricant can be allowed to fall on the tube, if the nurse prefers.

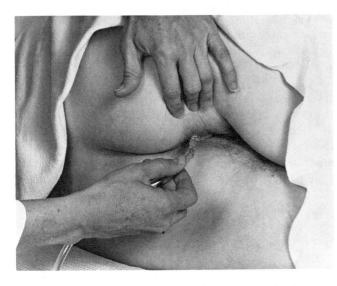

Figure 20-19 The nurse has exposed the anus and is about to insert the rectal tube at an angle that points toward the patient's umbilicus.

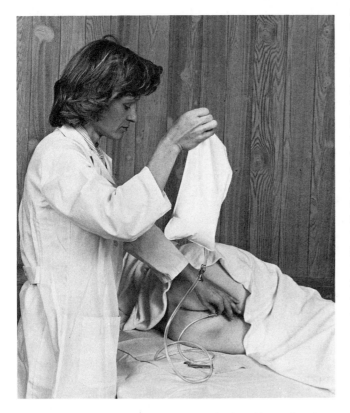

Figure 20-20 The nurse holds the rectal tube with one hand and holds the bag containing the solution with her other hand approximately 55 cm. or 18 inches above the patient's anus.

parts of a hardened, dry stool become lodged in the folds of the rectum.

Certain conditions predispose to fecal impactions, and the nurse will need to be alert to prevent their development. For example, patients who are required to maintain complete bed rest may find normal defecation difficult, and, unless some action is taken, constipation and fecal impactions may result. This may mean determining if the patient's food and fluid intake can be improved to aid defecation. Or, it may mean consulting the physician about the possibility of permitting the patient to use a commode or having a mild laxative or suppository daily.

Patients who are required to take constipating drugs over a period of time are also prone to develop fecal impactions; barium enemas for x-ray examinations of the colon are likely to cause fecal impactions if care is not taken to clean the colon of barium following examination.

Reports indicate that some fibrous foods, such as bran and fruit seeds have been found in fecal impactions, as have coated pills. Perhaps these substances were not the primary cause of the impaction, but they were contributing factors in susceptible persons.

The patient with a fecal impaction may complain of constipation, uncontrolled liquid fecal seepage or both. Usually, he experiences a frequent desire to defecate but is unable to do so. Rectal pain may be present. Very careful observation is needed to prevent fecal impactions. There is no particular time span associated with their formation. Some have been known to occur within 24 hours. There have been reports in the literature of impactions removed by surgical procedures. Prevention is based on observation of the stool as to amount, consistency, and frequency. If the patient is ambulatory, he will need to be instructed to make these observations. If he does not use the bathroom, nursing personnel or family members should assume this responsibility. If the causes are not eliminated, impactions are likely to recur. As with the prevention of constipation, all efforts to help a patient should be entered on the nursing care plan. When fecal impactions are not associated with circumstances beyond the nurse's control, such as antiperistaltic drugs or other therapy, the occurrence of an impaction usually is a sign of less than satisfactory nursing care.

When it has been determined that a fecal impaction is present, an oil retention enema is often used. This is followed by a cleansing enema two or three hours later. This may be followed by enemas twice a day if necessary until normal stools occur. If this procedure fails, often it is necessary to break up the impaction by digital manipulation.

To remove an impaction, the patient should be placed in the Sims' position if possible, the top bedding folded down to the foot of the bed, and the patient covered with a bath blanket; use protection for the bedding, such as a disposable pad or plastic sheeting, under the patient. The bedpan should be placed conveniently on the bed so that pieces of removed feces may be deposited in it. Clean gloves should be used. Lubricate the forefinger generously and insert it as gently as possible into the anal sphincter. The presence of the finger added to the mass already present in the rectum causes considerable discomfort to the patient. By carefully working the finger into the hardened mass, it is possible to remove pieces of it. Use plenty of lubricant in order to avoid irritating the mucous membrane or inducing bleeding. When a severe impaction exists, part of the impaction may need to be removed initially, possibly more oil instilled, and remaining parts removed at intervals of several hours. This will avoid extreme discomfort and possible harm to the patient.

Intestinal Distention

Excessive formation of gases in the stomach or the intestines is known as *flatulence*. When the gas is not expelled and accumulates in the intestinal tract, the condition is referred to as *intestinal distention* or *tympanites*.

Any disturbance in the ability of the small intestine to absorb gases or in its ability to propel gas along the intestinal tract usually will result in distention. Irritating foods, such as beans and cabbage, often predispose to flatulence and distention. Constipation is a frequent cause of distention. Certain drugs, morphine sulfate for example, tend to decrease peristaltic action which allows gas accumulation and thus causes distention. Swallowing large amounts of air while eating and drinking can cause distention. Persons who are tense often can be observed to be swallowing large amounts of air, especially when taking fluids. This habit can be overcome by purposely training oneself to eat and drink without swallowing air. Usually, air swallowers will eructate a great deal, and much air escapes in this manner before it reaches the intestines.

Distention can be noted by the presence of a swollen abdomen. Gentle percussion with the fingers produces a drumlike sound. In addition, usually the patient will complain of cramplike pain, and if distention is sufficient to cause pressure on the diaphragm and the thoracic cavity, shortness of breath and dyspnea may result.

Acting on the cause usually will relieve the distention. Movement in bed or ambulation will often promote escape of the flatus. Temporary relief may be afforded the patient by placing a heating pad on the abdomen and by inserting a rectal tube. The heating pad should be regulated on the lowest setting and should not be used on any patient for whom the treatment is contraindicated, such as the very young or persons with diabetes mellitus. Some health agencies do not allow the use of heating pads which means this measure cannot be used.

The sizes of rectal tubes used most frequently for the relief of distention in adults range from No. 22 to No. 32 Fr. Smaller sizes are used for children. The tips of rectal tubes also vary—some have smoothly rounded tips with an opening on the side of the tube near the tip, others have an opening at the tip as well as on the side of the tube. The distinct advantage of the rubber or plastic tube for rectal treatments is that it is flexible, and, with good lubrication and careful insertion, it can be introduced with relative ease beyond the anal canal into the rectum.

After lubricating the rectal tube, it should be carefully inserted for approximately 10 cm. or 4 inches. However, since fluids are not being introduced, it is possible to insert it a bit farther if no resistance is encountered and if it is noted that no flatus is being removed.

The rectal tube may be attached to a piece of connecting tubing of sufficient length to reach well into a small collecting container which can be attached to the bed frame. Water then can be put into the collecting container to cover the end of the tubing to determine whether or not the patient is expelling flatus; air bubbles indicate that gas is being removed.

A rectal tube should be left in place for a short time; usually 20 minutes is sufficient. Leaving the tube in place for long periods reduces the responsiveness of the sphincters. There is more likelihood of stimulating the sphincters and peristalsis if the rectal tube is reinserted every two to three hours as necessary. If the tube is inserted repeatedly over a period of several hours and no gas is removed, and the patient remains distended, the observation should be reported to the physician immediately.

Enemas and medications are also often used to prevent and relieve distention.

Diarrhea

Diarrhea is the passage of excessively liquid and unformed stools. Frequent bowel movements do not necessarily mean that diarrhea is present, although patients with diarrhea usually will pass stools at frequent intervals. Diarrhea often is associated with intestinal cramps. Nausea and vomiting may be present, as may be the presence of blood in the stools. Diarrhea is protective in nature when its cause is the presence of irritants in the intestinal tract.

Diarrhea may have a functional basis. The patient may have allergies to ingested food or drugs. The abuse of cathartics, and also certain dietary indiscretions, may cause diarrhea. Some persons know that, for them, certain foods and fluids such as rich pastries, coffee, or alcoholic beverages may produce temporary diarrhea. Avoidance of the factor causing it usually remedies the situation easily.

Diseases in parts of the body other than the intestinal tract may be at the root of the trouble. Examples include uremia and certain cardiac and neurological disorders.

Diarrhea may be caused by certain intrinsic conditions existing in the intestine itself. These include viral, bacteriological, fungal, protozoan, or metazoan invasion; alterations in the normal bacterial flora of the intestine; antimicrobial therapy; fistulas; inflammatory conditions such as ulcerative colitis; and tumors in the intestinal tract.

If the cause of diarrhea is psychic in nature, the nurse may be able to play an important part in assisting the patient to understand the cause. Situations in daily living may be disturbing to him. However, diarrhea may be associated with deep-seated emotional problems that require the help of a psychiatrist.

Whatever the cause of diarrhea, if it persists, the patient should be instructed to seek the advice of a physician. Most of the diarrhea commonly seen in adults is self-limiting. Many physicians feel that short-term or 24-hour diarrhea should be allowed to run its course since the gastrointestinal tract will purge itself. Medications are not ordinarily prescribed. Severe infectious diarrheas, especially in children and the elderly, will usually require appropriate therapy.

Diarrhea is often an embarrassing and usually a painful disturbance. Local irritation of the anal region and possibly the perineum and the buttocks from frequent watery stools is not uncommon. To help prevent irritation, the nurse may need to initiate special hygienic measures, such as washing the area after each stool, drying it thoroughly, and possibly applying a medicated skin cream or powder. Also, it may be necessary to caution the patient to use only very soft toilet tissue to reduce irritation.

When a person has diarrhea it is often impossible to control the urge to defecate for very long, if at all. Therefore, when it is known that a hospitalized patient has diarrhea, a comment to this effect should appear on the nursing care plan. This will alert nursing personnel to watch for his signal light. Or, it may be necessary to place the bedpan within easy reach for the patient, but yet out of sight to prevent embarrassment.

Table 23–3 in Chapter 23 illustrates how very frequently diarrhea leads to or is involved in fluid and electrolyte disturbances. Large amounts of fluids and electrolytes may be lost relatively quickly in the presence of diarrhea. This is especially true with infants; if neglected, such loss may easily place a baby's life in jeopardy. Parenteral fluids may be necessary when diarrhea is present. If oral intake is possible, cold fluids and rich foods, especially sweets, should be avoided.

Anal Incontinence

Anal incontinence is the inability of the anal sphincter to control the discharge of fecal and gaseous material. Usually, the cause of incontinence is an organic disease resulting either in a mechanical condition that hinders the proper functioning of the anal sphincter or in an impairment in the nerve supply to the anal sphincter.

While anal incontinence rarely is a menace to life, incontinent patients suffer embarrassment and may become disturbed emotionally. They require much emotional support and understanding as well as special nursing care to prevent odors, skin irritation, and soiling of the linen and the clothing.

Too often, incontinence is accepted as an inescapable situation. This attitude should not exist until every effort has been made to determine if continence can be achieved. While the condition itself is distressing to the patient, some of the nursing measures may be equally disturbing if not managed with tact, since they are not too different from those used with children before they gain bowel control.

Typical nursing measures follow. Note if there is a time of day when incontinence is more likely to occur, such as after a meal. If so, the patient may be placed on a bedpan at such times. If there is no pattern to the incontinence, place the patient on a bedpan at frequent intervals, such as every two or three hours. The patient's attempts at trying to use the pan may be successful and may lead to better muscular control. Consult with the physician about the advisability of using suppositories or a daily enema. For some patients, the problem is so severe that moisture-proof undergarments may be necessary in order to limit soiling of the patient and the bed linen. Disposable bed pads are available and convenient to use. Diapering the patient should be avoided because of its distressing psychological effect.

Anal control depends ultimately on proper functioning of the anal sphincter, and nursing or medical therapeutic measures depend on the cause. In certain instances, functioning of impaired anal sphincters can be improved with a planned program of bowel training. For these patients, aid in regaining bowel control becomes an important part of nursing care.

Bowel Training.   The matter of planning a regimen for bowel training is certainly a mutual proposition involving the physician, the patient, his family, and the nurse. As might be expected, it has great psychological implications for the patient, since almost every lucid individual desires normal control of this body function. The feasibility of initiating such a program must first be determined. Is there any possibility for success? It could be psychologically detrimental to the patient if even partial success was impossible. As a plan is being developed, and once it has been established, it should be a conspicuous part of the patient's nursing care plan, since interruptions may jeopardize the progress being made.

Before beginning bowel training, the patient will need to determine what time of day is best for him to have a bowel movement. This can be decided in terms of his past pattern of elimination and after he has considered his schedule at home and the facilities available. It is also essential that the nurse review the diet, the amount of exercise permitted, and the medications being administered.

Arrangements then should be made so that the patient can try to have a bowel movement at the time of day selected. If possible, the patient should be on a toilet or a commode, since in this position gravity and more effective muscular contraction aid defecation.

If the patient is paralyzed frequently the external sphincter is relaxed, but the training of the internal sphincter is possible, The patient should be encouraged to bear down as is done in a normal bowel movement. However, straining or persistent bearing down should be discouraged because of the possibility of inducing hemorrhoids.

A time limit for trying should be set, such as 15 to 25 minutes. If the patient had any previous habits that seemed to be associated with bowel elimination, these should be included. Frequently, patients state that hot coffee or a glass of water upon arising helps. Reading has some value in the procedure for certain patients. There is merit in taking advantage of any of the patient's suggestions and wishes concerning his previous bowel habits.

The physician may need to be consulted about using suppositories. Inserting one or two suppositories is often a satisfactory means of helping to create stimulation and subsequent emptying of the rectum. The results from the suppositories may not be obtained until several hours later, so that, during the early training period, the patient may be having results at other than the desired elimination time.

Because of the many discouraging aspects to such a program, especially the long time span before any progress is evident, the patient will need much encouragement to continue. He should also receive praise for his efforts.

There is no usual span of time which can be estimated for a bowel-training program. The rapidity with which a satisfactory pattern can be established depends on the patient's condition and often on the perseverance shown by both the patient and the nurse. If the patient becomes discouraged, the nurse may need to modify the procedure from time to time so that the patient has a feeling of some gain.

The Colostomy Irrigation

Patients who have cancer of the colon or other serious health problems may require surgery to create an opening in the abdominal wall for fecal elimination. The intestinal mucosa is brought out to the abdominal wall and a stoma is formed by suturing the mucosa to the skin. This artificially created opening for waste excretion is known as an *ostomy*. An *ileostomy* allows fecal content from the ileum to be eliminated through the stoma. A *colostomy* permits feces from the colon to exit through the stoma.

An ileostomy or a colostomy may be either temporary or permanent. Temporary ostomies are usually done to allow the intestine to repair itself following inflammatory disease, after some types of intestinal surgery, or following injury. Permanent ostomies are usually done because of debilitating intestinal disease or cancer of the colon or rectum.

As with surgery for urinary diversion, following

surgery, the patient will need physical and psychological support. This support can come from persons close to the patient, as well as from members of the health team and persons who have had similar experiences. The ostomy requires specific physical care for which the nurse is initially responsible. Keeping the patient clean and odor-free are especially important. Allowing opportunities for the patient to become acquainted with his new body image and new needs must be a nursing priority. It is generally expected that the patient will experience emotional depression during the early postoperative period. The nurse can generally help the patient to cope by listening, explaining, being available, and being supportive. Overt cheerfulness will usually not help the patient because he is facing a serious crisis and cannot initially see any positive aspects of his condition.

Immediately after surgery, the ostomy is generally covered with a sterile dressing. As the ostomy becomes functional, it is cared for by using clean technique. A protective substance is often applied to the surrounding skin. Several layers of fluffy gauze are put over the stoma. Then, several heavy abdominal pads are applied so that they will absorb the fecal drainage. The dressing should be thicker on the lateral and lower aspects since the drainage will flow by gravity in a downward direction. The dressing is held in place by reusable adhesive ties so that the ties do not have to be changed with each dressing. The nurse should make various observations during the dressing change, such as the appearance of the skin and stoma and the amount, color, and consistency of the feces. The observations are then recorded on the patient's record.

After a few days, an external appliance is generally applied over the stoma. If the ostomy is performed at or proximal to the splenic flexure of the colon, most patients will generally have to wear an external appliance at all times. Control of fecal elimination is usually not possible. If the ostomy involves the colon distal to the splenic flexure, some patients can achieve control over the exit of feces by regular irrigations and habitual emptying of the colon at a certain time each day. This control may be achieved within two months or less postoperatively. If control is achieved and the patient feels comfortable, he does not have to wear the appliance. He may choose to wear only a gauze pad over the stoma.

Irrigations may be used to help in regulating some colostomies. Ileostomies are generally not irrigated since the fecal content of the ileum is liquid which cannot be controlled in this way. Varying factors, such as site of the ostomy in the colon and the patient's and physician's preferences, determine whether a colostomy is irrigated. If an irrigation is to be done, the nurse should familiarize the patient with the technique to be used. She should explain the procedure, demonstrate the irrigating equipment and how it is inserted into the stoma, and demonstrate the way in which the return fluid can be directed into a bedpan or commode. It can also be helpful to have a family member learn the irrigation procedure in case there are times when the patient cannot do the irrigation himself.

A small flexible plastic or rubber catheter has traditionally been used to instill the solution for a colostomy irrigation. A cone-shaped tip also has been advocated as a replacement for the catheter. The use of the cone is felt to be more effective, easier to use, and safer. The cone has the advantage of preventing backflow during the irrigation. In addition, it is easy to handle and cannot be inserted to the extent of causing intestinal damage. If a catheter is used, it should be introduced a maximum of 10 cm. or 4 inches for an adult. The catheter should never be forced. If an obstruction is met, gentle rotating or reangling of the catheter may be helpful. Whether the cone or catheter is used, both should be lubricated to reduce friction before insertion into the stoma.

During irrigation, a soft plastic sleeve is used to cover the stoma and direct the flow of returning irrigating solution and fecal material into the toilet or a collecting receptacle. The sleeve is held in place by a belt. Most sleeves have a small opening near the top for insertion of the cone or catheter. The bottom of the sleeve can be left open for direct emptying into the toilet or a receptacle or it can be closed for containing the return for later emptying. Some persons prefer to close the sleeve so that they can move about and engage in other activities while the irrigating solution is returning, since it may take 30 to 45 minutes.

Warm tap water is commonly used for the irrigating solution. Occasionally, normal saline may be used. The recommended temperature of the solution is the same as for an enema, that is, 40.5° to 49° C. or 105° to 110° F. From 500 ml. to 1,000 ml. is considered typical. The height of the solution container will vary depending on the person but it is generally about 30 cm. or 12 inches above the pelvis. The flow of solution should be relatively slow. It should take from five to ten minutes for instilling 1,000 ml. A clamp on the container tubing can be used to regulate the flow rate. A description of the colostomy irrigation is given on page 496.

The colostomy irrigation

The purpose is to promote emptying of feces from the colon.

SUGGESTED ACTION	RATIONALE
Obtain equipment: irrigating solution, container with tubing and clamp, irrigation cone or catheter, water-soluable lubricant, irrigation sleeve and belt. A drainage receptacle, bed protector, and soap and water will be needed if the irrigation is not performed in a bathroom. A fresh colostomy appliance is needed if the patient is accustomed to wearing one.	An organized procedure aids in conserving patient energy and in making patient teaching more effective.
Place absorbent padding under the patient if he is in bed or in a chair.	This will prevent soiling the bed or chair.
Position the patient comfortably as he prefers.	Since the irrigation may take an extended time the patient should be in a relaxed and comfortable position.
Clamp the tubing and fill the container with irrigating solution, usually luke warm tap water.	Cold water may cause cramping and hot water can injure the intestinal mucosa.
Run irrigating solution through the tubing and catheter or cone into the bedpan or commode.	Running irrigating solution prior to insertion removes air from the tubing or cone.
Gently remove the stoma covering or appliance. Figure 20–21 illustrates exposed stoma.	Careless handling of the covering or appliance can cause damage to the stoma or surrounding tissue.
Place the irrigation sleeve over the stoma and secure it with the belt. Position the sleeve to drain into the bedpan or commode.	The irrigation sleeve provides a means for directing the returning irrigating solution and feces into a collecting receptacle.
Lubricate the cone or catheter and pass it through the upper sleeve opening. Gently insert the cone or catheter into the stoma. The cone should fit snugly into the stoma. The catheter should be inserted a distance of 5 to 10 cm. or 2 to 4 inches. Neither should be forced. Hold the cone or catheter in place. Figure 20–22 illustrates a lubricated cone about to be inserted.	The lubricant reduces friction on insertion and, therefore, reduces the likelihood of mucosal trauma. A snugly fitting cone will prevent irrigating solution leakage from the stoma. Intestinal mucosa injury may occur if insertion is forced or too extensive. The cone or catheter may slip out of place if not held securely.
Place the container approximately 30 cm. or 12 inches above the patient's pelvis and allow the irrigating solution to flow slowly by using the clamp as necessary. Figure 20–23 illustrates.	Low pressure should be maintained so that the flow will not injure the intestinal mucosa or cause cramping.
After administering the prescribed among of irrigating solution, shut off the clamp, remove the cone or catheter, and close the top of the irrigation sleeve.	The returning irrigating solution can spill out of the sleeve opening if it is not closed securely.
Prepare for the return flow either by placing the sleeve in the toilet or collection receptacle, as Figure 20–24 illustrates, or by closing the sleeve at bottom.	The time required for return flow will vary from a few minutes to 45 minutes. Accommodation for the return flow can prevent soiling.
When the return flow has ceased, remove the belt and sleeve and clean the stoma and surrounding skin with soap and water.	The skin should be thoroughly cleaned to preserve its integrity.
Apply the gauze covering or prepare the skin for the application of fresh external appliance. Apply the appliance.	An external appliance or gauze may be worn over the stoma to contain any drainage. If an external appliance is worn the skin should be protected from the irritating effect of intestinal secretions and/or adhesives.
Clean the equipment and store in a ventilated area.	Removal of excrement is easier when done immediately. Air circulation will retard odor and deterioration of the equipment.

For patients who wear external appliances, there are disposable and reusable ones available. The appliance should be changed every day or every other day. If reuseable, it should be washed with soap and water, a vinegar solution, and rinsed and allowed to dry and air. The procedure for cleaning around the stoma and applying a fresh pouch are the same for all ostomies. Keeping the skin and appliance clean are important for controlling odor and preventing skin irritation.

Patients with ostomies should be educated to various methods of odor control. The chlorophyll content in dark green vegetables helps in deodorizing the feces when these vegetables are included in the diet. Bismuth subgallots can be purchased at drug stores and can be taken with meals to aid in lessening fecal odor. Commercial oral and appliance deodorants are also available. Ileostomy patients will usually have fewer problems with fecal odors than will colostomy patients.

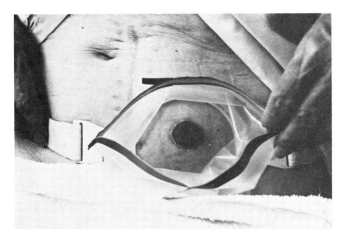

Figure 20–21   This photo shows an irrigation sleeve which is open to expose the colostomy stoma. The irrigating cone or catheter can be inserted through the opening. Note the plastic sleeve is held in place with an elastic belt.

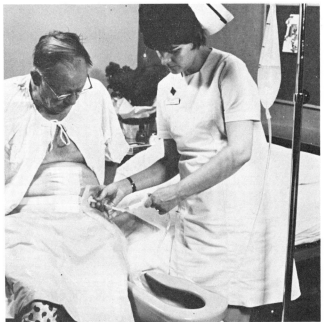

Figure 20–23   The nurse allows the irrigating solution to enter the colon from the elevated container.

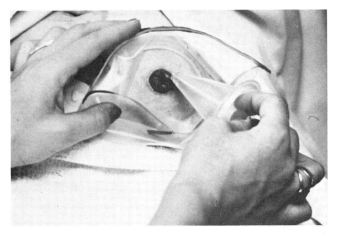

Figure 20–22   The lubricated cone is inserted into the stoma.

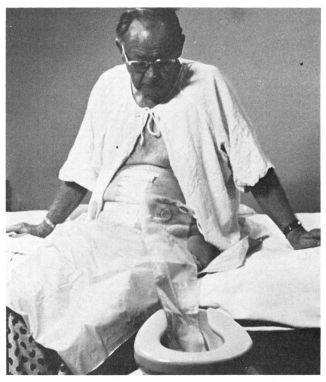

Figure 20–24   The irrigation sleeve is positioned in the bedpan for the return flow. As the patient becomes stronger, he can do the irrigation in the bathroom and allow the irrigation return to drain into the toilet.

Ostomy patients are usually encouraged to avoid foods high in fiber content initially and any other foods that they know cause them to have diarrhea or excessive amounts of flatus. By gradually adding new foods, the ostomy patients can generally build up to a normal diet. He may choose to avoid some foods he finds bothersome.

A new ileostomy surgical approach is being developed similar to the new urinary diversions. For selected persons, an internal reservoir for collecting liquid fecal material is being created. The person then inserts a small tube through the stoma into the reservoir for periodic drainage three to four times each day. An external appliance may not be necessary for persons having this type of surgery, or it may be worn for added security if the patient wishes.

The ostomy patient can live an active and useful life. He should be aware of community resources to assist him, such as home visit nurses, special clinics, and ostomy clubs. More details about the nursing care of the patient with an ostomy can be found in clinical texts.

MEASURING AND RECORDING THE PATIENT'S OUTPUT

A relative balance between fluid intake and output is essential for well-being and for life itself. Especially during illness, a record of the patient's fluid intake and output is maintained. The record may be used as an indicator of change in the patient's condition and as a guide to therapy. Intake and output is often abbreviated I and O. Measurement of intake was discussed in Chapter 19. The exact amounts of urine, suction tube drainage, and emesis are measured and recorded as output. Stool, especially if it is liquid, and wound drainage may also be measured, although estimates are generally satisfactory.

The patient who is having an output record maintained must use a urinal, bedpan, or other receptacle for urination. Then, the urine is poured into a calibrated container for measurement before discarding it. If he has an indwelling catheter, the amount of urine is noted before it is discarded. Usually, a form is kept at the patient's bedside or in the bathroom for recording each urination or defecation. In most agencies, the cumulative output is calculated at the end of each 8- and 24-hour period and entered on the patient's record, along with remarks about any significant observations.

For seriously ill patients, urine output may be calculated on an hourly basis. In such instance, the patients have indwelling catheters and calibrated collection receptacles.

Some patients and family members are taught to maintain output records. They need to be helped to understand the measurement technique and to establish a schedule for totaling the output. In the home, any convenient hour is satisfactory for totaling output as long as it is done at a consistent time during each 24-hour period.

To assure accuracy, the same container should be used for measuring output. In the home, any calibrated

	Date	7-3	3-11	11-7	Remarks
Intake	Oral	630	830	220	*No nausea or vomiting*
	I.V.	1000	—	—	
	Total	1630	830	220	
Output	Urine	1450	520	200	
	Drainage	—	—	—	
	Stool	E	0	0	*Large amount soft, formed*
					brown stool from 800 ml.
	Total	1450	520	200	*tap water enema*
	24 Hr. Intake	*2650 ml.*			
	24 Hr. Output	*2170 ml.*			

Stool
No stool - 0
Stool - ✓
Enema - E
Urine
Foley Cath - F
Voiding - ✓
Not Voiding - 0

Figure 20-25   This is a sample intake and output record.

household container of adequate capacity is satisfactory.

The alert patient and his family should be helped to understand the purpose, importance, and technique of output measurement. Their cooperation may be especially important for accuracy. Involving the patient who is able in this aspect of his care is also a means of promoting his independence.

Various forms are used in health agencies to maintain fluid output records. Figure 20–25 illustrates one type of an intake and output form. The patient at home can be assisted to adapt this type of form to meet his needs.

PROMOTING URINARY AND INTESTINAL ELIMINATION AND THE NURSING PROCESS

The information to be gathered will depend on the circumstances of each individual. Answers to the following questions help provide helpful information as the nurse collects data. What are the characteristics of the person's habits of urinary and intestinal elimination? Does he defecate and urinate at regular times? Does he have any discomfort associated with elimination? Does he identify any problems or concerns with urinary and intestinal elimination? What are the characteristics of his stools and urine? Has he noted any changes in his patterns of elimination? Does he use any urinary or intestinal appliances? Does he take any drugs which influence his urinary and intestinal elimination? Does he have any practices he finds helpful to promote urinary and intestinal elimination? Such questions can help to identify information which can be used in planning the patient's care.

Appropriate standards for assessing data pertaining to urinary and intestinal elimination will depend on the nature of the information. Some norms which could serve as standards have been presented in this chapter. Others can be found in various clinical references. The patient himself can provide important standards for assessing some aspects of elimination since normal variation exists among individuals. Many times, a change in the elimination pattern or characteristics of the excrement is more significant than the particular pattern.

Planning nursing care for the person with a problem with urinary or intestinal elimination depends on the nature of the particular problem. Since elimination has significant psychological implications and because involvement and cooperation of the individual is nearly always essential to success of the plan, participation of the person in establishing the objectives and selecting the nursing measures to be used is important. In many instances, participation of the patient's family is also useful.

Nursing intervention for a particular person is based on the nursing care plan. Many specific intervention measures have been discussed in this chapter. A summary of nursing measures for the person with a problem with urinary or intestinal elimination follows.

- Consider psychological as well as physiological factors when dealing with problems of urinary or intestinal elimination. Since elimination is a sensitive subject in our culture, persons with problems are often uncomfortable and hesitant about acknowledging and discussing them.

- Observe characteristics of the excrement carefully. These characteristics can be significant indicators of the health state of the patient.

- Encourage good general health habits. Food and fluid intake, exercise, and elimination routines can affect urinary and intestinal functioning. A poorly balanced diet, inadequate fluids, minimum physical activity, and poor defecation and urination habits can contribute to problems of elimination. The establishment of more healthful daily habits can often minimize or overcome problems of elimination even when pathology exists.

- Encourage proper positioning for elimination whenever possible. Positioning which allows the use of auxiliary muscles and organs facilitates elimination. For example, having the trunk elevated allows the abdominal organs to exert pressure on the bladder and thus makes urination easier. Being in a sitting position with the knees flexed allows the back and abdominal muscles to help in the act of defecation. The amount of energy required for elimination in these positions is believed to be significantly less than when the person is in abnormal positions.

- Provide privacy for elimination and for conducting procedures related to the urinary and intestinal systems. Since relaxation is conducive to the process of elimination, providing comfort and privacy contribute to ease of elimination and to the comfort of various diagnostic and therapeutic procedures.

- Keep the skin free of excrement. Besides being aesthetically disturbing, feces and urine can have a damaging effect on the skin within a short time. The intestinal enzymes in feces and the ammonia product of urine decomposition are highly irritating to the skin. In addition, moisture, warmth, and darkness are conducive to the growth of organisms.

- Observe good practices of medical and surgical asepsis.

Whether dealing with patients with urinary or intestinal elimination problems, the nurse is a key person in infection control. By consistently practicing handwashing, the nurse also serves as an example for patients. In addition to handwashing, careful attention to the handling of equipment and observing practices of medical and surgical asepsis are imperative.

- Be prepared to provide support and assistance for persons learning new elimination habits. Bladder and bowel training, ostomy irrigations, and external appliance care all require time before success is achieved and the person feels secure. Generally, the person initially feels uncomfortable, experiences some accidents, and has periods of discouragement. The nurse's continued support and interest can be an important factor in the patient's persisting with efforts required for success.

- Teach the importance of seeking professional help when problems occur. Since cancer of the rectum and sigmoid colon are diseases primarily of middle and advanced age, persons in these age groups are encouraged to seek medical attention when symptoms of intestinal disease are present. It is estimated that as many as 70 percent of rectal and low colon lesions can be visualized with the proctosigmoidscope. Therefore, persons past middle age are urged to have a routine endoscopic examination as part of an annual physical examination.

The parts of the nursing process and of the process as a whole are evaluated as described in Chapter 4.

CONCLUSION

Urinary and intestinal elimination are essential physiological processes. The nurse assists patients often by observing elimination patterns and by promoting normal elimination. Her functions in elimination frequently involve extensive teaching of the patient and his family. Her goal is to maintain or restore as near normal body elimination as is possible.

SUPPLEMENTAL LIBRARY STUDY

1. The following articles report the results of two studies conducted with patients who had problems of intestinal elimination. Compare the two reports according to subjects, treatments used, and results.

Bass, Linda, "More Fiber—Less Constipation." *American Journal of Nursing*, 77:254–255, February 1977.

Habeeb, Marjorie C. and Kallstrom, Mina D. "Bowel Program for Institutionalized Adults." *American Journal of Nursing*, 76:606–608, April 1976.

Assuming that the investigations were carefully conducted, how can you explain both approaches being successful when they used opposing dietary regimens?

2. The incidence of nosocomial infections caused by catheterization has been emphasized. This article gives some helpful pointers on reducing urinary tract infections.

DeGroot, Jane. "Catheter-Induced Urinary Tract Infections: How Can We Prevent them?" *Nursing 76*, 6:34–37, August 1976.

Test your practical knowledge on the care of patients with catheters by formulating your own answers to the questions on page 37 before reading the author's responses. How did your answers compare with the author's responses to these questions?

3. Collecting and transmitting urine and fecal specimens for laboratory analyses are often nursing responsibilities. Recommendations for assuring the most accurate and rapid results are described in the following two articles.

McGucklin, Maryanne. "Microbiologic Studies: Part 1. Urine Cultures-Key to Diagnosing Urinary Tract Infections." *Nursing 75*, 5:10–11, December 1975.

McGucklin, Maryanne. "Microbiologic Studies: Part 4. What You Should Know About Collecting Stool Culture Specimens." *Nursing 76*, 6:22–23, March 1976.

What information does the author recommend be included on the requisition slip accompanying the specimen and why? How should fecal specimens from patients with suspected or confirmed hepatitis be handled?

4. Irrigation of the colostomy was nearly universal in the past. In recent years, irrigations are not always used. The author of the article given below describes situations in which irrigation is generally desirable and when it is not.

Watt, Rosemary C. "Colostomy Irrigation—Yes or No?" *American Journal of Nursing*, 77:442–444, March 1977.

After reading the article, list factors which influence whether or not an irrigation will be done.

5. The articles below describe exercises for relieving flatus and the technique for administering an enema.

Blackwell, Ardith K. and Blackwell, William. "Relieving Gas Pains." *American Journal of Nursing*, 75:66–67, January 1975.

Hogstel, Mildred. "How to Give a Safe and Successful Cleansing Enema." *American Journal of Nursing*, 77:816–817, May 1977.

Identify the laws of physics basic to the effectiveness of the prescribed exercises and to the height of the enema solution container, as described in these articles.

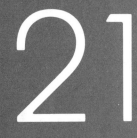

21

BEHAVIORAL OBJECTIVES

*When the content in this chapter has been mastered,
the student will be able to*

Define the terms appearing in the glossary.

Define and describe the preparation of a patient for
common diagnostic examinations of the respiratory
tract, including pulmonary function tests, blood gas
analysis, sputum collection, laryngoscopy,
bronchoscopy, skin testing, chest x-ray, and
bronchography.

Explain the purpose and proper use of common
measures for promoting normal respiratory
functioning.

Summarize the characteristics of oxygen by
describing the general actions taken when it is used
therapeutically.

Differentiate between the routes of oxygen
administration by describing the nursing care
involved in providing oxygen with a nasal cannula,
nasal catheter, face mask, and tent.

Illustrate how the removal of respiratory tract
secretions can be facilitated by postural drainage
and cupping and by tracheal suctioning.

Describe nursing measures for improving the
respiratory airway, including techniques for caring for
the person with a tracheotomy and with an
endotracheal tube.

Explain common methods for assisting ventilation,
including breathing exercises, intermittent positive
pressure breathing, and the use of self-inflating bag
and mask devices.

Describe the use of drugs in improving respiratory
functioning by identifying the purpose, actions, and
precautions for cough suppressants, expectorants,
lozenges, nasal decongestants, and bronchodilators.

Describe the nursing care of a person with a
problem with respiratory functioning, using the
nursing process as a guide.

Promoting Respiratory Functioning

GLOSSARY

Aerosolization: The suspending of medication droplets in a gas.

Anaerobic: Having the ability to live without air.

Atelectasis: The partial or total lack of expansion of the lungs.

Atomizer: A device for breaking a drug into comparatively large particles for inhalation.

Blood Gas Analysis: The examination of arterial blood to determine oxygen and carbon dioxide levels and pH.

Bronchography. A radiologic examination of the bronchi following injection of a radiopaque contrast substance.

Bronchoscope: A lighted tubular instrument used for visually examining the bronchi.

Bronchoscopy: A visual examination of the bronchi.

Congestion: The presence of excessive fluids or secretions in an organ or body tissue.

Cupping: The manual percussion of lung areas to loosen pulmonary secretions.

Dry Cough: A forceful expiratory effort. Synonym for nonproductive cough.

Endotracheal Tube: An artificial airway inserted through the nose or mouth into the trachea to facilitate breathing.

Expectorant: A drug that facilitates the removal of respiratory tract secretions.

Expiratory Reserve Volume: The additional amount of air which can be exhaled beyond tidal volume. Abbreviated ERV.

Forced Vital Capacity: The maximum amount of air that can be inhaled followed by a maximum, fast exhalation with maximum effort. Abbreviated FVC.

Hemoptysis: Blood in respiratory tract secretions.

Inspiratory Reserve Volume: The additional amount of air which can be inspired beyond tidal volume. Abbreviated IRV.

Intermittent Positive Pressure Breathing: A mechanical means of providing a specific amount of gases, water, and/or medication under increased pressure to the respiratory tract. Abbreviated IPPB.

Laryngoscope: A lighted tubular instrument used for visually examining the larynx.

Laryngoscopy: A visual examination of the larynx.

Lozenge: A small, solid medication intended to be held in the mouth until it dissolves.

Nebulizer: A device for breaking a drug into small particles to produce mist or fog for inhalation.

Nonproductive Cough: A forceful expiratory effort. Synonym for dry cough.

Oxygen Therapy: The provision of therapeutic oxygen.

Perfusion: The passing of fluid through tissue.

Phlegm: Thick respiratory secretions.

Postural Drainage: The utilization of gravity to drain secretions from the lungs.

Productive Cough: A cough which produces respiratory tract secretions.

Rales: The intermittent sounds heard as air passes through moisture in the trachea, bronchi, or alveoli.

Rebound Effect: Pronounced opposite results to the intended effect.

Residual Volume: The air remaining in the lungs following maximum exhalation. Abbreviated RV.

Rhonchi: Continuous sounds produced by air passing through respiratory passages narrowed by secretions. Synonym for wheezes.

Spirometer: A device used for measuring inhalation and exhalation volumes.

Suppressant: A drug which depresses a body function.

Sympathomimetic Agent: A drug which mimics the action of the sympathetic nervous system.

Tidal Volume: The amount of air inspired and expired in a normal respiration. Abbreviated TV.

Tracheostomy: An incision made into the trachea for insertion of a tube. Synonym for tracheotomy.

Tracheotomy: An incision made into the trachea for insertion of a tube. Synonym for tracheostomy.

Trendelenburg's Position: A position in which the head and chest are lower than the hips and legs.

Ultrasonic Nebulization: The use of high-frequency sound waves to break a drug into minute particles fo inhalation.

Ventilation: The exchange of gases.

Vital Capacity: The maximum amount of air which can be expelled from the lungs following a maximum inspiration. Abbreviated VC.

Wheezes: Continuous sounds produced by air passing through respiratory passages narrowed by secretions. Synonym for rhonchi.

INTRODUCTION

Respiration involves the exchange of gases in which oxygen from the air is delivered to the tissue cells and carbon dioxide is removed. Maintenance of the complex processes involved in this gas exchange is essential to life. In the past, many persons did not consider respiratory maintenance in the total picture of health care. It was taken for granted and did not command the attention that other activities directed toward health promotion did. For example, weight loss diets, concern about intestinal elimination, and taking tranquilizers to reduce tension have received more public attention than has respiration.

In the past few years, a national campaign to publicize the effect of air pollutants on respiration has resulted in more consideration being given to this physiological process. The prevalence of chronic lung diseases and cancer of the respiratory tract has also resulted in increased attention on measures to reduce and treat these serious pathological states. Mounting evidence supporting the detrimental effects of smoking on breathing has resulted in the initiation of various antismoking programs.

The factors mentioned, along with newly developed methods of prevention and treatment, have caused the nurse to focus increased attention on respiratory functioning also. Vast new areas of preventive teaching about and physical treatment of respiratory diseases exist. There are various types of educational programs for preparing nurses for highly specialized work in respiratory functioning.

Some of the physiological factors of respiration were discussed in Chapter 15 and will not be repeated here. The techniques of respiratory care when specific pathology is present are found in clinical texts containing descriptions of diseases and their treatment. Some commonly used diagnostic tests and the nurse's role in the testing will be discussed here. In addition, nursing measures for use with persons predisposed to or having common respiratory difficulties are presented.

GENERAL PRINCIPLES OF RESPIRATORY FUNCTIONING

Respiration is the exchange of gases between the living organism and its environment. Oxygen is inhaled and carbon dioxide discharged when internal respiration occurs at the cellular level.

All living body cells require oxygen. It follows then that the means by which the body receives this necessity of life should be kept in the best possible state.

The air passageway must remain patent for respiration to occur. Respiratory gases are transported from the nose to the alveoli and returned. Obstruction in any area of the normal passageway will impede respiration. Obstruction can occur from a foreign substance, such as a piece of food, a coin, a toy or other small object, or liquids, as in the case of the drowning victim. Obstruction can also arise from tissues or secretions within the body. For example, excessive or thickened secretions, tumor growths, or edema in the respiratory tract can cause an obstruction.

Muscle movements provide the physical force essential for respiration. The diaphragm and the intercostal muscles are responsible for normal inspiration and expiration. Accessory muscles of the abdomen and back are used to maintain respiratory movements at times when breathing is difficult. The condition of the body musculature can therefore affect the process of respiration.

The pressure changes resulting from expansion and contraction of the thoracic cavity produce the pulmonary gas exchange. Partial or total lack of lung expansion, known as *atelectasis*, prevents the pressure changes and gas exchange. Therefore, atelectic areas of the lung cannot fulfill one function of respiration. Atelectasis can result from obstruction caused by foreign bodies, mucus, or external compression by tumors or enlarged blood vessels.

Adequate fluid intake is essential to respiratory functioning. Fluid is essential to the production of the watery mucus which is normally present in the respiratory tract and is being constantly propelled towards the upper respiratory tract by ciliary action. This is an important mechanism because it helps remove foreign particles and debris from the lungs. This covering of mucus also protects the underlying tissues from irritation and infection. A few millimeters of fluid is also found between the pleural surfaces. The presence of this fluid allows the lungs to move easily along the chest wall as they expand and contract. In its absence, filling and emptying of the lungs are more difficult.

Not all lung tissue is active to the same degree with each respiration. Ventilation depends on the extent of perfusion in the area. *Ventilation* is the exchange of gases, while *perfusion* is the passing of fluid, in this case, the blood, through tissue. The amount of blood flow through the lungs is a factor in the amount of oxygen and other gases which are exchanged. Blood flow in the lungs is influenced by gravity. Therefore, the amount of blood present in any given area of lung tissue depends partially on whether the person is sitting up or lying down, prone, supine, or on either side. The perfusion of lung tissue also depends on activity. Greater activity results in increased cellular oxygen need and cardiac output and, consequently, increased blood return to the lungs. Like all other body tissues, use of healthy lung alveoli helps to maintain them in optimum condition. The implication for patients who are bedfast or generally sedentary is that they should be encouraged to increase their pulmonary activity with conscious effort.

Anatomically, the respiratory system consists of the nose, pharynx, larynx, trachea, the bronchial tree (bronchi with its ciliated cells, bronchioles), and the lungs. The lungs contain many alveoli and blood vessels. Gas exchange takes place in the vascular pulmonary tissue. Because all parts are interdependent, it is toward the maintenance of the entire system that nursing measures in this chapter are directed. Other measures, such as exercise, frequent turning and changing of position also are related and are discussed in other parts of this text.

COMMON DIAGNOSTIC MEASURES

Early detection is one of the prevention measures with which the nurse is often involved. Observations of the breathing rate and respiratory characteristics were described in Chapter 15. The nurse may also assist in diagnostic measures by preparing the person and by gathering specimens. In some industrial and office settings, the nurse may conduct certain diagnostic tests of the respiratory tract. However, in most instances, the diagnostic examinations are conducted by other health personnel, such as x-ray, laboratory, and respiratory therapy technicians. Regardless of who performs the examinations, the results of diagnostic tests found in the patient's record provide the nurse with data basic to nursing care planning and intervention. Many kinds of examinations can be used to determine breathing adequacy and respiratory tract problems. Pulmonary function testing, tissue, blood and secretion examination, skin testing, and radiography are discussed briefly here.

Pulmonary Function Tests

Pulmonary function tests are usually a part of health screening examinations and may be done as part of a preoperative evaluation. They are also done on persons with known respiratory diseases for comparative studies of disease progression and effectiveness of treatment. Pulmonary function testing provides information about the status of the respiratory process in the body, but it does not by itself provide definitive diagnostic information. There are numerous complex tests which can be done; the basic ones are described below.

A *spirometer* is the device commonly used for measuring inhalation and exhalation volume. The spirometer is equipped with a mouthpiece and a mechanism which measures air displaced by the person's respiratory effort. The person breathes through his mouth while being tested and generally wears a nose clip to prevent air leakage. As the air is displaced, the amounts are recorded. The following air volumes are commonly measured.

Tidal volume is the amount of air inspired and expired in a normal respiration. It is abbreviated TV. *Inspiratory reserve volume* is the additional amount of air that can be exhaled beyond tidal volume. It is abbreviated IRV. *Expiratory reserve volume* is the additional amount of air which can be exhaled beyond tidal volume. It is abbreviated ERV. *Residual volume* is the air remaining in the lungs following a maximum expiration. RV is the abbreviation. The residual air is important to prevent atelectasis. For example, even when alveoli are obstructed, the blood continues to absorb air from them. The residual volume provides a reserve available to the blood. If the obstruction can be relieved in a reasonable amount of time, atelectasis will be avoided. *Vital capacity* is the maximum amount of air which can be expelled from the lungs following a maximum inspiration. It is abbreviated VC.

Forced vital capacity is the maximum amount of air that can be inhaled followed by a maximum, fast exhalation with maximum effort. It is abbreviated FVC. The FVC differs from the VC in that the VC does not require a forced expiration; the person exhales slowly. The FVC is considered to be one of the most important diagnostic measurements and is often noted at one, two, and three second intervals.

Preparation of the patient for spirometry testing includes an explanation of the purpose of the test and careful instructions to secure his cooperation. The patient should understand that breathing through the mouth is essential, as is forced inspiration and expiration. Demonstration by the nurse and practice of the maximum respiration before testing may be helpful for some. The testing is not painful but it may be fatiguing. If the patient takes medications affecting respiratory functioning, this should be noted since they can influence interpretations of test results.

The norms for pulmonary function tests are calculated from computations which consider age, sex, race, and height. An individual patient's test results are compared with these norms. Norms also consider body temperature, barometric pressure, and water vapor in the air.

Blood Analysis

Since there is a direct relationship between pulmonary functioning and gas constituents of the blood, examination of blood specimens provides an indirect indication of lung physiology. Arterial blood is used to determine oxygen and carbon dioxide levels and pH. Examination of blood specimens for these purposes is commonly called *blood gas analysis.* Venous blood is more commonly used to determine the blood bicarbonate levels and respiratory acidosis and alkalosis, as will be discussed in Chapter 23. Venous blood is also used for analysis of cells, electrolytes, and enzymes.

Blood gases are commonly examined to determine the partial pressure of oxygen and carbon dioxide, the oxyhemoglobin saturation, and the arterial blood pH. The partial pressures of a mixture of gases indicate the proportion of pressure being exerted by each gas. These pressures differ from atmospheric pressure. The arterial blood pH is an indication of the hydrogen ion concentration of the blood. It is discussed further in Chapter 23. Normal blood gas values at sea level are listed in Table 21–1.

Preparation for blood gas analysis includes an explanation to the patient that an artery will be entered for the purpose of removing a specimen of blood. Commonly, arteries in the arm are used. In some instances, the femoral artery may be used. The blood is collected in an anaerobic syringe. *Anaerobic* means having the ability to live without air and is usually used to describe microorganisms that can live without free oxygen. An anaerobic syringe is air-free.

On completion of the arterial puncture, pressure is applied to the site for a minimum of five minutes to be certain that bleeding is controlled. Repeated observations for evidence of bleeding should be made over a number of hours. The patient having an arterial puncture should be made aware that the procedure is generally more painful than a venipuncture or other injection.

Respiratory Secretions

Secretions from the respiratory tract are often secured for diagnostic examination. As mentioned in Chapter 15, the nurse may be responsible for securing nasal and throat secretion specimens. The nurse may also collect sputum specimens. Sputum specimens are examined for cells, pus, bacteria, and blood. When collecting a sputum specimen, the nurse will encourage the patient to cough deeply so that the secretions are actually raised from the lungs. Merely collecting saliva from the mouth is not satisfactory. Early-morning specimens are generally easier to obtain, and usually approximately a teaspoonful is needed for most laboratory tests. Special specimen containers are supplied by the laboratory, and the patient expectorates directly into them. Care should be taken that the outside of the container does not become contaminated. Mechanical suction is sometimes used to secure a sputum specimen from a patient who is unable to raise sputum. Gastric washings are also occasionally used; a tube is inserted into the stomach to secure sputum the patient has swallowed.

Respiratory Tract Tissue

Specimens of respiratory tract tissue are examined generally to determine the presence of a malignancy. Such specimens are obtained by the physician, usually with special instruments. A *bronchoscope* is a lighted tubular instrument used for visually examining the bronchi while the *laryngoscope* is a similar instrument used to visualize the larnyx. Specimens are obtained at the time of viewing. A visual examination of the bronchi is called a *bronchoscopy,* and of the larnyx, a *laryngoscopy.*

A bronchoscopy or laryngoscopy is usually done with the patient in a fasting state. The physician will generally order a sedative for the patient prior to the examination. A local or general anesthetic is also used. When a local anesthetic is used, the patient's gag reflex is absent during and following the procedure until the effects of the anesthesia disappear. Following the examination, the patient's respirations should be observed for indications of progressive edema. Dyspneic signs

TABLE 21–1   Normal arterial blood gas values at sea level

PARAMETER	NORMAL VALUE
pO_2	80 to 100 mm. Hg
pCO_2	35 to 45 mm. Hg
O_2 saturation	96 to 98%
pH	7.35 to 7.45

should be reported. _Hemoptysis,_ that is, blood in respiratory tract secretions may be expected if a biopsy is performed.

The patient should be prepared with an explanation of the procedure. He should be made aware in advance that if he has a local anesthesia, the cough and gag reflexes will be stimulated by its administration. In addition, he may feel that his tongue and throat are swollen and he will have difficulty swallowing. He should know mechanical suctioning will be used throughout the procedure to remove the secretions. He should be assured that his airway will be maintained and that breathing will not be impaired. Following the procedure, food and fluids may be withheld for several hours until the effects of anesthesia have subsided. Local swelling and discomfort usually exist and may last for several days after a bronchoscopy or laryngoscopy.

Skin Tests

Skin tests are commonly used to detect the presence of antibodies against organisms commonly causing lung infections. Since the sensitivity of the body is increased following contact with the organism, an antigen-antibody reaction is induced. A small amount of dilute antigen prepared from the organism or its secretions is generally injected intradermally, that is, between the skin layers. The patient is observed at specified periods for a reaction which indicates the presence of antibodies resulting from previous contact with the antigen.

Skin testing is commonly part of the diagnostic procedure for tuberculosis, histoplasmosis, and coccidiodomycosis. The technique for intradermal injections will be discussed in Chapter 24. If the nurse is responsible for administering the test, she should explain its purpose to the patient and be careful to help him understand that a positive reaction is only an indication of the presence of antibodies, and not necessarily a current infection.

Skin testing is also used to identify substances which cause allergic respiratory symptoms. Intradermal scratch tests are usually done on a large body area, such as the skin of the upper back.

Radiography

X-ray examination of the lungs is another commonly used diagnostic method. The x-ray examination of the chest can demonstrate the size and shape of the lungs. This examination is most often used to detect densities produced by space-occupying lesions and infectious processes. No special preparation is necessary for the patient.

Bronchography is the radiologic examination of the bronchi following injection of a radiopaque contrast material. Usually following sedation and local anesthesia, a rubber catheter is inserted into the bronchus followed by the introduction of contrast material. The patient is asked to inhale deeply to spread the contrast material throughout the lung. The patient is placed in varying positions to visualize all areas of the bronchial tree. Following the films, the patient is returned to a sitting position and asked to cough vigorously to expectorate the contrast material. Another x-ray film may be taken to determine if the material is removed. Its retention in the lung can cause atelectasis or pneumonia. Oral intake is not permitted until the gag reflex has returned. The patient should be closely observed for signs of respiratory dysfunction for several days.

Preparation for bronchography includes having the patient in a fasting state. He should be aware that the examination is uncomfortable and fatiguing. The introduction of the local anesthesia and the catheter generally cause extensive retching and coughing. Removal of the contrast material requires maximum coughing.

COMMON MEASURES TO PROMOTE NORMAL RESPIRATORY FUNCTIONING

Deep Breathing

Habits of breathing that are not in the best interests of bodily functioning are common in well and ill persons. Some persons, for one reason or another, develop a pattern of shallow breathing or walk with a "caved-in" chest. The result may be decrease of lung distensibility. A means of combating this is taking deep breaths (hyperinflation). Daily periodic hyperinflation is essential for such persons.

Involuntary deep breathing often occurs during sleep. Persons who snore, although a problem to those who have to listen, may benefit by their condition in that they frequently take deeper breaths.

Positioning for ease of breathing is important. Helping an incapacitated patient assume a position that allows for the free movement of the diaphragm and expansion of the chest wall promotes ease of respiration. Sitting in a slumped position that permits the abdominal contents to push upward on the diaphragm will result in less lung expansion during inspiration.

Persons with dyspnea are more comfortable in a Fowler's or sitting position because the accessory muscles can be used more readily.

Because incisional discomfort following chest and abdominal surgery usually results in the person's unconsciously or consciously minimizing his respiratory movements, secondary pulmonary complications can occur. Teaching breathing and coughing exercises and encouraging the patient to practice before surgery, even sometimes before he enters the hospital, have been found to be very helpful in promoting a faster convalescence. Support of the incisional area with the hands, a pillow, or a folded blanket can minimize the patient's discomfort during the exercises. Teaching breathing and coughing exercises to members of the patient's family can help them to be able to provide encouragement and support for the patient.

Although there are some variations in what is considered to be *the* best method for therapeutic deep breathing, physiological principles guide the actions that are essential. For one, the person should be instructed to inhale slowly and evenly to the greatest chest expansion possible for him. Next, he should hold his breath for at least three seconds. Studies indicate that a longer period does not produce any more benefit than the three-second hold. Then the person permits normal recoil of the chest. Five successive breaths of this type are generally recommended. As to the frequency with which this should be done, the patient's condition is the best guide. For some persons two or three times every two or three hours is satisfactory. Patients in danger of pulmonary complications may need to deep breathe as often as every hour.

The person with known lung pathology needs to learn more specific exercises. Persons with chronic pulmonary diseases, in particular, profit by developing the auxiliary respiratory muscles through exercises. Some of these exercises will be discussed later in this chapter.

Coughing

Voluntary Coughing. The cough mechanism consists of an initial irritation, a deep inspiration, a quick tight closure of the glottis together with a foreceful contraction of the expiratory intercostal muscles, and the upward push of the diaphragm. This causes an explosive movement of air from the lower to the upper respiratory tract. To be effective, a cough should have enough muscle contraction to force air to be expelled and to propel a liquid or a solid on its way out of the respiratory tract. The cough is a cleaning mechanism of the body. It is an effective means of assisting the cilia keep the airway clear of secretions and other debris. When a cough does not occur as a result of reflex stimulation of the cough-sensitive areas, it can be induced voluntarily.

Patients who are susceptible to airway collections of secretions, such as persons following general anesthesia, are taught to cough voluntarily. Coughing is most effective when the patient is in a sitting position and when he is sufficiently well-hydrated so that the viscosity of the secretions permits their movement. Deep exhalation and inhalation followed by a forceful coughing expiration, using the abdominal and other accessory respiratory muscles, is generally effective. The nurse may have to demonstrate and have the patient practice several times before his cough is effective.

For the patient who is unable to cough voluntarily, manual stimulation over the trachea and prolonged exhalation can be helpful. If neither of these methods is successful, mechanical endotracheal stimulation with a catheter is sometimes used.

Although the actual teaching of preventive respiratory exercises, such as deep breathing and coughing, is relatively easy, experience has shown that it is difficult to have the patient follow through and do them. Frequent reminders throughout the day are necessary for most patients. Having a specific schedule on the nursing care plan is also useful. Figure 21–1, 21–2, and 22–3 illustrate breathing exercises.

Involuntary Coughing. Involuntary coughing is a frequent accompaniment of respiratory tract infections and irritations. As indicated earlier, coughing is a cleaning mechanism of the body and not desirable unless it is ineffective or becomes so frequent as to cause fatigue. Many persons find a cough annoying and want it suppressed. For this reason, many kinds of cough preparations are available for over-the-counter purchases. Nurses are often asked about them. The nurse may need to help the person understand the useful effects of a cough and explain that it is a symptom of some respiratory irritation which may need medical attention. However, noneffective coughing can be harmful because of its fatiguing effect or because the cough is inefficient for removing the secretions. In either case, medications may be helpful. Observations of the characteristics of breathing and coughing are necessary to determine the appropriate type of medication.

A *nonproductive cough* is a forceful expiratory effort caused by irritation which produces no secretions. It is

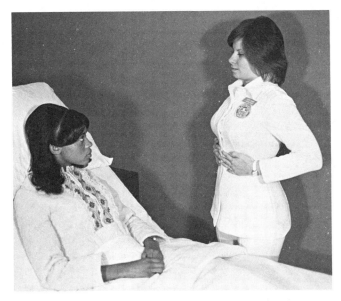

Figure 21-1 The nurse is preparing the patient for deep breathing and coughing postoperatively by explaining and asking her to practice prior to surgery. Here, the nurse is demonstrating that you can feel the chest expand and contract on deep inhalation and exhalation.

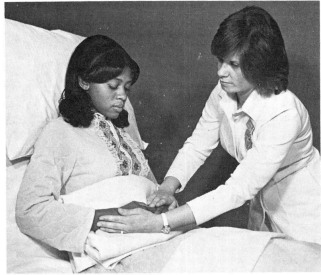

Figure 21-3 The nurse is showing the patient how a folded bath blanket can be used as an abdominal support to splint the incisional area before deep breathing and coughing.

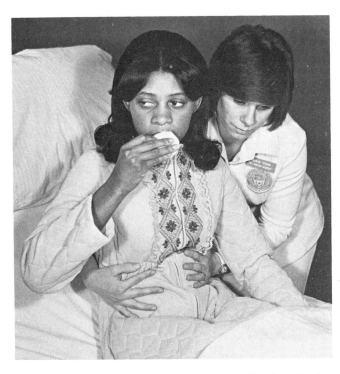

Figure 21-2 The nurse is using her hands to splint the patient's upper abdominal area as the patient coughs.

also called a *dry cough.* Thick respiratory secretions are sometimes called *phlegm.* A *productive cough* is one which produces respiratory tract secretions.

The presence of excessive fluids or secretions in an organ or body tissue is called *congestion.* A person with secretions or fluid in his lungs is said to have congested lungs. If his cough is dry, he is said to be congested with a nonproductive cough. If his cough is productive, he is referred to as being congested with a productive cough. If he is coughing with no congestion or secretions produced, he is described as being dry or noncongested with a nonproductive cough.

Suppressants and Expectorants. Two of the major types of cough preparations are suppressants and expectorants. *Suppressants are drugs which depress a body function,* in this case, the cough reflex. Codeine, which is present in many cough preparations, is generally considered the preferred cough suppressant ingredient. However, codeine can be addictive. Because of its abuse, many states require a physician's prescription for its use. Dextromethorphan hydrobromide is considered by some authorities to be as effective a cough suppressant ingredient as codeine without the addicting qualities. Diphenhydramine hydrochloride, a potent antihistamine, is an effective cough suppressant. However, it has the common side effect of other antihistamines, which is drowsiness. Therefore, it may not be safe to use when the individual must remain alert, such as when driving a car.

An irritating nonproductive cough in persons without congestion may be appropriately treated with suppressants. Inappropriate suppression of the cough in a person with respiratory congestion can result in harmful retention of the secretions.

Expectorants are drugs that facilitate the removal of respiratory tract secretions. They act by reducing the secretion viscosity. Patients with extremely tenacious secretions may need to have secretions liquified in order for the cough to remove them effectively. In that way, the nonproductive cough of a person with lung congestion can become productive. An expectorant used by a person who does not have congestion is inappropriate.

Ammonium chloride, terpin hydrate, and epicac have been widely used as expectorants in cough preparations. However, recent studies are questioning their value. Adequate fluid intake and air humidification are deemed to be equally effective as expectorants by some authorities.

Since cough preparations are so readily available and persons who purchase them are usually eager for relief, they sometimes take excessive amounts of more than one type. The nurse can often provide health teaching about the appropriate choice of cough preparations. She is also frequently in a position to help individuals to understand and adhere to the recommended directives. For example, some cough preparations can be harmful to some persons. Cough syrups with a high-sugar or alcohol content can disturb the metabolic balance of persons with diabetes mellitus. Preparations containing antihistamines have an anticholinergic action which can cause serious complications for persons with glaucoma, or cause urinary retention in males with prostate enlargement. Similarly, other cough preparations can be detrimental to persons with hypertension and with thyroid and cardiac diseases. In addition, prolonged use of self-prescribed cough preparations can result in concealing more serious health problems which should be evaluated by a health practitioner.

Lozenges. Mild nonproductive coughs in persons without congestion can often be relieved by lozenges. A *lozenge* is a small, solid medication intended to be held in the mouth until it dissolves. Lozenges generally control coughs by the local anesthetic effect of benzocaine. The local anesthetic can act on sensory and motor nerves by controlling the primary irritation and inhibiting afferent and efferent impulses.

Adequate Hydration

In addition to ridding the lungs of accumulated secretions through deep breathing and coughing, attention should be given to adequate hydration to minimize the viscosity of secretions. The patient's fluid intake should be increased to the maximum that his health state will tolerate. The patient who has an elevated temperature, is breathing through his mouth, or coughing, or is losing excessive body fluids in other ways should have special attention focused on his intake. The systemic implications of fluid deficit will be discussed in Chapter 24. Nursing measures to help increasing fluid intake were were discussed in Chapter 19.

In some circumstances in which the air is dry, that is, the humidity is low, artificial means for humidification may be necessary. The inspiration of dry air further removes the normal moisture in the respiratory passages which is essential for protection from irritation and infection. Room humidifiers may be helpful for some patients. Electric vaporizers which produce steam or cool mist are available. Authorities feel the therapeutic value of one over the other has not been demonstrated. A cool mist vaporizer does not present dangers with burns because it does not generate heat or hot water. However, it can provide the medium for pathogen growth if not cleaned adequately. The steam vaporizer does not present this problem.

IMPAIRED RESPIRATORY FUNCTIONING

Oxygen is essential for life, and the body has no reserve of it. Therefore, when there is insufficient oxygenation of the blood, oxygen must be added to inhaled air in order to sustain life. Respiratory therapists are available in many hospitals to provide different types of respiratory care. However, in many instances, the nurse is also responsible for initiating and maintaining respiratory therapies.

Supplying the body with optimum amounts of oxygen depends on a number of factors. They can be summarized as follows:

- The availability of appropriate concentrations of oxygen.
- The movement of air into and out of the lungs.
- The movement of air from the lung alveoli to the hemoglobin of the blood.
- The movement of blood containing oxygen, carbon dioxide and wastes between the lungs and other body tissues.

- The exchange of oxygen and carbon dioxide and other wastes between blood and tissue cells.

If a problem exists in any part of the respiratory process, hypoxia may occur. Environmental or pathological factors can be the cause of the problem. For example, high altitude or the presence of toxic fumes can alter the availability of oxygen. Depression of the respiratory center or pulmonary congestion can prevent the normal movement of air into and out of the lungs. Inadequate or abnormal hemoglobin can impede the passage of oxygen to the blood. An insufficient blood volume or depressed pumping action of the heart can prevent normal blood movement. Metabolic abnormalities of tissue cells can alter gas exchanges. A combination of factors can also exist which may influence several parts of the process of oxygenation.

Depending on the cause, various nursing measures and respiratory therapies may be helpful for the person experiencing hypoxia. Providing a supplemental supply of oxygen can increase the concentration of inspired oxygen when the amount in the atmospheric air is insufficient. Movement of air into and out of the thorax can be facilitated by the person's positioning. An upright position with the head back makes a straight and unimpeded respiratory passageway. A sitting or Fowler's position allows for the auxiliary chest, abdominal, and back muscles to assist with respiration. Various mechanical devices, techniques, and drugs can improve the movement of air into and out of the lungs by decreasing secretions. Artificial airways can bypass obstructions. Positioning, exercises, and mechanical devices can also assist or substitute for the inspiration and expiration processes and, thus, promote air movement.

Respiratory therapies are not generally helpful in relieving problems with the movement of oxygen between the alveoli, hemoglobin, and body tissues. Other types of therapies must be used to treat the causes of these problems. However, as indicated earlier, various parts of the process of oxygenation may be involved at one time. Therefore, respiratory therapy may be used when the primary cause of the hypoxia is not of a respiratory origin. For example, the cause may be of a cardiac or neurological nature, or blood volume may not be normal. In these instances, respiratory therapy is supplemental to the therapy used to treat the primary cause of the problem.

The most common symptoms of hypoxia are dyspnea, increased pulse and respiratory rates, and paleness or cyanosis. More detailed discussions of these and other signs of hypoxia as they relate to specific pathological conditions are included in clinical references.

PROVIDING SUPPLEMENTAL OXYGEN

The amount of oxygen available for inspiration can be increased by providing a supplemental supply. The provision of therapeutic oxygen is called *oxygen therapy*. Oxygen therapy must sometimes be instituted with such speed that there is little time for explanation to the patient. However, depending on the situation, some concurrent instructon is generally possible. If there is an emergency, once the patient is out of danger and is breathing easily he should be told about the device and the essentials necessary to serve him effectively. It is a terrifying experience to be unable to breathe, and the patient needs the support and comfort of feeling that everything possible is being done for him.

Supplemental oxygen is delivered to the respiratory tract artificially under pressure. Therefore, excessive drying of the mucous membrane lining the tract occurs unless the oxygen is humidified. Since oxygen is only slightly soluble in water, it can be readily passed through solution with little loss. Regardless of the method of administration, oxygen administered therapeutically should be humidified by water, saline, or a medicated solution before entering the respiratory tract.

There are patients who must become proficient in administering oxygen to themselves. They may have asthma or chronic lung ailments or impaired cardiac functioning and have oxygen at home for self-administration.

Oxygen, which constitutes approximately 20 percent of normal air, is a tasteless, odorless and colorless gas. It is heavier than atmospheric air. In addition to its vital importance in sustaining life, it has a chemical characteristic which requires careful consideration. Oxygen supports combustion. Therefore, open flames and sparks must be kept away from the area where oxygen is being stored or administered. This precaution cannot be emphasized enough since periodically tragic accidents occur as a result of this hazard. "No Smoking" signs should be placed in many prominent places in the patient's room and the patient and his visitors taught the necessity of observing this regulation. The patient and family should be taught to use similar precautions at home.

Other fire precautions should also be taken. Electrical devices, such as heating pads, electric bell cords, razors, and radios, should be checked carefully to be certain they are not emitting sparks. It is also recommended that synthetic fabrics which build up static electricity should be generally avoided around oxygen. Oil, including oil on clothing, should not be permitted around oxygen sources because oil can ignite spontaneously.

In most hospitals, oxygen is piped into each patient unit and is immediately available from an outlet in the wall. This piped-in oxygen is a valuable asset: it increases the patient's safety by eliminating the delay in transporting oxygen in tanks and the constant vigil on the gauge to check on the amount of oxygen remaining in the tank. When oxygen is not available from a wall outlet, it is obtained in portable cylinders.

The flow rate of oxygen is measured in liters per minute. In the past, this rate was used to regulate the amount of oxygen made available to the patient. The rate varied, depending on the condition of the patient and the route being used to administer oxygen. Now, more precise dosages are being prescribed in percent of inspired oxygen. The flow rate does not necessarily reflect the oxygen concentration actually inspired by the patient due to leakage and mixing with atmospheric air. Therefore, analysis of samples of the air mixture the patient is actually inhaling is recommended for regulating oxygen concentration accurately. Several types of commercial oxygen analyzers are available. The technique for their use varies with the manufacturer. Some are designed to measure the oxygen concentration continually while others measure it intermittently. It is recommended that oxygen concentrations be measured at least every three to four hours for persons receiving continuous oxygen therapy.

The nurse should note and record the administration route and the amount of oxygen the patient is receiving. The character of his respirations and his reaction to oxygen administration should also be noted.

Sources of Oxygen

Therapeutic oxygen is supplied from two sources: wall outlet or portable cylinder. As noted previously, the wall outlet source for oxygen can be prepared for use quickly. The oxygen is supplied from a central source through a pipeline, usually at 50 to 60 pounds per square inch of pressure. A specially designed flowmeter is attached to the wall outlet. The flowmeter opens the outlet and a valve makes possible regulation of the oxygen flow. Careful handling of the flowmeter is necessary to prevent damage and resulting oxygen loss. Figure 21–4 shows a flowmeter.

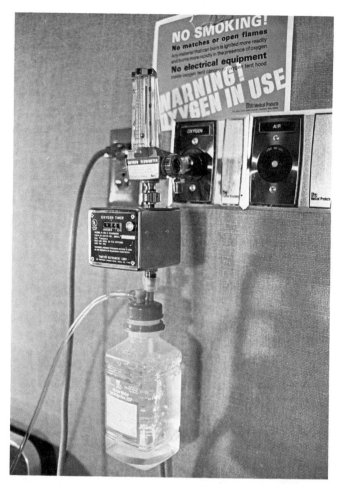

Figure 21–4 This photo illustrates piped-in oxygen equipment. The flowmeter or regulator determines the rate of flow of the oxygen which is bubbled through the humidifier bottle and passes through the plastic tubing to the patient. The sign indicating oxygen is in use is displayed at the patient's bedside and on the door entering the patient's room.

When not piped in, oxygen usually is dispensed under pressure in steel cylinders or tanks. The tank is delivered with a protective cap to prevent accidental force against the cylinder outlet. When a standard, large-sized cylinder is full, its contents are under more than 2,000 pounds per square inch of pressure. The force behind an accidentally partially opened outlet could cause the tank to take off like an uncontrolled, jet-propelled monster. Smaller cylinders are available for emergency, ambulatory, and home use. The principles and precautions in their use are the same as with the large cylinders.

To release the oxygen safely and at a desirable rate, a regulator is used. The regulator valve controls the rate of oxygen output. The regulator has two gauges. The one nearest the tank shows the pressure or amount of oxygen in the tank. The other gauge indicates the number of liters per minute of oxygen being released. Figure 21–5 shows an oxygen tank with its regulator.

Because of the nature of oxygen, caution must be used in handling the oxygen cylinder and the regulator. The oxygen cylinder should be transported carefully, preferably strapped onto a wheeled carrier to avoid possible falling and breaking of the outlet. Once the cylinder is located, it should be stabilized by securing it in a properly fitting stand.

Because of the possibility of dust or other particles becoming lodged in the outlet of the tank and being forced into the regulator, the tank is "cracked" before a regulator is applied. This calls for slightly turning the

handle on the tank which releases the oxygen so that a small amount of oxygen may be released, thus "flushing out" the outlet. The force with which the oxygen is released from this opening causes a loud hissing sound which usually startles anyone who is not aware of what it is. For this reason, it is recommended that oxygen tanks be "cracked" away from the patient's bedside. If this is not possible, the patient should be prepared for the noise by proper explanation. The oxygen can be released slowly and the sound reduced if both hands are placed on the handle. One hand helps control the movement of the other.

The Administration of Oxygen by Nasal Cannula

Usually the simplest method and the one best tolerated by the patient for the administration of oxygen, is via the nasal cannula. The cannula is a disposable plastic device with two protruding prongs for insertion into the nostrils. It is held in place by an elastic strap around the head. Before the oxygen is delivered to the cannula, it is bubbled through a humidifier containing distilled water. This method of administration is used in health agencies and home settings.

The cannula prongs should be lubricated with a water-soluble lubricant before insertion. The patient should be observed for signs of pressure from the positioning or tightness of the cannula. Periodic movement and gauze padding under the cannula may be helpful. Figure 21–6 shows a patient receiving oxygen through a nasal cannula. The technique for using the nasal cannula is described in the chart on page 514.

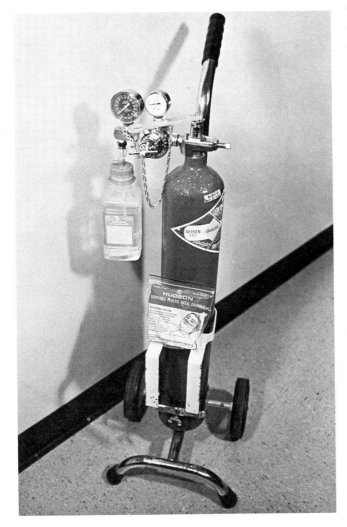

Figure 21–5 A small cylinder of oxygen is in readiness for an emergency. The regulator and humidifier bottle are attached and ready for use.

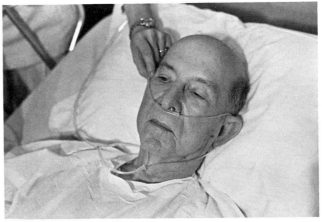

Figure 21–6 The nurse is adjusting the elastic head band for a patient receiving oxygen by nasal cannula.

The administration of oxygen by means of a nasal cannula

The purpose is to administer a therapeutic concentration of oxygen into the nostrils.

SUGGESTED ACTION	RATIONALE
Take actions to minimize fire hazards, such as checking electrical appliances and posting "No Smoking" signs.	Oxygen supports combustion.
Attach the humidifier bottle to the regulator or flowmeter.	Oxygen forced through a water reservoir is humidified before it is delivered to the patient, preventing dehydration of the mucous membrane.
Attach the nasal cannula to the connecting tube of the water reservoir. Lubricate the cannula prongs with a water-soluble lubricant and start the flow of oxygen at approximately 2 to 4 liters per minute.	Lubricant reduces irritation to the nasal mucosa. Having the oxygen flowing will provide for supplemental oxygen to be immediately available to the patient.
Place the prongs in the patient's nostrils. Secure the cannula strap and adjust it so that it is comfortably snug. Use gauze pads as necessary for comfort.	Correct placement of the prongs and the cannula strap will facilitate oxygen administration and comfort.
Adjust the oxygen flow to the rate specified.	Inadequate oxygen flow will not be therapeutic. Excess oxygen flow can cause drying and irritation of the nasal mucosa.
Instruct patient to breathe through his nose.	Mouth breathing can result in oxygen loss.
Remove and clean cannula and nares at least every eight hours. Apply lubricant to nostrils as necessary.	The continued presence of the cannula causes irritation and dryness to the mucous membrane. Lubricant can help to counteract the drying effect of the oxygen flow.

The Administration of Oxygen by Nasal Catheter

A nasal, or oropharyngeal, catheter is a more efficient means for administering oxygen. It is somewhat more uncomfortable for the patient than the nasal cannula but it delivers a higher concentration of oxygen. Moisturization of the oxygen is accomplished through a humidifier bottle attached to the flowmeter. The catheter is inserted into the nostril and passed until it is in full view at the back of the tongue as one looks into the mouth. It should be in the oropharynx. The horizontal distance from the nasal opening to the earlobe may be used as a guide for determining the length of catheter to be inserted. If the catheter is inserted too far, there is danger of insufflating the stomach; if it is not inserted far enough, much of the oxygen will escape before it is inhaled. Figure 21–7 shows the proper location of the nasal catheter. After being properly positioned, the catheter should be secured in place with tape.

Irritation of the mucous membrane by the catheter is minimized when the catheter is lubricated prior to insertion with a water-soluble lubricant. An oily substance used as a lubricant could be harmful if aspirated into the lungs. Nasal catheters should be removed for cleaning at least once every eight hours. A fresh catheter should be inserted and the alternate nostril used as indicated.

Frequent nasal and mouth care generally adds to the patient's comfort. Oxygen administered at too high a flow will dry the mucous membrane and the patient may complain of a sore throat. The chart on page 516 describes the insertion of the catheter.

The Administration of Oxygen by Face Mask

Various types of face masks have been devised for administering oxygen. The oronasal mask is designed to cover both the nose and the mouth and is necessary if the patient is a mouth breather. It presents problems in eating, drinking, and talking, however. The nasal mask covers the nose and permits the patient's mouth to be exposed. If it is possible for the patient to use it, this mask is more comfortable and convenient.

When a mask is used to administer oxygen, it must be fitted carefully to the patient's face to avoid leakage. Disposable and reusable masks are available in plastic and rubber. The mask should be comfortably snug but not tight against the patient's face. Frequent care of the face, including washing and powdering, will help to prevent irritation from the mask. In addition, the mask should be kept clean. Frequent washing helps to reduce the odors absorbed by the rubber.

Five types of face masks are available. The simple mask is the least expensive. It is usually plastic and disposable and has open vents for the elimination of exhaled air. It cannot deliver precise oxygen concen-

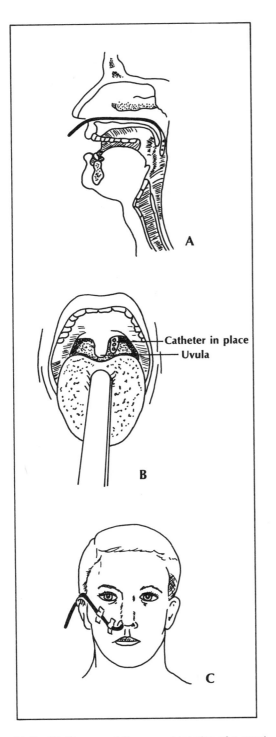

Figure 21-7 (A) Diagram of the correct location of a nasal catheter in the nose and the oropharynx.

(B) To make certain that the catheter is placed properly, it is necessary to ask the patient to open his mouth. The tip of the catheter should be located opposite the uvula.

(C) The catheter should be taped close to the nares and on the cheek. It can then drape over the ear. This provides freedom of movement of the lips and reduces pull on the catheter.

trations but is suitable in many noncritical situations.

Concentration masks are designed to supply specific concentrations of oxygen up to 40 percent. These masks dilute the 100 percent supplemental supply with atmospheric air. The oxygen is calibrated according to the oxygen concentration desired. Side vents allow for the escape of exhaled air. This type of mask permits the most precise administration of low concentrations of oxygen. It is also generally considered more comfortable because of the cooling effect of the high flow of the oxygen and atmospheric air.

The partial rebreathing mask is equipped with a reservoir bag for the collection of the first part of the patient's exhaled air. This air is primarily oxygen and is mixed with 100 percent oxygen for the next inhalation. The remaining exhaled air exits through vents. The use of this type of mask permits the conservation of oxygen.

The total rebreathing mask also has a reservoir bag but it has no opening to the atmosphere. The exhaled carbon dioxide is absorbed by a chemical and the reservoir bag supplies other gases. This type of mask is generally used for the administration of oxygen and anesthetic gases.

The nonrebreathing mask is similar to the partial rebreathing mask, except that it does not conserve the exhaled air. The reservoir bag is filled with oxygen which enters the mask on inspiration. Exhaled air escapes through side vents. This mask may also be used for administering gas mixtures.

Providing increased humidity with the face mask is generally recommended. However, in some instances, the water vapor from the patient's expirations will provide adequate humidity. Figure 21-8 on page 516 shows one type of face mask. The chart on page 517 describes the use of a face mask.

The Administration of Oxygen by Tent

The oxygen tent is a light portable structure made of clear plastic and attached to a motor-driven unit. The motor aids in circulating and cooling the air in the tent. The cooling device functions on the same principles as an electric refrigeration unit. A thermostat in the unit keeps the temperature in the tent at the degree considered most comfortable by the patient. The oxygen tent is used only occasionally today because it is very difficult to maintain a satisfactory oxygen concentration. Because oxygen is heavier than atmospheric air, it concentrates at the lower part of the tent and

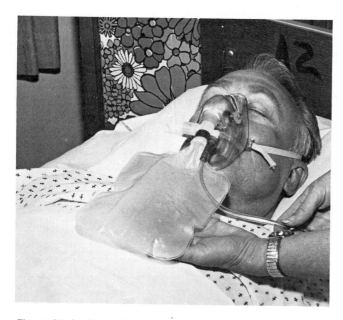

Figure 21–8   This patient is receiving oxygen through a face mask with a reservoir bag.

escapes easily at the bottom or through the openings in the tent. The temperature and humidity can be readily regulated. Therefore, the tent may be used for patients needing a cool or highly humidified air flow, such as febrile children with lung congestion.

An oxygen tent fits over the top part of the bed so that the patient's head and thorax are in the tent. It has side openings through which nursing care can be administered. The tent is sealed by tucking the sides under the mattress and by wrapping the front flap into a piece of bed linen. Patients may be frightened by the appearance of an oxygen tent since it frequently is associated with critical illness. However, if the patient is prepared adequately as to its purpose, few object to its use.

One disadvantage of which the nurse should be aware is the possibility of too great air movement in the tent. Many tents are constructed so that there is a complete exchange of air in the tent every few seconds, in order to prevent an increase in carbon dioxide content. The air movement may create a draft on the patient to the point of real discomfort. The discomfort can be avoided by protecting the patient's head, neck, and shoulders with a combination hood and shawl or a blanket. The temperature within an oxygen tent can be regulated within a desired range and should be maintained at a level that is comfortable for the patient.

A word of caution is necessary as a reminder that the tent is not soundproof. Usually, the patient is able to hear normal conversation from outside the tent. Speak to the patient in normal conversational tones unless he indicates that he cannot hear. It is distressing to the patient to have people outside of the tent shouting at him.

A signal cord that is not electric is generally preferred for use in the oxygen tent. A small hand bell is an example. This added precaution is generally taken although an electric call system should be grounded and safe.

The chart on page 518 describes the use of any oxygen tent.

REMOVING RESPIRATORY TRACT SECRETIONS

If the lungs are congested, moist sounds can be heard with each respiration. With minimum congestion, the sounds may be heard only upon auscultation. Sounds heard intermittently as the air passes through moisture in the trachea, bronchi, or alveoli are called *rales*. Rales generally are heard only on inspiration and can change with coughing.

Continuous sounds produced by air passing through respiratory passages narrowed by secretions are called *rhonchi* or *wheezes*. They can also be caused by narrowing due to swelling or tumors. With auscultation, they can be heard on both inspiration and expiration, but usually are louder on expiration.

Some persons can raise and expectorate their respiratory secretions by coughing. Others need to have them removed mechanically. Whether respiratory secretions are expectorated or mechanically removed, they should be observed and recorded. The color, amount, viscosity, and odor should be noted.

Humidification

The importance of adequate humidification to alleviate dehydration of the respiratory mucous membrane which accompanies some respiratory diseases has been emphasized. The dryness of the mucous membrane is accompanied by a drying of the respiratory secretions which make them more viscid. The increased viscosity of the secretions makes them more difficult to move and thus contributes to congestion of the upper and lower respiratory tract. Moisture promotes the liquification of the secretions and ease of their removal.

The administration of oxygen by means of a nasal catheter

The purpose is to administer a therapeutic concentration of oxygen into the oropharynx.

SUGGESTED ACTION	RATIONALE
Observe precautions to prevent fire, such as checking electrical appliances and posting "No Smoking" signs.	Oxygen supports combustion.
Attach the humidifier bottle to the regulator or flowmeter.	Oxygen forced through a water reservoir is humidified before it is delivered to the patient, preventing dehydration of the mucous membrane.
Attach a nasal catheter, No. 8 to No. 10 Fr., to the connecting tube on the water reservoir.	Using a small catheter minimizes discomfort for the patient.
Measure the catheter by holding it in a horizontal line from the tip of the nose to the earlobe. Mark it with a narrow strip of tape.	The distance from the tip of the nose to the earlobe usually places the tip of the catheter in the oropharynx when inserted.
Moisten the catheter with a water-soluble lubricant making certain that the openings are not obstructed.	Friction irritates the mucous membrane. The lubricant reduces friction. Obstructed catheter openings can impede the oxygen flow.
Start the oxygen flow at a rate of 2 to 3 liters per minute.	Some supplemental oxygen will compensate for partial obstruction of the airway caused by the catheter insertion technique. Too high a flow rate will irritate the mucosa as the catheter is being inserted.
Hold the tip of the patient's nose up and insert the tip of the nasal catheter into the nares downward. Move the catheter along the floor of the nose until the marking on the catheter is reached.	Direct connection from the nares to the oropharynx is made most easily by passing the catheter beneath the concha inferior.
Check the position of the tip of the catheter by depressing the tongue carefully with a tongue blade.	If the catheter has been inserted too far, it may stimulate the gag reflex.
Adjust the catheter as necessary so that the tip is visible opposite the uvula.	The oxygen stream can be inspired easily at this point.
Adjust the oxygen flow to the rate specified.	Excessively high rates of oxygen flow produce a forceful stream against the mucous membrane which is irritating and drying.
Secure the catheter with tape to the side of the patient's face.	The weight of the catheter and the moist surface of the mucous membrane will cause the catheter to slip out if not anchored.
Instruct patient to breathe through his nose.	Mouth breathing can result in oxygen loss.
Provide mouth and nostril care every two to three hours.	The continuing presence of the catheter and oxygen flow is irritating and drying to the mucous membrane. Mouth and nostril care helps to relieve the discomfort.
Insert a clean catheter in alternate nostrils as often as necessary and at least every eight hours.	The mucous membrane is irritated by continued presence of a foreign object. Prolonged irritation of the mucous membrane can cause ulceration.

The administration of oxygen by means of a face mask.

The purpose is to administer a therapeutic concentration of oxygen to the nose or nose and mouth.

SUGGESTED ACTION	RATIONALE
Observe precautions to prevent fire.	Oxygen supports combustion.
If used, attach a water humidifier bottle to the oxygen regulator or flowmeter.	Forcing oxygen through a water humidifier before it is delivered to the patient prevents dehydration of the mucous membrane. Due to their construction, a humidifier bottle is not used with some types of masks. For some patients, the water vapor in their exhalations may provide sufficient humidification.
Attach the face mask to the oxygen source or water reservoir. Start the flow of oxygen at approximately 10 to 12 liters per minute or at the specified rate if a concentration mask is used.	Having the oxygen flowing will provide supplemental oxygen for the patient immediately. This action tends to reduce his fear of suffocation.
Position the face mask over the patient's nose or nose and mouth. Adjust it to fit snugly on his face.	A loose- or poorly fitting mask will result in oxygen loss and decreased therapeutic value.
Adjust the liter flow to the rate specified. Check the concentration with an oxygen analyzer and readjust as necessary.	The proper concentration of oxygen is necessary for optimum therapeutic results.
Instruct the patient to breathe through his nose if a nasal mask is being used.	Mouth breathing can result in oxygen loss.
Remove and clean the face and mask every two to three hours if the oxygen is running continuously.	The tight-fitting mask and moisture from exhalations can cause irritation of the skin of the face.

The use of an oxygen tent

The purpose is to manage an oxygen tent so that the patient receives therapeutic oxygen, humidity, and temperature.

SUGGESTED ACTION	RATIONALE
Check or remove electrical appliances from the immediate area, including the electric signal cord.	Electric appliances may produce sparks and oxygen supports combustion.
Bring the tent unit to the bedside, plug in the motor, and start the unit. Turn on the oxygen flow. Check the oxygen flow inlet in the tent and exhaust outlet. Set the temperature control.	Testing the mechanical aspects of the tent reduces the possibility of causing further respiratory distress for the patient in the event of mechanical defect.
Close all openings of the hood. Seal the bottom opening of the hood by bringing the sides together and folding over several times, or by tying, so that the upper half of the hood is flooded with oxygen at 15 liters per minute.	For immediate benefit for the patient, the air in the tent should contain an oxygen content of at least 30 to 40 percent. Oxygen is heavier than air; therefore, flood the area which is to be over the patient's head.
Flood the tent for two to five minutes while the hood is closed.	A therapeutic concentration usually is established in this length of time.
Move the unit directly into position near the bed before opening the hood.	Having the unit in place prevents oxygen loss when the hood is placed over the patient.
Open the bottom of the hood and place the hood over the patient. Leaving some slack, tuck the part at the head of the bed well under the mattress as far as it will go.	The hood must be long enough to allow the head of the bed to be lowered if desired.
Tuck the sides of the hood well under the mattress as far as they will go.	A tightly closed hood prevents oxygen seepage.
Enclose the part of the hood which goes over the patient's thighs in a piece of linen and arrange so that open spaces between the hood and the bedding are closed. Tuck the ends under the mattress to hold them securely.	Oxygen, being heavier than air, will escape through open areas at the edge of the hood. Linen facilitates sealing the openings and also keeps the edge of the hood in place.
Test inside the tent for drafts by placing the hand in various locations near the patient's head. Protect the patient's head with a hood or other suitable covering as necessary.	Forced entrance of the oxygen and provision for withdrawal of air in the tent produce air motion in the tent.
Check the oxygen gauge and reduce flow to prescribed rate per minute. Check the concentration with oxygen analyzer at least every three to four hours. Regulate as necessary.	The rate of oxygen should be determined by the patient's need. Since oxygen loss is prevalent, frequent regulation of the flow is necessary to maintain a therapeutic amount.
Check the temperature indicator frequently until the temperature in the tent is stabilized. Adjust to the temperature most comfortable for the patient.	A comfortable environmental temperature varies with the patient and his state of health.
Empty the drainage near the base of the motor unit as often as recommended, usually once every 24 hours.	Moisture in the air which has been withdrawn from the tent condenses. There is also some condensation from the refrigeration unit.

Several methods of increasing inhaled moisture have been discussed. Increased moisture is also provided to some patients by various ventilation devices which are discussed later. Commercial face tents are also available for this purpose.

Drugs are available to help in the liquification of respiratory secretions so that they can be removed more readily. However, some authorities are now recommending that water or saline achieve the purpose as well as medications and do not have the undesirable side effects that most drugs do.

Increased humidification of the air breathed by patients with viscid respiratory secretions is essential. The nurse should be alert so that she may arrange for adequate moisture for these patients.

Postural Drainage and Cupping

Postural drainage is the utilization of gravity to drain secretions from the lungs. The person is positioned in a way that promotes the drainage of small pulmonary branches into larger ones where they can be removed by coughing.

A high Fowler's position will promote drainage of the upper lobes of the lungs. Changing positions from the lateral recumbent to supine to opposite lateral recumbent position will encourage middle lobe drainage. The lower lobes can be drained most effectively with the person in the *Trendelenburg position,* a position in which the head and chest are lower than the hips and legs. In the Trendelenburg position, the abdominal contents tend to push the diaphragm upward and promote drainage. For the patient who can tolerate it, an effective way to assume the Trendelenburg's position is to lie with the hips and legs horizontally across the bed. The head and chest hang over the edge of the bed. The person supports himself with his head resting on his folded arms on a pillow placed on the floor or on a chair if the bed is too high. For patients who cannot assume this position, pillows positioned to make the hips higher than the head and chest are often helpful in draining the lower lobes. Figures 21–9 and 21–10 show the Trendelenburg's and modified Trendelenburg's positions.

Postural drainage positioning is usually scheduled two to four times daily for periods of 20 to 30 minutes, depending on the patient's condition. Some persons with cardiac and vascular pathology, traction, some recent surgical procedures, extreme pain, and mechanical ventilators may not be able to assume postural drainage positions.

Pulmonary cupping is performed in conjunction with postural drainage for some persons. *Cupping* is manual percussion of lung areas to loosen pulmonary secretions. Cupping is performed with the hand held in rigid dome-shaped position, as shown in Figure 21–11. The cupped hand is used to strike over the lobe to be drained. A hollow sound is produced. The vibration of the percussion loosens the secretions from the bronchi. Cupping is not done on bare skin, nor should it be painful for the patient. The areas below the ribs or over the spine or breasts should not be cupped because soft tissue damage could result. The patient can learn to cup

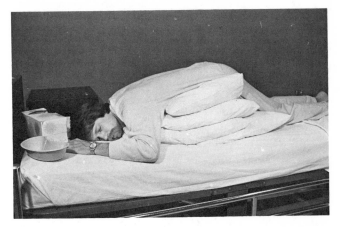

Figure 21–10 The modified Trendelenburg's position for postural drainage is demonstrated in this photo. The patient's hips are positioned to be higher than his chest and head to permit gravity drainage of the lower lobes of his lungs.

anterior surfaces himself. Family members are often taught to cup posterior surfaces.

When cupping is used, it generally precedes postural drainage of the cupped lobe. Cupping is generally performed for 30 to 60 seconds over an area.

Postural drainage and cupping are generally followed by deep breathing and coughing to expectorate the drainage and loosen secretions. If a patient doing postural drainage and cupping is receiving supplemental oxygen, it should not be discontinued during these procedures. The efforts to remove bronchial secretions are strenuous in themselves and a patient with hypoxia will generally need the additional oxygen supply.

Tracheal Suctioning

Some persons with excessive respiratory tract secretions are not able to raise and expectorate them. For these

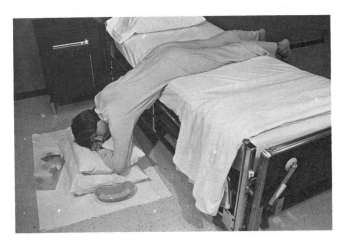

Figure 21–9 This patient has been assisted into the Trendelenburg's position to facilitate postural drainage of the lower lobes of his lungs.

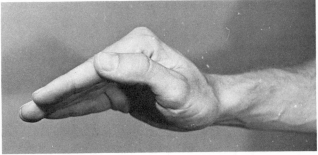

Figure 21–11 This photo illustrates the dome-shaped positioning of the hand for cupping or percussion of the chest wall to loosen pulmonary secretions.

persons, mechanical suctioning is often used. The negative pressure used for suctioning can be piped in and made available from a wall unit, as illustrated in Figure 21–12, or provided with a portable suction machine.

A sterile plastic or rubber catheter is used for respiratory suctioning. A size 14 to 18 Fr. catheter is generally appropriate for adults. The nurse should wash her hands carefully and put on a sterile glove before handling the catheter. The respiratory tract is not normally sterile but suctioning can introduce pathogens not normally present.

One outlet of a Y-connector is used for attaching the catheter to the tubing which joins the negative pressure source. The other outlet of the Y-connector allows the nurse to control the suction by closing it off with her thumb.

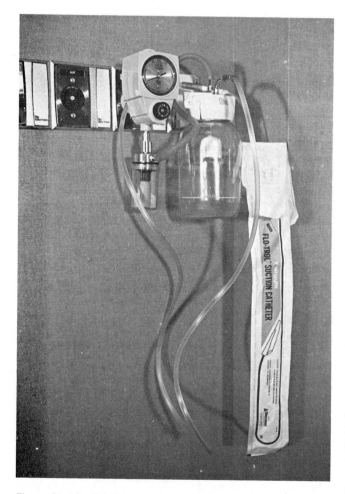

Figure 21–12   Piped-in negative pressure is available for performing tracheal suctioning. The pressure regulator, receptacle, and suction catheter are in readiness.

After moistening the catheter with sterile water, it is gently introduced into a nostril or the mouth through the pharynx and into the trachea. Entry into the trachea will usually initiate coughing which may help to raise secretions from the lungs. After the catheter is in place, the open outlet of the Y-connector is obstructed and the suction is initiated. Suctioning while the catheter is being inserted can cause trauma to the mucous membrane. The catheter is rotated as it is slowly withdrawn. Suctioning should not exceed 10 to 15 seconds because oxygen is being removed along with the secretions by the negative pressure. If necessary, the suctioning can be repeated after a two-to-three-minute rest period for the patient. The nurse should note and record secretions obtained and the patient's reaction to the suctioning. The technique for suctioning is given in the chart on page 521. Frequent oral hygiene is recommended for patients with excessive respiratory tract secretions.

IMPROVING THE RESPIRATORY AIRWAY

Tracheotomy

A *tracheotomy* or *tracheostomy* is an incision into the trachea for insertion of a tube to facilitate breathing. A tracheotomy is usually done to provide an airway which bypasses an obstruction in the upper respiratory tract. It may also be done to provide mechanical ventilation for supplying supplemental oxygen or other gases or to facilitate the removal of excessive or tenacious respiratory secretions. Care of the tracheotomy is a nursing responsibility. A person who has a permanent tracheotomy usually learns to care for it by himself.

The tracheotomized patient is unable to speak, except in a hoarse whisper. Therefore, his care should include consideration of his impaired ability to communicate. The patient is also frequently fearful and anxious, at least initially. He needs the reassurance and support of explanations and anticipation of his needs and concerns. Being unable to speak and having difficulty breathing are very frightening conditions. The nurse should make a conscious effort to decrease the individual's anxiety as she goes about activities related to the care of a tracheotomy.

A curved tube approximately 5 to 7.5 cm. or 2 to 3 inches in length is inserted into the tracheotomy opening. The tube may be made of metal or plastic. Some tracheotomy tubes have two cannulas. The outer can-

Nasotracheal or orotracheal suctioning

The purpose is to remove excess secretions from the trachea, pharynx, mouth, and/or nose.

SUGGESTED ACTION	RATIONALE
Prepare supplies: the suction device with Y-connector and sterile catheter, glove(s), and water.	Sterilization can be maintained more easily if the supplies are arranged in advance.
Attach the catheter to the Y-connector by touching only the end connecting to the adapter outlet. Turn on the suction. Put on sterile glove(s).	Touching the suctioning end of catheter with the hands would contaminate it. Suction should be ready to minimize the time loss. Sterile glove(s) makes it possible to handle the catheter without contamination.
Handling the catheter with the gloved hand, moisten it with sterile water. Gently insert the catheter, without suction, through the nostril or mouth, until vigorous coughing is induced.	Keeping the catheter sterile minimizes the introduction of pathogens. Water helps to lubricate the catheter and reduce friction. Suction upon insertion can cause trauma to the mucous membrane. Vigorous coughing is generally induced when the trachea is stimulated. The coughing helps to raise secretions.
Cover the open outlet of the Y-connector and rotate the catheter gently as it is gradually removed.	Covering the open outlet of the Y-connector will cause negative pressure and suction in the catheter. Rotation of the catheter allows for removal of secretions on all sides of the upper respiratory tract. Gentle handling of the catheter reduces trauma to the mucosa. Suctioning for more than 10 to 15 seconds can induce significant hypoxia.
If it is necessary to repeat suctioning, wait two to three minutes.	Breathing during the rest period helps to compensate for the induced hypoxia.

nula remains in place in the trachea while the inner cannula is removed for cleaning, as illustrated in Figure 21–13, and for suctioning secretions.

Many tracheotomy tubes used today have inflatable cuffs on the lower part of the tube. The distended cuff seals the opening around the tube against air leakage and the entrance of foreign bodies. Care should be taken to avoid overinflation of the cuff and to schedule routine cuff deflation to avoid tracheal edema or ne-

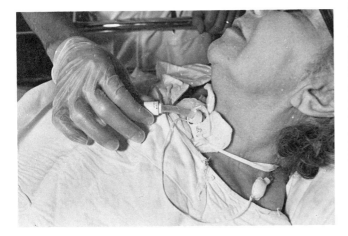

Figure 21–13 The nurse is removing the inner cannula of the patient's tracheotomy tube. Note the small tube and balloon with adapter lying against the patient's neck. The adapter is used for inflating and deflating the tracheotomy cuff. The balloon indicates the degree of cuff inflation.

crosis of the mucous membrane. In some instances, the cuff may be deflated as often as every hour. Cuffs that mechanically deflate and inflate regularly are available which relieves the nurse of this responsibility. However, the nurse remains responsible for checking to note whether the equipment is functioning properly. There are also low-pressure cuffs that exert minimum pressure on the tracheal mucosa. This type does not ordinarily require periodic deflation.

Since the tracheotomy tube serves as the patient's airway, care must be taken to prevent the inspiration of foreign material into the unprotected tracheotomy tube. For this reason, cotton balls, loose threads from gauze, or other small foreign bodies must be kept away from the tracheotomy opening. Because the nasal passages are being bypassed, the normal humidification process must be artificially provided for the patient with a tracheotomy. This may be accomplished by placing a moist gauze pad over the tracheotomy opening, keeping a humidifier at the bedside, or attaching a humidifier device.

Suctioning is used to remove secretions from the tracheotomy tube. The frequency of the suctioning varies with the amount of secretions present, but it should be sufficiently frequent to keep the patient's breathing as effortless and comfortable as possible.

Tracheotomy suctioning is carried out with sterile technique. The nurse wears a sterile glove and uses a fresh sterile catheter for each suctioning. Studies have demonstrated that tracheal suctioning in health agencies when only clean technique was used was a common cause of pulmonary infections. Careful handwashing before handling the tracheotomy is also recommended. The suctioning catheter should be approximately one-half the size of the tracheotomy tube. For adults, a size 10 to 12 Fr. is usually satisfactory. A size 8 to 10 Fr. catheter is generally used for children. It may be difficult to remove tenacious secretions if the catheter is too small while a catheter which is too large may obstruct too much of the tracheotomy tube and further impede the patient's breathing. A Y-connector is used to connect the catheter to the negative pressure source, as was described earlier in relation to nasotracheal suctioning. Figure 21-14 illustrates a nurse ready to suction a tracheotomy.

The inner cannula is removed before suctioning the double-cannula tracheotomy tube. Before suctioning the cuffed tracheotomy tube, the cuff is slowly deflated to allow the secretions to be forced upward by the positive pressure.

It is recommended that some patient's lungs be hyperinflated and hyperoxygenated before suctoning because of the hypoxia caused by the suctioning procedure. The negative pressure of suction removes oxygen as well as secretions from the airway. Some patients, especially those with cardiac disabilities, cannot tolerate even this temporary hypoxia. A breathing bag or increased oxygen flow can be used for hyperinflation and hyperoxygenation.

If the secretions are tenacious or copious, 5 to 10 ml.

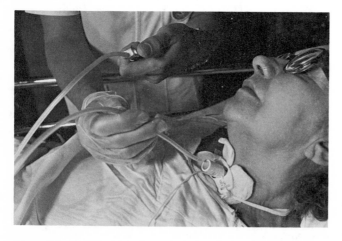

Figure 21-14 The nurse is ready for suctioning the tracheotomy. He uses his sterile gloved hand to handle the end of the sterile catheter. His thumb is ready to obstruct the negative pressure outlet to initiate the suction when he has the catheter in place.

of sterile normal saline solution may be instilled directly into the tracheotomy opening immediately before suctioning. The saline helps to decrease the viscosity of the secretions. The catheter is lubricated with sterile water and inserted without suction. The depth for inserting the catheter depends on the condition of the patient. In some instances, the catheter is inserted into each bronchus. Having the patient turn his head as far as possible to the left will facilitate entering the right bronchus and turning to the right will make entrance into the left bronchus easier.

When the desired depth is reached, suction is applied by putting the thumb over the Y-connector outlet as the catheter is rotated and slowly withdrawn. It is recommended that the suctioning take a maximum of ten seconds because of the effect of the hypoxia. If repeated suctioning is necessary, there should be an interval of two to three minutes and the hyperinflation and hyperoxygenation are repeated until they are no longer necessary.

The inner cannula is cleaned with a sterile solution, generally hydrogen peroxide. Its oxidizing action releases secretions adhering to the cannula. A lint-free brush or pipe cleaner may also be used to assist with the cleaning. The tube is rinsed in sterile water before inserting it and then it is secured in place. The technique for suctioning a tracheotomy is described in the chart on page 523.

The nature and amount of the secretions obtained by suctioning and the character of the patient's respirations should be noted and recorded by the nurse. If the patient is alert, his reaction to the tracheotomy should also be recorded periodically.

Oxygen can be administered directly into the tracheotomy tube via a special oxygen adaptor, as Figure 21-15 on page 524 illustrates. The general practices described in the section on oxygen therapy in this chapter apply to the tracheotomized patient also. Further discussion of these practices will be found in the references at the end of this unit.

Endotracheal Tube

An *endotracheal tube* is an artificial airway inserted through the nose or mouth into the trachea to facilitate breathing. It is generally inserted by a physician or a clinical nurse specialist. However, the nurse caring for the patient is responsible for the tube while it is in place. Endotracheal tubes are used most frequently when tracheal edema or obstruction of the airway from the tongue exists or is anticipated. They are often used to administer oxygen and other gases, especially

The suctioning of a tracheotomy

The purpose is to remove excess secretions from the tracheotomy tube or tracheotomy tube and bronchi.

SUGGESTED ACTION	RATIONALE
Have the sterile supplies in readiness: suction catheter, glove(s), saline and water, and a suction device with tubing and Y-connector. Sterile cleaning solution for the inner cannula may also be necessary.	Sterilization can be maintained more easily if supplies and equipment are arranged in advance.
Hyperoxygenate and hyperinflate the patient's lungs if his condition deems it necessary.	Preliminary hyperoxygenation and hyperinflation of the lungs decrease the effect of the induced hypoxia.
Attach the catheter to the Y-connector, touching only the end connected to the Y-connector outlet. Turn on the suction. Put on sterile glove(s).	Touching of suctioning end of the catheter without sterile glove(s) would contaminate it. Suction should be ready to minimize the time loss after the catheter is inserted.
When the cuffed tracheotomy tube is present, suction the nasal and/or oral pharyngeal area. Change sterile gloves and the catheter.	Removal of pharyngeal secretions prevents them from being aspirated when the cuff is deflated. Separate sterile gloves, catheters, and solution prevent the introduction of mouth, nose and pharyngeal organisms into the lungs.
Remove the inner cannula, if present, and place it in the cleaning solution. Slowly deflate the tracheotomy cuff, if present.	Soaking the inner cannula while suctioning will make cleaning easier. Slow deflation of the cuff will allow secretions to be forced upward.
Instill the sterile saline into tracheostomy opening. Handling the catheter with the gloved hand, moisten it with sterile water.	Saline helps to liquify secretions. Water helps to lubricate the catheter and facilitate its insertion.
Insert the catheter, without suction, into the tube for the specified distance. Ask the patient to turn his head to the side and elevate the chin if entering the bronchus.	Suction upon insertion of the catheter can damage the respiratory mucosa. Turning the head can facilitate entering of the opposite bronchus.
With the thumb over the open outlet of the Y-connector, rotate the catheter quickly and gently as it is removed.	Covering the open outlet of the Y-connector will cause negative pressure and suction in the catheter. Rotation of the catheter allows for removal of secretions on all sides of the tube and/or bronchus. Gentleness in handling the catheter reduces trauma to the mucosa. Significant hypoxia can result if suction is applied for longer than ten seconds.
If it is necessary to repeat suctioning, wait an interval of two to three minutes. Repeat hyperinflation and hyperoxygenation as appropriate. Have the patient turn his head in the opposite direction and repeat the technique.	Breathing during the interval helps to compensate for the induced hypoxia, as do hyperinflation and hyperoxygenation. The opposite bronchus can be entered more easily with the head turned.
Clean secretions from the inner cannula if used, rinse in sterile water, shake excess water from the cannula, reinsert and secure it in place.	Secretions can obstruct the tracheotomy airway. Cleaning solutions or excess water irritates the respiratory tract. If not secured in place, the inner cannula can be displaced by a cough.
Slowly reinflate the tracheotomy tube cuff if one is used, until audible leakage is faint or can no longer be heard. Usually 7 to 10 ml. of air is sufficient for the average-sized adult.	Too great cuff pressure can cause tracheal edema and necrosis. Too little pressure allows oxygen loss.

during surgical procedures. The endotracheal tube does not facilitate the removal of excessive or tenacious secretions as easily as does the tracheotomy tube. However, suctioning can be done in the same general manner.

The cuffed endotracheal tube is commonly used to prevent air leakage and bronchial aspiration of foreign bodies. The nurse must take precautions against excessive and prolonged inflation of the cuff to avoid tracheal edema and necrosis, as with the cuffed tracheotomy tube. Periodic deflation of the cuff should be scheduled in consultation with the physician and included in the nursing care plan.

Nasal Decongestants and Bronchodilators

Nasal decongestants and bronchodilators are two types of drugs which are commonly used to help improve the airway. Nasal decongestants act primarily by constricting the arterioles of the nasal mucosa. This reduces the blood flow to the area. The relief of congested vessels results in an increase in the diameter of the nasal passageway and a less obstructed airway. Many persons with common colds and allergic conditions find nasal decongestants helpful.

Sympathomimetic agents, those which mimic actions of

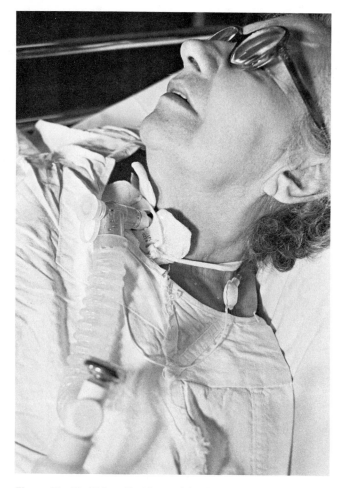

Figure 21–15 This patient is receiving humidified oxygen directly to her tracheotomy through the large plastic tubing.

the sympathetic nervous system, are often used in nasal decongestants. Phenyliphrine and phenylpropanolamine are common sympathomimetic agents. Many products usually available in drug stores contain these substances, along with other ingredients. They are available in capsules, tablets, nasal sprays, and nose drops. The primary advantage of the oral preparations is that they have a longer-lasting action. However, because they achieve their effect through systemic circulation, they also exert their influence elsewhere in the body. For some persons, the systemic effect can aggravate other health problems. Hence, it is recommended that persons who have hypertension, diabetes mellitus, and some types of heart and thyroid diseases avoid taking oral nasal decongestants unless a physician has been consulted.

The nasal sprays and drops have a rapid, but gener-

ally short action. When used as recommended for three to four days, their effect is generally satisfactory. However, if used for a long time, a *rebound effect,* that is, pronounced opposite results to those intended, often occurs. The local constriction of the blood vessels produced by the drugs is followed by secondary congestion of the vessels. The rebound effect is thought to result from the body's compensation for the decreased oxygen supplied to the tissues because of the vasoconstriction. The rebound effect can lead to a vicious cycle because it leads to more frequent use of the substance which caused it. Therefore, a person using nasal decongestant sprays or drops should follow the directions carefully.

Bronchodilators promote relaxation of the smooth muscle of the tracheobronchial tree and, thus, increase the lumen of the bronchioles and aveolar ducts. Some authorities also believe bronchodilators act to relieve spasms of the bronchi which in turn, increases their size. The relaxed bronchi provide less resistance to air flow and provide an enlarged respiratory passageway. Persons with various chronic lung diseases, such as emphysema and asthma, and who have infections, such as pneumonia, usually find relief with bronchodilators.

Sympathomimetic agents, such as epinephrine, ephedrine, and theophylline, are among the most common ingredients in bronchodilators. Some of these substances which can be administered orally and by inhalation, are available without a prescription. They also are available by prescription for rectal and injection administration. All forms of ephedrine, epinephrine, and theophylline have some undesirable side effects and should be used with care and according to directions.

Inhalation bronchodilators are administered in a mistlike spray. The liquid drug is divided into minute particles and carried into the lung on a stream of air or gas. Devices called *atomizers* and *nebulizers* are used to break the drug into fine particles. Generally, an atomizer produces larger particles than does a nebulizer. The smallest particles are produced by high-frequency sound waves; this is called *ultrasonic nebulization.* Suspending the droplets in a gas is called *aerosolization.* The finer the particles, the farther they will travel into the respiratory tract. The mist is generally inhaled through the mouth.

There are several ways in which a spray may be produced. The hand atomizer or nebulizer uses a bulb attachment which, when compressed, forces air through the container holding the drug in the solution. The increased pressure in the unit forces solution into a specially constructed strictured device. The force with which the solution is made to move through this stricture and to leave the container is sufficient to break the large droplets of fluid into a fine mist.

Bronchodilators and other inhalation drugs are available in commercially prepared aerosol containers. These are helpful for home use since no external source of pressure is necessary.

Nebulization can also be accomplished by using the force of an oxygen stream or compressed air to be passed through the fluid in a nebulizer or an atomizer. This method is valuable for patients who require inhalations of a special drug several times a day. The hand atomizer or nebulizer could prove to be quite fatiguing. The oxygen stream is also useful in the production of vapors when high humidity is needed continuously for long periods of time. One of the most common means of administering oxygen and the nebulized drug is the intermittent positive pressure breathing machine, which is discussed later in this chapter.

Ephedrine is available for oral administration and generally has a slower and more prolonged action than epinephrine and theophylline. Therefore, it is commonly used in milder forms of pulmonary obstruction. However, it does produce side effects of nervousness, excitability, and insomnia.

Epinephrine is only effective when administred by injection or inhalation. Most over-the-counter inhalation products which produce bronchodilation contain epinephrine. They act quickly, usually in five to ten minutes, but the duration of the effect is short, about 30 to 40 minutes. They produce side effects similar to ephedrine.

Theophylline is a potent bronchodilator. It is available for administration by mouth, rectum, or injection. Side effects of nausea, vomiting, and gastric irritation are common with all routes.

Ephedrine, epinephrine, and theophylline have systemic vascular effects. Because they are available in products without prescription, persons using them should be instructed to follow the directions. Persons with cardiac diseases, diabetes mellitus, and hypertension should be cautioned to avoid their use without a physician's advice.

As indicated, some nasal decongestants and bronchodilators are readily available. Because their misuse can have unpleasant and serious results, the nurse is encouraged to become familiar with these products and to use opportunities which arise for health teaching. Often, persons using these substances do so on their own initiative and the nurse becomes aware of it only accidentally.

Even though precautions are included with the products, many persons do not heed them unless their importance is emphasized.

Removal of Foreign Bodies

Obstruction of the respiratory airway can result from the presence of a foreign body. The removal of the foreign substance is essential to improving the airway. A recommended technique for removal is the Heimlich maneuver which will be discussed in Chapter 25.

ASSISTING VENTILATION

Various methods and devices are used to assist with ventilation. Some are supplementary to the patient's own pulmonary activities; others are substituted when the patient is unable to ventilate himself. Breathing exercises, intermittent positive pressure breathing, and the use of the Ambu bag are discussed here. Many commercial machines are available. The more complex ones are used in the care of critically ill patients and are discussed in clinical texts.

Breathing Exercises

Exercises to improve the quality of breathing are often taught by physical or respiratory therapists or by nurses who are clinical specialists. However, all nurses should understand the general purpose and technique of breathing exercises so that they can provide support for the patient as necessary.

The purpose of breathing exercises is to develop improved diaphragm control, use of abdominal muscles, and efficiency of expiration. While specific breathing programs are designed according to the needs of the patient, most programs include certain components. Initially the patient usually assumes the sitting position, although other positions may be assumed as he progresses. The patient is encouraged to inhale slowly through his nose while relaxing the abdominal muscles. As he exhales, he is encouraged to become aware of the distention of the abdomen. Exhalation should be through the mouth with the lips partially closed. The goal is for the exhalation to be two to three times longer than the inspiration. As he exhales, the patient should feel the abdominal muscles gradually tighten. The number of times the breathing exercises are done and their frequency depends on the condition of the patient.

Intermittent Positive Pressure Breathing

Intermittent positive pressure breathing, abbreviated IPPB, is a mechanical means of providing a specific amount of air; air, oxygen and water; or air, oxygen, and/or medication under increased pressure to the respiratory tract. The device forces deeper inspiration by positive pressure inhalation and then permits passive exhalation. The amount of pressure varies according to the patient's needs.

The IPPB apparatus can assist ventilation by being set so that the patient's natural inspiration is the stimulus for the pressure increase. Or, it can control the patient's ventilation by having a preset cycle. Assisted ventilation is used for persons who have respiratory disorders when periods of deeper inhalation would be helpful to further aerate the lungs or to move secretions. Controlled ventilation is used for patients who have no spontaneous respiratory movements, as in brain injuries or respiratory paralysis.

Pressure for the IPPB is supplied by a compressed air or oxygen source. The air or oxygen is forced through a nebulizer containing distilled water or medication and then is directed to the patient. The patient who is having assisted ventilation inhales the mist through a mouthpiece or a face mask. If a mouthpiece is used, the patient seals his lips tightly around the device and breathes only through his mouth. Nose clips can be used if he has difficulty with mouth breathing. If the face mask is used, it should fit tightly to avoid air leaks. Controlled ventilation is usually provided through a tracheotomy tube.

In many instances, the patient controls the rate of the machine by his breathing and the machine turns off automatically when his lungs are filled. In some instances, the rate is controlled by the machine. The patient should be instructed to inhale slowly and deeply and allow his lungs to be filled, then exhale as completely as possible before the next inspiration.

Having the patient in a sitting position for maximum respiratory movement is helpful. Depending on the amount of lung secretions, the IPPB treatment will usually induce productive coughing following its use. The patient should be encouraged to raise and expectorate as much of the secretions as he is able. Figure 21–16 shows a patient using an IPPB machine.

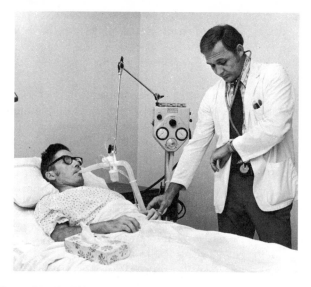

Figure 21–16   This patient is being given an intermittent positive pressure breathing treatment by the inhalation therapist.

The physician or the respiratory therapist determines the amount of positive pressure, medications and dosages, and frequency of treatments. Improper pressure or inappropriate medications can cause pulmonary tissue damage. Most often the treatments are done at least upon rising and before bedtime, but they may be done at more frequent intervals for some patients. Treatments should be avoided immediately preceding or following meals because the productive coughing may depress the appetite or induce vomiting.

Intermittant positive pressure breathing treatments are frequently recommended for persons with acute and chronic respiratory tract diseases. Many persons with long-term illnesses have the equipment to continue their treatment at home. Both manual and automatic equipment is available for home use. Treatments are also used for patients without specific lung pathology, especially following surgery, as a means of promoting respiratory ventilation and preventing complications. Deep breathing, coughing, and postural drainage are often used in conjunction with IPPB.

Adequate cleaning and disinfection or sterilization of the IPPB equipment following use is essential to prevent respiratory tract infections. Various sterilization methods are recommended, but steam under pressure is the preferred method for health agency use. Disinfectants are generally considered to be adequate for home use.

Other Means of Ventilation

For use in emergency situations, most health agencies have self-inflating bag and mask devices. The Ambu bag, as shown in Figure 21–17, is a common example. These devices are used for patients whose respirations have ceased. With the patient's head back, jaw pulled forward, and the airway cleared, the mask is held tightly over the patient's mouth and nose. The bag is compressed with the operator's other hand at a rate which approximates the normal respiratory rate of 16 to 20 breaths per minute in an adult. The respiratory rates of children are more rapid. The one-way valve in the mask allows for exhaled air to escape. The artificial ventilation can be sustained until spontaneous breathing starts, other mechanical assistance is available, or death is confirmed.

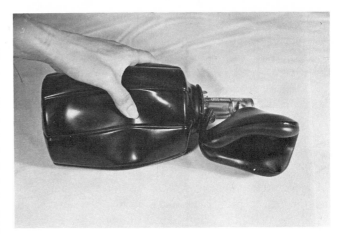

Figure 21–17 This is a self-inflating bag and mask used for assisting ventilation in emergency situations.

Most bag and mask ventilators can accommodate an oxygen tube to increase the oxygen supply to the patient. Many also have adaptors which allow them to be directly connected to a tracheotomy or endotracheal tube for manual ventilation of an intubated patient.

When heart function has ceased along with respirations, cardiopulmonary resuscitation is used. The technique involved will be described in Chapter 25.

Mechanical ventilators are also available for continuously assisting respirations. These devices are most often used with critically ill patients in conjunction with cuffed tracheotomy or endotracheal tubes. Their use is discussed in clinical texts.

PROMOTING RESPIRATORY FUNCTIONING AND THE NURSING PROCESS

Patient's problems with respiratory functioning can range from uncomfortable but minor congested nasal passageways to the inability to breathe independently. As with other health problems, precise data about the patient which should be collected vary with the circumstances. Answers to the following questions may help to provide information that can be useful in giving nursing care. What are the characteristics of the patient's respirations, coughing, breath sounds, mucous membrane of the respiratory tract, secretions, and skin color? Does he smoke? Does he have respiratory allergies, a chronic lung disease, or other pulmonary pathology? Does the patient indicate he has difficulty

with respiratory functioning? Are the results of diagnostic examinations of the respiratory tract available? Are diagnostic tests planned? Does he use supplemental oxygen? Does he use drugs, mechanical devices, positioning, or exercises to assist respiratory functioning? Does he have a knowledge of normal respiratory functioning? If he is receiving therapy related to pulmonary functioning, does he know how it relates to respirations?

Assessment of data requires comparing them with norms. The appropriate norms will depend on the specific data collected. Some norms for comparing respiratory data were included in Chapter 15, as well as in this chapter. Other norms can be found in physiology, pathology, pharmacology, and clinical references.

Planning for meeting the needs of patients with respiratory problems will depend on the characteristics of the specific problem. However, regardless of the nature of the problem, patient participation in the planning is important when the health state of the patient will permit. Since respiratory functioning is essential for life, any condition which influences it in a detrimental way creates some degree of anxiety for the patient. By involving him in planning for improving his respiratory functioning, some of the worry can usually be relieved. Cooperation in the use of therapy is more prevalent when the patient has participated in the planning.

Nursing intervention will include the measures which have been specifically planned for the patient. Many nursing measures for dealing with problems of respiratory functioning have been discussed in this chapter. The following statements will serve as guidelines.

- Explain normal respiratory tract functioning. If the patient and his family have an understanding of the normal process of respiration and the roles various anatomical parts play, understanding therapies is generally easier. An understanding of the purpose of therapy usually produces more satisfactory results.

- Provide reassurance for persons who are having difficulty breathing. The anxiety accompanying dyspnea generally makes respirations even more difficult. Remaining with the patient, being calm, using touch as a means of communication, and talking slowly and quietly are ways of allaying anxiety. Therapeutic measures, such as a noseclip or face mask, may engender fear of suffocation, and, hence, the use of these devices should be explained carefully. The dyspneic patient may need as much attention given to his fear as to the physical cause of his breathing difficulty.

- Provide adequate moisture. Patients who have symptoms of respiratory dysfunction or are receiving most respiratory therapies generally need increased moisture to keep their mucous membrane hydrated and mucus secretions from becoming viscid. An increased fluid intake, unless contraindicated, is usually recommended. Increased humidity of the inhaled air is also helpful in most instances. Regardless of the severity of the dysfunction, increased moisture usually eases the patient's respiratory efforts.

- Teach patients about the actions and correct use of drugs. It is generally recommended that patients and family members learn about the actions and side effects of all drugs they take. Many drugs which affect the respiratory system are commonly available without prescription. Patients with chronic respiratory tract diseases often take medications over long periods of time. Misuse of drugs frequently results. The abuse of these drugs can have uncomfortable and serious side effects. The nurse is often in a position to help patients learn to use drugs properly. In this way, she can contribute to the maintenance of the person's health.

- Use positioning to enhance a patient's respiratory processes. For example, a sitting position can increase the efficiency of muscles involved with inspiration and expiration. Various positions help in moving secretions from different parts of the respiratory tract. By using deliberate positioning, the nurse can help to decrease the patient's fatigue and to improve his respirations.

- Provide alternate means of communication for the tracheotomized and severely dyspneic patient. Since these patients are unable to speak or speak only with great difficulty, they need to have other means of communication available to them. A pad and pencil, a preprinted communication board, or a slate which can be erased easily can be useful. Constant access to a call system is vital. In addition, frequent checks by the nursing staff can alleviate some of the anxiety associated with a breathing problem compounded by the inability to speak easily.

The parts of the nursing process and of the process as a whole are evaluated as described in Chapter 4.

CONCLUSION

Adequate respiratory functioning is essential for life. The nurse can assist patients by promoting measures that prevent many respiratory problems as well as those that institute therapeutic measures. Because many persons take breathing for granted, preventive respiratory teaching is an important need for many individuals. Persons who have difficulty breathing are generally anxious and fearful. The nurse can play a major role in helping to alleviate their psychological distress which is often as significant to improved respirations as specific physical means.

SUPPLEMENTAL LIBRARY STUDY

1. An IPPB treatment can be a confusing and frightening experience for an uninformed patient. The authors of the following article stress that ". . . IPPB should be taught not given." They provide an outline for patient teaching.

   Rau, Joseph and Rau, Mary. "To Breathe or be Breathed: Understanding IPPB." *American Journal of Nursing,* 77: 613–617, April 1977.

   After reviewing the suggestions, role play by teaching a friend or family member who is not familiar with IPPB about it. Ask him to offer a critique of your teaching. Even though a respiratory therapist may initiate the treatments, there are many instances when the nurse must be prepared to provide supplementary explanations to the patient.

2. Respiratory tract suctioning is an anxiety-producing experience for the patient as well as for the inexperienced nurse. These authors give some practical tips to make it easier.

   Sandham, Gayle and Reid, Barbara. "Some Q's and A's About Suctioning . . . With an Illustrated Guide to Better techniques." *Nursing 77,* 7:60–65, October 1977.

   After reading this chapter, answer the question in boldface

type on pages 60 and 61. Test yourself before you check the answers provided by the authors.

3. Postural drainage, cupping, deep breathing, and coughing involve specific techniques to achieve maximum benefit. Study the directives and pictures in the article given below.

Moody, Linda E. "Primer for Pulmonary Hygiene." *American Journal of Nursing,* 77:104–106, January 1977.

Ask a friend to practice each technique with you until you are sure you can perform it satisfactorily. Be sure to check that you are achieving the intended purpose of each technique with minimum stress and discomfort for the patient.

4. Some persons are at greater risk for developing respiratory problems than others. The following article focuses on pneumonia.

Taylor, Carol M. "Pneumococcal Pneumonia: Your Patient's Second Threat?" *Nursing 76,* 6:30–38, March 1976.

What persons does the author suggest are especially prone to develop pneumonia? How can you use this information in the data collection and assessment parts of the nursing process?

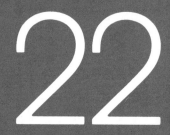

22

BEHAVIORAL OBJECTIVES

When content in this chapter has been mastered, the student will be able to

Define the terms appearing in the glossary.

Describe the stages of a local inflammatory reaction, phases of wound healing, and types of wound healing.

Identify four general principles of tissue healing and provide an example of a nursing measure which applies to each.

List two purposes of cleaning a wound and show how these purposes are achieved by the techniques of preoperative skin preparation and eye, ear, throat, vaginal, and wound irrigations.

Identify four principles involved when dressing a draining wound and indicate how they can be implemented in the wound-dressing technique.

Explain four principles used in the application of bandages and binders.

Summarize the general care of a patient with a cast and include four observations the nurse makes to determine the circulatory and neurological status of the casted area.

List five principles related to the body's reaction to heat and cold and indicate how each of these principles is employed when therapeutic heat and cold applications are used.

Describe the nursing care of a person with tissue damage, using the nursing process as a guide.

Promoting Tissue Healing

GLOSSARY

Abrasion: A wound that results from scraping or rubbing off skin or mucous membrane.

Abscess: A localized collection of pus.

Bandage: A piece of gauze or other material used to cover a wound.

Binder: A type of bandage, usually designed to fit a large body area.

Capillary Action: The process by which a liquid at the point of contact with a solid will rise. Synonym for capillarity.

Capillarity: The process by which a liquid at the point of contact with a solid will rise. Synonym for capillary action.

Closed Fracture: A break in a bone without an open wound. Synonym for simple fracture.

Closed Reduction: The approximation of bone fragments without an open wound.

Closed Wound: An injury in which there is no break in the skin.

Cold: A relative state meaning the absence of heat.

Compound Fracture: A break in a bone involving an open wound. Synonym for open fracture.

Compress: Several layers of moist absorbent cloth or gauze folded to cover a small body area.

Contusion: A bruise.

Debridement: The cleaning away of infected and devitalized tissue from a wound.

Diathermy: High-frequency currents used to produce heat in body tissue.

Dressing: The protective covering placed over a wound.

Fibrinous: Containing large amounts of fibrinogen.

Fracture: A break in the continuity of the bone.

Granulation Tissue: New tissue composed of fibroblasts and small blood vessels.

Heat: The energy of the motion of molecules of a material.

Hemorrhagic: Containing or mixed with blood. Synonym for sanguinous.

Hip Bath: A special type of bath which applies heated water to the pelvic area. Synonym for sitz bath.

Hyperemia: An increased blood supply to an area.

Incision: A wound made with a sharp, cutting instrument.

Insulator: A substance that is a poor conductor.

Laceration: A wound caused by a blunt instrument or object that tears tissue.

Many-Tailed Binder: A type of bandage with multiple tails. Synonym for scultetus binder.

Open Fracture: A break in a bone involving an open wound. Synonym for compound fracture.

Open Reduction: The approximation of bone fragments through a surgical incision.

Open Wound: An injury characterized by a break in the continuity of the skin.

Pack: Moist cloths or dressings applied to a large body area.

Puncture Wound: An injury caused by an object that penetrates the tissue. Synonym for stab wound.

Purulent: Containing pus.

Reduction: The act of restoring to a normal position.

Sanguinous: Containing or mixed with blood. Synonym for hemorrhagic.

Scar: The connective tissue which fills a wound area.

Scultetus Binder: A type of bandage with multiple tails. Synonym for many-tailed binder.

Serous: Resembling blood serum.

Shave Prep: Shaving the hair from an operative area.

Simple Fracture: A break in a bone without an open wound. Synonym for closed fracture.

Sitz Bath: A special type of bath which applies heated water to the pelvic area. Synonym for hip bath.

Stab Wound: An injury caused by an object that penetrates the tissue. Synonym for puncture wound.

Sterile Prep: Shaving and cleaning the skin under surgical aseptic conditions.

Suppuration: The process of pus formation.

Trauma: An injury.

INTRODUCTION

The tissues of the body are remarkably resistive to injury. When tissue injury or damage does occur, the restorative powers of the body are amazing. The healing process is partially the result of the body's response mechanisms to the trauma. The response is systemic; that is, the total body as well as the local area is involved. Although both trauma and the responses to it can be psychic as well as physiological, in this chapter the discussion will be limited to the local physical response to trauma.

The body's response to injury and the healing process are both normal protective mechanisms, and modern science has found no way to improve on them. Nevertheless, there are some actions that can be taken to support or assist these mechanisms. The body's reactions and ways in which the nurse can support the healing processes of soft tissues and bone will be discussed in this chapter.

THE BODY'S REACTION TO TRAUMA

Trauma is a general term meaning an injury. Tissue injury can occur from a variety of causes, such as physical pressure or force, temperature extremes, chemical substances, radiation, and pathogenic organisms. An injury or wound may be open or closed. An *open wound* is characterized by a break in the continuity of the skin. When there is no break in the skin, the wound is said to be a *closed wound.*

Wounds may be either accidental or intentional. An accidental wound is an injury due to a mishap, while an intentional wound is purposely created by the surgeon for therapeutic purposes.

The most common closed accidental wound is a *contusion,* or a bruise. Occasionally open wounds may exist along with contusions. Contusions usually occur as the result of force being applied to the tissue. There may be extensive soft tissue damage with ruptured blood vessels. The escape of blood into the subcutaneous tissue is what gives the characteristic bluish color to the injury. Contusions may occur in readily visible parts of the body, or they may occur internally when other signs indicate their presence. Brain contusions, for example, may follow a head injury with no external evidence of trauma. The same may be true of some abdominal organ injuries.

Open wounds may be classified according to the nature of the break in the continuity of normal tissue. An *incision* is a wound made with a sharp cutting instrument. It is the kind of wound that is made by the surgeon when he cuts tissue to enter the field of operation. Incised wounds also may occur by accident, as when one is cut with a knife, a sharp piece of glass, or a razor.

An *abrasion* is a wound that results from scraping or rubbing off skin or mucous membrane. A "floor or carpet burn" is a typical abrasive wound.

A *puncture* or *stab* wound is caused by an object that penetrates the tissue. Injuries from nails and bullets result in puncture wounds. A surgeon may also make a puncture wound to promote drainage.

A *laceration* is a wound caused by a blunt instrument or object that tears tissue. Falls against angular surfaces or cuts with irregular edges of broken glass frequently result in lacerated wounds.

Any combination of these last three types of wounds may also occur. Falling on broken glass may result in a wound that has lacerations as well as punctures and abrasions.

Fractures are generally the result of physical trauma. A *fracture* is a break in the continuity of the bone. If there is no open wound associated with the break, it is called a *closed* or *simple* fracture. If the fracture involves an open wound, it is called an *open* or *compound fracture.* Fractures are further classified according to the type of alteration in the bone continuity. Figure 22–1 indicates various types of fractures.

Both open and closed wounds of soft tissue or bone can be invaded by pathogens and an infection can result. The entrance of microorganisms into an accidental open wound can easily occur from contamination by the object causing the injury. Pathogens in an intentional wound generally occur as the result of poor aseptic technique. An infection in a closed wound is usually the result of the presence of pathogens in the blood. Tissue damage lowers the body's normal defenses against infection, and, in addition, the escaped blood of a contusion provides a site favorable for the growth of organisms. The body's normal reaction to any kind of wound is inflammation.

Inflammation

Inflammation is the defensive local response of the body to injury. Injury can be a major stressor for the body that also initiates the general adaptation syndrome or a systemic reaction. The patient who sustains

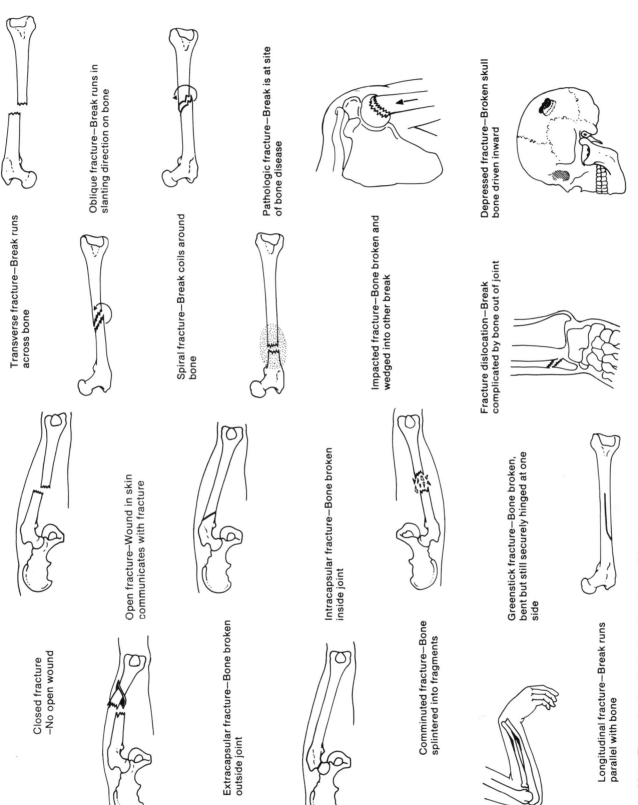

Transverse fracture—Break runs across bone

Oblique fracture—Break runs in slanting direction on bone

Spiral fracture—Break coils around bone

Pathologic fracture—Break is at site of bone disease

Impacted fracture—Bone broken and wedged into other break

Fracture dislocation—Break complicated by bone out of joint

Depressed fracture—Broken skull bone driven inward

Closed fracture —No open wound

Open fracture—Wound in skin communicates with fracture

Extracapsular fracture—Bone broken outside joint

Intracapsular fracture—Bone broken inside joint

Comminuted fracture—Bone splintered into fragments

Greenstick fracture—Bone broken, bent but still securely hinged at one side

Longitudinal fracture—Break runs parallel with bone

Figure 22–1 These sketches illustrate various types of fractures.

a wound or some type of injury often has both a general and a local response. The general and local adaptation syndromes were described by Selye and were discussed in Chapter 10. The following information deals with the immediate tissue area. Inflammation works to limit the tissue damage, remove the injured cells, and repair the traumatized tissue. This local tissue response is an example of the local adaptation syndrome. The inflammatory response is thought to occur in three stages: vascular, exudative, and reparative.

Vascular Stage. The vascular stage of inflammation is characterized by an immediate and brief constriction of the vessels in the area following the trauma. Then the vessels quickly dilate. The increased blood supply to the area is called *hyperemia* and causes the characteristic redness and warmth of the area. The resulting changes due to the filtration pressure of the blood and the increased permeability of the capillaries allow for the movement of plasma, blood cells, and antibodies into the interstitial spaces. The phagocytic process whereby leukocytes engulf the foreign substances and damaged cells is initiated.

Exudative Stage. The exudative stage is characterized by the formation of the fluid exudate. The exudate is made up of the fluid and cells from the blood, the damaged tissue cells, and any foreign bodies. The amount of exudate varies with the extent of the injury. In minor injuries very little exudate will form while in extensive injuries large quantities will collect. In a mild injury, such as a blister, the exudate will be *serous;* that is, it resembles blood serum. When the wound is infected, the exudate is described as *purulent* and is called pus. The process of pus formation is called *suppuration.* An extensive injury can result in an exudate containing large amounts of fibrinogen and is called a *fibrinous* exudate. Or, if erythrocytes are found in the exudate, it is called a *hemorrhagic* or *sanguinous* exudate. The collection of the exudate in the interstitial spaces will cause swelling and localized pain. Depending on the location and extent of the injury, the exudate collection can also cause loss of function of the part.

Reparative Stage. The reparative stage of the inflammatory process is characterized by the replacement of the damaged tissue cells by the regeneration of new cells or by scar tissue. This particular stage is often called wound healing.

Wound Healing

Although authorities differ in their descriptions of wound healing, it is usually said to consist of three phases. Generally, it is difficult to characterize any particular wound because the phases can be occurring simultaneously in various parts of the wound. The three phases are lag, fibroblastic, and contraction.

The lag phase occurs first, when blood, serum, and red blood cells form a fibrin network in the wound. The edges of the wound are glued together by this network, or scab, as it usually is called. If the damaged tissue is then healed by replacement of the tissue cells by similar cells, the healing is said to be by regeneration.

The fibroplasia phase is characterized by the growth of fibroblasts along and in the fibrin network. As this occurs, the fibrin network is gradually absorbed. These fibroblasts and accompanying small blood vessels are called *granulation tissue,* which grows to restore the continuity of the injured tissue. It is very friable, soft, and pinkish red in color. Epithelial cells then commence to grow from the edges to cover the wound. Depending on the extent of the wound, connective tissue cells then fill in the area and become the *scar* which is considerably stronger than the granulation tissue. This is known as replacement healing.

The phase of contraction is characterized by the disappearance of the small blood vessels in the new tissue and by a shrinkage of the scar. This phase may last indefinitely.

The strength of the wound is slight until it has progressed well into the fibroplasia phase. Scar tissue is strong, but it does not have the elasticity of normal tissue; therefore, it is desirable that healing occur with a minimum of scar formation, especially in an area where tension and pressure normally are present.

If a large area has been denuded, for example, when a large area of skin has been removed as a result of either an accident or surgery, it may be difficult or even impossible to approximate the edges of a wound. It has been observed that epithelium from the periphery of a wound continues to grow for only a certain distance and then stops. When the process of repairing a wound halts, a chronic ulcer or unhealed area develops on the denuded surface. This often becomes the site of infection, and tissue debris accumulates. Cleaning of an area of this sort is called *débridement.* It is done primarily to remove necrotic tissue and foreign material and to improve drainage from the wound in order to promote further wound healing. If healing still does not occur following débridement, it may be necessary to close the wound by using skin grafts.

Healing by First Intention.   Healing by first intention is the return of the tissues to normal with minimum inflammation and scarring. This process occurs when no infection is present and when the edges of the wound are well-approximated. Sutures or various adhesive materials may be used to keep the edges of the wound together. Suture materials are either absorbable or nonabsorbable by body tissues. The most common absorbable suture material is catgut. Silk and wire are nonabsorbable suture material. Some surgeons are now using metal staples to approximate the skin edges. Pressure may be used also by the proper application of materials that will secure dressings in place and aid approximation of the wound edges.

Few accidental wounds heal by first intention. Surgeons strive for and usually attain healing of a surgical incision by first intention.

Healing by Second Intention.   Secondary intention healing occurs when infection is present. The process of healing is prolonged. There is usually more extensive tissue injury and a purulent exudate, and approximation of the edges of the wound is dificult or even impossible. Extensive granulation tissue is required to fill the wound.

Healing by Third Intention.   Third intention healing occurs when secondary wound closure is necessary. The extensiveness of the wound or the exudate may necessitate leaving the edges unapproximated for repeated débridement or drainage, or occasionally the approximated wound edges may disrupt. In either case, when the final tissue approximation is delayed or must be repeated, the process is called secondary closure. Following the wound closure, healing then occurs by secondary intention. Figure 22–2 shows types of wound healing.

Fracture Reduction.   *Reduction* is the act of restoring to normal position. Fractures may be reduced by closed reduction or open reduction. *Closed reduction* is the approximation of bone fragments without an open wound. *Open reduction* of a fracture requires a surgical incision. An internal fixation device, such as special pins, screws, or nails, may be used to stabilize the fracture when an open reduction is performed. Exter-

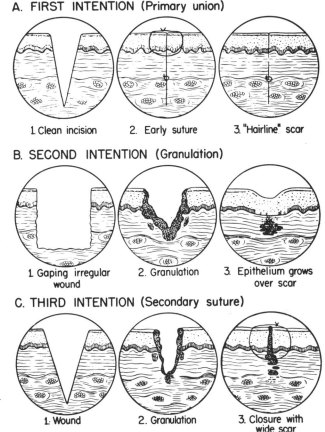

A. FIRST INTENTION (Primary union)

1. Clean incision   2. Early suture   3. "Hairline" scar

B. SECOND INTENTION (Granulation)

1. Gaping irregular wound   2. Granulation   3. Epithelium grows over scar

C. THIRD INTENTION (Secondary suture)

1. Wound   2. Granulation   3. Closure with wide scar

Figure 22–2   Chronologic course of wound healing by first, second, and third intention. In the final stage of second-intention healing it is to be noted that the underside of the epithelium is smooth and not serrated as normally. In the healing by second intention, the important role of contraction, which occurs in the patient in 3 dimensions and in the illustrations in 2 (B-2 and B-3), is shown. Contraction also plays a role in third-intention healing (C-2 and C-3). In C-3 an early phase is shown. Later the granulation tissue will be incorporated as a wide fibrous scar. (Rhoads et al.: Surgery: Principles and Practice, ed. 4, Philadelphia, J. B. Lippincott, 1970.)

nal immobilization may be used to maintain the correct alignment following open or closed reduction. The immobilization is achieved by splints, casts, or traction.

GENERAL PRINCIPLES OF TISSUE HEALING

The healthy body has an innate capacity to protect and restore itself. Increasing the blood supply to the damaged area, walling off and removing cellular and foreign debris, and initiating the cellular development are parts of the healing process. It occurs normally without assistance, although there are some medical and nursing actions that can help to support the process. The body's ability to respond to the tissue trauma is affected by the extent of the damage and the person's general state of health. The healthy individual who sustains a massive injury, the person with a chronic disease, or the very young and very old who experience minimum injury frequently will have some limitations on their capacity to deal adequately with the insult. The promotion of wellness is, of course, partially directed toward maintaining adequate body reserves to deal with traumatic occurrences. The person will respond more adequately to injury if he has fluid and electrolyte balance, proper nourishment, and adequate rest.

The body responds systemically to trauma of its parts. It has been stated earlier that physiological functioning of the body cannot be separated from the psychological. Similarly, local physical responses to an injury cannot be separated from an overall bodily reaction. For example, an injured foot or hand or an abdominal incision can cause a variety of systemic reactions that include an increase in body temperature, heart and respiratory rates, anorexia or nausea and vomiting, skeletal muscle tension throughout the body, and harmful hormonal changes. Because the body's response to injury is systemic, supportive or therapeutic measures should be directed toward the whole person. Adequate rest, relief of emotional tensions, and sufficient nutrients and fluids are particularly important for the person undergoing a response to trauma. Local measures for promoting desirable tissue responses will be discussed later in this chapter.

The blood is the means for transporting substances essential for effective trauma response to and from body cells. An adequate blood supply is fundamental to the body's normal response to any local injury. The blood brings increased erythrocytes, leukocytes, and platelets to the site. Antibodies are also carried by the plasma. The removal of toxins and debris and the supplying of nutrients, oxygen, and other cellular-building materials are provided by increased circulation to the damaged site. Any preexisting condition, such as cardiac or vascular pathology or anemia, or a factor from the injury which results in circulatory impairment, such as extensive blood loss, can inhibit normal response to trauma.

Intact skin and mucous membrane serve as first lines of defense against harmful agents, and a break in the skin continuity increases the likelihood of pathogen entry. Because the person's primary protective barrier is weakened when skin or mucous membrane breaks, the need for artificially preventing microorganism invasion becomes paramount. Careful handwashing before caring for the wound is probably the single most effective method for preventing secondary infection. While it is not possible to sterilize the skin, surgical asepsis is used with persons who have an open wound to minimize the possibility of pathogen entry. Precautions are also taken for persons with closed wounds because of the lowered resistance of the damaged tissue to infection and the possibility of pathogenic organisms being present.

Normal healing occurs when the wound is free of foreign bodies. The reparative stage will generally not start until foreign bodies are removed from the wound. Excessive exudate, dead or damaged tissue cells, pathogenic organisms, or imbedded fragments of bone, metal, glass, or other substances can all act as foreign bodies. The body's own rejection mechanisms generally are sufficient to remove many foreign substances. However, sometimes mechanical means may be employed to assist the process. There are situations in which the body walls off a collection of pus or another foreign body and healing occurs around it. This localized collection of pus is called an *abscess*. Usually it can be expected that the individual will develop symptoms at the unhealed site, although they may be delayed in their appearance.

MEASURES TO PROMOTE TISSUE HEALING

The inflammatory and healing processes normally occur spontaneously. However, measures have been developed that support and facilitate the desirable aspects of these processes.

The presence of pathogens increases the probability of a wound infection. Cleaning the area can help to remove pathogens in and adjacent to the wound. Since healing is also impeded by the presence of foreign bodies in the wound, cleaning can also help remove any debris that may be present.

While exudate formation is normal, the presence of excessive exudate can impede healing by obstructing the wound-healing phases. Techniques which promote the removal of excessive amounts of body fluids, serum, or pus from a wound have been developed to facilitate healing.

Protecting a wound from further injury and from

pathogens also promotes the restorative powers of the body. The major ways of providing protection are coverings, support, and immobilization of the wound area. Dressings, positioning, and physical devices are used for these purposes.

Circulation is important in both inflammation and healing. Temperature changes can affect circulation. Heat and cold applications are used to induce therapeutic circulation changes which are conducive to tissue healing.

CLEANING THE WOUND AREA

It has been stated that infections hinder optimum healing. An attempt is often made to reduce the number of pathogens and remove tissue debris to promote rapid, uncomplicated healing. In the case of an intentional wound, the skin and/or mucous membrane is prepared by reducing the number of pathogens in the area before the break in the tissue is made, such as before a surgical incision. When caring for such a wound, sterile technique and antiseptics are used to avoid the accidental introduction of pathogens. An accidental and open wound is generally cleaned at the earliest opportunity and also cared for while using sterile technique to avoid further pathogen entry. A closed wound is often cleaned with an irrigation to remove debris. Local heat to promote healing may be applied. Occasionally, open wounds may also be irrigated; sterile technique is used.

Preoperative Skin Preparation

Because hair shafts can harbor microorganisms which can enter a wound, the skin is often prepared for a surgical incision by removing the hair in the area. Shaving the hair from an operative area is frequently called a *shave prep*. Because the area adjacent to the actual incision can cause wound contamination, usually a much larger area than the actual size of the incision is prepared. For example, for an abdominal incision, the area from the nipple line to the pubis is usually prepared. The practice of extensive shave preps has decreased in recent years for some areas of the body. The exact areas vary depending on the practice of the health agency and the preference of the surgeon. Many persons do not realize that a human being has hair on all areas of his body except for the palms of the hands and the soles of the feet. Some of the hair may be so fine and light in color that it is difficult to see. The patient

needs an explanation of the purpose of the skin preparation and the reason for its extensiveness to avoid causing him undue anxiety.

The actual skin shaving may be performed by operating room personnel or by the nurse responsible for the care of the patient. The necessary supplies generally are dispensed from a central supply unit. Disposable prep trays are available commercially. While the equipment may vary somewhat, it generally includes a razor and a new blade, basins for soap solution and water, gauze or cotton applicators, and towels for draping the patient and protecting the bed. In addition, good lighting is essential for proper performance of this procedure.

After draping and soaping the area, long gentle strokes of the razor are used. The razor is moved in the direction the hair grows. The nurse may wish to hold the skin taut with one hand to facilitate the razor's movement. Great care must be taken to avoid breaking the patient's skin; this is especially important over bony prominences. Careful inspection of the skin with direct lighting is necessary to assure that the area is free of hair. Following completion of the shaving, the area is rinsed of soap residue and dried.

In some situations, especially preceding orthopedic (bone) surgery, a sterile prep may be done. A *sterile prep* is the technique used to shave and clean the skin under surgical aseptic conditions. Actually, the term is a misnomer because the skin cannot be sterilized. In a sterile prep, the supplies that come in contact with the surgical area are sterile, for example, the soap solution, water, razor, applicators, and drapes. The person carrying out the technique wears sterile gloves. After the area is shaved, it may be cleaned with an antiseptic or soap solution before it is wrapped in sterile towels.

In other situations, skin preparation for surgery may consist of a thorough cleaning of the area with a soap solution or an antiseptic. The shave prep may be omitted.

Irrigations

An irrigation is the cleaning of an area with a flowing solution. The purpose of an irrigation may be to clean the area or to apply local heat or an antiseptic.

Eye, ear, throat, and vaginal tissues are most commonly irrigated. Open wound irrigations are sometimes done to promote debridement.

The type of wound determines the type of solution that is used. Water, saline, and antiseptic solutions are commonly used. Generally, if the wound is closed, nonsterile solutions are used; if the wound is open, a sterile irrigating solution is needed.

Conjunctival Irrigations.

A conjunctival irrigation, frequently called an eye irrigation, usually is done for cleaning purposes to remove secretions from the conjunctival sac. Mild antiseptic solutions may be prescribed if an infection is present.

For cleaning purposes, normal saline usually is prescribed. The solution is administered at body temperature unless specified otherwise. The amount of solution will depend on the situation and may be as little as 30 ml. or as much as 250 ml. or more.

Several methods may be used for irrigating the conjunctival sacs. An eyedropper is satisfactory when small amounts of solution are used. For larger amounts, a soft rubber bulb syringe is appropriate.

In an emergency, an eye irrigation can be done to remove chemicals that may burn the eye. Copious amounts of tap water should be used to remove chemicals. The irrigation should continue for at least 15 minutes and then a physician should be consulted.

Following the irrigation, the patient should be asked to close the lids, and the excess fluid is wiped off gently from the inner canthus to the outer canthus. Any additional solution in the area around the eye is also wiped away gently with a cotton ball.

The technique for a conjunctival irrigation is described in the chart below.

Irrigation of the External Auditory Canal.

Irrigation of the external auditory canal generally is done for cleaning purposes. Usually normal saline is used, although any number of antiseptic solutions may be used for their local action. The amount of solution needed depends on the purpose of the irrigation, but approximately 500 ml. usually is adequate. The solution is prepared so that it is approximately body temperature when it enters the ear. Colder or hotter solutions are uncomfortable for the patient, since the endolymph is set in motion, and dizziness and nausea may result.

Irrigations may be used also for applying heat to the ear. An irrigating container with tubing and an ear tip generally is used. The height of the container should be just enough to have the solution flow gently. The glass or plastic ear tip fits easily into the external canal and has two extensions projecting from it: one for the solution to enter the canal and the other for it to leave the canal and drain into a receiving basin. A soft rubber bulb syringe may be used, but it is not as comfortable for the patient, because the flow of solution must be interrupted during the irrigation while the syringe is refilled.

The technique for an external auditory canal irrigation is described in the chart on page 539.

Administering an irrigation of the eye

The purpose is to clean the lower conjunctival sac.

SUGGESTED ACTION	RATIONALE
Have the patient sit or lie with his head tilted toward the side of the affected eye so that solution will flow from the inner canthus of the affected eye toward the outer canthus.	Gravity will aid the flow of solution away from the unaffected eye.
Clean the lids and the lashes with normal saline or the solution ordered for the irrigation.	Materials lodged on the lids or in the lashes may be washed into the eye.
Place a curved basin at the cheek on the side of the affected eye to receive the irrigating solution.	Gravity will aid the flow of solution.
Expose the lower conjunctival sac.	The conjunctival sac is less sensitive than the cornea.
Direct the flow of the irrigating solution from the inner canthus to the outer canthus along the conjunctival sac.	Solution directed toward the outer canthus helps to prevent the spread of contamination from the eye to the lacrimal sac, the lacrimal duct, and the nose.
Irrigate. Use only sufficient force to remove secretions from the conjunctiva gently.	Directing solutions with force may cause injury to the tissues of the eye, as well as to the conjunctiva.
Avoid touching any part of the eye with the irrigating tip.	The eye is injured easily. Touching the eye is uncomfortable for the patient.
Have the patient close his eye periodically during the procedure.	Movement of the eye when the lids are closed helps to move secretions from the upper conjunctival sac to the lower.
Continue irrigating the lower conjunctival sac until the purpose achieved.	Irrigation of the lower conjunctival sac is more comfortable for the patient.

Administering an irrigation of the external auditory canal

The purpose is to clean the external auditory canal.

SUGGESTED ACTION	RATIONALE
Have the patient sit up or lie with his head tilted toward the side of the affected ear. Have the patient support a basin under his ear to receive the irrigating solution.	Gravity causes the irrigating solution to flow from the ear to the basin.
Clean the pinna and the meatus at the auditory canal as necessary with normal saline or the irrigating solution.	Materials lodged on the pinna and at the meatus may be washed into the ear.
Fill the bulb syringe with solution. If an irrigating container is used, allow air to escape from the tubing.	Air forced into the ear canal is noisy, and therefore unpleasant for the patient.
Straighten the auditory canal by pulling the pinna down and back for an infant and up and back for an adult.	Straightening the ear canal aids in allowing solution to reach all areas of the canal easily.
Direct a steady slow stream of solution against the roof of the auditory canal, using only sufficient force to remove secretions.	Solution directed at the roof of the canal aids in preventing injury to the tympanic membrane.
Do not occlude the auditory canal with the irrigating nozzle.	Continuous in-and-out flow of the irrigating solution helps to prevent pressure in the canal.
At completion of the treatment have the patient lie on the side of the affected ear.	Gravity allows the remaining solution in the canal to escape from the ear.

Throat Irrigations. Throat irrigations are used primarily for loosening and removing secretions in the throat and for applying heat to the area. Mild antiseptics and normal saline are used most frequently. Sodium bicarbonate solution also is effective, especially when the secretions are tenacious.

Usually, the solution is used as hot as the patient can tolerate it, but a temperature above approximately 49° C. (120° F.) is likely to cause tissue damage. If the irrigation is done primarily for applying heat, it is necessary to prepare sufficient solution so that the irrigation will continue for a time. Approximately 1,500 to 2,000 ml. given slowly generally is sufficient. The total amount should not be used if the patient becomes fatigued during the procedure. An irrigating container with a clamp on the tubing and an irrigating nozzle are used. It is convenient to use a pole on which to hang the irrigating container.

It is preferable if the patient assists during a throat irrigation by handling the nozzle himself and directing the flow of solution to various areas of the throat. The nurse should make certain that all areas in the throat are being irrigated. She shows the patient how to discontinue the flow of solution.

The technique for a throat irrigation is presented in the chart below.

Administering a throat irrigation

The purpose is to clean the throat and/or to apply heat.

SUGGESTED ACTION	RATIONALE
Arrange the container of irrigating solution on a pole at the bedside so that the base is only slightly above the level of the patient's mouth.	The gag reflex can be stimulated by a forceful stream of water into the throat. Keeping the level of the solution low minimizes pressure. Gravity will cause the solution to flow as long as the irrigating tip is below the base of the fluid.
Place the patient in a sitting position with his head tilted directly over a basin placed in front of him.	Gravity causes the solution to flow back out into the basin.
Instruct the patient to hold his breath while the solution is flowing.	Breathing while the solution is flowing into and out of the mouth may result in aspirating some of the solution.
Insert the nozzle into the mouth, being careful not to touch the base of the tongue or the uvula. Direct the flow so that all parts of the throat are irrigated.	The gag reflex can be stimulated by touching the uvula or the tongue.
Clamp the tubing to interrupt the irrigation at regular intervals to permit the patient to breathe and rest.	Holding the breath interrupts normal physiological functions of respiration.

Throat Gargles. Gargles are sometimes used for the same purposes as throat irrigations. However, a gargle may be more uncomfortable, since gargling places strain and tension on an area that usually is already swollen, irritated, and painful. Also, a gargle generally is unsatisfactory for reaching all parts of the throat tissues; therefore, an irrigation is often preferred. A gargle generally is satisfactory for cleaning the mouth and the oral pharynx.

Many persons believe that gargling with a strong antiseptic is an almost sure way of preventing sore throats and upper respiratory infections. There is no scientific evidence to support this belief. If done often enough and with full-strength antiseptic solutions, the normal defenses in the mouth and the oropharynx may be destroyed, and more harm than good is done.

Vaginal Irrigations. A vaginal irrigation generally is called a douche. The irrigation is often done simply to clean the area, as mentioned in Chapter 16. It may also be used to apply heat or an antiseptic to the area. The solution of choice is normal saline or tap water when the irrigation is for cleaning or for applying heat. Any number of antiseptic solutions may be used, but for cleaning purposes they are actually not necessary.

Usually, a quantity of about 1,500 ml. of solution is prepared, but smaller or larger amounts may be indicated, depending on the purposes of the irrigation. The vagina tolerates relatively high temperature, but the membranes and the skin around the meatus do not. Therefore, solutions are prepared so that they are introduced at approximately 38° C. (100° F.), or approximately 43° C. (110° F.) if the effect of heat is desired.

An irrigating container connected with tubing to an irrigating nozzle is used. Irrigating nozzles are curved to fit the normal contour of the vagina and may be made of glass or plastic. The nozzle should be handled carefully and examined before use to prevent injury should the nozzle be cracked or chipped.

If a woman is to do vaginal irrigations as a part of a therapeutic regimen to be carried out at home, the nurse may be expected to provide appropriate teaching for this procedure.

As Chapter 16 indicated, a vaginal irrigation may be done at home with the woman lying in a bathtub; the irrigating container is suspended at the proper height on a towel rack or on a chair at the side of the tub. Some women may prefer using a douche pan or a bedpan when carrying out this procedure.

The technique for a vaginal irrigation is described in the chart on page 541.

Open Wound Irrigation. As indicated earlier, open wounds are occasionally irrigated for the cleaning effect of the flowing solution. Generally tissue debris exists and its mechanical removal with solution will hasten healing.

Sterile technique should be used when the skin or mucous membrane is broken because of the danger of introducing pathogens. This is true even in the presence of an existing infection.

The type and amount of solution varies with the tissue involved and the condition of the wound. Sterile saline, water, antiseptic, or occasionally antibiotic solutions are used. Hydrogen peroxide may also be the solution of choice because its oxygen-releasing ability has an effective cleaning effect.

A sterile, large-volume syringe is often used to hold the solution. Care should be taken so that the solution flows directly into the wound and not over a contaminated area before entering the wound. Following the irrigation, a sterile dressing is generally applied to the wound.

The technique for a wound irrigation is presented in the chart on page 541.

PROTECTING THE TRAUMATIZED TISSUE

The tissue of both open and closed wounds is more susceptible to further injury than normal tissue. Prevention of further injury and the promotion of healing are two goals of wound care. Protection from mechanical or microorganism trauma and reduction of strain on the part can assist the physiological healing process. Tissues of most closed and some open wounds are left uncovered and supported or immobilized to promote healing. Open wound tissues are frequently covered as well as supported or immobilized. The protective covering placed over a wound is commonly called a *dressing*. Binders and bandages are usually used to secure dressings and to immobilize and support parts. Casts, splints, braces, and prostheses of various sorts may also be used to immobilize or support body parts. This section of this chapter will discuss the use of dressings, bandages, and binders. Other clinical texts, especially those discussing the care of the orthopedic patient, contain information on such supportive mechanisms as casts, braces, and so on.

The Undressed Wound

Some authorities subscribe to the practice of leaving an open wound undressed if it has sealed itself and can be protected from trauma and irritation. This is true even

Administering a vaginal irrigation

The purpose is to clean the vagina.

SUGGESTED ACTION	RATIONALE
Have the patient void before beginning the treatment.	A full bladder interferes with distention of the vagina by the nozzle and the solution.
Have the patient in the dorsal recumbent position. Remove all but one pillow from under the patient's head and place her on a bedpan if the patient is in bed. A waterproof support may be necessary if a bathtub is used.	Gravity will cause the solution to flow into the distal portion of the vagina.
Arrange the irrigating container at a level just above the patient's hips so that the solution flows easily yet gently.	The greater the distance between the level of the fluid and the outlet in the tubing, the greater will be the force of the solution as it leaves. Undue force could drive solution and contamination into the cervical os.
Clean the vulva by separating the labia and allowing the solution to flow over the area. If this does not seem to be sufficient, wash it with a soap or detergent solution.	Materials lodged around the vaginal meatus can be introduced into the vagina.
Permit some solution to run through the tubing and out over the end of the nozzle to lubricate it.	Moist surfaces have less friction when moved against each other.
Insert the nozzle gently into the vagina while directing it down and back.	In the dorsal recumbent position, normally the vagina is directed down and back.
Gently rotate the nozzle in the vagina during the treatment.	Movement of the nozzle aids in directing the solution against all surfaces of the vagina.
Wash and dry the perineal area after the irrigation.	Debris removed by the irrigation can adhere to the perineal skin where it can cause odor and irritation if not removed.

of wounds that have been surgically induced and sutured. Or, there may be occasions when a wound may be undressed for most of the day and then covered at bedtime. Many small cuts and abrasions heal more quickly if left undressed.

There are several reasons for leaving some wounds undressed, all based on the principles mentioned earlier: the body has resources for healing itself; friction and irritation destroy epithelial cells; and dark, warm, moist areas are suitable for the growth of microorganisms. Therefore, a dressing applied to skin in such a fashion that it produces friction can break the scab which has formed. In addition, the normal flora on the skin can be rubbed into the wound, and if the area is moist and dark, bacterial growth can take place.

Some surgical wounds are left uncovered because it is felt exposure to the air and lack of impediment of circulation caused by a dressing promote faster healing. One approach to the care of extensive burns is the open or no-dressing method.

Administering an open wound irrigation

The purpose is to clean the wound.

SUGGESTED ACTION	RATIONALE
Place the patient in a position so the solution will flow from the wound down to a clean basin held below the wound.	Gravity causes the flow of liquids. Contaminated solution flowing over the wound could introduce microorganisms into the wound.
Irrigate the wound generously but carefully with the solution, being sure to irrigate pockets in the wound.	The solution washes away organisms, tissue debris, and drainage.
Clean the skin around the wound to remove irrigating solution. Be careful not to touch the wound.	Microorganisms are normally present on the skin.
A bland ointment may be applied on the skin immediately surrounding the wound if drainage is present.	An emollient on the skin prevents drainage from irritating the epithelium.
Cover the wound with sterile dressings and secure it in place.	Well-secured sterile dressings protect the wound from trauma, minimize the danger of organisms entering the wound, and absorb secretions.

The Dressed Wound

Dressings serve several purposes. If used properly, dressings and the materials used for securing them help to prevent pathogens from entering the wound, absorb exudate, protect the area from trauma, and restrict motion that tends to disrupt the approximation of the wound edges. They also may be applied with pressure to reduce blood flow or stasis and to aid in approximating edges of the wound. For aesthetic reasons, a dressing serves to cover an area of disfigurement.

Changing the Dressing. Some patients are taught to change their own dressings when they are able, or in other situations the physician or nurse may change the dressing. Some dressings are changed at the hospitalized patient's bedside. In other instances, a special room set aside for this purpose may be used. When infection control is a major concern or anesthesia for the patient is necessary, the operating room may be used for the dressing change. In clinics or offices, an examining room is usually used.

In the past, some agencies had dressing carts which contained a variety of dressing supplies that were wheeled from one patient to another. Since carts can provide a vehicle for pathogen transmission among patients, and in a number of cases, had been shown to be involved in cross-contamination, the common dressing cart is generally not recommended. The preferred method is to use commercially prepared and individually packaged disposable supplies that are selected according to the patient's needs and taken to him. Another common approach is to have individual dressing trays containing necessary equipment. These trays are returned to a central supply unit for sterilization between patients.

Since dressing changes are a common cause of nosocomial infections, the person changing the dressing should use careful handwashing technique before and after the procedure. In some instances, special antiseptics may be recommended for handwashing before dressing changes.

The patient should be prepared for the dressing change by an explanation of what will be done before the procedure is initiated. Consideration should be given to providing privacy for the patient and to the possibility that he may be disturbed by the sight of the wound. In some instances, patients do not wish to look at their wounds, and they should not be encouraged to do so nor chided about it. This is particularly true of patients whose wounds involve change in their bodily functions or appearance, such as the removal of a breast, the amputation of a foot or a leg, or the placement of a tube in the abdominal wall.

The patient should be helped to assume a comfortable and safe position that is also convenient for the person changing the dressing. If the procedure is likely to produce considerable discomfort, an analgesic medication may be given before the procedure is begun.

When preparing to change a dressing, it is necessary to have a means for removing the old dressing without contaminating the wound or the fingers of the person removing it and also equipment for cleaning the wound, dressing it adequately, and securing it. Sometimes, masks and gowns are worn by persons changing the patient's dressings.

Sterile instruments may be used to remove the dressings adhering to a wound and for treating it. In some instances, as with an amputation, sterile gloves are worn. When the instruments are removed after use, they should be handled so that they do not contaminate otherwise clean objects or surfaces, such as overbed tables, utility room counters and carts. Some spray-on, plasticlike transparent dressings are removed with special solvents.

A safe method should be used for disposing of the old dressing and the gauze or the cotton used to clean the wound. The best practice is to discard them in a moistureproof bag which can be closed and discarded for burning.

The antiseptic used to clean the wound is a matter of agency policy or the physician's preference. If the wound is to be irrigated, the prescribed solution, a sterile irrigating syringe, and a basin to collect returns will also be needed.

Dressing materials usually are made of gauze folded into various sizes and shapes. Some gauze sponges are filled with absorbent cotton. Some dressings have a nonadherent surface. The size, the number, and the types of dressings used depend on the nature of the wound. In some instances, a clear spray or collodion may be used to cover the wound and act as a dressing. Cotton balls are useful for cleaning; but are generally not used as a dressing on a wound, for the cotton tends to stick to the wound and becomes difficult to remove.

Individual instrument and dressing packs afford the ultimate in safety for the patient. Surgical dressings and instruments kept in common containers cannot be counted on to be sterile after the container is opened.

Items for securing the dressing will also vary, depending on the extent and nature of the wound.

Securing the Dressing. This reponsibility often demands considerable ingenuity and resourcefulness on the part of the nurse. It requires consideration of such factors as the size of the wound, its location, whether drainage is present, the nature of the drainage, the frequency with which the dressing needs changing, and the activities of the patient.

For securing a very small dressing on a wound with little or no drainage, liquid adhesive or collodion may be used effectively. The edges of the outer piece of gauze that are cut to fit over the dressing are painted with the liquid adhesive or collodion and then glued to the skin.

Strips of tape are used most frequently for securing dressings. Tape is dispensed in various widths, and the length is cut according to the need. Adhesive, paper, and elasticized tapes are common. Adhesive tape has been the most frequently used but paper tape causes a minimum amount of skin irritation and has become more popular. Elasticized tape allows for more movement of a body part without pull on adjacent tissues.

Because adhesive tape often causes skin irritation, especially when dressings must be changed frequently, it is good practice to apply a protective coating to the skin before applying the tape. A preparation frequently used is compound benzoin tincture which is painted on the skin immediately before the tape is applied. When adhesive tape is removed, some of the gummy substance may remain on the skin. A mild solvent followed by thorough rinsing should be used to clean the area.

Some patients are allergic to adhesive mixtures; therefore, the nurse should investigate any complaint of discomfort caused by adhesive tape. Patients who have endured the discomforts of the adhesive for a period of days have been known to need treatment for months following its removal. Various kinds of nonallergenic tapes are available on the market today.

When removing tape, loosen the end and then gently remove it by pulling parallel with the skin surface and toward the wound. Pulling at a right angle or away from the wound can disturb the healing tissue. When tape is used on areas with hair growth, whenever possible, remove the tape by pulling it in the direction the hair grows. Pulling the tape in this direction reduces the discomfort caused by pulling the hair.

When dressings must be changed frequently, it is advisable to consider the use of Montgomery straps for securing the dressing, since they do not require changing with each dressing as tape strips do. These can be made easily or are available commercially. The adhesive end of the strap is placed on the skin well away from the wound. The end of the strap near the wound remains free since the adhesive side has been turned back upon itself. Gauze or woven strips passed through eyelets are tied over the wound to secure the dressing. When the dressing is changed, the strips are untied and turned back to allow for wound care. After the fresh dressing is applied, the strips are retied to hold the dressing in place. Figure 22–3 shows the use of Montgomery straps.

When a dressing is being secured, the tape should be pressed in place with gentle pressure exerted away from the wound. This practice helps to avoid applying tape with tension only in one direction. When one-way tension exists, the resulting traction and skin distortion can cause irritation and blistering. Tape should not be applied to irritated skin. The dressing should be secured well enough so that it does not slip out of place when the patient moves.

The chart on page 544 describes the technique for changing a dressing.

When tape cannot be used safely and effectively, various types of binders and bandages may be used for securing dressings. A description of various types of binders and bandages and their application follow later in this chapter.

Frequency of Changing Dressings. The frequency with which dressings should be changed cannot be stated

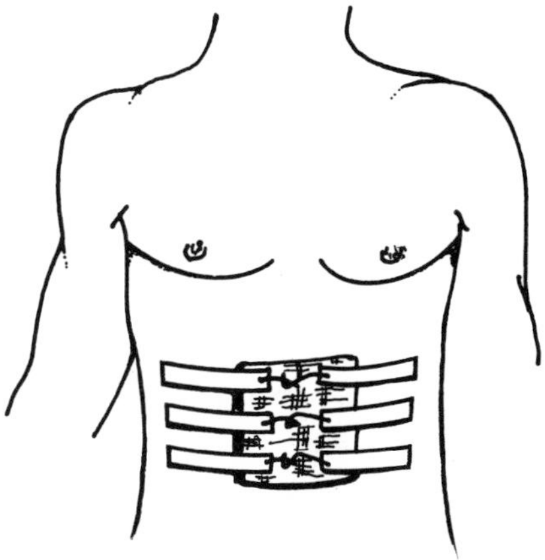

Figure 22–3 Montgomery straps serve as a means for securing dressings that must be changed frequently. By untying the strips, a fresh dressing can be applied without the irritation of repeated removal of the tapes.

The care of a dressed wound

The purpose is to remove a soiled dressing, clean the wound, and apply a sterile dressing.

SUGGESTED ACTION	RATIONALE
Undo materials securing the dressing. Lift the dressing off by touching the outside portion only. If it is soiled, use individual forceps.	Microorganisms can be transferred by direct contact.
If the dressing adheres to the wound, moisten it with sterile water, normal saline, or hydrogen peroxide. Remove when completely loose.	An intact scab is a body defense mechanism and can be damaged if not handled gently.
Drop the soiled dressing into a waterproof bag for later burning.	Burning destroys microorganisms. Confined microorganisms cannot be transmitted by air currents or by contact.
Clean the wound carefully with an antiseptic of the physician's or the agency's choice. Sterile gloves or a sterile forceps may be used to hold cotton balls.	Cleaning aids in removing organisms, tissue debris, and drainage. Sterile supplies reduce the danger of contaminating the wound.
Start from either directly on or adjacent to the wound and work away from it.	Microorganisms are normally present on the skin and could be transferred to the area which is to be kept most clean.
Discard the gauze or the cotton used for cleaning after each stroke over the wound.	Microorganisms removed from one area can be applied to another by direct contact.
Cover the wound with sterile dressings handled with sterile gloves, a sterile forceps, or touched only on the outer surface. Secure the dressings.	A contaminated dressing can introduce pathogens into the wound. Well-secured dressings protect the wound from trauma and absorb drainage.

categorically; it will depend on the physician's preference, the nature of the wound, and whether drainage is present. Some surgeons may wish to leave a clean wound untouched for several days, in which case dressings are left unchanged. They generally believe that a frequent change of dressings on a clean, nondraining wound is a possible source of contamination. In their opinion, it is best if the wound's own protective seal is left undisturbed. Other physicians prefer to have the dressings changed frequently, even several times a day, because close observations of changes in the wound can be made this way.

Recording the Care of the Wound. The nurse caring for a wound is responsible for observing it and for noting factors that may be interfering with the process of healing. She is expected to call the physician's attention to anything unusual in the process of healing as well as to its progress.

On the patient's record, the nurse records each time wound care is given, the nature of the care given, and the appearance of the wound. If drainage is present, it is described. If the patient has a rather complicated dressing, details for caring for the wound should be described on the patient's nursing care plan. Often, the patient who has an extensive wound has preferences as to the time the dressings are changed and how they can be arranged best. Also, patients can become distressed if one nurse uses one method and another nurse a different one, even if both employ proper technique.

Care of Draining Wounds

In order to promote exudate drainage, a rubber or plastic tubular drain is sometimes placed in a wound during surgery. If a drain is in a wound, care must be exercised so that it is not dislodged while dressings are changed. The physician may order that a straight drain be shortened each day. This can be done by grasping the end of the drain with sterile forceps, pulling it out a short distance while using a twisting motion and cutting off the end of the drain with sterile scissors. If the drain is in the abdominal cavity, a large sterile safety pin often is placed at the end of the drain so that it cannot slip down out of sight. Other drains may be attached to suction devices to remove exudate.

The skin around a draining wound quickly becomes irritated and excoriated unless precautions are taken. Keeping the skin clean is of prime importance. This requires that dressings be changed often enough so that drainage-soaked dressings are not left on the skin for long periods of time. The skin surrounding the wound is washed, preferably with a warm soap or detergent solution, and rinsed thoroughly with water or normal saline. A thorough cleaning is accomplished by the emulsifying and mechanical actions involved in this method. An antiseptic solution may be used on the skin after foreign materials have been washed off thoroughly and the skin dried properly. Some antiseptics are not effective if used on moist skin surfaces. Even if antiseptics are not used, the skin should be dry.

In order to prevent skin irritation and excoriation, a protective ointment or paste may be applied so that drainage cannot contact the skin. This may be particularly important when it is anticipated that the drainage period will be prolonged or when the person's skin is especially susceptible to irritation.

When a protective ointment or paste has been used on the skin, it is important to remove it at regular intervals, at least daily, and clean the skin under it. Ointments prepared in a water-soluble base may be removed with a soap-and-water or detergent solution. Oil-based ointments and pastes can be removed with mineral oil and then the skin cleaned with soap and water. Care must be exercised when ointments and pastes are removed so that the friction created by rubbing is kept at a minimum. Friction may destroy epithelial cells, causing skin irritation.

A dressing placed on a draining wound is more effective and comfortable when basic principles are observed.

The property of surface tension exhibited by liquids and the forces of cohesion and adhesion cause a column of liquid to rise in a fine tube or on a hair. This is called *capillary action* or *capillarity*. For example, absorbent cotton allows for greater capillarity than untreated cotton; therefore, sponges lined with the former material soak up more liquid. Loosely packed gauze, the threads of which act as numerous wicks, enhances capillarity and will allow for drainage to be directed upward and away from its source. Fluffed and loosely packed dressings, then, are more absorbent than tightly packed dressings and will carry drainage up and away from the wound.

Evaporation occurs more readily when there is circulation of air. Prolonged heat and moisture on the skin deteriorate epithelial cells. These principles are utilized when the nurse applies dressings and secures them so that circulation of air is possible. Loosely packed dressings secured with materials that allow for air circulation promote evaporation of moisture and dissipation of heat to the environment, both of which help to protect the skin. To protect the patient's clothing and bed linen, waterproof material, such as a plastic, can be used on the bed when a wound is draining profusely. Waterproofing should generally be avoided over the dressing because it reduces the circulation of air through the dressings, and the skin and the wound may be injured due to an accumulation of heat and moisture.

Gravity causes liquids to flow from a high to a low level. Dressings on a draining wound should be arranged according to the patient's position and the expected direction of flow. For example, when a patient with a draining abdominal wound is ambulatory, a heavy application of dressings should be placed at the base of the wound and secured so that the drainage does not escape under the dressings and onto the patient.

Gravity should be kept in mind when observing the patient's dressing for evidence of bleeding. The top part of a dressing may be dry, but blood may be draining from the wound by gravity. Therefore, when checking an abdominal dressing, look at the bed linen under the patient near the wound. When checking a dressing at the throat, such as the patient will have following the removal of the thyroid gland, check under the patient's neck and on the pillow for evidence of bleeding.

Contamination can occur through a moist medium. If a sterile dressing remains in place until it is saturated or drainage has been absorbed through an entire area of the dressing, microorganisms from the external surface can move through the dressing to the wound. For this reason, dressings should not be allowed to become saturated. They should either be replaced with fresh dressings or reinforced before drainage causes saturation.

Teaching the Patient to Dress His Wound

Today, patients with wounds are often not hospitalized or they return home before wounds are healed. Therefore, they or family members often need to learn to care for the wound. The nurse may teach in the physician's office, a clinic, in the patient's home, or in a hospital. The nurse can promote health maintenance in all of these settings. Health maintenance includes teaching consumers how to cope with minor abrasions and injuries, as well as with some surgical wounds.

The nature and the amount of teaching needed to help a person care for a wound will depend on individual circumstances. Nurses have observed that patients usually are concerned about odor from dressings, discomfort, and fear of soiling clothing when drainage is present. Other disturbing factors include fear that the dressings will slip out of place and cause infection, concern for the reaction of friends and family to the appearance of the dressings, and the cost of dressings.

The patient and his family should understand the basic steps in the procedure for the care of a dressed wound described on page 544. Allowing the patient or family member to practice the technique under the supervision of the nurse prior to dismissal from a health agency is helpful.

If specific antiseptics have not been prescribed, a variety of substances can be purchased. Any mild soap for cleaning is satisfactory. At this point, studies do not indicate that soaps which claim antiseptic properties are superior to others in destroying organisms. The use of soap and water to remove drainage is important to prevent skin irritations.

Isopropyl alcohol and povidone-iodine preparations are useful as antiseptics for treating minor wounds. Hydrogen peroxide is an effective antiseptic for open wounds. Its oxidizing action has a cleansing effect in the presence of organic material. However, its use is of doubtful value when skin is intact because the release of oxygen is too slow to be effective.

Antibiotic substances in ointment or liquid forms are available without prescription for treating wounds and controlling infections. Bacitracin, gramicidin, neomycin, and polymyxin B sulfate are prepared alone or in combination with each other for such use. Products that contain vitamins A and D and zinc oxide are also commonly used as protectants to prevent or treat skin irritations due to moisture. The patient should be directed to follow the directions as they are stated on the containers of the antibiotic and protective agents.

Individually packaged sterile dressings are available at surgical supply stores and some drug stores. While it remains important to use appropriate materials for wound care, the nurse should also assist the patient in choosing materials that are not unreasonably expensive. Occasionally, the patient may need financial assistance for the purchase of dressings and an appropriate community agency may be asked to help. Or, the patient may be referred to a local health organization that distributes dressings at a nominal cost or free of charge. The nurse who uses ingenuity based on appropriate principles can help the patient to keep the cost within a reasonable range and still carry out the procedure effectively.

Attention to aseptic technique and to the disposal of the old dressings and supplies is particularly important in controlling the spread of infection. The nurse should emphasize the need for the person handling the dressing to wash his hands prior to and following the procedure. A specific plan for appropriate discarding of the soiled dressings should be discussed by the nurse in her teaching. The interested patient or family member can be helped to learn independent and effective care of wounds.

IMMOBILIZING AND SUPPORTING THE WOUND

Bandages and Binders

A *bandage* is a piece of gauze or other material used to cover a wound. Usually, bandages are dispensed in rolls of various widths. A *binder* is a type of bandage specifically designed to fit a large body area, such as the abdomen, the chest, or the breasts. Some texts use the terms synonomously, although in the strictest sense they are not.

Bandages and binders are used for several purposes: to create pressure over an area, to immobilize a part of the body to restrict its motion, to support a part of the body, to prevent or reduce swelling, to correct a deformity, and to secure a limb to a splint. They are used also to hold dressings in place.

Usually, gauze fabric is used for bandages. It is light and soft and can be adjusted readily to fit a body part comfortably. Because it is porous, it is cool and allows for circulation of air. Gauze bandage is relatively inexpensive. It rarely can be reclaimed for repeated use because it frays very easily.

Muslin and flannel are materials also used for bandages. Being strong and firm, they are useful when pressure and immobilization are desired. Flannel is more absorbent than muslin and molds easily to fit the contours of the body. Flannel also helps to keep the area warm, which may be an advantage or a disadvantage depending on individual circumstances. Self-adhering, synthetic bandages are also available. Binders are made of muslin, flannel, or synthetics. Muslin or flannel bandages are suited to home use because they can be washed and reused. Synthetic binders are often elasticized and some are self-adhering.

Various types of elastic webbing can be purchased which are particularly effective when bandaging is needed for firm support and immobilization and for preventing swelling in extremities. The webbing is strong and molds well because of its elastic quality. It can be washed and used repeatedly.

One type of elastic webbing has an adhesive surface on one side. This can be used like adhesive and has the advantage of molding well to body contours. It does not withstand washing and therefore cannot be reclaimed for repeated use.

Ribbed cotton material dispensed as stockinet is used for bandaging. It has an elastic quality, is inexpensive, and can be reclaimed for repeated use, but it is not as sturdy and strong as elastic webbing.

General Principles of Applying Bandages and Binders

A well-applied bandage or a binder will promote healing, prevent damage to wounds and skin, and offer the patient comfort and security. Certain general principles guide action in the application of bandages and binders and aid in attaining these objectives.

Unclean bandages and binders may cause infection if applied over a wound or a skin abrasion. This fact guides what may seem like rather obvious action; that is, that bandages and binders should be kept clean and free of contamination. Medical asepsis is observed when applying bandages and binders. Skin abrasions and wounds are first covered with sterile dressings before clean bandages and binders are applied in order to protect the wound from trauma and contamination. Certain bandages and binders may be used repeatedly, but only after they have been washed and sterilized between patients.

When objects in contact move in opposition to each other, friction occurs which opposes motion, and can destroy or damage epithelial cells. Applying a small amount of fine talcum powder to the unbroken skin helps to keep it dry and decreases friction, but care must be exercised to prevent powder from entering the open wound, if one is present. No two skin surfaces should be allowed to touch each other. This is another measure to decrease friction on the skin and prevent moisture from accumulating in body crevices. Use absorbent material between fingers and toes, in the axilla, and under the breast, to absorb moisture and to prevent surfaces of skin from touching each other. A bandage or a binder should be applied securely so that it will not shift about when the patient moves, causing friction that may result in chafing and skin abrasions.

Prolonged heat and moisture on the skin may cause its epithelial cells to deteriorate. It will be recalled that this principle is observed when dressings are applied to a wound. When bandages and binders are used, it indicates to the nurse that the area to be covered should be cleaned and dried thoroughly before applying a bandage or a binder. An unnecessarily thick or extensive bandage should be avoided so that the part being covered does not become excessively warm. Porous materials are preferable to nonporous in order to allow air to circulate so that perspiration can evaporate.

Placing and supporting the part to be bandaged in the normal functioning position prevents deformities and discomfort and enhances the circulation of blood in the part involved. This principle has been used as a guide for action throughout this text in the discussions of the importance of proper body mechanics and body alignment. It is equally important when bandages and binders are being used. Since bandages and binders usually restrict some motion and often are intended to immobilize a part of the body, it is important that the part involved first be placed at rest and comfortably in the position of normal functioning so that deformities and impaired circulation will not result. For example, when the foot is bandaged, it should be supported so that the bandage will not force it into footdrop.

Blood flow through the tissues is decreased by applying excessive pressure on blood vessels. The healing process is impaired, and tissue cells may die if the blood supply is inadequate to remove wastes and bring nourishment to the part involved. These are well-known physiologic facts that guide action in several ways. The bandage or the binder is applied with sufficient pressure to provide the amount of immobilization or support desired, to remain in place, and to secure a dressing if one is present. However, pressure should not be great enough to impede circulation of blood in the part involved.

Weakened veins, especially those of the lower extremities, can usually function more effectively when their walls are supported. Sufficient pressure to support the distended veins without impairing blood flow can be helpful in preventing edema.

The tension of each bandage turn should be equal, and unnecessary and uneven overlapping of turns should be avoided to prevent undue and uneven pressure. Bony prominences over which bandages and binders must be placed are padded. Hollows in the body contour may be filled with padding to provide comfort and to aid in maintaining equal pressure from the bandage or binder. An extremity is bandaged *toward the trunk* to avoid congestion and impaired circulation in the distal part. After a bandage or a binder has been applied, the part is observed frequently for signs of impaired circulation. For example, when an extremity is bandaged, the toes and the fingers are left exposed, if possible, so that circulation in the nailbeds and signs of beginning swelling, which often indicate that circulation has been impaired, can be observed. A bandage placed over a wet dressing or a draining wound is applied less tightly since shrinkage of the material may cause the bandage to become too tight to allow for adequate circulation when it dries. In addition to being dangerous, a bandage or a binder applied too tightly is usually very uncomfortable for the patient.

Pins and knots, often used to secure a bandage or a binder, are placed well away from a wound or a tender and inflamed area. Care is observed so that pins, knots, and seams will not cause undue pressure or cause the patient discomfort. Movement often causes binders and bandages to loosen so they should be inspected and reapplied at regular intervals.

A well-applied bandage or binder will be comfortable for the patient, durable, neat, and clean. This is important for the patient's mental security as well as for promoting the best possible physiological functioning of the body.

Application of Common Types of Bandages and Binders

Many types of commercial bandages and binders are available for use today. There are variations in the techniques of applying and in the type of binder or bandage; some of the more common ones will be described here.

Roller Bandages. A roller bandage is a continuous strip of material wound on itself to form a cylinder or roll. Roller bandages are made in various widths and lengths. They are the most commonly used type of bandage and usually are made of gauze, although any other type of material may be used also. Elastic webbing is dispensed usually as a roller bandage. Kerlix and Kling are two types of commercial roller bandages that are stretchable. They are particularly useful for securing a dressing on an irregularly shaped body part, such as an extremity or around the head.

The free end of the roller bandage is the initial portion, while the terminal end is in the center of the roll. The rolled portion is called the body. The outer surface of the bandage is the surface toward the outside of the body of the bandage. The inner surface is toward the inside or the center of its body. The outer surface is placed next to the patient's skin and dressing. When the bandage is begun, the initial end is held in place with one hand while the other hand passes the roll around the part. Once the bandage is anchored, usually with two circular turns, its body may be passed from hand to hand, being careful that equal tension is being exerted with each turn around the part. It is easier to keep tension equal by unwinding the bandage gradually and only as it is required. Several basic turns are used to apply bandages, the selection of the turn depending on the part to be bandaged.

Circular Turn. When using the circular turn, the bandage is wrapped around the part with complete overlapping of the previous bandage turn. It is used primarily for anchoring a bandage where it is begun and where it is terminated. Figure 22–4 illustrates this turn to anchor a bandage before beginning a spiral turn.

Spiral Turn. When using the spiral turn, the bandage ascends in spiral fashion so that each turn overlaps the preceding one by one-half or two-thirds the width of the bandage. The spiral turn is useful when the part being bandaged is cylindrical, such as the area around the wrist, the fingers, and the trunk. Figure 22–5 illustrates this turn.

Spiral-Reverse Turn. A spiral-reverse turn is a spiral turn in which reverses are made halfway through each turn. Spiral-reverse turns are particularly effective for

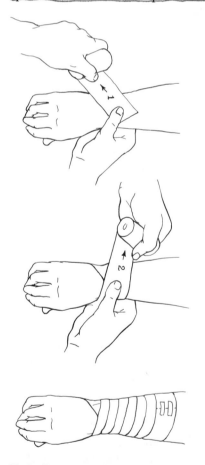

Figure 22–4   The top two sketches illustrate how the circular turn is used to anchor a roller bandage. The bottom sketch illustrates a spiral turn which was performed after the bandage was anchored.

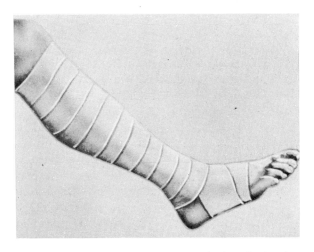

Figure 22–5   This photo illustrates an elastic roller bandage applied to the leg, using spiral turns. (Becton, Dickinson & Co., Rutherford, N.J.)

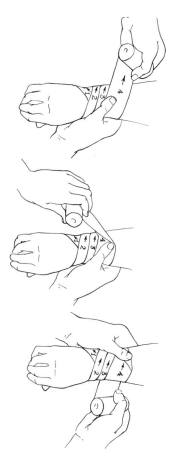

Figure 22–6   From top to bottom, these sketches illustrate the technique for making the spiral-reverse turn.

bandaging a cone-shaped part, such as the thigh, the leg, or the forearm. Figure 22–6 illustrates the spiral-reverse turn. The position of the nurse's thumb on the bandage on the patient's arm shows the manner in which the reverse is made.

Figure-of-Eight Turn.   The figure-of-eight turn consists of making oblique overlapping turns that ascend and descend alternately. Each turn crosses the one preceding it so that it appears like the figure eight. Figures 22–7 and 22–8 illustrate how this turn is made. It is effective for use around joints, such as the knee, the elbow, the ankle, and the wrist. It provides a snug bandage and therefore is used often for immobilization.

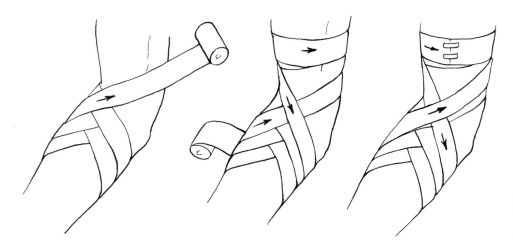

Figure 22–7   From left to right, these sketches illustrate the technique for making the figure-of-eight turn.

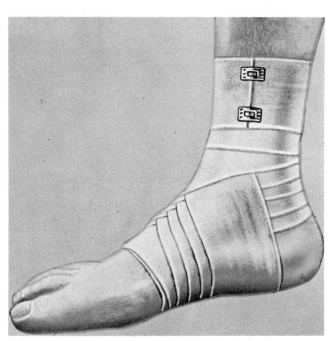

Figure 22–8   This photo illustrates the figure-of-eight turn when used to apply elastic bandage to the ankle. (Becton, Dickinson & Co., Rutherford, N.J.)

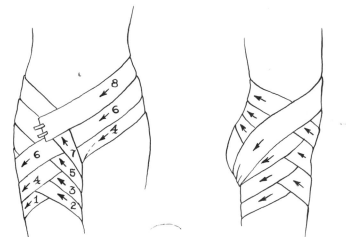

Figure 22–9   This sketch illustrates the technique for making the spica bandage.

Spica.   The spica consists of ascending and descending turns with all turns overlapping and crossing each other to form an angle. It is particularly useful for bandaging the thumb, the breast, the shoulder, the groin, and the hip. Figure 22–9 illustrates its application.

Recurrent Bandage.   Sometimes this type of bandage is called a stump bandage. It is used for fingers and for the stump of an amputated limb. After a few circular turns to anchor the bandage, the initial end of the bandage is placed in the center of the part being bandaged, well back from the tip to be covered. The body is passed back and forth over the tip, first on the one side and then on the other side of the center piece of bandage. Figure 22–10 illustrates the manner of applying a recurrent bandage to a stump and of using the figure-of-eight turn to finish the bandage. Figure 22–11 shows an elastic bandage applied to a stump. Recurrent bandages also are used effectively for head bandages.

Whichever turn is being used, care should be taken to provide even overlapping of one-half to two-thirds the width of each bandage, except for the circular turn. All surfaces of the skin should be covered by the fin-

ished bandage to prevent pinching the skin between turns of the bandage. The bandage is completed well away from the wound or inflamed and tender areas. The terminal end of the bandage may be secured with adhesive, special clamps, by tying a knot or with a safety pin, being careful to avoid undue pressure.

Removing Roller Bandages.   In order to prevent too much movement, it is best to cut a roller bandage with a bandage scissors when removing it. Cutting should be done on the side opposite the injury or the wound, from one end to the other, so that the bandage can be folded open for its entire length. If it is an elastic bandage and is to be reused, it may be unwound by keeping the loose end together and passing it as a ball from one hand to the other while unwinding.

T Binders.   A T binder is so named because it looks like the letter T. A single T binder has a tail attached at right angles to a belt. A double T binder has two tails attached to the belt. T binders are particularly effective for securing dressings on the rectum and perineum and in the groin. The single T is used for females, and the double T for males. The belt is passed around the waist and secured with safety pins. The single or the double tails are passed between the legs and pinned to the belt.

Many-Tailed Binders.   Many-tailed binders are also called *scultetus binders.* The binder consists of a rectangular piece of fabric which has vertical tails, each about 5 cm. or 2 inches wide, attached to the sides of the rectangu-

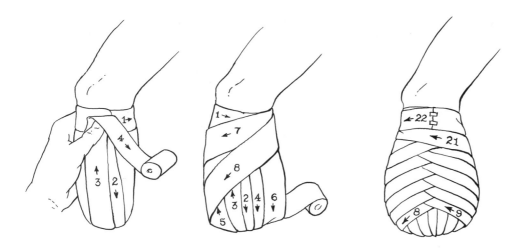

Figure 22-10 From left to right, these sketches illustrate the technique for making a recurrent bandage to cover a stump.

lar piece. They are used to support the abdomen or hold dressings on it or on the chest. When a scultetus binder is applied to the abdomen, the patient lies on his back and on the center of the binder. The lower end of the binder is placed well down on the hips, but not so low that it will interfere with the use of a bedpan or with walking. The tails are brought out to either side on the patient's body with the bottom tail in position to wrap around the lower part of the abdomen first. A tail from each side is brought up and placed obliquely over the abdomen until all tails are in place. The last tails are fastened with safety pins. Figure 22-12 on page 552 illustrates the application of a scultetus binder to the abdomen.

Sling. A sling is used for the support of an upper extremity. Health care agencies generally have

commercial strap slings or sleeve slings available for use. In the home, a large piece of cloth folded in a triangle can be used as a sling. Figure 22-13 on page 552 illustrates a sling used as an arm support and shows the method of applying it. The open sling or triangle is placed on the chest, and then the affected arm is placed across the sling. One end of the sling is placed around the neck on the side of the unaffected arm. The other end is placed over the affected arm, and the ends are tied off to the side of the neck so that the knot does not rub over the cervical vertebrae. The material at the elbow is folded neatly and may be secured with a pin placed behind the sling so that it will be out of sight.

Straight Binders. This straight piece of material usually is about 15 to 20 cm. or 6 to 8 inches wide and long enough to more than circle the torso. It generally is used for the chest and the abdomen. Straight binders must be applied to fit the contours of the body. This usually is done by making small tucks in the binder as necessary. In some instances, these tucks can be secured with safety pins. A straight binder for the chest often is provided with shoulder straps so that it will not slip down on the trunk. *Triangular*

Stockinet. Stockinet is a stretchable tubular bandage, constructed so that a body part may be inserted into it, such as a finger, a foot, or an arm. It is dispensed in various widths or diameters. It has advantages over the roller bandage in that it remains in place better, applies a uniform pressure and is extremely simple and quick to use.

Stockinet is useful for making caps for securing dressings on the head. The desired length is cut from a roll of an appropriate width, usually 15 cm. or 6 inches

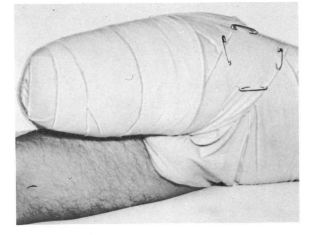

Figure 22-11 This photo illustrates an elastic bandage used to dress a stump. (Becton, Dickinson & Co., Rutherford, N.J.)

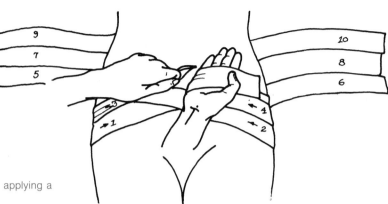

Figure 22-12 This sketch illustrates the technique for applying a many-tailed binder.

wide. The stockinet is placed over the head and folded back on itself at the forehead for extra security. The opposite end is tied or pinned at the top of the head. Stockinet as a bandage on the head seems to offer more security than other types; therefore, it is also more comfortable for the patient.

Stockinet in a narrow width is appropriate for finger bandages. An applicator is dispensed with the stockinet so that it can be slipped over the finger with ease.

Elasticized Stockings. Some persons may need to have pressure applied to their legs, for example, persons with varicose veins, those with circulatory disturbances, or women during pregnancy. Many patients routinely wear elasticized stockings following major surgery or when they are confined to bed for long periods. The

stockings help to promote venous blood return and to avoid stagnation of blood and possible clot formation. Several manufacturers produce men's and women's hose which are capable of applying pressure to the leg from the foot to the midthigh. Some apply mild pressure, while others are capable of applying pressure equivalent to an elastic bandage. They are available in a variety of colors so another stocking is not required underneath or over them for the ambulatory patient. They are more expensive than regular stockings, which may make them prohibitive for some patients. However, they wear well, and many persons who are on their feet or remain in one position a great deal of the time, such as homemakers, nurses, salespersons, and businesspersons, find them very useful. The mild sustained pressure helps to prevent the accumulation of

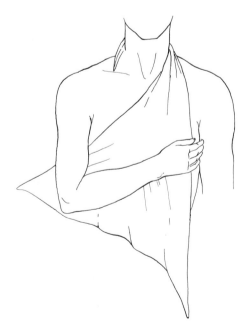

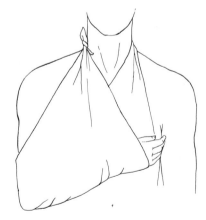

Figure 22-13 This sketch illustrates a sling that is used to support the arm. The sling is made from a triangular piece of cloth.

tissue fluid in the feet and the lower leg. Many patients can benefit from such stockings, and the nurse should be prepared to advise about their correct use. The stockings should be correctly fitted to the measurements of the individual. Also, they should be applied immediately upon awakening before getting out of bed and before the legs are in a dependent position. Immobilized patients who wear them continuously should have them removed and their legs inspected and bathed at least daily. Figure 22–14 illustrates a nurse teaching a patient about elasticized stockings.

Breast binder

Casts

The purpose of a cast is to immobilize a part of the body to provide protection and support. A cast is generally used to hold bone fractures in place until healing occurs. In order to prevent movement, a cast is usually applied so that it includes the joint above and below the affected area. A physician generally applies a cast, but the nurse is responsible for the care of the hospitalized patient after it is in place. Frequently she is also responsible for teaching the patient how to care for the cast at home.

Most casts are made of bandages impregnated with plaster of Paris. They are moistened and then applied to a body area that has been covered with padding material, such as webril, felt, or stockinette. A cast may take several hours or several days to dry, depending on the type of cast and the environmental conditions. As the cast dries, the plaster of Paris releases heat, which can ordinarily be felt by the patient. Some casts are also made of plastic material.

The cast should be kept uncovered while drying. Exposure to warm circulating air hastens drying. The patient with a new cast should be placed on firm, moisture-proof pillows while the cast dries. A wet cast should not be placed on a hard surface because the cast may become flat on the posterior surface. This can produce pressure on the underlying tissue.

A casted extremity should be positioned so that each distal joint is higher than the preceding joint. This positioning facilitates venous return and reduced edema of the injured area. Proper body alignment should be maintained to prevent injury to other body areas. Figure 22–15 on page 554 shows the positioning of a casted extremity.

The nurse caring for the patient in a cast must make careful observations regarding the casted area to prevent complications. Neurological and circulatory status of the area should be observed at regular and frequent intervals. Changes in color, temperature, pulsations, or sensations in tissues adjacent to the cast can indicate that the cast is causing pressure against the underlying tis-

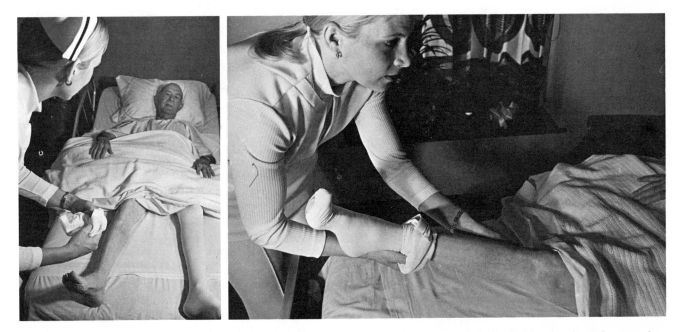

Figure 22–14   In the photo on the left, the nurse is teaching the patient about the purpose of elastic stockings as she gathers one in her hand before putting it on the patient's foot. In the photo on the right, the elastic stocking is pulled up on the patient's leg while his foot is elevated.

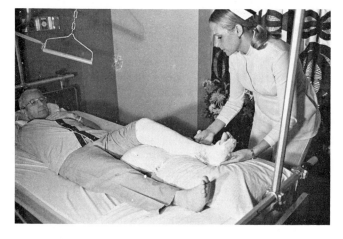

Figure 22–15   This patient has had a cast applied from his foot to above his knee for a fractured ankle. Note that the toes have been left exposed to be accessible for circulatory and neurological observations. The nurse is positioning the cast with the foot elevated to control edema.

sues. Pallor, coolness to touch, or weak or absent pulses distal to the cast can be indicative of circulatory problems. Sensations of pressure, burning, tingling, numbness, or constant pain under or distal to the cast can be symptomatic of neurological or circulatory impairment. Most authorities recommend that the casted area be observed for these changes every hour for the first 24 hours following a cast application. Thereafter, observations are usually made every four hours for the next two to three days.

Trauma from the wound can cause edema to occur under the cast. The application of ice bags to the wound site may be useful in preventing or controlling edema. Edema under the cast can create circulatory or nerve impairment.

If there is an open wound, bleeding can occur under the cast. Any blood that seeps through the cast should be encircled, timed, and dated to make comparisons possible. In the event that the seepage progresses rapidly, the physician should be notified.

After a cast is dry, the cast edges should be finished by pulling the stockinette over the edges or placing adhesive tape around the edges. The skin around the edges of the cast should be inspected for irritation and appropriate padding applied if needed. The skin should be kept clean and lotions to protect the skin are used.

Positioning the patient in a cast can be difficult and should be carefully planned. When moving the patient in a cast, he should be turned toward the unaffected side. This prevents undue pressure on the affected area

and is more comfortable for the patient. Sufficient pillows should be available to provide adequate support for comfort and to avoid pressure from the cast. Turning a patient with a large cast requires coordinated efforts by nursing personnel to reduce the patient's anxiety and the possibility of injury. The casted extremity should be supported under joints during the turning process to prevent the cast from cracking. The patient in a cast should have his position changed every two hours if he is immobilized, at which time the nurse should observe for indications of pressure areas.

In addition to turning and positioning, the nurse should encourage active range of motion exercises for the unaffected extremities. When ambulation is started, the patient should have assistance to provide the necessary support to prevent injury. Casts are heavy and those used on the lower extremities can cause problems with balance until the person becomes accustomed to it.

A cast that is near the perineal area requires special consideration to maintain cleanliness. Positioning of the bedpan can be enhanced by the use of pillows under the cast and body for support and to prevent soiling. Fracture bedpans may also be helpful. For a small child or an incontinent adult, the perineal area of the cast may be covered with small strips of plastic to prevent soilage. If the cast is soiled, it can be cleaned with a damp cloth.

Isometric exercises can be taught to the patient to maintain strength in muscles under the cast. The activities that are allowed should be emphasized and an explanation should be given when some activities are to be curtailed.

Itching under the cast is a common problem when a cast has been in place for a time. The nurse should emphasize that small objects should not be used to scratch under the cast because they can become lodged there and cause pressure on underlying tissues. If plaster of Paris particles fall into the cast, a vacuum cleaner on low suction can be used to remove these particles. This should be done for a few seconds only and the nozzle should not be placed down into the cast.

Many persons are fearful about having a cast removed. Casts are removed with vibrating devices called cast cutters. The cast is opened on two sides and spread apart to remove the extremity. The patient needs to be reassured that removal of the cast is not painful and that his skin will not be touched by the cast cutter. Often the extremity will tingle or feel stiff after the cast is removed. In addition, the skin may appear scaly and be dry.

Many patients with casts are discharged from health care facilities soon after cast application. If so, the nurse needs to teach the patient or a family member how to care for the casted extremity. The teaching plan should include reporting to health personnel any evidence of numbness, tingling, loss of sensation, and temperature or color changes in the casted extremity. A discussion of the signs of infection should be included so that the patient can report these promptly. These signs include a musty odor under the cast, fever, increase in pain or pressure, and drainage on the cast. The patient should know how to position the cast and to clean the skin around it. He should also know that casts should be kept dry. The reader is directed to orthopedic or clinical texts for more comprehensive information on special types of casts and their care.

HEAT AND COLD APPLICATIONS

Until late in the eighteenth century, heat was believed to be a kind of fluid that could flow from one substance to another. This theory was refuted when it was found that heat was related to motion. *Heat* is defined as the average kinetic energy, or the energy of the motion of molecules of a material.

Cold is a relative term. It is used to mean that a material has a relatively low temperature, that is, little or no warmth. In other words, as the motion of molecules decreases, the heat is less, and the material is said to be cool or cold. Absolute zero is the temperature at which molecular motion ceases. Theoretically, this occurs at a hypothetical point 273° below zero on the Celsius scale. The important thing to realize is that for all practical purposes, heat is present in all material, therefore, discussions concerning the nature of heat apply also to those of cold. However, the *effects* of applying something warm to the human body are different from the effects of applying something cool, as will be discussed later.

General Principles Related to the Body's Reaction to Heat and Cold

It will be recalled that cells in the hypothalamus act as a thermostat to regulate body temperature. The anterior cells of the hypothalamus are vasodilating and heat-dissipating while the posterior or caudal cells are vasoconstricting and heat-conserving. These cells receive impulses through somatic and visceral neurons in the brain and the spinal cord. The skin plays an important role in maintaining body temperature through the activity of its sweat glands and its pilomotor muscles. When one is exposed to warm surroundings, the sweat glands secrete perspiration. The body cools when the perspiration changes from liquid to vapor. Evaporation requires heat; hence, heat is released. When exposed to cold surroundings, the pilomotor muscles contract and make the hair stand on end in animals and cause "gooseflesh" in man. This phenomenon is the body's attempt to conserve internal body heat. Shivering, also under hypothalamus regulation (lateral cells), generates considerable body heat by agitating the muscles.

The caliber of the cutaneous blood vessels also plays an important role in maintaining body temperature. The smaller the caliber, the smaller will be the quantity of heat brought by the blood to the surface of the skin and lost to the environment. The larger the caliber, the larger the quantity of heat brought to the surface and lost. This phenomenon can be observed when the skin appears flushed as the body becomes too warm, and pale as the body becomes too cool. The blood vessels in the skin are capable of containing large or small quantities of blood, and their caliber increases or decreases as the local and the general needs of the body change. The change in caliber of the blood vessels is regulated by the vasomotor centers in the medulla oblongata of the brain stem, under hypothalamic influence. The local exposure of body areas to heat and cold produces changes in blood vessel sizes and influences blood flow to the area. This response is the basis for the therapeutic use of heat and cold applications.

When receptors for heat and cold are stimulated, they set up impulses that are carried to the hypothalamus and the cerebral cortex via the somatic afferent fibers. The conscious sensation of temperature is aroused in the cerebral cortex, while the hypothalamus serves as a reflex center to integrate somatic and visceral motor responses to maintain a normal temperature.

Receptors for cold lie superficially, while those for heat are located deeper in the skin. The density of receptors varies; in some parts of the body they are more numerous than in others. The cold receptors, for example, are particularly numerous on the thorax and the upper limbs. The cold receptors are estimated to be approximately eight to ten times more numerous than receptors for heat.

There is difference of opinion on receptors for high temperatures. It is more generally agreed that, when hot stimuli are received by the skin, the pain receptors are also stimulated, and the sensation of burning is the result of this double stimulation of receptors. A less widely accepted theory is that a second type of heat receptor in the skin with a very high threshold is stimulated when hot objects touch the skin.

Heat and cold receptors adjust readily if the stimulus is not extreme. For example, if the arm is placed in warm water, the sensation of warmth soon diminishes because of the adaptability of the heat receptors. The same phenomenon occurs if cool water is used. It is important to remember the ability of receptors to adapt to heat and cold when using hot and cold applications. Once the receptors adapt, the patient may become unaware of temperature extremes until tissue damage occurs.

The temperature that the skin can tolerate varies with individuals. Some can tolerate warmer and colder applications more safely than can others. Certain areas of the skin are also more tolerant of temperature variations than are other areas. Those parts of the body where the skin is somewhat thinner generally are more sensitive to temperature variations than exposed areas where the skin is often thicker. Therefore, it is important to apply warm and cold applications well within the generally known safe limits of temperature variations. But, in addition, the skin should be observed so that persons who are more sensitive to temperature changes will not receive tissue damage, even though applications have been applied within recommended temperature range.

Water is a better conductor of heat than air. This fact is used in guiding action whenever heat or cold is applied to the skin, since the skin will tolerate greater extremes of temperature if the heat or the cold is dry rather than moist. For example, a moist hot dressing should be applied at a lower temperature than a cloth-covered hot water bag in order to prevent burning the skin. The reason is that the air between cloth fibers acts as an insulator.

The body tolerates greater extremes in temperature when the duration of exposure is short. When duration is lengthy, the temperature range that the body can tolerate safely is narrower. The area involved is also important. In general, the larger the area to which heat or cold is applied, the less tolerant is the skin to extremes in temperature.

The condition of the patient is an important factor to consider when heat and cold are being applied to the body. Certain patients are sensitive to physical agents and tolerate heat and cold poorly. Special care also is indicated for patients who are debilitated, unconscious, or insensitive to cutaneous stimulation. Patients who have disturbances in circulation are more sensitive to

heat and cold. Broken skin areas are also more subject to tissue damage, since the subcutaneous tissue is less tolerant of heat and cold, and the temperature and pain senses may be impaired and unable to heed warning stimuli.

Transfer of Heat. As discussed in Chapter 15, heat is transferred by radiation, convection, and conduction. For example, the heat felt by the hand near a light bulb has been transferred to the hand by radiation. Convection explains the phenomenon of wind because the unequal heating of the earth's surfaces produces air currents. Local applications of heat and cold transfer heat to and from the body by conduction.

A poor conductor is called an *insulator*. Many of the actions that nurses take when applying heat or cold to the body are guided by a knowledge of the transmission of heat by conduction.

If hot water bags were made of metal, they would conduct heat so rapidly that the patient would be burned since metals are good conductors of heat. Even rubber is a fairly good conductor; therefore, hot water bags and other rubber heating devices are covered with cloth before being applied to the patient's skin. The cloth covering serves as an insulator.

Before hot wet packs are applied to an area, the skin may be lubricated with petrolatum. It acts as an insulator since it slows down the transmission of heat.

Water is a better conductor of heat than air. This fact is used to guide action whenever heat or cold is applied to the skin since the skin will tolerate greater extremes of temperature if the heat is dry rather than moist. Thus, a moist hot dressing should be applied at a lower temperature than a cloth-covered hot water bag in order to prevent burning of the skin. The reason is that the air between cloth fibers acts as an insulator.

Effects of Local Application of Cold. When cold is applied to the skin, the first visible reaction is vasoconstriction; that is, the caliber of the cutaneous vessels decreases. The skin becomes cool and pale. The skin receptors for cold are stimulated, the impulses are carried to the hypothalamus and the cerebral cortex, and the body reacts to conserve heat. The constriction of blood vessels reduces circulation in the skin in order that heat may be conserved by preventing loss of heat from the blood to the environment. This vasoconstriction limits the reaction of the vascular stage in the inflammatory process.

In addition to vasoconstriction, there is a decrease in

sealed containers that are filled with an alcohol-base solution. The ice bags are maintained in freezing units generally located in central supply rooms and are available on request.

A cover should be placed on the ice bag to make it more comfortable for the patient and also to provide for absorption of the moisture which condenses on the outside of the bag.

To be effective as a local application, the ice bag should be applied for one-half to one hour and removed for approximately one hour. In this way the tissues are able to react to the effects of the cold.

Cold Compress.

A *compress* is several layers of moist absorbent cloth or gauze folded to cover a small area. Moist, cold, local applications usually are called cold compresses. They might be used for an injured eye, headache, tooth extraction, and in some situations, for hemorrhoids. The texture and the thickness of the material used will depend on the area to which it is to be applied. For example, eye compresses could be prepared from surgical gauze compresses which have a small amount of cotton filling. A washcloth makes an excellent compress for the head or the face.

The material used for the application is immersed in a clean basin, appropriate for the size of the compress, that contains pieces of ice and a small amount of water. The compress should be wrung thoroughly before it is applied to avoid dripping, which is uncomfortable for the patient and may also wet the bed or clothing. The compresses should be changed frequently. Usually, the patient can feel when they have become warm, and many patients like to apply their own compresses. The application should be continued for 15 to 20 minutes and repeated every two to three hours. Ice bags or commercial devices for keeping the compresses cold decrease the frequency with which the compresses must be changed.

Alcohol or Cold Sponge Bath.

Hypothermia is the artificial lowering of body tissue temperature. Occasionally, an alcohol or a cold sponge bath is recommended for reducing a patient's elevated temperature. Alcohol added to tepid water is tolerated more easily than a cold bath by most patients. Alcohol vaporizes at a relatively low temperature and therefore removes heat from the skin surfaces rapidly. Cold water very often produces a strong initial reactionary effect which elevates the temperature further.

When an alcohol or a cold sponge bath is given, it is essential that it be continued until the initial reaction of chilliness, or shivering, is overcome and the body has adjusted to the temperature. Therefore, it is considered preferable that the procedure lasts for at least 25 to 30 minutes. Each extremity should be bathed for at least five minutes, and then the entire back and the buttocks for an additional five to ten minutes.

During the procedure, place moist, cool cloths over large superficial blood vessels, as in the axilla and the groin as a further aid in lowering the temperature. A warm water bottle placed at the feet helps to overcome a sensation of chilliness. To help prevent congestion and to provide comfort, an ice bag is applied to the head.

Mechanical hypothermia blankets or mattresses and plastic pads through which a thermostatically controlled solution is circulated are available for use with patients who need prolonged hypothermia.

Therapeutic Applications of Heat

The optimum temperature for applying local hot applications cannot be stated. As has been pointed out, the condition of the skin, the size of the area being covered, the duration of the application, the method of applying heat (moist or dry), the condition of the patient, and the differences in heat tolerances need to be considered when determining optimum temperatures for applying heat. When the temperature of the skin surpasses approximately 43° C. (110° F.), many individuals are likely to suffer burns.

The temperature of water used for applications is described usually as neutral or warm, hot, and very hot. The temperature ranges stated frequently are as follows:

Warm or neutral	Approximately 34° to 37° C. (93° to 98° F.)
Hot	Approximately 37° to 41° C. (98° to 105° F.)
Very hot	Approximately 41° to 46° C. (105° to 115° F.)

The common methods for applying heat discussed later in this chapter state the temperature ranges for applications which have been found satisfactory for most persons. However, checking the condition of the patient's skin is still necessary in order to avoid possible tissue damage.

Effects of Very Hot Applications.

If very hot applications are applied to the skin for short periods, the reaction is similar to that of cold; that is, the cutaneous vessels may contract and decrease the blood supply. The reason is that the body is protecting itself against excessive loss of internal heat when exposed to an extreme of temperature in the environment. Muscles may fail to relax. Warm applications, on the other hand, lead to relaxation of muscles and increased blood supply. The effects of a warm bath and of a hot shower illustrate this difference in reaction of the body when warmth and heat are used. Contraction of small vessels is a desired reaction when hemorrhage is present, but cold rather than very hot applications are used more commonly to aid in checking bleeding.

There is logic in this when one recalls that cold increases the viscosity of blood. Increased viscosity slows the speed of flow, and blood clotting is facilitated by lower speed of circulation with vasoconstriction resulting from the cold.

Electric Heating Pads.   The electric heating pad is a popular means for applying dry heat locally. It is easy to apply, provides constant and even heat, and is relatively safe to use. Nevertheless, careless handling can result in injury to the patient or the nurse as well as damage to the pad.

The heating element of an electric pad consists of a web of wires that convert electric current into heat. Crushing or creasing the wires may impair proper functioning, and portions of the pad will overheat. Burns and fire may result. Pins should be avoided for securing a pad, since there is danger of electric shock if a pin touches the wires. Pads with a waterproof covering are preferred, but they should not be operated in a wet or moist condition because of danger of short-circuiting the heating element and consequent shock.

Heating pads for home use have a selector switch for controlling the heat. After the heat has been applied and a certain amount of depression of the peripheral nerve endings has taken place, the patient often increases the heat because the pad does not feel sufficiently warm. Many persons have been burned in this manner.

The nurse should instruct the patient not to place a heating pad under a portion of the body or an extremity. If the heating pad is between the patient and the mattress, there may be inadequate heat dissipation. These circumstances could lead to burning the patient or bed linens. The heating pad should be placed anteriorly or laterally to a body part.

Like other devices for applying dry heat, electric pads should be covered with flannel or similar material. This helps to make the heat therapy more comfortable for the patient. The pad can be used repeatedly when the cover is washed after each patient's use. However, it is important not to cover the pad too heavily, for heavy covering over an electric pad prevents adequate heat dissipation.

Because of problems with burning, some health agencies do not allow the use of electric heating pads. If a patient insists on using one, he is asked to sign a form freeing the agency of liability should he sustain a burn from its use. Electric heating pads with a preset temperature control are used in some health agencies to help prevent accidents with burning. An electric heating pad can be dangerous when not used properly and carefully.

Plastic pads with tubular inner construction which can be filled with water are also available for providing local heat. One is illustrated in Figure 22–17. An electric control unit attached to the pad heats the water and keeps it at an even temperature. The temperature is set prior to operation and the patient cannot change it because it requires a key. Such pads are useful on wet dressings when heat must be applied.

Hot Water Bags.   When electric heating pads are not available, frequently the hot water bag is used. Hot water bags have disadvantages in that they may leak, and their weight makes them less comfortable than the electric pad. However, they are less expensive and may be safer for some patients.

To help to prevent burning the patient, it is considered essential to test the temperature of the water accurately with a thermometer before pouring it into the bag. A safe temperature range for infants under two years of age is from 41° to 46° C. (105° to 115° F.); for children over two years of age and for adults, from 46° to 52° C. (115° to 125° F.).

In order to keep the bag as light as possible in weight and easy to mold to the body area, it should be filled about two-thirds full. The air remaining in the bag can be expelled in one of two ways: by placing the bag on a flat surface and permitting the water to come to the opening and then closing the bag; or by holding the bag up and twisting the unfilled portion to remove the air and then closing it. After the bag has been filled, hold it upside down to test it for leaks. Apply the flannel cover to the bag securely before placing it on the body part. In order that the patient may feel warmth immediately, the cover can be warmed before it is placed on the hot water bag. Otherwise, it will

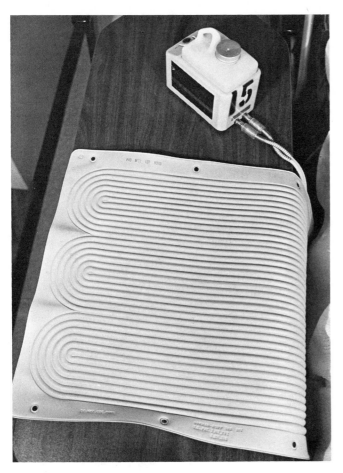

Figure 22–17   This electric device can be set to maintain water at a constant temperature and circulate it through the coils of the plastic pad. The pad can be used to provide dry heat or it can be placed over a moist dressing to provide moist heat.

take time for the heat of the bag to be transmitted through the covering.

The temperature ranges given above will produce the desired local effects if the bag is filled properly and the cover warmed. However, many patients will tend to think that the water is not hot enough. Unless the patient receives an explanation beyond simply telling him that the temperature will not burn him, it is likely that the bag may be filled from the hot water tap when the nurse is not around. If the patient cannot do it, a visitor or another patient may oblige.

Hot Moist Packs and Compresses. Moist cloths or dressings applied to a large body area are called *packs*. Packs usually are applied to a more extensive area than compresses. Packs and compresses are generally applied as hot as the patient can tolerate them comfortably.

Depending on the situation, a pack or compress may be applied using sterile technique. If so, all materials and the solution must be sterile and the person applying the pack or compress wears sterile gloves.

If the compress or pack is to remain in place for an extended period, the frequency of the change of the application will depend on the thickness of the material used for the application and the amount of protection used for maintaining the temperature. A warm water bottle, a heating pad, or a mechanical heating device can be used to maintain the temperature of a pack or compress. However, since moisture increases the heat conduction, a lower temperature should be used than when dry heat is applied to avoid tissue damage.

Because of the effect of the moist hot applications on circulation, the patient is likely to feel chilly. Precautionary comfort measures should be taken during and following the treatment to keep the patient, and especially the area which has been treated, warm and free from drafts. Applyng a hot moist pack or compress is described in the chart on page 562.

Commercially prepared sterile premoistened compresses are available in many health agencies. These compresses are moistened either with sterile normal saline or sterile water. The exterior of the package is designed so that the compresses can be used for cold applications or heated by an infrared lamp for heat applications. The precautions and observations used in the traditional methods are applicable to this technique too.

Proper positioning of the patient is also important, especially if the pack is to be left in place for an extended time. Figure 22–18 on page 563 shows a patient with a leg pack supported in good alignment.

Hip or Sitz Baths. As a means of applying tepid or hot water to the pelvic area, patients are often placed in a tub filled with sufficient water to reach the umbilicus. These baths are called *hip* or *sitz baths*. Special tubs and chairs or basins which fit onto the toilet seat are available. Sitz tubs and chairs are designed so that the patient's buttocks fit into a rather deep seat which is filled with water of the desired temperature; the legs and the feet remain out of the water. The basin is smaller in size, and permits primarily the perineal area to be in contact with the water. The basins are disposable and economical for home or health agency use. A regular bathtub is not as satisfactory for a sitz bath because the heat is applied also to the lower extremities, and this alters the effect desired in the pelvic region.

If the purpose of the sitz bath is to apply heat, water

Appling hot moist compresses or packs to a body area

The purpose is to apply heat to an area to produce changes in the blood vessels and the underlying tissues.

SUGGESTED ACTION	RATIONALE
Prepare pieces of woolen, flannel, or gauze material sufficiently large to cover the area adequately.	Absorbent and loosely woven fibers hold moisture.
Prepare a hot water bag, heating pad, or other heating device to keep application hot.	External heat continually applied to the moist application will slow cooling.
Immerse the packs in hot water until they are saturated.	The woolen or flannel material absorbs the water slowly.
Prepare the patient's body area so that no time will be wasted in applying the pack after it is removed from the hot water. Place a dry pack and a waterproof cover under the extremity or near the area where the pack is to be applied. the dry pack will cover the moist one, and the waterproof cover will be on the outside.	Air will reduce the temperature of the pack. The dry pack and the waterproof cover will act as insulation and will prevent rapid heat and moisture loss from the wet pack.
Lubricate the skin in the area of application with petrolatum if desired and if the skin is unbroken.	Petrolatum delays the transmission of the heat from the pack to the skin.
Wring the hot wet packs until water does not drip from them.	Saturated packs are heavy and will lose water. Both can cause discomfort for the patient.
Shake once or twice.	Loss of steam helps to reduce temperature.
Place the pack on the skin lightly and, after a few seconds, lift the pack to inspect the patient's skin for degree of redness.	Degree of vasodilation indicates intensity of heat.
Wrap the pack around the area snugly and mold it to the skin surface.	Air is a poor conductor of heat. Air spaces between the skin and the pack will reduce the effect of the application.
Cover the moist pack tightly with the dry pack and waterproof covering. Secure in place with safety pins or ties.	Insulation and covering prevent heat and moisture loss.
Apply the hot water bottle, heating device, or heating pad to the area in a manner so the weight is not increased over the wound area.	External heat will help to maintain the pack temperature. Weight of the heat supply can cause fatigue and discomfort.

at a temperature of 43° to 46° C. (110° to 115° F.) for 15 minutes will produce relaxation of the parts involved after a short initial period of contraction. Warm water should not be used if considerable congestion is already present.

If the purpose of the sitz bath is to produce relaxation or to help to promote healing in a wound by cleaning it of discharge and debris, then water at a temperature of 34° to 37° C. (94° to 98° F.) is used. The temperature of the water should be tested frequently to prevent too great a deviation from the desired range from occurring.

Since a large body area is involved when a sitz bath is given, the patient should be observed closely for signs of weakness and faintness. The nature of the procedure also makes it necessary to protect the patient from exposure. Usually, a bath blanket is wrapped around the patient's shoulders and then draped over the tub. After the bath, the patient should be covered adequately and encouraged to remain out of drafts. If a warm sitz bath has been given, it may be best for the patient to lie down until normal circulation is resumed.

Sitz tubs and chairs are not adjustable to the comfort needs of patients, especially short patients. After the patient is in the tub or the chair, check to see whether or not there is pressure against the patient's thighs or legs. If the patient's feet do not touch the floor, and the weight of the legs is resting on the edge of the chair, a stool should be procured to support the feet and relieve the pressure on the vessels in the legs.

In addition to avoiding any pressure areas, it may be necessary to place a towel in the water to support the patient's back in the lumbar region. Fifteen to 20 minutes can seem like a very long time if one's body is not in good alignment and comfortable.

Soaks. The direct immersion of a body area into warm water or a medicated solution is called a soak. The purposes of soaks vary: to increase blood supply to a locally infected area, to aid suppuration, to aid in cleaning large sloughing wounds such as burns, to improve circulation, and to apply medication to a locally infected area. A soak has the added advantage of making manipulation of a painful area much easier, since the body part is buoyed up by the weight of water it displaces.

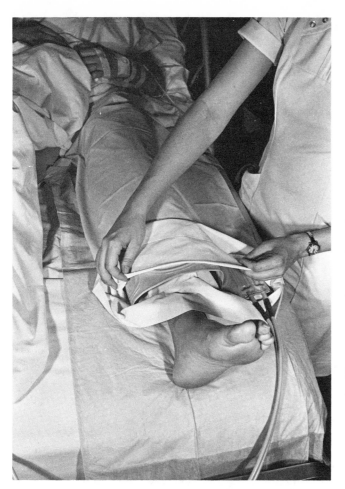

Figure 22–18 The nurse has changed the patient's dressing, positoned her leg, and is now arranging the heating pad before she replaces the footboard. Alignment and support of the extremity are important for preventing fatigue and muscle complications.

If a soak is prescribed for a large wound, such as might cover an entire arm or lower leg or even an area of the torso, a compromise with sterile technique usually is made. The container into which the body area is placed is sterilized before use if possible; if not, the container should be cleaned scrupulously. Tap water may be used for soaks, since it is accepted generally as being free from pathogens.

During the treatment, which is usually 15 to 20 minutes per soak, the temperature should be kept as constant as possible. This may be done by discarding some of the fluid every five minutes and replacing it, or by adding solutions at a higher temperature.

Care must be taken to avoid burning the patient. If hot solution is added and it is not stirred or otherwise agitated, it may not diffuse into the cooler solution quickly enough to prevent discomfort or tissue injury.

Unless the temperature of the soak is prescribed otherwise, a range of 41° to 43° C. (105° to 110° F.) is considered as being physiologically effective and comfortable for the patient.

The container holding the fluid should be positioned so that the part to be immersed is comfortable and the patient is in good body alignment. For example, an arm basin placed on top of the bedside stand may cause the patient's shoulders to be thrown out of alignment, and it may also cause pressure on the back of the patient's arm. Or, a hand basin may be so situated as to cause wrist fatigue. Whenever a soak basin is placed in position, the nurse should look for pressure areas and observe the patient's degree of comfort.

Diathermy. *Diathermy* is the production of heat in body tissue by the use of high-frequency currents. It is used generally for producing heat in deep tissues. Special equipment is used for diathermy; generally, trained technicians are responsible for giving diathermy treatments. The reaction of the deep tissue to the heat produced by diathermy is similar to that of the skin and more superficial tissue when heat is applied locally.

PROMOTING TISSUE HEALING AND THE NURSING PROCESS

The exact data to be collected when caring for a patient with a wound will be determined by the particular situation. However, the following questions suggest information which can be helpful in providing care. What is the nature of the patient's wound? Is it open or closed? Was it an accidental or intentional wound? What is the appearance of the wound? If inflammation is present, at what stage is it? If drainage is present, what are its characteristics? If healing is occurring, at what phase is it? How is the person responding to the wound physiologically and psychologically? Does the patient have any preexisting health problems or is he taking medications routinely which are known to delay healing? How is the wound protected? How is the wound immobilized?

Standards for assessing the data must be selected in accordance with the information gathered. General norms pertaining to inflammation and wound healing have been presented in this chapter. More precise standards for specific types of wounds can be found in clinical texts.

Planning for meeting the nursing needs of the person with a wound depends on the specific situation. As indicated, many persons care for their own wounds after being seen as an ambulatory patient or following hospital discharge. Therefore, planning for wound care should include teaching of the patient and the family. Like other aspects of nursing care, planning for wound care should also incorporate the preferences of the patient and his situation with the therapeutic measures being considered.

The precise nursing intervention for a patient is determined by his plan of care. Many nursing measures for care of a patient with a wound have been discussed in this chapter. The following statements will summarize the use of some of the measures in nursing intervention.

- Facilitate the body's normal defense mechanisms. Inflammation, suppuration, and healing are physiological processes normally carried out by the body. In most instances, cleaning, protecting, and immobilizing a wound is all that is necessary to promote the body's normal restorative processes. In some situations, drugs, applications of heat or cold, and the promotion of drainage may be additional measures which speed healing. The body heals itself and intervention measures at best only facilitate the normal processes.

- Support systemic body processes. Even though a wound may be localized, the patient responds as a whole to the injury. Therefore, therapy should be directed toward the whole person. Psychological support is important no matter how small the wound appears. For example, severe physiological shock can follow an accident when tissue injury is minor. Adequate nutrition and fluid intake play a major part in the body's response to a wound and to healing. Sufficient rest can permit the body to focus its energies on the injury. Reducing the exposure to pathogens can prevent not only wound infections but systemic infections due to the person's lowered resistance following trauma. Actions which are directed toward supporting and enhancing the person's general emotional and physiological reserves aid wound healing.

- Increase precautionary measures for persons who have slow or impaired healing processes. Generally, patients who are very young, old, have chronic diseases, or are receiving other therapy have slower wound healing and are more susceptible to complications. For this reason, special efforts to promote healing in these persons often need to be initiated immediately and before indications of problems exist. Special diets and means of assuring adquate nutrition and fluid intake can be instituted, strict

surgical asepsis should be practiced even on minor wounds, positioning and elastic stockings can be used to maintain adequate circulation, and active and passive range of motion exercises should be initiated to prevent the loss of muscle tone. By taking these and other precautionary measures, problems with wound healing can often be avoided.

- Avoid the entrance of microorganisms into open wounds. Nonpathogenic organisms which exist routinely on the skin without problem can cause infections or lower the resistance to pathogens when they enter a wound. For this reason, every precaution should be taken to maintain an open wound as free from organisms as possible. The larger the wound, the more imperative this becomes. The hands of health personnel are one of the most common means of introducing organisms into wounds. Therefore, careful handwashing both before and after handling wounds cannot be overemphasized.

- Provide explanations for all aspects of wound care. If the nurse develops the habit of providing an explanation for wound care each time she gives it, she can provide health teaching with little effort. Such teaching can help the patient learn to care for his existing wound and also help to prepare him for caring for future injuries and wounds.

- Anticipate that edema will generally occur adjacent to wounds. Depending on the extent of the wound, the maximum inflammatory reaction and associated edema will generally occur within the first 24 to 48 hours. In some instances, it may take longer. By anticipating the edema, the nurse knows she should check the wound site more frequently during the first several days to detect whether dressings, bandages, binders, casts, and other confining devices may become too tight and impair circulation. Loosening or altering the device may be necessary. Positioning is also important during this period to avoid a dependent position for the wound site and to assure maximum venous return. Applications of cold and heat may also be used for controlling edema.

The parts of the nursing process and of the process as a whole are evaluated as described in Chapter 4.

CONCLUSION

Tissue trauma is a common occurrence. The ability of the body to contain and heal an injury is truly remarkable. Nursing actions discussed in this and other chapters throughout this book can serve to promote the physiological processes of the body. Since many persons care for accidental injuries without ever seeking the assistance of health personnel, attempts to increase their knowledge of the body's defensive and restorative processes, and ways of supporting them can be classified as a means of health maintenance for the future. At the time of dealing with an existing injury, the patient is very often interested and motivated to learn.

SUPPLEMENTAL LIBRARY STUDY

1. The author of the following article suggests several methods for promoting wound healing.

   Castle, Mary. "Wound Care: Clear-Cut Ways to Speed Healing." *Nursing 75,* 5:40–44, August 1975.

   What ways are identified to deal with copious drainage? What technique is recommended to prevent inoculation of the wound with infecting organisms?

2. Casts have been a common way of immobilizing fractures for many years. These authors describe a new method of treating fractures.

   Deyerle, William M. and Crossland, Sharon A. "Broken Legs Are to be Walked On." *American Journal of Nursing,* 77:1927–1930, December 1977.

   What advantages do the thigh lacer and the cast brace have over the traditional plaster of Paris cast? What new nursing responsibilities arise with the use of these devices?

3. Proper first aid for open wounds makes an important contribution to minimizing complications for the injured person. The following article discusses some emergency techniques for dealing with wounds.

   Boericke, Peter H. "Emergency! Part 2: First Aid for Open Wounds, Severe Bleeding, Shock, and Closed Wounds." *Nursing 75,* 5:40–47, March 1975.

   Prepare a list of the steps involved in managing open wounds during an emergency situation.

4. Observation for early signs of complications when a patient has a fracture is an important responsibility of the nurse. This author refers to the most important observations as the five P's.

   Webb, Kenneth. "Early Assessment of Orthopedic Injuries." *American Journal of Nursing,* 74:1048–1052, June 1974.

   What are the P's? What specific changes in each P would you report.

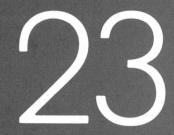

BEHAVIORAL OBJECTIVES

When content in this chapter has been mastered, the student will be able to

Define terms appearing in the glossary.

List primary functions of water in the body, indicate sources of body water, and describe how water is lost from the body.

Describe the compartments in which body fluids are normally found.

Explain how the hydrogen ion is used to develop a standard of chemical activity or combining power and list the four most common cations and the six most common anions in the body.

Describe the five most common ways in which body fluids are delivered to and from intracellular compartments.

Indicate how acid-base balance is maintained by the body's carbonic acid-sodium bicarbonate buffering system; the protein buffering system; and the phosphate buffering system.

Explain briefly how the lungs and kidneys; the circulatory, endocrine, and nervous systems; and the gastrointestinal tract function to help maintain fluid and acid-base balance.

List nine principle electrolytes of the body and describe the primary role of each in the body. Indicate the primary sources from which the body obtains each and the system or organ primarily responsible for regulating its level of concentration.

List four common water, eight common electrolyte, and four common acid-base imbalances; indicate common signs/symptoms of each; and list several conditions that typically lead to imbalances.

Indicate normal ranges of the principle electrolytes in plasma; of hemoglobin and hematocrit levels; and of partial pressure of carbon dioxide and oxygen in arterial blood. Indicate differences, when they occur, among children, men, and women.

Indicate normal ranges of the pH level of plasma and of urine, and of the specific gravity of urine.

Identify eight common signs and symptoms of fluid imbalances manifested in body tissues, in behavior, and in measurements for which the nurse should be alert.

Summarize fluid balance and imbalance, using the nursing process as a guide.

Fluid Balance and Common Imbalances

GLOSSARY

Acid: A substance containing a hydrogen ion that can be liberated or released.

Acidosis: The condition characterized by a proportionate excess of hydrogen ions in the extracellular fluid in which the pH falls below 7.35.

Active Transport: The movement of substances, including electrolytes, against a concentration gradient where energy is required.

Alkali: A substance that can accept or trap a hydrogen ion. Synonym for base.

Alkalosis: A condition characterized by a proportionate lack of hydrogen ions in the extracellular fluid concentration, in which the pH exceeds 7.45.

Anion: An ion which carries a negative electrical charge.

Base: A substance that can accept or trap a hydrogen ion. Synonym for alkali.

Body Fluid: The liquid part of the body consisting of both water and its solutes.

Body Water: The liquid part of the body consisting of water only.

Buffer: A substance that prevents body fluid from becoming overly acid or alkaline.

Cation: An ion which carries a positive electrical charge.

Cellular Fluid: Fluid within the cell. Synonym for intracellular fluid.

Colloid Osmotic Pressure: Pressure exerted by plasma proteins on permeable membranes in the body. Synonym for oncotic pressure.

Crenation: The process of losing fluid from a red blood cell which eventually results in a shrunken, knobbed cell due to loss of intracellular water.

Dehydration: Decreased extracellular water volume.

Diffusion: The tendency of solutes to move freely throughout a solvent from an area of higher concentration to an area of lower concentration until equilibrium is established.

Electrolyte: A substance capable of breaking into ions and developing an electrical charge when dissolved in solution.

Extracellular Fluid: Fluid outside the cells. Abbreviated ECF. It includes intravascular and interstitial fluids.

Filtration: The passage of a fluid through a permeable membrane whose spaces do not allow certain solutes to pass. Passage is from an area of higher pressure to one of lower pressure.

Filtration Pressure: The difference between colloid osmotic pressure and blood hydrostatic pressure.

Fluid Balance: The state in which water and its solutes in the body are in normal proportions and concentrations and are in appropriate body compartments.

Fluid Imbalance: The state in which water and its solutes in the body are in improper proportions and concentrations and/or are improperly located in body compartments.

Hemolysis: The freeing of a red blood cell of its hemoglobin by destruction of the cell membrane.

Hydration: The union of a substance with water. The term is often used as the opposite of dehydration, in which case it means that there is normal intra- and extracellular water volume.

Hydrostatic Pressure: The force exerted by a fluid against the container wall.

Hypercalcemia: An excess of calcium in extracellular fluid.

Hyperkalemia: An excess of potassium in the extracellular fluid.

Hypermagnesemia: An excess of magnesium in extracellular fluid.

Hypernatremia: An excess of sodium in extracellular fluid.

Hypertonic: Having a greater concentration than the solution with which it is being compared.

Hypervolemia: An excess of fluid in extracellular areas.

Hypocalcemia: An insufficient amount of calcium in the extracellular fluid.

Hypokalemia: An insufficient amount of potassium in the extracellular fluid.

Hypomagnesemia: An insufficient amount of magnesium in the extracellular fluid.

Hyponatremia: An insufficient amount of sodium in the extracellular fluid.

Hypoproteinemia: An insufficient amount of protein substances in the extracellular fluid.

Hypotonic: Having a lesser concentration than the solution with which it is being compared.

Hypovolemia: A deficiency in fluid in the extracellular fluid.

Insensible Water Loss: Nonperceptible water being lost from the body as moisture through the breath and by evaporation from the skin.

Interstitial Fluid: Fluid between the cells.

Intracellular Fluid: Fluid within the cell. Abbreviated ICF. Synonym for cellular fluid.

Intravascular Fluid: Fluid within the vascular system. Synonym for plasma.

Ion: An atom or molecule carrying an electrical charge in solution.

Ionization: The process by which substances dissociate to form ions.

Isotonic: Having approximately the same concentration as the solution with which it is being compared.

Liter: A metric standard of measurement for liquids. Abbreviated L. One liter contains 1,000 milliliters.

Lysis: The disintegration of any cell.

Metabolic Acidosis: A proportionate deficiency of bicarbonate ions in the extracellular fluid.

Metabolic Alkalosis: A proportionate excess of bicarbonate ions in the extracellular fluid.

Milliequivalent: A unit of measurement to describe electrolyte chemical activity. Abbreviated mEq. One milliequivalent is equivalent to the activity of 1 milligram of hydrogen.

Milliliter: One-thousandth of a liter. Abbreviated ml.

Nonelectrolyte: Molecules which remain intact and do not ionize. Synonym for undissociated molecules.

Oncotic Pressure: Pressure exerted by plasma proteins on permeable membranes in the body. Synonym for colloid osmotic pressure.

Osmolality: The total number of dissolved particles in a solution; it describes concentration of solutes in a solvent.

Osmosis: The passage of a solvent through a semipermeable membrane from an area of lesser concentration to an area of greater concentration until equilibrium is established.

Osmotic Pressure: The drawing power for water or the attraction for water exerted by solute particles.

Osteomalacia: Softening of the bones due usually to a deficiency or loss of calcium salts from the body.

Overhydration: Above normal amounts of water in extracellular spaces.

pH: An expression of hydrogen ion concentration and resulting acidity of a substance.

Phagocytosis: The cell's engulfing of substances in order to destroy them.

Pinocytosis: The cell's taking in of substances by invagination of the cell membrane.

Plasma: The liquid constituent of blood. Synonym for intravascular fluid.

Preformed Water: Water in food.

Respiratory Acidosis: A proportionate excess of carbonic acid in the extracellular fluid.

Respiratory Alkalosis: A proportionate deficiency of carbonic acid in the extracellular fluid.

Semipermeable Membrane: A selectively permeable membrane which allows water to pass through it but is either impermeable or very selectively permeable to solutes.

Solute: The substance that is dissolved in a solution.

Solvent: A liquid holding a substance in solution.

Total Body Water: The total amount of water in the body expressed as a percentage of body weight. Abbreviated TBW. The term total body fluid, abbreviated TBF, is also used; fluids are usually considered to include water and electrolytes.

Turgor: Normal tension within a cell.

Undissociated Molecules: Molecules that remain intact and do not ionize. Synonym for nonelectrolytes.

INTRODUCTION

Fluid balance is essential for health. The body with its remarkable adaptive ability, maintains balance normally by integrated physiological processes which result in a relatively constant but dynamic cell environment. The task is indeed formidable. We ingest a wide variety of materials of various quantities, often unmatched with body needs, and dispose of wastes and excesses as a result of intricate mechanisms to maintain a relatively small range of normality. This ability of the body to maintain fluid balance is homeostasis, a term that was discussed in Chapter 10. When balance cannot be attained, assistance must be offered since serious imbalances may become a threat to life itself.

Some conditions in the healthy person and virtually all illnesses threaten fluid balance. For example, participating in extensive outdoor physical activity on a hot day, going for a long time without an adequate water intake, or eating a poorly balanced diet for an extended period can cause disturbances in fluid balance. Conditions resulting in vomiting, diarrhea, and an elevated body temperature, or illness states such as diabetes mellitus and burns, surgical procedures, and infectious processes frequently upset fluid balance. Therapeutic regimens also may upset fluid balance. The use of diuretics and of some of the adrenal cortex hormones upset the balance if not used judiciously.

BODY WATER

Many authors and clinicians differentiate between the terms, body fluid and body water. *Body water* refers to water only. *Body fluid* includes both water and its solutes. A *solute* is the substance that is dissolved in a solution, and a *solvent* is a liquid holding a substance in solution. *Fluid balance* means that water and its solutes in the body are in normal proportions and concentrations and are in their appropriate compartments. *Fluid imbalance* means that water and its solutes in the body are in improper proportions and concentrations and/or are inappropriately located. In almost all instances, it is appropriate to use the term body fluids, even when only body water is in question, because all body liquids contain both the solvent water and its various solutes.

Water has various functions in the body. It serves as a medium for transporting nutrients to cells and for excreting cell wastes. Within the cell, it is important for cellular metabolism. It acts as the solvent for both electrolytes and nonelectrolytes. In addition, water serves to help maintain body temperature, to aid digestion, and to promote elimination. It transports such substances as hormones, enzymes, red and white blood cells, plus many other substances.

Fluids are located in various compartments or spaces in the body. There is fluid in each of the cells which is called *intracellular fluid*, abbreviated ICF, or *cellular fluid*. This fluid serves as the internal medium necessary for the cell's proper chemical functioning. *Extracellular fluid*, abbreviated ECF, is all fluid outside of the cells. It acts to transport nutrients to and wastes from the cells. Extracellular fluid consists of the body's plasma which is called *intravascular fluid*. *Plasma* is the liquid constituent of blood. Extracellular fluid also consists of the fluid in which tissue cells are bathed; it is called *interstitial fluid*.

In health, normal *total body water,* often abbreviated

TABLE 23–1 Average percentages of water in relation to body weight in persons of different ages in the various water compartments of the body

| WATER COMPARTMENT | INFANT | ADULT | | ELDERLY |
		MALE	FEMALE	
Extracellular				
Intravascular	4%	4%	5%	5%
Interstitial	25%	11%	10%	15%
Intracellular	48%	45%	35%	25%
TOTAL BODY WATER	77%	60%	50%	45%

TBW, comprises approximately 45 to 75 percent of the body's weight. The letters, TBF, refer to total body fluid. The variations depend on several factors, as is shown in Table 23–1.

Note that Table 23–1 describes amounts of body water in an infant. Because infants have a higher basal metabolism rate, a proportionately greater body surface, and a larger percentage of body water than an adult, they suffer from deficits more quickly than older persons. Also, infants normally require relatively greater water intake in proportion to body weight than do adults. By the time a child reaches adolescence, the total body water and its distribution in the various compartments approximate that of an adult.

Table 23–1 also illustrates that the elderly person has a lesser amount of body water than the younger adult. This can be observed in the elderly by dry skin, dry hair, and wrinkles. Hence, just as with youngsters, elderly persons suffer from water deficits more quickly than do younger adults.

Total body water also depends on the build of a person. Because fat tissues contain a small amount of water, the more obese the person, the smaller the percentage of total body water when compared with body weight. In an obese male, total body water can be as little as 50 percent of body weight; in an obese female, total body water can be as little as 42 percent of body weight.

Water for the body is derived from the ingestion of liquids and food and from metabolic oxidation. The amount of water available to the body tissues varies with the individual but average daily amounts have been established for the healthy adult. Figure 23–1 on page 570 shows these amounts.

As can be observed in Figure 23–1, oral ingestion of liquids makes up the largest amount of fluid normally taken into the body. Personal habits and circumstances are responsible for the variations.

Water in food, or *preformed water,* makes up the next largest water source. This also varies extensively de-pending on the dietary items that are eaten. Melons and citrus fruits have a high-water content while cereals and dried fruits have a relatively low-water content.

When food is oxidized during metabolism, water is one of the end products. Water made available through metabolic oxidation varies with nutrients. Metabolism of 100 Gm. of fat produces 107 Gm. of water while 100 Gm. of carbohydrate will yield 55 Gm. of water, and 100 Gm. of protein will produce 40 Gm. of water. Therefore, a person eating a high-fat diet will have a proportionately greater amount of water resulting from his metabolic process than a person having a high-protein diet.

Average daily amounts of water necessary for balance in children is based on various formulae using body weight or body surface areas. The age of the child in itself is not a reliable indicator for calculating fluid requirements. Texts dealing with the care of children contain various formulae used for estimating fluid requirements for children of different ages.

Like water intake, losses vary with the individual and his circumstances and no absolute standards can be given. However, average amounts have been established and are also given in Figure 23–1. Water is lost from the body normally through the kidneys with urine, through the intestinal tract with feces, and through the skin as perspiration. Water is also lost in insensible ways. *Insensible water loss is water loss that is nonperceptible.* For example, in addition to perspiration which is perceptible, an invisible amount of water is lost from the skin constantly through evaporation. Insensible loss from the lungs is moisture exhaled through the breath.

Authorities indicate a range of 1,500 ml. to 3,500 ml. daily is a desirable adult fluid intake and loss. The majority of individuals have a 2,000 ml. average intake and loss per day. While these figures are helpful as guidelines, the person's balance between his actual intake and loss must be considered when assessing nursing needs. An individual's intake should normally

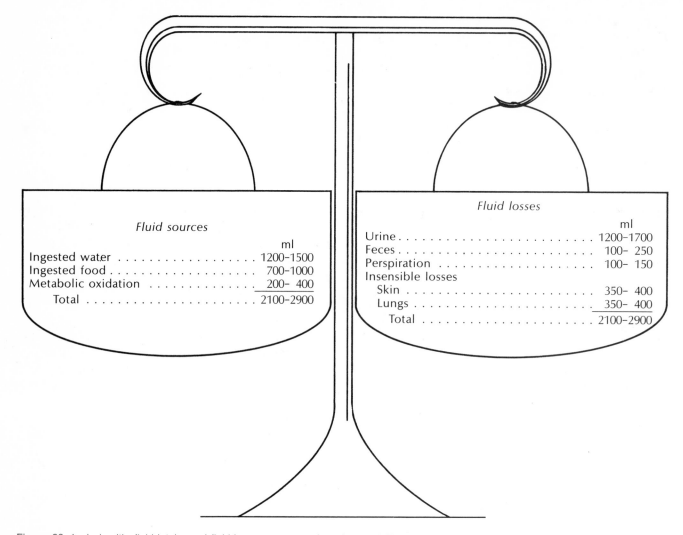

Figure 23–1   In health, fluid intake and fluid losses are approximately equal. The amounts indicated are average adult daily fluid sources and losses.

be approximately balanced by his output or fluid loss. A general rule is that in the healthy adult, the output of urine normally approximates the ingestion of liquids; and the water from food and oxidation is balanced by the water loss through the feces, the skin, and the respiratory process. The intake should be within the desirable average range. The intake-output balance may not always exist in a single 24-hour period but should normally be achieved within two to three days.

Marked deviations from this approximate balance of intake and output alert the nurse to impending and possibly preventable imbalance. They may be symptomatic of illness. For example, two symptoms of diabetes

mellitus are excessive urinary output and excessive thirst; a symptom of a urinary tract infection is frequent urination; and disinterest in fluid and food intake occurs frequently in the presence of many infections.

The body is in a state of peril when water imbalances occur. The nurse needs to be aware of factors which influence a patient's water intake and output in order to plan care that helps the patient maintain water balance. A person may retain water in abnormal amounts which results in edema. Edema, to be discussed later in this chapter, is a common symptom in persons with certain heart diseases. On the other hand, a person may have an increased water loss because of an elevated environmental temperature, decreased relative humidity in the environment, increased physical activity, or an extended period of mouth breathing. Table 23–2 illustrates how an adult's fluid losses vary with certain changing circumstances. An elevated body temperature, vomiting, diarrhea, kidney malfunction, blood loss, or wound drainage also influence fluid loss. The body's homeostatic mechanisms will attempt to conserve water loss from one exit route when the loss is increased from another. Thus, the person who is perspiring profusely will ordinarily have less urinary output. But in many circumstances, the body needs help to maintain balance when water is either retained or lost in abnormal amounts. Hence, the nurse has the responsibility of helping to increase or decrease the patient's intake of water when retention or losses are greater than normal.

ELECTROLYTES AND NONELECTROLYTES

Chemical compounds in solution tend to behave in one of two ways. If molecules remain intact, they are called undissociated or nonelectrolytes. In the human body, urea and glucose are undissociated.

Other compounds in solution dissociate to form ions by the process of ionization. An ion is an atom or molecule carrying an electrical charge in solution. Substances capable of breaking into electrically charged ions when dissolved in solution are called electrolytes. Some ions develop a positive electrical charge and are called cations. Others develop a negative charge and are called anions. Water is the solvent in the body that makes up solutions with solutes; the solutes are electrolytes and nonelectrolytes.

Measurements for water and electrolytes in the body have been universally adopted. The metric system is used for water. One liter, abbreviated L., is the standard for water. A liter is slightly larger than the common household measure of 1 quart. One liter contains 1,000 milliliters, abbreviated ml. In some instances, a cubic centimeter, abbreviated cc., has been used as an equivalent of 1 milliliter. The centimeter is a linear measurement and, hence, milliliter which is a liquid measurement, is preferred.

Electrolytes are dynamic chemicals. The unit of measure used to describe electrolytes is expressed in terms of their chemical combining power, or chemical activity. From chemistry one learns that the weight of an ion is not related to its combining ability. As an analogy, assume one wishes to compare the physical prowess of two persons. Their prowess is not necessarily related to their weight so in order to describe prowess, a standard by which one wishes to compare the two persons needs to be established.

The standard used to describe the chemical activity of electrolytes is the chemical activity of one milligram of hydrogen. The milliequivalent, abbreviated mEq., has been adopted as the unit of measure to describe the chemical activity of an electrolyte. One milliequivalent is chemically equivalent to the activity of 1 milligram of hydrogen. Stated inversely, 1 milligram of hydrogen exerts 1 milliequivalent of chemical activity. This is true whether the comparison with hydrogen is made with a cation or an anion. Hence, 1 milliequivalent of any cation is equivalent to 1 milliequivalent of any anion.

Using the milliequivalent system, the total cations in the body are normally equal to the total anions, as Figure 23–2 illustrates. Fluids in various compartments of the body differ from one another. For example, intravascular fluid contains more protein than intersti-

TABLE 23–2 Average daily water losses of healthy adults under varying circumstances

EXIT ROUTE	WHEN BODY TEMPERATURE IS NORMAL	WHEN AN ELEVATED TEMPERATURE IS PRESENT	FOLLOWING PROLONGED EXERCISE
Urine	ml.	ml.	ml.
Urine	1,400	1,200	500
Feces	200	200	200
Perspiration	100	1,400	5,000
Insensible loss			
Skin	350	350	350
Lungs	350	250	650
TOTAL	2,400	3,400	6,700

Adapted from Shepard, R. S., *Human Physiology*. p. 390. Philadelphia, J. B. Lippincott, 1971.

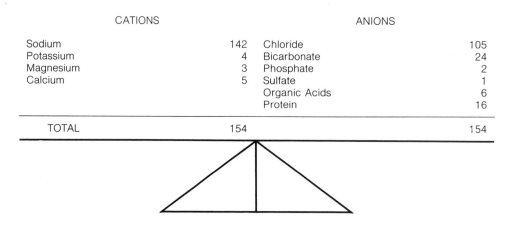

CATIONS		ANIONS	
Sodium	142	Chloride	105
Potassium	4	Bicarbonate	24
Magnesium	3	Phosphate	2
Calcium	5	Sulfate	1
		Organic Acids	6
		Protein	16
TOTAL	154		154

Figure 23-2 Intravascular electrolytes in milliequivalents per liter.

tial fluid; intracellular fluid has higher concentrations of potassium, phosphate, and protein than extracellular fluid. Figure 23–3 illustrates differences in the electrolyte composition of various body fluids.

Plasma is used to study the electrolytes in the body since plasma is easily accessible. Samples of blood are drawn for laboratory study of electrolyte composition in the plasma.

In a healthy person, the milliequivalents per liter for electrolytes vary within a narrow range. Just as was true of water, when electrolytes are not in normal balance, the person is in a state of jeopardy. Ranges of normal electrolyte values in plasma will be given later in this chapter.

METHODS OF TRANSPORTING BODY FLUIDS

Each body cell is nourished and gets rid of unwanted substances through the extracellular fluid. These exchanges which normally result in fluid balance and homeostasis are essential to life itself. There are several methods of transporting materials to and from intracellular compartments.

Osmosis

The membranes of cells have selective permeability; that is, these membranes are *semipermeable* because they allow water to pass through but are either impermeable or very selectively permeable to solutes. *Osmosis* is the passage of a solvent through a semipermeable membrane. When there are two solutions of different concentrations separated by a semipermeable membrane, the solvent (water) will pass from the area of lesser concentration to the area of greater concentration until equilibrium is established.

The term *osmolality,* often used to describe solution concentration, is defined as the total number of dissolved particles in a solution. When using this term, osmosis can be described thus: when two solutions of different osmolality are separated by a semipermeable membrane, water moves from the solution of higher to the solution of lower osmolality until equilibrium is established.

The electrolyte sodium, which is a constituent of table salt (NaCl), plays a critical role in water balance in the body. Assume three salt solutions of different concentrations are prepared and a red blood cell is placed in each solution. One solution is *isotonic;* that is, it has approximately the same concentration as the solution with which it is being compared. In the case of the red blood cell, an isotonic solution has the same concentration as the intracellular red blood cell fluid. A sodium chloride solution of 0.9 percent is isotonic when compared with body fluids and is usually called normal saline. If the solution into which the red blood cell is placed has a higher concentration than the intracellular fluid, the solution is said to be *hypertonic.* If the solution into which the red blood cell is placed has a lower concentration than the intracellular fluid, the solution is *hypotonic.* Figure 23–4 illustrates osmosis when the red blood cell was placed in isotonic, hypertonic, and hypotonic solutions. The figure also demonstrates the saying, "Water goes where salt is."

As the water molecules move through a semipermeable membrane from an area of lesser concentration to

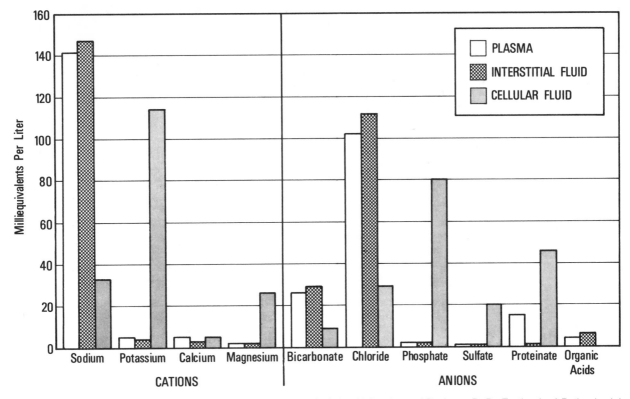

Figure 23-3   Electrolyte composition of normal body fluids. (From Snively, W. D., Jr., and Beshear, D. R.: Textbook of Pathophysiology, p. 136. Philadelphia, J. B. Lippincott Company, 1972.)

one that is higher, the volume of the more concentrated solution will increase and the volume of the weaker solution will decrease. The difference in volume produces pressure called *osmotic pressure* which can be defined as the drawing power for water or the attraction for water exerted by solute particles. The greater the difference in the concentration of two fluids on each side of a semipermeable membrane, the greater the osmotic pressure. In part A of Figure 23-4, there is no osmotic pressure; that is, the concentration of solutions in the beaker and in the cell are equal. Osmotic pressure will exist in parts B and C until the concentration of solutions in the cell and in the beaker is equal, unless the cell membrane eventually bursts, as illustrated in part B or until the fluid within the cell is depleted, as illustrated in part C.

Knowledge of osmosis is important when, for example, the patient receives intravenous fluids. Distilled water which is hypotonic is rarely used and hypertonic solutions are used with great care for intravenous therapy because of the danger of causing blood cells either to swell and burst or to shrink and shrivel. Intravenous fluids will be discussed further in Chapter 24.

Lysis is a general term meaning the disintegration of any cell. *Hemolysis* means the freeing of a red blood cell of its hemoglobin by destruction of the cell membrane. *Crenation* is the process of losing fluid from a red blood cell which eventually results in a shrunken, knobbed cell due to loss of intracellular water.

Osmosis is of great importance in the body. Water shifts, and, hence, fluid balance, depend heavily on this mode of transport.

Diffusion

Diffusion is the tendency of solutes to move freely throughout a solvent. The solute moves from an area of higher concentration to an area of lower concentration until equilibrium is established.

A typical chemistry laboratory experiment shows diffusion, as Figure 23-5 illustrates. When copper sulfate is placed in a beaker of water, the particles disperse equally throughout the solvent. The molecules bump about and against each other until they have scattered uniformly. Gases also move about by diffusion. For example, if an open pan of water is left in a room,

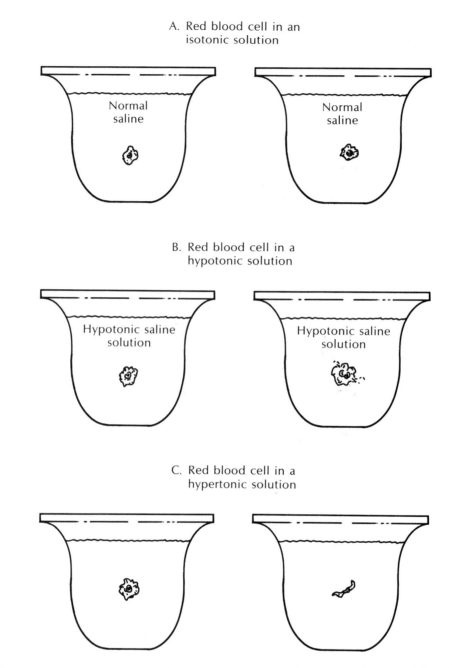

A. Red blood cell in an
isotonic solution

Normal
saline

Normal
saline

B. Red blood cell in a
hypotonic solution

Hypotonic saline
solution

Hypotonic saline
solution

C. Red blood cell in a
hypertonic solution

Figure 23–4 A. Although there will be exchanges of fluid between the red blood cell and the isotonic solution, there will be a balance; that is, the solvent will neither swell nor deplete the cell of its normal amount of water. B. After a red blood cell has been in a hypotonic solution, water will pass into the cell through its semipermeable membrane. Hence, the red blood cell will swell and eventually rupture, thus liberating hemoglobin. This process is called hemolysis. C. After a red blood cell has been in a hypertonic solution, water will pass out of the cell through its semipermeable membrane. Hence, the red blood cell will shrink and shrivel. This process is called crenation. Water goes where salt is, while each electrolyte particle strives for its fair share of available water.

evaporation occurs as the water molecules disperse themselves about the room. Oxygen and carbon dioxide exchange in the alveoli and in tissue cells occurs by diffusion.

Active Transport

When substances move from areas of lesser concentration to areas of higher concentration, active transport

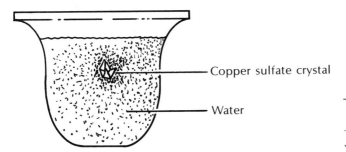

Figure 23-5 The copper sulfate crystal goes into solution when placed in water and the solute disperses equally eventually throughout the solvent. The solute moves from a higher concentration to a lower one. This tendency is called diffusion.

occurs. *Active transport* is the movement of substances, including electrolytes, against a concentration gradient where energy is required. Although the process is not completely understood, the energy requirement is affected by characteristics of the cell membrane, specific enzymes, and concentrations of ions. This process explains the so-called pump mechanism. It is illustrated in Figure 23-6 using sodium and potassium as examples. If diffusion can be called "coasting down hill," active transport can be called "pumping uphill." The following substances are believed to use active transport: amino acids; glucose but in certain places only, such as in the kidneys and intestines; and ions of sodium, potassium, hydrogen, phosphate, calcium, and magnesium.

Filtration

Filtration is the passage of a fluid through a permeable membrane whose spaces do not allow certain solutes to pass. Passage is from an area of higher pressure to one of lower pressure. It is important to know the process of filtration in order to understand how blood leaves the arterioles and enters the venules in the body's circulatory system.

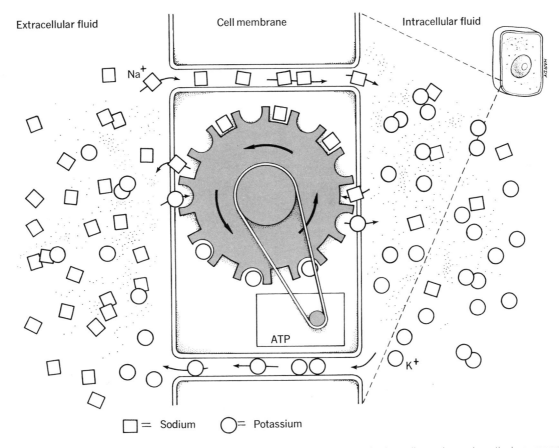

Figure 23-6 Active transport. Sodium (□) that diffuses into the cell through a pore in the cell membrane is actively pumped out of the cell by a carrier system, represented by the wheel. A similar fate awaits potassium (○) that diffuses out of the cell as it is actively pumped back into the cell.

Certain substances—those with high molecular weights, such as the plasma proteins—exert what is called *colloid osmotic pressure* or *oncotic pressure* which is exerted by plasma proteins on permeable membranes in the body. <u>*Hydrostatic pressure* is force exerted by a fluid against the container wall.</u> Blood hydrostatic pressure is the pressure of plasma and blood cells in the capillaries; it depends primarily on arterial blood pressure on the arteriolar side of capillaries and on venous blood pressure on the venular side of capillaries. From physiology, one recalls that arterial pressure is greater than venous pressure. <u>*Filtration pressure* is the difference between colloid osmotic pressure and blood hydrostatic pressure.</u>

These pressures are significant when describing how fluid leaves arterioles, enters the interstitial compartment, and eventually returns again to the venules. The filtration pressure is positive in the arterioles and, hence, helps force or filtrate fluids into interstitial spaces; it is negative in the venules and, hence, helps fluid enter at the venules. This is illustrated in Figure 23–7.

Filtration is also involved in the proper functioning of the glomeruli of the kidneys.

Pinocytosis and Phagocytosis

Pinocytosis and phagocytosis come from Greek roots which mean <u>drinking</u> and <u>eating by cells</u>. <u>*Pinocytosis* can be defined as the cell's taking in of certain substances by invagination of the cell membrane.</u> For example, protein molecules with variable amounts of fluid enter a cell through the mechanism of pinocytosis, as is illustrated in Figure 23–8. <u>*Phagocytosis* is the cell's engulfing of substances in order to destroy them.</u> It occurs in the same manner as pinocytosis, but the term is used when larger particles, such as bacteria and cell fragments, are engulfed.

These various ways of transporting water, electrolytes, and nonelectrolytes make it possible for tissue cells to be nourished and cleared of wastes. Simultaneously, the various fluid compartments retain their constituents in balance.

ACID-BASE BALANCE

Body fluids must also maintain a normal acid-base balance in order to sustain health and life. Acidity or alkalinity of a solution is determined by its concentration of hydrogen (H^+) ions and hydroxyl (OH^-) ions. <u>An *acid* is a substance containing hydrogen ions that can be liberated or released.</u> <u>An *alkali* is a *base* which is a substance that can accept or trap a hydrogen ion.</u> Equation 1 illustrates an acid. Equations 2 and 3 illustrate a base.

Equation 1.

$$H_2CO_3 \longrightarrow H^+ + HCO_3^-$$

Carbonic acid   releases   hydrogen   to form a   bicarbonate base

Equation 2.

$$HCO_3^- + H^+ \longrightarrow H_2CO_3$$

Bicarbonate base   traps   hydrogen   to form   carbonic acid

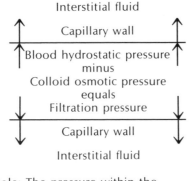

Arteriole: The pressure within the arteriole is *positive* and hence, fluid is forced into interstitial fluid.

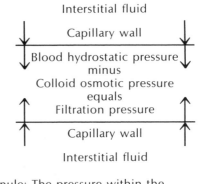

Venule: The pressure within the venule is *negative* and hence, fluid is forced into the venule.

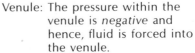

Figure 23–7 This illustrates filtration which is the tendency of solutes to move from an area of higher pressure to an area of lower pressure.

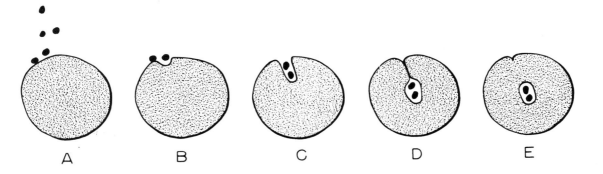

Figure 23–8 Mechanism of pinocytosis. Two protein molecules become adsorbed to the surface of a cell membrane. A position of the membrane then invaginates, carrying the protein with it.

Equation 3.

$$OH^- \quad + \quad H^+ \quad \longrightarrow \quad H_2O$$

Hydroxyl   traps   hydrogen   to form   water
ion from
a base

The unit of measure when acid-base balance is described is *pH*, which is an expression of hydrogen ion concentration and the resulting acidity of a substance. The pH scale ranges from 1 to 14. Neutrality of a solution is 7.0; an example is pure water. Because pH is based on a negative logarithm, as the hydrogen ions increase and a solution becomes more acid, the pH becomes less than 7.0. When the concentration of the hydroxyl ions exceeds the concentration of hydrogen ions, the solution is alkaline and the pH is greater than 7.0. Gastric secretions which are strongly acid have an approximate pH of 1.0 to 1.3, while strongly alkaline pancreatic secretions have an approximate pH of 10.0.

Normal blood plasma is slightly alkaline and has a normal pH range of 7.35 and 7.45. When the normal pH range is exceeded in either direction, the person develops signs and symptoms of illness and if the condition goes on unabated, death will result. *Acidosis* is the condition characterized by a proportionate excess of hydrogen ions in extracellular fluid in which the pH falls below 7.35. *Alkalosis* occurs when there is a proportionate lack of hydrogen ions and the pH exceeds 7.45. Figure 23–9 illustrates normal pH, acidosis, and alkalosis and also the points at which death can be expected to occur. Note that acidosis is used to describe the condition when pH is between 6.80 and 7.35. Actually, the extracellular fluid of most patients who are clinically described as being in a state of acidosis is still alkaline since the fluid will be between 7.0 and 7.35. When the fluid acidity falls below 7.0, the person is gravely ill or dying.

The narrow range of normal pH is achieved by the body's buffer systems, carbon dioxide excretion by the lungs, and the selectivity of ion secretion by the kidneys. A *buffer* is a substance that prevents body fluids from becoming overly acid or alkaline. The body has three buffer systems, the most important of which is the carbonic acid-sodium bicarbonate system. If a strong acid, such as hydrochloric acid, is added to the base, sodium bicarbonate, the response given in Equation 4 results.

Equation 4.

$$HCl \quad + \quad NaHCO_3 \quad \longrightarrow \quad NaCl \quad + \quad H_2CO_3$$

Strong   added   sodium   yields   salt   and   weak
hydrochloric   to   bicarbonate   carbonic
acid   base   acid

When a strong base is added to an acidic buffer, the reaction in Equation 5 results.

Equation 5.

$$NaOH \quad + \quad H_2CO_3 \quad \longrightarrow \quad NaHCO_3 \quad + \quad H_2O$$

Strong   added   carbonic   yields   weak   and   water
sodium   to   acid   sodium
hydroxide   buffer   bicarbonate
base   base

The processes described in Equations 4 and 5 occur frequently and very rapidly in the body and carry a major responsibility in maintaining normal acid-base balance.

The ratio of carbonic acid to the base bicarbonate is important for acid-base balance. Normal extracellular fluid has a ratio of 20 parts bicarbonate to one part carbonic acid. The exact quantities are unimportant for acid-base balance as long as they remain in a 20 to 1 ratio.

The lungs are the primary controller of the body's

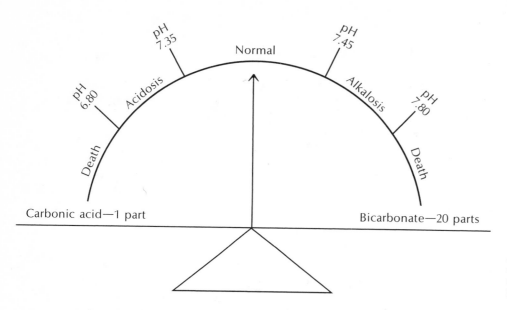

Figure 23-9 An illustration of acid-base balance. A tilt will occur if carbonic acid is added or subtracted, or, if bicarbonate is added or subtracted.

carbonic acid supply. Carbon dioxide is constantly produced by cellular metabolism and enters the extracellular fluid. As it does, the carbon dioxide and water are acted upon by the enzyme, carbonic anhydrase, to produce carbonic acid, as illustrated in Equation 6.

Equation 6.

$$CO_2 \underset{\text{dioxide}}{\underset{\text{Carbon}}{}} + H_2O \underset{\text{water}}{\underset{\text{and}}{}} \xrightarrow[\text{yields}]{\text{(carbonic anhydrase)}} H_2CO_3 \underset{\substack{\text{carbonic}\\\text{acid}}}{}$$

The carbonic anhydrase can also break down the carbonic acid into carbon dioxide and water, as Equation 7 illustrates.

Equation 7.

$$H_2CO_3 \underset{\substack{\text{Carbonic}\\\text{acid}}}{} \xrightarrow[\text{yields}]{\text{(carbonic anhydrase)}} H_2O \underset{\text{water}}{} + CO_2 \underset{\substack{\text{carbon}\\\text{dioxide}}}{\underset{\text{and}}{}}$$

The carbon dioxide of Equation 7 can be excreted by exhalation. As the amount of carbon dioxide in the blood increases, the sensitive respiratory center of the medulla is stimulated to increase the rate and depth of respirations in order to eliminate more carbon dioxide. When the blood level of carbon dioxide is below normal, the center will decrease the rate and depth of respirations to retain the carbon dioxide so that carbonic acid can be formed and the delicate balance maintained. This total respiratory process also occurs frequently and nearly as rapidly as the buffering action in the carbonic acid-sodium bicarbonate system described earlier.

Cellular, plasmatic, and hemoglobinic proteins have buffering ability. One portion of the protein molecule can accept hydrogen ions while another can give up hydrogen ions. The protein buffer system is the most plentiful in the body and with its great versatility, acts as an acid or a base as the situation in the body demands.

The concentration of bicarbonate in the plasma is regulated by the kidneys through the excretion of hydrogen ions and by forming additional bicarbonate as needed. When the pH of the plasma reaches the lower range of normal, hydrogen ions are eliminated and bicarbonate is formed and retained. When plasma pH is elevated or above normal, hydrogen ions are retained and bicarbonate excesses are excreted. The kidneys regulate hydrogen and bicarbonate ions in three ways: reabsorbing bicarbonate, forming ammonium salts, and forming phosphate salts. A sodium ion combines with bicarbonate to form sodium bicarbonate which is reabsorbed by the plasma in the kidney tubule cells. Thus, bicarbonate is conserved. This reaction is illustrated in Equation 8.

Equation 8.

$$Na^+ \underset{\text{Sodium}}{} + HCO_3^- \underset{\text{bicarbonate}}{\underset{\text{and}}{}} \xrightarrow[\text{yields}]{} NaHCO_3 \underset{\substack{\text{sodium}\\\text{bicarbonate}}}{}$$

As a result of amino acid metabolism, ammonia (NH_3) is formed in the kidney tubule cells and is secreted into the tubule where it unites with hydrogen to form an ammonium ion (NH_4^+). Ammonium further unites with chloride (Cl^-) to form ammonium chloride (NH_4Cl) which is excreted. These reactions are illustrated in Equations 9 and 10.

Equation 9.

$$\underset{\text{Ammonia}}{NH_3} + \underset{\text{hydrogen}}{H^+} \xrightarrow{\text{and}} \underset{\text{ammonium}}{\text{yields}} \underset{\text{ammonium}}{NH_4^+}$$

Equation 10.

$$\underset{\text{Ammonium}}{NH_4^+} + \underset{\text{chloride}}{Cl^-} \xrightarrow{\text{and}} \underset{\text{ammonium}}{\text{yields}} \underset{\text{chloride}}{NH_4Cl}$$

Phosphate salts are formed by exchanging a sodium ion for a hydrogen ion in the conversion of alkaline sodium phosphate (Na_2HPO_4) to acid sodium phosphate (NaH_2PO_4). The acid sodium phosphate is then excreted. This is called the phosphate buffering system and is illustrated in Equation 11.

Equation 11.

$$\underset{\substack{\text{Alkaline}\\\text{sodium}\\\text{phosphate}}}{Na_2HPO_4} + \underset{\text{hydrogen}}{H^+} \xrightarrow[\text{yields}]{\text{and}} \underset{\substack{\text{acid}\\\text{sodium}\\\text{phosphate}}}{NaH_2PO_4} + \underset{\text{sodium}}{Na^+}$$

Acid-base regulation by the kidneys is a vast combination of chemical processes and it occurs more slowly than the carbonic acid-sodium bicarbonate system or by the respiratory regulation. It may take up to three days for fluid pH to be restored by the kidneys. The pH of urine varies depending on the ions which are being excreted, but generally it is in the 4.5 to 8.2 range.

Acid-base balance and imbalance can be assessed by using plasma findings. The pH of plasma will indicate balance or impending acidosis or alkalosis. But in addition, a study of the blood's oxygen and carbon dioxide gases are important. The partial pressures of these gases, or their tensions, are determined by the use of a nomogram which reflects the chemical and physical activities of the two gases. The partial pressure of carbon dioxide is abbreviated pCO_2; for oxygen, it is pO_2. When the pO_2 is low, hemoglobin is carrying less oxygen; when the pO_2 is high, the hemoglobin carries more oxygen. The pCO_2 is influenced almost entirely by respiratory activity. If the pressure exceeds normal, carbonic acid formation has increased as follows:

$$CO_2 + H_2O \longrightarrow H_2CO_3$$

If the pressure is below normal, carbon dioxide of carbonic acid is leaving the body in excessive amounts as follows:

$$H_2CO_3 \longrightarrow CO_2 + H_2O$$

Normal levels of pCO_2 and pO_2 are given later in this chapter. There is additional discussion of blood gases in the section dealing with acid-base imbalances later.

There are special laboratory methods used to measure bicarbonate levels. However, they measure these levels indirectly by determining carbon dioxide content in the blood. Even though the results are stated as carbon dioxide content, they are used to assess bicarbonate levels, not carbon dioxide levels.

PRIMARY ORGANS OF FLUID HOMEOSTASIS

Almost every body system and organ help in some way to maintain fluid homeostasis.

Lungs

Proper functioning of the lungs regulates the oxygen and carbon dioxide levels in the body. Earlier, the very crucial role of carbon dioxide in acid-base balance was described, and the lungs are primarily responsible for regulating the body's level of this gas. Insensitive amounts of water are lost with breathing. Anything that interferes with normal respirations can influence fluid balance and particularly the body's acid-base balance.

Kidneys

The kidneys are often called the master chemists of the body. They selectively retain electrolytes and water to maintain balance, and excrete wastes and excesses that have been indiscriminately absorbed in the body.

The kidneys are the chief means by which water balance is maintained. The relationship between the kidneys and the endocrine system is involved in this complex process. The antidiuretic hormone, usually abbreviated ADH, is released by the posterior pituitary and acts primarily on the kidney tubules to regulate the amount of water that is reabsorbed. When the amount of ADH is increased, the permeability of the collecting ducts of the kidneys is increased which promotes greater water reabsorption and, thus, less urine formation. When ADH is decreased, the collecting ducts reabsorb less water, and hence, the urine output is increased. The stimulus for ADH release is generally thought to be the osmotic pressure of the extracellular fluid which is determined by its electrolyte and water relationship. Thus, we see that the composition of extracellular fluid itself influences water balance throughout the body. The diuretic hormone, usually abbreviated DH, is released by the anterior lobe of the pituitary gland. There is little known about DH, but it functions to increase urinary output. The antidiuretic hormone and DH function cooperatively but in opposite ways.

Thirst is a normal regulatory mechanism related to water balance. Thirst is a subjective experience and an important factor in determining water intake, and eventually, output through the kidneys. The mechanism responsible for thirst is poorly understood. Psychological as well as physiological factors are involved, but it is particularly important for the nurse to remember that the person who is unable to respond to the thirst stimulus as well as the person who seems to have no stimulus may need professional assistance in relation to proper water intake.

Circulatory System

The circulatory system is vital for the transportation of blood to all body cells. The blood's quantity and constituents and its hydrostatic and colloid osmotic pressure created within the system all influence proper cell functioning.

Just as with all other tissues, the kidneys depend on adequate circulation for proper functioning. Patients with circulatory problems should be observed closely since they very often experience fluid imbalances when renal circulation is impaired. An example is a patient with congestive heart failure whose fluid imbalance due to poor renal circulation may result in pulmonary edema which is an accumulation of fluid in the lungs.

Endocrine System

The primary hormones involved in fluid balance are the antidiuretic hormone, the diuretic hormone, aldosterone, and the thyroid and parathyroid hormones. The antidiuretic hormone and diuretic hormone have already been mentioned.

Aldosterone is secreted by the adrenal cortex. It acts on renal tubules and influences primarily sodium, potassium, and chloride excretion and absorption. Thus, the hormone influencing these three electrolytes also plays a significant role in water balance. Aldosterone is often called the great conserver of sodium, and because of this, water is conserved. The hormone adrenocorti-

cotropin, abbreviated ACTH, stimulates the release of aldosterone, among other things. Adrenocorticotropin is produced by cells in the anterior lobe of the pituitary gland.

Thyroxin, released by the thyroid gland, increases blood flow in the body. This in turn increases renal circulation which results in increased glomerular filtration and urinary output.

The parathyroid hormone, abbreviated PTH, is a homeostatic regulator for calcium and phosphate ions. It acts primarily on the kidneys, the gastrointestinal tract, and the bones.

Gastrointestinal Tract

It is through the gastrointestinal tract that water and electrolytes normally enter the body. Here, water and electrolytes are absorbed to replace those that are lost. Also, water and electrolytes move back and forth across the intestinal mucosa constantly and rapidly. Because of the role of the gastrointestinal tract in water and electrolyte balance, it can be seen that anything that upsets normal gastrointestinal functioning or interferes with the normal intake of nutrients and water can quickly place the body in states of imbalance.

Nervous System

The nervous system acts as a switchboard and inhibits and stimulates mechanisms that influence water and electrolyte balance. It functions chiefly as the regulator of sodium and water intake and excretion.

The thirst center is located in the hypothalamus. The role of thirst in helping to maintain water balance was discussed earlier.

PRINCIPLE ELECTROLYTES OF THE BODY

Previous material in this chapter has already indicated some of the functions of electrolytes in the body, how they are transported, and organs that are primarily responsible for maintenance of certain electrolyte balances. This section will briefly summarize information concerning the most prevalent electrolytes in the body.

The cation sodium is the chief electrolyte of extracellular fluid. It is found in much smaller quantities within the cell, as Figure 23–3 illustrated. It moves easily between the intravascular and interstitial spaces and its concentration is primarily responsible for helping to maintain isotonicity of body fluids. When sodium intake is low, the resulting hypotonicity of body fluids causes an increase in water loss. It was previously thought that sodium could not move out of a cell but the pump mechanism of active transport described earlier demonstrates that it does.

Sodium also plays a role in acid–base balance and is instrumental in many chemical reactions, particularly within nervous and muscle tissue cells. Sodium excesses are eliminated primarily by the kidneys; small amounts are also normally lost in the feces and perspiration. The kidneys are very effective in conserving sodium through reabsorption stimulated by aldosterone and, hence, the body fluid levels are relatively easy to maintain under normal conditions.

Sodium is normally found in many foods, such as bacon, ham, many sausages, catsup, mustard, relishes, and processed cheese. It is found in the drinking water in some areas of the country. Sodium is ingested by most persons also in the form of table salt added to foods for seasoning. The average American diet includes 3 to 7 Gm. of sodium daily, an amount which more than adequately meets the daily minimum requirements.

Potassium is the major cation of the intracellular fluid. Its main function is comparable to the task of sodium in extracellular fluid. It is the chief regulator of intracellular electrolyte balance. Potassium also plays an integral part in many physiological processes, such as the transmission of electrical impulses, particularly in nerve, heart, skeletal, intestinal, and lung tissue; protein and carbohydrate metabolism; and cellular building. A small amount of potassium is normally also found outside of the cells. The gastrointestinal secretions are normally rich in potassium. Some is also found in perspiration and saliva.

Potassium is excreted primarily by the kidneys in urine. Unlike sodium, the kidneys do not have an effective method for conserving potassium. Therefore, if the excreted amounts are not replaced, a deficiency will develop readily. Because of the high-potassium content of gastrointestinal secretions, large losses of these secretions will quickly cause a deficit, such as when diarrhea is present. Normal adult values of extracellular potassium is normally in the 4.0 to 5.6 mEq. per L. but the normal adult value of intracellular potassium is between 155 and 160 mEq. per L. Potassium is found in many foods and is ordinarily readily available in a well-balanced diet. Certain fruits, for example, bananas, peaches, and figs; meats; whole milk; and orange, tomato, and grapefruit juice, are good sources

of potassium. The average daily dietary intake contains 2 to 4 Gm. of potassium which is adequate to replace losses under normal conditions.

Chloride is the chief extracellular anion. It plays an important role in maintaining the normal plasma pH. The highest concentration of chloride is found in gastric secretions. Chloride is excreted primarily by the kidneys in combination with sodium, and like sodium, the major part of chloride is conserved and reabsorbed. It is taken into the body primarily in foods to which table salt has been added.

Calcium is a very versatile electrolyte as well as the most abundant one in the body. It is found mainly in bones and teeth in a nonunion form. If plasma levels fall, the body will take calcium from the bones and teeth. A small amount is normally found in both extracellular and intracellular fluids. Calcium is necessary for nerve impulse transmission, blood clotting, and muscle contraction, and it acts also as a catalyst for many chemical activities of cells. Dairy products are the most prevalent natural source of calcium.

The major anion in the body is phosphate. There is a small amount in plasma and it is particularly important for helping to maintain acid–base balance. Phosphorus is present in most foods. When calcium needs are met by milk intake, so too will phosphorus needs. Excesses are excreted by the kidneys.

Most of the body's magnesium is found in the cells. It is especially important for the metabolism of carbohydrates and proteins. It is believed to have an effect on tissue irritability and to function as a co-factor in certain enzyme reactions. Magnesium is abundant in green vegetables.

The bicarbonate molecule is essential for proper acid–base balance because of its role, along with carbonic acid, in the body's primary buffering system. Its proper concentration depends principally on kidney functioning. It is ordinarily readily available as a result of the formation of carbon dioxide in the process of metabolism.

Sulfate is found primarily within cells and in association with cellular protein. Excesses are excreted by the kidneys.

Organic acid anions are a normal intermediary in cell metabolism. The major one in the body is lactic acid.

The protein anion functions in the process of diffusion to move substances to and from the capillaries, as described earlier. Plasma proteins include albumin, globulin, and fibrinogen.

There are still other electrolytes that are also essential

for proper cell functioning but they are found only in traces in the body. One example is chromium. A well-balanced diet will ensure an adequate supply of these substances.

Cellular and extracellular fluids are making constant changes and these are reflected in each other. As previously mentioned, cellular fluid is not readily available for examination. Hence, extracellular fluid which is easily accessible as plasma is used for laboratory analysis when assessing fluid status. Table 23–5 gives normal ranges of laboratory findings that are most commonly used to assess fluid balance in the body. This table appears on page 588.

COMMON FLUID IMBALANCES

As discussed earlier, fluid balance is essential to health. In some circumstances, the body's compensatory mechanisms are not able to maintain the homeostatic state, and imbalance occurs. Imbalances can relate to either volume or distribution disturbances of the water or electrolytes. While in actual situations, the imbalances frequently occur in combination, for purposes of clarity, the major ones are presented here individually. Table 23–3 lists the most common disturbances with examples of common nursing observations and causes of the disturbances.

TABLE 23–3 Various water and electrolyte disturbances, problems likely to produce them, and common nursing observations

CLINICAL ENTITY	EXAMPLES OF PROBLEMS LIKELY TO LEAD TO DISTURBANCE	COMMON NURSING OBSERVATIONS
Extracellular fluid volume deficit Hypovolemia	Insufficient water intake Vomiting Diarrhea Elevated body temperature	Dry skin and mucous membranes Scanty urine Weight loss Lassitude and fatigue Longitudinal tongue furrows Low urinary output Rapid pulse and respiratory rates Depressed fontanels in infants Elevated red blood count, hemoglobin, and hematocrit
Extracellular fluid volume excess Hypervolemia	Excessive ingestion or injection of fluids with sodium chloride or sodium bicarbonate Renal malfunction Congestive heart failure disease Malnutrition	Puffy eyelids Shortness of breath Dyspnea Moist rales Edema Weight gain Bounding pulse Engorged peripheral veins Decreased red cell count, hemoglobin, and hematocrit
Plasma to interstitial fluid shift Hypovolemia	Burns Massive crushing injuries Perforated peptic ulcer Intestinal obstruction	Fast, weak pulse Pallor Cold extremities Hypotension Apprehension and disorientation Unconsciousness—coma Elevated red cell count, hemoglobin, and hematocrit
Interstitial fluid to plasma shift Hypervolemia	Excessive infusion of hypertonic solutions Compensation following hemorrhage Recovery phase of plasma to interstitial fluid shift	Early—hypertension Late—hypotension Air hunger Moist rales Bounding pulse Engorged peripheral veins Pallor Weakness Decreased red cell count, hemoglobin, and hematocrit
Metabolic acidosis (base bicarbonate deficit)	Decreased food intake Systemic infections Renal insufficiency Diabetic acidosis Ketogenic diet Salicylate intoxication	Disorientation-stupor Deep rapid breathing—may not be present in infant Unconsciousness when severe Plasma pH below 7.35 Plasma bicarbonate below 25 mEq./1 Urine pH below 6

TABLE 23-3 (*Continued*)

Metabolic alkalosis (base bicarbonate excess)	Vomiting Excessive ingestion of alkalies Gastric suction Adrenal cortex hormone administration	Depressed shallow respirations Hypertonic musculature Tetany Plasma pH above 7.45 Plasma bicarbonate above 29 mEq./1 Urine pH above 7
Respiratory acidosis (carbonic acid excess)	Pneumonia Emphysema Respiratory suppression Asthma Respiratory obstruction	Disorientation Respiratory embarrassment Rapid, deep breathing when body is compensating Coma Weakness Plasma pH below 7.35 Plasma bicarbonate below 25 mEq./1 Urine pH below 6
Respiratory alkalosis (carbonic acid deficit)	Unconsciousness Tetany Oxygen lack Elevated body temperature Extreme emotion Salicylate intoxication	Deep rapid breathing Deliberate overbreathing Convulsion Slow, shallow respirations when body is compensating Plasma pH above 7.45 Plasma bicarbonate below 25 mEq./1 Urine pH above 7
Sodium deficit Hyponatremia	Excessive perspiration and drinking water Gastrointestinal suction and drinking water Repeated use of water enemas Infusions with electrolyte-free solutions Diuretic administration	Apprehension—anxiety—confusion Abdominal cramps Rapid weak pulse Fingerprinting over sternum Cold, clammy skin Hypotension Convulsions Scanty urine with low specific gravity Plasma sodium below 135 mEq./1
Sodium excess Hypernatremia	Inadequate water intake and excessive sodium chloride intake Diarrhea Pyrexia with rapid breathing	Dry, sticky mucous membrane Thirst Firm tissue turgor Flushed skin Rough, dry tongue Scanty urine with high specific gravity Convulsions Elevated body temperature Plasma sodium above 147 mEq./L.
Potassium deficit Hypokalemia	Diarrhea Intestinal disease Emotional, physical stress Burns Diuretic administration Metabolic alkalosis	Weak and faint pulse Falling blood pressure Malaise Anorexia; vomiting Distention Soft, flabby musculature Prominent U wave on electrocardiogram Plasma potassium below 4 mEq./L.
Potassium excess Hyperkalemia	Burns Crushing injuries Kidney disease Excessive infusion of potassium Adrenal insufficiency Metabolic acidosis	Nausea Irritability Muscle General muscle weakness Scanty to no urine Intestinal colic Diarrhea Irregular pulse Ventricular fibrillations Plasma potassium above 5.6 mEq./1
Calcium deficit Hypocalcemia	Sprue Excessive infusion of citrated blood Subcutaneous infections—massive Peritonitis Removal of parathyroid glands Diarrhea Rapid or overcorrection of acidosis Magnesium excess	Tingling of fingers and in circumoral area Abdominal muscle cramps Tetany Convulsions Carpopedal spasm Plasma calcium below 4.5 mEq./1

Table 23–3 (*Continued*)

Calcium excess Hypercalcemia	Prolonged bed rest Tumor—parathyroid gland Excessive vitamin D intake Overactivity of parathyroid glands Excessive milk or hard water intake	Relaxed musculature Flank pains Kidney stones Nausea and vomiting Stupor and coma Deep bone pains, as "shin splints" Plasma calcium above 5.8 mEq./1

Protein deficit
  Hypoproteinemia
	Hemorrhage—chronic bleeding
	Draining wounds or ulcers
	Burns
	Inadeqaute protein intake
		Mental depression
		Fatigue
		Pallor
		Weight loss
		Loss of muscle tone
		Edema
		Decreased hemoglobin and
		  hematocrit

Magnesium deficit Hypomagnesemia	Chronic alcoholism Vomiting Diarrhea Impaired intestional absorption Enterostomy drainage Severe renal disease	Disorientation—hallucinations Hypertension Tremors—tetany Hyperactive deep reflexes Convulsions Rapid pulse rate Plasma magnesium below 1.4 mEq./1

The body has a desirable balance for fluids in all three spaces: intravascular, interstitial, and intracellular. Constant extracellular and intracellular exchanges mean that extracellular disturbances have implications for intracellular functioning. This fact, plus the relative availability for study of the extracellular fluid, results in fluid imbalances being diagnosed and treated in relation to extracellular levels. Also, diagnosis and treatment takes into account that while the body attempts to maintain a balance in all fluid spaces, if circumstances demand, the intravascular fluid will usually be protected at the expense of interstitial and then intracellular fluids.

As the term implies, extracellular fluid deficit is a deficiency in the amount of both water and electrolytes in the extracellular fluid. The water and electrolyte proportions remain near normal. The state is commonly known as *hypovolemia*. Both osmotic pressure and hydrostatic pressure changes force the interstitial fluid into the intravascular space. As the interstitial space becomes depleted, its fluid will become hypertonic and cellular fluid will then be drawn into the interstitial space, leaving the cells without adequate fluid to function properly.

Dehydration is sometimes used as a synonym for hypovolemia but this is technically an inaccuracy. *Dehydration* refers only to a decreased volume of water. *Hydration* is a union of a substance with water. The term is often used to mean that there is normal water volume in the body, although strictly speaking, this is not entirely correct.

Fluid deficit occurs in persons with excessive body excretions or secretion losses when they are not replaced. It also occurs in persons who are too ill to help themselves to an adequate fluid intake or do not have a sufficient amount of fluids available. The very young and the elderly and those fatigued or weakened by illness are particularly susceptible. A weight loss of 5 percent for adults and 10 percent for infants can occur rapidly. A 5 percent weight loss is considered to be pronounced fluid deficiency and an 8 percent loss or more is considered severe. A 15 percent weight loss due to fluid deficiency usually has reached the point of threatening life.

Extracellular fluid excess is a surplus of fluid amounts while maintaining near normal proportions. It is called *hypervolemia*. Overhydration is commonly used as a synonym for hypervolemia, but strictly speaking, this is an inaccuracy. *Overhydration* refers only to above normal amounts of water in extracellular spaces. Malfunction of the kidneys causing an inability to excrete the excesses is the most common cause. However, cardiac and liver disturbances can also be influential. Since the kidneys are responsible for sodium excretion also, when water is retained in excessive amounts, so is sodium.

Because of the increased extracellular osmotic pressure from the retained sodium, fluid is pulled from the cells to equalize the tonicity. By the time the intracellular and extracellular spaces are isotonic to each other, an excess of both water and sodium are in the extracellular fluid while the cells are nearly depleted. This condition accounts for the typical signs and symptoms given in Table 23–3. The characteristic bubbling respiratory sounds are called rales. The excessive extracellular fluid may be stored in tissue spaces and is known as edema. Edema frequently can be seen around the eyes, the fingers, ankles, and the sacral area. It may result in a weight gain in excess of 5 percent. When the excess fluid remains in the intravascular space, the concentration of solids in the blood is decreased.

Plasma-to-interstitial shift describes the occasional movement of fluid from the blood to the spaces between the cells. It occurs most often following major tissue damage, as for example, when there has been a crushing or tearing injury or extensive second- or third-degree burns. The person develops symptoms of decreased intravascular fluid. Since the blood solids remain behind, and therefore, are in greater concentration, the laboratory examination of the blood will show an increase in the red blood count, hemoglobin, and hematocrit. This shift in fluid is also called hypovolemia; note that, just as in the case of extracellular fluid deficit, the intravascular compartment is deficient.

Interstitial-to-plasma shift is the movement of fluid from the space surrounding the cells to the blood. This shift is a compensatory response to volume or osmotic pressure changes of the intravascular fluid. This may occur when a replacement is needed for blood lost in hemorrhage or when excessive hypertonic solutions are administered intravenously. Intravascular increases will be demonstrated by venous engorgement, and blood pressure, cardiac, and pulse changes. The increased intravascular volume will cause laboratory examinations to show a decrease in the red cell count, hemoglobin, and hematocrit. This shift in fluid is also called hypervolemia; note that, just as in the case of extracellular fluid excess, there is excessive intravascular fluid.

Sodium deficit is an insufficient amount of sodium in the extracellular fluid. This condition is called *hyponatremia*. It can be caused either by an excessive sodium loss or an inadequate intake. An inadequate intake is usually the result of a poorly managed sodium-limited diet or merely an inadequate food intake. Excessive perspiration with associated drinking of a great deal of water, extensive loss of gastrointestinal secretions, kidney reabsorption malfunctions, adrenal cortex disturbance, and administration of diuretics or nonelectrolyte infusions are all fairly common causes of excessive sodium loss. An increase in aldosterone will stimulate the kidneys to reabsorb available sodium, and along with it chloride and water, so the urinary output is decreased. Osmotic pressure changes of the fluid will result in extracellular fluid moving into the cells.

When this occurs, a typical sign is fingerprinting over the sternum; an examiner's fingerprints tend to remain on the patient's skin over the sternum when pressure is applied with the fingers. The phenomenon results from tissue plasticity as fluid moves into cells. The extracellular fluid loss can also cause vascular changes, as a decrease in blood pressure and a weak pulse. The vascular changes may induce disturbances of concentration and thinking.

Sodium excess is a surplus of sodium in the extracellular fluid. This state is also called *hypernatremia*. The excess of sodium can be the result of either an increased intake or decreased elimination of the electrolyte. It can also occur as the result of a decreased intake or an increased loss of water. An excessive intake can be either by intravenous or oral routes. Kidney and adrenal cortex malfunctions were mentioned earlier as a cause of sodium retention and resulting extracellular fluid excess. Extreme water losses, such as may occur when hyperpnea or diarrhea are present, can cause a proportionate sodium excess. Because of the increased extracellular osmotic pressure, fluids move from the cells, leaving them in a poorly hydrated state.

Potassium deficit is an insufficient amount of potassium in the extracellular fluid. This state is known as *hypokalemia*. It can be caused by a decrease in potassium intake, intestinal absorption, or an increased loss. Since potassium is available in so many foods and malabsorption disorders of the intestine are generally treated effectively, excess loss is by far the most common cause of potassium deficiency. Kidney disturbances resulting in tubular malfunction or excessive aldosterone stimulation will cause increased potassium losses. Diuretics promote fluid and potassium excretion. Gastrointestinal secretion losses from vomiting, diarrhea, or mechanical removal by suctioning can be the cause of a deficiency. Tissue trauma resulting in cellular damage also causes potassium losses. When the extracellular potassium level falls, potassium moves out from the cell creating an intracellular potassium deficiency. Sodium and hydrogen ions are retained by the cells to maintain an ionic balance. These shifts not only influence normal cellular functioning but also influence the pH of the extracellular fluid. Muscle tissues are generally the first to demonstrate a potassium deficiency.

Potassium excess, also known as *hyperkalemia,* is an excess of potassium in the extracellular fluid. An excess of potassium can be the result of excessive administration or decreased excretion or a combination of the two. A decrease in urine output for any reason will minimize potassium excretion. Adrenal cortex malfunctions can cause the reabsorption of excessive potassium. Extensive tissue damage causes the movement of intracellular potassium to the extracellular space. Excessive administration of either oral or intravenous potassium, especially in the presence of kidney dysfunction, can cause an extracellular increase.

A calcium deficit in extracellular fluid is called *hypocalcemia*. If the condition is prolonged, calcium will be taken from the bones. This results in *osteomalacia* which is manifested by soft and pliable bones. Acute hypocalcemia is ordinarily treated with infusions of calcium gluconate. A high-calcium diet with oral supplements of calcium is usually used for mild deficits.

A calcium excess is called *hypercalcemia*. Hypercalcemia presents an emergency situation because the condition often leads to cardiac arrest. Treating the underlying cause is important. Sulfate and phosphate solutions are often administered intravenously because it has been found that they usually reduce the calcium level fairly promptly.

A magnesium deficit is called *hypomagnesemia*. The reason is unknown but alcoholism is very often linked with a magnesium deficit, even when the magnesium intake is within a normal range. Liver diseases and losses of gastrointestinal secretions, in combination, will almost always lead to a deficit. The body's potassium level also drops because the kidneys tend to excrete more potassium when magnesium is in poor supply. Hence, hypomagnesemia and hypokalemia very often occur together. Magnesium deficit is ordinarily treated with the administration of magnesium sulfate.

Magnesium excess is called *hypermagnesemia*. It is a rare condition but does occur when the kidneys fail to excrete excessive amounts or when excessive amounts are used therapeutically.

A protein deficit is called *hypoproteinemia*. The condition is often associated with potassium deficits since potassium is important for the proper utilization of proteins in the body. The recuperative powers of persons with a protein deficit are poor. Treatment is usually dietary, but when this is not possible, protein may be administered into the circulatory system.

Acid–base imbalances occur when the carbonic acid or bicarbonate levels become disproportionate. Two kinds of disturbances upset the balance. A metabolic disturbance alters the bicarbonate proportion. A respiratory disturbance alters the carbonic acid proportion. When there is a single primary cause, these disturbances are known as metabolic acidosis or alkalosis and respiratory acidosis or alkalosis.

Metabolic acidosis is a proportionate deficit of bicarbonate in the extracellular fluid. The deficit can occur as the result of an increase in acid components or an excessive loss of bicarbonate. Increased fat metabolism with resultant acidic ketone wastes, ingestion of large amounts of acidic salicylates, or kidney malfunctions which result in reabsorption disturbances are potential causes of metabolic acidosis. The lungs attempt to increase the carbon dioxide excretion by increasing the rate and depth of the respirations. The kidneys attempt to compensate by retaining bicarbonate and excreting more hydrogen; thus, the urine increases in acidity. If the body is unable to achieve normal balance, the person may lose consciousness as metabolic acidosis increases. If metabolic acidosis is uncorrected, death will eventually result. The blood and urine characteristically both have a lowered pH.

Metabolic alkalosis is a proportionate excess of bicarbonate in the extracellular fluid. This may be the result of excessive acid losses or increased base ingestion or retention. Loss of gastric secretions through vomiting or gastrointestinal suctioning decreases the body's acid component extensively. Drinking large amounts of plain water while a patient is undergoing gastric suctioning has the effect of "washing out" the stomach electrolytes along with the water, and thus, predisposes him to alkalosis. Large ingestions of sodium bicarbonate or other absorbable alkaline substances can disturb the balance. The body will attempt to compensate by retaining carbon dioxide. The respirations will become slow and shallow and apnea may even occur. The kidneys will attempt to excrete potassium and sodium with the excessive bicarbonate and will retain hydrogen in carbonic acid.

Respiratory acidosis is a proportionate excess of carbonic acid in the extracellular fluid. Any deficiency in respiratory ventilation can cause respiratory acidosis. As the plasma carbonic acid content increases, the lungs are stimulated to "blow off" more carbon dioxide through an increased rate and depth of respirations. The kidneys will attempt to retain more bicarbonate and increase their ammonium excretion.

Respiratory alkalosis is a proportionate deficit of carbonic acid in the extracellular fluid. It is the result of increased alveolar ventilation and, as a result, a decrease in carbon dioxide. An increase in respiratory rate and depth causes the carbon dioxide loss. Since the carbon dioxide is excreted faster than normal, the carbon dioxide combining power is lowered. Hysteria and anxiety may be causative factors. Pyrexia, anoxia (especially at higher altitudes), and some central nervous system diseases may also cause this excessive carbon dioxide loss. Because of the deficit of carbon dioxide which is a chemical respiratory stimulant, depression or cessation of respirations will eventually occur. The kidneys attempt to alleviate the imbalance by increasing the bicarbonate excretion and retaining more hydrogen. When respiratory alkalosis is present, the plasma and urine pH will increase and the plasma bicarbonate level will decrease.

To summarize acid-base imbalances, respiratory acidosis and alkalosis are the result of respiratory phenomena and the primary organs for compensation to restore balance are the lungs. Compensation occurs by either trying to conserve or trying to excrete more carbon dioxide which is available in weakly ionized carbonic acid. Thus,

Respiratory acidosis = high pCO_2 due to hypoventilation. Compensation requires hyperventilation.

Respiratory alkalosis = low pCO_2 due to hyperventilation. Compensation requires hypoventilation.

Metabolic acidosis and alkalosis are influenced almost entirely by metabolic processes. Compensation occurs by either trying to conserve or trying to excrete more bicarbonate. Thus,

Metabolic acidosis = low bicarbonate. Nonvolatile acid is present to use up HCO_3^- in disproportionate amounts, or HCO_3^- is being lost in disproportionate amounts.

Metabolic alkalosis = high bicarbonate. Nonvolatile acid is lost and not using up HCO_3^-, or HCO_3^- is being gained in disproportionate amounts.

As indicated earlier, these conditions may occur in various combinations in the body. Table 23–4 shows common imbalances resulting from body fluid losses.

LABORATORY FINDINGS THAT ASSIST IN ASSESSING FOR FLUID BALANCE AND IMBALANCE

In addition to the signs and symptoms presented by an individual, the laboratory offers help when determining whether fluid balance or imbalances exist. Table 23–5 on page 588 gives normal ranges for the most

TABLE 23–4 Imbalances resulting from fluid loss of specific body fluid*

FLUID BEING LOST	IMBALANCES LIKELY TO OCCUR
Gastric juice	Extracellular fluid volume deficit
	Metabolic alkalosis
	Sodium deficit
	Potassium deficit
	Tetany (if metabolic alkalosis is present)
	Ketosis of starvation
	Magnesium deficit
Intestinal juice	Extracellular fluid volume deficit
	Metabolic acidosis
	Sodium deficit
	Potassium deficit
Bile	Sodium deficit
	Metabolic acidosis
Pancreatic juice	Metabolic acidosis
	Sodium deficit
	Calcium deficit
	Extracellular fluid volume deficit
Sensible perspiration	Extracellular fluid volume deficit
	Sodium deficit
Insensible water loss	Water deficit (dehydration)
	Sodium excess
Wound exudate	Protein deficit
	Sodium deficit
	Extracellular fluid volume deficit
Ascites	Protein deficit
	Sodium deficit
	Plasma-to-interstitial fluid shift
	Extracellular fluid volume deficit

*From Snively, W. D. Jr., and Beshear, D. R: Water and electrolytes in health and disease. In Kintzel, K. C., ed.: Advanced Concepts In Clinical Nursing. p. 264. Philadelphia, J. B. Lippincott, 1971.

commonly used laboratory examinations that are used when assessing fluid balance.

IMPLICATIONS FOR NURSING

Health Promotion in Relation to Fluid Balance

Health promotion in relation to fluid balance should be directed toward assisting persons to maintain balance and to seek assistance when symptoms of imbalance occur. In health, an adequate fluid intake and a well-balanced, nutritious diet with appropriate adjustments throughout the life cycle are basic essentials. When homeostasis is functioning well, the body will maintain fluid balance automatically and can make necessary adjustments when occasional indescretions do occur.

From this chapter, it can be seen that there is little in daily living that does not influence fluid balance. Here are some of the basic items that the nurse needs to

TABLE 23–5 Laboratory Values

I. NORMAL RANGES

A. Blood Formed Elements*

	BIRTH	3 MO.	1 YR.	5 YR.	12 YR.	WOMEN	MEN
RBC—million/cu. mm.	4.1–5.7	3.1–4.7	3.9–4.7	4.0–4.8	4.3–5.1	4.2–5.0	4.8–6.0
Hemoglobin—Gm./100 ml.	14–20	9–13	11–12.5	12–14.7	13.4–15.8	13–16	15–18
Hematocrit—% Vol. of packed RBC/100 ml.	43–63	28–40	32–40	36–44	39–47	39–47	44–52

B. Plasma Chemical Constituents

Plasma Na^+	137–147 mEq./L.
Plasma K^+	4.0–5.6 mEq./L.
Plasma Ca^{++}	4.5–5.8 mEq./L.
Plasma Cl^-	98–106 mEq./L.
Plasma magnesium	1.4–2.3 mEq./L.
Plasma protein	6–8 Gm./100 ml.
Plasma HCO_3^-	Adults: 25–29 mEq./L.
	Children: 20–25 mEq./L.
Plasma Cl^- plus plasma HCO_3^-	123–135 mEq./L.
Plasma pH	7.35–7.45
Plasma HPO_4^-	1.7–2.6 mEq./L.

C. Urine Values

Urine pH	4.5–8.2
Urine specific gravity	1.010–1.030

D. Blood gases, arterial blood

pO_2—80–100 mm. Hg.
pCO_2—35–45 mm. Hg.

* Covers 94% of normal population.

consider to help promote health in relation to fluid balance.

- Thirst is a sensation related to fluid balance and normally functions throughout life. Heeding it will help maintain balance. Abnormalities, that is, excessive thirst or lack of it when not related to normal physiological functioning, require prompt attention.

- A well-balanced, nutritious diet is essential. Adjustments in diet throughout life are often necessary. For example, infants do not tolerate roughage; a person doing heavy labor requires more calories than does one with sedentary work; the elderly with dentures need adjustments concerning chewable food. But no matter what adjustments are made, the diet should still be well-balanced and consist of foods containing the essential constituents for proper nourishment.

- Fad diets that recommend food and fluid intake which are not consistent with proper nutritional and water needs are likely to cause imbalances and should be avoided. Guidance is recommended when persons wish to gain or lose considerable amounts of weight.

- Any condition which threatens balance needs careful watching and care. Examples include nausea and vomiting, diarrhea, abnormal urinary output, abnormal thirst, and so on.

- Self-medicating may threaten balance. Examples of over-the-counter pharmaceutical agents which may lead to imbalances include laxatives and cathartics, antacids, diuretics, and vitamins. Large doses of vitamin D may influence calcium balance.

- Heavy perspiring, when fluid and salt are not adequately replaced, can lead to fluid imbalances. Conditions that often result in excessive perspiration include strenuous exercising, outdoor labor in hot climates, an elevated body temperature, and prolonged exposure to the sun and wind.

- Symptoms of imbalances were summarized in Table 23–3. Teaching persons how to recognize common imbalances should include the more common symptoms, such as rapid weight gains or losses, swollen fingers and feet, swollen abdomen, puffy eyelids, muscle weakness, changes in skin sensations, and scanty or profuse urine production.

- Promoting balance includes being aware of the normal ways in which the body gains and loses water. When symptoms of imbalance occur, it is necessary to measure the patient's intake and output carefully. Measuring intake and output were discussed in Chapters 19 and 20.

- When a medical regimen has been prescribed, the nurse is responsible for monitoring the person and for helping him appreciate the importance of observing the regimen carefully. Making adjustments without guidance can lead to serious fluid imbalances in almost all instances.

- There is need to teach persons with chronic illnesses how to promote fluid balance. Examples include those with diabetes mellitus, chronic obstructive pulmonary disease, kidney and heart ailments, and alcoholism. Many of these people are taking medications and are not eating and taking fluids properly. Hence, they need help to learn how to maintain balance.

- It is ordinarily far easier to prevent fluid imbalances than to treat problems of fluid imbalance. Healthful living characterized by moderation in habits of daily living are important.

Prevention of Fluid Imbalances

The importance of observation in gathering data that the nurse uses as the basis for assessing fluid balances and imbalances cannot be overstressed. As indicated in Chapter 4, knowing when and what type of information should be collected is essential. In other words, the nurse must be alert to situations in which the potential for fluid disturbances is increased, and then she needs to know what information is pertinent.

It is essential that the nurse be familiar with the patient's health state, the history of any present illness, and the medical plan for therapy. She should be aware of the patient's needs in relation to his sex, age, and weight. Any one, or any combination, of these factors may predispose the patient to fluid imbalance. Because balance is maintained normally when compatibility exists between the intake of water and electrolytes on one hand and their output on the other, anything that upsets the scale on either side acts as a warning. Typical questions for which the nurse seeks answers include the following: Has the patient's normal food and fluid intake changed? If so, for how long has it differed? Have there been restrictions for any reason on what he could eat and drink? Has there been any abnormal loss of body fluids? What particular body fluid is involved? What is the patient's intake and output of fluids?

Any situation in which the person has lost excessive fluids is a potential hazard, such as extreme perspiration with or without pyrexia, vomiting or diarrhea, wound or body secretion drainage, or blood loss. Inadequate fluid and electrolyte intake can result from nausea, a poorly balanced diet, or the unavailability of food or fluids. Excessive ingestion or injection of either electrolytes or fluids can also be a problem. Because the young and the elderly have less effective physiological compensatory mechanisms at their disposal, they will tend to develop imbalances faster than adults and, therefore, are higher risks.

Once predisposing factors are known and highrisk persons are identified, the next step concerns prevention of fluid imbalance. Every measure, nursing as well as medical, is ordinarily taken to aid in maintaining balance in the first place. Drugs are ordered to handle many infectious processes that predispose to imbalance. Every effort is made to encourage patients to take adequate nourishment when lack of appetite or vomiting is a problem. Nursing measures were discussed in Chapter 19. When medications that increase the excretion of electrolytes are prescribed, dietary supplements are ordinarily indicated. For example, when diuretics that increase potassium output are used, foods high in potassium content are indicated in the diet. Fluid intake should be encouraged or guarded, depending on the circumstances. Efforts are taken, as described in Chapter 16, to avoid the development of decubitus ulcers, which, if allowed to occur, can result in exuding ulcers that may upset balance. The inactivity of bed rest often accompanying illness may result in such disturbances as an increased excretion of nitrogen. Hence, high protein diets often are prescribed for patients requiring prolonged bed rest. Calcium is mobilized from the matrix of bones during long periods in bed and excreted through the kidneys. Hence, nursing measures, such as those discussed in Chapter 17, are used to promote activity to the greatest extent possible. Additional measures were discussed in Chapter 20 in relation to elimination. Elderly persons in general, whose normal physiological functioning has become more fragile with age, need special monitoring to help prevent imbalances. This becomes especially important when the elderly person is taking medications for various reasons.

Because successful prevention of fluid imbalances must actively involve the patient, helping him to understand the significance of disturbances, their symptoms, and preventive measures is extremely important. The nurse may find that an extensive teaching program for the patient and his family may result in prevention of a serious illness for the patient and the conservation of her time in the long run.

The nurse's vigilance is extremely important in detecting the first signs of impending imbalance so that preventive measures can be intensified. The frequency of observation of high-risk patients should be increased because the signs of impending imbalances are often insidious. Once imbalance occurs, the nurse will observe common signs as described earlier. The reader's attention is called in particular to deviations in the vital signs, given in Table 23–3. Personnel other than nurses often assist in obtaining vital signs. When fluid balance is in jeopardy, the nurse is encouraged to make her own observations as well.

Common Signs and Symptoms of Fluid Imbalance

No single symptom is in itself necessarily indicative of fluid imbalance. All must be reviewed in relation to the patient's characteristics during health. Combinations of symptoms should be reviewed with possible disturbances in mind. Probably more important than any particular sign is how it compares with the person's normal or usual characteristic. In assessing data, then, the selection of standards pertinent to the individual's situation is extremely important. Data considered significant to fluid imbalances and to which the nurse needs to be alert are grouped here as tissue characteristics, behavioral manifestations, and measurements.

Tissue Characteristics   Tissue characteristics pertinent to the determination of fluid deficiency include dryness of the skin and mucous membrane. The mucosa of the mouth and lips may be covered with a whitish coating and/or may be cracked. Generally, the mucous secretions are increased in viscosity. The texture of the

tissues can be very significant. A depletion of tissue fluids will cause a characteristic sunken appearance of the eyes, because the supportive fat pads for the eyeballs have been dehydrated. In the infant, fontanels may be depressed. Figure 23–10 illustrates the appearance of an infant who has a depletion of body fluids. The tissue cells will lose some of their elasticity when interstitial fluid decreases; thus, the cells have decreased turgor. *Turgor* is the normal tension within a cell. When the skin is pinched up between the fingers, normally it resumes its original shape immediately upon release. In poor hydration states, it remains in folds or returns slowly to its normal posture. This is somewhat unreliable in the elderly whose skin normally returns to its original shape slowly. An excess of fluids in the tissues will cause increased tension and a characteristic firmness and/or swelling. This edema is often seen initially around the eyes, in the fingers, at the ankles, and in the sacral area. Edema is illustrated in Figure 23–11. Changes in muscle tissue are particularly prevalent with electrolyte imbalance. Because the neurological stimuli and/or the ability to respond may be disturbed, the muscle tissues may appear flaccid or limp, or they may be tense and actually twitch or cramp involuntarily.

Behavioral Manifestations   Behavioral manifestations of fluid disturbances vary extensively. They can range from lethargy and coma to disorientation, hallucinations, and hyperactivity. Extreme personality changes can occur. The normally quiet, reserved person can become very talkative and physically active, or the person who normally participates in mental and physical activities shows no interest and becomes withdrawn. A change in the normal behavior of the individual is the most significant factor. Speech changes can occur from a simple slurring to an actual voice change or hoarseness. When thirst is a factor, a person's behavior can be grossly affected. The patient can become so conscious of the thirst sensation that his actions are motivated by it alone. In such instances, patients have been known to drink intravenous fluids, water from flowers, and even urine.

Measurements   Measurements of various types have already been mentioned. Changes in the vital signs can be significant. An increase in body temperature usually accompanies fluid deficiencies. Respiratory rate and depth are directly affected by carbonic acid blood levels. Fluid disturbances can also influence the pulse rate and blood pressure. Pulse rate and changes in pulse quality are also influenced by potassium disturbances.

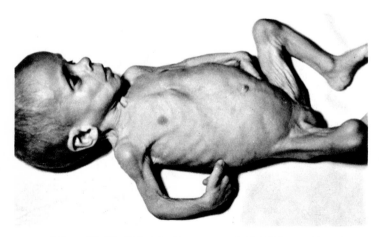

Figure 23–10   This infant has severe fluid deficiency. Note the sunken eyes and poor skin turgor.

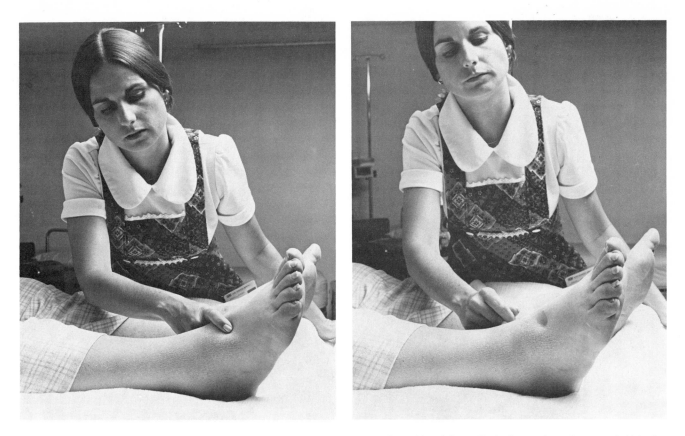

Figure 23–11   In the photo on the left, the nurse depresses an area near the ankle of the patient where edema is present. Note the indentation of edematous tissues after the nurse releases pressure, as illustrated in the photo on the right.

Weight changes, either a loss or increase, can result when there are fluid and/or sodium disturbances. Usually, the change must exceed 5 percent in a short time before it is considered to be fluid balance related. A gain or loss of 2.2 pounds (1 kilogram) is equivalent to a gain or loss of 1 liter of water. Peripheral veins normally empty or fill quickly. When a fluid deficit is present, the rate of filling decreases noticeably and the vein may even remain empty. Two procedures for checking peripheral vein filling are illustrated in Figure 23–12. With an increased fluid volume, the time for vein emptying is usually increased. Measurements which show a disproportion between fluid intake and output or which show an abnormally low intake and output even if they are in proportion to each other can be indicative of imbalance. Circulating blood volume and central venous pressure determinations are also useful. Another type of measurement useful for determining fluid imbalances is laboratory analysis of body fluids. Blood and urine test results, which indicate the quantity of their constituents, specific gravity, pH, and

other factors, provide important data. Laboratory findings were given in Table 23–5.

Measures to Help Correct Fluid Imbalances

Oral Measures.   When fluid imbalances are present, action must be taken to correct them. The degree of imbalance and the body's compensatory mechanisms will determine the type and intensity of the therapy involved. Planning and implementing the nursing care must therefore be based on the individual patient's situation. Because his active participation is highly desirable, whenever possible, the patient should be involved in determining the nursing care objectives and in selecting the actions to achieve the goals. Patient and family teaching is nearly always a key component of this care.

Some electrolyte deficiencies can be corrected by increasing the ingestion of the needed substance. Bananas and most fish are high in potassium and their

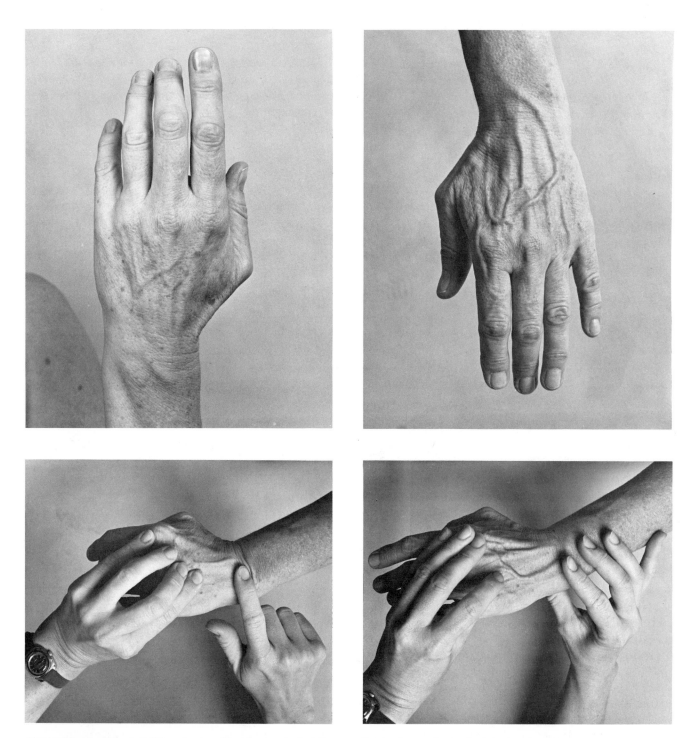

Figure 23–12 (Top, left) When the hand is raised, note that the superficial veins on the back of the hand are hardly visible. (Top, right) When the hand is dropped, the superficial veins on the back of the hand normally fill in a matter of a few seconds. (Bottom, left) A superficial vein on the back of the hand has been "milked" of blood while pressure is applied with the fingers at the end of the area where blood is removed from the vein. (Bottom, right) When pressure is released, the superficial vein on the back of the hand normally fills in a matter of a second or two.

inclusion in the diet might help overcome a potassium deficit. A sodium deficiency might be corrected by adding more salt to foods. Other examples were given in the section describing the principle electrolytes of the body. Supplementary forms of electrolytes are also commonly used to correct deficits.

Mild fluid deficiencies can be corrected by increasing the ingestion of water. The reader will recall that the average adult daily fluid intake is 2,100 ml. to 2,900 ml., but a person with a water deficit may need to take in more than this to correct the disturbance. Or, if his intake has been considerably less than this, a proportionate increase will be an improvement. Recalling that some foods contain more water than others, an increase in foods with high water content may be helpful. Since both food and fluids cause gastric expansion and a sensation of fullness, some persons can ingest larger volumes of liquids if they are spaced between meals. Whenever the patient's situation permits, encouraging as wide a variety of liquids as possible can help to prevent boredom and may make a larger volume more palatable.

Decreasing the oral intake of fluid and electrolytes may be necessary to correct imbalances. The foods that are high in excess electrolytes may need to be limited or eliminated; the restriction of sodium is a particularly common practice for persons with cardiovascular or renal diseases. The degree of restriction will vary depending on the patient's condition. Severe sodium limitations will require the use of distilled water in some parts of the country where the natural content is high. Potassium and calcium restrictions are also necessary for some persons.

Oral liquid limitations are less common, but are necessary for some people with cardiac or renal diseases. Securing the patient's understanding and cooperation is important, especially if the restrictions are severe, because it is nearly impossible to prevent a person who is up and about from securing fluids if he is motivated to do so, as indicated earlier.

Chapter 19 discussed various measures to assist patients obtain adequate nourishment and water and to help patients whose dietary or water intake requirements need adjustments.

Intravenous Measures. A relatively common form of therapy for handling fluid disturbances is the use of various solutions injected intravenously. Although the physician is responsible for prescribing the proper kind of solution and the amount to be used, the nurse is usually responsible for initiating and monitoring the therapy. The procedures will be discussed in Chapter 24. Additional material concerning intravenous therapy as a means of handling fluid disturbances will be found in the references at the end of this unit.

The variety of solutions on the market is almost without limit. There are maintenance solutions containing electrolytes in the proportion normally found in the body. There are replacement solutions with electrolyte content similar to fluids being lost. There are solutions containing amino acids, glucose, and vitamins as well as electrolytes. There is whole blood, as well as blood derivatives and replacements. There are isotonic, hypertonic, and hypotonic solutions. In some agencies, solutions are tailor-made to meet a particular patient's requirements. Should the nurse have questions concerning the selection of a particular solution, two good sources usually are readily available. The physician in charge of the therapy generally is glad to explain his selection. The pharmaceutical companies preparing the solution have excellent literature explaining the nature and common indications of each. Selection of the fluid is based on the patient's needs. Laboratory analysis of the patient's body fluids and clinical symptoms provide the guide for determining the appropriate solution.

There are several ways in which the amount of fluid to be infused is calculated. Although age and weight are important, either one in itself rarely gives sufficient knowledge to calculate amount. It is easy to see that a 40-year-old man weighing 200 pounds requires quite different amounts from a 40-year-old woman weighing 120 pounds. A combination of weight and age is often used as a guide.

Using the patient's weight to estimate his body surface area in square meters also is common. Charts that list estimates of surface area in relation to weight are available, although calculations still are necessary when the patient's body build deviates considerably from the average for his age.

Regardless of the method used—and the nurse will want to be familiar with it—another factor influences the physician's decision always, and that is the patient's clinical picture. A patient suffering from severe depletion or excess of fluids and/or electrolytes has needs different from one with moderate or mild imbalance. The need is still different from that of a patient with no indication of imbalance, who is placed on maintenance dosages because a condition exists that without care may lead to disturbances.

FLUID BALANCE AND THE NURSING PROCESS

Collecting data on the patient's state of fluid balance frequently begins with a study of the patient's fluid intake and his eating patterns. A review of Chapter 19, especially the section on the nursing process late in the chapter, and the section on nursing implications in this chapter, is advised. Specific questions to which the nurse will wish to seek answers were given. In addition, Table 23–3 in this chapter can serve as an excellent guide during data collection. The nurse will also wish to collect data on medications, prescription as well as nonprescription drugs, that the patient is taking. Obtaining a drug history will be discussed in Chapter 24 and it includes typical questions to which the nurse will wish to seek answers. Knowing the patient's health history and his reason for seeking care are important.

This chapter offered many standards that will be useful for assessing data. For instance, most illustrative material and tables give standards for assessment. Figure 23–12 illustrates normal vein filling and emptying. Figure 23–9 illustrates acid-base balance. Table 23–5 gives many laboratory values. And so on. In certain instances, clinical texts may be necessary for more detailed discussions of appropriate standards when particular pathological conditions are present.

Planning nursing care will be based on nursing diagnoses that were developed during assessment. The plan will be individualized and will depend on the patient's particular fluid imbalance or on specific factors the nurse identifies that present a threat to fluid balance.

After appropriate intervention measures are selected, they are then implemented. Many intervention measures were described earlier in this chapter. The following guidelines are ones which the nurse will wish to keep in mind.

- Remember that most disease conditions threaten fluid balance. The body normally has remarkable adaptive ability to maintain balance but normality falls within a relatively small range in many instances. Pathological conditions can sometimes upset balance quickly.

- Recall that many therapeutic regimens, such as the use of diuretics, can upset fluid balance. Knowing that a particular type of therapy is prescribed to help overcome a pathological condition does not relieve the nurse of responsibility to continue to observe for and use appropriate nursing measures to prevent fluid imbalance.

- Be alert to the patient's intake and output. Many times, in an effort to carry out measures to help restore health, inadequate attention may be paid to meeting normal nutritional and fluid needs. As a result, the most sophisticated care may be in vain. For example, a variety of drugs may be used to help a patient who has an overwhelming infection, or a complex surgical procedure may be needed to restore normal heart functioning. However, such therapy may be of no avail if the patient's daily need for nourishment and fluid are overlooked.

- Use laboratory findings to assist in assessment, planning care, and implementing care. While other observations are important to detect the status of fluid balance, laboratory findings serve as important objective evidence and often reveal imbalances before other signs and symptoms occur. Also, they often illustrate threatening imbalances and action can then be taken before the patient's condition deteriorates further.

- Use teaching opportunities to explain how to minimize threats to fluid balance and how to help overcome imbalances. As has been pointed out, even in health, certain activities can threaten fluid balance, such as exercise that results in excessive perspiration. Teaching should include common symptoms of imbalance.

- A knowledge of how the body functions to maintain fluid balance is essential in order to help prevent and overcome fluid imbalances. There is no one course of action to maintain and restore balance. Numerous factors and normal functioning of the entire body must be taken into account.

The parts of the nursing process and of the process as a whole are evaluated as described in Chapter 4.

CONCLUSION

As one author stated, water and electrolyte balances are "Much ado about something." This chapter presented fundamental information upon which the nurse can develop nursing care appropriate for the patient at risk or in a state of fluid imbalance and for teaching and using other nursing measures that will help promote fluid balance. Clinical and specialty texts are recommended for additional study.

SUPPLEMENTAL LIBRARY STUDY

1. In order to test your knowledge of certain acid-base disorders, take the pretest in the following article:

"Metabolic Acid-Base Disorders: Part 1. Chemistry and Physiology." (Programmed Instruction) *American Journal of Nursing,* 77:1619–1650, October 1977.

How does water act, as an acid or as a base, according to the footnote on P.I. page 9? According to the footnote on P.I. page 14, why is a normal saline solution neither an acid nor a base? After studying this article, take the final quizz on P.I. page 32 to determine your knowledge of the subject presented in this programmed instruction.

2. The following article describes several imbalances commonly seen in the care of persons in an emergency room:

Sweetwood, Hannelore. "Acute Respiratory Insufficiency. How to Recognize This Emergency . . . How to Treat It." *Nursing 77,* 7:24–31, December 1977.

What abnormality was found in each of the four patients described in this article? What measures are suggested by the author to detect trouble when respiratory insufficiency is present?

3. Ware, Alma Miller and Chelgren, Mary Nofziger, "When "Holding On" Brought Change: Selected Physiologic and Behavioral Parameters in Retrospect." *The Nursing Clinics of North America,* 6:125–134, March 1971.

What behavioral changes were symptoms of the patient's electrolyte imbalance? What supportive nursing actions might you have used to respond to the patient's "holding on?"

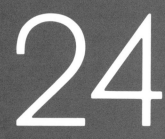

BEHAVIORAL OBJECTIVES

When content in this chapter has been mastered, the student will be able to

Define the terms appearing in the glossary.

List the seven parts of a drug order and indicate the importance of each.

Identify and discuss at least eight principles which are important for the safe preparation and administration of any drug.

Describe how to administer drugs orally, subcutaneously, intramuscularly, intravenously, and intracutaneously and how to inject relatively large amounts of solution intravenously and subcutaneously. Include a discussion of the various sites of the body into which drugs and solutions are injected and how these sites are properly identified.

Summarize how drugs are administered topically to the skin, eyes, ears, nose, throat, and vagina.

Discuss characteristics of human blood that make typing and crossmatching important when a blood transfusion is given and indicate the nursing responsibilities for the administration of blood and its common extracts.

Indicate nursing responsibilities for teaching individuals how to take their own drugs and for public education concerning drug abuse.

Describe how to administer therapeutic agents, using the nursing process as a guide.

The Administration of Therapeutic Agents

GLOSSARY

Agglutinin: An antibody which causes a clumping of specific antigens.

Antibody: A protein substance developed in the body in response to the presence of an antigen in the body.

Antigen: A substance which causes the formation of antibodies.

Bevel: The sloped edge of a needle.

Blood transfusion: The infusion of whole blood from a healthy person into a recipient.

Buccal: Pertaining to the cheek or mouth.

Crossmatching: Determining the compatibility of two blood specimens.

Cut-Down: The incision of a vein, most often for the purpose of administering an infusion.

Direct Transfusion: The infusion of blood while it is being taken from the donor.

Donor: A person who donates blood for giving to another person.

Drug: A substance that modifies body functions when taken into the living organism. Synonym for medication.

Embolism: The obstruction of a blood vessel by a foreign body or air.

Embolus: A foreign body or air in the circulatory system. The pleural form is emobli.

Enteral: Within the intestines.

Hyperalimentation: The intravenous infusion of solution that contains sufficient nutrients to support life and maintain normal growth and development. Synonym for Total Parenteral Nutrition, abbreviated TPN.

Hypodermic Injection: An injection into the subcutaneous tissue. Synonym for subcutaneous injection.

Hypodermoclysis: The injection of relatively large amounts of solution into subcutaneous tissues.

Indirect Transfusion: The infusion of blood from a container in which the donor's blood was received.

Infiltration: The escape of fluid into subcutaneous tissue.

Inhalation: The administration of a drug in solution via the respiratory tract.

Instillation: Pouring or dropping a liquid into a cavity or onto a surface.

Intraarterial Injection: An injection into an artery.

Intracardial Injection: An injection into heart tissue.

Intracutaneous Injection: An injection under the epidermis. Synonym for intradermal injection.

Intradermal Injection: An injection under the epidermis. Synonym for intracutaneous injection.

Intramuscular Injection: An injection into muscle tissue.

Intraosseous Injection: An injection into bone tissue.

Intraperitoneal Injection: An injection into the peritoneal cavity.

Intraspinal Injection: An injection into the spinal canal.

Intravenous Infusion: The injection of relatively large quantities of solution into a vein.

Intravenous Injection: An injection into a vein.

Inunction: Rubbing substances into the skin.

Irrigation: Flushing of a canal or cavity with liquid.

Medication: A substance that modifies body functions when taken into the living organism. Synonym for drug.

Oral Administration: Giving an agent by mouth.

O-T-C: The abbreviation for over-the-counter.

Parenteral: Outside of the intestines or alimentary canal. It is popularly used to refer to injection routes.

Pharmacist: A person licensed to prepare and dispense drugs.

Pharmacology: The study of actions of chemicals on living organisms.

Phlebitis: An inflammation of a vein.

Prescription: A physician's order.

Recipient: A person receiving another person's blood.

Rh: An inherited antigen.

Single Order: A directive to be carried out one time.

Standing Order: A directive to be carried out until canceled.

Stat Order: A directive to be carried out at once.

Subcutaneous Injection: An injection into subcutaneous tissue. Synonym for hypodermic injection.

Sublingual: The area in the mouth under the tongue.

Therapeutic Agent: A substance used to treat a pathological condition.

Thrombus: A blood clot. The pleural form is thrombi.

Topical Application: The application of a substance directly to a body site.

Total Parenteral Nutrition: The intravenous infusion of solution that contains sufficient nutrients to support life and maintain normal growth and development. Abbreviated TPN. Synonym for hyperalimentation.

Typing: Determining a person's blood type.

Unit Dose: A separate packing and labeling of an individual drug dose.

INTRODUCTION

A *drug* or a *medication* is any substance that modifies body functions when taken into the living organism. The study that deals with chemicals affecting the body's functioning is called *pharmacology*. A *pharmacist* is a person licensed to prepare and dispense drugs.

Blood and its derivatives and various fluid-electrolyte solutions administered intravenously are used for therapeutic purposes. These are physiological substances and not pharmaceutical agents. However, many principles used to guide the nurse when she administers these substances are similar to those used when administering drugs, and hence, the administration of intravenous substances will be discussed in this chapter.

When a person is receiving less than normal quantities of nutrient substances for whatever reason, supplements may be prescribed. Vitamins and minerals are two substances often used therapeutically as nutrient supplements. The procedure for administering such nutrient supplements is the same as that used for administering drugs. For ease of reading, the term nutrient supplements will not be repeated each time the words drug and medication are used in this chapter, although it should be recognized that these supplements are not correctly classified as drugs.

Therapeutic agents include drugs and physiological substances used to treat pathological conditions. This chapter is concerned primarily with the nurse's responsibilities for the administration of these agents. Information about specific drugs, their actions, and pharmaceutical toxicology are more appropriately discussed in pharmacology texts.

THE MEDICATION ORDER

Although many times the nurse supplies information to assist the physician to develop a therapeutic drug plan for his patients, the physician is legally responsible for prescribing therapeutic agents. He conveys directives for his plan to others by a physician's order or a *prescription*. Safe practice is to follow only a written order. A written order by the physician is least likely to result in error or misunderstanding. Under certain circumstances, a verbal order from the physician may be given to a registered nurse or pharmacist. The legal circumstances of dispensing and administering an agent without a written order vary, and the nurse is cautioned to be familiar with the exact agency policy wherever she is called upon to administer therapeutic agents.

Each health agency has a policy specifying the manner in which the physician writes his order. In most cases, orders are written on a form specifically intended for the physician's orders. This becomes part of the patient's permanent record or the pharmacy record, as was described in Chapter 5.

Types of Orders

There are several types of orders that the physician may prescribe. One type is called a *standing order* and is to be carried out as specified until it is canceled by another order. Occasionally, the physician writes a standing order and its cancellation simultaneously—that is, the physician specifies that a certain order is to be carried out for a stated number of days or times. After the stated period has passed, the order is canceled automatically. Some health agencies and pharmacies have policies that specify that standing orders must be reviewed and rewritten at regular intervals or they will be canceled.

A second type of order is called a *single order;* that is, the directive is carried out only once, either at early convenience or at a time specified by the physician. A *stat order* is also a single order, but it is one which is to be carried out at once. When a patient has had surgery or when he is transferred to another clinical service or another health agency, it is general practice that all orders related to drugs are discontinued, and new orders are written. To keep physicians aware of orders in effect, some hospitals specify a day of the week when orders are to be rewritten or they will be automatically discontinued.

It is usual hospital policy that when a patient is admitted, unless specific orders to the contrary are written, all drugs which the physician may have ordered while the patient was at home are discontinued. This may prove to be a problem when a patient brings his medications to the hospital. To avoid the possibility of having the patient continue taking his medications while receiving the same ones or others under new orders, all medications should be sent home with the family or removed from the patient's unit and placed in safekeeping. This will require an explanation to the patient and family of how the patient's drug plan will be implemented. However, in some inpatient facilities, patients keep their medications at their bedside and learn or continue to administer them as they would at home. It is felt that this approach helps to promote the independence of patients. The nurse should be aware when patients are allowed to take their own medications while hospitalized and should know the agent's purpose and possible undesirable side effects. Also, a notation should be made on the patient's plan of care so that everyone knows the patient has medications at his bedside.

Parts of the Drug Order

The drug order consists of seven parts: the name of the patient, the date the order is written, the name of the drug to be administered, the dosage, the route by which it is to be administered and special directives about its administration, the time of administration and/or frequency, and the signature of the person writing the order. Drug prescriptions to a pharmacist serving an outpatient may also specify whether or not the name of the drug should be included on the label and how many times the prescription can be refilled.

The *patient's full name* is used. The middle name or initial should be included to avoid confusion with other patients. Some health agencies have facilities to imprint the patient's name mechanically on the order form.

The *date* the order is written is given. In some situations, the *time* the order is written may also be included. Since the nursing staffs in inpatient facilities change several times during each 24-hour period, the date and the time help to prevent errors of oversight as different nurses take charge of a unit. When an order is to be followed for a specified number of days, the date and the time are important in order that the discontinuation date and time can be determined accurately. The time that an order for a narcotic remains valid is determined by law. Therefore, the date and the time the order was written are essential for determining when the order for a narcotic becomes invalid.

The *name of the drug* is stated in the order after the physician has indicated the patient for whom it is intended. Some agencies require that the physician use generic nomenclature. Certain trade names are well-known, but the practice of using the official name is the safest one. If the nurse is unfamiliar with a drug, she can investigate by referring to certain standard references. In this country, *The United States Pharmacopeia* (U.S.P.) and the *National Formulary* (N.F.) are official sources. Most other countries have similar references which describe official therapeutic agents. Many agencies also provide their own book listing the official drugs commonly used by the agency. The American Society of Hospital Pharmacists and the American Medical Association's Council on Drugs also publish helpful resources for drug information. The *Physician's Desk Reference to Pharmaceutical Specialties and Biologicals* (PDR), is another handy source of information. It is published by Medical Economics, Inc. from information supplied by pharmaceutical companies.

If a patient at home is taking a drug that does not have the name of the medication on the label, the nurse needs to contact the physician or pharmacist to determine the identity of the substance. It is unsafe to care for patients when the nurse does not know the name and prescribed dosage of drugs and the physician's directives to the patients for taking them.

The Council on Drugs of the American Medical Association has gone on record as favoring labeling of prescriptions. While it is agreed that, for some drugs and for some patients, the drug should be nameless, in most cases labeling is desirable for several reasons. It generally is felt the patient has a right to be informed about his health state and the drugs he is taking. With labeling there may be less likelihood of taking incorrect medications, especially when several persons in a home may have prescribed drugs on hand. In case of accident, emergency treatment can be facilitated when the exact content of the drug is known. With the trend toward teaching patients about their therapy, the patient usually is told what drugs he is receiving.

The *dosage* of a drug can be stated in either the apothecary or the metric system. With planned conversion of this country's measurements to the metric system, apothecary measurements are being used less frequently. Self-administered drugs are frequently labeled in household measurements to facilitate administration. Most agencies post a table of common equivalent dosages for persons who have learned to use one system and find that the agency in which they work uses the other system. Although these tables are convenient and useful, the nurse should be prepared to convert from one system to the other, since such tables are not available in every situation. The nurse should also be familiar with common equivalent measurements when using household equipment such as teaspoons, tablespoons, and so on, since usually the home is not equipped with special measuring devices. Table 24–1 on page 600 shows some of the common equivalents.

Certain standard abbreviations are used to indicate drug amounts. Before a nurse can administer drugs, she will be required to acquaint herself with these common abbreviations. Table 24–2 on page 600 indicates some of the most commonly used abbreviations.

The nurse also should be aware of common factors that influence dosage calculation; for example, a child's

TABLE 24–1   Approximate equivalents of fluid and weight measures

WEIGHTS (approximate)

METRIC	APOTHECARY	METRIC	APOTHECARY	METRIC	APOTHECARY	METRIC	APOTHECARY
0.2 mg. = 1/300 grain		3.0 mg. = 1/20 grain		60.0 mg. = 1 grain		1.0 Gm. = 15 grains	
0.3 mg. = 1/200 grain		6.0 mg. = 1/10 grain		0.12 Gm. = 2 grains		4.0 Gm. = 60 grains (1 dram)	
0.4 mg. = 1/150 grain		10.0 mg. = 1/6 grain		0.2 Gm. = 3 grains		6.0 Gm. = 90 grains	
0.5 mg. = 1/120 grain		15.0 mg. = 1/4 grain		0.3 Gm. = 5 grains		10.0 Gm. = 2½ drams	
0.6 mg. = 1/100 grain		25.0 mg. = 3/8 grain		0.5 Gm. = 7½ grains		15.0 Gm. = 4 drams	
1.0 mg. = 1/60 grain		30.0 mg. = 1/2 grain		0.6 Gm. = 10 grains		30.0 Gm. = 1 ounce	

LIQUID MEASURE (approximate)

METRIC	APOTHECARY	HOUSEHOLD	METRIC	APOTHECARY
0.06 ml.	= 1 minim	= 1 drop	30 ml.	= 1 fluid ounce
0.5 ml.	= 8 minims		250 ml.	= 8+ fluid ounces
1.0 ml.	= 15 minims		500 ml.	= 1+ pint
4.0 ml.	= 1 fluid dram	= 1 teaspoon	1,000 ml. (1 liter)	= 1+ quart

Adaptation courtesy Becton, Dickinson and Company, Rutherford, New Jersey.

dose for a drug is smaller than an adult's dose. Various formulae have been devised to calculate children's dosage by reducing adult dosages in proportion to the age or the weight of the child. One common formula is Clark's Rule, based on the assumption that the average adult weighs 150 pounds:

$$\text{Usual adult dose} \times \frac{\text{weight of child in pounds}}{150} = \text{child's dose.}$$

Weight is a factor in dosage calculation because, in general, the heavier the person, the larger the dosage of drugs he can tolerate.

The route of administration influences dosage calculations. Drugs given by mouth are adsorbed more slowly and less completely than those given intravenously. Hence, the dosage of a drug given intravenously generally is smaller than that of the same drug given orally.

TABLE 24–2   Common abbreviations for measures

ABBREVIATION	UNABBREVIATED FORM
ʒ	dram
gtt.	drop
gr.	grain
Gm.	gram
mg. or mgm.	milligram
ml.	milliliter
m or min.	minim
℥	ounce
tbsp.	tablespoon
tsp.	teaspoon

The general condition of the patient and his drug intolerances are also factors that may influence dosage calculations. Age and the patient's sex may also be significant. Generally, elderly persons and women require smaller dosages than younger adults and men.

The *route* to be used when administering the medication is stated clearly because some drugs can be given in more than one way and some may be used safely only via one route. If a route is not specified, it is generally understood to be an *oral* medication; that is, it is given by mouth.

As in the case of calculating dosages, there are several factors that influence the choice of route. These include the desired action of the drug, the speed of absorption and rapidity of response, the nature of the medication, and the condition of the patient.

The action of drugs can be either systemic or local. A systemic action occurs when the agent is absorbed by the bloodstream and is distributed throughout the tissues and the fluids of the body. For example, an antibiotic given by injection is absorbed by the blood and acts upon certain organisms wherever they may be harboring in body tissues or fluid.

A local action occurs when the agent is placed directly in contact with tissue and it is intended to act upon that specific tissue only. One type occurs with a drug for athlete's foot where the drug acts directly upon the diseased tissue and the causative organism. Other local actions include eyedrops containing drugs which can, when instilled, either dilate or contract the pupil, and local anesthetic agents.

Table 24–3 illustrates common routes by which

TABLE 24-3 Routes for administering drugs

ROUTE	HOW DRUG IS ADMINISTERED	TERM USED TO DESCRIBE ROUTE
Given by mouth	Having patient swallow drug	Oral Administration
Given via respiratory tract	Having patient inhale drug	Inhalation
Given by injection	Injecting drug into	Administration by injection
	1. Subcutaneous tissue	1. Hypodermic or subcutaneous injection
	2. Muscle tissue	2. Intramuscular injection
	3. Corium (under epidermis)	3. Intracutaneous injection
	4. Vein	4. Intravenous injection
	5. Artery	5. Intraarterial injection
	6. Heart tissue	6. Intracardial injection
	7. Peritoneal cavity	7. Intraperitoneal injection
	8. Spinal canal	8. Intraspinal injection
	9. Bone	9. Intraosseous injection
Given by placing on skin or mucous membrane	Inserting drug into	
	1. Vagina	1. Vaginal administration
	2. Rectum	2. Rectal administration
	Placing drug under tongue	Sublingual administration
	Placing drug between cheek and gum	Buccal
	Rubbing drug into skin	Inunction
	Placing drug into direct contact with mucous membrane	Instillation
	Flushing mucous membrane with drug in solution	Irrigation

therapeutic agents are administered. The *time* and *frequency* with which a drug is to be administered usually are stated in standard abbreviations in the medication order.

Common abbreviations used in writing prescriptions, including time and frequency, are listed in Table 24-4.

The nursing service department of inpatient facilities usually determines the hours at which routine drugs are given. For example, if certain drugs are to be given every four hours, the nursing service policy indicates the times. Every-four-hour administration may be at the times of 4 A.M., 8 A.M., 12 A.M. (noon), 4 P.M., 8 P.M., and 12 P.M. (midnight). Another agency may use the hours 5 A.M., 9 A.M., 1 P.M., 5 P.M., 9 P.M., and 1 A.M. If a drug is ordered to be given before or after meals, the time will depend on the hours at which meals are served.

If a drug is to be given only once or twice a day, the decision as to which hours to use will depend on the nature of the drug and the patient's plan of care. Whenever possible, there should be consideration for the patient's choice of time.

Drugs should be administered punctually as ordered. However, a nurse administering drugs to several patients cannot give all of them exactly on the hour indicated. Agency policies vary, but a common one is that drugs should be administered within a half hour before or after the indicated hour. Thus, a drug to be administered at 9 A.M. can be administered any time between 8:30 and 9:30 A.M., using this policy. This policy does not apply to all drugs. A preoperative medication ordered to be given at 7:30 A.M. should be administered at that hour since the time was planned in relation to the time surgery is to begin. This also holds true when patients are given drugs prior to certain diagnostic procedures and stat orders.

The *signature of the person writing the order* follows the order. The signature is of importance for legal reasons because the authority to prescribe drugs is defined by state laws. Also, should there be a question about the order, the signature indicates who should be contacted.

Questioning the Medication Order

The nurse is responsible for questioning a drug order if in her judgment the order is in error. The suspected error may be in the name of the patient, the medication prescribed, dosage, the time, or the frequency with which it is to be administered, or the route by which it is to be given. The legal implications are serious when there is an error in the medication order and when the nurse involved could be expected, from her knowledge and experience, to have noted the error. On occasion, the nurse may not feel that there is an error in the order, but she may not understand why the medication

TABLE 24-4 Common abbreviations used in prescribing drugs

ABBREVIATION	UNABBREVIATED FORM	MEANING
a.a.	ana	of each
a.c.	ante cibum	before meals
ad lib	ad libitum	freely
agit.	agita	shake
ante	ante	before
aq.	aqua	water
b.i.d.	bis in die	twice each day
c̄	cum	with
cap.	capsula	capsule
dil.	dilutus	dissolve or dilute
elix.	elixir	elixir
h.s.	hour of sleep	at bedtime
IM	intramuscular	into muscle
IV	intravenous	into a vein
non rep.	non repetatar	do not repeat
o.d.	oculus dexter	right eye
o.s.	oculus sinister	left eye
os	os	mouth
o.u.	oculus uterque	each eye
p.c.	post cibum	after meals
PO	per os	by mouth
p.r.n.	pro re nata	according to necessity
q	quaque	every
q.d.	quaque die	every day
q.h.	quaque hora	every hour
q.i.d.	quater in die	4 times each day
q.o.d.	quaque aliem die	every other day
q.s.	quantum satis	quantity sufficient
Rx	recipe	take
s̄	sine	without
s.o.s.	si opus sit	if necessary
ss.	semis	a half
stat.	statim	at once
subcu or subq	subcutaneous	into subcutaneous tissue
t.i.d.	ter in die	3 times a day
tinc.	tinctura	alcohol base solution

has been prescribed. In such an instance, the nurse should ask so that she may understand how the order relates to the patient's plan of care.

Occasionally, a nurse may have difficulty reading the order. *Guessing is gross carelessness;* rechecking with the person who wrote the order is the only safe procedure.

SAFEGUARDING DRUGS

In each health agency, there is at least one area where drugs are stocked and kept in readiness for dispensing to patients. The cabinet or room is usually locked, and only authorized personnel have access to the key to protect persons from unsafe drug use.

Drugs may be kept in a central area for all patients or they may be kept separately for individual patients.

Some inpatient facilities have locked wall cupboards near the entrance to each patient's room for drug storage. Other agencies have locked mobile cupboards which require an individually keyed card or key for access to each patient's supply.

Unit dose packaging, that is, the separate packaging and labeling of individual drug doses, has become popular and helps promote better drug control, fewer errors, and cleanliness. Pharmacies of some hospitals deliver the single dose of medication, which is ready for administration, to the nurse caring for the patient.

Patients often need to be taught the importance of safeguarding drugs at home. Keeping all medications out of the reach of children is especially important. The number of children who are poisoned from seemingly harmless aspirin and vitamin pills every year is alarmingly high.

Narcotics are kept in a double-locked drawer, box, or room. This precaution is observed as an additional safety measure. Narcotics may be ordered only by physicians registered with the Department of Justice, Bureau of Narcotics and Dangerous Drugs. According to federal law, a record must be kept for each narcotic that is administered. Health agencies provide forms for keeping such records, and these forms are kept with the narcotics. Although the forms differ, the following information generally is required: the name of the patient receiving the narcotic, the amount of the narcotic used, the hour the narcotic was given, the name of the physician prescribing the narcotic, and the name of the nurse administering the narcotic. It is common practice to check narcotics daily at specified intervals. In hospitals checking is usually done at each change of shift. The amount of narcotics on hand is counted, and each used narcotic must be accounted for on the narcotic record. A narcotic count which does not check must be reported immediately. The law requires these special precautions in the use of narcotics in order to aid in the control of drug abuse. The nurse administering narcotics has an important responsibility to see that the federal law is observed.

While in the past it was common practice for nurses to prepare and administer most drugs, today in many inpatient facilities, pharmacy personnel prepare medications and in some agencies may administer them also. This practice permits the persons most knowledgeable about drugs to deal with them and provides more time for nurses to spend with patients. Whether nurses actually prepare or administer drugs or not, they still have a responsibility to understand how the medications a patient receives fit into his total regimen of care, to observe their effects, and to teach patients and family members appropriately about the patient's drug therapy.

GENERAL PRINCIPLES OF PREPARING AND ADMINISTERING DRUGS

When the nurse is to give a drug, her first step is to follow the agency's policy specifying the manner in which the medication order is checked. Various systems are used. Some agencies use a card system. Others check with the original written order. Still others use a computer printout sheet. The nurse should be familiar with the system used and implement it correctly to minimize errors in administering medications.

Knowledge of the Patient and the Drug

Intelligent administration of drugs requires that the nurse understand the patient's health status and its relationship to the therapeutic agent. Without such knowledge, the nurse cannot observe the patient's responses so that they can be used to plan and adjust therapy according to changes in the patient.

The nurse should know the desired action, both local and systemic, of the drugs she administers, their toxic manifestations, and side effects. This type of information is described in pharmacology texts. In addition, these texts describe the various effects that may result when a person is taking several drugs at the same time. The nurse should have such knowledge about any drug she administers in order to guide her observation of patients receiving therapy.

Safety Measures for Preparing Drugs

An environment that promotes safety and good working habits contributes to accuracy in the preparation of drugs for administration. It is important that good lighting be available when preparing drugs. Also, while the nurse is preparing drugs, she should work alone. This practice helps prevent distractions and interruptions, which may lead to errors.

Once the nurse begins to prepare drugs for administration, she should not leave them. If it is imperative that she leave for a short time, the drugs which have been prepared should be placed carefully in a locked area until her return.

The label on the medication container should be read and checked *three times:* when reaching for the container of medication, immediately prior to pouring the medication, and when replacing the container on the shelf. The importance of checking three times cannot be overemphasized. The safe nurse does not allow automatic habits of preparing drugs to replace *constant thinking, purposeful action,* and *repeated checking* for accuracy.

Safety in Transporting Drugs

Drugs should be clearly identified. Special trays or carts on which to carry medications to the patient are provided. These trays are designed for individual or group use. They usually provide a means by which the identifying information and the medication container can be kept together safely. A medication cart is illustrated in Figure 24–1. If a large number of medications are to be given by injection, it is safer as well as convenient to have medication trays or carts which also hold syringes securely. During the time the nurse is administering the medications to the patients, the tray or cart should never be out of her sight. This is to prevent persons from taking medications not intended for them and accidental dislodging of cards or spilling of drugs.

When medications are to be given to more than one

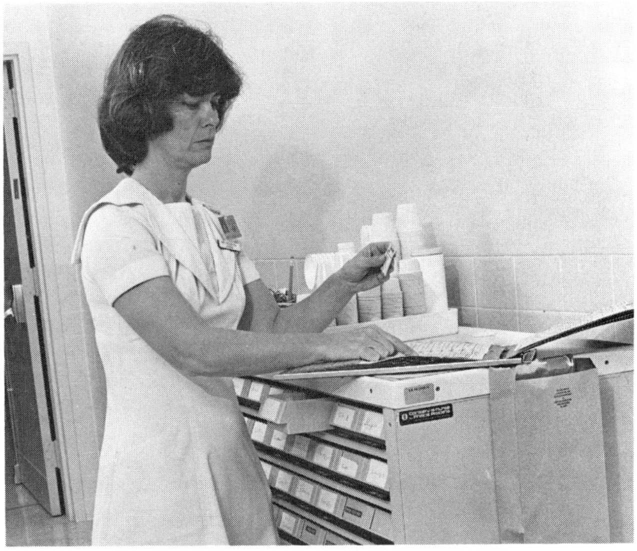

Figure 24–1 This mobile cart and the Kardex are taken to the patient's room when medications are given. Each patient's medications are stored in a separate drawer, numbered according to the patient's room. Note that the nurse carefully checks the medication she will give with the Kardex. The cart is stored between uses in a locked room near the nurses' station.

patient, it is efficient to arrange the medications in order of administration. This may be according to location of the patients or problems associated with the administration of drugs to certain patients. If a patient requires a great deal of assistance, it is recommended that all other medications be given first and only his medications remain on the tray.

Identifying the Patient

Positive identification of the patient is essential to safe drug administration. Before the nurse administers the drug, she checks carefully to see that she is giving the drug to the right patient. Patients in inpatient health agencies generally wear identification bracelets. The nurse is identifying the patient by checking her bracelet in Figure 24–2. All patients should be called by name. When calling the patient by name, accuracy and clear diction are important so that the nurse can be sure of proper identification. When the patient is unknown to the nurse, he should be asked to state his name. This is particularly important when patients have a language handicap or are confused. These patients may answer to a name other than their own without realizing it.

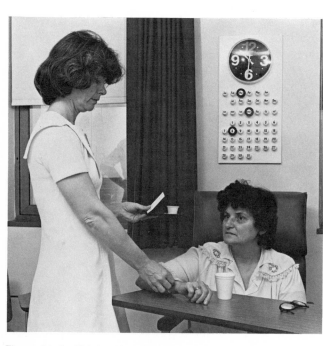

Figure 24–2   This health agency uses a card system for administering medications. The patient's name on her identification bracelet is checked with the name on the medication card in the nurse's hand. Whatever procedure is used, an essential step is to check the patient's identification bracelet carefully to avoid errors.

Administering a Drug

The nurse should remain with the patient and see that he takes the drug before she leaves. If the patient receives several drugs, offer them separately so that if one is refused or dropped, positive identification can be made and the drug recorded or replaced. Leaving medications for the patient to take later is considered unsafe practice. The patient may not take the drug after the nurse leaves. Also, the nurse should not record a drug as given unless the patient has actually received it. If the drug is harmful in large doses and the patient intends to harm himself, he may save a sufficient quantity to do so, such as with sleeping pills. This paragraph describes giving medications by mouth. However, the same general principle applies when using other routes as well; that is, a drug must be actually taken or administered for it to have an effect or in order to record it as taken or administered.

Recording the Administration of Drugs

Accurate record keeping makes review and evaluation of drug therapy possible. Every drug administered should be recorded on the patient's record. Most agencies have a special form and a specific policy for such recordings as was described in Chapter 5. While there are variations, the drug, its dosage, and route of administration are always included. The location of giving other than oral drugs may be required. Thus, policy may require that the nurse record that drops were placed in the right, left, or both ears, or that an injection was given into the left gluteus maximus or right deltoid muscle. Some agencies also require other specific information about the patient. For instance, the pulse rate may be recorded when administering some cardiac drugs or a description of the effects on the patient's pain when administering analgesics.

Omitted or Refused Drugs

Omitting a drug may influence successive drug actions. Inadvertent omission of a drug should be reported as soon as it is detected to determine whether a dose should be administered at that time. For example, a medication given daily might be given in the afternoon after it was discovered that it had been omitted in the morning. Generally, however, if the omission goes undetected until the following day, a double dose would not be given. A medication administered every six hours would probably be given if its omission was

The administration of oral medications

The purpose is to prepare and administer oral medications safely and accurately.

SUGGESTED ACTION	RATIONALE
After checking the order, read the label three times while preparing the drug.	Frequent checking helps to ensure accuracy and to prevent errrors.
When removing tablets or capsules from a bottle, pour the necessary number into the bottle cap and then place the tablets in a medication cup.	Pouring tablets or capsules into the nurse's hand is unsanitary.
Use the appropriate measuring device when pouring liquids and read the amount of medication at the bottom of the miniscus.	Accuracy is possible when the appropriate measuring device is used and then read accurately.
Pour liquids from the side of the bottle opposite the label.	Liquid that may drip onto the label makes the label difficult to read.
Place each medication in a separate container. Prepackaged single-dose medications are opened at the patient's bedside.	If drugs are spilled or refused, positive identification as to type or amount can be made.
Keep the medication card and drug together at all times.	Keeping drugs identified ensures proper administration of the correct drug to the correct patient.
Transport medications to the patient's bedside carefully and keep the medications in sight at all times.	Careful handling and close observation prevent accidental or deliberate disarrangement of medications.
Identify the patient carefully, using all precautions: check the bed card, look at the identification band, call the patient by name, or ask the patient to state his name.	Illness and strange surroundings often cause patients to be confused.
Assist the patient to an upright position if necessary.	Swallowing is facilitated by proper positioning.
If more than one drug is to be given at one time, administer each one separately.	Individual administration promotes accuracy.
Offer water or other permitted fluids with pills, capsules, tablets, and some liquid medications.	Liquids facilitate swallowing of solid drugs. Some liquid drugs are intended to adhere to the pharyngeal area, in which case, liquid is not offered with the medication.
Remain with the patient until each medication is swallowed. Unless the nurse has seen the patient swallow the drug, it cannot be recorded that the drug was administered.	The patient's chart is a legal record.
Offer the patient additional fluids as necessary, especially if drug tends to irritate mucosa.	Fluids help to dissolve and dilute solid drugs.
If the patient's intake is measured, record the fluid the patient took with the medication.	All fluid intake is to be recorded for accuracy in determining total intake.
Promptly record the medications given, refused, or omitted.	Prompt recording avoids the possibility of accidentally repeating the administration of the drug.

Preparing Drugs for Administraton by Injection

Drugs for administration by injection are marketed in several ways. Those that deteriorate in solution usually are dispensed as tablets or powders and placed in solution immediately prior to injection. If drugs remain stable in solution, usually they are dispensed in ampules, bottles, or vials in an aqueous or oily solution or suspension.

Some medications are available in syringes that are prefilled by the manufacturer. Drug companies specify the route intended for each medication and a drug should not be administered by any route other than the one for which it was specified. For example, a drug labeled for intramuscular use should not be given intravenously.

Drugs may be dispensed in single-dose glass ampules, single-dose rubber-capped vials, and multiple-dose rubber-capped vials.

Most single-dose glass ampules have a constriction in the stem of the ampule which facilitates opening it. Before preparing to open the ampule, make certain that all of the drug is in the ampule proper and not in the stem. The drug tends to be trapped in the stem, and it may be necessary to tap the stem several times with a snap of a finger to help bring the drug down. Ampules without a constriction do not present this problem.

A practice in some agencies is to wipe the outside of

the ampule with an antiseptic solution before it is opened. This practice has not been justified scientifically. Considering that the antiseptic is merely passed over the glass briefly, and that immediately thereafter it will be scored by an unsterile file, it would appear that this gesture adds nothing to the safety of the procedure.

When all the drug has been brought to the bottom of the ampule, gauze is used to hold the ampule firmly and to protect the nurse's fingers. Sterile gauze or other material is used because it will be in close proximity to the opening of the ampule when the stem is removed. A saw-tooth file is used to scratch the glass gently on the stem, well above the level of the medication. Scratching it on opposite sides helps to ensure a quick, even break. After the scratch marks have been made, the ampule is held in one hand, and the other is used to break off the stem. This is illustrated in Figure 24–3. Many single-dose ampules are prescored and do not require filing. These are identified by a colored marking at the neck of the ampule. However, there is still need to protect the fingers. A commercial ampule opener with a protective flange is also available.

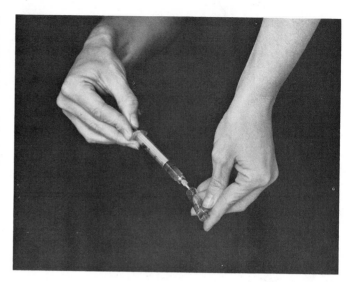

Figure 24–4 The nurse places the needle into the solution in an open ampule and withdraws the solution into the syringe. No air is injected into the ampule since it is an open vessel.

The medication in the ampule is now in an open vessel. To remove it, insert the needle into the ampule and withdraw the solution. Be careful not to touch the edge of the glass with the needle in order to prevent contamination. The fluid in the ampule is immediately displaced by air; therefore, there is no resistance to its withdrawal. The nurse in Figure 24–4 is removing medication from an ampule. With additional skill, it will be possible to pick up the ampule and hold it between two fingers of one hand and the syringe in the other hand. When removing the drug in this fashion, the trick lies in keeping the needle in the solution at all times, even as the ampule is inverted.

For safety in transporting and storing, the single-dose rubber-capped vial usually is covered with a soft metal cap which can be removed easily. The rubber part which then is exposed is the means of entrance into the vial. At the time of preparation, this rubber portion of the seal was sterilized, but many agencies specify that the cap be cleaned with an antiseptic before the needle is inserted. Use friction when cleaning. The rubber stopper should be entered with slight lateral pressure on the needle during piercing of the stopper to prevent a core of the stopper from entering the vial.

To facilitate the removal of the drug from the closed container, it is best to inject an amount of air comparable with the amount of solution to be withdrawn. This increases the pressure within the vial, and then the drug can be withdrawn easily, since fluids move from an area of greater pressure to an area of lesser pressure. If air is not injected first, an area of lesser pressure, that

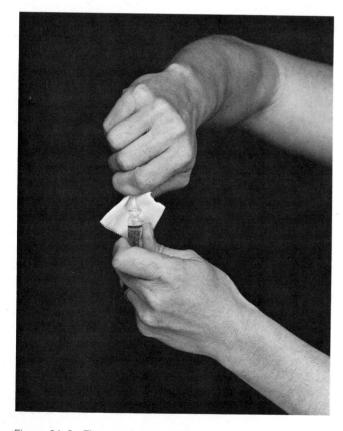

Figure 24–3 The ampule in this photo was prescored by the manufacturer. Note that the nurse uses a gauze square to protect herself from injury.

is, a partial vacuum, is created in the vial as fluid is withdrawn, because air cannot displace the fluid being removed. This area of lesser pressure exerts pull on the fluid, making it difficult to withdraw.

Some drugs are dispensed in vials containing several or multiple doses, such as an insulin vial. These are managed in the same manner as the single-dose sealed vial. The cap is cleaned by thorough rubbing with a cotton ball or a gauze pledget moistened with an antiseptic solution. An amount of air equivalent to the amount of solution to be withdrawn is injected. The air should be injected accurately, since not enough air will make withdrawal of the drug difficult, and increasing the pressure in the vial by adding too much air will interfere with the ease of preparing the correct dose by pushing solution into the syringe. Figure 24–5 illustrates a nurse injecting air in an amount equivalent to the amount of medication she will remove from a rubber-capped vial.

If the amount of fluid to be removed from a vial is rather large or several doses are to be removed in succession, a simple method is to insert a separate sterile needle through the cap. This will allow air to enter and replace the fluid as it is being withdrawn. This is illustrated in Figure 24–6.

Surgical and Medical Asepsis When Agents Are to be Injected

While details of methods for administering injections may vary from one agency to another, there is one

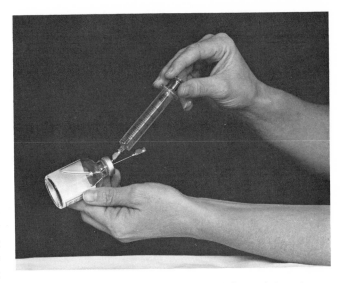

Figure 24–6 The second needle in the vial allows air to enter as solution is withdrawn.

basic principle which underlies all—strict asepsis minimizes the danger of injecting organisms into the patient's tissues or bloodstream.

All objects coming in contact with the drug and the patient's tissues should be sterilized prior to use by the most reliable means available. Findings related to types A and B viral hepatitis leave little doubt that it is transmitted easily via injection therapy. Many agencies take extra precautions by using disposable items, including syringes, needles, and single-dose cartridges for medications. Figure 24–7 on page 610 shows the parts of the syringe and needle that must be kept sterile.

If a drug must be prepared and then transported to the patient's unit, the needle must be kept sterile. Using the holder which protected the needle offers the greatest amount of safety.

Cleaning the skin before an injection has been considered a traditional part of the technique, although some studies indicate that it is unnecessary. However, until further evidence is gathered, most authorities continue to recommend thorough skin cleaning before an injection.

The choice of an antiseptic agent for cleaning the skin prior to injection therapy is of periodic concern to every health agency. However, as was pointed out, sterilization of the skin cannot be expected. Since sterilizing the skin is not possible, the purpose of cleaning the area is to make certain that it is free from gross contamination and dried skin cells. In cleaning the area, a circular motion is used, beginning at the point of injection and moving outward and away from it. This carries material away from the critical site. Hap-

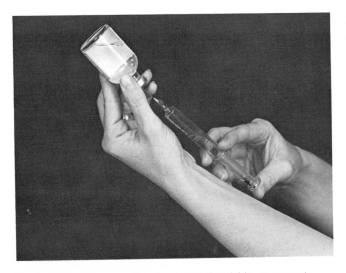

Figure 24–5 The nurse injects air into the vial in an amount equivalent to the amount of solution she will withdraw. This creates pressure within the vial so that the solution may be removed easily.

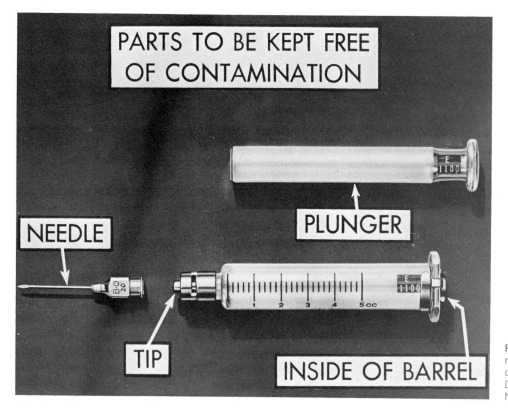

Figure 24-7 Syringe and needle-parts to be kept free of contamination. (Becton, Dickinson and Co., Rutherford, N.J.).

hazard up-and-down movements should be avoided, since they bring the material right back again. The correct action is accompanied by firm pressure so that mechanical cleaning is also accomplished. Individually packaged gauze moistened with an antiseptic is now in common use.

When the patient's skin is soiled from drainage or discharges, thorough cleaning with soap and water should precede cleaning with an antiseptic. This is especially true for incontinent patients who may need to have intramuscular injections. The point cannot be overstressed: the nurse should exercise careful judgment in the preparation of any body site for injection and not rely on the conscience-salving procedure of a superficial swipe with an antiseptic-soaked pledget.

Since many patients and their families are learning to administer injections, the problem of sterilization at home will arise. A person's home equipment is purchased for him and used only for him. Therefore, the possibility of cross-contamination between patients is eliminated. Boiling of syringes and needles in the home has been recommended for years and found to be safe, as long as the equipment is not shared.

For home technique, cotton used to clean the skin need not be sterile as long as the person is instructed

not to cover the needle with it. Since he will not have a needle protector, he will need to be shown how to keep the needle sterile. Usually, the person is advised to keep it off the edge of a table or surface on which he will place the syringe while preparing the skin. It should lie on the surface and be directed so that it cannot be touched accidently.

The cost of disposable equipment has been reduced and, therefore, more people are using such items for injections that are given at home.

Reducing Discomfort When Injecting Subcutaneously and Intramuscularly

The discomfort associated with injections sometimes is considered to be a disadvantage. However, skill in giving injections can greatly reduce discomfort.

One source of discomfort is the needle's passing through a cutaneous pain receptor. For the very sensitive or anxious patient, this discomfort can be minimized by applying cold compresses or by placing an ice cube on the area of injection for a short time immediately prior to the injection. Some physicians may also recommend spraying a volatile solution such as ethyl chloride on the site of injection. The use of cold and of volatile sprays numbs sensory receptors and therefore decreases pain.

It is of prime importance to use a sharp needle, free of burrs, and to select one of the smallest gauge that is appropriate for the site and for the solution to be injected. Today's disposable needles avoid the problems of dull and damaged needles.

The needle should be free of medication which often irritates superficial tissues as the needle is inserted. For example, when medications are removed from an open vial, there is likely to be solution remaining on the needle. Recommended procedure is to use two needles, one to remove the medication from the vial and a second to inject the medication.

Subcutaneous tissue is relatively insensitive, but if the needle distorts fascia of underlying muscle tissue, pain will result. The injection of nonirritating drugs in an isotonic solution is usually painless. A small amount of anesthesia, such as procaine hydrochloride, may be added to irritating drugs. Drugs irritating to subcutaneous tissues are ordinarily well-tolerated when administered intramuscularly.

Injecting a medication into relaxed musculature has been found to be less painful than injecting into a contracted muscle where there will be more pressure on tissues from the injected solution. For example, when using the dorsogluteal and ventrogluteal areas to inject a drug intramuscularly, it is preferable to have the patient lie on his abdomen. He should rotate his legs by pointing his toes inward. The rotation of the femur is controlled by the gluteus maximus muscles. When the toes are pointing outward, the gluteus maximus contracts; it relaxes when the leg is rotated inward. When using the side-lying position, the gluteus muscle will relax when the upper leg is flexed and placed in front of the lower leg.

Pain is minimized by inserting and removing the needle without hesitation and by injecting solutions slowly so that they may be dispersed into the surrounding tissues. Select a site where the skin appears free of irritation and danger of infection.

While removing the needle from an injection site, hold a gauze pledget firmly against the skin around the needle. The needle will not then pull on tissues as it is removed. Pulling on tissues increases discomfort.

Following an injection, firm pressure and massage of the injection site hastens absorption of the drug and relieves discomfort. Massage is not recommended after the injection of certain drugs given intramuscularly. One such drug is iron dextran (Imferon) because it is very irritating to subcutaneous tissue and massage may force some of the drug into subcutaneous tissue. If injections are being given often to a patient, rotating the site is necessary to avoid the discomfort of inserting the needle into an area recently injected. There will be further discussion concerning rotating injection sites later in this chapter.

ADMINISTERING DRUGS SUBCUTANEOUSLY

Sites for Subcutaneous Injections and Rotation of Sites

Although there is subcutaneous tissue all over the body, for convenience, a site on the upper arm is usually selected. The thigh, lower abdomen, and upper back are also common sites. Persons who give themselves subcutaneous injections generally find the thigh and abdomen the most convenient sites. Subcutaneous injections into the arm or leg are not ordinarily recommended when the patient's peripheral circulation is poor. Figure 24–8 on page 612 illustrates sites on the body where subcutaneous injections can be given.

If a patient is to receive frequent injections, it is necessary to rotate the sites. This helps prevent irritation and permits complete absorption of the solution. It is not uncommon for patients who receive injections repeatedly in one site to note an area of hardened and tender tissue. For rotating sites, it is necessary for a routine to be incorporated in the patient's plan of care. A marked diagram is most helpful for noting alternate sites. It is futile to rely on memory. Not even the patient will always be able to recall where he had the previous injection.

The amount of subcutaneous tissue underlying the skin is not the same for all individuals. Some persons may have very little and others, a great deal. For the average adult, it generally is recommended that the needle be injected at a 45° angle. However, for an obese patient, a needle injected at this angle may not reach subcutaneous tissue, while muscular tissue may be reached in a very thin and dehydrated patient. The angle and length of the needle must be adjusted to the individual patient. For example, a ⅝-inch needle held at a 90° angle is necessary to reach subcutaneous tissue in a large person; a 1-inch needle at a 45° angle for the same person will reach subcutaneous tissue. Some authorities recommend that insulin be administered while holding the needle at a 90° angle to be *sure* it reaches subcutaneous tissue.

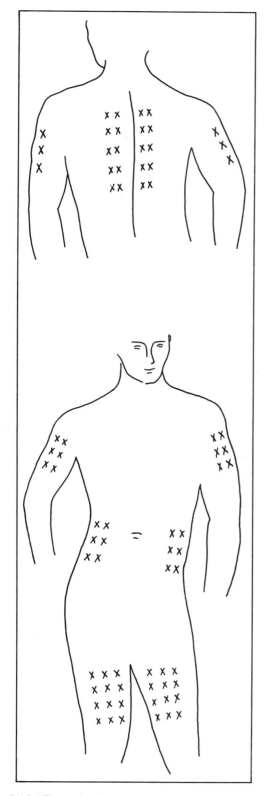

Figure 24–8   These sketches illustrate sites on the body where subcutaneous injections can be given.

Equipment Commonly Used for Subcutaneous Injections

The needle most commonly used for injecting into subcutaneous tissue is a 25-gauge, ⅝-inch needle. Needle gauge determines the size of the inner diameter or lumen of the needle. However, there are variations, and some patients need a shorter or longer needle, as was described above.

The needle must be in perfect condition and free from burrs on the point. Once a needle has been bent, it should not be forced straight for reuse. Because a needle is a delicately constructed item having a lumen, the shaft is weakened if the needle is bent and then forced back into place again. Weakening the shaft of the needle increases the possibility of its breaking in the patient's tissues if the patient moves or if other strain is placed on it.

Patients who have been taught to give their injections at home should be shown how to test the point of a reusable needle for burrs. This is done easily by running the point of the needle, both sides, over a piece of cotton or along the back of the hand before sterilizing it. If the point of the needle picks up cotton or scratches the hand, it requires sharpening. A needle with a burr on its point results in a painful injection.

Health agencies and persons at home are increasingly using disposable needles. Public health officials have cautioned all who use such needles to discard them appropriately. The needle should be bent or broken and covered to prevent accidental puncture wounds of those handling trash. This procedure should also be followed to prevent needles being retrieved by persons who are abusing injectable drugs.

Syringes for hypodermic injections are calibrated in both minims and cubic centimeters or milliliters. They are available in 2, 2½, and 3 ml. sizes. Reusable syringes are made of glass and disposable ones, of plastic.

When a very small dose of a drug must be measured, as when giving an allergen extract or a vaccine, a 1-ml. syringe calibrated in tenths and hundredths of a ml. and in minims is used. Such syringes provide for more accuracy than can be obtained from the usual syringe.

Previously, a variety of insulin syringes were in use according to the unit strength of the insulin being used. A U100 insulin is now available for use with U100 calibrated syringes and is intended for all patients regardless of their insulin dosage. This product replaces older U40 and U80 insulin and syringes. The U100 syringes are available in reusable and disposable types.

Loading gauges are available on the market that help the visually impaired diabetic measure correct dosages of insulin. These gauges come in various sizes to accommodate different dosages. The gauge, set at the appropriate dosage, is placed on the plunger and the barrel of the syringe, as is illustrated in Figure 24–9.

Hypodermic needles and syringes are dispensed in a variety of ways, some already assembled and others unassembled. If the needle is to be attached to the syringe, it should be held by the hub. A small sterile forceps can be used both to attach and to tighten the needle. However, the fingers can be used, provided that the hub does not contaminate a sterile surface following this, such as a needle protector or a sterile cotton ball.

The chart on page 614 describes the technique of giving a subcutaneous injection. The question of whether to remove all of the air from the syringe before injecting the medication is often raised. No harm will come from a small amount. In fact, a small air bubble is helpful to force medication remaining in the needle shaft into the injection site, and the technique is often recommended. The major concern caused by air in the syringe is to make certain that it does not cause an error in the measurement of the amount of medication. The air can be easily eliminated by holding the syringe in a vertical position and pushing gently on the plunger until the air is removed.

ADMINISTERING DRUGS INTRAMUSCULARLY

The intramuscular route often is used for drugs that are irritating, since there are few nerve endings in deep muscle tissue. If a sore or inflamed muscle is entered, the muscle may act as a trigger area, and severe referred pain often results. It is best to palpate a muscle prior to injection. Select a site that does not feel tender to the patient and where the tissue does not contract and become firm and tense.

Absorption occurs as in subcutaneous administration but more rapidly because of the greater vascularity of muscle tissue. Approximately 2 to 5 ml. of solution usually is given via this method. However, when as much as 5 ml. of a solution is ordered to be given intramuscularly, judgment should be used as to whether the dose should be divided and half given into one site and half into another. The pressure created by the introduction of such a quantity usually creates discomfort for the patient. If divided doses are not possible because of the frequency of subsequent ones, the injection should be given very slowly to allow for dispersal of the solution in the tissues.

Sites for Intramuscular Injections and Rotation of Sites

Because of the widespread use of intramuscular injections, it is not too surprising that complications have

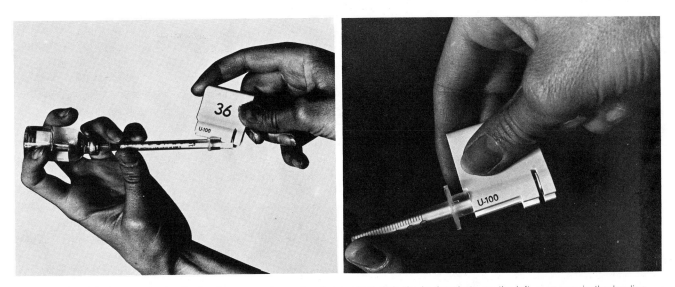

Figure 24–9   This is an example of a loading gauge for a visually impaired diabetic. In the photo on the left, a groove in the loading gauge is slipped onto the end of the plunger. The plunger is withdrawn for the width of the gauge, as shown in the photo on the right. This patient has measured 36 units of U-100 insulin. (Meditec Corporation, Englewood, Colorado)

The administration of a subcutaneous injection

The purpose is to inject a medication into subcutaneous tissue.

SUGGESTED ACTION	RATIONALE
Obtain the equipment and drug. Assemble the syringe and needle according to the manufacturer's directions. Keep the drug and sterile items in sight.	Sterile items that are out of sight are in danger of being contaminated accidentally.
Draw the drug into the syringe and protect the needle with a sterile needle cover or a sterile dry cotton ball until ready for injection.	Prolonged exposure to the air and/or contact with moist surfaces will contaminate the needle.
Carry the syringe to the patient on a tray or a medication carrier.	Keeping the prepared syringe on a flat, steady surface reduces the possibility of moving the plunger and thus possibly losing the drug.
Clean the area of skin around the injection site, as illustrated in Figure 24–10, by using firm, circular motion while moving outward from the injection site.	Friction helps clean the skin. A clean area is contaminated when a soiled object is rubbed over its surface.
Grasp the area surrounding the site of injection and hold it in a cushion fashion, as illustrated in Figure 24–11.	Cushioning the subcutaneous tissue helps to ensure having the needle enter subcutaneous tissue and helps prevent injecting muscle tissue.
Inject the needle quickly at an angle of 45° to 90°, depending on the amount and turgor of the tissue and the length of the needle, as illustrated in Figure 24–11.	Subcutaneous tissue is abundant in well-nourished, well-hydrated persons and sparse in emaciated, dehydrated, or very thin persons.
Once the needle is in place, release the grasp on the tissue.	Injecting the solution into compressed tissues results in pressure against nerve fibers and creates discomfort.
Aspirate by pulling back gently on the plunger of the syringe to determine whether the needle is in a blood vessel. If blood appears, the needle should be withdrawn and a new site selected.	Discomfort and possibly a serious reaction may occur if a drug intended for subcutaneous use is injected into a vein.
If no blood appears, inject the solution slowly.	Rapid injection of the solution creates pressure in the tissues, resulting in discomfort.
Withdraw the needle quickly while applying pressure against the injection site, as illustrated in Figure 24–12.	Slow withdrawal of the needle pulls the tissues and causes discomfort. Applying pressure around the injection site helps prevent pulling on the tissue as the needle is withdrawn.
Massage the area gently with the antiseptic pledget.	Massaging helps distribute the solution and hastens its absorption.

occurred, possibly even more frequently than the literature reports. Common complications have included abscesses, necrosis and skin slough, nerve injuries, lingering pain, and periostitis.

A crucial point in the administration of an intramuscular injection is the selection of a safe site, one that is away from large nerves and the large blood vessels.

Dorsogluteal Site. The dorsogluteal site, located on the buttock, was a common site for giving intramuscular injections. The classic method is to inject about 5.0 to 7.5 cm or 2 to 3 inches below the crest of the ilium in the upper outer quadrant of the buttock. Figure 24–13 illustrates the way in which the area is located. However, this site is losing favor because a common error is made when the upper landmark is merely identified by eye rather than by palpation of the iliac crest. The usual miscalculation is the result of the buttock being equated with the gluteus muscle and the injection is given too low. The result is that there is the danger of striking the sciatic nerve.

Another method for locating a site on the buttock is illustrated in Figure 24–14 on page 616. Locate a line from the posterosuperior iliac spine to the greater trochanter of the femur; an injection lateral and slightly superior to the midpoint of the line will also avoid the dangerous area.

A common error in locating a site is improper mapping of the area. Many people believe that the fleshy part of the buttock should certainly be the safest spot. Nothing could be more incorrect. Also, many incorrectly include the fleshy portion of the upper thigh, especially in obese patients, as a part of the buttock. The site is so important that no injection into the buttock should be given without good visualization of the entire area and careful mapping to locate the proper site. This necessitates adequate exposure by the lowering of undergarments. Merely raising one side of underclothing permits only a partial visualization of the area. It is recommended that the patient be in a prone position with the toes pointed inward or the side-lying position with the upper knee flexed and the upper leg

leg and the midlateral thigh on the side. The middle third of the muscle, measuring up from just above the knee and down from the greater trochanter, is recommended for injections. This provides space for a large number of injections. The patient may lie on his back or be sitting up with injection this site. Figure 24-16 illustrates and describes the location of this sight.

Deltoid and Posterior Triceps Muscles. These muscles also may be used for intramuscular injections. However, since they are relatively small, and a misplaced needle may injure the radial nerve, they are not often recommended. Also, many patients experience more discomfort and tenderness in this area than in others. The patient may lie on his back or be sitting up with injection of this site. Figure 24-17 illustrates this site and describes its location.

Rectus Femoris Muscle. This muscle is on the anterior part of the thigh. The site is used only when others are contraindicated, since many patients find it uncomfortable. However, some patients who must inject themselves at home use this site.

Because many drugs are given via the intramuscular route and therapy often calls for repeated injections, consideration should be given to the rotation of the sites used. The sites described earlier all may be used on a rotating basis.

Whatever pattern of rotating sites is used for a patient, a comment describing it should appear in the nursing care plan.

Equipment Commonly Used for Intramuscular Injections. As noted in the discussion of subcutaneous injections, the

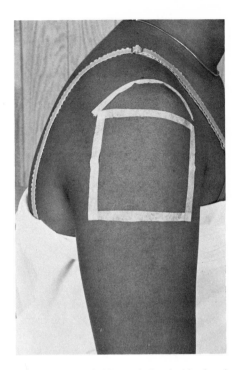

Figure 24-17 The mid-deltoid area is located by forming a rectangle. It is bounded by the lower edge of the acromion which is marked with a curved line in this photo. The lower boundary is about opposite the axilla. The two side boundaries are lines parallel to the arm one-third and two-thirds of the way around the outer aspect of the arm.

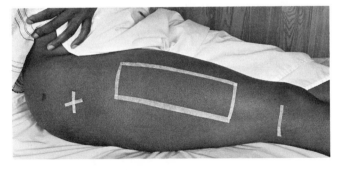

Figure 24-16 The area for injecting into the vastus lateralis is bounded by the midanterior thigh on the front of the leg, the midlateral thigh on the side, a hand's breadth from the greater trochanter which is marked with an X, and a hand's breadth above the knee which is marked by a line. The injection site is in the middle of this rectangle.

length of the needle necessary to reach the desired tissue varies with each individual. The one most commonly used for intramuscular injection is a 22-gauge, 1½-inch needle. However, for drugs of an oily nature, a larger gauge, such as a 20 gauge, is indicated. The length of the needle for an intramuscular injection should be determined by the site to be used and the condition of the patient. This is especially important if the patient is obese and the drug is irritating; 3-inch needles cause no more discomfort than 1½-inch needles, and, with proper injection, there is a greater likelihood of the drug being introduced into muscle. For children, a shorter needle is necessary, such as a ¾-inch or a 1-inch needle. In many instances, it is possible to use a hypodermic needle to give an intramuscular injection to an infant.

The age, the weight, the condition, and the tissue turgor of the patient should be taken into consideration rather than relying on a standard needle gauge for each type of injection.

The chart on page 618 describes an intramuscular injection. Just prior to injection, a small air bubble, approximately 0.2 to 0.3 ml., is included in the syringe with the solution to be injected. Figure 24–18 illustrates the air bubble in the syringe. As was the case with the subcutaneous injection, this air bubble will help to expel the remaining solution that is trapped in the shaft of the needle. Solution which remains in the shaft of the needle after the solution is injected is in danger of being pulled up through the tissues as the needle is withdrawn. If the drug is a particularly irritating one, this causes discomfort to the patient and may result in tissue damage. The air bubble also helps to trap the injected solution in the intramuscular tissue. There is no danger of an air embolus with this procedure.

Z-Track or Zigzag Technique for Intramuscular Injections. The Z-track or zigzag technique is used to inject medications that cause superficial tissue irritation and tissue bruising or staining when minute quantities of the solution escape from the injection site. The Z-track technique is accomplished as follows:

- Pull the skin and underlying tissue at the injection site to one side, about 1 inch laterally, and hold it in position with the left hand, for a right-handed person.

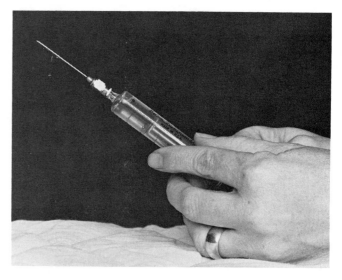

Figure 24–18   Approximately 0.2 to 0.3 ml. of air is drawn into the syringe. When the needle is injected, the air bubble will rise to the top of the solution in the syringe. The air serves to push the solution in the shaft of the needle into the muscle tissue and helps trap the solution in the tissue.

- Insert the needle while holding onto the syringe with the small, ring, and middle finger.

- Aspirate for blood with the thumb and index finger.

The administration of an intramuscular injection

The purpose is to inject a medication into the gluteus maximus muscle.

SUGGESTED ACTION	RATIONALE
Have the patient assume a position appropriate for the site selected.	Injection into a tense muscle causes discomfort.
Locate the site of choice according to directions given in this chapter.	Good visualization helps correct location of the site. The proper location of the injection site helps to avoid damage to tissues.
Place a small air bubble in the syringe.	The air bubble will force medication out of the needle shaft and helps trap the medication in the muscular tissue.
Clean the area thoroughly, using friction.	Pathogens present on the skin can be forced into the tissues by the needle.
Hold the syringe in a horizontal position until ready to inject.	Gravity may alter the position of the plunger in the syringe if held vertically, causing loss of drug.
With the needle as a 90° angle and while pressing down and holding the skin taut, as illustrated in Figure 24–19, quickly thrust the needle into the tissue.	Quick injection minimizes discomfort. A thrust helps insert the needle. Holding the skin taut and pressing down helps assure reaching muscular tissue.
As soon as the needle is in place, aspirate by slowly pulling back on the plunger to determine whether the needle is in a blood vessel. This is illustrated in Figure 24–20. If blood is aspirated, pull the needle back slightly and test again.	Discomfort and possibly a serious reaction may occur if a drug intended for intramuscular use is injected into a vein.
If no blood is aspirated, inject the solution slowly, followed by the air bubble.	Injecting slowly helps reduce discomfort by allowing time for the solution to disperse in the tissues.
Remove the needle quickly while applying pressure against the injection site with the antiseptic pledget.	Slow removal of the needle pulls tissues and may cause discomfort. Applying pressure around the injection site helps avoid pulling tissues with the needle as it is removed.
Massage the area with the antiseptic pledget.	Massaging helps the distribution and the absorption of the solution.

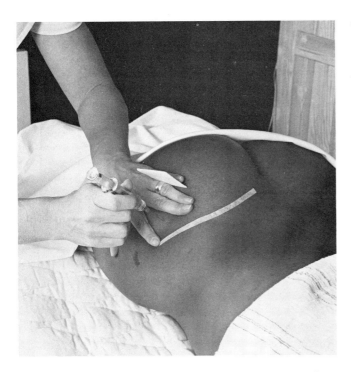

Figure 24–19 The nurse is giving an intramuscular injection into the ventrogluteal site. Note that she holds the syringe at a 90° angle and in a manner so that she can thrust the needle into the tissue. She presses down firmly on the patient's skin and holds the skin taut.

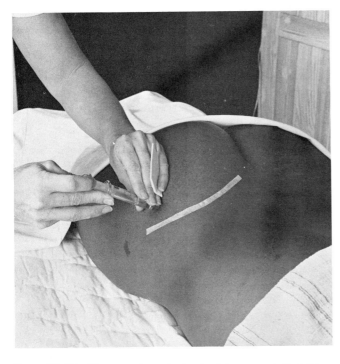

Figure 24–20 The nurse is aspirating to determine whether the needle is in a blood vessel.

- Push the plunger with the thumb to inject solution when it has been determined that the needle is not in a blood vessel.
- Withdraw the needle.
- Release the left hand so that the skin and underlying tissue return to normal position.
- Use light, steady pressure over the needle site. The area may be massaged unless the manufacturer's direction on the drug label state that massage is contraindicated.

ADMINISTERING DRUGS INTRAVENOUSLY

A variety of drugs is administered intravenously by introducing them directly into a vein. This is frequently called the intravenous "push." The technique allows immediate absorption of the drug and is often used in emergency situations.

There are essentially three ways to administer drugs by intravenous "push." A needle and syringe can be used. The vein is prepared and entered in the same manner as will be described later in this chapter when giving an intravenous infusion. The method is not ordinarily recommended when intravenous drugs must be given frequently because of the repeated need to puncture the skin and enter the vein.

A heparin lock provides a method to introduce intravenous medications at regular intervals without repeated injections because the needle is anchored and left in place between drug administrations. The needle has a short length of tubing attached to it which has a resealable injection site at its end. The needle is inserted as for an infusion. A small amount of the drug, heparin, is injected initially into the needle and tubing and then preceding and following each drug administration, or every eight hours if the drug is not given at least that often. Heparin helps prevent clotting of blood which could clog the needle between uses. The needle and tubing should be checked carefully and frequently. If heparin runs dry, blood will enter the needle and tubing and provide an excellent medium for the growth of bacteria. Irrigating the clogged needle and tubing causes the blood clots to circulate as emboli in the circulatory system. It is recommended that a heparin lock be changed every 72 hours and at any time when it is clogged with blood clots. A heparin lock is illustrated in Figure 24–21 on page 620.

A third way to introduce a drug directly into the bloodstream is to administer it through an injection site in the tubing of an intravenous infusion. The injection

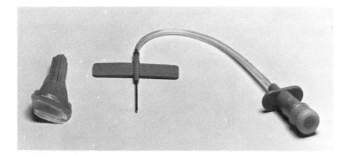

Figure 24–21 This is a heparin lock. The needle sheath has been removed. The flaps on either side of the needle are flexible and make the needle easy to handle and anchor. There is a sterile plug at the end of the tubing. When it is removed, a syringe containing a drug in solution can be attached and the medication is then injected.

site will differ, depending on the manufacturer, but the site is near the needle and offers an easy way to give drugs without subjecting the patient to repeated venipuncture. Figure 24–22 illustrates a nurse introducing a drug into a site on the patient's intravenous tubing.

Drugs administered intravenously by the methods just described should be given slowly and diluted as indicated by the drug's manufacturer. Otherwise, the drug may irritate the vein and cause it to become scarred or necrotic. Also, introducing a drug too rapidly may cause a toxic reaction by flooding blood-rich organs with high concentrations of the drug. It has been determined that it takes only approximately 15 seconds for a drug injected into a peripheral vein to reach the heart where it will be pumped to the brain.

Drugs may also be placed in a patient's infusion solution. The intravenous infusion will be described later in this chapter. A characteristic of this method of drug administration is that the patient receives the drug slowly and over a long period. While this can some-

times be an advantage, it is also a disadvantage when it is necessary for the patient to receive the drug relatively quickly. In addition, if for some reason all of the solution cannot be given intravenously, the patient will not receive the prescribed amount of drug. There is equipment available to overcome these disadvantages, as will be described later in this chapter.

ADMINISTERING DRUGS INTRACUTANEOUSLY

Solutions injected into the corium of the skin are called intracutaneous or intradermal injections. Solutions are absorbed slowly via the capillaries. Small amounts of solution are used—usually no more than several minims. A common site for injection is the inner aspect of the forearm, although other areas are also satisfactory. Intracutaneous injections generally are used for diagnostic purposes; examples are the tuberculin test, and tests to determine sensitivity to various substances. The advantage of the intracutaneous route for these tests is that the reaction of the body to these substances is easily visible, and, by means of comparative studies, degrees of reaction are discernible. Vaccination for smallpox is a therapeutic intradermal injection, although this also may be done by multiple skin punctures and scratches.

A fine needle is used, usually 26 gauge. It is injected bevel side up very superficially. The *bevel* of the needle is its sloped edge. It is illustrated in Figure 24–23. The lumen should barely be concealed by the skin. The medication is injected and forms a small raised area on the skin. The needle is removed quickly after the drug is injected. The area is not massaged after injection. Figure 24–24 illustrates a nurse giving an intracutaneous injection.

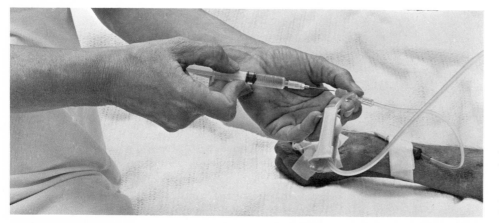

Figure 24–22 The needle is at the point in this intravenous tubing where a medication can be injected. Note that the site of injection is near the site where the needle enters the patient's vein.

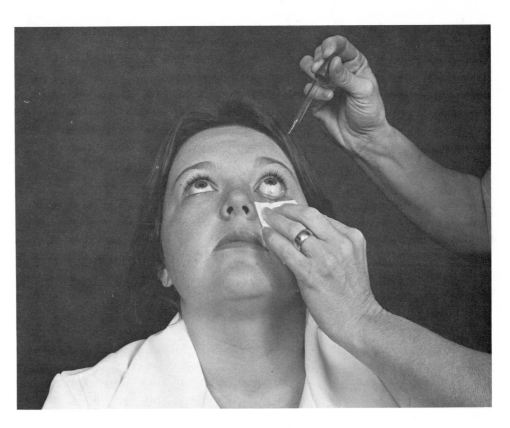

Figure 24–25 The nurse exposes the lower conjunctiva of the eye where she will place eyedrops by having the patient look up and by applying pressure downward with two fingers over the bony prominence of the check. The thumb may be used for applying pressure downward if it is more convenient for the nurse.

The eyelids and the eyelashes should be cleaned of secretions and crusts before applying the ointment. Eye ointments usually are dispensed in a tube. A small amount of the ointment is distributed along the conjunctival sac after everting the lower lid. The ointment is squeezed from the tube, but care should be taken to avoid touching the eye or the conjunctiva. Following the application, the eyelids should be closed. The warmth will help to liquefy the ointment. The patient should also be instructed to move his eye. This will aid in spreading the ointment under the lids and over the surface of the eyeball.

Ear Instillations

The ear contains the receptors for hearing and for equilibrium. It consists of the external ear, the middle ear, and the inner ear.

The external ear consists of the auricle or pinna and the exterior auditory canal. The auditory canal serves as a passageway for sound waves. Drugs or irrigations are instilled into the auditory canal.

In adults, the auditory canal is directed inward, forward, and down. The outer portion is cartilaginous, and the inner portion consists of osseous tissue. In an infant, the canal is chiefly cartilaginous and is almost straight, but the floor of the auditory canal rests on the tympanic membrane. The direction of the canal is important to consider when administering treatments to the ear. For solution to reach all parts of the canal, the pinna should be pulled down and back for infants; for adults, up and back. The ear is grasped on the cartilaginous portion of the pinna when straightening the canal. Figure 24–26 on page 624 illustrates a nurse instilling ear drops in an adult.

The lining of the auditory canal consists of modified epithelium. It contains ceruminous glands, which secrete wax found in the ear, and the hair follicles.

The tympanic membrane separates the external ear from the middle ear. Normally, it is intact and closes the entrance to the middle ear completely. If it is ruptured or has been opened by surgical intervention, the middle ear and the inner ear have a direct passage to the external ear. When this occurs, instillations and irrigations should be done with the greatest of care to prevent forcing materials from the outer ear into the middle ear and the inner ear, which may result in serious infection.

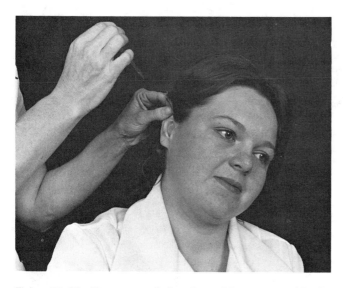

Figure 24–26 The nurse pulls the pinna of the ear up and back in order to straighten the ear canal in this adult patient. She then will place eardrops on the side of the canal.

Normally, the external ear is not a sterile cavity. However, if the tympanic membrane is not intact, surgical asepsis should be observed.

Drugs in solution are placed in the auditory canal for their local effect. They are used to soften wax, relieve pain, apply local anesthesia, destroy organisms, or destroy an insect lodged in the canal which can cause almost intolerable discomfort.

It is more comfortable for the patient when the solution is warmed to approximately body temperature. A dropper is used to instill the solution. The ear canal is straightened, and the drops are allowed to fall on the side of the canal. The patient lies on his side with the ear to be treated uppermost and remains in this position following instillation to prevent the drops from escaping from the canal. Occasionally, a loose cotton wick is inserted into the canal in order to maintain a continuous application of the solution instilled. A wick is never packed into the ear because it interferes with outward movement of normal secretions and could create excessive pressure.

Nasal Instillations

Besides serving as the olfactory organ, the nose also functions as an airway to the lower respiratory tract and protects the tract by cleaning and warming the air that is taken in by inspiration. Small hairs, called cilia, project on most of the surface of the nasal mucous membrane and are important in helping to remove particles of dirt and dust from the inspired air. The nose also serves as a resonator when speaking and singing.

The nose is divided into the right and the left chambers by the nasal septum. There are four pairs of nasal sinuses that communicate with the nasal fossa: the frontal, the ethmoid, the maxillary, and the sphenoid sinuses. Normally, these are filled with air and lined with mucous membrane similar to that which lines the nose.

Because of the position of the nose, secretions from it drain out easily when the person is in the upright position. Because of its connection with the upper respiratory tract and the mouth, secretions drain back into the area when the person is reclining.

Normally, the nose is not a sterile cavity. However, because of its connection with the sinuses, utmost caution should be taken when using nasal instillations.

Instillation of Nosedrops. Medications instilled into the nares are used primarily for the relief of nasal congestion. Most authorities recommend using a drug in normal saline solution, since oily solutions tend to interfere with the normal ciliary action in the nose and, if aspirated, may result in a pneumonitis. Anesthetics and antiseptics also may be instilled into the nose for their local effects.

Paper wipes should be provided for the patient. The patient is assisted to a sitting position with his head tilted back, or he lies in bed with his head tilted back over a pillow. This position allows the solution to flow back into the nares. Sufficient solution for both nares is drawn into a dropper. The dropper is placed just inside the nares, approximately 1 cm. or one-third inch and the number of drops prescribed is instilled. Touching the dropper to the nares may create a desire to sneeze. The patient should be instructed to keep his head tilted back for several minutes to prevent the escape of solution from the anterior nares. The patient usually will wish to expectorate solution that runs down into the oropharynx and the back of the mouth.

When instilling drops into the nares of an infant or an irrational patient, the tip of the dropper should be protected with a piece of soft rubber tubing to minimize the danger of injuring the nasal mucous membrane.

Nasal Spray. Solutions that are instilled by drops also may be applied to the nasal mucous membrane by using a spray. A small atomizer generally is used.

The end of the nose is held up, and the tip of the nozzle is placed just inside the nares and directed backward. Only sufficient force is used to bring the spray into contact with the membrane. Too much force may drive the solution and the contamination into the sinuses and the eustachian tubes.

Throat Applications

The throat, more properly called the pharynx, is divided into three portions: nasal, oral, and laryngeal. The pharynx communicates with the nasal cavity anteriorly, with the oral cavity below this, and with the laryngeal cavity below the oral pharynx. The eustachian tubes open into the nasopharynx. The pharynx is a muscular passageway and is lined with modified epithelium.

The pharynx is a passageway for air. The oral and the laryngeal portions also serve as a passageway for food.

The adenoids or pharyngeal tonsils are located in the nasopharynx. The palatine tonsils are in the oral pharynx. The tonsils and the adenoids are composed of lymphoid tissue and often become the seat of infections.

The throat is not a sterile area. However, practices of medical asepsis are observed, especially in caring for the equipment after use. The mouth harbors microorganisms that could be harmful to others.

Throat Sprays and Paints. Antiseptics and anesthetics may be applied to the throat by spraying and by painting the area. The patient's head is tilted back, and his tongue is held down with a tongue depressor. The solution is either sprayed or painted onto the tissues. A cotton applicator is effective for painting. When a spray is used, more force is necessary to reach tissues in the throat than is necessary when using a nasal spray.

Lozenges. Lozenges may contain drugs that are used for the local treatment of the mouth and the throat. Cough drops are an example. When sucked, the lozenge liberates the active ingredient, and, when the solution is swallowed, the mouth and the throat are bathed in it. The use of lozenges is unsatisfactory for reaching all parts of the throat. The patient should be instructed to suck the lozenge or place it between his cheek and gum for *buccal* administration. Chewing or swallowing it shortens the period of contact with the tissues and decreases its effectiveness.

Vaginal Applications

The vagina is a musculomembranous canal extending from the outside of the body at the vulva to the cervix uteri. It lies between the bladder and the rectum. The size and the shape vary, but it is capable of distending, such as during childbirth and sexual intercourse. Normally, the walls of the vagina are in contact with each other.

In health, the vagina contains few pathogens but many nonpathogenic organisms. The nonpathogens are important, since they protect the vagina from the invasion of pathogens. The normal secretions in the vagina are acid in reaction and further serve to protect the vagina from microbial invasion. Therefore, the normal mucous membrane is its own best protection.

Creams can be applied intravaginally, using a narrow tubular applicator with an attached plunger. Suppositories that melt when exposed to body heat are also prepared for vaginal insertion. Suppositories should normally be refrigerated for storage.

When a cream or suppository is used, the patient should lie on her back and flex and spread her knees. An applicator filled with cream is inserted into the vagina carefully as far as it will go comfortably. The plunger of the applicator is fully depressed to express the cream. While keeping the plunger depressed, the applicator is then removed. Gloves are worn when a suppository is inserted into the vagina by the nurse. The suppository should be placed well within the vaginal cavity. The techniques just described for applying creams and inserting suppositories help widespread distribution of the preparations in the vagina and minimize loss at the vaginal orifice. A perineal pad to avoid soiling clothing may be indicated after using vaginal creams or suppositories.

Rectal Applications

Rectal suppositories are used primarily for their local action, although some systemic effect does occur. Rectal installation are also occasionally used. The techniques for rectal applications were discussed in Chapter 20.

THE INTRAVENOUS INFUSION

A relatively common form of therapy for handling fluid disturbances is the use of various solutions injected intravenously. An *intravenous infusion* is the injection of relatively large quantities of solution into a vein. Although the physician is responsible for prescribing the kind and amount of solution to be used, the nurse is ordinarily responsible for initiating, monitoring, and discontinuing the therapy.

Mention of the large variety of solutions on the market for therapy was made in Chapter 23. Just as was true with drugs, the nurse should understand the patient's need for therapy, the type of solution being used, its desired effect, and untoward reactions that may occur.

Equipment Commonly Used for Intravenous Infusions

Because a vein is being entered, sterile technique is observed. Most health agencies use disposable infusion tubing and needles, thus eliminating many possible sources of contamination and reducing the cost of the aftercare of equipment.

For most intravenous infusions for adults, an 18-, 20-, or 22-gauge needle with a short bevel is used. Whenever possible, the needle size should be appreciably less than the vein to reduce the tissue trauma. However, the fluid viscosity and rate of flow will also have to be considered. A short bevel also reduces the extent of vein damage. Butterfly needles, which are short-beveled, thin-walled needles with plastic flaps, are also used extensively because of the ease in handling and stabilizing them. A butterfly needle was illustrated in Figure 24–21.

If an infusion is to run for an extended time, an intravenous catheter may be used. Catheters are specially prepared plastic tubes which have been mounted on a needle or are threaded through a needle for insertion. Because of the incidence of serious complications from this type of equipment, only experienced practitioners should attempt to use it.

Normally, the pressure in the patient's vein is higher than atmospheric pressure. Gravity is used to increase the pressure differential between the needle and the solution container, except when using an intravenous pump which will be discussed later. The solution is placed at a level approximately 45 to 60 cm. or 18 to 24 inches above the level of the vein or at a height where gravity is sufficient to overcome the venous pressure and to allow the solution to enter the vein. The bottle of solution is suspended on a pole, and the solution flows through the attached tubing and the needle directly into the patient. The height of the fluid container in relation to the patient will affect the pressure of the fluid and thus, the rate of flow. The higher the solution, the faster it will run. As the bottle is lowered, the flow will become slower.

The rate of flow of the solution is also manually controlled by a clamp or constricting device on the tubing. A device known as a dripmeter connects the solution bottle and tubing and permits the number of drops per minute of the solution to be counted.

Solutions for infusions are dispensed in either bottles or plastic bags. The bags collapse because of atmospheric pressure as the solution enters the patient's vein. Rigid containers cannot collapse, and hence, they have an air vent which allows air to replace fluid.

When there are substances added to the solution, such as drugs or electrolytes, it is recommended that this be done by the pharmacist, preferably under a laminar air flow hood. The danger of contamination has been shown to be reduced by the use of this filtered air screen device. Because of the complexity and incompatibility of some additives and the resulting dangers to the patient, having the pharmaceutical personnel prepare the solutions also decreases the likelihood of undesirable combinations being prepared. Any additives should be clearly labeled on the bottle as to type and amount.

In some hospitals, adding substances to intravenous solutions is a nursing responsibility. The importance of adhering to strict sterile technique cannot be overemphasized. The nurse should also check very carefully that only compatible substances are mixed together, and that only substances intended for intravenous use are added to the solution. The manufacturer's directions should be observed, but if there are any additional questions, a pharmacist should be consulted. The technique of placing the intravenous drug into the solution will depend on the equipment available to the nurse in the health agency in which she gives care. One additional precaution: the nurse should double-check that the substance is ordered to be added to the intravenous solution. Errors have occurred when the intent was to give the drug intravenously, using techniques described on page 619; or that the drug be given by techniques described later in this section.

The precise method of attaching the tubing to the solution varies with the design of the container being used, but sterile technique should be used to avoid contamination of the ends of the tubing and the solution. After the tubing has been connected to the bottle of solution, the bottle is elevated to allow the air to escape and the fluid to fill the tubing. When all the air is out of the tubing, it is clamped shut. The tip of the tubing can then be attached to the sterile needle.

Before the infusion is started, a final check should be made of the solution to make sure it is clear and contains no particles of any kind. Since some additives create precipitates, this check is especially important when substances have been added to the solution. In-line filters are commercially available also to filter the solution immediately before it enters the patient's vein.

Intravenous drugs may be placed in a special cham-

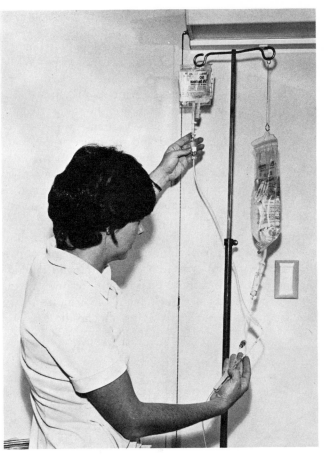

Figure 24-28 A medication in solution in the small container on the left side of the standard will enter the patient's vein before the solution in the larger container on the right.

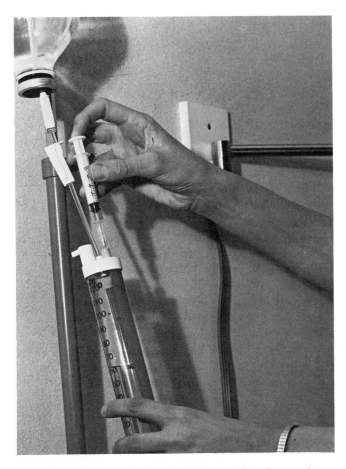

Figure 24-27 This nurse is using equipment that allows a drug to be injected with a needle and syringe into a chamber that is located between the bottle of solution and the patient. The patient will receive the medication more quickly in this manner than had the drug been mixed with the entire amount of solution in the bottle. Also, introducing the drug into the chamber eliminates needing to open the bottle of solution, thereby decreasing the danger of contaminating the solution with airborne organisms.

ber located between the bottle and patient. This chamber will empty and enter the patient's vein before the remainder of the solution in the container. One type of equipment for adding drugs in this manner is illustrated in Figure 24-27. Or, a second bottle containing a small amount of intravenous solution and drug can be arranged in a tandem manner. This is often called the "piggy back" method. It is illustrated in Figure 24-28. Both of these methods allow the drug to be introduced more quickly than had the drug been mixed with the entire amount of solution.

Since an infusion usually takes several hours to complete, the patient should be made comfortable. If the procedure is unusually long, the patient's position should be changed frequently if he is to remain in bed. If allowed to walk, proper precautions are taken to prevent the needle from slipping out of place. Figure

24–29 illustrates an ambulatory patient receiving intravenous therapy.

The arm to be used is abducted slightly from the body and placed on an arm board, if necessary. When veins on the back of the hand are used, an arm board may be unnecessary for many patients. When the arm is secured to an arm board, attention should be given to keeping it in good position. Very often it is possible to have the forearm pronated and the palm of the hand downward and in the grasping position over the edge of the arm board. This position more nearly resembles the normal anatomical position of the arm and is therefore more comfortable for the patient. Hyperextension of the elbow causes fatigue for the patient, often to the point where it may be impossible for him to move his forearm voluntarily after an infusion is discontinued. It takes assistance in flexing and extending the elbow passively to help regain "feeling" in the arm. If the area is hairy, such as a man's arm, it may be best to shave the area involving the needle site and adhesive, although some persons do not recommend shaving because of possible irritation to the skin at the entry site.

A tourniquet is applied to aid in distending the vein. The tourniquet is placed under the arm above the selected site and ready to tie. The arm is secured to the board with bandage or ties. Do not obstruct circulation or cause discomfort to the patient, but make the board snug enough to hold the arm securely. The skin over the vein where the needle will be introduced is cleansed thoroughly with antiseptic solution.

Sites for Intravenous Injections

Suitability of veins for intravenous infusions varies with individual situations. Selection should be determined after considering several factors: accessibility and condition of veins, type of fluid to be infused, and anticipated duration of the infusion.

Accessibility of a vein is partially determined by the condition of the patient. For example, a person with severe burns on both forearms will not have vessels in these areas available. Veins in a surgical area should not be used, nor usually even those adjacent to the area. For example, infusions in the arm should not be given on the same side as recent extensive breast surgery because of vascular disturbances in the area.

The most accessible veins are not necessarily the most desirable for infusion. The antecubital veins located at the inner aspect of the elbow are among the most accessible. However, often they are not a good choice for infusion because of the need to limit the patient's arm flexion for an extended period of time. Since there is danger of dislocation of the needle and vein trauma even with slight movement, damage to these vessels may limit later use of the lower arms and hand veins that are distal to it. These vessels are quite satisfactory for blood withdrawal or for small amounts of intravenous medication administration.

The lower cephalic vein, accessory cephalic vein, and the basilic vein are good sites for infusion. The superficial veins on the dorsal aspect of the hand can also be used successfully for some persons. The metacarpal veins, basilic veins, and cephalic veins are recommended good sites. Figure 24–30 illustrates these locations.

Veins of the legs are generally not recommended for infusions, unless other sites are not accessible, because of the danger of stagnation of peripheral circulation and possible serious complications. Scalp veins are often used for infants, because of their accessibility and relative ease of preventing dislocation of the needle.

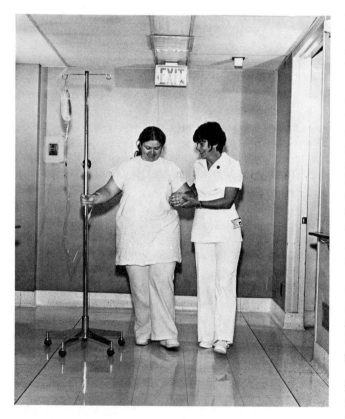

Figure 24–29 An ambulatory patient can be assisted to walk while receiving intravenous fluid. Note that the patient wears good walking shoes which affords her greater comfort and safety.

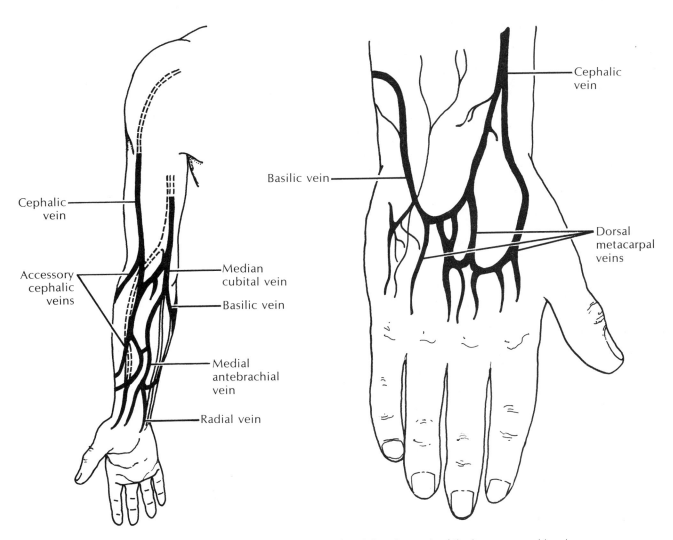

Figure 24–30 These sketches illustrate infusion sites on the ventral and dorsal aspects of the lower arm and hand.

Vein condition is an important consideration because it may determine the ease or difficulty of successive entry into the vein. Thin-walled and scarred veins, especially in some elderly patients, make continued infusion a problem. Experience will help the nurse acquire skill in palpating veins to determine their general condition.

The type of fluid to be administered is influential in vein selection because the solution should be compatible with the vein size. Hypertonic solutions, those containing irritating medications, those administered at a rapid rate, and those with a high viscosity should be given in a large vein to minimize vessel trauma and facilitate the rate of flow. Generally, the forearm veins are preferred over veins on the back of the hand for these solutions.

The anticipated duration of the infusion therapy becomes a more important factor in vein selection as the duration is extended. Comfort of the patient is facilitated when any restriction in movement is kept to a minimum. When joint immobility is prolonged, discomfort is common. Trauma from infusions does occur, at least temporarily, at the venipuncture site. Therefore, it is recommended that sites be changed frequently, starting with sites as distal as possible and moving in a proximal direction on the alternate arms.

Either arm may be used for intravenous therapy. If the patient is right-handed and both arms appear to be equally usable, usually the left arm is selected so that the right arm is then free for the patient's use.

The suggested technique for administering an intravenous infusion is described in the chart on page 630.

Administering an intravenous infusion

The purpose is to enter a vein to inject a solution.

SUGGESTED ACTION	RATIONALE
Have the patient in the supine position and the bed in semi-Fowler's position.	The supine position when venipuncture is performed permits either arm to be used while in good alignment.
Place the arm on the board with the tourniquet under the arm above the intended site of entry. Secure the arm to the board and fix it snugly enough to hold the arm securely. For some patients, an arm board is not necessary.	Arm motion will move the vein, causing a change in the position of the needle.
Look for and palpate for a suitable vein, as Figure 24–31 illustrates.	A palpable firm vein is relatively easy to enter with a needle.
Apply the tourniquet to obstruct venous blood flow; direct the tourniquet ends away from the site of entry.	Interrupting the blood flow back to the heart causes veins to distend. Interruption of arterial flow would impede venous filling. Distended veins are easy to see, palpate, and enter. The ends of the tourniquet could contaminate the area of injection.
Ask the patient to open and close his fist. Observe and palpate for a suitable vein.	Contraction of the muscles of the lower arm forces the blood along in the veins, thereby distending them further.
When the vein is not clearly visible, remove the tourniquet and arm board and apply warmth to the area.	Warmth helps dilate superficial veins, making them more clearly visible.
Using friction, clean the skin *thoroughly* at and around the site of entry.	Pathogens present on the skin can be introduced into the tissues or the blood with the needle.
Use the thumb to retract down on the vein and the soft tissue below the intended site of entry, as illustrated in Figure 24–32.	Pressure on the vein and the surrounding tissues aids in preventing movement of the vein as the needle is being introduced.
Hold the needle with the bevel up at about a 30° to 45° angle, in line with the vein at a point about 1.2 cm. or ½ inch away from intended site of entry, as Figure 24–32 illustrates.	The pressure needed to pierce the skin can be sufficient to force the needle into the vein at an improper angle and possibly through the opposite wall.
When the needle is through the skin, lower the angle of the needle until it is nearly parallel with the skin, following the same course as the vein, and insert into the vein.	Following the course of the vein prevents the needle from leaving the vein at another site because of the pressure needed to puncture the skin and vein simultaneously.
When the blood comes back through the needle into the tubing, insert the needle further into the vein about 1.7 to 2.5 cm. or ¾ to 1 inch.	The pressure of the patient's blood is usually greater than the pressure in the tubing causing automatic backflow. Having the needle placed well into the vein helps to prevent easy dislodgment of the needle. "Riding" the needle into the vein while it is distended helps to prevent pushing it through the wall.
Release the tourniquet.	An occluded vessel prevents the solution from entering circulation.
Start the flow of solution by releasing the clamp on the tubing.	Blood can clot readily if no fluid flow is present.
Support the needle with a small piece of dry gauze if necessary to keep it in proper position in the vein.	The pressure of the wall of the vein against the bevel of the needle will interrupt the rate of flow of the solution. The wall of the vein can be punctured easily by the needle.
Loop the tubing near the site of entry and anchor the tubing with tape to prevent pull on the needle, as Figure 24–33 illustrates.	The smooth structure of the vein does not offer resistance to the movement of the needle. The weight of the tubing is sufficient to pull the needle out of the vein.
Adjust the rate of solution flow according to the physician's order.	The physician specifies the rate of flow.

Monitoring and Discontinuing the Infusion

The monitoring of the infusion is the nurse's responsibility and involves maintaining the flow rate while assuring the comfort and safety of the patient. The flow rate is determined by the physician's order. He may indicate the amount to be infused in an 8- or a 24- hour period. The rate is calculated on the basis of drops of solution infused per minute. The following formula can be used to determine the flow rate:

$$\text{Drops per minute} = \frac{\text{Total volume infused} \times \text{drop factor (drops/ml.)}}{\text{Total time of infusion in minutes}}$$

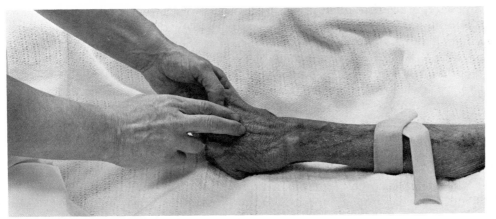

Figure 24–31 The nurse palpates for a suitable vein on the back of the patient's hand. She has the tourniquet in place but untied.

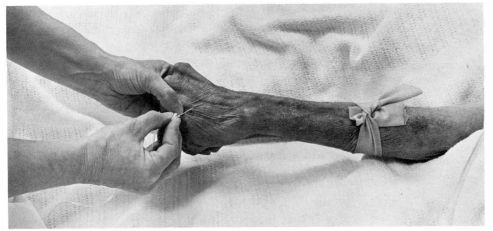

Figure 24–32 The tourniquet is secured. The needle, bevel side up, is near the intended site of entry and held at about a 30° angle. Note that the nurse steadies the vein she will enter below the site of entry with her left thumb.

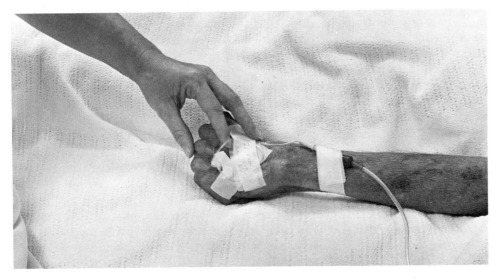

Figure 24–33 The tourniquet has been removed, the fluid is flowing, the needle is in place, and it and the tubing are well-anchored. In this health agency, the nurse prints her initials, the date, and the solution on the tape used to anchor the needle.

The drop factor, or drops per milliliter, is determined by the size of the opening in the infusion apparatus.

There is no standard size opening; it varies with the commerical company producing the product. Most health agencies use the products of a single company; thus, the nurse should familiarize herself with the products used in her agency. The more common drop factors are 15 drops per ml., 20 drops per ml., and 60 drops per ml. The small opening required for 60 drops per ml. is used most frequently when small fluid volumes are important, as in infants and small children. There are also adapters available which make it possible to reduce the drop size. If 3,000 ml. are to be infused over a period of 24 hours, and the drop factor is 20 drops per ml., the flow rate would be determined as follows:

$$\frac{3{,}000 \text{ ml.} \times 20}{60 \times 24} = \frac{60{,}000}{1440}$$
$$= 42 \text{ drops per minute}$$

It is also relatively simple to determine the desired hourly infusion amount rate. The following formula can be used:

$$\frac{\text{Total infusion volume}}{\text{Total number of hours}} = \text{ml. per hour}$$

In the above example, the hourly rate would be calculated as follows:

$$\frac{3{,}000 \text{ ml.}}{24 \text{ hours}} = 125 \text{ ml. per hour}$$

Many factors can alter the rate of flow of an intravenous infusion. The height of the container in relation to the patient, the patient's blood pressure, and the patient's position are influential. The nurse needs to know the desired rate and then adjust the infusion as necessary to achieve the rate. Her task can be facilitated by calculating the hourly flow rates and by marking them on the bottle. She then regulates the drop per minute rate by timing the flow. As she periodically checks on the infusion, she can determine quickly by glancing at her marking if the solution is being infused at the proper hourly rate. If it is not, she again regulates the flow. Because the patient's movements, disturbances of the regulation mechanism, or change in the height of the infusion bottle or bed can alter the flow rate, even after it is regulated, the nurse needs to continue to check on the infusion at regular intervals. It has been reported that standard intravenous administration sets lose up to one-half of their initial flow rate

during the first hour of infusion because of tubing flexibility, and therefore the rate needs adjustment.

Maintenance of the flow rate is important because of the implications relative to the patient's fluid balance. Too slow a flow may result in either the occurrence of deficits because the input is not balancing the loss, or in delaying the restoration of the balance. Infusing intravenous fluid too rapidly can overtax the body's capacities to adjust to the increase in the water volume or the electrolytes it contains. Nurses who allow infusions to get behind schedule and increase the rate to catch up may be seriously insulting the patient's compensatory mechanisms and jeopardizing the patient's well-being.

Devices which limit the amount of fluid which can be infused at any one time are available on the market. There are also battery-operated rate meters which quickly calculate the milliliter per hour flow rate of a solution as it is infusing. Some agencies use infusion pumps which automatically regulate the flow rate at preset limits and notify the nurse by an alarm system when the solution level of the bottle is getting low. Some models also sound an alarm when there is air in the tubing. These pumps bring solution to the vein by exerting positive pressure, either on the fluid or on the intravenous tubing. Syringe pumps are also available. They deliver small amounts of fluid, 100 ml. or less, and are particularly useful with children. There are portable models on the market also which are handy for the ambulatory patient. An infusion pump is shown in Figure 24–34.

After the initial tissue penetration, most intravenous infusions should not create discomfort for the patient. If the patient is uncomfortable, the nurse should check to see that the infusion is entering the vein as intended, that the flow rate is not too rapid, and that the patient's position is satisfactory. Anxiety over the implications of an infusion can also cause discomfort for the patient.

Dislodging the needle or penetration of the vessel wall can cause the fluid to pass into the subcutaneous tissue and result in swelling, pallor, coldness, or pain at the site. This escape of fluid into the subcutaneous tissue is known as *infiltration*. The frequently used method of lowering the solution bottle below the infusion site so the vein pressure is higher than the pressure in the tubing, and then looking for blood to enter the tubing, is not a foolproof way of determining if the needle is in the vein. Blood can return in the tubing when the needle has penetrated only partially through the vessel wall. A backflow of blood in the tubing can then occur even though fluid is passing into the tissue. The needle bevel can be lodged against the vessel wall,

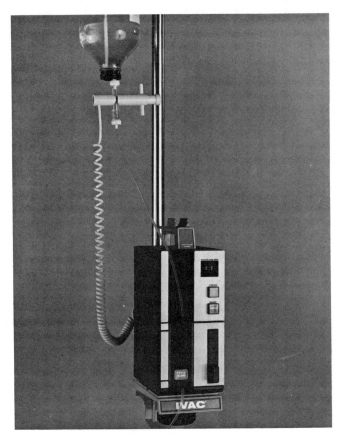

Figure 24–34 This is an example of an infusion pump. It is a positive pressure pump that automatically regulates the flow rate. The alarm on this model is activated by an empty fluid container, occluded tubing, or unobtainable drop rate. (Ivac Corporation, San Diego, California)

a blood vessel by a foreign body or air. Serious damage can result if vital vessels are obstructed and tissues are deprived of blood.

While normally well-handled infusions do not permit air to enter the vein, it can occur when negative pressure exists in the vein and a solution bottle is allowed to become empty. Negative pressure may occur when the extremity used for the infusion is kept at a higher elevation than the heart. The quantity of air which would be fatal to humans is not known, but animal experimentation indicates that it is much larger than usually depicted in murder mysteries. Estimates vary from 35 ml. to 350 ml. of intravenous air as being necessary to cause the death of a person. The average infusion tubing holds about 5 ml. of air. Patients, however, are often frightened when they see air in the infusion tubing, and every effort should be made to avoid this happening. When there is air in the intravenous system, it should be removed.

If more than one bottle of solution is ordered for the patient, the nurse attaches the additional bottles. The method by which this is done will depend on the procedure of the agency. Some intravenous equipment is designed to simplify the procedure by making it possible to attach additional bottles with a tandemlike arrangement. Because infusions often are continued after the responsibility for a patient's care changes from one nurse to another, it is a good practice to agree on one common method for managing infusions. Without such uniformity, serious errors can occur, or valuable time is lost in checking and rechecking.

When the amount of solution the physician has ordered has been absorbed, the nurse assumes responsibility for discontinuing the infusion. The adhesive strips are removed, the needle is removed quickly, in line with the vein, and pressure is applied immediately to the site. If the patient is able to do so, he may be asked to hold the pressure dressing for a minute or more.

If the patient's arm or leg has been immobilized for several hours or longer, the nurse should manipulate it carefully in an attempt to put the joint through range-of-motion and passively move the muscles of the area.

The following information is recorded when the infusion has been completed: the date and the time the infusion was started and completed, the kind and the amount of solution infused, the name and the amount of any drugs added, and the name of the person starting and discontinuing the infusion.

Symptoms of reaction are recorded as well as any treatment which the physician may prescribe for it.

and, therefore, no blood backflow will occur when the bottle is lowered even though the needle is in the vessel. Swelling and discomfort at the infusion site or continued flow of the infusion while a tourniquet occludes the veins are the best indications of infiltration. The needle should be removed when infiltration occurs.

Phlebitis is an inflammation of the vein. It is another potential hazard of intravenous infusions. Mechanical trauma or chemical irritation causes a painful inflammation along the vein. The application of moist heat will usually relieve the condition. Further use of the vein should be avoided.

Blood clots, called *thrombi,* can form at the end of the needle or catheter from tissue trauma. When the thrombus is dislodged and circulates in the blood, it is called an embolus. An *embolus* is a foreign body or air in the circulatory system. *Embolism* is the obstruction of

Symptoms of desired effects are also recorded. Intravenous catheters are recommended to be changed every 48 hours. The intravenous site should also be changed every 48 to 72 hours. These practices are observed to help control contamination and the problem of possible introduction of microorganisms into the bloodstream.

It has been general policy to change tubing and bottles every 24 hours when patients receive intravenous infusions over a period of time. However, the Center for Disease Control has recently challenged this policy and reports that according to its findings, 48 hours is satisfactory and does not increase the risk of infection or phlebitis.

The method just described is the most common one for administering an intravenous infusion. Another method for entering a vein in order to infuse a solution is called a *cut-down*. A cut-down is an incision into a vein for the purpose of administering a solution. It may be necessary when the superficial veins are not readily accessible. An incision is made by the physician into the skin over a vein. This procedure is carried out under surgical asepsis since it constitutes minor surgery. The physician wears sterile gloves, and many agencies specify that the physician and the nurse wear masks. Radiopaque plastic tubing is threaded through the needle and placed into the vein. It is held in place with a suture. The infusion is conducted as described previously. When the plastic tubing is removed, a stitch or two is placed in the skin at the site of incision.

Hyperalimentation

Infusing intravenous solutions containing sufficient nutrients to sustain life and maintain normal growth and development is called *hyperalimentation*. This form of therapy is also called *total parenteral nutrition* and is abbreviated TPN. It is a means of providing amino acids along with glucose, vitamins, and electrolytes for persons who cannot ingest nutrients normally for an extended period and for whom standard infusions are not adequate. The method is used generally for seriously ill patients and is discussed in more detail in clinical texts. At the present time, a physician is responsible for initiating and discontinuing the therapy. The hypertonic solution is infused into the superior vena cava through a special tubing threaded through the subclavian or internal jugular vein. The superior vena cava, with its large volume of blood, is needed for the rapid dilution of the hypertonic solution. Various chemical and volume tests are used frequently to adjust the solution components and flow rate to meet the patient's needs.

HYPODERMOCLYSIS

Hypodermoclysis, which is the injection of relatively large quantities of solution into subcutaneous tissue, is used infrequently because the intravenous method is more efficient. It can be used to administer electrolyte-containing solutions when the oral and the intravenous routes are unsatisfactory. The fluid is injected slowly into subcutaneous tissue where absorption occurs via the blood capillaries. The solution usually used is isotonic or occasionally hypotonic. Hypertonic solutions may cause water and salt depletion and damage to the subcutaneous tissue.

To hasten the rate of absorption, hyaluronidase or a similar product is used. The drug dissolves cellular protective substances and thus makes it possible for the solution to enter the circulatory system more rapidly. It is effective for this procedure as well as for speeding the absorption of hematomas and certain drugs that ordinarily are absorbed slowly from the tissues.

For the adult patient, the most common sites of injection are the anterior thighs. However, for the adult female, the area directly below the breasts can be used. For children, the sites directly over the scapulae are usually used.

THE BLOOD TRANSFUSION

A *blood transfusion* is the infusion of whole blood from a healthy person into a recipient's vein. The person receiving the blood is called the *recipient* while the person giving the blood is called the *donor.* Blood may be given either by direct or indirect transfusion. In *indirect transfusion,* blood is infused after it has been collected from a donor; this is the most commonly used method. The technique is similar to that for giving an intravenous infusion. In *direct tranfusion,* the blood is infused as it is being taken from the donor. This method is rarely used except in emergencies and will not be discussed here.

Whole blood is used most frequently when a patient has sustained acute blood loss, such as following a hemorrhage.

Typing and Crossmatching

Before blood may be given to a person, it must be determined that the blood of the donor and that of the recipient are compatible. If they are not, clumping and hemolysis of the recipient's blood cells will result. The laboratory examination to determine a person's blood type is called *typing*. The process of determining compatibility between blood specimens is known as *cross-matching*.

Human blood is most often classified according to the ABO system into four major groups: O, A, B, and AB. Some of these groups have been broken down into still more groups. Sophisticated laboratory techniques are used to determine blood groupings and their compatability with other bloods.

An *antigen* is a substance which causes the formation of antibodies. An *antibody* is a protein substance developed in the body in response to the presence of an antigen which has in some way gained access to the body. An *agglutinin* is an antibody which causes a clumping of specific antigens. Individuals who have type A blood have an A antigen on their red blood cells; those with type B blood have B antigens on their cells; those in the AB groups have A and B antigens; and type O persons have neither A or B antigens on their red blood cells. Persons in each blood group have the agglutinins to the red cell antigens that they lack. Group A persons have the agglutinin for B; group AB persons have no agglutinins for A and B while group O persons have both A and B agglutinins in their blood serum. Assume a person with type O blood is transfused with blood from either a person with group A or B blood. There would be destruction of the recipient's red cells since his anti-A or anti-B agglutinins would react with the A or B antigens in the donor's red cells. From this example, it can be seen why group AB persons are often called universal recipients because persons in this blood group have no agglutinins for either A or B antigens, and group O persons are often called universal donors because they have neither A or B antigens.

The determination of the Rh factor in blood dates back several decades when it was discovered why receiving blood from certain persons produced transfusion reactions even when the donor's and recipient's blood were in the same blood group. The Rh factor was found to be the culprit. The Rhesus system was developed and so-called because of its relationship to substances in the red blood cells of Rhesus monkeys.

The *Rh factor* is an inherited antigen in human blood. There are five antigens in the Rh system but the one designated D is of first concern. A person whose blood contains a D antigen is called Rh positive; an Rh negative person lacks D. It is important that an Rh negative person receive blood from another Rh negative person. If Rh positive blood is injected into an Rh negative person, the recipient will develop anti-Rh agglutinins. Subsequent transfusion with Rh positive blood may cause serious reactions with clumping and hemolysis of red blood cells.

The Rh factor is of special importance during pregnancy since Rh incompatability between mother and fetus is often the problem when an infant has hemolytic disease. It is estimated that approximately 15 percent of the Caucasian population and about 5 percent of the black population in the United States are Rh negative.

The selection of blood donors must be done with care. Not only must the donor's blood be accurately typed, but it is also important to determine whether or not the donor is free from diseases, such as type A or B hepatitis. The virus causing these diseases can be transmitted to the recipient. Persons who have allergies usually are not used; nor those with a history of a chronic disease, such as tuberculosis. As a further precaution, some blood banks will not accept blood from a donor who has been immunized recently because of a possible allergic reaction to the blood.

Also, the donor is examined carefully at the time of donation and is permitted to give blood only if his heart and chest sounds, blood count, temperature, pulse and respiratory rates, and blood pressure are within normal ranges.

Equipment Commonly Used for a Blood Transfusion and Initiating the Transfusion

Sterile technique is used when administering a blood transfusion. The equipment necessary for the procedure is similar to that used for an intravenous infusion by the gravity method. The drip chamber in a transfusion set contains a filter. The filter is essential for removing any particulate matter that may be injurious to the patient, and it should be changed as necessary. A slightly larger needle, usually 18 gauge, is used because of the viscosity of blood. If the patient is sensitive to the pain of the larger needle as it pierces the skin, a small amount of local anesthesia given intradermally at the site of the injection or a volatile spray for numbing the pain receptors may be used.

Isotonic saline solution with a connection between it and the blood container is ordinarily used to start the transfusion. The saline solution makes the blood backflow into the tubing upon vein entry easy to determine; if blood is already present in the tubing, it is extremely difficult to detect the patient's blood backflow. Glucose or dextrose solutions should not be used with blood because hemolysis may occur. These same solutions given intravenously do not cause hemolysis because of the rapidity with which it is dispersed in the patient's bloodstream.

The blood is dispersed in bottles by a blood bank or a laboratory and is ready for use. Or, it may be dispensed in disposable polyvinyl bags. These bags expand when blood is collected and collapse as blood is administered. Disposable tubing and needles are ordinarily used with either bottles or plastic bags. The bag should not be punctured with a needle or a similar instrument for an air vent because of the danger of introducing microorganisms. Furthermore, an air vent is unnecessary since the bag collapses as the blood is given.

The blood container, either a bottle or a plastic bag, is the one used for obtaining the blood from the donor and contains acid-citrate-dextrose (ACD), or a similar anticoagulant, to prevent the donor's blood from clotting.

The safe storage of fresh whole blood has been limited to 21 days. After this time, too large a proportion of red blood cells have deteriorated and having released their potassium. If old blood is transfused, the recipient's blood potassium level may become too high and his life would be in danger because of the possibility of cardiac arrest.

Blood may be frozen and kept for three years or longer although some authorities recommend it not be used after one year. Plasma is first extracted and the red blood cells are then coated with glycerol to prevent damaging the cells during freezing. The glycerol is removed after thawing by a special machine and it is then reconstituted. This frozen blood, as it is called, offers several advantages: blood from donors with rare blood types can be readily available when necessary; blood can be kept for longer periods; and transmitting the hepatitis virus with frozen blood appears to be negligible or absent.

Fresh whole blood should be administered within 30 minutes after it leaves the blood bank or laboratory. The desirable temperature range to prevent blood cell deterioration is small. Therefore, storage areas are equipped with precise temperature controls. Refrigerators in nursing units normally do not provide these controls and for this reason, blood which has been dispensed from the laboratory is generally not permitted to be returned.

Blood is not warmed before administration in order to prevent cell damage. The blood is warmed sufficiently by the time it passes through the length of the tubing and enters the vein. Exceptions to this are occasionally made in emergency situations when large amounts of blood are transfused rapidly. In order to reduce the adjustment of the patient's body to an extreme volume of low temperature blood, heat exchange coil units or special microwave units are used to warm the blood. *Hot water should not be used to warm blood.*

Occasionally, when small amounts are being given, as for children, the syringe method is used. The necessary equipment is the same as that used for intravenous injections.

Every precaution should be taken to avoid mistaken identity before administering blood. *All personnel handling blood should check and double-check the labels, the numbers, the Rh factor, and compatability.* After identifying information on the patient's record is checked, identification of the patient should be reaffirmed at the bedside.

The blood should be inspected carefully before administration. It should be discarded if gas bubbles which may indicate that bacterial growth has occurred, hemolysis, clotting, or any other abnormal appearance is present.

Gentle inversion of the blood container will resuspend red blood cells before the transfusion. Blood should not be vigorously shaken because of the possibility of causing damage to the red cells. The procedure for initiating the transfusion is the same as that for starting an intravenous infusion.

Monitoring the Transfusion and Observing the Patient for Signs of a Reaction

The nurse should stay with the patient for at least the first five minutes after blood has started to enter the vein. Serious reactions often occur very soon after blood starts entering the patient. Blood is administered slowly during this period at approximately 30 or 40 drops per minute. If no signs or symptoms of a transfusion reaction occurs, the rate is increased to as fast as 60 to 100 drops per minute according to the physician's prescription. Monitoring the patient should occur regularly and frequently, at least every 5 to 10 minutes. The blood container may need to be gently agitated occasionally when the red blood cells settle.

When rapid infusion of blood is indicated, the blood may be pumped with a pressure bulb until the patient's immediate need for the whole blood has ceased.

Reactions to transfusion occur even when every precaution has been observed in selecting the blood and in sterilizing and preparing the equipment. The nurse should be prepared to recognize the signs and the

- What is the purpose of his taking each of these agents? Does the patient understand these purposes and how do the agents meet their intended purpose?

- Has the patient been taking these medications accurately with regard to dosage and frequency and time of day, and for how long has he taken them? Has he been omitting taking any of these drugs for a time, and if so, why and for how long?

- Have the medications been accomplishing the purposes for which they were intended?

- Has the patient experienced any untoward side effects and, if so, what symptoms did he experience?

- Are his medications compatible with each other? Are any of them likely to cause untoward interreactions?

- Is the procedure the patient uses to take his medications appropriate? Is he observing proper techniques of medical and surgical asepsis?

- Is there evidence of drug abuse?

The nurse will gather information concerning the patient from a variety of sources, as described in Chapter 4. She will wish to use literature dealing with pharmacology when she has questions about the nature of therapeutic agents.

The nurse will compare data she has gathered with her knowledge of pharmacology, normal health, and the pathophysiology influencing the patient's state of health. When she is unfamiliar with appropriate standards for assessing, she will turn to the numerous sources of information available to her.

The plan of nursing care for therapeutic agents the patient is receiving is developed and built upon nursing diagnoses and the strengths exhibited by the patient that were noted during data gathering and assessment. Including the patient when developing his plan of care is important. This is also important when teaching the patient to take his own therapeutic agents.

The various commonly used techniques for administering therapeutic agents have been described in this chapter. Administering any therapeutic agent is a nursing responsibility that cannot be taken lightly or carried out in an automatic or routine manner. Errors can add to the patient's health problems and can also threaten the patient's life. In addition to the proper administration of therapeutic agents, the following are additional guidelines which the nurse will wish to use:

- While the importance of using proper techniques for administering therapeutic agents cannot be overemphasized, an injustice is being done when concern with a skill becomes more important than concern for the patient. The uniqueness of each patient and the health problems with which he must deal remain of utmost importance.

- Teaching the patient about the therapeutic agents indicated for him, including how to administer his own medications, is an important intervention measure.

- Education of the public in general is a significant nursing responsibility, especially in view of the widespread misuse and abuse of drugs.

- The nurse teaches well when she observes high personal standards of conduct in relation to the use of therapeutic agents.

- Here are some important "do's" and "don't's" as a summary concerning teaching about the taking of drugs:

Don't be casual about taking drugs.

Don't take drugs you don't need.

Don't overbuy and keep drugs for long periods.

Don't combine drugs carelessly.

Don't continue taking O-T-C drugs if symptoms persist.

Don't take prescription drugs not prescribed specifically for you.

Do read and follow directions for use.

Do be cautious when using a drug for the first time.

Do dispose of old prescription drugs and outdated O-T-C medications.

Do seek professional advice before combining drugs.

Do seek professional advice when symptoms persist or return.

Do get medical checkups regularly.

The nurse has an important responsibility for seeing that laws on drugs are observed.

The nurse works cooperatively with other health personnel as the patient's advocate and contributes to decision-making on the use of therapeutic agents through her observations.

The parts of the nursing process and of the process as a whole are evaluated as described in Chapter 4.

CONCLUSION

Therapeutic agents are an important part of both health maintenance and health restoration. The nurse's knowledge and resulting judgment, observational ability, and technical skills are all important to the patient's therapeutic regimen.

Therapies are continually being introduced, and hence, the nurse's education can never stop in this area. With many patients receiving a number of agents simultaneously, her awareness of the incompatability is of particular importance.

SUPPLEMENTAL LIBRARY STUDY

1. The nurse has an excellent opportunity for teaching when persons talk about medications they have been taking at home.
    "Patient Counseling: The Commonsense Home Medicine Chest." *Nursing Update,* 7:1, 13–15, January 1976.
    List at least ten types of drugs which this article discusses and the recommendations given for the home use of each. According to this article, what six articles should be considered for stocking in a home medicine chest and what telephone numbers should be taped to the medicine chest?

2. The following article includes a short quiz on drugs and mathematics:
    Carr, Joseph J., et al. "How To Solve Dosage Problems in One Easy Lesson." *American Journal of Nursing,* 76:1934–1937, December 1976.
    Take the quiz on page 1937. If you answered any items incorrectly, study the article in order to determine how you made your errors.

3. The following article offers advice on drug errors:
    Newton, Marion and Newton, David W. "Guidelines for Handling Drug Errors." *Nursing 77,* 7:62–68, September 1977.
    Describe specific techniques the authors recommend for

preventing errors. The authors admit that to err is human. But what advice do they give on the course of action when an error is made? What three types of evidence were deemed necessary to prove negligence, according to the case described on page 68, when an error in administering drugs was made?

4. The nurse who wrote the following letter offers a method to apply cold to the area where an injection will be made:

   Wing, Donna M. "A Different Approach to IM Injections." (Letters) *American Journal of Nursing,* 76:1239–1240, August 1976.

   Upon what two principles did the author base her technique? What advantage does Ms. Wing's suggestion have over applying, for example, cold compresses to the area to be injected? In your opinion what possible disadvantage does her technique have?

5. Note the drug cards illustrated on pages 2192 and 2193 of the following article:

   Deberry, Pauline, et al. "Teaching Cardiac Patients to Manage Medications." *American Journal of Nursing,* 75:2191–2193, December 1975.

   Is there any additional information you would wish to add to a card, such as those illustrated, when teaching patients how to manage their medications at home? Describe how the pretest given on page 2191 could be modified and used to take a medication history. What information on drugs did these authors find was most difficult for patients to learn?

   In this same issue of the *American Journal of Nursing,* December 1975, on page 2216, there is a description of a device to be carried in a wallet for persons who take medications on a regular basis. What information is included in this device and why is it considered as necessary information to be kept with the person at all times?

25

BEHAVIORAL OBJECTIVES

When content in this chapter has been mastered, the student will be able to

Define the terms appearing in the glossary.

Describe several typical situations in which cardiopulmonary resuscitation is and is not recommended.

Discuss briefly how a rescuer determines the need for administering cardiopulmonary resuscitation.

Indicate how cardiopulmonary resuscitation administered to infants and children differs from cardiopulmonary resuscitation administered to adults.

Describe the administration of cardiopulmonary resuscitation and list at least ten errors associated with cardiopulmonary resuscitation and discuss the effects they have on a victim.

Summarize recommendations for the termination of basic life support.

Explain when the precordial thump is used, how it is administered, and what contraindications there are for its use.

Describe the removal of a foreign body from a victim's upper airway when using finger sweeping of the victim's mouth and upper throat, a blow to the victim's back, and the Heimlich maneuver.

Describe basic life support, using the nursing process as a guide.

Providing Basic Life Support

GLOSSARY

Advanced Life Support: Measures of basic life support plus additional adjunctive therapy to stabilize the condition of a victim who has suffered a sudden and unexpected cardiac arrest.

Basic Life Support: Measures that provide respiratory and cardiac functioning by artificial means for a person who has suffered a sudden and unexpected cardiac arrest.

Cardiac Arrest: A cessation of functional circulation.

Cardiopulmonary Resuscitation: Techniques to open and maintain a patent airway and to provide artificial ventilation and circulation for a person who has suffered a sudden and unexpected cardiac arrest. Abbreviated CPR.

External Cardiac Compression: The rhythmic administration of pressure on the sternum to produce artificial circulation.

Heimlich Maneuver: A technique to remove a foreign body from the upper respiratory tract by placing pressure on the residual air in the lungs to pop out the debris.

Precordial Thump: The administration of a blow to the sternum that acts as a stimulus to start a heartbeat.

Precordium: The area on the anterior of the body that lies over the heart and its great vessels.

Rescue Breathing: Artificial ventilation of the lungs with a rescuer's breath.

INTRODUCTION

A great variety of measures have been used in the past to resuscitate persons who had just died or who were near death. As knowledge of the functioning of the body, especially of the cardiopulmonary system, increased, better procedures of resuscitation were developed. It has been estimated that as many as 600,000 to 700,000 sudden and unexpected deaths each year are being prevented when proper care is started immediately after cardiopulmonary failure.

In 1973, a National Conference on Standards for Cardiopulmonary Resuscitation and Emergency Cardiac Care described basic and advanced life support measures. This chapter will discuss basic life support. *Advanced life support* is more appropriately discussed in speciality texts and includes such therapies as intubation of the respiratory tract; internal cardiac compression; defibrillation; the use of drugs, oxygen, and intravenous solutions; and monitoring.

Basic life support includes measures that provide respiratory and cardiac functioning by artificial means. *Cardiopulmonary resuscitation,* abbreviated CPR, is used for basic life support. Cardiopulmonary resuscitation consists of opening and maintaining a patent airway and providing artificial ventilation and circulation. The purpose is to maintain functioning of the vital centers in the central nervous system by providing them with sufficient oxygen to sustain cell integrity and life.

The term *rescue breathing* is often used for artificial ventilation of the lungs. It means using the rescuer's breath to revive someone who is unable to breathe for himself. *Cardiac arrest* is a sudden cessation of functional circulation. Circulation is maintained artificially when cardiac arrest occurs by *external cardiac compression* which consists of the rhythmic administration of pressure on the chest wall. It has been found that the systolic pressure will peak as high as 100 mm. Hg in the carotid arteries and about one-fourth to one-third the usual amount of blood will enter the brain when cardiac compression is properly executed.

Cardiopulmonary resuscitation is recommended when sudden and unexpected death occurs. It is ordinarily not recommended when a person is terminally ill and death is anticipated, or when there has been such a prolonged cardiac arrest that resuscitation efforts are judged to be futile. An example is the person who has been found dead and signs indicate that he has been dead for a time. When the approximate time of death is unknown but signs of death are not pronounced, the victim is given the benefit of the doubt and resuscitation efforts are ordinarily made.

INDICATIONS FOR BEGINNING BASIC LIFE SUPPORT

When a person suddenly and unexpectedly stops breathing or his heart ceases to function, a crisis exists. It can be expected that there is usually considerable anxiety present in this emergency. The rescuer must work speedily, make spur-of-the-moment decisions, and carry out intervention measures deftly and quickly. Helter-skelter running about is likely to add to the victim's problem at a time when death already threatens. Logical and deliberate thinking and acting are required. Ideally, *only seconds should elapse between recognizing the victim's needs for resuscitation and starting it.*

When a person suddenly collapses and/or is unconscious, the rescuer immediately notes whether breathing and circulation are adequate or absent. If the victim is not breathing but a pulse can be felt, rescue breathing becomes necessary. If there is no evidence of a pulse, artificial circulation must be started along with rescue breathing.

Respiratory failure can be noted when efforts to breathe are absent. There is no air movement through the nose or mouth and the chest and abdomen do not move. If there is doubt about whether the victim is breathing, rescue breathing is started. It can do no harm, but grave consequences may result if it is not done when necessary. When the airway is partially obstructed, the victim demonstrates labored breathing and retraction of soft tissues in the areas between the ribs and above the sternum and clavicles. Every accessory muscle of respiration will be called into action. There will be discussion later in this chapter on the removal of foreign bodies in the upper airway.

Cessation of breathing can be of cardiac or pulmonary origin. If the heart stops, breathing usually stops within 30 to 45 seconds. If cessation of breathing is of respiratory origin, the heart may continue to beat but it will become more and more feeble, and, unless action is taken, it will stop too. Breathing cessation of respiratory origin occurs when a person's airway is blocked by a foreign body, such as a piece of food.

When cardiac arrest occurs, the victim does not breathe, is pulseless, and appears ashen. The carotid artery is recommended for checking the pulse. It is an easily accessible artery when clothing about the neck is removed. Also, peripheral arteries may be pulseless while a pulse can still be felt at the large carotid artery even when a heartbeat is of poor quality. A femoral artery is satisfactory but is ordinarily not as accessible as the carotids. If the victim is an infant or small child, it is recommended that the rescuer feel for the apical

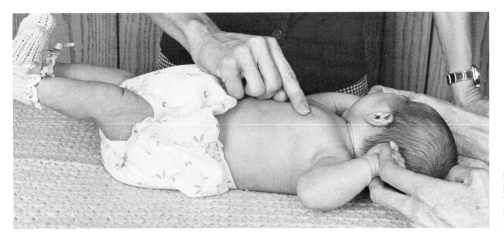

Figure 25-1 The nurse has placed her index finger under the nipple and to the left of the sterum to feel for this infant's apical pulse.

pulse in the precordium which is under the nipple line and just to the left of the sternum. This is illustrated in Figure 25-1. The *precordium* is the area on the anterior of the body that lies over the heart and its great vessels.

A person who is not breathing and is pulseless can sustain integrity of the body cells for only a matter of minutes. Brain damage is reported unlikely when cardiopulmonary resuscitation is started within four minutes of cardiac arrest. It is probable after four to six minutes, and after ten minutes, permanent brain damage is almost a certainty.

ADMINISTERING CARDIO-PULMONARY RESUSCITATION

The procedure of cardiopulmonary resuscitation is often described as the A, B, C's of basic life support:

A for airway
B for breathing
C for circulation

These three steps should be started as quickly as possible and in that order after a victim suddenly collapses. The letter A means that the respiratory tract must be opened in order that air can enter and leave the victim's lungs. The letter B means that if the victim does not start to breathe spontaneously after the airway is opened, artificial ventilation must be started. The letter C means that if the victim is pulseless, artificial circulation must be started along with rescue breathing.

The chart on page 646 describes cardiopulmonary resuscitation when using either one or two rescuers. Table 25-1 describes common errors that may occur when cardiopulmonary resuscitation is being administered and the effects they have on the victim.

When there are two rescuers, they may switch positions during cardiopulmonary resuscitation to relieve fatigue. At a given signal and immediately after a rescue breath has been given, the rescuer administering artificial ventilation moves to the side of the victim opposite the second rescuer. The first rescuer positions his hands properly over the hands of the rescuer administering cardiac compression. He then takes over chest compression while the other rescuer moves to the victim's head to perform rescue breathing. There should be no break in the rhythm and regularity of rescue breathing and cardiac compression during this switch in positions.

Many health and professional organizations have recommended and supported widespread efforts to teach cardiopulmonary resuscitation to both health personnel and laypersons. Health agencies ordinarily have infant and adult mannikins for practice. So also do many chapters of the American Heart Association and the National Red Cross. The procedure should be well-rehearsed and reviewed periodically so that cardiopulmonary resuscitation can be administered quickly and correctly without hesitation when an emergency arises.

CARDIOPULMONARY RESUSCITATION IN INFANTS AND CHILDREN

The techniques for administering cardiopulmonary resuscitation to infants and children are essentially the same as those for adults with these important exceptions:

- Since the neck of the very young child is pliable, tilt the head backward to maintain a patent airway gently and without exaggeration.

Administering cardiopulmonary resuscitation (CPR)

The purpose is to provide respiratory and cardiac functioning by artificial means.

SUGGESTED ACTION	RATIONALE
Two Rescuers	
Place the victim on a flat, firm surface, such as the floor, ground, litter, or wooden board. Legs may be slightly elevated.	During cardiac compression, the firm surface upon which the victim lies prevents dissipation of pressure on the sternum. There will be inadequate blood flow to the brain if the victim is in a vertical position. Lying flat with the legs slightly elevated promotes blood flow to the brain.
Place one rescuer on one side of the victim near the victim's head; this rescuer will provide artificial ventilation. Place the second rescuer on the victim's opposite side near his chest; this rescuer will provide artificial circulation.	Having the rescuers positioned as described allows for maximum efficiency when administering artificial ventilation and circulation.
First Rescuer	
Tilt the victim's head backward as far as possible by placing one hand under the victim's neck and the other hand on the victim's forehead. Lift up with the hand under the neck and press down with the hand on the forehead. This is illustrated in Figure 25–2.	Tilting the victim's head backward opens the airway by extending the neck and lifting the tongue and mandible from the throat.
OR	
If the airway does not open with the above maneuver, the jaw thrust maneuver should be used. Move to the top of the victim's head and place the fingers behind the victim's jaws. Forcefully push the jaw forward while tilting the head backward; use the thumbs to retract the lower lip. This is illustrated in Figure 25–3.	
When breathing does not start spontaneously with either of the above two maneuvers, one rescuer does artificial ventilation while the second rescuer does cardiac compression.	
While keeping the head tilted backward with one hand under the victim's neck and one on the forehead, pinch the victim's nose shut with a finger and thumb on the hand which is on the victim's forehead, as illustrated in Figure 25–4.	Keeping the head tilted backward helps maintain an open airway. Pinching the nose shut allows maximum ventilation with no dissipation of air through the nostrils.
Take a deep breath, seal lips around the victim's widely opened mouth and blow breath forcefully. Lift face away from the victim and allow him to exhale passively. The chest should rise visibly and then fall.	The force of rescue breathing needs to be sufficient so that the chest visibly rises when it is forced into the victim's mouth, and then visibly falls with the victim's passive exhalation. The rescuer will note resistance in his own airway and can hear and feel air leave the victim when rescue breathing is administered properly.
Repeat the above procedure four times without allowing time for the victim's lungs to deflate completely between breaths.	An initial four quick breaths provides the victim with a quick supply of oxygen.
When it is not possible to develop a good seal around the victim's mouth, the nose may be used. In such instances, the rescuer's mouth should provide a good seal around the victim's nose. The rescuer then proceeds to administer ventilation as described above. The victim's lips may need to be opened between rescue breaths to allow the escape of air.	
Continue with one rescue breath every five seconds without pause as long as the victim shows respiratory inadequacy by quickly interspersing one breath after each five cardiac compressions and without interrupting regular cardiac compressions.	The rate of 12 regularly spaced rescue breaths per minute has been found to supply the victim with sufficient oxygen to maintain cell integrity.
Continue to tilt the victim's head backward during all of artificial ventilation.	Keeping the head tilted throughout artificial ventilation helps maintain a patent airway.
Second Rescuer	
Place the width of the heel of one hand, the part near the wrist, over the long axis of the lower half of the sternum but 2.5 to 3.8 cm. or 1 to $1\frac{1}{2}$ inches from the xiphoid process.	Keeping pressure off the xiphoid process at the tip of the sternum prevents possible rupture of the liver and internal hemorrhaging.
Place the second hand over the first hand; preferably the fingers should interlock. Bring the shoulders directly over the hands and keep the elbows and arms straight. This is illustrated in Figure 25–5.	Interlocking the fingers helps keep them off the victim's ribs where pressure may cause fractures of the ribs. This position with the elbows and arms straight allows for best exertion of pressure on the sternum over the heart.

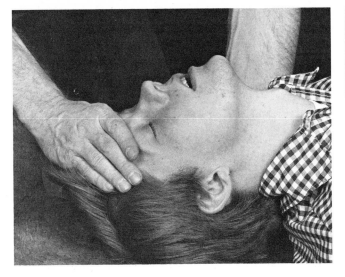

Figure 25–2 Lifting up on the victim's neck with one hand and pressing down on the forehead with the other hand, a maneuver frequently called the head tilt, opens the victim's airway.

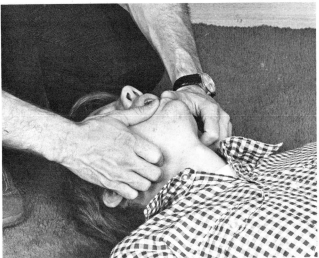

Figure 25–3 The jaw thrust also helps open the airway. The rescuer's fingers are placed behind the victim's jaws and the jaws are pushed forward with the rescuer's thumbs.

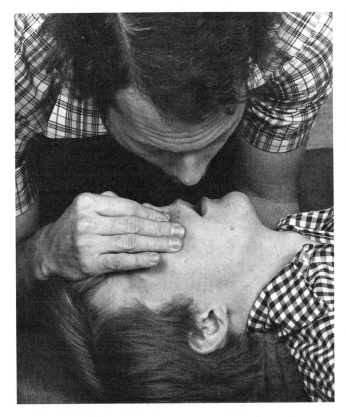

Figure 25–4 The head remains tilted, the victim's nose is pinched shut, and the rescuer takes a deep breath in readiness to administer a rescue breath.

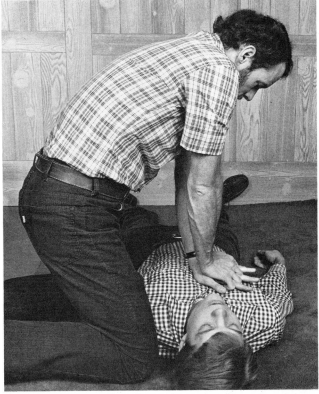

Figure 25–5 The rescuer has his fingers interlaced, has the heel of his lower hand on the victim's sternum about 2.5 to 3.0 cm. or 1 to 1½ inches from the xiphoid process,and has brought his shoulders over his hands. The rescuer is in position to apply pressure over the heart and begin external cardiac compressions.

Exert pressure on the sternum by rocking forward slightly so that pressure is applied almost vertically downward. Depress the sternum a minimum of 3.8 to 5.0 cm. or 1½ to 2 inches and then relax the pressure immediately.

The depression of the sternum with pressure causes the heart to be compressed and forces blood into the aorta and pulmonary arteries. Relaxation of pressure allows the heart to expand and refill.

Keep the hands in proper position and on the victim's chest wall between compressions.

Keeping the hands in place over the sternum helps administer regular and even compressions.

Continue with compressions and relaxations, each equal in length of time, regularly and without pause at the rate of 60 per minute as long as the victim's heart does not beat spontaneously.

Compressions of 60 per minute will maintain adequate blood pressure and flow to maintain cell integrity.

Check the effectiveness of CPR after the first minute and then regularly every few minutes by noting whether the pupils respond to light, whether there is pulsation at the carotid artery, and whether the victim's color has improved.

When pupils constrict in the presence of light, adequate blood flow with oxygenated blood is reaching the brain. The carotid artery is large, centrally located, and ordinarily readily accessible. Color will improve and pulsation will return spontaneously when the victim's heart begins to beat on its own.

Check the effectiveness of CPR without interrupting artificial ventilation and circulation. This is done by the rescuer administering artificial ventilation or preferably, by a third person.

It is important to carry out CPR without interruption to assure adequate blood flow with oxygenated blood to maintain cell integrity.

The procedure for CPR is as described above when there is only one rescuer to perform artificial ventilation and circulation, *except*
   Administer two quick rescue breaths after each 15 cardiac compressions. Do not allow the victim time for complete passive exhalations in order to be able to administer 60 cardiac compressions per minute between the rescue breaths.
   Administer cardiac compressions at the faster rate of 80 per minute in order that the victim will receive a total of 60 cardiac compressions each minute between rescue breaths.

TABLE 25–1   Common errors that may occur when cardiopulmonary resuscitation is being administered and their effects on the victim

ERROR	EFFECT
The airway is not patent.	Air cannot enter the lungs in sufficient quantity to sustain life when the airway is not open.
The head is tilted back too far and with too much force when a cervical injury is present.	The head tilt may cause damage to the victim's spinal cord in the area of the injury. A modified head thrust is recommended; that is, the head is maintained in a neutral position rather than tilted backward.
The seal made by the rescuer's mouth over the victim's mouth or nose is broken.	Sufficient air will not enter the victim's lungs when the seal formed by the rescuer's mouth is not secure.
The rescue breaths are of insufficient force to cause the victim's chest to rise with each rescue breath.	When the victim's chest does not visibly rise and fall with each complete rescue breath, sufficient air for adequate ventilation is not entering the lungs.
Artificial ventilation is too forceful or it is administered when there is an airway obstruction.	There will be distention of the stomach if artificial ventilation is too forceful. This occurs more commonly in children than in adults. The danger is that distention tends to cause vomiting and predisposes to aspiration, and it causes the diaphragm to rise and interfere with proper artificial ventilation and circulation. Figure 25–6 illustrates a technique to relieve gastric distention.
The fingers of the rescuer who is placing pressure on the sternum rests on the ribs of the victim during compression.	Pressure on the rib cage caused by the fingers of the rescuer may result in fractures of the ribs.
The xiphoid process is depressed during cardiac compression.	Depression of the xiphoid process may rupture the liver and cause internal hemorrhaging.
Some pressure is maintained between cardiac compressions on the victim's chest wall.	When complete relaxation after each cardiac compression is not maintained, the heart cannot adequately fill with blood.
The sternum is depressed less than the recommended distance.	Blood flow and pressure will be insufficient to maintain cell integrity.
The rescuer administering cardiac compression is not properly positioned directly over the victim and/or his elbows are bent.	The thrust of compression will be ineffective when the rescuer is improperly positioned. Also, the rescuer will tire more quickly.
Sudden, irregular, or jerking movements are made during cardiac compressions.	Sudden, irregular, and jerking movements tend to cause injuries and are ineffectual for maintaining good blood flow and pressure.
CPR is interrupted for more than five seconds. If a victim *must* be intubated or moved, the interruption should not exceed 15 seconds.	Ventilation and circulation quickly become inadequate and cell integrity will suffer when CPR is interrupted.

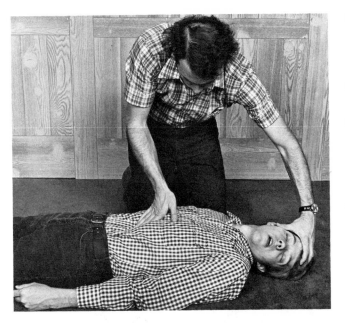

Figure 25–6 To decompress the stomach when it is distended, the rescuer exerts moderate pressure over the victim's upper abdomen with his fingers. His fingers are between the victim's lower rib margin and the naval. The victim's head is turned to help fluid from the stomach escape from the mouth.

TERMINATING BASIC LIFE SUPPORT

When a victim begins ventilation and circulatory efforts on his own, cardiopulmonary resuscitation is discontinued. If the victim has not already been taken to a health agency, he is ordinarily transported at this time where advanced life support is used. Rescuers are relieved of their responsibilities when professional personnel take over their work.

Moving a victim to a hospital or life support unit as quickly as possible after cardiac arrest is ideal. The victim may be transferred during the administration of cardiopulmonary resuscitation provided basic life support continues without interruption.

- Cover both the mouth and the nose with the mouth of the rescuer during artificial ventilation. Some authorities recommend covering the mouth of the rescuer with a handkerchief while administering rescue breathing.

- Use small breaths and less force than when ventilating adults.

- For small children, compress the sternum with one hand only. For infants, compress with the index and middle finger only; or encircle the thorax with two hands and compress the sternum with the thumbs. These two methods for an infant are illustrated in Figure 25–7.

- Exert pressure about midway on the sternum, as shown in Figure 25–7, since the heart lies higher in the chest cavity in infants and children than it does in adults. The liver also lies high and under the lower sternum and xiphoid process, and hence, danger of liver laceration is increased when compression is applied too low on the sternum.

- Compress the sternum 1.3 to 1.9 cm. or ½ to ¾ inches for infants and for young children, 1.9 to 3.8 cm. or ¾ to 1½ inches.

- Compress an infant's chest 80 to 120 times per minute with a quick rescue breath after each five to eight compressions; and 60 to 80 times per minute for an older child with a rescue breath after each five to seven compressions.

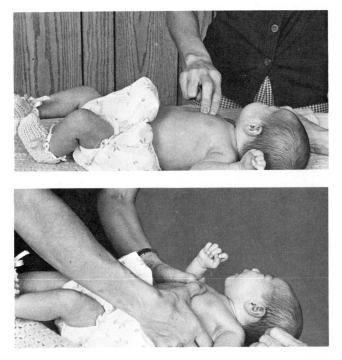

Figure 25–7 In the photo at the top, the nurse uses her index and middle finger to exert pressure on the infant's midsternum. In the photo at the bottom, the nurse has encircled the infant's thorax with two hands and compresses the infant's midsternum with her two thumbs.

It is recommended that any victim requiring cardio-pulmonary resuscitation also have at least some advanced life support measures.

If the victim does not respond to resuscitation, remains unconscious, and the pupils are dilated even in the presence of light for as long as 30 minutes, further resuscitation efforts will probably be of no avail. However, the final decision concerning further resuscitation efforts is ordinarily left up to a physician. In the meantime, the victim is given the benefit of the doubt since, in some instances, persons have been reported to have survived without permanent brain damage even after signs of death were present for as long as an hour or two. This has been found to be the case with some children and with some persons suffering from hypothermia, such as victims who have been in very cold water.

THE PRECORDIAL THUMP

When a cardiac arrest is *observed* in an adult and the person is noted to be pulseless, a *single* precordial thump is recommended. A *precordial thump* is the administration of a blow to the sternum which acts as a stimulus to start a heartbeat. The thump produces a small electrical impulse. When administered within the first minute of the cardiac arrest, the electrical impulse is often an effective stimulus for starting spontaneous heat action.

The procedure for administering the blow is as follows:

• Tilt the head backward to open the airway and determine that the victim is pulseless by feeling at the carotid artery.

• Make a fist with one hand. Hold it between 20 to 30 cm. or 8 and 12 inches above the victim's chest wall, as illustrated in Figure 25–8, and administer one sharp blow over the midsternum area with the fleshy part of the fist.

If the carotid pulse and voluntary breathing do not return, administer cardiopulmonary resuscitation as described earlier in this chapter, beginning with four quick rescue breaths.

At this time, the precordial thump is not recommended for children and infants. Nor is it recommended for an unwitnessed arrest when hypoxia of heart tissue is almost certainly present. If heart tissues are already suffering from lack of sufficient oxygen, a thump may cause the heart to go into rapid and ineffectual contractions.

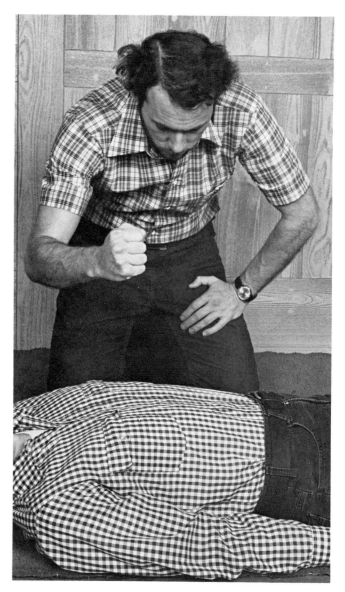

Figure 25–8 The rescuer is about to administer a precordial thump with his fist. He holds his hand about 30 cm. or 12 inches above the victim's chest wall in this photo.

REMOVING FOREIGN BODIES FROM THE UPPER AIRWAY

When cardiopulmonary resuscitation is indicated, it is recommended that the rescuers not take time to look for foreign bodies in the upper airway unless there is strong suspicion that one is present. If believed to be present, the victim should be quickly rolled to his side and his mouth should be forced open. The rescuer should then use his index and middle finger to sweep the entire mouth and the upper throat to remove the foreign body. If this maneuver is unsuccessful, a sharp blow should be delivered with the heel of one hand between the victim's shoulder blades. When the victim is a small child, it is better to invert the youngster over the rescuer's arm and deliver the blow with a flat hand between the victim's shoulder blades. Or, a small child or infant can be momentarily suspended by the ankles as the blow to the back is delivered.

The *Heimlich maneuver* has often been recommended when a person is choking to death because of a foreign body stuck in the upper airway. The maneuver is most often used when the foreign body is a piece of food, but it may be used to remove other foreign bodies as well. The choking person will be speechless, turn pale and then blue, and will collapse if not given immediate emergency care.

The Heimlich maneuver uses residual air in the lungs to pop out the debris in the upper respiratory tract. The procedure is as follows:

- The rescuer stands behind the victim and places his arms around the victim, as illustrated in Figure 25-9.

- The rescuer makes a fist with one hand which he grabs with his other hand, as shown in Figure 25-9. He places his fist against the victim's abdomen, slightly below the rib cage and above the navel.

- The victim is allowed to fall forward with his head, arms, and upper chest over the rescuer's arms, as illustrated in Figure 25-10 on page 652.

- The rescuer then presses his fist into the victim's abdomen with a forceful upward thrust.

- The maneuver is repeated if necessary.

The Heimlich maneuver can also be done while the victim lies flat on his back. The rescuer kneels over the victim while facing in the direction of the head. He places one leg on each side of the victim's hips. The rescuer places his hands on top of each other between the victim's rib cage and navel. Figure 25-11 on page 652 illustrates. He then performs the forceful upward thrust with the heel of the bottom hand.

BASIC LIFE SUPPORT AND THE NURSING PROCESS

Time is of essence when a victim is in need of resuscitation, and hence, the nurse must focus on essentials in order not to waste precious moments. Details must

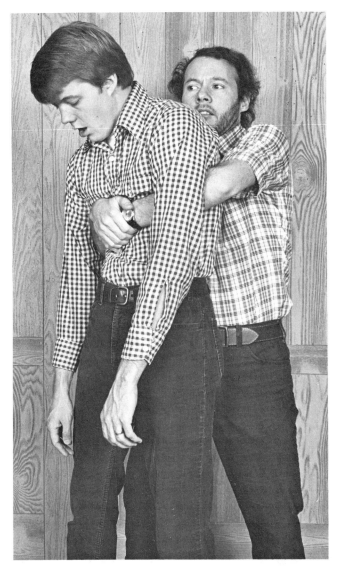

Figure 25-9 This rescuer is about to use the Heimlich maneuver to help the victim. He has placed his arms around the victim, made a fist with one hand which he has grabbed with his other hand, and placed his fist against the victim's abdomen.

wait until the urgency of sustaining life has subsided. The collecting of data consists of determining immediately and quickly whether breathing and circulation are adequate or absent.

Assessment of the victim is based on knowledge that a person who is not breathing and is pulseless cannot sustain cell integrity for more than a matter of minutes.

The immediate plan of care for a victim is to start basic life support. While basic life support measures are being used, a plan to move the victim to a health

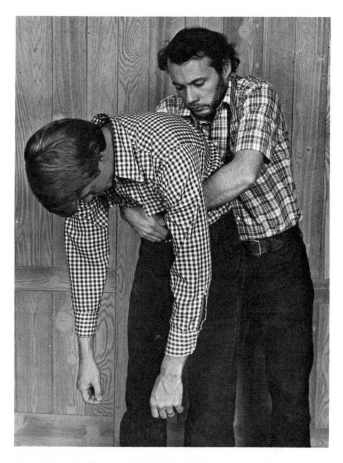

Figure 25–10 To complete the Heimlich maneuver, the victim falls forward with his head, arms, and upper chest over the rescuer's arms. The rescuer presses his fist into the victim's abdominal wall with a forceful upward thrust.

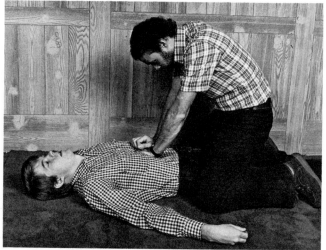

Figure 25–11 This is another way to perform the Heimlich maneuver when a victim has a foreign body in his upper respiratory passage. The rescuer straddles the victim, places his hands on top of each other between the victim's rib cage and navel, and then performs a forceful upward thrust with the heel of his bottom hand.

agency that can administer advanced life support should be arrived at. Other persons at the scene of the emergency can be asked to call for help, such as for an ambulance to transport the patient.

Intervention measures to provide respiratory and circulatory functioning artificially have been described in this chapter. The following are some general guidelines that the nurse will wish to keep in mind:

- Time is of the essence when a victim requires basic life support. The rescuer who is thoroughly familiar with indications for its use and with the techniques of sustaining life artificially is best able to function effectively when a victim suffers with cardiopulmonary failure. The nurse is admonished to practice regularly so that she remains skillful in administering basic life support.

- At present, there is a concerted effort in this country to teach large numbers of people, laypersons as well as health personnel, how to administer basic life support. Not only should every nurse know how to administer basic life support, but she should be ready as necessary to teach others how to do so. A mannikin should be used for demonstration and practice. Fortunately, mannikins are readily available on the market and most health agencies and many community associations and organizations have them on hand for teaching purposes.

- Even though all efforts are focused on saving a life when sudden cardiopulmonary failure occurs, psychological care is important to help the victim as he regains consciousness and to offer support to relatives and friends. The presence of a rescuer who demonstrates technical skills offers relatives and friends comfort in itself. But when time permits after the victim's care has been turned over to other health personnel, emotional support should be offered or provided for, depending on the circumstances.

- Giving another person mouth-to-mouth breathing sometimes is difficult psychologically for the rescuer when the victim has been vomiting, has infected and draining wounds, is unshaven and dirty, smells of alcohol, is already dead, and is otherwise repellent. Some persons who have worked with such victims report that the overwhelming need to offer life-saving measures helps overcome any psychological aversion. A handkerchief or piece of cloth may be placed between the rescu-

Care for the Patient With a Terminal Illness

GLOSSARY

Autopsy: An examination of organs and tissues of the body after death.

Bereavement Program: A program designed to offer assistance to those who have lost a loved one to death.

Brompton Mixture: A mixture for pain control consisting of morphine or heroin, codeine, ethyl alcohol, and a flavoring agent. A modified Brompton mixture does not contain codeine.

Cryonics: The freezing of dead human bodies.

Euthanasia: Painless or mercy killing.

Hospice: A way-station for travelers; a health agency specifically designed for the care of persons having terminal illnesses.

Living Will: A description of a person's wishes with regard to the use of artificial means or heroic measures when there is no reasonable expectation of recovery from a physical or mental disability.

Terminal Illness: An illness from which recovery is beyond reasonable expectation.

Thanatology: The study of death and its medical and psychological effects.

INTRODUCTION

A *terminal illness* is one from which recovery is beyond reasonable expectation. The illness may be due to a disease or the result of an accident. Errors in judgment concerning recovery sometimes are made. Persons who have been predicted to be dead in days or weeks have lived months and even years. Also, during the course of an illness, medical science may bring forth a means of saving a life. Hence, there is reason to remain hopeful while caring for terminally ill patients. The patient and his family often find courage and support in knowing that everything possible is being done and the hope for recovery is never completely abandoned.

The inevitability of death is nowhere better expressed than in Ecclesiastes 3:1-2—"To everything there is a season, and a time to every purpose under the heaven; A time to be born, and a time to die; . . ." Everyone has the privilege of and the right to meet death serenely and comfortably, and the nurse can do much to provide care which allows the individual to meet death peacefully and in his own way.

In addition to the continuing research during the last decade or two to find ways to prevent death from specific pathology, there has been increased interest in the process of dying and death *per se*. *Thanatology* is the study of death and its medical and psychological effects.

The questions, both scientific and ethical, surrounding dying and death are extensive and complex. Health personnel, bioengineers, lawyers, social scientists, philosophers, biologists, theologians, and laypersons are among those involved in the discussion and investigations. The increased use of organ transplants and bioengineering techniques that make it possible to sustain life in persons who previously would have died, the liberalization of abortion laws, the desire for some persons to control the end of their life, and research on life after death are some of the factors that have stimulated increased attention on death.

The concept that death is a natural part of life and not just a failure in medical science has become more prevalent today. In the past, health workers and agencies held as their top priorities, cures, health maintenance, and restoration so that death was often viewed as a personal failure on the part of health personnel. Unfortunately as a result, the terminally ill patient was frequently avoided, except for essential physical care.

Health personnel received little formal educational preparation for care of the dying person. There was generally a reluctance on the part of health personnel to discuss or acknowledge feelings about death with a patient or family members or even in professional conferences, let alone with oneself.

Today, death and dying are commonly the focus of literature, conferences, and investigations, and are included as a part of virtually all curricula designed to prepare health personnel. Public education through television, radio, periodicals, books, and newspapers is in increased evidence. There are varied programs offered to family members both during the terminal illness of patients and following death in some areas. In addition, in some agencies, routinely scheduled health team conferences for dealing constructively with health workers' feelings and for planning improved patient care are indications of other changes which have occurred and which are generally improving the care of terminally ill persons.

The nurse is often a key person in the care of the patient who is dying and is in contact with his family, regardless of whether the patient is at home or in a health agency. Both the patient and the family often turn to her for support and assistance. In order to provide effective care, the nurse must have reconciled some of her own feelings about death. She needs to understand the phases of grieving and dying and be able to recognize their manifestations. Perhaps most of all, she needs to be able to accept and support the individuality of the person, whether or not his beliefs or behavior coincide with her own. Provision of care may be easier if the nurse sees her purpose as that of assisting the patient to meet his physical and psychological needs, just as with any other patient. Her goal is to provide the support and assistance necessary to help the patient die in comfort and dignity.

The Code for Nurses of the American Nurses' Association includes in the elaboration of its first statement a summary of some of the ideas just expressed.

> The nurse's respect for the worth and dignity of the individual human being extends throughout the entire life cycle, from birth to death, . . . the young and the old, the recovering patient as well as the one who is terminally ill or dying. In the latter instance the nurse should use all the measures at her command to enable the patient to live out his days with as much comfort, dignity, and freedom from anxiety and pain as possible. His nursing care will determine, to a great degree, how he lives this final human experience and the peace and dignity with which he approaches death.*

The Division on Geriatric Nursing Practice of the American Nurses' Association has included a statement on the nurse's responsibility regarding the dying pa-

---

* "Code for Nurses." *American Journal of Nursing,* 68:2582, December 1968.

tient. "The nurse seeks to resolve her conflicting attitudes regarding aging, death, and dependency so that she can assist older persons, and their relatives, to maintain life with dignity and comfort until death ensues." *

THE NURSE'S FEELINGS ABOUT DYING AND DEATH

Understanding others through understanding oneself is an often-repeated psychological principle, the importance of which probably would be argued by few. Since impending death is accompanied by fear of the unknown and the natural instinct of all creatures to cling to life, it becomes particularly important for the nurse to understand her own feelings about terminal illness, death, and its usual accompanying grief in order to help to meet the needs of patients for whom she is caring. This understanding is essential to her own professional development. Investigations have shown that most nurses know how to give physical care to the terminally ill patient but fail to give psychosocial care because of their own uncomfortable feelings about death.

Because in our culture, youth and productivity are highly valued in contrast to illness, aging, and dying, the nurse brings these influences with her when caring for terminally ill patients. The orientation of society and her educational background are strongly directed toward health and life. These experiences make dealing with death a difficult occurrence. For example, a student in nursing may never have viewed a body or observed or experienced the grief that accompanies the death of a loved one. She may never have spoken with a dying person. The nurse must also deal with her views and feelings regarding prolongation of life by artificial means and regarding *euthanasia*, that is, painless or mercy killing.

The nurse who neglects to deal with her feelings about life, dying, and death is in a questionable position for being able to analyze and consider the needs of patients who are facing death. Therefore, one's own feelings play a major role in determining how one cares for a patient with a terminal illness. Everyone, not only the nurse, experiences emotion when death is pending. The easy way to react is to ignore the feelings of the patient and his family. Sadly enough, as a result, the

* "Standards for Geriatric Nursing Practice." *American Journal of Nursing,* 70:1897, September 1970.

dying person and his family are often emotionally abandoned and left to face a lonesome situation alone.

Discussing one's feelings and views with others is one of the most effective ways of developing increased insight and learning to handle personal emotions related to dying and death. This may be done in a health team or a nursing team conference, with friends or relatives, or with a clergyman. Also, the patient himself can often help the nurse to clarify how she feels about death and dying, as will be discussed later in this chapter.

The following are some questions, the answers to which often help the nurse to clarify feelings about her own finiteness:

- If I could control the events that result in my death, where would I want to be? What cause of death would I choose? Whom would I want to have present during my terminal illness?

- What fears do I have about death?

- How would I answer these same questions for a patient for whom I have been caring?

- How could I improve the quality of care for a patient for whom I am caring and who is terminally ill?

- If I were a member of the patient's family, what things would I want nurses to do for me?

HELPING TO MEET THE PSYCHOSOCIAL NEEDS OF THE TERMINALLY ILL PATIENT

While every person reacts to the knowledge of impending death or to loss in his own unique way, there are similarities in the psychosocial responses to the situation. The world renown authority, Dr. Elisabeth Kübler-Ross, has studied the responses to death and dying in depth and her findings have been used extensively by nursing and other helping professions.

When persons speak of their fears of death, responses typically include fear of the unknown, pain, separation, leaving loved ones, loss of dignity, unfinished business, and so on. However, Kübler-Ross believes that there is still another more overwhelming and more significant fear that is often repressed and unconscious. She describes this fear as the catastrophic destructive force that has befallen a person and that the person cannot change; the person is helpless in being able to do anything about it.

Kübler-Ross points out that terminally ill persons

communicate this fear of a destructive force but largely through symbolic language. The person may use non-verbal language, such as a facial expression, a particular kind of hand clasp, or in the case of children, through drawings and manner of play with toys. Verbal communication may also be used symbolically. Kübler-Ross gave an example of a dying youngster in an oxygen tent who asked what would happen if there were a fire in her tent. In this case, the destructive force over which the child felt she had no control was her death, but she described it symbolically in terms of a fire.

Many authorities, including Kübler-Ross, believe that the more persons in the helping professions listen to dying persons, the more they will learn how to come to grips with the death of others and the more comfortable they become with their own death. Repeatedly, Kübler-Ross stresses the word *listen*. Her investigations have convinced her that dying persons do want and are able to talk about their death and are also able to communicate about when they will die. To deny them the opportunity to talk and to fail to listen and perceive what is being said leave the dying person isolated and alone. Health workers often tend to be struggling with their own needs when caring for the terminally ill. It is they, not the patient, who do not want to speak of death. Listening to the patient helps to put the spotlight on the patient's needs rather than on those of the nurse or other health workers.

Communication is an essential vehicle for persons to find self-identity and as Chapter 9 pointed out, the need for self-identity is lifelong, even up to the moment of death. Developing meaningful communications with a patient requires that the nurse have a trusting relationship with the patient. This relationship was explored in Chapter 6. Nurses, as well as others, may find it difficult to communicate with terminally ill patients about their death and often for good reason. The subject of death has been taboo for many years; health workers have placed much more emphasis on cure and prevention of disease than on the care of the terminally ill, and death is usually a stressful and emotional experience for everyone. Also, many health workers have used giving the patient the best possible physical care as an escape from guilt when unable to offer psychosocial care. Certainly physical care is important. But until the nurse can listen and pick up verbal and nonverbal cues to help her identify the real needs of the patient, the nurse will have missed an important opportunity to assume a therapeutic role when caring for the terminally ill.

An especially important means of communicating with the terminally ill patient is touch. One need not always say something to show support, concern, and care. Touch with silence can often communicate far more than any spoken word. Nearly all of the illustrations in this chapter use this form of communication and health personnel who work with the dying patient continually emphasize the importance of touch as a means of communication. Touch can also be used effectively when helping to support relatives and friends of the person who is dying.

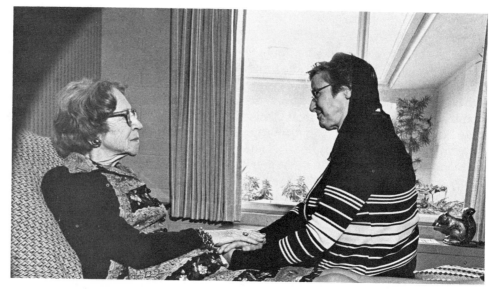

Figure 26–1 The nurse and the patient exchange communications by touch and the nurse listens while the terminally ill patient speaks. This hospice resident has brought several personal possessions from home and chooses to wear her own street clothes.

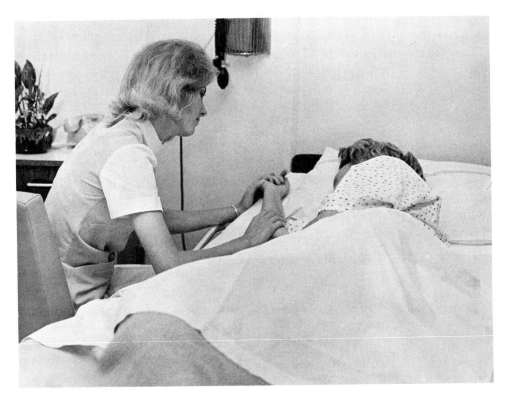

Figure 26–2 The nurse can often communicate her concern and support for the patient by simply silently remaining at the patient's side. Touch is among the most effective means for communicating care for the terminally ill patient.

The Stages of Dying

Kübler-Ross has described stages of dying. The stages do not always follow one another or they may overlap. Sometimes a patient may go through a stage but later move back to it again. The duration of any stage can vary from as little as a few hours to as long as a period of months. When a particular stage is very brief, unless the nurse pays particular attention, it may even appear that the patient has skipped a stage.

The first stage is one of shock and denial. It is characterized by the comment, "No, not me." During this stage, the patient is really saying that death happens to others but not to him. The patient is usually so overcome with his denial that he hears little of the facts that may be described to him. He may even repress what he hears. Or, he may seek help from a variety of professional and nonprofessional sources as he tries to escape the truth of his impending death.

The second stage is characterized by rage and anger. Now the person is saying, "Why me?" It is often difficult for the nurse to cope with the patient during this stage. The patient is very likely to be critical of everyone and everything. He is easily enraged by health workers and with whatever they try to do.

Kübler-Ross states that this stage is a blessing for the patient rather than a curse. Anger is the patient's defense mechanism, but his real anger lies with health and life, the two things health workers represent. This is a time when the nurse must guard against being judgmental and recognize anger and rage as normal reactions to death that need expressing.

Next follows the stage of bargaining. The patient is saying, "Yes, me, but . . ." Anger has ordinarily subsided and the patient may even appear to be at peace with what is happening to him. However, the stage of bargaining is a time for truce and the patient now tries to barter for more time. He will often make promises to God if he is a believer, such as promising to lead a better life in exchange for more time. He will make requests that will give him a longer life. For example, a mother may say that she will do anything for enough time to see her children reared or her grandchildren born. It is during the bargaining phase that many persons tend to get their houses in order before death and will take care of such things as making a will and providing for the loved ones they will leave. The recommendation is that during bargaining, as many requests as can be fulfilled, should be. This is part of the unfinished business to be taken care of before death.

Stories are told of patients who have one last request to see a sporting event, visit a particular relative, see the newest grandchild, go on one last trip to dinner, and so on. Meeting these requests is advised because bargaining helps persons step into later stages, even though they tend to continue to add one more request.

The fourth stage is one of depression as the patient is saying, "Yes, me." This tends to be a very sad time because the patient is in a state of mourning over past losses and the present loss of his own life, along with the good things he enjoyed in the past. Patients tend not to speak much during this stage and may often cry. It is a time for the nurse to sit by quietly as the patient goes through his own period of grieving before death.

The last stage of dying is marked by acceptance of death. The patient has by now taken care of unfinished business and may not wish to talk because he really has said all that needs saying. Bargaining is over and it is a period of peace and tranquility. Kübler-Ross states that having reached this stage does not necessarily mean that death is near. A person may live in a stage of acceptance for a long time. She also points out that this is not resignation which is defeat. In other words, resignation to death is not acceptance of death. In her examples, Kübler-Ross tells of patients who appear calm and at peace and will make statements, such as "Let death take me soon for I am ready," when they are expressing only defeat. She states that she was of the opinion from her observations that the majority of patients in nursing homes are resigned to die. They have not accepted death but, rather, have no purpose in living. She believes that people who are resigned but have not accepted death need to have love and care as well as to love and to care for others.

Sometimes, a patient may mask his true feelings about death or may not really want to face the truth. The patient may claim to be unafraid and prepared for death when he really is fearful and just trying to appear brave. Patience, careful observation, and listening in order to learn true feelings are a prerequisite if the nurse desires to give sincere comfort and support to the dying patient.

What can the nurse do as patients move through these five stages of dying? The following are some suggestions that can be gleaned from Kübler-Ross's investigations. It is important to allow patients to go through these stages of dying and to act as a catalyst so that the patient can proceed to the final stage of acceptance. Recognize the patient's needs, not one's own, and attempt to meet them. Allow and encourage the patient to talk and to express his emotions freely in a nonjudgmental environment. Be available to the patient, especially at night when it seems most patients waken and want to talk. Respect the patient's behaviors for they are his defense mechanisms; to strip him of his defenses as he dies leaves him open to additional anguish and psychological pain. If one is not sure whether the patient wishes to talk, ask the patient a straightforward question, such as "Do you want to talk about it?" and then listen and perceive what he is trying to say.

A registered nurse who knew she was dying wrote these words for her peers:

1. Kübler-Ross is accurate. What she says happens, and it happens exactly the way she says it happens. If they doubt my word, they can talk to someone else who is dying.

2. It is *normal* for the dying person to use denial, become angry, depressed, try to make deals, et cetera. You *really* have a problem if your dying patient doesn't do these things.

3. You learn to interact with dying people by interacting with dying people. I suspect that anyone who suggests this skill can be learned by role playing or other "games" is strongly denying death herself. It also seems to me that a teacher, of all people, should be made aware of this.

I offer two simple hints to those who are anxious about contact with the dying:

1. All of you send strong nonverbal cues to us, the dying, about your degree of comfort with the subject of death. The dying person will sense your comfort or discomfort and proceed accordingly. If he doesn't bring up the subject, he either senses your discomfort or else simply doesn't have a need to talk about it at that time. So relax!

2. We, the dying, are not all that fragile or so easily devastated. Don't get so hung up about saying or doing the wrong thing. No lasting harm will be done if you reinforce our denial, retaliate when we are angry, or urge us to cheer up when we are depressed.

We understand. We were once in your shoes and we know exactly where you are coming from.*

The Will to Live or to Die

Kübler-Ross feels that hope should not be abandoned while caring for the terminally ill. Hope is a desire accompanied by a feeling of anticipation or expectation. Without hope, despair exists. Hope, no matter how minimal, usually occurs in the patient, his family, and in the nurse. However, very often, the patient's hope, the family's hope, and the nurse's hope are not the same. As the patient begins to face impending death

---

*Hammack, Joyce L. "We, the Dying, Are Not All That Fragile or So Easily Devastated." (Letters) *American Journal of Nursing,* 77:40, January 1977.

and accepts the fact that cure or prolongation of life is no longer probable, he may hope to be free of pain or nausea or to be able to walk down the hall one more time. His family may still be hoping for a miraculous cure while the nurse may be at some point in between. It is the patient's hope which should be identified and supported if it is realistic. The patient usually is quick to identify expressions of unrealistic hopes for cures.

The will to live or to die has been observed to be a powerful force during a terminal illness. Patients with overwhelming pathological involvement that made life seem impossible lived to see still one more relative, to return to their place of birth, to see a child graduate from college, to celebrate a birthday or anniversary, and so on. On the other hand, others may die when they so wished, without pathological reason. It has been noted that during certain times in the year, natural death rates drop, such as during a holiday season or near national holidays. Some persons have predicted their own death with great accuracy. When the patient is the focus of care, his wishes to live or die become apparent, and at times, no type of intervention appears able to change the course of events.

What to Tell the Terminally Ill Patient

The question usually arises concerning what to tell the terminally ill patient about his prognosis. It is the physician who usually is responsible for deciding what and how the patient shall be told. Usually he makes this decision after discussing the problem with the patient's family and after assessing the patient individually. The nurse, social worker, clergyman, or others in helping professions may also be involved in making the decision and in discussing it with the patient.

Kübler-Ross found in her studies that the majority of patients wished to know their prognosis as early as possible so that they had time to come to grips with it. They asked for continued hope even though cure and prolongation of life appeared improbable. They pleaded not to be deserted and left alone to die.

It is now generally considered unkind and unjust to permit such a patient to die without his having known the seriousness of his condition. By not knowing, he may have had the time denied him to arrange important business affairs, papers, finances, and so on. Many people, especially those who have responsibilities to others, such as their children, find comfort in the fact that, should they die, "their house is in order."

From many observations, it has been seen that most patients realize without being told that they are suffer-

ing from an incurable illness. The nonverbal communication of the patient's family and the health personnel often speak louder than their words. Patients often feel even more isolated, lonely, and rejected when the truth is withheld, especially when falsehoods are told them. After the prognosis has been discussed in an open and frank manner, health personnel must be prepared to offer the patient support. But usually the patient finds solace eventually in knowing and realizing that he will not be left to meet death alone.

The important thing for all involved persons is to know exactly what the patient and family have been told. Patients and families often direct questions to the nurse concerning prognosis. Unless all persons are aware of what the patient has been told, they may be working at cross-purposes. It is up to the nurse to take the initiative to discuss the problems with other health team members in circumstances in which uncertainty exists.

Health team members caring for dying patients need a close working relationship. A type of camaraderie will often develop as a result of the stress usually involved when helping patients and families cope with a difficult situation. Mutual trust and respect among health care personnel can promote a climate which provides additional security for the patient and his family. Physicians will often depend on the nurse for care suggestions because the physician may no longer have an active medical regimen to implement.

As has been stated earlier in this text, the patient should be permitted to retain as much independence and decision-making capacity as he is able. When

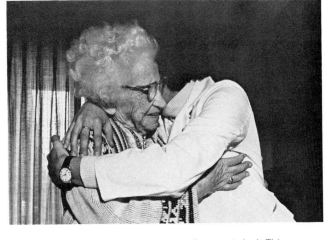

Figure 26–3 Sometimes a hug can tell a great deal. This nurse and her patient, a hospice resident, embrace as they exchange feelings of caring and trust.

physical abilities fail, determining when he wishes his medication, for example, may be all the control of his life he retains.

The adult patient has the ultimate right to refuse treatment. In dealing with the person with an incurable illness, health personnel sometimes find the patient's desire not to have further surgery or extensive treatments difficult to accept. At other times, the patient has ambivalent feelings and needs to be permitted time and the support necessary to explore those feelings.

Many terminally ill patients find great comfort in the support that they receive from their religious faiths. It is important to aid in obtaining the services of a clergyman as each situation indicates. In some instances, the nurse may offer to call a clergyman when the patient or family has not expressed a desire to see one, but this must be handled tactfully and in good judgment so that the patient is not frightened by the suggestion. However, it must be remembered that a religious faith is not an insurance policy guaranteeing security from the loneliness of death. The chaplain's visit does not replace the kind words and the gentle touch of the nurse. Rather, he should be considered as one of the team assisting the patient to face terminal illness.

Many patients make decisions to donate various body organs after death to organ banks for possible transplantation. The patient may ask the nurse questions about the technique or about her views. He may be seeking information or he may wish to explore his feelings aloud. The nurse should assist the patient in these conversations rather than focus on her own beliefs. Legal documents permitting organ removal are available from most health agencies. Care should be taken to see that they are accurately completed if it is the patient's desire to donate organs.

HELPING TO MEET THE PHYSICAL NEEDS OF THE TERMINALLY ILL PATIENT

Unless death occurs suddenly, there are certain problems concerning the patient's physical needs that the nurse usually can expect to encounter.

Meeting Nutritional and Fluid Needs

The patient who is terminally ill usually has little interest in food and fluids. His appetite fails, and often the physical effort to eat or drink is too great for him.

Meeting nutritional and fluid needs may in itself help to prolong life and it also helps to make the patient more comfortable. Dehydration and malnutrition predispose to exhaustion, infection, and other complications, such as the development of decubitus ulcers. Therefore, maintaining the nutritional state of the patient plays an important part in sustaining energy and preventing additional discomfort. When the patient is unable to take fluids and food by mouth, the physician may order intravenous therapy or other means of maintaining nutrition.

When death is pending, the normal activities of the gastrointestinal tract decrease. Therefore, offering the patient large quantities of food may predispose to distention and added discomfort.

If the swallowing reflex is intact, offering sips of water at frequent intervals is helpful. As swallowing becomes difficult, aspiration may occur when fluids are given. The patient can suck on gauze soaked in water or on ice chips wrapped in gauze without difficulty because sucking is one of the last reflexes to disappear as death approaches.

Caring for the Mouth, Nose, Eyes, and Skin

If the patient is taking foods and fluids without difficulty, oral hygiene is similar to that offered other patients. However, as death approaches, the mouth usually needs additional care. Mucus that cannot be swallowed or expectorated accumulates in the mouth and the throat and may need to be aspirated. The mouth can be wiped out with gauze, or, if indicated, suctioning may be necessary to remove mucus. Positioning the patient on his side very often helps in keeping the mouth and the throat free of accumulated mucus.

The mucous membrane should be kept free of dried secretions. Lubricating the mouth and the lips is helpful as well as comfortable for the patient.

The nostrils should be kept clean also and lubricated as necessary.

Sometimes, secretions from the eyes accumulate. The eyes may be wiped clean with wipes or cotton balls moistened in normal saline. If the eyes are dry, they tend to stay open. The instillation of a lubricant in the conjunctival sac may be indicated to prevent friction and promote comfort.

As death approaches, the patient's temperature usually is elevated above normal. But, as peripheral circulation fails, the skin feels cold, and the patient often perspires profusely. It is important to keep the bed linens and the bed clothing dry by bathing the patient and changing linens as necessary. Using light bed linen and supporting it so that it does not rest on the patient's body usually give additional comfort. The patient often is restless and may be observed to pick at his bed linen. This may be due to the fact that he feels too warm; sponging him and keeping him dry often promote relaxation and quiet sleeping.

Promoting Elimination

Some patients may be incontinent while others may need to be observed for retention of urine and for constipation, both of which are uncomfortable for the patient. Cleansing enemas may be ordered for relieving and preventing constipation and distention, but it should be remembered that, if the patient is taking little nourishment, there may be only small amounts of fecal material in the intestine.

Catheterization at regular intervals, or indwelling catheters, may be necessary for some patients. If the patient is incontinent of urine and feces, care of the skin becomes particularly important to prevent odors and decubitus ulcers. Waterproof bed pads are easier to change than all of the bed linens; they make keeping the bed clean and dry less of a problem.

Positioning the Patient and Protecting Him from Harm

The dorsal recumbent position often is associated with the dying patient. However, good nursing care provides for varied positions with frequent changes in position. The patient may not be able to express a desire to have his position changed, or he may feel that the effort is too great. Even though the patient appears to be unconscious, proper positioning is important. Poor positioning without adequate support is fatiguing as well as uncomfortable.

Sometimes the nurse is confronted with the problem of a patient who experiences intractable pain except when in one position. She must weigh the consequences of constant pressure, impaired circulation, and tissue breakdown against the patient's comfort.

When dyspnea is present, the patient will be more comfortable when supported in the Fowler's position. Stertorous or noisy breathing frequently is relieved when the patient is placed on his side. This position helps to keep the tongue from obstructing the respiratory passageway in the oropharynx. Proper positioning

has been discussed earlier in this text, and the same principles that were discussed then guide action in positioning the terminally ill patient.

The terminally ill patient may be restless. In these instances, special precautions are necessary to protect the patient from harm. The use of siderails may be indicated. Restraining the patient usually is undesirable but may be necessary in extreme cases. If relatives of the patient offer to remain with him so that he does not injure himself, the nurse may give them simple guidelines about talking softly to the patient and reassuring him with gentle touch. Family members of the patient should not be left with the complete burden of the patient's safety. The nurse should check the patient frequently because the responsibility for the patient's welfare is hers. Well-meaning, but unprepared, fatigued, and stressed family members sometimes use poor judgment in protecting the patient. Feeling the responsibility of care, or guilt if some unexpected occurrence results in injury, is an unfair price to expect family members to pay. If relatives or friends do stay with the patient, the nurse should see that they are relieved periodically. Remaining with a confused and restless terminally ill person can be both physically and emotionally taxing.

Caring for the Environment

It is economical of nursing time to place the hospitalized patient in a room that is convenient for giving nursing care and for observing him at frequent intervals. Very often, the patient is placed in a private room to avoid distressing other patients. However, this experience in itself may be upsetting to the patient. Social deprivation can be distressing, even when the patient cannot express this.

Having familiar objects in view can help to make the patient feel more comfortable and secure. The family can be encouraged to make his room meaningful to him. Pictures, books, and other significant objects can be very important. Whether the patient is at home or in a health agency, it is desirable to have the environment reflect his preferences. Once the environment is pleasing to the patient, it can remain as it is unless he chooses to make alterations. In this way, the self-esteem of the patient may be supported by giving him some degree of control over his environment when he has lost control of most other aspects of daily living. The home environment is generally not difficult to maintain according to the patient's wishes. However, the hospital or nursing home setting can be an austere, neat room conveying a regimented and impersonal environment unless a concerted effort is made to avoid it.

Normal lighting should be used in the patient's room. Terminally ill patients may experience increased loneliness, fear, and poor vision when in a darkened room. The room should be well-ventilated, and the patient protected from drafts.

While conversing near the patient's bedside, it is preferable to speak in a normal tone of voice. Whispering can be annoying to the patient and may make him feel that secrets are being kept from him. It generally is believed that the sense of hearing is the last sense to leave the body, and many patients retain a sense of hearing almost to the moment of death. Therefore, care should be exercised concerning topics of conversation. Even when the patient appears to be unconscious, he may hear what is being said in his presence. It

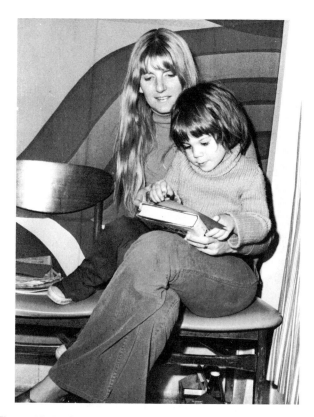

Figure 26–5   Observing the normal activities of a four-year-old helped his father remain part of the family. Note the mural on the wall in the background. It was painted by the patient's wife to individualize the hospital room and to add a note of cheer too.

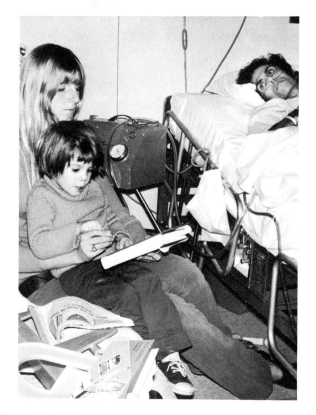

Figure 26–4   The practice of this health agency encourages families of terminally ill persons to spend as much time as possible with the patient. This patient was comforted because his wife and son were nearby and they shared the majority of the last weeks with him. The agency encouraged the family to decorate and arrange the room in as homelike a fashion as possible when the patient's condition necessitated his being hospitalized. The wife remained with her husband constantly and the child visited for several hours each day.

generally is comforting to the patient for others to say things which he may like to hear. Even when he cannot respond, it is kind and thoughtful to speak to him. It also remains important for the nurse to explain to the patient what she is going to do when giving nursing care or working in the unit so that the patient does not misunderstand her actions or become fearful.

Keeping the Patient Comfortable

Efforts to meet the physical needs of a terminally ill patient may still fall short of keeping him comfortable, and then it becomes necessary to consider the use of medications that relieve pain, restlessness, and anxiety. In most instances, a narcotic is prescribed for relieving pain. Although such medications should be administered with the usual precautions, there appears to be little excuse for withholding their use until the patient suffers from discomfort. When pain is intense, analgesia is more difficult to attain. Therefore, it is better to keep pain in remission. A tranquilizer or antidepressant may be prescribed in conjunction with an analgesic. When used appropriately with analgesics, pain can be controlled without heavy sedation.

It has been observed that complaints of pain sometimes are a camouflage for fear. In such instances, the pain may appear to be disproportionate to the patient's pathology. However, pain is less likely to be overrated when the nurse has gained the patient's confidence. Persons working with the terminally ill have noted that patients experiencing good emotional support require less analgesic drugs.

Some patients prefer and are able to control their own medication regimen. They can tolerate discomfort with greater ease when they know they can administer the next dose, rather than being dependent on someone else to bring it. Other persons may find tolerating pain more acceptable than the clouding of mental alertness and loss of awareness that come with use of more potent analgesics.

As peripheral circulation fails, the absorption of drugs given subcutaneously is impaired, and other routes of administering the drug may become necessary.

Health personnel working exclusively with the termminally ill, especially those working in hospices, have developed pain control programs which have proven to be very effective. These health workers point out that chronic, intractable pain is among the greatest fears of terminally ill patients, especially those with malignant diseases. It is more than a physical pain; it also has emotional, social, religious, and economic overtones. Each aspect of pain must be handled on an individual basis, but experience has shown that the person who receives emotional support from caring persons tends to require fewer analgesics than terminally ill patients without this type of care.

An oral analgesic known as the *Brompton mixture* was developed in British hospices. This mixture contains morphine, or heroin, cocaine, ethyl alcohol, and a flavoring, such as grenadine syrup. A modified Brompton mixture does not contain cocaine. The Brompton and modified Brompton mixtures are given on a preventive schedule for patients with chronic pain. The elixir is given around the clock whether the patient is in pain or not. This method of administration provides for a continuous level of tissue analgesia. It has been found that the maintenance dose for pain relief is lower than when a drug is offered as needed on a p.r.n. basis. Simultaneously, the patient experiences less anxiety and more confidence than when he is allowed to experience pain first before a drug is given, according

to investigations. Non-narcotics can be used when discomfort is mild, and appropriate drugs for depression and marked anxiety are often used along with the analgesia.

Hospice personnel report several advantages to the use of the elixir of morphine. It is an oral medication, and, hence, the added discomfort of repeated injections is avoided. The amount of morphine in the elixir can be increased or decreased without the patient's concern about the number of injections or tablets he takes. Other drugs, such as those to control nausea, can be easily added to the elixir to meet specific needs of the patient.

According to studies, there has been no significant amount of tolerance developed with the use of the Brompton and modified Brompton mixtures. Increased dosages are observed to be related to progression of the disease rather than to tolerance. Addiction also is not a practical problem when caring for the terminally ill, according to these health workers. They believe that psychological dependence on narcotics is rare since the purpose of the drug is for the relief of pain rather than the euphoric effects which the classical drug addict seeks.

SIGNS OF APPROACHING DEATH

Death is a progressive process—the body does not die suddenly. During this process, there are signs that usually indicate rather clearly that death is imminent.

Motion and sensation are lost gradually; this usually begins in the extremities, particularly the feet and the legs. The normal activities of the gastrointestinal tract begin to decrease, and reflexes gradually disappear. As peristalsis slows, the patient may become distended.

Although the patient's temperature usually is elevated, he feels cold and clammy, beginning with his extremities and the tip of his nose. His skin is cyanosed, gray or pale. The pulse becomes irregular, weak, and fast.

Respirations may be noisy, and the "death rattle" may be heard. This is due to an accumulation of mucus in the respiratory tract which the patient is no longer able to raise and expectorate. Cheyne-Stokes respirations occur commonly.

As the blood pressure falls, the peripheral circulation fails. Pain, if it has been present, usually subsides, and there is mental cloudiness. The patient may or may not lose consciousness—the amount of mental alertness varies among patients, which is important to remember when giving care to the patient who appears to be dying. It has been noted by some observers that some patients see visions just prior to death.

The jaw and the facial muscles relax and the patient's expression, which may have appeared anxious, becomes one of peacefulness. The eyes may remain partly open. The lower jaw tends to drop.

Even though these signs may be present, the nurse will realize that neither she nor any other member of the health team can predict the amount of time before death actually occurs. The family of a dying patient, because of fears and concerns, may ask the nurse how long she thinks the patient will live. The nurse's role at this time is to be supportive and to indicate that she is unable to give a realistic answer to the question. Keeping families aware of changes that are occurring is generally helpful to assist them to prepare themselves for the patient's death.

SIGNS OF DEATH

In the past, the person was considered dead when no pulse and respirations could be determined for a period of several minutes, even with auscultation. In death, the pupils remain dilated and fixed. With the extensive use of artificial means to maintain cardiac and respiratory activity, other means of determining death have had to be developed. The absence of all reflexes and no brain wave activity, reflected as a flat electroencephalogram, for a period of 24 hours are generally considered as positive indications of death.

The increasing incidence of sustaining life by mechanical means and the use of organs for transplant have resulted in continued efforts to refine determinants of death. In general, authorities agree that death is a gradual process, its progress depending on the varying ability of tissues to live without oxygen. The electroencephalograph currently is the most helpful diagnostic tool to support clinical judgment in determining death.

The legal profession has asked for more specific guidelines than now exist concerning when death occurs. The American Medical Association has taken the position that a statutory definition of death is not desirable at this time. It recommends that death be determined on a case-by-case basis and that advances in medical science should guide the physician's judgment.

THE DYING PERSON'S BILL OF RIGHTS

What rights do dying persons have? The following bill of rights developed by nurses helps to answer the question:

THE DYING PERSON'S BILL OF RIGHTS

I have the right to be treated as a living human being until I die.

I have the right to maintain a sense of hopefulness however changing its focus may be.

I have the right to be cared for by those who can maintain a sense of hopefulness, however changing this might be.

I have the right to express my feelings and emotions about my approaching death in my own way.

I have the right to participate in decisions concerning my care.

I have the right to expect continuing medical and nursing attention even though "cure" goals must be changed to "comfort" goals.

I have the right not to die alone.

I have the right to be free from pain.

I have the right to have my questions answered honestly.

I have the right not to be deceived.

I have the right to have help from and for my family in accepting my death.

I have the right to die in peace and dignity.

I have a right to retain my individuality and not be judged for my decisions which may be contrary to beliefs of others.

I have the right to discuss and enlarge my religious and/or spiritual experiences, whatever these may mean to others.

I have the right to expect that the sanctity of the human body will be respected after death.

I have the right to be cared for by caring, sensitive, knowledgeable people who will attempt to understand my needs and will be able to gain some satisfaction in helping me face my death.

This Bill of Rights was created at a workshop on "The Terminally Ill Patient and the Helping Person," in Lansing, Mich., sponsored by the Southwestern Michigan Inservice Education Council and conducted by Amelia J. Barbus, associate professor of nursing, Wayne State University, Detroit.*

*Whitman, Helen H. and Lukes, Shelby J. "Behavior Modification for Terminally Ill Patients." *American Journal of Nursing,* 75:99, January 1975.

HELPING THE PATIENT'S FAMILY

Words of comfort for the family of a terminally ill person may be hard to find. It may be best to say nothing and to be a listener if the relatives wish to express their thoughts. Relatives often find comfort in feeling that they are assisting the patient during his terminal illness, that everything possible is being done for him, and in knowing that he is being kept comfortable. Also, they need to be offered hope. They derive little comfort from efforts to cheer them and suggestions that they try to forget and think of something else. Sometimes, allowing a willing member of the family to assist with aspects of nursing care is comforting to the patient as well as to the relative. If family members do give care to the patient, the nurse needs to check the patient frequently to determine his condition as well as the relative's ability to cope with the situation. The nurse should provide necessary explanations and help the relative to feel he can call for assistance at any time. The family member needs to feel that when she leaves the patient or is too tired to give care, a nurse will intervene. Some family members may not want to provide care, but they may need help in knowing what to expect and what to say to the patient. The nurse's explanations and support can be helpful here too.

The considerate nurse will remember that as relatives become tired, they may also become critical of nursing care. The families may well be correct in their assessment, as research has shown that the dying patient's call light is frequently answered last. At any rate, the nurse should spend time with the relative to determine the cause of critical comments. This technique may be further broadened by a nursing team conference with the family member present. The relative may view this gesture as one of sincere concern by all those caring for the patient. In addition, the staff will gain insight and understanding of the patient's family unit.

There are instances when the nurse spends more time with the relatives than she does the patient. Frequently, this may occur when the patient becomes comatose. It takes less nursing time to turn and position the patient than it does to be sufficiently supportive to the family waiting at the bedside.

Family members may need to be reminded to get rest and to eat. Occasionally, a family member will want to spend the night with the patient. When permitted, the nurse should provide as much comfort as possible for the relative.

Children too play an important role in the family of a dying person. When allowed to visit the hospitalized patient, they may help brighten his day. Children also

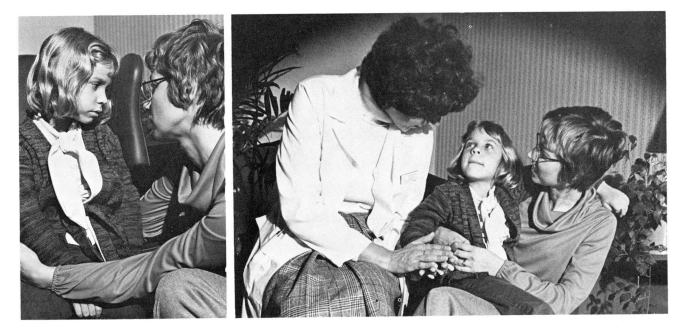

Figure 26-6 Children need to know about death too. This youngster's grandfather was terminally ill and her mother is helping to prepare her daughter for the loss of a loved one. In the photo on the right, the nurse is helping to explain. Note the use of touch in both of these photos.

usually benefit from seeing and knowing where the parent or grandparent is. Just as adults, children need honest information about what is happening.

Too many visitors may tire the patient, and, when explanations are offered, relatives usually understand this readily. When they wish to remain at the hospital, it is desirable to direct them to a place where it is quiet and they may relax.

An example of the significance of a relative spending time with a patient is demonstrated by Mr. H. Mr. H. was an elderly man hospitalized in the terminal stages of a malignancy. He was observed to sleep all day. His wife visited daily from early morning until late afternoon and sat quietly at his bedside as he slept. Nurses noted that Mr. H. awakened about 5:30 P.M. in time for supper and then spent the remainder of the evening watching television. Throughout the night he read and talked with the nurses when they were available. When his wife appeared in the early morning, she, along with the daylight, provided the security and comfort that allowed Mr. H. to fall asleep, less frightened of dying. His wife's presence did more for Mr. H. than any number of skillful nurses might have.

Sometimes the patient's close family members encounter problems when extended family members or friends are informed of the patient's condition. These persons may accept the information and offer sympathy and support. But they may also challenge the diagnosis and question the competency of the health team. This type of behavior describes denial and may add additional distress to close family members. The alert nurse will recognize such conflicts and allow family members to speak openly of their problem.

During terminal illness, the patient's family members are often required to take on different responsibilities as the family role of the dying member shifts to other persons. A financial strain, when present, forces the family to address an economic burden as well.

When hospitalization is temporary due to an exacerbation of a terminal illness, planning requires thinking of the future. Is home care needed? Will the patient return to the health agency for terminal care? The nurse can serve to share information about available community resources with the family.

When a terminally ill person reaches his final stage of illness, a crisis of sorts occurs with unconsciousness. The family may interpret the loss of consciousness as a sign of impending death. Some patients experience a period of unconsciousness for weeks and since the family members are not usually prepared for this, they may need extra help from health team members.

The lack of communication with the unconscious person is a barrier to family relationships. When family members have not come early enough to say goodbye, the regret over this missed experience may hinder resolution of grief for a long time.

Issues Related to Prolonging Life

Family members of terminally ill patients are often asked to participate in making a decision about the sustaining of life when many artificial means are being used. The physician usually initiates this discussion with the family, but relatives often involve the nurse in their decision-making. The nurse's role may be one of providing information, helping relatives explore their feelings and ideas, and offering support. The nurse should not advise or persuade.

The issue of allowing death to occur without aggressive intervention took on significance for many persons when the news media publicized controversies over prolonging the life of certain unconscious persons when recovery appeared improbable. No clear-cut guidelines have developed and each case is being handled on an individual basis. But the tendency is to respect the wishes of the closest relatives in relation to prolonging life by artificial means.

Many persons are now planning ahead before trauma or terminal illness occurs by seeking an alternative to prolonging their life unnecessarily. One method for facilitating an objective personal decision on prolonging life is for the person to prepare a living will. A *living will* describes a person's wishes with regard to being kept alive by artificial means or heroic measures when there is no reasonable expectation of recovery from a physical or mental disability. The Euthanasia Educational Council has prepared a form for a living will and offers it to anyone upon request. It is illustrated in Figure 26–7. The physician notes on the patient's chart when resuscitation and life-prolonging measures are not to be used for these patients. The nurse may sometimes be ambivalent in her feelings about not resuscitating, but as with other health care measure, the right of a competent, rational, adult person to make decisions concerning his own death is becoming more and more accepted.

Living wills are not currently legally binding except in California, but momentum to legislate so-called death with dignity is being well-fueled by public opinion. Many states have bills presently under consideration. California's law exempts the physician and other health professionals from liability when they act on

immediately instigated to save a life. In many instances, the health team is overwhelmed with demands to meet the patient's physical needs as it tries to save a life. Unfortunately, distraught relatives and friends are left to wait without emotional support or information. Ideally, a private room is available and persons not involved with the physical care of the person, such as trained volunteers, social workers, or clergymen, help family members. Family members should not be left along during an emergency.

The question most often asked by relatives of the emergency victim concerns whether he will live. Just as with chronically ill patients, it is important to allow for some hope even when the prognosis is grim. A comment explaining that the health team will not give up and will fight to save a life using every possible means possible is often helpful.

The family that loses a member in a sudden, unexpected death has not had the opportunity to experience any of the grieving process before death occurs. These persons are especially in need of emotional support that includes allowing them to express their grief and listening to them as they vent their feelings. They should not be rushed from the room or health agency but should be given the time they need to overcome the initial reaction to a shocking experience. Discussing plans for the care of the body can wait temporarily.

The survivors may request seeing the body of the deceased. Authorities generally agree that the request should be granted after the body is cleaned and mutilated areas, if present, are covered. It is believed survivors need this opportunity to view and touch the body in order to experience the reality of the death. Sedating especially distraught survivors is generally not recommended since this delays progress in the grieving process. However, such survivors should not be allowed to leave alone because overwhelming emotional reactions to sudden, unexpected death may precipitate suicidal tendencies.

A *bereavement program* is a program designed to offer assistance to those who have lost a loved one to death. They are especially helpful when sudden, unexpected death occurs. Remaining in touch with survivors and offering whatever supportive care is indicated are invaluable means for helping them progress through the grieving process. Often, family and friends remain close at hand at times of an emergency. Shortly, they tend to leave, especially when they judge survivors as being slow in overcoming the pain of the death or when they feel uncomfortable in the situation. Then especially, the nurse can fill a void by follow-up care of the bereaved. This departure of others, leaving the close survivors to face their problems alone, often happens when death is expected also.

When Children Die

Studies have indicated that children have a much better understanding of death than most adults realize. Toddlers and infants are believed to have no concept of death. But as early as age three, it is believed a child can understand a death concept in terms of loss of objects. Up until about age five, a child may be more curious than concerned about death and may even view it as reversible. Their fear is primarily fear of separation from mother, should they become terminally ill. Beginning at about school age, it appears that most children see death as an irreversible, final, personal experience. By about 10 or 12 years of age and on, it is believed that the youngster and adolescent view death much as an adult.

Surprisingly enough, investigations have shown that most terminally ill children become aware of their impending death even when not told, just as do most adults. Although it is a very difficult task, authorities in general are recommending that children over about five should be told their prognosis. This is an especially difficult time for parents when they wish not to inform the child. The result is that this leaves the child alone and unable to express his fears, anxieties, and sadness. In such instances, the child often turns to a mother substitute for help. When this is the nurse, as it so often is, she has an important role in offering support which family members may simply feel unable to give at the time. The family members also need help in such situations so they too become aware of the child's need for them.

The death of a child is usually a devastating experience for the family. It is an emotional crisis and makes coping with grief difficult. Earlier discussion in this section on helping these persons applies here as well. The family of a child needs time to accept the reality of the situation, opportunities to talk and to be listened to, and the experience of expressing themselves behaviorally in a nonjudgmental environment.

The nurse will note that the family of a terminally ill child may express feelings of guilt for wondering if members were responsible for the impending death. They may cling to their child and be hostile toward health personnel as their psychological pain reaches high levels. They may then progress to depression and finally, to a stage of accepting the inevitable. Some authors describe this process before death as anticipatory grief which prepares them for grieving after the death of a loved one. Prior to death, allowing the family every opportunity to be with the child and planning meetings with other families with terminally ill children have been found helpful to promote the resolution of grief.

HEALTH TEAM MEMBERS AND GRIEF

Health team members have been observed to experience grief too when persons for whom they are caring die. Just as with family members, health team members need the time to go through the grieving process and the opportunity to express their emotions. Health team and nursing team conferences are recommended to discuss the feelings of members. Anger, frustration, and despair which many health team members experience are better expressed than repressed.

Occasionally, a team member may have lost a loved one to death relatively recently and finds helping families of the terminally ill patient especially difficult and painful. Kübler-Ross recommends that such a person may need reassignment until sufficient time has elapsed for grief to be resolved.

Caring for the patient with humanness and compassion almost always involves some personal emotional investment. It is unrealistic and unfair to expect that health personnel handle circumstances surrounding death without feelings. The best policy appears to be taking the time to explore one's feelings, express them, discuss them with others, and expect that health workers often grieve also.

HOME CARE OF THE TERMINALLY ILL PATIENT

In some cases, the terminally ill patient remains at home, and the family assumes responsibility for his care. Various health agencies offer services for the care of the terminally ill at home. The nurse in the hospital may anticipate this need and assist the family in obtaining such services. Some hospitals permit nursing staff members to make home visits between hospitalizations to provide support and a continuity of the care. The community health nurse may provide some aspects of care, teach necessary skills to family members, promote the use of other community services, and provide support and guidance to the patient and his family.

In past decades, it was customary for persons to die at home. With increasing specialization of hospitals, the trend has been for terminally ill patients to be hospitalized. The availability of community services supportive to families and criticisms of the impersonal hospital environment now seem to be increasing the tendency for more persons to remain in their homes as long as it is possible.

When the terminally ill person is surrounded by his familiar home environment and has family members nearby, he usually feels more secure. He often can have his own routines maintained, have food that is familiar, and can maintain some degree of his family role. Family members have time to demonstrate their feelings of love without concern for institutional regulations. Guilt feelings may be lessened by family members caring for the person. Children can participate more extensively in the last days and can be helped to understand death with less fear. Since the process of dying generally is a gradual one, the family members can have the opportunity to work through some of the beginning phases of grieving that are often more difficult when the patient is in a health agency.

The nurse will want to remember that the care needed by some patients is too complex or demanding for family members. Some patients and family members find security in the facilities of a health agency. Families may have neither the physical nor emotional strength to deal with the terminally ill person in the home. The nurse must be careful that she does not unintentionally make the family feel guilty about not having the person at home.

THE HOSPICE MOVEMENT

Dr. Cicely Saunders is given credit for developing a philosophy of care for the terminally ill at St. Christopher's Hospice in London several decades ago. The word *hospice* means a way-station for travelers. Saunders used the term to mean a way-station where people in a caring environment can live out their final days with dignity and meaningfulness.

The type of care offered by a hospice is essentially the same as that described in this chapter. One major difference is that its services are offered in an autonomous unit. The unit may be a separate facility or be related to or be part of a hospital for the acutely ill. The separateness of the physical environment for the terminally ill focuses attention entirely on the needs of these patients. When they were in hospitals for the acutely ill, it was believed that their care was often inadequate since health personnel tended to neglect them in preference to helping patients who were expected to recover. In addition, since health workers in a hospice care only for the terminally ill, their skills become highly developed to meet the needs of the terminally ill person.

Some hospices offer day or night care, home care, and bereavement care, in addition to 24-hour, inservice care. Hospices provide emotional support and physical care and comfort for patients for whom therapy is no longer being actively pursued since cure is considered improbable. The goal is to allow the person to experience a natural death that is as tranquil and dignified as possible. The patients are assured that they will not be left to die alone and will be kept as free of pain as is possible. The pain control program used by hospices was described earlier in this chapter and reportedly, has been very effective for keeping patients comfortable. Philosophically, the hospice is as committed to the family as to the terminally ill person. As one author described it, the "patient" in a hospice is the terminally ill patient *and* his family.

There is a great flexibility in hospices in order to meet the patient's individual needs. This flexibility includes having unlimited visiting hours, allowing children and pets to visit, offering food on demand, and allowing the use of alcoholic beverages. Patients may wear their own clothing if they wish and are encouraged to bring favorite possessions from home if they desire. Every effort is made to comply with patients' last wishes. As an example, one hospice resident said her last request was to see the city from a helicopter. This was arranged by hospice personnel and when she returned, she said, "And now everything is complete. Do you understand?"

The philosophy upon which the hospice was developed is experiencing wide acceptance both in Europe and in this country. At present, the number of such facilities and the services they offer are on the increase throughout the United States.

CARE OF THE BODY AFTER DEATH

After the physician has pronounced the patient dead, the nurse is usually responsible for preparing the body for discharge from the health agency. The nurse will be guided by local procedure. Although these procedures vary with agencies and morticians, there are certain commonalities.

To prevent discoloration from the pooling of blood, the body should be placed in normal anatomical position. Soiled dressings are replaced and tubes removed. Inasmuch as the body is washed by the mortician, a complete bath is unnecessary except as individual situations indicate. A shampoo is unnecessary, but hairpins should be removed to avoid scratching the face. Most morticians prefer that dentures *not* be replaced. It generally is considered better for the mortician to place the teeth in position in order to minimize possible trauma, should they become situated oddly in the mouth. The nurse should see to it that dentures, properly identified, are given to the mortician when he calls for the body.

Double identification of the body is advised. One tag should be fastened securely to the shroud or garment in which the body is wrapped or covered. The second one should be tied to the ankle. If it is tied to the wrist, the wrist should be padded first and the tag tied loosely around the padding to avoid damaging tissue from a tight band. *The importance of proper and complete identification of the body cannot be overstressed.* Mistakes which have occurred can cause embarrassment and added sorrow for all concerned.

The arms are placed on the abdomen. Tying them in place may result in tissue damage. The legs may be tied together at the ankles. The body is then wrapped with a shroud or other garment provided by the agency. To facilitate moving the body from the bed, placing a full sheet around the body and tucking it securely in place prevents the extremities and head from falling out of place and minimizes tissue damage. Most morticians ask that the body be cooled as soon as possible. Morticians may take the body from the patient's room, or it may be removed to the hospital morgue refrigerator from where it will be taken to the mortuary.

When death occurs following certain communicable diseases, the body requires special handling to aid in preventing the spread of the disease. The requirements are specified by local law and policy. The measures taken will depend on the causative organism, the mode of transmission, the viability, and the other characteristics.

No special preparation is usually recommended for persons who have died at home.

Relatives of patients occasionally ask about a form of body preservation after death known as *cryonics,* which is freezing the dead human body. While freezing will slow tissue deterioration, there is no means at this time to prevent irreversible cell structure damage or to restore whole organs or bodies.

AUTOPSY

An *autopsy* is an examination of the organs and tissue of a human body following death. Consent for autopsy is a legal requirement. The person authorized to give approval varies. Generally the closest surviving family member or members have the authority to determine whether or not an autopsy is performed.

It is generally the physician's responsibility to obtain permission for an autopsy. Sometimes the patient may grant this permission before he dies. When permission is being sought from relatives of the patient, the nurse often can assist by helping to explain the reasons for an autopsy. This requires tact and good judgment, but many relatives will find comfort when they are told that an autopsy may help to further the development of medical science as well as establish proof of the exact cause of death.

If death is caused by accident, suicide, homicide, or illegal therapeutic practice, the coroner must be notified according to law. The coroner may decide that an autopsy is advisable and can order that one be performed even though the family of the patient has refused to consent. In many cases, a death occurring within 24 hours of admission to the hospital is reportable to the coroner.

TISSUE AND ORGAN REMOVAL

Body organs and tissues are often used for transplants or for medical research and study. Permission must be secured for the removal of body parts such as the heart, liver, eyes, kidneys, skin, brain, and bone. Prior to death, patients may grant such permission. However, in many states, after death the next of kin still must sign a permit and have it properly witnessed before tissue or organs can be removed from the body. The opportunity to sign a permit for organ removal is available when obtaining a driver's license in many states. This procedure allows the person to decide objectively prior to terminal illness concerning organ removal. The nurse will want to acquaint herself with local laws on transplant permits to aid in avoiding the unpleasantness of possible legal action.

THE DEATH CERTIFICATE

The laws of this country require that a death certificate be prepared for each patient who has died. The laws specify the information that is needed. Death certificates are sent to local health departments, which compile many statistics from the information that become important in identifying needs and problems in the fields of health.

The mortician assumes responsibility for handling and filing the death certificate with proper authorities. However, the physician's signature is required on the certificate, as well as that of the pathologist, the coroner, and others in special cases. The death certificate also carries the mortician's signature, and, in some states, his license number as well.

THE CARE OF VALUABLES

Each agency has policies on the care of valuables when patients are admitted to the institution. Those which the patient has chosen to keep with him, usually rings, a wristwatch, money, and so on, require careful handling after death. Occasionally, the patient's family may take the valuables home when death becomes imminent, and this should be noted on the form sheet which the agency specifies. If valuables are still with the patient at the time of death, they should be identified, accounted for, and sent to the appropriate department for safekeeping until the family claims them. If it is impossible to remove jewelry, such as a wedding ring, the fact that it remained on the body should be noted, and, as a further safeguard, the article should be secured with adhesive so that it becomes impossible for it to slip off and be lost. Loss of valuables is serious and can result in a legal suit against the hospital. The nurse owes it to the patient's family as well as to the agency in which she works to use every precaution to prevent loss and misplacement of valuables.

CARING FOR THE TERMINALLY ILL AND THE NURSING PROCESS

Data gathering begins by knowing the patient and his family. Who is the patient and what condition places his life in jeopardy? What treatment plan is in progress, if any? What evidence is there concerning his knowledge of his prognosis and in what stage of dying is he? Is he in pain? Are his family members aware of his prognosis and if so, how are they reacting to it? To what philosophy of life and death do the patient and his family subscribe? These are typical questions to which the nurse will wish to seek answers.

Various standards were given in this chapter which

can be used appropriately for assessing the patient with a terminal illness as well as his family members. For example, the nurse can use the stages of dying to assess in what stage the patient is. Similarly, she can assess the patient's family in relation to phases of grieving. A knowledge of various philosophies of life and death becomes important too when assessing the patient and his family. Signs of death become a standard when assessing the patient as his life ends.

This text emphasized the importance of including the patient when planning his care. It continues to be essential when caring for a terminally ill patient, and including the family members is equally important. Stages of dying and grief when patients and families are often critical and hostile were described. Nurses have found that while such behavior can be assessed as typical during certain stages of dying and grief, including the patient and family in planning nursing care very often helps them to express their hostilities. Thus also, it helps them to progress to later stages of dying and grief. Both patients and families tend to find comfort when they know everything possible is being done. Sharing the planning of nursing care with them often helps accomplish this goal. When nurses respect the right of the patient to make choices and decisions about his illness and the circumstances surrounding his last days of living and when they strive to share that final experience with the patient, including him in planning becomes imperative.

Giving care to terminally ill patients and to their families often requires extraordinary skills for meeting both physical and psychosocial needs. The following are some guidelines that the nurse will wish to keep in mind when administering nursing care to dying patients and to their families:

- Authorities on dying and death emphasize the need for health workers to explore their own philosophies of life and death and their feelings about death and dying. They question the ability of a nurse or any other health worker to offer high-quality care to terminally ill persons until feelings are thoroughly explored. Kübler-Ross points out that the patient is a marvelous teacher and can help us to understand ourselves too if we will but listen. Some authors have described what they refer to as the "nonaccountability of psychosocial care." They suggest that health workers in general fail to meet the psychosocial needs of patients because of inadequate team work among health personnel, lack of education for meeting the psychosocial needs of dying persons, and failure to explore their own feelings and to develop a personal philosophy of life and death.

- The importance of maintaining hope was discussed. Without hope, the patient despairs. With it, even when cure is considered improbable, a better quality of life tends to result. However, false hope is not condoned since the patient will almost always sense its falsity and feel victimized, alone, and isolated. Kübler-Ross empha-

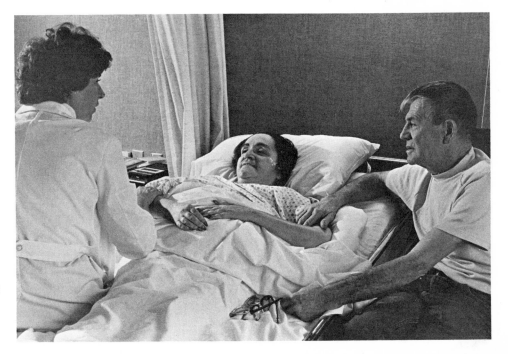

Figure 26–8 Including the family in planning nursing care for the terminally ill patient is important. The nurse is conferring with the patient and her husband, both of whom are aware of the patient's prognosis.

sizes using the word *improbable* rather than the word *impossible* when caring for the terminally ill. The difference in the two words may be technically subtle but they remain important from a psychosocial point of view.

- Giving top priority to the quality of survival for a dying person means shifting precedence from prevention and cure to *care,* that is, care for the psychosocial well-being of the person. Such care has its roots in human compassion and involves working *with* a patient and offering care in a nonjudgmental environment. The behavior of a person and his family members may not conform to what the nurse holds to be correct. But her actions must be guided by the patient's and family's feelings, not hers. Such care respects the right of the patient to be involved with the conditions surrounding the last days of his life and to meet death in his own way.

- The preoccupation of many dying persons is not death per se but isolation and aloneness. In addition, there is a significant fear concerning a destructive force over which he has no control. Possibly the three most effective tools the nurse can use to help the terminally ill patient are to be there, to allow the patient to talk, and to listen. Listening includes perceiving what the patient, who may use nonverbal and symbolic language, is really saying. It is rarely too late to talk with a patient *now,* but it may be later. Assuming he is too sick, too tired, or too weak often suggests that the nurse is uncomfortable with her own feelings about death. Keeping communication channels open and using every skill of communication are important. The importance of touch was discussed and illustrated in this chapter. There appears to be little that can replace the need for opportunities to experience verbal release from the awesome experience of dying and death and receive support through nonverbal communication, including touch.

- Most patients fear the intractable pain so often associated with terminal illness, especially when illness is due to a malignancy. There tends to be a general fear of addiction in our society which is understandable. But judgment must be exercised when caring for the terminally ill so that fear of addiction as well as fear of giving an analgesic because the patient may then expire, do not stand in the way of proper pain control.

- Meeting the patient's physical needs is an important nursing responsibility until the moment of the patient's death. It has been observed that giving skilled physical care often promotes the patient's psychosocial well-being also. Although it cannot replace psychosocial care, physical care also plays an important part in the control of

discomforts and enhances drug therapy that is being used in the patient's pain control program.

- Caring for the terminally ill person includes offering his family support while a loved one is dying as well as after death through bereavement programs. The philosophy of the hospice which considers its "patients" to be a terminally ill person *and* his family is a sound one for the nurse to observe wherever she is caring for patients whose death is imminent.

- One author's comments help to summarize:

The nurses and health-care workers who seem to have the least difficulty and the most job satisfaction in interacting with dying patients seem to have some or all of the following characteristics:

1. Comfort with their own philosophy of life, religion, or value system.
2. Comfort with their concept of their own body image and sexuality.
3. Sense of humor that is not buried too deep in their seriousness of purpose.
4. Ability to converse nonjudgmentally with patients who have a variety of value systems.
5. Ability to listen actively, encouraging expressive feelings of the patient.
6. Lack of overreactiveness to strong odors, malformed bodies; no restricton of "hands on" interventions to bodies so needful of touch.
7. Ability to diagnose sources of physical discomfort and anxiety and to propose interventions or solicit help from other disciplines.
8. Ability to bear with the coping mechanisms of patients or calmly sit out agitated or angry behavior.*

The parts of the nursing process and of the process as a whole are evaluated as described in Chapter 4.

CONCLUSION

Care of the patient who is dying requires delicate and demanding skill on the part of the nurse. She must be capable of giving supportive psychosocial and physical care. She is called upon to assist family members as well. In order to meet the patient's needs, she must come to grips with her own feelings about life and death. While care of the person who is dying may not always be easy, skillful nursing can contribute extensively to the comfort of both the patient and his family and can provide satisfaction for the nurse too.

---

*Williams, Shirley L. "The Nurse as Crisis Intervener." In Earle, Ann M., et al, editors. *The Nurse as Caregiver for the Terminal Patient and His Family.* Columbia University Press, New York, 1976, p. 47.

SUPPLEMENTAL LIBRARY STUDY

1. For a description of several hospices in the United States, read the following article:

    Plant, Janet. "Finding a Home for Hospice Care in the United States." *Hospitals, Journal of the American Hospital Association,* 51:53, 55, 57, 58, 61, July 1, 1977.

    What does the author mean when she wrote that the hospice is an amalgam of reactions and responses? What pros and cons of the hospice movement were presented? Indicate how the title of this article is related to its contents.

2. Read how Jory Graham speaks out about disease and death: "A Time to Write: A Plucky Woman Speaks Out About Disease and Death." *Time,* 110:94–96, November 14, 1977.

    Why does Ms. Graham reprimand physicians concerning their role in the care of a patient who lives under a shadow of death? What advice does she give about distraction and perception when with a person with a life-threatening illness? How did she eventually answer the question, "Why me?"

3. Who should decide how long life should be sustained artificially?

    Lestz, Paula. "Ethics: A Committee to Decide the Quality of Life." *American Journal of Nursing,* 77:862–864, May 1977.

    What four policies are presently being observed concerning sustaining life artificially? Which policy does the author believe to be the poorest? What does she consider as the key to solving the problem of determining quality of life?

4. The following article discusses the ability to control the process of dying:

    Burgess, Karen E. "The Influence of Will on Life and Death." *Nursing Forum,* 15:238–258, Number 3 1976.

    Describe how the "giving-up-given-up" complex is presented to illustrate a loss of will to live. How does the author describe "social death" and what is its relationship to physiological death? Describe "psychic death," and its relationship to curses, clairvoyance, premonitions, and so on. What physiological phenomenon did Cannon, who developed the fight-or-flight theory of fear, describe in persons who experienced voodoo deaths?

5. What do you do if a patient asks you if he will die shortly? Read the following article:

    "Nurse-Patient Relations: Helping the Elderly Cope with Bad News." *Nursing Update,* 7:1, 14–16, February 1976.

    List eight basic counseling principles described in this article. What suggestions are offered when a patient must be transferred to a nursing home, whether he is terminally ill or not?

References For Unit V

CHAPTER 15

Bates, Barbara. *A Guide to Physical Examination.* J. B. Lippincott Company, Philadelphia, 1974, 375 p.

Beaumont, Estelle. "Product Survey: Diagnostic Kits." *Nursing 75,* 5:28–33, April 1975.

Blainey, Carol Gohrke. "Site Selection in Taking Body Temperatures." *American Journal of Nursing,* 74:1859–1861, October 1974.

Blount, Mary, et al. "Obtaining and Analyzing Cerebrospinal Fluid." *The Nursing Clinics of North America,* 9:593–609, December 1974.

Corns, Rebecca H. "Maintenance of Blood Pressure Equipment." *American Journal of Nursing,* 76:776–777, May 1976.

Eymontt, Michael J. and Eymontt, Daina. "Preparing Your Patient for Nuclear Medicine." *Nursing 77,* 7:46–49, December 1977.

Graas, Suzanne. "Thermometer Sites and Oxygen." *American Journal of Nursing,* 74:1862–1863, October 1974.

Greenfield, Diane, et al. "Children Can Have High Blood Pressure, Too." *American Journal of Nursing,* 76:770–772, May 1976.

Jarvis, Carolyn Mueller. "Perfecting Physical Assessment: Part 1." *Nursing 77,* 7:28–37, May 1977.

Jarvis, Carolyn Mueller. "Perfecting Physical Assessment: Part 2." *Nursing 77,* 7:38–45, June 1977.

Jarvis, Carolyn Mueller. "Perfecting Physical Assessment: Part 3." *Nursing 77,* 7:44–53, July 1977.

Jarvis, Carolyn Mueller. "Vital Signs: How to Take Them More Accurately . . . And Understand Them More Fully." *Nursing 76,* 6:31–37, April 1976.

Lancour, Jane. "How to Avoid Pitfalls in Measuring Blood Pressure." *American Journal of Nursing,* 76:773–775, May 1976.

LeMaile-Williams, Robert L. "The Clinical and Physiological Assessment of Black Patients," in Dorothy Luckraft (Editor), *Black Awareness: Implications for Black Patient Care.* The American Journal of Nursing Company, New York, 1976, pp. 16–26.

McVan, Barbara. "What the Nose Knows: Odors." *Nursing 77,* 7:46–49, April 1977.

Malasanos, Lois, et al. *Health Assessment.* The C. V. Mosby Company, Saint Louis, 1977, 526 p.

Milligan, Carol, et al. "Screening for Cervical Cancer." *American Journal of Nursing,* 75:1343–1344, August 1975.

Overfield, Theresa. "Biological Variation: Concepts from Physical Anthropology." *The Nursing Clinics of North America,* 12:19–26, March 1977.

Roach, Lora B. "Color Changes in Dark Skin." *Nursing 77,* 7:48–51, January 1977.

Roberts, Sharon L. "Skin Assessment for Color and Temperature." *American Journal of Nursing,* 75:610–613, April 1975.

Skydell, Barbara and Crowder, Anne S. *Diagnostic Procedures: A Reference for Health Practitioners and a Guide for Patient Counseling.* Little, Brown and Company, Boston, 1975, 248 p.

Sparks, Colleen. "Peripheral Pulses." *American Journal of Nursing,* 75:1132–1133, July 1975.

Tom, Cheryl K. "Nursing Assessment of Biological Rhythms." *The Nursing Clinics of North America,* 11:621–630, December 1976.

Van Meter, Margaret and Lavine, Peter G. "What Every Nurse Should Know About EKG's: Part 1." *Nursing 75,* 5:19–27, April 1975.

CHAPTER 16

"A Better Water Bed." (Medical Highlights) *American Journal of Nursing,* 75:657–658, April 1975.

"And Now . . . A Towel Bath." *Nursing 75,* 5:44, December 1975.

Berecek, Kathleen H. "Etiology of Decubitus Ulcers." *The Nursing Clinics of North America,* 10:157–170, March 1975.

Berecek, Kathleen H. "Treatment of Decubitus Ulcers." *The Nursing Clinics of North America,* 10:171–210, March 1975.

"Better Decubitus Care." *Nursing 76,* 6:13, April 1976.

Block, Philip Lloyd. "Dental Health in Hospitalized Patients." *American Journal of Nursing,* 76:1162–1164, July 1976.

"Contaminated Cosmetics." (Nurse's Notebook) *Nursing 77,* 7:66, February 1977.

"Dental Flaws: Open Wide, Please, Should Not Include the Wallet." (Medicine) *Time,* 110:44, September 5, 1977.

DeWalt, Evelyn M. "Effect of Timed Hygienic Measures on Oral Mucosa in a Group of Elderly Subjects." *Nursing Research,* 24:104–108, March/April 1975.

Dornburg, Jo Anne L. "Decubiti's Demise." (Tips & Timesavers) *Nursing 75,* 75:82, September 1975.

Gould, Herman. "How to Remove Contact Lenses from Comatose Patients." *American Journal of Nursing,* 76:1483–1485, September 1976.

Gruis, Marcia L. and Innes, Barbara. "Assessment: Essential to Prevent Pressure Sores." *American Journal of Nursing,* 76:1762–1764, November 1976.

"Hairy "Staph" Trouble." (Medical Highlights) *American Journal of Nursing,* 74:1330–1331, July 1974.

"Higher Income, More Caries." (Medical Highlights) *American Journal of Nursing,* 76:2002, December 1976.

Kavchak-Keyes, Mary Anne, Consultant. "Four Proven Steps for Preventing Decubitus Ulcers." *Nursing 77,* 7:58–61, September 1977.

Lang, Christine and McGrath, Anne. "Gelfoam for Decubitus Ulcers." *American Journal of Nursing,* 74:460–461, March 1974.

Larsen, George. "Removing Cerumen with a Water Pik." *American Journal of Nursing,* 76:264–265, February 1976.

Maurer, Jean. "Providing Optimal Oral Health." *The Nursing Clinics of North America*, 2:671–685, December 1977.

Michelsen, Dana. "Giving a Great Back Rub." *American Journal of Nursing*, 78:1197–1199, July 1978.

Miller, Marian E. and Sachs, Marvin L. *About Bedsores: What You Need to Know to Help Prevent and Treat Them.* J. B. Lippincott Company, Philadelphia, 1974, 46 p.

Reitz, Marie and Pope, Wilma. "Mouth Care." *American Journal of Nursing*, 73:1728–1730, October 1973.

Spencer, Sue. "Decubiti—The Endless Problem." *Nursing 76*, 6:72, June 1976.

Van Ort, Suzanne Rowe and Gerber, Rose M. "Topical Application of Insulin in the Treatment of Decubitus Ulcers: A Pilot Study." *Nursing Research*, 25:9–12, January/February 1976.

Wallace, Gladys and Hayter, Jean. "Karaya for Chronic Skin Ulcers." *American Journal of Nursing*, 74:1094–1098, June 1974.

Zucnick, Martha. "Care of an Artificial Eye." *American Journal of Nursing*, 75:835, May 1975.

CHAPTER 17

Bilger, Annetta J. and Greene, Ellen H., Editors. *Winter's (sic) Protective Body Mechanics: A Manual for Nurses.* Springer Publisher Company, Inc., New York, 1973, 108 p.

Cooper, Kenneth H. *The New Aerobics.* Bantam Books, Inc., New York, 1970, 191 p.

Dayhoff, Nancy. "Soft or Hard Devices to Position Hands?" *American Journal of Nursing*, 75:1142–1144, July 1975.

Delaney, James E. "Health and Vitality Throughout the Day." *AORN Journal*, 25:669–677, March 1977.

Ford, Jack R. and Duckworth, Bridget. "Moving a Dependent Patient Safely, Comfortably: Part 1—Positioning." *Nursing 76*, 6:28–36, January 1976.

Ford, Jack R. and Duckworth, Bridget. "Moving a Dependent Patient Safely, Comfortably: Part 2—Transferring." *Nursing 76*, 6:58–65, February 1976.

Gordon, Janet E. "CircOlectric Beds: Circumventing the Trauma of Positioning." *Nursing 77*, 7:42–47, February 1977.

Hefferin, Elizabeth A. and Hill, Betty J. "Analyzing Nursing's Work-Related Injuries." *American Journal of Nursing*, 76:924–927, June 1976.

Hirschberg, Gerald G., et al. "Promoting Patient Mobility and Other Ways to Prevent Secondary Disabilities." *Nursing 77*, 7:42–47, May 1977.

Hogan, Leola and Beland, Irene. "Cervical Spine Syndrome." *American Journal of Nursing*, 76:1104–1107, July 1976.

Jensen, J. Trygve. *Physics for the Health Professions.* Edition 2. J. B. Lippincott Company, Philadelphia, 1976, 249 p.

Jungreis, Sidney W. "Exercises for Expediting Mobility (and Decreasing Disability) in Bedridden Patients." *Nursing 77*, 7:47–51, August 1977.

Kukuk, Helen M. "Safety Precautions: Protecting Your Patients & Yourself. Part One." *Nursing 76*, 6:45–51, May 1976.

Kukuk, Helen M. "Safety Precautions: Protecting Your Patients & Yourself. Part Two." *Nursing 76*, 6:49–52, June 1976.

Long, Barbara C. and Buergin, Patricia S. "The Pivot Transfer." *American Journal of Nursing*, 77:980–982, June 1977.

O'Dell, Ardis J. "Hot Packs for Morning Joint Stiffness." *American Journal of Nursing*, 75:986–987, June 1975.

Olson, Edith V. "The Hazards of Immobility." *American Journal of Nursing*, 67:779–797, April 1967.

Peters, Ruanne K., et al. "Daily Relaxation Response Breaks in a Working Population: I. Effects on Self-reported Measures of Health, Performance, and Well-being." *American Journal of Public Health*, 67:946–953, October 1977.

Rottkamp, Barbara C. "An Experimental Nursing Study: A Behavior Modification Approach to Nursing Therapeutics in Body Positioning of Spinal Cord-Injured Patients." *Nursing Research*, 25:181–186, May/June 1976.

Snyder, Mariah and Baum, Rebecca. "Assessing Station and Gait." *American Journal of Nursing*, 74:1256–1257, July 1974.

Wilson, Robin L. "An Introduction to Yoga." *American Journal of Nursing*, 76:261–263, February 1976.

Young, Sr. Charlotte. "Exercise: How to Use It to Decrease Complications in Immobilized Patients." *Nursing 75*, 5:81–82, March 1975.

CHAPTER 18

Bakan, Paul. "The Right Brain is the Dreamer." *Psychology Today*, 10:66–68, November 1976.

Brunner, Lillian Sholtis and Suddarth, Doris Smith. *Textbook of Medical-Surgical Nursing.* Edition 3. J. B. Lippincott Company, Philadelphia, 1975, pp. 141–153.

Cashatt, Barbara. "Pain: A Patient's View." *American Journal of Nursing*, 72:281, February 1972.

Davitz, Lois J. and Davitz, Joel R. "How Do Nurses Feel When Patients Suffer?" *American Journal of Nursing*, 75:1505–1510, September 1975.

Fass, Grace. "Sleep, Drugs, and Dreams." *American Journal of Nursing*, 71:2316–2320, December 1971.

Johnson, Marion. "Pain: How Do You Know It's There and What Do You Do?" *Nursing 76*, 6:48–50, September 1976.

Kales, Anthony, Editor. *Sleep: Physiology and Pathology: A Symposium.* J. B. Lippincott Company, Philadelphia, 1969, 360 p.

Karlins, Marvin and Andrews, Lewis M. *Biofeedback: Turning on the Power of Your Mind.* Warner Paperback Library, New York, 1972, 190 p.

Leidig, Ruth M. "Narcolepsy: Jody's Story." *American Journal of Nursing*, 73:491–493, March 1973.

"Little Sleep or Many Awakenings?" (Medical Highlights) *American Journal of Nursing*, 77:884, 886, May 1977.

Long, Barbara. "Sleep." *American Journal of Nursing*, 69:1896–1899, September 1969.

McCaffery, Margo. *Nursing Management of the Patient With Pain.* J. B. Lippincott Company, Philadelphia, 1972, 248 p.

McCaffery, Margo and Hart, Linda L. "Undertreatment of Acute

Pain with Narcotics." *American Journal of Nursing,* 76:1586–1591, October 1976.

McCaffery, Margo and Moss, Fay. "Nursing Intervention for Bodily Pain." *American Journal of Nursing,* 67:1224–1227, June 1967.

Moss, Fay T. and Meyer, Burton. "The Effects of Nursing Interaction Upon Pain Relief in Patients." *Nursing Research,* 15:303–306, Fall 1966.

Narrow, Barbara W. "Rest Is . . ." *American Journal of Nursing,* 67:1646–1649, August 1967.

"Night Owls and Early Risers." *Human Behavior,* 6:31, March 1977.

Nordmark, Madelyn T. and Rohweder, Anne W. *Scientific Foundations of Nursing.* Edition 3. J. B. Lippincott Company, Philadelphia, 1975, pp. 182–186; 251–260.

Pace, J. Blair. "Helping Patients Overcome the Disabling Effects of Chronic Pain." *Nursing 77,* 7:38–43, July 1977.

"Pain and Suffering." (A Special Supplement) *American Journal of Nursing,* 74:489–520, March 1974.

"Pain Without Suffering." *Human Behavior,* 6:23–24, August 1977.

Rosno, Suzanne. "Can Sleeping be Dangerous?" *Nursing 76,* 6:16–17, September 1976.

Sobel, David. "Love and Pain." *American Journal of Nursing,* 72:910–912, May 1972.

Stewart, Elizabeth. "To Lessen Pain: Relaxation and Rhythmic Breathing." *American Journal of Nursing,* 76:958–959, June 1976.

Wiener, Carolyn L. "Pain Assessment on an Orthopedic Ward." *Nursing Outlook,* 23:508–516, August 1975.

Williams, Donald H. "Sleep and Disease." *American Journal of Nursing,* 71:2321–2324, December 1971.

CHAPTER 19

"Attacking the Starvation Habit." (Public Welfare) *Human Behavior,* 6:51, September 1977.

Caghan, Susan B. "The Adolescent Process and the Problem of Nutrition." *American Journal of Nursing,* 75:1728–1731, October 1975.

Caly, Joan C. "Helping People Eat for Health: Assessing Adults' Nutrition." *American Journal of Nursing,* 77:1605–1609, October 1977.

Dansky, Kathryn H. "Assessing Children's Nutrition." *American Journal of Nursing,* 77:1610–1611, October 1977.

Erlander, Darlene. "Dietetics—A Look at the Profession." *American Journal of Nursing,* 70:2402–2405, November 1970.

"Evaluating Your Patient's Taste and Smell Disturbances." *Nursing Update,* 6:1, 9–11, June 1975.

Freiermuth, Donna. "Dieting Decor." (Personal File) *Human Behavior,* 6:16, November 1977.

Literte, Jean Willacker. "Nursing Care of Patients with Intestinal Obstruction." *American Journal of Nursing,* 77:1003–1006, June 1977.

McConnell, Edwina A. "Ensuring Safer Stomach Suctioning with the Salem Sump Tube." *Nursing 77,* 7:54–57, September 1977.

Nelson, Alice H. "Self-Recorded Diet Histories." *American Journal of Nursing,* 72:1601, September 1972.

Nordmark, Madelyn T. and Rohweder, Anne W. *Scientific Foundations of Nursing.* Edition 3. J. B. Lippincott Company, Philadelphia, 1975, pp. 78–111.

Rosenberg, Frances H. "Lactose Intolerance." *American Journal of Nursing,* 77:823–824, May 1977.

Shumway, Sandra and Powers, Marjorie. "The Group Way to Weight Loss." *American Journal of Nursing,* 73:269–272, February 1973.

Snell, Barbara and McLellan, Connie. "Whetting Hospitalized Preschoolers' Appetites." *American Journal of Nursing,* 76:413–415, March 1976.

Waechter, Eugenia H. and Blake, Florence G. *Nursing Care of Children.* Edition 9. J. B. Lippincott Company, Philadelphia, 1976, pp. 175–176.

Wellborn, Stanley N. "Are You Eating Right?" *U.S. News & World Report,* 83:39–43, November 28, 1977.

"When Vomiting Signals a Geriatric Emergency." *Nursing Update,* 6:12–15, June 1975.

Williams, Eleanor R. "Making Vegetarian Diets Nutritious." *American Journal of Nursing,* 75:2168–2173, December 1975.

CHAPTER 20

Altshuler, Anne, et al. "Even Children Can Learn To Do Clean Self-Catheterization." *American Journal of Nursing,* 77:97–101, January 1977.

Beaumont, Estelle. "Product Survey: Diagnostic Kits." *Nursing 75,* 5:28–33, April 1975.

Bellfy, Luanne C. "You Can Improve Your Catheterized Patient's Care." *RN,* 40:33–35, April 1977.

Broadwell, Debra C. and Sorrells, Suzanne L. "Loop Transverse Colostomy." *American Journal of Nursing,* 78:1029–1031, June 1978.

Center for Disease Control. *National Nosocomial Infections Study Quarterly Report.* First and Second Quarters 1973, Issued July 1974, pp. 20–27.

Center for Disease Control. *National Nosocomial Infections Study Quarterly Report.* Third and Fourth Quarters 1973, Issued March 1974, pp. 19–28.

Champion, Victoria L. "Clean Technique for Intermittent Self-Catheterization." *Nursing Research,* 25:13–18, January/February 1976.

Connors, Melba. "Ostomy Care: A Personal Approach." *American Journal of Nursing,* 74:1422–1425, August 1974.

Corman, Marvin L., et al. "Cathartics." *American Journal of Nursing,* 75:273–279, February 1975.

DeGroot, Jane. "Urethral Catheterization—Observing 'Niceties' Prevents Infections." *Nursing 76,* 6:51–55, December 1976.

Dobbins, Janet and Gleit, Carol. "Experience with the Lateral

Position for Catheterization." *The Nursing Clinics of North America*, 6:373–379, June 1971.

Dudas, Susan, Guest Editor. "Symposium on Care of the Ostomy Patient." *The Nursing Clinics of North America*, 11:389–478, September 1976.

Hyman, Eleanor, et al. "The Pouch Ileostomy—New Nursing Applications of Time-Tested Techniques." *Nursing 77*, 7:44–47, September 1977.

Jorow, Marie. "How to Teach Patients to Catheterize Themselves." *RN*, 38:19–21, December 1975.

Lamanske, Jacqueline. "Helping the Ileostomy Patient to Help Himself." *Nursing 77*, 7:34–39, January 1977.

Mahoney, Joanne M. "What You Should Know About Ostomies: Guidelines For Giving Better Postop Care." *Nursing 78*, 8:74, 76, 78, 80, 82, 84, May 1978.

Maney, Janet Yost. "A Behavioral Therapy Approach to Bladder Retraining." *The Nursing Clinics of North America*, 11:179–188, March 1976.

Moore, Dianne S. and Bauer, Carolyn Sleeter. "Effect of Prepodyne® as a Perineal Cleansing Agent for Clean Catch Specimens." *Nursing Research*, 25:259–261, July/August 1976.

Schauder, Marilyn R. "Ostomy Care: Cone Irrigations." *American Journal of Nursing*, 74:1424–1427, August 1974.

Schumann, Delores. "Tips for Improving Urine Testing Techniques." *Nursing 76*, 6:23–27, February 1976.

Watt, Rosemary C. "Urinary Diversion." *American Journal of Nursing*, 74:1806–1811, October 1974.

Wentworth, Arlene and Cox, Barbara. "Nursing Management of the Patient with a Continent Ileostomy." *American Journal of Nursing*, 76:1424–1428, September 1976.

Whyte, John F. and Thistle, Nancy A. "Male Incontinence: The Inside Story on External Collection." *Nursing 76*, 6:66–67, September 1976.

Woodrow, Mary, et al. "Suprapubic Catheters, Part 1: A Direct Line to Better Drainage." *Nursing 76*, 6:40–45, October 1976.

Woodrow, Mary, et al. "Suprapubic Catheters, Part 2: A Direct Line to Better Drainage." *Nursing 76*, 6:40–42, November 1976.

CHAPTER 21

Affonso, Dyanne and Harris, Thomas. "Continuous Positive Airway Pressure." *American Journal of Nursing*, 76:570–573, April 1976.

Amborn, Sylvia Arlene. "Clinical Signs Associated with the Amount of Tracheobronchial Secretions." *Nursing Research*, 25:121–126, March/April 1976.

Codd, John and Grohar, Mary Ellen. "Postoperative Pulmonary Complications." *The Nursing Clinics of North America*, 10:5–15, March 1975.

Felton, Cynthia L. "Hypoxemia and Oral Temperatures." *American Journal of Nursing*, 78:56–57, January 1978.

Foley, Mary, et al. "Pulmonary Function Screening Tests in Industry." *American Journal of Nursing*, 77:1480–1484, September 1977.

Johnson, Marion. "Outcome Criteria to Evaluate Postoperative Respiratory Status." *American Journal of Nursing*, 75:1474–1475, September 1975.

Lawless, Carolyn A. "Helping Patients with Endotracheal and Tracheostomy Tubes Communicate." *American Journal of Nursing*, 75:2151–2153, December 1975.

Laycock, Joan. "Nursing the Patient on the Ventilator." *The Nursing Clinics of North America*, 10:17–25, March 1975.

Libman, Robert H. and Keithley, Joyce. "Relieving Airway Obstruction in the Recovery Room." *American Journal of Nursing*, 75:603–605, April 1975.

Malkus, Bobby L. "Respiratory Care at Home." *American Journal of Nursing*, 76:1789–1791, November 1976.

Tinker, John H. "Understanding Chest X-rays." *American Journal of Nursing*, 76:54–58, January 1976.

Tinker, John H. and Wehner, Robert "The Nurse and the Ventilator." *American Journal of Nursing*, 74:1276–1278, July 1974.

Traver, Gayle A., Guest Editor. "Symposium on Care in Respiratory Disease." *The Nursing Clinics of North America*, 9:97–207, March 1974.

Waterson, Marian, Consultant. "Teaching Your Patients Postural Drainage." *Nursing 78*, 8:50–53, March 1978.

CHAPTER 22

Beaumont, Estelle. "Product Survey: Hypo/Hyperthermia Equipment." *Nursing 74*, 4:34–41, April 1974.

Johnson, Jean E., et al. "Altering Children's Distress Behavior During Orthopedic Cast Removal." *Nursing Research*, 24:405–410, November/December 1975.

Knight, Marie Ray. "A 'Second Skin' for Patients with Large, Draining Wounds." *Nursing 76*, 6:37, January 1976.

Laughlin, Victor C. "Stopping the Constant Drip of Draining Wounds." *Nursing 74*, 4:26–27, December 1974.

LeMaitre, George D. and Finnegan, Janet A. *The Patient In Surgery: A Guide for Nurses*. Edition 3. W. B. Saunders Company, Philadelphia, 1975, 506 p.

Manson, Helen. "Exorcising Excoriation from Fistulae & Other Problems." *Nursing 75*, 5:52–55, October 1975.

O'Dell, Ardis J. "Hot Packs for Morning Joint Stiffness." *American Journal of Nursing*, 75:986–987, June 1975.

Rinear, Charles E. and Rinear, Eileen E. "Emergency Bandaging: A Wrap-Up of Better Techniques." *Nursing 75*, 5:29–35, January 1975.

Ross, Russell. "Wound Healing." *Scientific American*, 220:40–50, June 1969.

Ryan, Rosemary. "Thrombophlebitis: Assessment and Prevention." *American Journal of Nursing*, 76:1634–1636, October 1976.

"Standards for Preoperative Skin Preparation of Patients." *AORN Journal*, 23:974–975, May 1976.

"Wound Suction—Better Drainage With Fewer Problems." *Nursing 75*, 5:52–55, October 1975.

CHAPTER 23

del Bueno, Dorothy J. "Electrolyte Imbalance: How to Recognize and Respond To It. Part 1." *RN,* 38:52–54, 56, February 1975.

del Bueno, Dorothy J. "Electrolyte Imbalance: How to Recognize and Respond To It. Part 2." *RN,* 38:54–55, March 1975.

Elbaum, Nancy. "Mg++: Detecting and Correcting Magnesium Imbalance." *Nursing 77,* 7:34–35, August 1977.

Grant, Marcia M. and Kubo, Winifred M. "Assessing a Patient's Hydration Status." *American Journal of Nursing,* 75:1306–1311, August 1975.

Keyes, Jack L. "Basic Mechanisms Involved in Acid-Base Homeostasis." *Heart and Lung: The Journal of Critical Care,* 5:239–246, March/April 1976.

Keyes, Jack L. "Blood-Gas Analysis and the Assessment of Acid-Base Status." *Heart and Lung: The Journal of Critical Care,* 5:247–255, March/April 1976.

Kubo, Winifred, et al. "Fluid and Electrolyte Problems of Tube-Fed Patients." *American Journal of Nursing,* 76:912–916, June 1976.

Lee, Carla A., et al. "Extracellular Volume Imbalance." *American Journal of Nursing,* 74:888–891, May 1974.

Lee, Carla A., et al. "What To Do When Acid-Base Problems Hang in the Balance." *Nursing 75,* 5:32–37, August 1975.

Metheny, Norma Milligan and Snively, W. D. Jr. *Nurses' Handbook of Fluid Balance.* Edition 2. J. B. Lippincott Company, Philadelphia, 1974, 313 p.

Mutton, C. J. "Blood pH—1. The ABC of Acid-Base Chemistry." *Nursing Times,* 71:968–971, June 19, 1975.

Mutton, C. J. "Blood pH—2. Acidosis and Alkalosis." *Nursing Times,* 71:1010–1012, June 26, 1975.

Rogenes, Paula R. and Moylan, Joseph A. "Restoring Fluid Balance in the Patient With Severe Burns." *American Journal of Nursing,* 76:1952–1957, December 1976.

Sharer, Jo Ellen. "Reviewing Acid-Base Balance." *American Journal of Nursing,* 75:980–983, June 1975.

CHAPTER 24

Beaumont, Estelle. "The New I.V. Infusion Pumps." (Product Survey) *Nursing 77,* 7:31–35, July 1977.

Beaumont, Estelle and Claypool, Shirley, Editors. "Student Nurse Practitioners Learn How to Advise on Over-The-Counter Drugs." (Innovations in Nursing) *Nursing 75,* 5:38, July 1975.

Boyles, Virginia A. "Injection Aids for Blind Diabetic Patients." *American Journal of Nursing,* 77:1456–1458, September 1977.

Conway, Alice and Williams, Tamara. "Care of the Critically Ill Newborn: Parenteral Alimentation." *American Journal of Nursing,* 76:574–577, April 1976.

Conway, Barbara, et al. "The Seventh Right." *American Journal of Nursing,* 70:1040–1043, May 1970.

DeMarco, Carl T. "Breach of Duty: When Are You Liable for Drug-Related Injuries?" *Nursing 76,* 6:103–104, 106, April 1976.

Galton, Lawrence. "Drugs and the Elderly: What You Should Know About Them." *Nursing 76,* 6:38–43, August 1976.

Geolot, Denise H. and McKinney, Nancy P. "Administering Parenteral Drugs." *American Journal of Nursing,* 75:788–793, May 1975.

Hanson, Robert L. "Heparin-Lock or Keep-Open I.V.?" *American Journal of Nursing,* 76:1102–1103, July 1976.

Hays, Doris. "Do It Yourself the Z-Track Way." *American Journal of Nursing,* 74:1070–1071, June 1974.

"How To Help Your Patients Know Their Meds." (Innovations in Nursing) *Nursing 77,* 7:23, October 1977.

"IV Nutrition: Sustaining Life Through TPA." *Nursing Update,* 6:1–9, September 1975.

Kurdi, William J. "Refining Your I.V. Therapy Techniques." *Nursing 75,* 5:41–47, November 1975.

Lang, Susan Havens, et al. "Reducing Discomfort From IM Injections." *American Journal of Nursing,* 76:800–801, May 1976.

Lowenthal, Werner. "Factors Affecting Drug Absorption." (Programmed Instruction) *American Journal of Nursing,* 73: 1391–1408, August 1973.

Norcross, Marilyn B. "Calibrating I.V. Fluids." (Ideas That Work) *American Journal of Nursing,* 75:2003, November 1975.

Plumer, Ada Lawrence. *Principles and Practice of Intravenous Therapy.* Edition 2. Little, Brown and Company, Boston, 1975, 349 p.

"Profile: Daniel A. Hussar, PhD." *Nursing 75,* 5:10, June 1975.

Schwartz, Doris. "Safe Self-Medication for Elderly Outpatients." *American Journal of Nursing,* 75:1808–1810, October 1975.

Snider, Malle Avolaid. "Helpful Hints on I.V.'s." *American Journal of Nursing,* 74:1978–1981, November 1974.

Ungvarski, Peter J. "Parenteral Therapy." *American Journal of Nursing,* 76:1974–1977, December 1976.

CHAPTER 25

Cardiopulmonary Resuscitation. The American National Red Cross, Washington, D.C., 1974, 42 p.

CPR in Basic Life Support for Unwitnessed Cardiac Arrest. Committee on Emergency Cardiac Care, American Heart Association, Dallas, Texas, 1977, 8 p.

Hart, Romaine, "What to do When You're Number 1: CPR Review," *Nursing 78,* 8:48–53, June 1978.

Molyneux-Luick, Marilee. "The ABC's of Multiple Trauma." *Nursing 77,* 7:30–36, October 1977.

Palen, Charity S. "The Passage." *American Journal of Nursing,* 75:2004–2005, November 1975.

"Standards for Cardiopulmonary Resuscitation (CPR) and Emergency Cardiac Care (ECG)." *The Journal of the American Medical Association,* 227:837–868, February 18, 1974.

Ungvarski, Peter J., et al. "CPR: Current Practice Revised." *American Journal of Nursing,* 75:236–241, February 1975.

Waechter, Eugenia H. and Blake, Florence G. "Emergency Care: Nursing Care in Cardiopulmonary Resuscitation," in *Nursing Care of Children.* Edition 9. J. B. Lippincott Company, Philadelphia, 1976, pp. 796–797.

CHAPTER 26

Adams, Nancy R. "Prolonged Coma: Your Care Makes All the Difference." *Nursing 77,* 7:20–27, August 1977.

Anastasia, Sister. ". . . The Living Will . . . Some Potential Problems." (Letters) *American Journal of Nursing,* 76:554, 556, April 1976.

Beauchamp, Joyce M. "Euthanasia and the Nurse Practitioner." *Nursing Forum,* 14:56–73, Number 1, 1975.

Burgess, Karen E. "The Influence of Will on Life and Death." *Nursing Forum,* 15:238–258, Number 3, 1976.

Cawley, Michele Anne. "Ethics: Euthanasia: Should It Be a Choice?" *American Journal of Nursing,* 77:859–861, May 1977.

Copp, Laurel Archer. "The Spectrum of Suffering." *American Journal of Nursing,* 74:491–495, March 1974.

Craven, Joan and Wald, Florence S. "Hospice Care for Dying Patients." *American Journal of Nursing,* 75:1816–1822, October 1975.

Earle, Ann M., et al., Editors. *The Nurse as Caregiver for the Terminal Patient and His Family.* Columbia University Press, New York, 1976, 252 p.

Engel, George L. "Grief and Grieving." *American Journal of Nursing,* 64:93–98, September 1964.

Freihofer, Patricia and Felton, Geraldene. "Nursing Behaviors in Bereavement: An Exploratory Study." *Nursing Research,* 25:332–337, September/October 1976.

Goleman, Daniel. "We Are Breaking the Silence About Death." *Psychology Today,* 10:44–47, 103, September 1976.

Griffin, Jerry J. "Family Decision: A Crucial Factor in Terminating Life." *American Journal of Nursing,* 75:794–796, May 1975.

Hampe, Sandra Oliver. "Needs of the Grieving Spouse in a Hospital Setting." *Nursing Research,* 24:113–120, March/April 1975.

Jaffe, Lois and Jaffe, Arthur. "Terminal Candor and the Coda Syndrome." *American Journal of Nursing,* 76:1938–1940, December 1976.

Johnson, Priscilla. "Ethics: The Gray Areas—Who Decides?" *American Journal of Nursing,* 77:856–858, May 1977.

Kavanaugh, Robert E. "Dealing Naturally With The Dying." *Nursing 76,* 6:22–29, October 1976.

Kobrzycki, Paula. "Dying With Dignity at Home." *American Journal of Nursing,* 75:1312–1313, August 1975.

Koch, Joanne. "When Children Meet Death." *Psychology Today,* 11:64–66, 79–80, 82, August 1977.

Kübler-Ross, Elisabeth. *Coping With Death and Dying.* A Psychology Today Library Cassette, 1973, Five tapes.

Kübler-Ross, Elisabeth. *On Death and Dying.* The Macmillan Company, New York, 1969, 289 p.

Lande, Shellie. "A Gift of Hope." *American Journal of Nursing,* 77:639–640, April 1977.

LeRoux, Rose S. "Communicating With the Dying Person." *Nursing Forum,* 16:144–145, Number 2, 1977.

Lewis, Frances Marcus. "A Time to Live and a Time to Die: An Instructional Drama." *Nursing Outlook,* 25:762–765, December 1977.

Nietzke, Ann. "The Miracle of Kübler-Ross." *Human Behavior,* 6:18–27, September 1977.

Pennington, Elisabeth A. "Postmortem Care: More Than Ritual." *American Journal of Nursing,* 78:846–847, May 1978.

Popoff, David and *Nursing 75.* "What Are Your Feelings About Death and Dying? Part 1." *Nursing 75,* 5:15–24, August 1975.

Popoff, David and *Nursing 75.* "What Are Your Feelings About Death and Dying? Part 2." *Nursing 75,* 5:55–62, September 1975.

Sobel, David E. "Death and Dying." *American Journal of Nursing,* 74:98–99, January 1974.

Sonstegard, Lois, et al. "The Grieving Nurse." *American Journal of Nursing,* 76:1490–1492, September 1976.

Ufema, Joy K. "Dare to Care for the Dying: An Affirmation from a Nurse Who Does Care." *American Journal of Nursing,* 76:88–90, January 1976.

Wentzel, Kenneth B. "The Dying Are The Living." *American Journal of Nursing,* 76:956–957, June 1976.

Williams, Jane C. "Understanding the Feelings of the Dying." *Nursing 76,* 6:52–56, March 1976.

Index

NOTE: Page numbers in italics indicate illustrations. Page numbers followed by t indicate tabular material.